Caplan's Stroke

A Clinical Approach

Fifth Edition

Edited by

Louis R Caplan

Beth Israel Deaconess Medical Center and Harvard Medical School, Boston, MA, USA

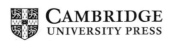
CAMBRIDGE
UNIVERSITY PRESS

CAMBRIDGE
UNIVERSITY PRESS

University Printing House, Cambridge CB2 8BS, United Kingdom

Cambridge University Press is part of the University of Cambridge.

It furthers the University's mission by disseminating knowledge in the pursuit of education, learning and research at the highest international levels of excellence.

www.cambridge.org
Information on this title: www.cambridge.org/9781107087293

Fifth edition © Cambridge University Press 2016

First published in 1993 by Elsevier
Fourth edition: 2009 by Elsevier
Fifth edition: 2016 by Cambridge University Press

Printed in the United Kingdom by Clays, St Ives plc

A catalogue record for this publication is available from the British Library

Library of Congress Cataloguing in Publication data
Caplan, Louis R, editor. | Caplan's stroke.
Preceded by (work):
Caplan's stroke : a clinical approach / edited by Louis R Caplan.
Stroke
Fifth edition. | Cambridge ; New York : Cambridge University Press, 2016. | Preceded by Caplan's stroke / Louis R. Caplan. 4th ed. Philadelphia : Elsevier/Saunders, c2009. | Includes bibliographial references and index.
LCCN 2016005752 | ISBN 9781107087293 (hardback)
| MESH: Stroke – diagnosis | Stroke – therapy | Cerebrovascular Disorders – diagnosis | Cerebrovascular Disorders – therapy
LCC RC388.5 | NLM WL 356 | DDC 616.8/1–dc23
LC record available at http://lccn.loc.gov/2016005752

ISBN 978-1-107-08729-3 Hardback

Contents

Colour plates are to be found between pp. 342 and 343.

v

Preface

Although this is the fifth edition of my Stroke book, in many ways it represents a completely new endeavor. This edition is both single and multi-authored – a somewhat new concept. I have continued to control the organization, writing style, and patient-oriented focus of the book and each of the chapters. The new aspect is that I have chosen respected experienced experts who have reviewed each chapter in their particular area of expertise. They have corrected prior mis-statements, elaborated on aspects they feel were incompletely covered, and updated each chapter with new information that has accrued since the fourth edition was published in 2009. After receiving the input of the chapter co-authors, I have re-reviewed the chapters, added information and references, and ensured that the finalized chapter preserves the goals, style, and main content of the book.

Three observations stimulated this new approach. (1) Critics of the last edition opined that the topic of stroke has become much too large for any one person to cover well. The basic science and clinical stroke literature has expanded exponentially during the last decade. There is much truth to this criticism. (2) After writing and rewriting and re-editing the same chapters for decades, an individual (myself) loses the ability to be critical about their own writing and coverage of a subject. One just wants it to be finally done and sent in. Others can view the coverage freshly and critically much better than the original author. So, broadening the authorship, I believe, gives this edition more credibility and depth than prior editions. (3) The lack of genetic information in prior editions. A new chapter on genetics has also been added in this edition written by Dr Stéphanie Debette a clinical neurologist and geneticist.

At the same time what made this book different from multi-authored texts was the simplicity, patient focus, uniform organization, clinical emphasis, writing style, and clarity of the four prior editions. The previous books were all organized to be read from cover to cover to teach about clinical stroke. They were also organized so that information would be easily read by both novitiates and stroke specialists. I strove to maintain these aspects while still broadening the content by seeking the inputs of many others.

Louis R Caplan, MD
Boston, MA, USA

Contributors

Pierre Amarenco, MD PhD
Professor, Department of Neurology, Bichat University
Hospital, Paris, France

Fernando Barinagarrementeria, MD
División de Ciencias de la Salud, Universidad del Valle
de México, Hospital Ángeles de Querétaro, Querétaro,
Mexico

José Biller, MD FACP FAAN FAHA
Department of Neurology, Loyola University Stritch School of
Medicine, Maywood, IL, USA

Marie-Germaine Bousser, MD
Professor, Department of Neurology, Lariboisière Hospital,
Paris, France

Bruce Campbell, MBBS(Hons) BMedSc PhD FRACP
Department of Medicine and Neurology, Royal Melbourne
Hospital, University of Melbourne, Parkville, VIC,
Australia

Louis R Caplan, MD
Senior Neurologist, Beth Israel Deaconess Medical Center,
Professor of Neurology, Harvard Medical School, Boston,
MA, USA

Steven C Cramer, MD
Professor of Neurology, University of California Irvine, Irvine,
CA, USA

Marie Dagonnier, MD
Research Fellow at the Florey Institute of Neuroscience and
Mental Health, Melbourne, VIC, Australia

Stephen Davis, MD FRCPEd FRACP
Professor of Neurology, The Melbourne Neuroscience
Center, The Royal Melbourne Hospital, Parkville, VIC,
Australia

Stéphanie Debette, MD
Department of Neurology, Bordeaux University Hospital,
Bordeaux, France

Michael DeGeorgia, MD FCCM FNCS
Maxeen Stone and John A Flower Professor of Neurology at
Case Western Reserve University School of Medicine, Director,
Center for Neurocritical Care, Neurological Institute, University
Hospitals Case Medical Center, Cleveland, OH, USA

Gabrielle deVeber, MD
Professor of Neurology, The Hospital for Sick Children,
Toronto, ON, Canada

Geoffrey Donnan, MBBS MD FRACP FRCP (Edin)
Professor of Neurology, University of Melbourne, Director at
The Florey Institute of Neuroscience and Mental Health,
Parkville, VIC, Australia

Philip B Gorelick, MD MPH FACP
Professor at the Department of Translational Science and
Molecular Medicine, Michigan State University College of
Human Medicine, Medical Director at Mercy Health
Hauenstein Neurosciences, MI, USA

Tudor Jovin, MD
Associate Professor of Neurology and Neurosurgery Director,
UPMC Stroke Institute Director, UPMC Center for
Neuroendovascular Therapy, President, Society of Vascular
and Interventional Neurology (SVIN), University of
Pittsburgh, PA, USA

Carlos S Kase, MD
Department of Neurology, Boston University Medical Center,
Boston, MA, USA

Jong S Kim, MD PhD
Professor of Neurology at the Asan Medical Center, University
of Ulsan, Seoul, Korea

Sandeep Kumar, MD
Department of Neurology, Beth Israel Deaconess Medical
Center, Boston, MA, USA

David S Liebeskind, MD
Professor of Neurology and Director, Neurovascular
Imaging Research Care, UCLA, Department of Neurology, USA

Ayrton R Massaro, MD
Department of Neurology, Hospital Siro-Libanês, Sao Paulo, Brazil

Jeffrey Saver, MD
Professor of Neurology, Geffen School of Medicine at UCLA, Los Angeles, CA, USA

Aneesh B Singhal, MD
Department of Neurology, Massachusetts General Hospital, Boston, MA, USA

Lawrence Wechsler, MD
Henry B Higman Professor and Chair, Department of Neurology, University of Pittsburgh, and Vice President for Telemedicine, University of Pittsburgh Medical Center, Pittsburgh, PA, USA

Introduction and perspective

Louis R Caplan

It was then that it happened. To my shock and incredulity, I could not speak. That is, I could utter nothing intelligible. All that would come from my lips was the sound ab which I repeated again and again ... Then as I watched it, the telephone handpiece slid slowly from my grasp, and I, in turn, slid slowly from my chair and landed on the floor behind the desk ... At 5:15 in that January dusk I had been a person; now at 6:45 I was a case. But I found it easy to accept my altered condition. I felt like a case.
Eric Hodgins[1]

"Cheshire Puss ... Would you tell me, please, which way I ought to go from here?"
"That depends a great deal on where you want to get to," said the Cat.
"I don't much care where –," said Alice.
"Then it doesn't matter which way you go," said the Cat.
"– so long as I get *somewhere*," Alice added ...
"Oh, you're sure to do that," said the Cat, "if you only walk long enough."
Lewis Carroll[2]

The past is always with us, never to be escaped; it alone is enduring; but, amidst the changes and chances which succeed one another so rapidly in this life, we are apt to live too much for the present and too much in the future.
William Osler[3]

Numbers

In the United States, according to 2014 statistics, 795 000 individuals have a stroke each year (610 000 are first strokes).[4] In 2010, one of every 19 deaths was attributed to stroke; on average a stroke occurred every 40 seconds and someone died of stroke about every 4 minutes. At any one time, there are approximately two million stroke survivors living in the United States. In China, approximately 1.5 million people die each year because of stroke.[5] Stroke affects three times as many women as breast cancer and yet receives much less public attention. For a long time, stroke has been the third leading cause of death in most countries in the world, surpassed as a killer only by heart disease and cancer. Strokes are an even more important cause of prolonged disability. Survivors of strokes are often unable to return to work or to assume their former effectiveness as spouses, parents, friends, and citizens. The economic, social, and psychological costs of stroke are enormous. In the United States, each ischemic stroke costs on average $140 000, and costs related to stroke nationwide was estimated to be $62.7 billion in 2007.[5]

Important medical and historical figures who had strokes

The history of the world has undoubtedly been altered by stroke. Many important leaders in science, medicine, and politics have had their productivity cut prematurely short by stroke. Marcello Malpighi, discoverer of capillaries and the microscopic anatomy of the lungs, kidneys, and spleen, died of an apoplectic right hemiplegia.[6] Louis Pasteur, at age 46 years, had a stroke that caused a left hemiparesis, although he continued to make important advances until additional strokes impaired his function at age 65.[6]

Three important figures in twentieth century neurology – Russell DeJong,[7] the first editor of the journal *Neurology*; Raymond Escourolle, the French neuropathologist; and H. Houston Merritt, longtime Columbia professor and writer of *Merritt's Neurology* –were severely disabled by multiple strokes in their later years. Two important political leaders during the early twentieth century, Vladimir Lenin and Woodrow Wilson, had intellectual impairment owing to stroke while they were at the helms of their countries at critical times in history. Lenin, at age 52 years, had the sudden onset of dysarthria and right hemiparesis. An observer noted that "often as he spoke, the words were slurred, and he paused several times like a man who has lost the thread of his argument."[8] Wilson, the architect of the League of Nations, had a series of small strokes that left him pseudobulbar and with a left hemiparesis at a time when he was ardently working for world peace and cooperation. The heads of state who met at Yalta and elsewhere to divide up the spheres of influence after the Second World War, Franklin D Roosevelt, Winston Churchill, and Joseph Stalin, (shown in Figure 1.1) all had severe cerebrovascular disease at the time.[8] Roosevelt subsequently died of a fatal stroke after years of severe hypertension.[9] History might have been different if the brains of these leaders had not been addled by strokes. Public awareness of stroke increased dramatically when President

Caplan's Stroke: A Clinical Approach, 5th Edition, ed. Louis R Caplan. Published by Cambridge University Press. © Cambridge University Press, 2016.

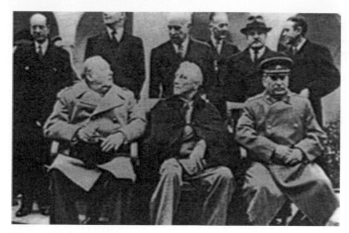

Figure 1.1 A photograph taken at the Yalta conference after the Second World War showing (from left to right in the front row) Winston Churchill, Franklin D Roosevelt, and Joseph Stalin. From Toole JF. *Cerebrovascular Disorders*, 4th ed. New York: Raven Press, 1990.

Dwight Eisenhower developed acute dysarthria, when Richard Nixon died after a large embolic cerebral hemisphere infarction, and when Ariel Sharon the Prime Minister of Israel was left unconscious after a series of cerebrovascular events.

The personal tragedy of stroke

The mortality, morbidity, and economic toll of stroke is impressive. Knowledge that government leaders may have brains damaged and even riddled with brain infarcts and hemorrhages is undoubtedly sobering. Yet even more important, in my own opinion, is the effect of stroke on the individual. What could be worse than the sudden inability to speak, move a limb, stand, walk, see, read, or feel, or become unable to understand spoken language, write, think clearly, or remember? Loss of function is often instantaneous and totally unanticipated; impairments may be transient or permanent, slight or devastating. The first common term for stroke, apoplexy, literally meant in Greek "struck suddenly with violence."[10] The word stroke refers to being suddenly stricken. Stroke patients tell graphically about the personal tragedy of their illness. Eric Hodgins, the popular author of *Mr. Blandings Builds His Dream House*, wrote an autobiographical account of his stroke that he titled *Episode*, from which I quoted at the beginning of this chapter.[1] He changed from a functioning human in one moment to a helpless, dumb invalid, "a case" in the next instant. Imagine an articulate author dependent for his livelihood on his use of language becoming totally unable to speak. Surely, the brain is wholly responsible for intelligence, capability, character, wit, humor, personality, and most of the characteristics that make us recognizable as individuals and as humans. Losing brain function can be dehumanizing and often makes individuals dependent on others. For these reasons, most individuals fear stroke more than any other disease, with the possible exception of cancer. Everyone would like to exit this life with their capabilities and mind intact, despite the inevitable aging of their bodies.

When I conjure in my own mind the personal tragedy of stroke, I picture one of my own patients, Dr Herman Blumgart, an extremely gifted physician, teacher, and investigator. He was, for many years, physician-in-chief at the Beth Israel Hospital in Boston.[11] His early investigations in coronary artery disease were landmark advances in the understanding of vascular disease of the heart.[12,13] He gave the annual introductory lecture to incoming Harvard Medical School students about the joys and responsibilities of being a physician. I recall his vivid, articulate lectures and bedside demonstrations. He was, in many ways, the model physician. He was also a vocal advocate on behalf of patients. His lecture "Caring for the Patient," presented in 1963 and reported in the *New England Journal of Medicine*, remains a model exposition on doctoring, as valid today as when it was originally delivered.[14] Tragically, this master of communication became in an instant, severely aphasic. His Wernicke-type aphasia was so severe that he could barely communicate verbally his basic needs and could hardly understand the queries and spoken and written statements of others. He could no longer read, eliminating one of his lifelong joys. As a junior staff neurologist, I was one of his physicians. The angst and frustration of his plight showed clearly on his face each time I saw him. This personal disaster was palpable and dramatic.

A brief history of stroke

In any human endeavor, the future is heavily influenced by the past. As the Wonderland dialogue between Alice and the Cheshire Cat (quoted at the beginning of this chapter)[2] teaches, if you want to get somewhere, you must know where you are going. If clinicians are to know where they are headed, they must know where they are, and where they and their predecessors have been. History adds an important dimension to knowledge. The past helps focus and broaden the perspective of the present and the future. Osler, and most other important medical innovators, were aware of their debt to history and of their inevitable entanglement with the past as well as the present and future.[3] I begin with a review of the history of stroke. Space necessitates inclusion of only a brief review of some important people and milestones to convey a sense of the historical context of the present state of knowledge about stroke. Of course, the following view of history is eclectic and personal and should be recognized as such.

Early observers: Hippocrates to Morgagni

Hippocrates (c. 400 BC) was probably the first to write about the medical aspects of stroke.[6,10] He and his followers were mostly interested in prognosis, predicting for the patient and family the outcome of an illness.[15–17] Hippocrates was a keen observer and urged careful observation and recording of phenomenology. Hippocrates wrote in his aphorisms on apoplexy, "persons are most subject to apoplexy between the ages of forty and sixty,"[16] and attacks of numbness might reflect "impending apoplexy."[10] He astutely noted, "when persons in good health are suddenly seized with pains in the head and straightaway are laid down speechless and breathe with stertor, they

die in seven days when fever comes on."[6,17] This description of subarachnoid hemorrhage shows the Hippocratic emphasis on observation and prognosis. Hippocrates also observed that there were many blood vessels connected to the brain, most of which were "thin," but two (the carotid arteries) were stout. The Greeks recognized that interruption of these blood vessels to the brain could cause loss of consciousness, and so they named the arteries *carotid*, from the Greek word Karos, meaning "deep sleep."

A few hundred years after Hippocrates, Galen (131–201 AD) described the anatomy of the brain and its blood vessels from dissections of animals. Although his early writings emphasized observation and experimentation, much of his later works combined mostly theorizing and speculation, in which he attributed disease to a disequilibrium between putative body humors and secretions such as water, blood, phlegm, bile, and so forth.[15] Galen and his voluminous writings dominated the 1300 years after his death. During the ensuing Dark and Middle Ages, persons who called themselves physicians gained their knowledge solely from studying the Galenic texts, considered at the time to be the epitome of all medical wisdom. Dissection, experimentation, and personal observations were discouraged and not considered scholarly.

Andreas Vesalius (1514–1564) challenged the Galenic tradition by dissecting humans and relying on his own personal observations instead of Galen's writings. Vesalius could not find the rete mirabile of blood vessels that Galen had described (presumably in a lower animal).[15] Vesalius's dissections were published in a volume entitled *De Humani Corpis Fabrica* (usually referred to as the *Fabrica*), which contained the detailed drawings his young artist and collaborator Jan Kalkar reproduced as woodcuts and copper plates.[6,18] The seventh book of the *Fabrica* contains 15 diagrams of the brain. These were the most detailed neuroanatomical studies up to that time.[6] By all accounts, Vesalius had a great flair for lecturing and teaching, and his works and personage stimulated much interest in anatomy and in the brain.[15]

During the last half of the seventeenth century, two important physicians, Johann Jakob Wepfer (1620–1695) and Thomas Willis (1621–1675), made further anatomical and clinical observations. Wepfer wrote a popular treatise on apoplexy that was originally published in 1658 and had five subsequent editions.[6,19] Wepfer performed meticulous examinations of the brains of patients dying of apoplexy. He described the appearance of the carotid siphon and the course of the middle cerebral artery in the sylvian fissure. Obstruction of the carotid and vertebral arteries was recognized as a cause of apoplexy (the blockage preventing sufficient blood from reaching the brain).[19,20] Wepfer was the first to show clearly that bleeding into the brain was an important cause of apoplexy. Thomas Willis (shown in Figure 1.2), a physician and neuroanatomist best known for his *Cerebri Anatome*, which contained a description of a circle of anastomotic vessels at the base of the brain, was also a well-known clinician and an astute observer. Willis was born soon after the deaths of William Shakespeare and Queen Elizabeth I when Great Britain was still basking in the artistic bloom of Elizabethan

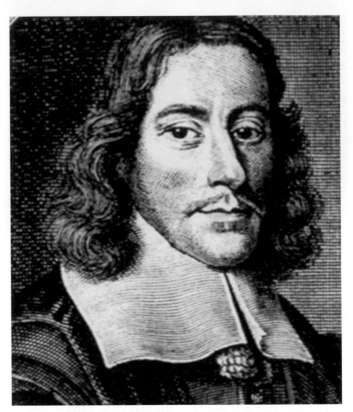

Figure 1.2 Sir Thomas Willis (1621–1675).

England. Willis recognized transient ischemic attacks and the phenomenology of embolism, as well as the existence of occlusion of the carotid artery.[20–25] Willis described clearly the collateral circulation in the head and neck: "The cephalic arteries, whether they be carotid or vertebrals, communicate one with the other reciprocally in various ways . . . This we have demonstrated by injecting dark substances in only one branch and observing that the whole brain becomes colored."[22] Willis was able to recruit a remarkable group of coworkers to Oxford, England, including the illustrator and architect Christopher Wren, and the physicists Robert Hooke and Robert Boyle.[24,25] These investigators were an important stimulus for science in post-Elizabethan England.[24]

During the eighteenth century, one of the true giants in medical history, Giovanni Battista Morgagni (1682–1771), was able to focus attention on pathology and the cause of disease. Up to that time, anatomy and prognostic formulas had prevailed. Morgagni, a distinguished professor of anatomy at the University of Padua, had a vision that the secret to understanding disease was to carefully perform necropsies on humans with illnesses and then to correlate the pathological findings with their symptoms during life.[15] Although the clinicopathological method is now taken for granted, this was a new approach for physicians in the eighteenth century. Morgagni labored his entire career to meticulously collect material for his epic work, *De Sedibus et Causis Morborum per Anatomen Indagatis*, which was published when he was 79 years old.[15,26] *De Sedibus* is a 5-volume work organized in the form of 70 letters to a young man describing the cases

collected. The first volume was titled *Disease of the Head*. Morgagni's clinical descriptions of patients were detailed but contained no formal physical or neurological examinations because these were not performed during his lifetime.

One of Morgagni's descriptions illustrates the style and content of the book:

> A certain man, who was a native of Genoa, blind of one eye, and liv'd by begging, being drunk, and quarreling with other drunken beggars, receiv'd two blows by their sticks; one on his hand which was slight, and another violent one at the left temple so that blood came out of the left ear. Yet soon after, the quarrel being made up, he sat down at the fire with them ... and again fill'd himself with a great quantity of wine, by way of pledge of friendship being renewed; and not long after, on the same night, he died.[15]

Necropsy showed a large epidural hematoma. Morgagni also described cases of intracerebral hemorrhage and recognized that paralysis was on the side of the body opposite to the brain lesion. Morgagni's work shifted the emphasis from anatomy alone to inquiry about diseases and their pathology, causes, and clinical manifestations during life.

The nineteenth and early twentieth centuries: Atlas makers, Virchow and Foix

During the early years of the nineteenth century, an influential treatise on apoplexy was written by a prominent Irish physician John Cheyne (1777–1836). Cheyne's book, which appeared in 1812, was titled *Cases of Apoplexy and Lethargy with Observations upon the Comatose Diseases*.[27] In it, he sought to separate the phenomenology of lethargy and coma from apoplexy. Cheyne's description of the neurological abnormalities was more detailed than those of his predecessors, and the "morbid appearances" of the patients' brains were emphasized after the example of Morgagni. One illustrative patient was a woman of 32 years who was near the end of her pregnancy. After a headache she became less responsive. Cheyne found that "she preserved the power of voluntary motion of the left side, but the right was completely paralytic. She seemed perfectly conscious, attempted to speak, but could not articulate; she signified by pointing with her left hand that she desired to drink."[27] After describing her case history, Cheyne discussed the available treatments (blood-letting, emetics, purges, and external applications) and then described 23 other cases. The pathological findings included clear descriptions of brain softenings and intracerebral and subarachnoid hemorrhages.[27] After Cheyne, developments were made concurrently in the clinical, anatomic, and pathological aspects of stroke.

John Abercrombie contributed a more detailed clinical classification of apoplexy in his general text published in 1828.[28] Abercrombie used the presence of headache, stupor, paralysis, and outcome to separate apoplectics into three clinical groups. In the first group, which he termed primary apoplexy, the onset was sudden, unilateral paralysis; rigidity and stupor were present, and the outcome was poor. These patients probably had large intracerebral hemorrhages or large

brain infarcts. In the second group, patients had the sudden onset of headache, vomiting, and either faintness or falling but no paralysis. Undoubtedly, these patients had subarachnoid hemorrhages. In the third group, there was unilateral paralysis, often with abnormal speech, but neither stupor nor headache was present. This group must have had small infarcts or parenchymatous hemorrhages. Abercrombie also speculated on etiological mechanisms, mentioning spasm of vessels, interruption of the circulation, and rupture of diseased vessels causing hemorrhage.[10,28]

During the middle of the nineteenth century, dissemination of knowledge about the pathology of stroke came with the publication of four atlases, each containing plates of brain and vascular lesions. Hooper's atlas, published in 1828, clearly illustrated pontine and putaminal hemorrhages and a subdural hematoma.[29] Cruveilher (1835–1842),[30] Carswell (1838),[31] and Bright (1831)[32] also published atlases containing lithographs of systemic and neuropathological lesions. Bright, better known for his work on nephritis, collected more than 200 neuropathological cases and included illustrations of 25 nervous system specimens, including cerebrovascular cases, in his volume on nervous system disorders.[32]

During the latter half of the nineteenth century, the most important experimental and pathological information about vascular disease was published by Rudolf Virchow (1821–1902) (Figure 1.3), a pathologist working in Berlin.[15] He described the phenomenology of in-situ antemortem thrombosis with subsequent embolism. In a remarkable series of observations and experiments, Virchow analyzed the relationship between thrombi and infarction, locally and at a distance. Among 76 necropsies performed in 1847, Virchow found thrombi in extremity veins in 18 patients and within the pulmonary arteries in 11, and reasoned that the bloodstream emanating from these veins must have been the conduit for transportation of the thrombi to distant sites such as the

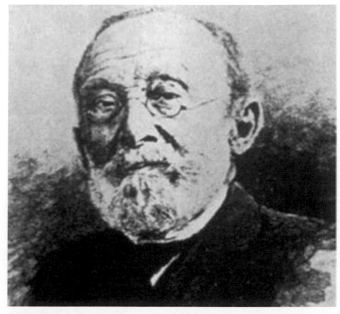

Figure 1.3 Rudolf Ludwig Carl Virchow (1821–1902).

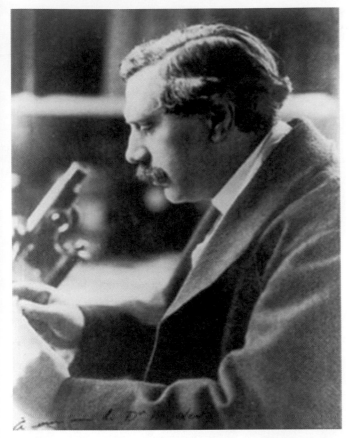

Figure 1.4 Charles Foix (1882–1927).

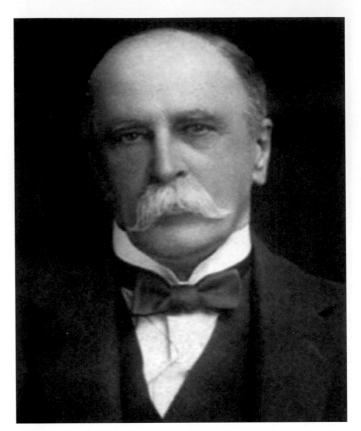

Figure 1.5 Sir William Osler (1849–1919).

arteries of the lung.[33,34] Virchow then used animal experiments to study the fate of foreign materials placed in veins. He later sought and found obstruction of brain, splenic, renal, and limb arteries at necropsy in patients who had cardiac valve disease and left atrial thrombi. Virchow showed systematically that in-situ thrombosis and embolism were the cause of infarction and that the process was unrelated to inflammation, the predominant theory at that time. Virchow described his classic triad of vascular thrombosis: (1) Stasis of blood in a vessel; (2) injury to the wall of the blood vessel; and (3) an abnormality in the balance between blood procoagulant and anticoagulant factors. Before Virchow's studies and reports, blood factors and thrombosis were given little attention.

During the later part of the nineteenth and the early years of the twentieth centuries, the anatomical details of the arteries supplying the brain were studied carefully. Detailed observations of the distribution of the arteries and veins in the cranium were made by Düret, a French neurosurgeon, first working in Charcot's laboratory;[35,36] by Stopford in Britain;[37] and later by Foix, who dissected pathological specimens at the Salpetrière in France.[38–41] Foix (Figure 1.4) made many key anatomical and clinical observations. Also during this same period, clinicians gathered more information on the clinical findings in patients with strokes that involved various brain regions. The bulk of these data involved clinical descriptions, with little interest concerning pathogenesis, laboratory confirmation, or treatment. The general medical and neurological texts of Osler,[42] Gowers,[43] and Wilson[44] contained detailed descriptions of the clinical findings and prognosis of many stroke syndromes. Sir William Osler (Figure 1.5), a famous internist, writer, and teacher, noted in detail the neurological findings in patients with bacterial endocarditis and described brain embolism in patients with rheumatic carditis. Osler first described the findings in patients with hemorrhagic telangiectasia (Osler, Weber, Rendu disease). The clinicopathological method culminated in descriptions by Foix and his colleagues of the syndromes of infarctions in the regions of the middle cerebral artery,[40,41] posterior cerebral artery,[41,45] anterior cerebral artery,[41,46] and vertebrobasilar arteries.[39,41]

Mid twentieth century and Miller Fisher

After Foix, a Canadian and American neurologist, C Miller Fisher (Figures 1.6–1.8), did much to awaken clinical interest in stroke. Fisher enlisted in the Canadian army during World War II and was captured and spent years in a prisoner-of-war camp. After the war, he was determined to make important contributions to medicine. His interest in stroke was tweaked by encounters with patients. One particular patient described in detail his episodes of transient monocular blindness that had heralded a hemisphere stroke. Fisher reviewed the literature and found scant reference to transient episodes before stroke. Fisher took meticulous thorough histories from patients hospitalized with stroke at a Veterans hospital in Canada and found that transient prodromal episodes were quite common. In patients with transient monocular blindness preceding stroke, Fisher reasoned that the causative occlusive process

5

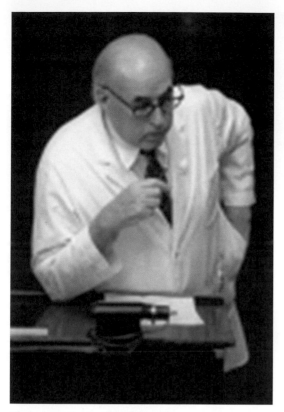

Figure 1.6 Charles Miller Fisher giving a presentation in 1978.

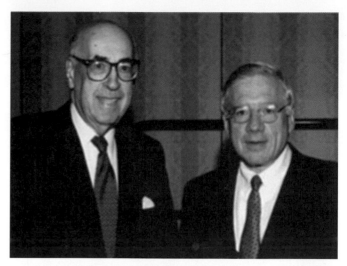

Figure 1.7 Charles Miller Fisher with Louis R Caplan in 1998.

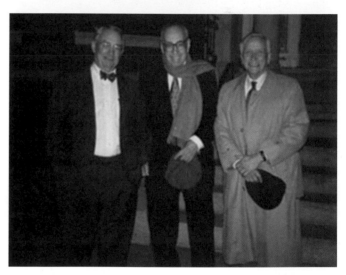

Figure 1.8 Jay P Mohr, Charles Miller Fisher, and Robert Ackerman.

was likely in the internal carotid artery in the neck or head. A patient with transient monocular blindness then died suddenly. After death, Fisher dissected the neck and found, as predicted, that the internal carotid artery was occluded.[47] He then collected and reported series of patients with internal carotid artery occlusions and described in detail the clinical histories and neurological findings.[48,49] Fisher emphasized the frequent occurrence of warnings before stroke that he later dubbed transient ischemic attacks. "Prodromal fleeting attacks of paralysis, numbness, tingling, speechlessness, unilateral blindness, or dizziness often preceded and warned of impending strokes in patients with carotid artery disease."[9]

Fisher, like Foix, was both a pathologist and a clinician. During his early career in Canada, and later in Boston, he thoroughly examined at necropsy the neck and cranial arteries and their microscopic-sized branches. He obtained specimens of arteries from their origins from the aorta to their major intracranial branches. During the 1950–1990 period, Fisher made many major pathological and clinical observations on the pathological and clinical features of carotid artery disease;[48–52] the pathological and clinical aspects of intracerebral hemorrhage;[53–56] the pathological and clinical syndromes related to lacunar brain infarction;[57–59] and the clinical and pathological features of various posterior circulation neurological signs and brain and vascular lesions.[60–66] Before Fisher's major stroke publications, Raymond Adams, his mentor, had written a classic clinicopathological descriptive report with Charles Kubik on basilar artery occlusion.[67]

Fisher developed the first stroke fellowship in the United States and mentored many now senior stroke neurologists. I was fortunate to serve as his stroke fellow during 1969–1970. Figure 1.7 is a recent picture of Miller Fisher and I. Dr Jay P Mohr, who worked with me in developing and maintaining the Harvard Stroke Registry in the early 1970s, and a leader in the field of stroke trials, was another of Dr Fisher's stroke fellows. Dr Robert Ackerman, a pioneer in the early field of PET scanning and stroke, and in the non-invasive evaluation of stroke risk was a trainee and later colleague of Dr Fisher and was the organizer of the Boston Stroke Society for three decades. Mohr, Fisher, and Ackerman are shown in Figure 1.8. Ackerman also trained stroke fellows including several future leaders in the field: Geoffrey Donnan and Steven Davis (Australia); Jean-Claude Baron (France and UK), and James Grotta and Viken Babikian (United States).

Fisher's reports contained meticulous descriptions of the signs and symptoms found in patients with infarcts and

hemorrhages in various vascular and brain distributions. Elegant and thorough as these descriptions were, their limitations included: (1) Reliance on only the fatal cases because precise diagnosis was not possible during life; (2) predominance of anecdotal cases, with few data on the incidence and frequency of findings in large series of patients with the specific described conditions; (3) insufficient availability of technology to allow accurate diagnosis or clarification of the pathogenesis or pathophysiology of the vascular lesions and their effects on the brain; and (4) little information about the effectiveness of various treatments.

1975 to present

During the last quarter of the twentieth century, there was an explosive growth of interest in and knowledge about stroke. Advances in technology allowed better visualization of the anatomy and functional aspects of the brain and of vascular lesions during life. Databases and registries of large numbers of well-studied stroke patients helped identify and quantify the most common clinical and laboratory findings in patients with various stroke syndromes. Epidemiological studies identified more accurately the risk factors for stroke and suggested prevention strategies. New surgical and medical treatments were now possible. Therapeutic trials began to evaluate systematically the efficacy and safety of some of these treatments. Physicians began to explore the use of devices that could be introduced through the arterial system to treat various arterial lesions including atherosclerotic stenoses, aneurysms and vascular malformations. Other devices could be used to retrieve thromboemboli that blocked arteries in the neck and head. Thrombolysis became a reality and strokes were considered a medical emergency requiring urgent attention. Stroke units were formed in many hospitals and greatly improved the care of stroke patients.

Advances in diagnostic technology

The technological revolution probably began with the work of the Portuguese neurosurgeon Egas Moniz (1874–1955). Moniz surgically exposed and temporarily ligated the internal carotid artery in the neck and then rapidly injected by hand a 30% solution of sodium iodide, taking skull films later at regular time intervals.[68] He first used the technique for studying patients suspected of having brain tumors, but he later studied stroke patients. By the time of his monograph on angiography in 1931,[69] Moniz had studied 180 patients; had switched to another opaque-contrast agent, Thorotrast, because of convulsions that had occurred after the injection of sodium iodide; and had demonstrated the occurrence of occlusion of the internal carotid artery during life.[68,69] Modern angiography began with the work of Seldinger in Sweden, who devised a technique by which a small catheter could be inserted into an artery over a flexible guidewire after withdrawing the needle.[70,71] Catheter angiography of selected vessels in the carotid and vertebral circulations was then possible without surgical incisions. Newer dyes and

filming techniques have since made angiography safer and more definitive.

Hounsfield of the research laboratories of Electrical Musical Instruments (EMI) in Britain originated the concept of computed tomography (CT) during the mid 1960s. The instrument was first tried at the Atkinson-Morley Hospital in London.[6] CT scanners were first introduced to North America in 1973. Films from first-generation scanners were quite primitive, but by the late 1970s, third-generation scanners had made CT a useful, almost indispensable, diagnostic technique. By the mid 1980s, CT was readily available throughout North America and most of Europe. CT allowed clear distinction between brain ischemia and hemorrhage and allowed definition of the size and location of most brain infarcts and hemorrhages. The advent of magnetic resonance imaging (MRI) into clinical medicine in the mid 1980s was a further major advance. MRI proved superior to CT in showing old hemosiderin-containing hemorrhages and in imaging vascular malformations, lesions abutting on bony surfaces, and posterior fossa structures. MRI also made it easier to visualize lesions in different planes by providing sagittal, coronal, and horizontal sections. Improved filming techniques have made it possible to image the brain vasculature through the techniques of magnetic resonance angiography[72] and CT angiography.[73]

Ultrasound was introduced into medicine in 1961 by Franklin and colleagues, who used Doppler shifts of ultrasound to study blood flow in canine blood vessels.[6,74] B-mode ultrasound was soon used to provide images of the extracranial carotid arteries non-invasively. By the early 1980s, B-mode, continuous-wave (CW), and pulsed-Doppler technology could reliably detect severe extracranial vascular occlusive disease in the carotid and vertebral arteries in the neck. Sequential ultrasound studies allowed physicians to study the natural history of the development and progression of these occlusive lesions and to correlate the occurrence and severity of disease with stroke risk factors, symptoms, and treatment. In 1982, Aaslid and colleagues introduced a high-energy bidirectional pulsed-Doppler system that used low frequencies to study intracranial arteries, termed transcranial Doppler ultrasound (TCD).[75] TCD made possible non-invasive detection of severe occlusive disease in the major intracranial arteries during life, as well as sequential study of these lesions.[76]

Introduction of echocardiography and ambulatory cardiac rhythm monitoring in the 1970s and 1980s greatly improved cardiac diagnoses and detection of cardiogenic sources of embolism. By the early 1990s, clinicians could safely define the nature, extent, and localization of most important brain, cardiac, and vascular lesions in stroke patients. Accurate diagnosis using modern technology facilitated clinical-imaging correlations in patients with non-fatal strokes, and this paved the way for monitoring the effects of various treatments. By the end of the twentieth century, advanced brain imaging with CT, MRI, and newer magnetic resonance (MR) modalities,

including fluid-attenuated inversion recovery (FLAIR) images, diffusion, perfusion, and functional MRI, and MR spectroscopy, were able to show clinicians the localization, severity, and potential reversibility of brain ischemia. Vascular lesions could be quickly and safely defined using CT angiography, MR angiography, and extracranial and transcranial ultrasound. During the first decades of the twenty-first century, high-resolution MR and CT studies of lesions imaged in cross-section could better define the nature of atherosclerotic plaques and other arterial wall abnormalities. Cardiac and aortic sources of stroke were studied using transesophageal echocardiography. More sophisticated hematological testing led to new insights into the role of altered coagulability in causing or contributing to thromboembolism. Clinicians were finally able to recognize and quantify quickly and accurately the key data elements needed to logically treat patients with brain ischemia and hemorrhage.

Data banks and stroke registries

During the middle years of the twentieth century, clinicians had advanced knowledge of clinical phenomenology by personally studying and describing small groups of patients. In 1935, Aring and Meritt studied a group of patients coming to necropsy at the Boston City Hospital to clarify the differential diagnosis between brain hemorrhages and infarcts.[77] Fisher and his colleagues and students studied and described the clinical findings in small numbers of patients with various cerebrovascular syndromes. During the 1970s and 1980s, the technological advances described made it possible to define the clinical and laboratory features of non-fatal, even minor, strokes and pre-stroke vascular lesions. With better knowledge of clinical and morphological features, clinicians naturally sought more quantitative data. How often did intracerebral hemorrhages or lacunar infarcts occur? How often did each of the clinical symptoms and signs occur in each subtype of stroke? Clinicians recognized that valid, statistically meaningful data could not be collected unless large numbers of patients with a wide spectrum of representative cases were studied and analyzed. The advent of computers in medicine in the 1970s greatly facilitated the storage and analysis of large quantities of complex data. Collection of data on large numbers of stroke patients began with the series of Dalsgaard-Nielsen in Scandinavia[78] and with series of patients seen by clinicians at the Mayo Clinic in Rochester, Minnesota.[79,80] The Harvard Cooperative Stroke Registry in the early 1970s was the first computer-based registry of prospectively studied stroke patients.[81] Other stroke registries and databases were developed around the world and provided more quantitative information about clinical and laboratory phenomena and diagnoses.[82–89] Community-based studies in south Alabama[90]; Framingham, Massachusetts[91]; Oxfordshire in Great Britain[92]; the Lehigh Valley in Pennsylvania[93]; and various regions in North Carolina, Oregon, and New York[94] generated important epidemiological data. Computer-based registries and data banks have undoubtedly assisted collection and analysis of a wide variety of clinical, radiological, pathological, and epidemiological information.[95,96] Especially important has been recognition

of various risk factors that predispose to stroke. The present text relies heavily on data from these studies, especially those in which I was personally involved.[81,83,85]

Stroke units, stroke specialists, and stroke nurses

During the nineteenth and the first two-thirds of the twentieth century nearly all acute stroke patients were cared for in the general wards and rooms of hospitals. There were very few stroke specialists and no stroke nurse specialists. Some rehabilitation units, almost entirely outside of acute hospitals did specialize in stroke rehabilitation. During the 1960s and 1970s Neurology departments began to be split off from Departments of Internal Medicine within academic medical centers in the United States and Europe. When this occurred, hospitals with neurology departments began to place stroke patients and other patients with neurological diseases on neurology wards and private rooms while other stroke patients continued to be treated on medical services scattered throughout the hospitals. During the 1970s and 1980s, hospitals placed very sick patients requiring frequent monitoring and care into specialized intensive care units (ICUs). Cardiac, surgical, and medical ICUs were first formed. Neurosurgeons and neurologists in large medical centers were successful in creating Neuroscience ICUs manned with nurses specially trained to care for very ill and acute neurological disorders including stroke. A new neurological specialty – neurology intensivists began to grow.

A number of factors during the 1980s and 1990s conspired to promote the development and proliferation of specialized stroke units. CT, MRI, ultrasound, and vascular imaging capabilities made it clear that strokes were complex and composed of very diverse etiologies and pathophysiologies. Moreover specific diagnosis could be made rather quickly and safely but required special training, expertise, and experience. Funding for trials made it possible in academic medical centers to hire nursing coordinators. The development of managed care strategies in hospitals in the United States forced more rapid and efficient care and throughput of stroke patients. Newer therapies, surgeries, percutaneous interventions, and especially thrombolysis made it advantageous to segregate stroke patients in ICUs and specialized stroke units.

These specialized units were composed of nurses with experience and training in stroke, internists, and stroke neurologists. These stroke units were able to deliver: specialized nursing care; attention to management of blood pressure, fluid volumes, and other physiological and biochemical factors; protocols and practices to facilitate rapid and thorough evaluation and treatment, monitor treatment, carry out randomized therapeutic trials, and prevent complications; education about stroke and its prevention to patients and their families and caregivers.[97–100] They also promoted an up-beat optimistic view of stroke recovery in contrast to the situation previously present on medical wards where stroke patients were often considered undesirable patients with hopeless outcomes.

Once these units began to proliferate especially in Europe, it became clear that they were an important major advance.

Dedicated stroke units have been convincingly shown to decrease mortality, limit stroke morbidity, and allow more patients to retain their independence and to return home after stroke.[101-103] Between the carrying out of the two large European thrombolytic trials (ECASS I and ECASS II),[104,105] neurologists in the hospitals engaging in these trials developed dedicated stroke units. These units attended to the general medical care of the stroke patients and prevention of complications. As a result the morbidity in both the thrombolytic treatment group and the placebo groups improved dramatically in the ECASS II trial and the good results in the placebo-treated group exceeded that of any prior thrombolytic trial. The milieu and the care in dedicated stroke units leads to better outcomes. Mortality is reduced. More patients return home and less are transferred to chronic hospitals and nursing homes. Short-term and long-term functional outcomes are also improved. There is no longer any doubt that stroke units work. One of the the most important therapeutic advances during the last decades of the twentieth century in the treatment of patients with acute stroke was the development of stroke services, stroke nurses, stroke specialists, and stroke units.

Advances in medical and surgical therapy and randomized trials

During the first half of the twentieth century, researchers discovered the anticoagulant effects of warfarin and heparin compounds. McLean, a medical student at Johns Hopkins, first isolated an anticoagulant compound from body tissues.[6,106] Howell and Holt extended Mclean's research and named the new compound heparin.[6,107] Link and colleagues found that a natural coumarin compound found in hay was transformed during spoilage into a substance that led to bleeding in cattle.[6,108] Link crystallized dicumarol in 1939, and soon thereafter many laboratories synthesized related warfarin-type compounds that could be used therapeutically.[6] During the 1950s clinicians began to give these anticoagulants to patients with various clinical syndromes mostly based on the tempo of brain ischemia – transient ischemic attacks, progressing stroke, completed stroke, etc.

One of the first randomized therapeutic trials concerned the effectiveness of anticoagulant therapy in patients with various ischemic syndromes.[109] This trial, which was reported in 1962, contained only 443 patients, 219 of whom were anticoagulated.[109] The methodology and analysis used in this trial would be considered rather primitive by today's standards. Treatment was open label, not blinded, the number of patients in each ischemic group was very few, and the endpoints varied depending on the nature of the group; for example, in patients entered in the group "thrombosis-in-evolution" (128 patients) the investigators analyzed progression of infarction and mortality. This study antedated CT scanning so that estimates of progression of infarction were only clinical. During the last decades of the twentieth century many trials studied the utility of anticoagulation in a variety of causes of brain ischemia, especially prevention of stroke in patients with atrial fibrillation.[110-113]

Sparked by clinical observations, clinicians in the mid twentieth century turned to drugs that affect platelet functions as an alternative to heparin and coumadin. Probably the first clinical observations on the potential anticoagulant functions of aspirin were made by Craven who noted that dental patients bled more if they had used aspirin.[6] He urged friends and patients to take 1 or 2 aspirin tablets a day and later published the effectiveness of this strategy in preventing coronary and cerebral thrombosis among 8000 men in articles during the mid 1950s in the *Mississippi Valley Medical Journal*.[114,115] Case reports from the United States and Britain on the effectiveness of aspirin in preventing attacks of transient monocular blindness brought the subject to more general attention.[116,117] The American[118] and Canadian[119] aspirin trials soon followed during the 1970s. These studies were the first of many trials of various antiplatelet agents almost invariably studied in large numbers of patients lumped together as having transient ischemic attacks or minor strokes.

Subsequent trials studied the relative safety and efficacy of aspirin versus warfarin in preventing stroke recurrence in a large numbers of ischemic stroke patients, the WARSS (Warfarin–Aspirin Recurrent Stroke Study) trial,[120] and in patients who had brain ischemia attributable to severe intracranial arterial stenosis, the WASID (Warfarin–Asprin Symptomatic Intracranial Disease) trial.[121] Physicians became increasingly aware that warfarin compounds were difficult to use in practice. These vitamin K inhibitors worked indirectly on the coagulation system, were affected by other medications and foods, and were difficult to keep in target range of optimal anticoagulation. As a result many patients were intermittently under anticoagulated and at risk for brain ischemia, and bleeding was an important problem. Multiple frequent blood tests were needed to monitor anticoagulation. Because it took time for warfarin to become clinically effective, heparin was customarily used until patients were effectively anticoagulated with warfarin. Pharmaceutical companies placed on the market newer anticoagulants that were direct thrombin inhibitors (dabigatran) and factor Xa inhibitors (apixaban, rivaroxaban, edoxaban). These agents were all taken orally, worked quickly so that heparin was not needed initially, had fixed doses so that long-term blood test monitoring was not essential, and were not as affected by other agents and foods as the vitamin K inhibitors. Trials of these agents tested their safety and efficacy versus warfarin in patients with atrial fibrillation, a known important cause of brain embolism.[122-125] These newer anticoagulants caused less intracranial bleeding and were at least as effective as warfarin in stroke prevention.

Miller Fisher in his seminal reports on carotid artery disease in the early 1950s predicted that one day in the future surgery would be feasible on the internal carotid artery to prevent stroke.[47,49] During the 1950s, surgeons reported their experience with surgery on the internal carotid[126-128] and other extracranial arteries.[6,129-131] In order to study the effectiveness of surgery on the extracranial arteries, a host of neurologists and adventurous surgeons led by Dr William S Fields organized and carried out a large surgical trial during the 1960s.[132,133] The trial was entitled the Joint Study of

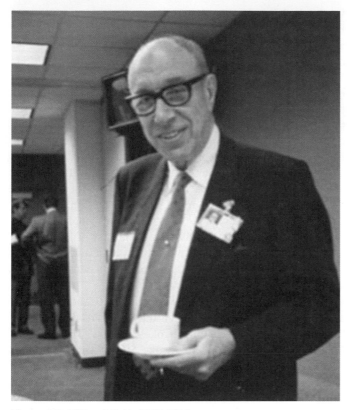

Figure 1.9 William S Fields (1913–2004).

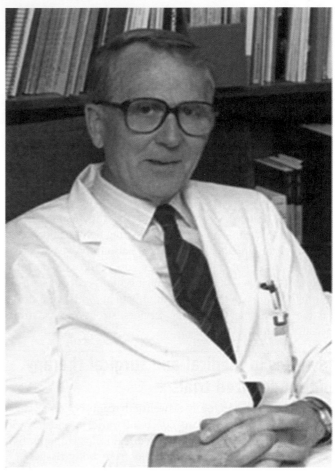

Figure 1.10 Sir Henry J M Barnett. From Barnett HJM (ed), *Cerebrovascular Disease*, Neurological Clinics Vol 1, No. 1. Philadelphia: W B Saunders, 1983.

Extracranial Arterial Occlusions and was supported by the National Heart Institute. This was the first surgical versus medical treatment trial carried out in the United States in which 6535 patients were randomly assigned to surgical versus non-surgical treatment. Mortality in this trial was equal in the medical and surgical groups and death was most often cardiac. Fields (Figure 1.9) was a pioneer in the study of cerebrovascular diseases, hosted and published many conferences in Houston about various stroke conditions, and was the principal investigator and organizer of pioneering stroke trials.[6,134,135]

During the 1960s and early 1970s Donaghy and his colleagues devised a microsurgical technique to anastamose small arteries together.[136,137] One of their trainees, Gazi Yasargil, was mostly responsible for bringing this technique into clinical practice when he created surgical extracranial-to-intracranial (EC-IC) shunts to treat patients with occlusive vascular disease who had brain ischemia.[138–140] By 1977 bypass procedures usually anastamosing the superficial temporal artery to branches of the middle cerebral artery were being performed widely in the United States and Europe. Henry Barnett (Figure 1.10) organized and performed a trial of these EC-IC bypass procedures, and showed that the procedure as performed at the time was less successful than medical treatment.[141] The results of this trial, published in 1985, drastically reduced the number of these procedures performed. Because neurologists and surgeons continued to posit that some patients with symptomatic atherosclerotic internal carotid artery occlusion and hemodynamic cerebral ischemia were at high risk for subsequent stroke when treated medically,

a trial was carried out testing the efficacy of bypass in patients with cerebral ischemia identified by ipsilateral increased oxygen extraction fraction as measured by positron emission tomography (PET).[141,142] The trial was terminated early for futility because of the high rate of ipsilateral ischemic strokes within 30 days of creation of the surgical bypass.[141,142]

Alarmed that the number of carotid endarterectomy cases was growing out-of-hand, Henry Barnett organized a trial of surgical versus medical treatment for patients with symptomatic carotid artery disease. This North American Symptomatic Carotid Endarterectomy Trial (NASCET)[143,144] and the concurrent European Carotid Surgery Trial (ECST)[145,146] showed the effectiveness of carotid endarterectomy in selected patients with selected lesions performed by surgeons who had low surgical mortality and morbidity results. Trials of carotid surgery in patients who had no related symptoms soon followed in both the United States[147] and Europe.[148,149] Carotid surgery and stenting were later compared in the CREST (Carotid Revascularization Endarterectomy Versus Stenting) Trial in the USA.[150,151]

During the last decades of the twentieth century there was an almost religious zeal for randomized clinical trials. Some enthusiasts saw the future dominated by doctors searching computer databases of trials to choose what to do

for their individual patients,[152-154] while some clinicians including myself remain very skeptical about this vision of the future.[155,156]

Thrombolysis

Beginning in the late 1950s, a few clinicians reported very small series of thrombolytic treatment of stroke patients.[157-160] These early investigators used bovine or human thrombolysins or streptokinase. During the early 1960s, John Sterling Meyer and his colleagues in Detroit randomized 73 patients with progressing strokes to receive streptokinase intravenously and/or concomitant anticoagulants within 3 days of stroke onset.[161,162] Clots were lysed in some patients, but 10 patients treated with streptokinase died, and some patients developed brain hemorrhages. After these studies, streptokinase and other thrombolytics were considered to be too dangerous to be given to stroke patients. The use of streptokinase for systemic and cardiac thromboembolism was considered contraindicated in the presence of brain lesions or past strokes.

The successful use of thrombolytic agents for the treatment of coronary artery thrombosis reawakened an interest in stroke thrombolysis during the 1980s. A group of neurologists in Aachen, Germany, led by Klaus Poeck, Hermann Zeumer, Werner Hacke, Andreas Ferbert, Berndt Ringelstein, and Helmut Bruckmann, began to treat patients with both anterior and posterior circulation thromboembolism using intra-arterial thrombolytic agents.[163,164] The early results were published in *Neuroradiology* journals. Then Hacke and colleagues published a landmark paper in the journal *Stroke* in 1988 that convincingly showed the benefit of intra-arterial thrombolysis in patients with acute basilar artery thromboembolism when the artery was successfully recanalized.[165] Following this a consortium of investigators that included Hacke and the Aachen group, Michael Pessin and I at the New England Medical Center in Boston, Tony Furlan at the Cleveland Clinic, Gregory del Zoppo at the Scripps Clinic in la Jolla California, and Etsuko Mori from Japan began studies, one of which was sponsored by the Burroughs-Welcome Company, on intravenous thrombolysis.[166,167] These investigators and others during the late 1980s and early 1990s performed many, usually small observational studies concerning the utility and risk of intravenous and intra-arterial thrombolysis. In these studies an angiogram was performed after CT scan had excluded hemorrhage and the catheter was not removed from the patient; the thrombolytic drugs – streptokinase, urokinase, or recombinant tissue plasminogen activator (rt-PA) – were then given either intravenously or intra-arterially to patients whose arteriogram had shown an intracranial arterial occlusion. A follow-up angiogram was then performed after thrombolysis to determine if the occluded artery had recanalyzed. In most studies thrombolytic drugs were given within 6–8 hours or longer after symptom onset. The results of these preliminary observational, non-randomized studies were reviewed by Drs Pessin, del Zoppo, and Furlan at the Nineteenth Princeton Vascular Disease Conference.[168] In 1990, a group of investigators convened the first meeting on stroke thrombolysis in Heidelberg Germany.[169] The proceedings of this meeting were published and succeeding international stroke thrombolytic meetings have occurred, at first every 2 years and, more recently, annually. The results of these early angiographically controlled series showed that: recanalization correlated with outcome; patients who recanalized often improved; recanalization was better after intra-arterial treatment than intravenous treatment; manipulation of the clot during intra-arterial treatment abetted recanalization, and brain hemorrhage was an important complication, more commonly noted after intravenous treatment, which involved a larger dose of thrombolytic agent.

Stimulated by these early encouraging results studies were planned and launched in the United States (supported by the National Institute of Neurological Disease and Stroke (NINDS) and aided by Genentech)[170] and in Europe[104,105]. In contrast to the prior smaller observational series, these studies were randomized and controlled, had larger patient numbers, no suggested or mandated vascular studies, and shorter time intervals from symptom onset were used – 90, 180, and 360 minutes. Publication of the positive results of the NINDS study in the prestigious *New England Journal of Medicine*[170] gave momentum to a movement in the United States to quickly introduce intravenous thrombolysis into the treatment of patients with acute ischemic strokes. During the summer of 1996, about 6 months after the publication of the NINDS rt-PA study, the US Federal Drug Administration (FDA) approved the use of rt-PA for the treatment of stroke patients when the drug was given within the first 3 hours. Subsequent published treatment protocols adopted by committees of the American Heart Association[171] and the American Academy of Neurology[172] recommended intravenous administration of rt-PA according to the methods and inclusion–exclusion criteria of the NINDS trial. The drug authorization authorities in Canada and Europe released rt-PA for clinical use much later than the US FDA. In 2008, a European Registry confirmed the effectiveness of tissue plasminogen activator (tPA) administered between 3.0 and 4.5 hours after stroke symptom onset.[173] Authorities in Europe and other areas provided a license for giving tPA in this extended time interval. Intravenous tPA (IV-tPA) was often used during a longer time window (6–8 h) with effectiveness in some patients with documented basilar artery occlusions.[174,175] Efforts to administer IV-tPA sooner after symptom onset has stimulated research into the feasibility of delivering treatment at the time patients are collected by specialized ambulances that contain CT scanning equipment.

During the 1990s, clinicians and investigators launched randomized controlled trials of intra-arterial thrombolysis using pro-urokinase. These trials were carried out in the United States and Canada.[176,177] The larger Prolyse in Acute Cerebral Thromboembolism (PROACT II) study included 180 patients with angiographically shown middle cerebral artery occlusions treated intra-arterially within 6 hours.[177] The study showed unequivocally that the treatment was

effective but inexplicably the US FDA failed to approve intra-arterial thrombolysis. Clinicians however, impressed by the results, continued to treat selected patients intra-arterially. When clot retrieval devices became available, interventional intra-arterial delivery of thrombolytic agents was often accompanied by or replaced by mechanical clot extraction through catheters placed within the arteries.

During the last few years of the twentieth century clinicians and investigators began to use intravenous and intra-arterial thrombolysis and to accrue results. Unfortunately less than 5% of acute stroke patients were treated. Clinicians began to explore ways to establish more stroke centers, ways to get patients to these stroke centers more quickly, and to devise protocols for more rapid evaluation and treatment. They also explored ways to extend the window of treatment by using modern brain and vascular imaging (MRI/MR angiography (MRA), CT/CT angiography (CTA), and neck and transcranial ultrasound) to identify the presence and extent of infarction and the presence and nature of occluded supply arteries. Research continues in determining which treatments (intravenous or intra-arterial thrombolytics with or without mechanical clot removal) should best be given to which patients at what ages and with what comorbidities with which arterial occlusive lesions at what timing after symptom onset.

Mechanical devices

The two most popular treatment-related buzz-words used during the last quarter of the twentieth century were "evidence-based" and minimally invasive surgery." During the 1970s physicians began to explore non-surgical means of obliterating cerebral aneurysms and vascular malformations. Much credit should go to Serbenenko, a Russian neurosurgeon who pioneered the use of detachable latex balloons introduced through the arterial system.[178] Serbenenko used the balloons to obliterate arteries feeding aneurysms and to occlude aneurysms sparing the feeding artery. He also used the balloons to occlude arteries supplying arteriovenous malformations (AVMs). Later, interventionalists began to use silicone detachable balloons.[179] Balloons, however, had limited utility in treating aneurysms since many of the balloons were unable to conform to the shape of the lumens of aneurysms and they exerted force on the walls of the aneurysm. A major advance was the development of fibered platinum coils that could be delivered through the neck of the aneurysmal sacs to obliterate aneurysms. Guglielmi, an Italian radiologist, deserves credit for developing electrolytically detachable coils that are still much in use today to obliterate aneurysms.[180] Later stents were introduced to help ensure that coils would be directed into the aneurysmal sac. Endovascular coiling was performed after stent deployment through a microcatheter; the coils were advanced through the stent struts or had been placed inside the aneurysm sac before the stents were introduced and jailed between the stent and the vessel wall.[181,182] Still later, during the first decade of the twenty-first century, flow-diverting stents were introduced into treatment of large intracranial aneurysms. These flow diverters disrupted flow near the neck

of aneurysms inducing thrombosis in the aneurysmal sac while preserving physiological blood flow in the parent vessel and in adjacent branches.[183,184] These were mostly used to treat large aneurysms. Observational studies and trials later showed that interventional treatment of aneurysms was at least as effective as surgery and was associated with less mortality and morbidity. Neurosurgeons began to train in interventional treatment as the twentieth century ended. The number of neurosurgeons, neurologists, and neuroradiologists trained to provide interventional transvascular treatments has grown dramatically during the past two decades. As a result now 60% or more of intracranial aneurysms are treated in the United States and Europe through an endovascular approach.

During the last half of the twentieth century physicians also explored a variety of techniques to treat brain vascular malformations.[185] Luessenhop and Spence used silastic beads introduced from extracranial intra-arterial catheters to try and obliterate arteries that fed AVMs and reported the first case in 1960.[186] Subsequently neurosurgeons and interventional radiologists began to use a wide variety of materials introduced through intra-arterial catheters to obliterate AVMs – microcatheters, glues and tissue adhesives, beads and other particles, microcoils, sutures, and balloons.[185] During the last decade of the twentieth century, interventional treatment, radiation, and surgery were often used sequentially and selectively depending on the features of the malformations.

During the 1960s and early 1970s researchers explored the use of catheter systems that dilated arteries in animals. Andreas Gruentzig deserves great credit for introducing angioplasty into clinical practice in man. In 1978 Gruentzig reported the results from the first 5 coronary balloon angioplasties,[187] and a year later, reported the results from the first 50 patients so treated.[188] Stimulated by the successful use of angioplasty in the coronary arteries, researchers and clinicians began to explore angioplasty in the arteries that supplied the brain. Endovascular treatment of carotid artery disease with balloon angioplasty began in 1980.[189] Kerber and colleagues reported the first use of angioplasty for treatment of carotid artery stenosis.[190] A second small series was later published in 1983 by Bockenheimer and Mathias.[191] In 1987, Theron and colleagues published the first sizable series of extracranial stenosis patients treated with angioplasty (48 patients); the technical success rate was 94% and the major stroke morbidity was 4.1%.[192] Carotid artery angioplasty became quite popular and by 1995 it was possible to publish a review that included a worldwide experience among 523 patients.[189,193] The development of stenting in conjunction with balloon angioplasty for carotid artery stenosis was based on studies that showed improved outcomes during coronary percutaneous interventions when stents were used.

By the end of the twentieth century, stenting for extracranial carotid artery stenosis threatened to supplant surgical endarterectomy and trials began to compare the two treatment strategies. In a large randomized trial, the results of carotid endarterectomy and carotid artery stenting proved very similar, with surgery slightly better for older patients and stenting slightly more reasonable for younger

individuals.[150,151] Interventionalists also began to use angioplasty and stents to treat intracranial arterial stenotic lesions,[194] and to angioplasty vasoconstricted arteries in patients with subarachnoid hemorrhages. Devices began to be made and employed that could help retrieve clots. In patients with acute stroke related to thromboemboli, interventionalists could use chemical (thrombolytics) or mechanical means to retrieve thrombi within arteries, and angioplasty and stenting could be performed during the same procedure to maintain arterial patency. Many different specialists including neurologists, neuroradiologists, neurosurgeons, vascular surgeons, and cardiologists were trained to perform interventional treatments. The equipment available to the interventionalist looked more like a hardware store than a usual medical equipment tray. At the end of the century, physicians also explored the use of filters placed in the aorta to catch aortic and other debris generated during cardiac surgery, and to use balloons placed in the aorta to augment cerebral blood flow in patients with brain ischemia due to occlusive cerebrovascular disease and vasoconstriction after subarachnoid hemorrhage.

Stroke as a model example of brain and vascular disease

Stroke is the prototype of a focal, well-circumscribed brain lesion. Miller Fisher was fond of saying that neurology is learned "stroke by stroke." Knowledge of the symptoms and signs in patients with focal brain infarcts and hemorrhages has been instrumental in developing an understanding of the functioning of various brain structures and regions. Awareness of the clinical findings in patients with frontal-lobe hemorrhages has undoubtedly helped clinicians to recognize tumors, focal infections, atrophies, and other disease processes located in the frontal lobes. The ability to localize infarcts and hemorrhages precisely with CT and MRI has greatly facilitated study of anatomic-physiological correlations. Study of stroke patients and stroke animal models has improved understanding of brain electrophysiology, chemistry, pharmacology, and overall physiology.

Stroke also provides a model for the study of vascular diseases. Atherosclerosis, embolism, and thrombosis are all systemic disorders that affect many critical organs in addition to the brain. Information about the morphology, development, and etiology of lesions in the cerebrovascular bed has undoubtedly influenced knowledge of vascular conditions that affect the coronary, renal, and limb arteries. Of course, the corollary is also true; stroke clinicians clearly can and should gain from clinicians and researchers who study vascular diseases affecting these other body regions.

Similarly, study of patients with cardioembolic strokes has advanced knowledge about the heart and its diseases.[195] Stroke patients often have abnormalities of blood coagulation. Elucidation of clotting and bleeding dysfunction underlying stroke has advanced general knowledge about the formed and serological elements of the blood and the vascular endothelium and about their functions in coagulation.

Stroke care

It is not possible to overemphasize that the care of strokes is not the same as the care of individual stroke patients. Most strokes result from systemic illnesses such as hypertension, atherosclerosis, cardiac diseases, and coagulopathies. These conditions profoundly affect other body organs and general health, as well as the brain and central nervous system. Specialists sometimes only see and treat one portion of the body and ignore the general problem, similar to the proverbial blind men feeling isolated parts of the elephant. As physicians, we must be sure that the general systemic disorders, such as hypertension and atherosclerosis, receive deserved detailed and long-term attention. As entry portals into the healthcare system, clinicians seeing stroke patients can and should become key figures in preventing disease and in correcting unhealthy practices.

Strokes create other health problems. These include not only the acute complications but also problems such as increased wear and tear on the joint structures of the hip, knee, and ankle because of altered gait; aspiration and recurrent bronchopulmonary infections; and poor bladder emptying, with an increased frequency of urinary tract infections. Complications are discussed in Chapter 19. Strokes also have profound social, psychological, and economic effects on stroke patients and their families and friends. Physicians caring for stroke patients must consider all of the multiple facets of the condition and must liberally use other medical and ancillary health personnel. The family often needs as much attention, education, and compassion as the patient. In other books, written for physicians[196] and for the general public,[197–199] I have devoted considerable attention to the general approach toward and care of patients, especially those with stroke and other neurological illnesses.

The other organs exist to keep the brain functioning normally. Any change in the brain's function and activity profoundly affects living. No medical task exists that is more complex, more multifaceted, more important, and potentially more rewarding than caring for a stroke patient.

References

1. Hodgins E. *Episode: Report On the Accident Inside My Skull.* New York, NY: Atheneum, 1964, pp 7–14.

2. Carroll L. *Alice's Adventures in Wonderland.* New York, NY: Dutton, 1929, pp 93–94.

3. Osler W. Aequanimitas. In *Aequanimitas With Other Addresses to Medical Students,* *Nurses and Practitioners Of Medicine.* Philadelphia, PA: Blakiston, 1932, pp 8–9.

4. Go AS, Mozaffrian D, Roger VL et al. Executive summary: Heart disease and stroke statistics – 2014 update: A report

from the American Heart Association. *Circulation* 2014;**129**(3):399–410.

5. Rosamond W, Flegal K, Friday G et al. Heart disease and stroke statistics – 2007 update: A report from the American heart Association Statistics Committee and Stroke Statistics Committee. *Circulation* 2007;**115**(5):e69–e171.

6. Fields WS, Lemak NA. *A History Of Stroke: Its Recognition and Treatment.* New York, NY: Oxford University Press, 1989.

7. Gilman S. Russell N DeJong. 1907–1990. *Ann Neurol* 1991;**29**:108–109.

8. Friedlander WJ. About three old men: An inquiry into how cerebral atherosclerosis has altered world politics. *Stroke* 1972;**3**:467–473.

9. Bruenn HG. Clinical notes on the illness and death of president Franklin D. Roosevelt. *Ann Intern Med* 1970;**72**:579–591.

10. McHenry LC Jr. *Garrison's History Of Neurology.* Springfield, IL: Charles C Thomas Publisher, 1969.

11. Linenthal AJ. *First a Dream: The History of Boston's Jewish hospitals, 1896 to 1928.* Boston, MA: Beth Israel Hospital, 1990, pp 276–294.

12. Blumgart HL, Schlesinger MJ, Davis D. Studies on the relation of the clinical manifestations of angina pectoris, coronary thrombosis, and myocardial infarction to the pathological findings. *Am Heart J* 1940;**19**:1–9.

13. Blumgart HL, Schlesinger MJ, Zoll PM. Angina pectoris, coronary failure, and acute myocardial infarction. *JAMA* 1941;**116**:91–97.

14. Blumgart HL. Caring for the patient. *N Engl J Med* 1964;**270**:449–456.

15. Nuland S. *Doctors, Bibliography Of Medicine.* Birmingham, AL: Libraries of Gryphon Editions, 1988.

16. Adams F. *The Genuine Works of Hippocrates: Translated from the Greek.* Baltimore, MD: Williams & Wilkins, 1939.

17. Clark E. Apoplexy in the Hippocratic writings. *Bull Hist Med* 1963;**37**:301–314.

18. Vesalius A. *De Humani Corporis Fabrica.* Basileae, Italy: J Oporini, 1543.

19. Wepfer JJ. *Observationes Anatomicae, Ex Cadaveribus Eorum, Quos Sustulit Apoplexia, Cum Exercitatione De Ejus Loco Affecto.* Schaffhausen, Germany: Joh. Caspari Suteri, l658.

20. Gurdjian ES. History of occlusive cerebrovascular disease: I. From Wepfer to Moniz. *Arch Neurol* 1979;**36**:340–343.

21. Willis T. *The London Practice Of Physick.* London: Thomas Basset at the George in Fleet Street and William Crooke at the Green-Dragon without Temple-Bar, 1685.

22. Willis T. *Cerebri Anatome: Cui Accessit Nervorum Descriptio Et Usus.* London: J Flesher, 1664.

23. Willis T. Instructions and prescripts for curing the apoplexy. In *The London Practice of Physic* (Portage S, ed.), 1679.

24. Zimmer C. *Soul Made Flesh: The Discovery Of the Brain and How It Changed the World.* New York, NY: William Heinemann (Random House), 2004.

25. Caplan LR. Posterior circulation ischemia: Then, now, and tomorrow. The Thomas Willis lecture – 2000. *Stroke* 2000;**31**:2011–2023.

26. Morgagni GB. *The Seats and Causes Of Disease Investigated By Anatomy.* Translated by B Alexander. London: Millar and Cadell, 1769. Birmingham: Classics of Medicine Library, 1983.

27. Cheyne J. *Cases of Apoplexy and Lethargy With Observations Upon the Comatose Diseases.* London: J Moyes Printer, 1812.

28. Abercrombie J. *Pathological and Practical Researches On Diseases Of the Brain and Spinal Cord.* Edinburgh: Waugh and Innes, 1828.

29. Hooper R. *The Morbid Anatomy Of the Human Brain Illustrated By Coloured Engravings Of the Most Frequent and Important Organic Diseases To Which That Viscus Is Subject.* London: Rees, Orme, Brown & Green, 1831.

30. Cruveilher J. *Anatomie Pathologique Du Corps Humain: Descriptions Avec Figures Lithographiées Et Caloriées Des Diverses Alterations Morbides Dont Le Corps Humain Est Susceptible.* Paris: J B Bailliere, 1835–1842.

31. Carswell R. *Pathological Anatomy: Illustrations Of the Elementary Forms Of Disease.* London: Longman, 1838.

32. Bright R. *Reports Of Medical Cases, Selected With a View Of Illustrating the Symptoms and Cures Of Diseases By a Reference To Morbid Anatomy.* London: Longman, Rees, Orme, Brown & Green, 1831.

33. Fisher CM. The history of cerebral embolism and hemorrhagic infarction. In *The Heart and Stroke* (Furlan A, ed.), Berlin: Springer-Verlag, 1987, pp 3–16.

34. Virchow R. Ueber die akut entzundung der arterien. *Virchows Arch Path Anat* 1847;**1**:272–378.

35. Duret H. Sur la distribution des arteres nouricieres du bulbe rachidien *Arch Physiol Norm Pathol* 1873;**2**:97–113.

36. Duret H. Recherches anatomiques sur la circulation de l'encephale. *Arch Physiol Norm Pathol* 1874;**3**:60–91,316–353.

37. Stopford JS. The anatomy of the pons and medulla oblongata. *J Anat Physiol* 1928;**50**:225–280.

38. Foix C, Hillemand P. Irrigation de la protuberance. *C R Soc Biol (Paris)* 1925;**92**:35–36.

39. Foix C, Hillemand P. les Arteres de l'axe encephalique jusqu'au diencephale inclusivement. *Rev Neurol (Paris)* 1925;**41**:705–739.

40. Foix C, Levy M. les Ramollissements sylviens. *Rev Neurol (Paris)* 1927;**43**:1–51.

41. Caplan LR. Charles Foix – the first modern stroke neurologist. *Stroke* 1990;**21**:348–356.

42. Osler W. *The Principles and Practice Of Medicine* (5th ed). New York, NY: D Appleton, 1903.

43. Gowers WR. *A Manual Of Disease Of the Nervous System.* London: J & A Churchill, 1893.

44. Wilson SAK, Bruce AN. *Neurology* (2nd ed). London: Butterworth–Heinmann, 1955.

45. Foix C, Masson A. Le Syndrome de l'artere cerebrale posterieure. *Presse Med* 1923;**31**:361–365.

46. Foix C, Hillemand P. Les syndromes de l'artere cerebrale anterieure. *Encephale* 1925;**20**:209–232.

47. Estol CJ. Dr C Miller Fisher and the history of carotid artery disease. *Stroke* 1996;**27**:559–566.

48. Fisher CM. Occlusion of the internal carotid artery. *Arch Neurol Psychiatry* 1951;**65**:346–377.

49. Fisher CM. Occlusion of the carotid arteries. *Arch Neurol Psychiatry* 1954;**72**:187–204.

50. Fisher CM, Ojemann RG. A clinico-pathologic study of carotid endarterectomy plaques. *Rev Neurol* 1986;**142**:573–589.

51. Fisher CM. Observations of the fundus oculi in transient monocular blindness. *Neurology* 1959;**9**:333–347.

52. Fisher CM. Facial pulses in internal carotid artery occlusion. *Neurology* 1970;**20**:476–478.

53. Fisher CM. The pathology and pathogenesis of intracerebral hemorrhage. In *Pathogenesis and Treatment Of Cerebrovascular Disease* (Fields WS, ed.), Springfield, IL: CharlesThomas Publishers, 1961, pp 295–317.

54. Fisher CM. Clinical syndromes in cerebral hemorrhage. In *Pathogenesis And Treatment Of Cerebrovascular Disease* (Fields WS, ed.), Springfield, IL: CharlesThomas Publishers, 1961, pp 318–342.

55. Fisher CM. Pathological observations in hypertensive cerebral hemorrhage. *J Neuropathol Exp Neurol* 1971;**30**:536–550.

56. Fisher CM, Picard EH, Polak A, Dalal P, Ojemann R. Acute hypertensive cerebellar hemorrhage: Diagnosis and surgical treatment. *J Nerv Ment Dis* 1965;**140**:38–57.

57. Fisher CM, Lacunes: Small deep cerebral infarcts. *Neurology* 1965;**15** 774–784.

58. Fisher CM. The arterial lesions underlying lacunes. *Acta Neuropath (Berlin)* 1969;**12**:1–15.

59. Fisher CM. Pure motor hemiparesis of vascular origin. *Arch Neurol* 1965;**13**:30–44.

60. Fisher CM, Karnes W, Kubik CS. Lateral medullary infarction. The pattern of vascular occlusion. *J Neuropath Exp Neurol* 1961;**20**:323–379.

61. Fisher CM. A new vascular syndrome – "the subclavian steal". *N Engl J Med* 1961;**265**:912.

62. Fisher CM, Caplan LR. Basilar artery branch occlusion: a cause of pontine infarction. *Neurology* 1971;**21**:900–905.

63. Fisher CM. The posterior cerebral artery syndrome. *Can J Neurol Sci* 1986;**13**:232–239.

64. Fisher CM. Ocular bobbing. *Arch Neurol* 1964;**11**:543–546.

65. Fisher CM. Some neuro-opthalmological observations. *J Neurol Neurosurg Psychiatry* 1967;**30**:383–392.

66. Fisher CM. The "herald hemiparesis" of basilar artery occlusion. *Arch Neurol* 1988;**45**:1301–1303.

67. Kubik CS, Adams RD. Occlusion of the basilar artery: A clinical and pathological study. *Brain* 1946;**69**:73–121.

68. Moniz E. l'Encephalographie artèrielle, son importance dans la localization des tumeurs cérébrales. *Rev Neurol (Paris)* 1927;**2**:72–90.

69. Moniz E. *l'Angiographie Cérébrale.* Paris: Masson, 1931.

70. Gurdjian ES, Gurdjian ES. History of occlusive cerebrovascular disease: II. After Moniz with special reference to surgical treatment. *Arch Neurol* 1979;**36**:427–432.

71. Seldinger SI. Catheter replacement of the needle in percutaneous arteriography. *Acta Radiol* 1953;**39**:368–376.

72. Edelman RC, Mattle HP, O'Reilly GV, et al. Magnetic resonance imaging of flow dynamics in the circle of Willis. *Stroke* 1990;**21**:56–65.

73. Knauth M, von Kummer R, Jansen O, et al. Potential of CT angiography in acute ischemic stroke. *Am J Neuroradiol* 1997;**18**:1001–1010.

74. Franklin DL, Schlegel WA, Rushner RF. Blood flow measured by Doppler frequency shift of back-scattered ultrasound. *Science* 1961;**134**:564–565.

75. Aaslid R, Markwalder TM, Nornes H. Non-invasive transcranial Doppler ultrasound recording of flow velocity in basal cerebral arteries. *J Neurosurg* 1982;**57**:769–774.

76. Caplan LR, Brass LM, DeWitt LD, et al. Transcranial Doppler ultrasound: Present status. *Neurology* 1990;**40**:696–700.

77. Aring CD, Meritt HH. Differential diagnosis between cerebral hemorrhage and cerebral thrombosis. *Arch Intern Med* 1935;**56**:435–456.

78. Dalsgaard-Nielsen T. Survey of 1000 cases of apoplexia cerebri. *Acta Psychiatr Neurol Scand* 1955;**30**:169–185.

79. Whisnant JP, Fitzgibbons JP, Kurland LT, et al. Natural history of stroke in Rochester, Minnesota, 1945 through 1954. *Stroke* 1971;**2**:11–22.

80. Matsumoto N, Whisnant JP, Kurland LT, et al. Natural history of stroke in Rochester, Minnesota, 1955 through 1969: An extension of a previous study 1945 through 1954. *Stroke* 1973;**4**:20–29.

81. Mohr JP, Caplan LR, Melski JW, et al. The Harvard Cooperative Stroke Registry: A prospective registry. *Neurology* 1978;**28**:754–762.

82. Kunitz S, Gross CR, Heyman A, et al. The Pilot Stroke Data Bank: Definition, design, and data. *Stroke* 1984;**15**:740–746.

83. Caplan LR, Hier DB, D'Cruz I. Cerebral embolism in the Michael Reese Stroke Registry. *Stroke* 1983;**14**:530–536.

84. Chambers BR, Donnan GA, Bladin PF. Patterns of stroke: An analysis of the first 700 consecutive admissions to the Austin Hospital Stroke Unit. *Aust N Z J Med* 1983;**13**:57–64.

85. Foulkes MA, Wolf PA, Price TR, et al. The Stroke Data Bank: Design, methods, and baseline characteristics. *Stroke* 1988;**19**:547–554.

86. Bogousslavsky J, Mille GV, Regli F. The Lausanne Stroke Registry: An analysis of 1,000 consecutive patients with first stroke. *Stroke* 1988;**19**:1083–1092.

87. Moulin T, Tatu L, Crepin-Leblond T, Chavot D, Berges S, Rumbach T. The Besancon Stroke Registry: An acute stroke registry of 2,500 consecutive patients. *Eur Neurol* 1997;**38**(1):10–20.

88. Heuschmann PU, Kolominsky-Rabas PL, Misselwitz B, et al.; German Stroke Registers Study Group. Predictors of in-hospital mortality and attributable risks of death after ischemic stroke: The German Stroke Registers Study Group. *Arch Intern Med* 2004;**164**:1761–1768.

89. Vemmos KN, Takis CE, Georgilis K, Zakopoulos NA, Lekakis JP, Papamichael CM, Zis VP, Stamatelopoulos S. The Athens stroke registry: Results of a five-year hospital-based study. *Cerebrovasc Dis* 2000;**10**:133–141.

90. Gross CR, Kase CS, Mohr JP, et al. Stroke in south Alabama: Incidence and diagnostic features-a population based study. *Stroke* 1984;**15**:249–255.

91. Wolf PA, Kannel WB, Dauber TR. Prospective investigations: The Framingham study and the epidemiology of stroke. *Adv Neurol* 1978;**19**:107–120.

92. Oxfordshire Community Stroke Project. Incidence of stroke in Oxfordshire: First year's experience of a community stroke registry. *BMJ* 1983;**287**:713–717.

93. Alter M, Sobel E, McCoy RC, et al. Stroke in the Lehigh Valley: Incidence based on a community-wide hospital registry. *Neuroepidemiology* 1985;**4**:1–15.

94. Yatsu FM, Becker C, McLeroy K, et al. Community hospital-based stroke programs: North Carolina, Oregon, and New York: I. Goals, objectives, and data collection procedures. *Stroke* 1986;**17**:276–284.

95. Mohr JP. Stroke data banks [editorial]. *Stroke* 1986;**17**:171–172.

96. Caplan LR. Stroke data banks, then and now. In *Basis For a Classification Of Cerebrovascular Disease* (Courbier R, ed.). Amsterdam: Excerpta Medica, 1985, pp 152–162.

97. Caplan LR. Caplan's short rendition of stroke during the 20th century: Part 2. A short history. *Int J Stroke* 2006;**1**:228–234.

98. Indredavik B, Bakke F, Solberg R et al. Benefit of a stroke unit: a randomized controlled trial. *Stroke* 1991;**22**:1026–1031.

99. Indredavik B, Slordahl SA, Bakke F, Rokseth R, Haheim LL. Stroke unit treatment. Long term effects. *Stroke* 1997;**28**:1861–1866.

100. Diez-Tejedor E, Fuentes B. Acute care in stroke: Do stroke units make the difference? *Cerebrovasc Dis* 2001;**11**(Suppl 1):31–39.

101. Birbeck GL, Zingmond DS, Cui X, Vickrey BG. Multispecialty stroke services in California hospitals are associated with reduced mortality. *Neurology* 2006;**66**:1527–1532.

102. Stroke Unit Trialists' Collaboration. Collaborative systematic review of the randomized trials of organised in-patient (stroke unit) care after stroke. *BMJ* 1997;**314**:1151–1159.

103. Stroke Unit Trialists' Collaboration. How do stroke units improve patient outcomes? A collaborative systematic review of the randomized trials. *Stroke* 1997;**28**:2139–2144.

104. Hacke W, Kaste M, Fieschi C et al. Intravenous thrombolysis with recombinant tissue plasminogen activator for acute hemispheric stroke. The European Cooperative Acute Stroke Study (ECASS). *JAMA* 1995; **274**:1017–1025.

105. Hacke W, Kaste M, Fieschi C et al. for the Second European-Australasian Acute Stroke Study Investigators. Randomised double-blind placebo-controlled trial of thrombolytic therapy with intravenous alteplase in acute ischaemic stroke (ECASS-ll). *Lancet* 1998;**352**:1245–1251.

106. McLean J. The thromboplastic action of cephalin. *Am J Physiol* 1916;**41**:250–257.

107. Howell WH, Holt E. Two new factors in blood coagulation – heparin and pro-antithrombin. *Am J Physiol* 1918;**47**:328–341.

108. Link KP. The discovery of dicumarol and its sequels. *Circulation* 1959;**19**:97–107.

109. Baker RN, Broward JA, Fang HC, et al. Anticoagulant therapy in cerebral infarction. Report on cooperative study. *Neurology* 1962;**12**:823–835.

110. The Boston Area Anticoagulation Trial for Atrial Fibrillation Investigators. The effect of low-dose warfarin on the risk of stroke in patients with nonrheumatic atrial fibrillation. *N Engl J Med* 1990;**323**:1505–1511.

111. Petersen P, Godtfredsen J, Boysen G et al. Placebo-controlled, randomized trial of warfarin and aspirin for prevention of thromboembolic complications in chronic atrial fibrillation: The Copenhagen AFASAK study. *Lancet* 1989;**1**:175–179.

112. The Stroke Prevention in Atrial Fibrillation Investigators. The stroke prevention in atrial fibrillation study: Final results. *Circulation* 1991;**84**:527–539.

113. EAFT (European Atrial Fibrillation Trial) Study Group. Secondary prevention in non-rheumatic atrial fibrillation after transient ischaemic attack or minor stroke. *Lancet* 1993;**342**:1255–1262.

114. Craven LL. Experiences with aspirin (acetylsalicylic acid) in the nonspecific prophylaxis of coronary thrombosis. *Mississippi Valley Med J* 1953;**75**:38–44.

115. Craven LL. Prevention of coronary and cerebral thrombosis. *Mississippi Valley Med J* 1956;**78**:213–215.

116. Mundall J, Quintero P, von Kaulla K, et al. Transient monocular blindness and increased platelet aggregability treated with aspirin – a case report. *Neurology* 1971;**21**:402.

117. Harrison MJG, Marshall J, Meadows JC, et al. Effect of aspirin in amaurosis fugax. *Lancet* 1971;**2**:743–744.

118. Fields WS, LeMak NA, Frankowski RF, Hardy RJ. Controlled trial of aspirin in cerebral ischemia. *Stroke* 1977;**8**:301–316.

119. The Canadian Cooperative Study Group. A randomized trial of aspirin and sulfinpyrazone in threatened stroke. *N Engl J Med* 1978;**299**:53–59.

120. Mohr JP, Thompson JLP, Lazar RM et al. for the Warfarin-Aspirin Recurrent Stroke Study Group. A comparison of warfarin and aspirin for the prevention of recurrent ischemic stroke. *N Engl J Med* 2001;**345**:1444–1451.

121. Chimowitz MI, Lynn MJ, Howlett-Smith H, et al. Comparison of warfarin and aspirin for symptomatic intracranial arterial stenosis. *N Engl J Med* 2005;**352**:1305–1316.

122. Connolly SJ, Ezekowitz MD, Yusuf S, et al. RELY Steering Committee and Investigators. Dabigatran versus warfarin in patients with atrial fibrillation. *N Engl J Med* 2009;**361**:1139–1151.

123. Granger CB, Alexander JH, McMurray JJ, et al. ARISTOTLE Committees and Investigators. Apixaban versus warfarin in patients with atrial fibrillation. *N Engl J Med* 2011;**365**:981–992.

124. Patel MR, Mahaffey KW, Garg J, et al. ROCKET-AF Investigators. Rivaroxaban versus warfarin in nonvalvular atrial fibrillation. *N Engl J Med* 2011;**365**:883–891.

125. Giugliano RP, Ruff CT, Braunwald E, et al. ENGAGE AF-TIMI 48 Investigators. Edoxaban versus warfarin in patients with atrial fibrillation. *N Engl J Med* 2013;**369**:2093–2104.

126. Eastcott HHG, Pickering GW, Rob CG. Reconstruction of internal carotid artery in a patient with intermittent attacks of hemiplegia. *Lancet* 1954;**2**:994–996.

127. DeBakey ME. Successful carotid endarterectomy for cerebrovascular insufficiency. Nineteen years follow-up. *JAMA* 1975;**233**:1083–1085.

128. Carrea R, Molins M, Murphy G. Surgical treatment of spontaneous thrombosis of the internal carotid artery in the neck. Carotid–carotideal anastamosis. *Acta Neurol Latinoamer* 1955;**1**:71–78.

129. Cooley DA, Al-Naaman YD, Carton CA. Surgical treatment of arteriosclerotic occlusions of common carotid artery. *J Neurosurg* 1956;**2**:1265–1267.

130. Cate WR Jr, Scott HW. Cerebral ischemia of central origin. Relief by subclavian–vertebral artery thrombendarterectomy. *Surgery* 1959;**45**:19–31.

131. Thompson JE. The evolution of surgery for the treatment and prevention of stroke: The Willis lecture. *Stroke* 1996;**27**:1427–1434.

132. Fields WS, North RR, Hass WK et al. Joint Study of Extracranial Arterial Occlusion as a Cause of Stroke: Organization of study and survey of patient population. *JAMA* 1968;**203**:955–960.

133. Hass WK, Fields WS, North R et al. Joint Study of Extracranial Arterial Occlusion. II. Arteriography, techniques, sites, and complications. *JAMA* 1968;**203**:961–968.

134. Fields WS (ed). *Pathogenesis and Treatment Of Cerebrovascular Disease*. Springfield, IL: Charles C Thomas Publisher, 1961.

135. Fields WS, Sahs AL (eds). *Intracranial Aneurysms and Subarachnoid Hemorrhage*. Springfield, IL: Charles C Thomas Publisher, 1965.

136. Maroon JC, Donaghy RMP. Experimental cerebral revascularization with autogenous grafts. *J Neurosurg* 1973;**38**:172–179.

137. Hunter KM, Donaghy RMP. Arterial micrografts. An experimental study. *Can J Surg* 1973;**16**:23–27.

138. Yasargil MG, Krayenbuhl HA, Jacobson JH. Microneurosurgical arterial reconstruction. *Surgery* 1970;**67**:221–233.

139. Yasargil MG (ed). *Microsurgery Applied To Neurosurgery*. Stuttgart: George Thieme Verlag, 1969.

140. EC/IC Bypass Study Group. Failure of extracranial–intracranial arterial bypass to reduce the risk of ischemic stroke: results of an international randomized trial. *N Engl J Med* 1985;**313**:191–200.

141. Powers WJ, Clarke WR, Grubb RL et al. for the COSS Investigators. Extracranial–intracranial bypass surgery for stroke prevention in hemodynamic cerebral ischemia. The Carotid Occlusion Surgery Randomized Trial. *JAMA* 2011;**306**(18):1983–1992.

142. Caplan LR. Bypassing trouble. *Arch Neurol* 2012;**69**(4):518–520.

143. North American Symptomatic Carotid Endarterectomy Trial (NASCET) Collaborators. Beneficial effects of carotid endarterectomy in symptomatic patients with high-grade carotid stenosis. *N Engl J Med* 1991;**325**:445–453.

144. Barnett HJM, Taylor DW, Eliasziw et al. For the North American Symptomatic Carotid Endarterectomy Trial Collaborators. Benefit of carotid endarterectomy in patients with symptomatic moderate or severe stenosis. *N Engl J Med* 1998;**339**:1415–1425.

145. European Carotid Surgery Trialists' Collaborative Group. MRC European Carotid Surgery trial: Interim results of symptomatic patients with severe (70–99%) or with mild (0–29%) carotid stenosis. *Lancet* 1991;**1**:1235–1243.

146. European Carotid Surgery Trialists' Collaborative Group. Randomized trial of endarterectomy for recently symptomatic carotid stenosis: Final results of the MRC European Carotid Surgery Trial (ECST). *Lancet* 1998;**351**:1379–1387.

147. Asymptomatic Carotid Atherosclerosis Study Group. Carotid endarterectomy for patients with asymptomatic carotid artery stenosis. *JAMA* 1995;**273**:1421–1428.

148. Halliday AW, Thomas DJ, Mansfield AO. The asymptomatic carotid surgery trial (ACST). *Int Angiol* 1995;**14**:18–20.

149. Halliday A, Mansfield A, Marro J. Prevention of disabling and fatal strokes by successful carotid endarterectomy in patients without recent neurological symptoms: Randomised controlled trial. *Lancet* 2004;**363**:1491–1502.

150. Brott TG, Hobson RW II, Howard G, et al.; CREST Investigators. Stenting vs. endarterectomy for treatment of carotid-artery stenosis. *N Engl J Med* 2010;**363**(1):11–23.

151. Caplan LR, Brott TG. Of horse races, trials, meta-analyses, and carotid artery stenosis. *Arch Neurol* 2011;**68**(2):157–159.

152. Meinert CL. *Clinical Trials: Design, Conduct, and Analysis*. New York, NY: Oxford University Press, 1986.

153. Sackett DL. Evidence-based medicine: What it is and what it isn't. *BMJ* 1996;**312**:71–72.

154. Sackett DL, Rosenberg W. On the need for evidence-based medicine. *Evidence-based Medicine* 1995;**1**:5–6.

155. Caplan LR. Editorial. Evidence based medicine: concerns of a clinical neurologist. *J Neurology Neurosurg Psychiatry* 2001;**71**:569–576.

156. Caplan LR. Evidence and the effective clinical neurologist. The 2009 H Houston Merritt Lecture. *Arch Neurol* 2011;**68**(10):1252–1256.

157. Sloan MA. Thrombolysis and stroke: Past and future. *Arch Neurol* 1987;**44**:748–768.

158. Sussman BJ, Fitch TSP. Thrombolysis with fibrinolysin in cerebral arterial occlusion. *JAMA* 1958;**167**:1705–1709.

159. Herndon RM, Meyer JS, Johnson JF et al. Treatment of cardiovascular thrombosis with fibrinolysisn. *Am J Cardiol* 1960;**30**:540–545.

160. Clark RL, Clifton EE. The treatment of cerebrovascular thrombosis and embolism with fibrinolytic agents. *Am J Cardiol* 1960;**30**:546–551.

161. Meyer JS, Gilroy J, Barnhart ME et al. Anticoagulants plus streptokinase therapy in progressive stroke. *JAMA* 1963;**189**:373.

162. Meyer JS, Gilroy J Barnhart ME et al. Therapeutic thrombolysis in cerebral thromboembolism. Randomized evaluation of intravenous streptokinase. In *Cerebral Vascular Diseases*. (Millikan CH, Siekert R, Whisnant JP, eds), New York, NY: Grune & Sratton, 1964, pp 200 213.

163. Zeumer H, Hacke W, Ringelstein EB. Intra-arterial thrombolysis in vertebrobasilar thromboembolic disease. *AJNR Am J Neuroradiol* 1983;**4**:401–404.

164. Zeumer H, Hundgen R, Ferbert A et al. Local intra-arterial fibrinolyic therapy in inaccessible internal carotid occlusion. *Neuroradiology* 1984;**76**:315–317.

165. Hacke W, Zeumer H, Ferbert A, Bruckmann H, del Zoppo G. Intra-arterial thrombolytic therapy improves outcome in patients with acute vertebrobasilar occlusive disease. *Stroke* 1988;**19**:1216–1222.

166. del Zoppo GJ, Poeck K, Pessin MS et al. Recombinant tissue plasminogen activator in acute thrombotic and embolic stroke. *Ann Neurol* 1992;**32**:78–86.

167. Wolpert SM, Bruckmann H, Greenlee R et al. Neuroradiologic evaluation of patients with acute stroke treated with recombinant tissue plasminogen activator. The rt-PA Acute Stroke Study Group. *AJNR Am J Neuroradiol* 1993;**14**:3–13.

168. Pessin MS, del Zoppo GJ, Furlan AJ. Thrombolytic treatment in acute stroke: Review and update of selected topics. In *Cerebrovascular Diseases, 19th Princeton Conference, 1994.*

Boston, MA: Butterworth–Heinemann, 1995, pp 409–418.

169. Hacke W, del Zoppo GJ, Hirschberg M (eds). *Thrombolytic Therapy In Acute Ischemic Stroke*. Berlin: Springer-Verlag, 1991.

170. The National Institute of Neurological Disorders and Stroke rt-PA Study Group. Tissue plasminogen activator for acute ischemic stroke. *N Engl J Med* 1995;**333**:1581–1587.

171. Adams HP, Brott TG, Furlan AJ et al. Use of thrombolytic drugs. A supplement to the guidelines for the management of patients with acute ischemic stroke. A statement for Health Care Professionals from a special writing group of the Stroke Council American Heart Association. *Stroke* 1996;**27**:1711–1718.

172. Quality Standards Subcommittee of the American Academy of Neurology. Practice advisory: Thrombolytic therapy for acute ischemic stroke – summary statement, *Neurology* 1996;**47**:835–839.

173. Hacke W, Kaste M, Bluhmki E et al. for the ECASS Investigators. Thrombolysis with alteplase 3 to 4.5 hours after acute ischemic stroke. *N Engl J Med* 2008;**359**:1317–1329.

174. Lindsberg P, Soinne L, Tatlisumak T et al. Long-term outcome after intravenous thrombolysis of basilar artery occlusion. *JAMA* 2004;**292**:1862–1866.

175. Lindsberg PJ, Mattle HP. Therapy of basilar artery occlusion: A systematic analysis comparing intra-arterial and intravenous thrombolysis. *Stroke* 2006;**37**:922–928.

176. del Zoppo GJ, Higashida RT, Furlan AJ et al. PROACT: A phase II randomized trial of recombinant pro-urokinase by direct arterial delivery in acute middle cerebral artery stroke. *Stroke* 1998;**29**:4–11.

177. Furlan AJ, Higashida RT, Wechsler L et al. Intra-arterial prourokinase for acute ischemic stroke. The PROACT II Study: A randomized controlled trial. *JAMA* 1999;**282**:2003–2011.

178. Serbenenko FA. Balloon catheterization and occlusion of major cerebral vessels. *J Neurosurg* 1974;**41**:125–145.

179. Introcaso JH, Uske A. Endovascular treatment of intracranial aneurysms. In *Cerebrovascular Disease* (Batjer HH, Caplan LR, Friberg L et al., eds), Philadelphia, PA: Lippincott-Raven, 1996, pp 915–927.

180. Guglielmi G, Vinuela F, Sepetka I et al. Electrothrombosis of saccular aneurysms. Neurosurgery via endovascular approach. I. Electrochemical basis, technique, and experimental results. *J Neurosurg* 1991;**75**:1–7.

181. Fiorella, Albuquerque FC, Woo H et al. Neuroform stent assisted aneurysm treatment: evolving treatment strategies, complications and results of long term follow-up. *J Neurointerv Surg* 2010;**2**:16–22.

182. Geyik S, Yavuz N, Yurttutan N, Saatci I, Cekirge HS. Stent-assisted coiling in endovascular treatment of 500 consecutive cerebral aneurysms with long-term follow-up. *AJNR Am J Neuroradiol* 2013;**34**:1–6.

183. D'Urso PI, Lanzino G, Cloft HJ, Kallmes DF. Flow diversion for intracranial aneurysms: A review. *Stroke* 2011;**42**:2363–2368.

184. Chalouhi N, Tjoumakaris S, Starke R et al. Comparison of flow diversion and coiling in large unruptured intracranial saccular aneurysms. *Stroke* 2013;**44**:2150–2154.

185. Latchaw RE, Madison MT, Larsen DW, Silva P. Intracranial arteriovenous malformations: Endovascular strategies and methods. In *Cerebrovascular Disease* (Batjer HH, Caplan LR, Friberg L et al., eds), Philadelphia, PA: Lippincott-Raven, 1996, pp 707–725.

186. Luessenhop AJ, Spence WT. Artificial embolization of cerebral arteries. Report of use in a case of arteriovenous malformation. *JAMA* 1960;**172**:1153–1155.

187. Gruentzig A. Transluminal dilatation of coronary artery stenosis. *Lancet* 1978;**1**:263.

188. Gruentzig AR, Senning A, Siegenthaler WE. Nonoperative dilatation of coronary artery stenosis: percutaneous transluminal coronary angioplasty *N Engl J Med* 1979;**301**:61–68.

189. Meyers PM, Schumacher HC, Higashida RT, Leary MC, Caplan LR. Use of stents to treat extracranial cerebrovascular disease. *Annu Rev Med* 2006;**57**:437–454.

190. Kerber CW, Cromwell LD, Loehden OL. Catheter dilatation of proximal carotid stenosis during distal bifurcation endarterectomy. *AJNR Am J Neuroradiol* 1980;**1**:348–349.

191. Bockenheimer SA, Mathias K. Percutaneous transluminal angioplasty in arteriosclerotic internal carotid artery stenosis. *AJNR Am J Neuroradiol* 1983;**4**:791–792.

192. Theron J, Raymond J, Casasco A, Courtheoux F. Percutaneous angioplasty of atherosclerotic and postsurgical stenosis of carotid arteries. *AJNR Am J Neuroradiol* 1987;**8**:495–500.

193. Kachel R. Results of balloon angioplasty in the carotid arteries. *J Endovasc Surg* 1996;**3**:22–30.

194. Meyers PM, Schumacher C, Tanji K, Higashida RT, Caplan LR. Use of stents to treat intracranial cerebrovascular disease. *Ann Rev Med* 2007;**58**:107–122.

195. Caplan LR, Manning W (eds). *Brain Embolism*. New York, NY: Informa Healthcare, 2006.

196. Caplan LR, Hollander J. *The Effective Clinical Neurologist* (3rd ed). Shelton, CT: People's Medical Publishing House, 2011.

197. Hutton C, Caplan LR. *Striking Back At Stroke: A Doctor–Patient Journal*. Washington, DC: Dana Press, 2003.

198. Caplan LR. *Stroke*. St. Paul, MN: AAN Press, 2005.

199. Caplan LR. *Navigating the Complexities of Stroke*. New York, NY: Oxford University Press, 2013.

Pathology, anatomy, and pathophysiology of stroke

Louis R Caplan and David S Liebeskind

Introduction

Stroke is quite heterogeneous and not a single entity. Disorders as different as rupture of a large blood vessel that causes flooding of the brain with blood and occlusion of a tiny artery with softening in a small but strategic brain site both qualify as strokes. These two pathological caricatures of stroke subtypes are as divergent as grapes and watermelons, two very different substances that fit in the general category of fruit. Stroke refers to any damage to the brain or the spinal cord caused by an abnormality of the blood supply. The term *stroke* is typically used when the symptoms begin abruptly, whereas *cerebrovascular disease* is a more general term that carries no connotation as to the tempo of brain injury. Of course, many patients with severely diseased blood vessels have no injury to brain tissue, largely due to compensatory mechanisms such as collateral circulation. A blood or cardiovascular abnormality precedes and subsequently leads to the brain injury. Recognition of the cardiac or cerebrovascular lesion or hematological disorder before the brain becomes damaged offers clinicians a window of opportunity during which brain damage can be prevented. At times, even when brain injury has occurred, the patient is unaware of any symptoms and neurologists may not be able to detect any abnormality on neurological examination. Sophisticated neuroimaging techniques have taught clinicians that such "silent strokes" are common, now posing an additional target for stroke prevention efforts

Diagnosis and treatment of stroke patients require a basic understanding of the anatomy, physiology, and pathology of the major structures involved – the brain and spinal cord, the heart and blood vessels that supply blood to these structures, and the blood itself. To be effective, clinicians caring for stroke patients must be intimately familiar with: (1) the appearance of the normal brain and its various lobes and regions; (2) the appearance of brain tissue damaged by various vascular disorders; (3) the usual locations and course of arteries supplying the brain and spinal cord and veins that drain blood from these regions; and (4) the frequency, location, and appearance of diseases of the cerebrovascular system. Note that this discussion includes a number of words related to vision. Many of the diagnostic tests used, especially imaging of the brain and blood vessels, produce pictures. Clinicians must be able to visualize what the structures and diseases look like. For this reason, this chapter relies heavily on illustrations.

This chapter offers succinct and basic coverage of the topics just mentioned. We begin the chapter by introducing the various mechanisms of brain damage in stroke. These stroke mechanisms are the major players, the key actors in the drama of stroke. Their characterization, recognition, and treatment form the core of this book. Normal vascular anatomy and distribution are then described and illustrated. Next, the usual distribution and frequency of these various mechanisms in the blood vessels and in the brain are discussed and diagrammed. The chapter closes with a discussion of stroke pathophysiology, the dynamics of the functional response of the vascular system and brain to the primary injuries.

Pathology: mechanisms of cerebrovascular damage to brain tissue

The first questions that the clinician should ask about a stroke patient are "What caused the brain dysfunction?" and "What pathological process is active in this patient?" There are two major categories of brain damage in stroke patients: (1) ischemia, which is a lack of blood flow depriving brain tissue of needed fuel and oxygen; and (2) hemorrhage, which is the release of blood into the brain and into extravascular spaces within the cranium or skull contents. Bleeding damages the brain by cutting off connecting pathways and by causing localized or generalized pressure injury to brain tissue; biochemical substances released during and after hemorrhage also may adversely affect nearby vascular and brain tissues.[1,2]

Ischemia

Ischemia can be further subdivided into three different mechanisms: thrombosis, embolism, and decreased perfusion or blood flow in a region of the brain. An analogy to a simple plumbing situation illustrates the differences among the mechanisms. Suppose that a homeowner calls a plumber and tells him that when the faucet in the second-floor bathroom at the right is turned on, water does not flow (Figure 2.1). The plumber finds that the pipe feeding the sink is rusty and has become blocked. The plumber repairs the local pipe, and water

---

Caplan's Stroke: A Clinical Approach, 5th Edition, ed. Louis R Caplan. Published by Cambridge University Press. © Cambridge University Press, 2016.

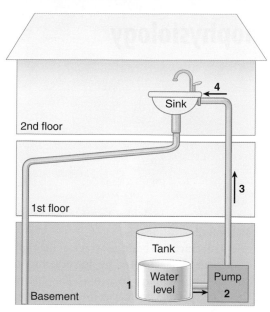

Figure 2.1 Cartoon of home plumbing illustrating possible problem areas: (1) insufficient water in the tank; (2) low pump pressure; (3) low water pressure in the pipes; and (4) rust build-up or blockage in a pipe leading directly to the sink.

flow is restored. The local occlusive process in the pipe, in vascular terms, would qualify as *thrombosis*, meaning a process that occurs in situ within a blood vessel. Suppose instead that the pipe had been blocked by material that originated in the water tank and simply became lodged in the pipe to the sink, occluding the pipe. This obstruction by material originating from afar is referred to as *embolism*. Fixing the local pipe would not prevent additional material from getting into the system and blocking other pipes. Suppose instead that the plumber finds that the water pressure is intermittently low and the flow to all the sinks and showers is deficient because of a leak in the water tank or low water pressure in the house's entire plumbing system. This situation is akin to systemic *hypoperfusion*, low blood flow; there is no local problem with the pipe to a single sink but instead a general circulatory problem or factor limiting the delivery of blood flow. Clearly, these three situations dictate different management by the plumber, and that is the main reason for separating them into the three mechanisms. This analogy will also be referred to in Chapter 6 when treatment is discussed

Thrombosis

By convention, *thrombosis* refers to an obstruction of blood flow due to a localized occlusive process within one or more blood vessels. Although this implies that thrombus or clot is the cause of the blockage, such an obstruction can also be caused by atherosclerotic plaque with superimposed thrombotic occlusion. The lumen of the vessel is narrowed or occluded by an alteration in the vessel wall or by superimposed clot formation. Figure 2.2A shows a normal artery, Figure 2.2B shows plaque encroaching on the arterial lumen, and Figure 2.2C shows occlusion of the artery by a red thrombus which has formed on top of a white platelet–fibrin thrombus.

The most common type of vascular pathology is atherosclerosis, in which fibrous and muscular tissues overgrow in the subintima, and fatty materials form plaques that can encroach on the lumen. Next, platelets adhere to plaque crevices and form clumps that serve as nidi for the deposition of fibrin, thrombin, and clot.[3,4] Figure 2.3 is a cartoon that shows the development of plaque in a carotid artery in the neck with subsequent occlusion of the artery by thrombus and embolization of the clot intracranially, causing a large brain infarct in the distribution of that carotid artery. Figure 2.4 is a photograph of a necropsy specimen that shows a large thrombus in an internal carotid artery; the lumen of the artery was nearly occluded by atherosclerotic plaque. Atherosclerosis affects chiefly the larger extracranial and intracranial arteries.[5,6] Occasionally, a clot forms within the lumen because of a primary hematological problem, such as polycythemia, thrombocytosis, or a systemic hypercoagulable state. The smaller, penetrating intracranial arteries and arterioles are more often damaged by hypertension than by atherosclerotic processes.[7,8] In such cases, increased arterial tension leads to hypertrophy of the media and deposition of fibrinoid material into the vessel wall, a process that gradually encroaches on the already small lumen. Small atheromatous deposits, often referred to as *microatheromas*, can obstruct the orifices of penetrating arteries.

Less common vascular pathologies leading to obstruction include: (1) fibromuscular dysplasia,[9] an overgrowth of medial and intimal elements that compromises vessel contractility and luminal size; (2) arteritis, especially of the Takayasu[10] or giant-cell type[11]; (3) dissection of the vessel wall,[12] often with a luminal or extraluminal clot temporarily obstructing the vessel; and (4) hemorrhage into a plaque,[13] leading to acute or chronic luminal compromise. At times, the focal vascular abnormality is a functional change in the contractility of blood vessels. Intense focal vasoconstriction can lead to decreased blood flow and thrombosis. Dilatation of blood vessels also alters local blood flow and clots often form in dilated segments.[14]

Embolism

In embolism, material formed elsewhere within the vascular system lodges in an artery and blocks blood flow. Blockage can be transient or may persist for hours or days before moving distally. In contrast to thrombosis, embolic luminal blockage is not caused by a localized process originating within the blocked artery. The material arises proximally, most commonly from the heart; from major arteries such as the aorta, carotid, and vertebral arteries; and from systemic veins (Figure 2.5). Cardiac sources of embolism include the heart valves and clots or tumors within the atrial or ventricular cavities.[15] Artery-to-artery emboli are composed of clots, platelet clumps, or fragments of plaques that break off from the proximal or upstream vessels.[16] Clots originating in systemic veins travel to the brain through venous to arterial shunts including cardiac defects such as an atrial septal defect or a patent foramen ovale, a process termed *paradoxical embolism*.[17] Also, occasionally air, fat, plaque material,

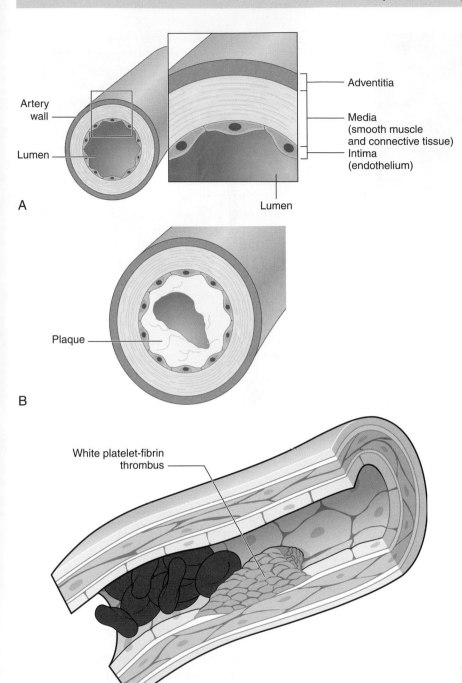

Artery wall

Lumen

Adventitia

Media
(smooth muscle
and connective tissue)

Intima
(endothelium)

Lumen

A

Plaque

B

White platelet-fibrin
thrombus

C

Figure 2.2 (A) The drawing shows a normal brain-supplying artery. The insert shows the various layers within a normal artery. (B) Atherosclerotic plaque within an artery narrowing the lumen. (C) White and red thrombi occluding a longitudinal segment of an artery.

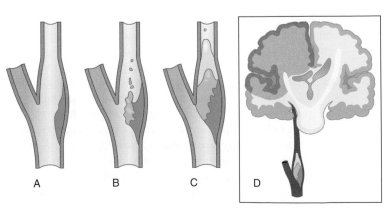

A   B   C   D

Figure 2.3 Internal carotid artery atherosclerotic lesions: (A) plaque; (B) plaque with platelet–fibrin emboli; (C) plaque with occlusive thrombus; (D) recent ischemic cerebral infarct due to embolization of the internal carotid artery thrombus.

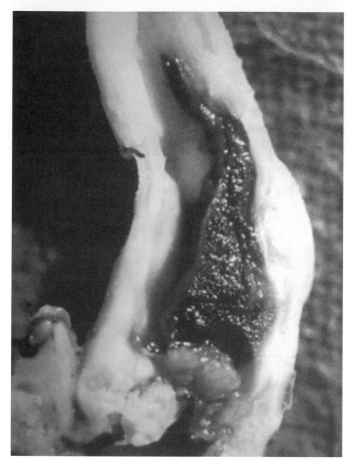

Figure 2.4 Carotid artery removed at necropsy. The internal carotid artery origin is nearly occluded by an atherosclerotic plaque. A long thrombus protrudes from the plaque and extends far rostrally within the arterial lumen. A part of this thrombus had embolized intracranially to cause a fatal brain infarct. Courtesy of Dr Pierre Amarenco.

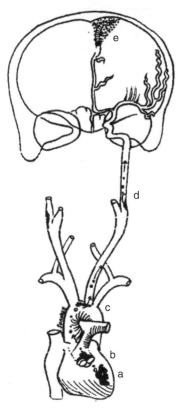

Figure 2.5 Examples of potential sources of embolism: (a) cardiac mural thrombus; (b) vegetations on heart valve; (c) aortic plaque (d) emboli from carotid plaque. Label (e) shows infarcted cortex in area supplied by terminal anterior cerebral artery due to embolism.

particulate matter from injected drugs, bacteria, foreign bodies, and tumor cells enter the vascular system and embolize to brain arteries.[18] The three main components in embolism are: the donor source, the embolic material, and the recipient artery. An embolic mechanism is often inferred from the pattern of ischemic brain injury on imaging studies and the location and appearance of arterial occlusion on vascular imaging, but proof of embolism requires demonstration of material traversing the blood vessels from a proximal to downstream location or from material found in the recipient artery that only could have arisen proximally.

Decreased systemic perfusion

In systemic hypoperfusion, diminished flow to brain tissue is caused by low systemic perfusion pressure. The most common causes are cardiac pump failure (most often due to myocardial infarction or arrhythmia) and systemic hypotension (due to blood loss or hypovolemia). In such cases, the lack of perfusion is more generalized than in localized thrombosis or embolism and affects the brain diffusely and bilaterally. Poor perfusion is most critical in borderzone or so-called watershed regions at the periphery of the major vascular supply territories (Figure 2.6, compare B with

both A and C).[19-21] Asymmetric effects can result from pre-existing vascular lesions causing an uneven distribution of hypoperfusion.

Venous occlusions and venous hypertension

Although the veins are always involved in the regulation of blood flow through a region of the brain, consideration of stroke pathophysiology typically focuses on the arterial delivery or interruption of blood flow to the brain. In a small fraction of patients with strokes, the veins are the main or initiating site of pathophysiology. Venous hypertension may cause both ischemia and hemorrhage due to backup or impaired drainage of blood from an area of the brain. Venous patterns of injury are defined by the venous anatomy, much as arterial territories are determined by arterial anatomy. Due to the complexity, redundancy, and extensive capacity of venous collaterals to redistribute blood in the brain, venous patterns are often more difficult to recognize. In Figure 2.7, the main damage is in the distribution of the vein of Labbé. Knowing that the occlusive pattern is venous is important in choosing treatment. The mechanisms of venous hypertension cause injury by first preventing drainage or engorging an area of the brain, which typically leads to hemorrhage. If the mass effect from such engorgement and hemorrhage becomes excessive, then ischemia is caused when the arterial inflow pressure does not exceed the venous pressure. This sequence of events is

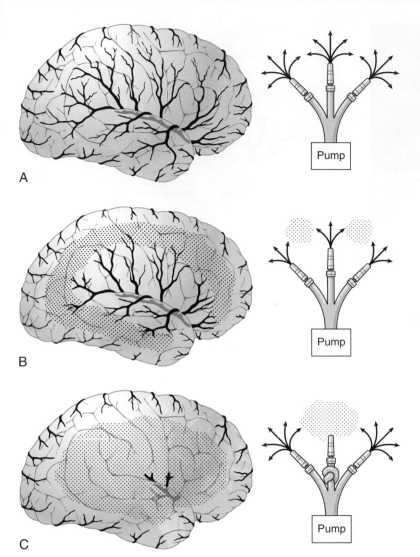

Figure 2.6 In heart (pump) failure and watershed infarction: (A) normal pump and arterial circulation; (B) low pump pressure and borderzone ischemia. Water goes to the center of hoses (arteries), and stippled areas show poor flow. In contrast, with (C) "blocked hose" and middle cerebral artery infarction, water flow is deficient in the center of supply (stippled area).

markedly different than arterial ischemia where hemorrhage occurs after ischemia is maximal.

Damage caused by ischemia

The three mechanisms of brain ischemia are illustrated in Figure 2.8. All may lead to temporary or permanent tissue injury. Permanent injury is termed *infarction*. Capillaries or other vessels within the ischemic tissue may also be injured, so that reperfusion can lead to leakage of blood into the ischemic tissue, resulting in hemorrhagic infarction.[22] The extent of brain damage depends on the location and duration of the poor perfusion and the ability of collateral vessels to perfuse the tissues at risk. The systemic blood pressure, blood volume, and blood viscosity also affect blood flow to the ischemic areas. Brain and vascular injuries may lead to brain edema during the hours and days after stroke. In the chronic phase, glial scars form, and macrophages gradually ingest the necrotic tissue debris within the infarct, leading to shrinkage of the volume of the infarcted tissue or to formation of a frank cavity.

Hemorrhage

Hemorrhage can be further subdivided into four subtypes: subarachnoid; intracerebral; subdural; and epidural (Figure 2.9). These subtypes have different causes, pose different clinical problems, and have different management.

Subarachnoid hemorrhage

In subarachnoid hemorrhage, blood leaks out of the vascular bed onto the brain's surface and is disseminated quickly via the spinal fluid pathways into the spaces around the brain (see Figure 2.9, top left).[23,24] Bleeding most often originates from aneurysms or arteriovenous malformations, but bleeding diatheses or trauma can also cause subarachnoid bleeding. A ruptured aneurysm releases blood rapidly at systemic blood pressure, suddenly increasing intracranial pressure, whereas bleeding from other causes is usually slower and at lower pressures. The blood within the subarachnoid space often contains substances that promote vasoconstriction of the basal arteries that are bathed in cerebrospinal fluid.

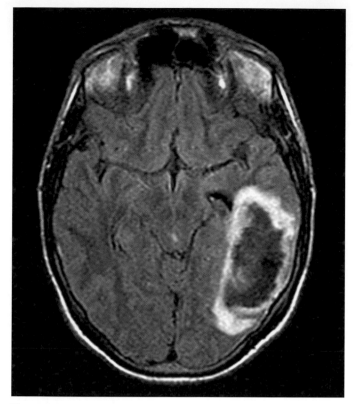

Figure 2.7 Axial FLAIR MRI revealing hemorrhagic infarction of the left temporal and parietal lobes dues to occlusion of the vein of Labbé.

Intracerebral hemorrhage

The terms *intracerebral* and *parenchymal hemorrhage* describe bleeding directly into the brain substance. It is important to distinguish such primary hemorrhagic strokes from hemorrhagic transformation, where bleeding occurs into an area of brain tissue shortly after ischemic stroke due to disruption of the blood–brain barrier and/or reperfusion. The cause of primary intracerebral hemorrhage is most often hypertension, with leakage of blood from small intracerebral arterioles damaged by the elevated blood pressure.[25–29] Bleeding diatheses, especially from the prescription of anticoagulants or from trauma, drugs, vascular malformations, and vasculopathies (such as cerebral amyloid angiopathy), also cause bleeding into the brain. Intracerebral hemorrhages occur in a localized region of the brain (see Figure 2.9, top right). The degree of damage depends on the location, rapidity, volume, and pressure of the bleeding.

Intracerebral hemorrhages are at first soft and dissect along white matter fiber tracts. When bleeding dissects into the ventricles or onto the surface of the brain, blood is introduced into the cerebrospinal fluid. The blood in the hematoma clots and solidifies, causing swelling of adjacent brain tissues. Later, blood is absorbed, and after macrophages clear the debris, a cavity or slit forms that may disconnect brain pathways (Figure 2.10). The intracranial cavity is a closed system. The bony skull and dura mater act as a fortress protecting the brain from outside injury. In adverse situations, such as swelling or hemorrhage arising inside the fortress, these structures can

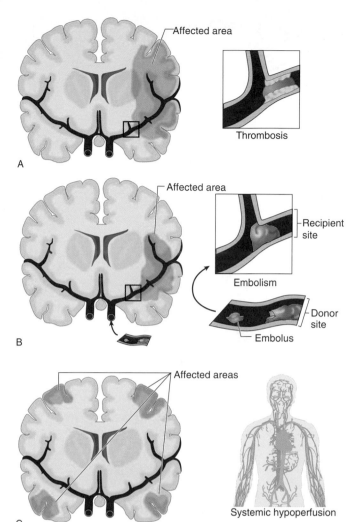

Figure 2.8 Illustrations of the three major causes of brain ischemia. Thrombosis: (A) the insert shows a thrombus in an atherosclerotic artery leading to a brain infarct. Embolism: (B) a thrombus that originated in a donor source embolized to the recipient site (shown in the insert) causing an embolic brain infarct, and (C) systemic hypoperfusion. Infarcts are in borderzone regions.

function as a prison, restricting and strangulating their enclosed contents and forcing herniation of tissue from one compartment to another.[30–32]

Subdural and epidural hemorrhages

These hemorrhages are typically caused by head trauma. Subdural hemorrhages arise from injured or torn bridging veins that are located between the dura mater and the arachnoid membranes. The bleeding is most often slow and accumulates during days, weeks, and even a few months. When a large vein is lacerated, bleeding can develop more rapidly over hours to days. Epidural hemorrhages are caused by tearing of meningeal arteries, most often the middle meningeal artery. Blood accumulates rapidly over minutes to hours between the skull and the dura mater. Both subdural and epidural hemorrhages cause symptoms and signs by compressing brain tissue and increasing intracranial pressure (see Figure 2.9, bottom).

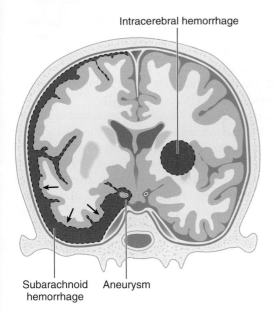

Intracerebral hemorrhage

Subarachnoid hemorrhage Aneurysm

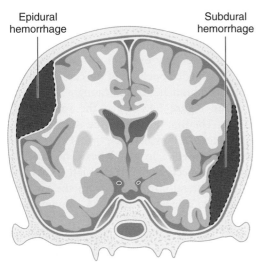

Epidural hemorrhage

Subdural hemorrhage

Figure 2.9 Illustrations of the main types of brain hemorrhages: intracerebral; subarachnoid; subdural; and epidural.

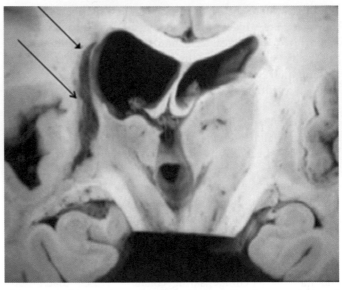

Figure 2.10 Brain specimen showing a slit-like cavity adjacent to the lateral ventricle. A large putaminal hematoma had been present at this site. There is also a butterfly-shaped infarct adjacent to the IIIrd ventricle that resulted from herniation caused by the mass effect of the putaminal hemorrhage. The patient survived for some time after the hemorrhage.

Recognition of the stroke mechanism guides treatment

The problems in these five major subtypes of stroke – thrombosis, embolism, decreased systemic perfusion, subarachnoid hemorrhage, and intracerebral hemorrhage – are quite distinct and require different treatment strategies. Identifying the etiology and underlying stroke mechanism is essential to guide rational therapy, both in the early or acute stage and to prevent recurrence. Some therapies suitable for ischemia would be disastrous if the problem were hemorrhage (e.g., using anticoagulants or opening a blood vessel to diminish supposed ischemia would augment hemorrhage). Even within the various subcategories of ischemia, treatment depends on the subtype or specific cause. For example, in a patient with embolism arising from the heart, operating on a recipient artery for supposed local thrombosis would certainly be ineffective in preventing subsequent embolism. The origin of an embolus

also affects treatment: Embolism arising from the heart requires different therapeutic strategies than embolism arising from localized vessel plaques. In regard to systemic hypoperfusion, pump failure or hypovolemia owing to intestinal bleeding needs urgent attention, which would be needlessly delayed by inappropriate angiography or a futile search for a localized extracranial vascular lesion.

In subarachnoid hemorrhage, the major aim of treatment is to prevent the next aneurysmal leak, whereas in intracerebral hemorrhage, rebleeding is rare and treatment is aimed at controlling and limiting the bleeding and pressure effects of the hemorrhage. When subdural and epidural hemorrhages are sizable, surgical drainage is the main treatment.

To treat the stroke patient optimally, it is imperative that the physician identify the correct mechanism of stroke. Because it is not always possible to be absolutely certain of the single true mechanism, the clinician often must consider the possibility of more than one mechanism, such as thrombosis and embolism, and must evaluate for each. At times, more than one mechanism is operant. For example, in subarachnoid hemorrhage, the blood may cause spasm of blood vessels and thus induce local ischemia, and a thrombus obstructing a carotid artery can also fragment and lead to distal artery-to-artery embolism. Furthermore, local hypoperfusion and embolic events often coexist.

Anatomy: common anatomical sites of vascular and brain lesions

Clinical neurology differs from most medical specialties in its emphasis on, and even obsession with, the complex and unique anatomy of the cerebral circulation. To localize and repair damage to water pipes, the effective plumber must be aware

of exactly where the pipes are, what they supply, and where they are most likely to be damaged by various hazards. Abnormal neurological signs and symptoms depend more on the localization of the brain injury than on its mechanism. Although all portions of the lung or liver look and function identically, different regions within the brain appear and act differently. The nervous system is a world of uncountable individual nerve cells and networks, each with quite different and unique characteristics and chemical messengers. Each of the various mechanisms of stroke just reviewed has its own preferences for anatomical brain locations. Identification of the location of the stroke depends on analysis of the abnormal neurological symptoms and signs and on interpretation of brain imaging. A major important question in every stroke patient is – where is the brain and vascular problem located? Even once a specific region of the brain is implicated, questions remain regarding the specific arterial or venous distribution and the role of compensating collateral vessels that modify potential injury.

This section reviews the important anatomical facts about the extracranial and intracranial vessels,[33] their normal or typical regions of supply or drainage, and the most common locations for various vascular pathologies. Differences in the anatomy of extracranial and intracranial arteries are outlined. Next, the anatomical predilections of the major stroke mechanisms within the brain are discussed. Aspects of the anatomy and localization of various lesions are reviewed more extensively in the second part of this book, where specific stroke syndromes are addressed. Much as there is anatomical variation in the normal vascular anatomy of the brain, there are many collateral flow patterns arising from neighboring vessels that may be encountered with different stroke syndromes.

Normal vascular anatomy

Arterial circulation

The common carotid arteries (CCAs) bifurcate in the neck, usually opposite the upper border of the thyroid cartilage, into the internal carotid arteries (ICAs), which are located posteriorly as a direct extension of the CCA, and into the external carotid arteries (ECAs), which course more anteriorly and laterally. The ICAs travel behind the pharynx; they give off no branches in the neck. Figure 2.11A shows the carotid arteries in the neck. Figure 2.11B shows the branches of the ECA, which supplies the face and major cranial structures except for the brain. The ICAs then enter the skull through the carotid canal within the petrous bone and form an S-shaped curve. The ICA within this curve is usually referred to as the *carotid siphon*. There are three divisions of the ICA within the siphon – an intrapetrous portion, an intracavernous portion within the cavernous sinus, and a supraclinoidal portion[34] (Figure 2.11C). The siphon portion of the ICAs (usually the clinoidal segment but occasionally the intracavernous segment) gives rise to ophthalmic artery branches that exit anteriorly. The ICAs then penetrate the dura mater and give rise to anterior choroidal and posterior communicating arteries, which arise and course posteriorly from their proximal supraclinoid portions. The termination of the intracranial ICAs (the so-called T-portion because of its shape) is the bifurcation into the anterior cerebral arteries (ACAs), which course medially, and the middle cerebral arteries (MCAs), which course laterally. Figure 2.12 shows the major intracranial branches of the ICA.

The ECAs have two major vascular channels that ordinarily supply the face that can act as collateral circulation if the ICAs occlude: the facial arteries, which course along the cheek toward the nasal bridge, where they are termed the *angular arteries*, and the preauricular arteries, which terminate as the superficial temporal arteries. The internal maxillary artery and ascending pharyngeal branches of the ECAs also can contribute to collateral circulation when an ICA occludes. The internal maxillary arteries give off the middle meningeal artery branches, which penetrate into the skull through the foramen spinosum. Another important arterial supply of the face involves the frontal and supratrochlear branches that originate from the ophthalmic arteries (ICA system), which supply the medial forehead above the brow. When an ICA occludes, these ECA branches can be an important source of collateral blood supply.

The ACAs course medially until they reach the longitudinal fissures and then run posteriorly over the corpus callosum. They supply the anterior medial portions of the cerebral hemispheres and give off deep branches to the caudate nuclei and the basal frontal lobes. Figure 2.13 shows the small artery branches of the ACAs. The first portion of the ACA is sometimes hypoplastic on one side, in which case the ACA from the other side supplies both medial frontal lobes. The anterior communicating artery connects the right and left ACAs and provides a means of collateral circulation from the anterior circulation of the opposite side when one ACA is hypoplastic or occludes.

The main stem of the MCAs course laterally, giving off lenticulostriate artery branches to the basal ganglia and internal capsule (Figure 2.14). Although most often the lenticulostriate penetrating branches arise from the mainstem MCA, when the mainstem is short, the lenticulostriate branches may arise from the superior division branch. Similarly, lenticulostriate perforators may also arise from the terminal ICA or proximal ACA. As they near the sylvian fissures, the MCAs usually trifurcate into an early anterior temporal branch that courses inferiorly and then relatively larger superior and inferior divisions that arise from the most distal portion of the horizontal segment of the MCA as it reaches the sylvian fissure near the insula. There is marked variability in such branching patterns and angiographic descriptions have either utilized branch points as landmarks to distinguish various segments of the MCA or alternatively, named MCA segments based on the location of adjacent brain regions. The superior division supplies the lateral portions of the cerebral hemispheres above the sylvian fissures, and the inferior division supplies the temporal and inferior parietal lobes below the sylvian fissures. Figure 2.15 is a view of the lateral surface of the left cerebral hemisphere showing the MCA branches and the supply of the superior and inferior divisions of the left MCA. Figure 2.16 is a drawing of the paramedian sagittal surface of the cerebral

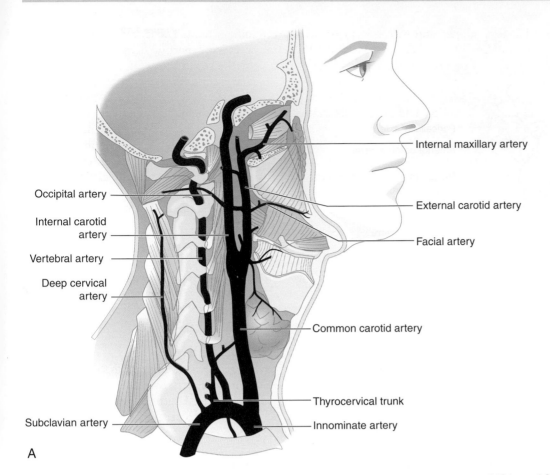

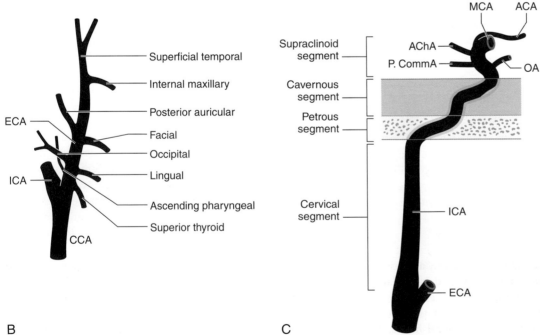

Figure 2.11 Drawings of the major right-sided neck arteries. (A) The innominate artery gives rise to subclavian and CCA branches. The right vertebral artery is shown originating from the right subclavian artery. The common carotid artery bifurcation into internal and external carotid arteries is also shown. The external carotid artery and its branches (B), and (C) the segments of the ICA are shown in relation to their relationships with the adjacent skull structures. ACA, anterior cerebral artery; AChA, anterior choroidal artery; CCA, common carotid artery; ECA, external carotid artery; ICA, internal carotid artery; MCA, middle cerebral artery; OA, occipital artery; P.CommA, posterior communicating artery.

hemispheres showing the distribution of the ACA and posterior cerebral artery (PCA) branches.

The anterior choroidal arteries (AChAs) are relatively small arteries that originate from the ICAs after the origins of the ophthalmic and posterior communicating arteries. The ophthalmic artery projects anteriorly into the back of the orbit, whereas the anterior choroidal and posterior communicating arteries project posteriorly from the ICA. The AChAs course posteriorly and laterally running along the optic tract. They straddle territory between components of the anterior (internal carotid) and posterior circulations (vertebrobasilar system).[35] The AChAs give off penetrating artery branches to the globus pallidus and posterior limb of the internal capsule. They then give branches laterally to the

A-P view

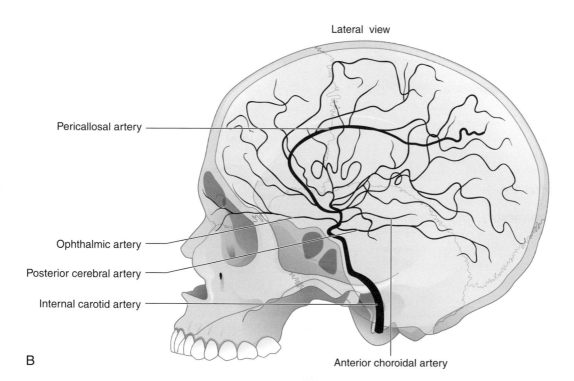

Pericallosal artery

Anterior cerebral artery

Recurrent artery of Heubner

Anterior choroidal artery

Middle cerebral artery

Ophthalmic artery

Internal carotid artery

A

Lateral view

Pericallosal artery

Ophthalmic artery

Posterior cerebral artery

Internal carotid artery

B

Anterior choroidal artery

medial temporal lobe, and medial branches supply a portion of the midbrain and the thalamus. The AChAs end in the lateral geniculate body where they anastamose with lateral posterior choroidal artery branches of the PCAs and in the choroid plexus of the lateral ventricles near the temporal horns. The AChAs have a characteristic shape because of this meandering trajectory that crosses from medial to lateral, inferior to superior, and anterior to posterior reaches. Figure 2.17 is a drawing of the course of the AChA. Figure 2.18 shows a drawing of a coronal section of the cerebral hemispheres showing the distribution of the supply of the MCA, ACA, PCA, and the AChA. More detailed maps of the distribution of the blood supply in the cerebral hemispheres have been published.[36]

By convention, the carotid artery territories just described are referred to as the *anterior circulation* (front of the brain), whereas the vertebral and basilar arteries and their branches are termed the *posterior circulation* (because they supply the back of the brain). Each ICA supplies roughly two-fifths of the brain by volume, whereas the posterior circulation accounts for approximately one-fifth of the total. Despite its much smaller size, the posterior circulation contains the brainstem, a midline strategically critical structure without which consciousness, movement, and sensations cannot be preserved. The posterior circulation is constructed quite differently from the anterior circulation and consists of vessels from each side (the vertebral and anterior spinal artery branches),

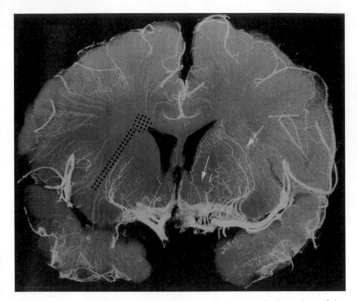

Figure 2.13 Coronal post-mortem angiogram showing the branches of the anterior cerebral arteries (ACAs) (white arrows). The black dot region (left of drawing) indicates the internal borderzone region. From Pullicino P, Lenticulostriate arteries. In Bogousslavsky J, Caplan LR (eds). *Stroke Syndromes*, 2nd ed. Cambridge: Cambridge University Press, 2001, pp 428–437.

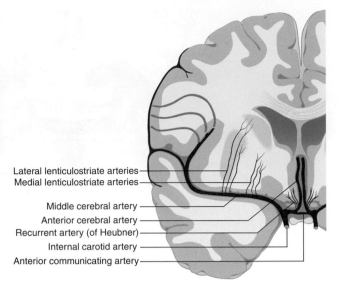

Figure 2.14 Drawing of a coronal section of the cerebral hemispheres showing one mainstem middle cerebral artery and its lenticulostriate artery branches.

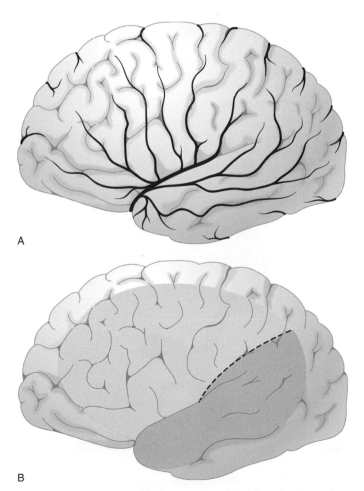

Figure 2.15 (A) Drawing of the lateral surface of the left cerebral hemisphere showing the usual branches of the middle cerebral artery (MCA). (B) The superior division MCA supply is mainly suprasylvian (pink) and the inferior division mainly infrasylvian supply is shown in darker pink.

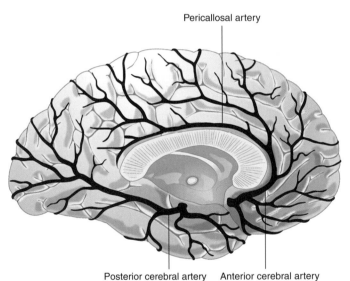

Figure 2.16 Drawing of sagittal-section paramedian view of cerebral hemispheres showing branches of the anterior (ACA) and posterior (PCA) cerebral arteries.

which unite to form midline arteries that supply the brainstem and spinal cord. Within the posterior circulation, there is a much higher incidence of asymmetric, hypoplastic arteries; of variability of supply; and of retention of fetal circulatory patterns.[37,38] This occurs due to incomplete fusion of two lateral opposed vascular conduits to form the single posterior circulation later in development. The proximal portions of the posterior circulation on the two sides differ. On the right, the subclavian artery arises from the innominate artery, a common channel supplying the anterior and posterior circulations. On the left side, the subclavian artery usually arises directly from the aortic arch after the origin of the left CCA.

The first branch of each subclavian artery is the vertebral artery (VA) (Figure 2.19; see also Figure 2.11). The VAs course upward and backward until they enter the transverse foramens

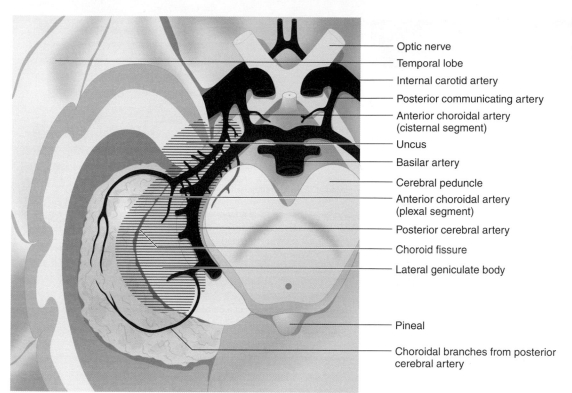

Figure 2.17 Drawing of vascular supply territory of the anterior choroidal artery (AChA).

- Optic nerve
- Temporal lobe
- Internal carotid artery
- Posterior communicating artery
- Anterior choroidal artery (cisternal segment)
- Uncus
- Basilar artery
- Cerebral peduncle
- Anterior choroidal artery (plexal segment)
- Posterior cerebral artery
- Choroid fissure
- Lateral geniculate body
- Pineal
- Choroidal branches from posterior cerebral artery

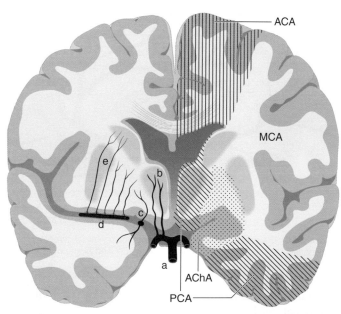

Figure 2.18 Drawing of a coronal view of the cerebral hemispheres showing the vascular supply territories: The right side depicts territories supplied by the anterior cerebral artery (ACA), middle cerebral artery (MCA), posterior cerebral artery (PCA), and anterior choroidal artery (AChA). The left side depicts individual vessels: (a) basilar artery; (b) thalamoperforators, which originate in the PCA; (c) AChA; (d) MCA; (e) lenticulostriate arteries.

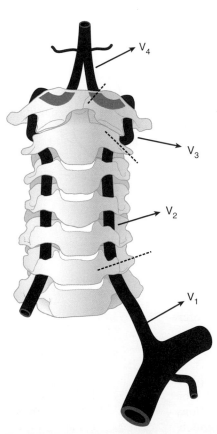

Figure 2.19 Drawing showing portions of the vertebral artery (VA) and their relation to the bony vertebral column.

of the sixth or fifth cervical vertebra and run within the intravertebral foramina, exiting to course behind the atlas before piercing the dura mater to enter the foramen magnum. Their intracranial portions end at the medullopontine junction, where the two VAs join to form the basilar artery. Figure 2.19 shows the divisions of the VAs: the first portion before entry into the bony vertebral column (V_1), the portion within the vertebral columns (V_2), the portion of the artery

after exit from the vertebral column that arches behind the atlas and before entry into the cranium (V_3), and the intracranial portion (V_4). In the neck, the VAs have many small muscular and spinal branches.

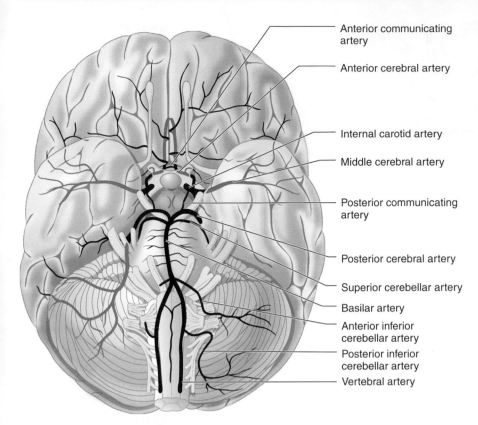

Anterior communicating
artery

Anterior cerebral artery

Internal carotid artery

Middle cerebral artery

Posterior communicating
artery

Posterior cerebral artery

Superior cerebellar artery

Basilar artery

Anterior inferior
cerebellar artery

Posterior inferior
cerebellar artery

Vertebral artery

Figure 2.20 Drawing of a basal view of the brain showing the intracranial branches of the vertebral and basilar arteries and the basal branches of the circle of Willis and the carotid arteries.

The intracranial portions of the VAs give off posterior and anterior spinal artery branches, penetrating arteries to the medulla and the large posterior inferior cerebellar arteries (PICAs). The basilar artery runs in the midline along the clivus, giving off bilateral anterior inferior cerebellar artery (AICA) and superior cerebellar artery (SCA) branches before dividing at the pontomesencephalic junction into terminal PCA branches (Figure 2.20). The major arterial branches of the intracranial vertebral and basilar arteries as they appear on angiograms are shown on Figure 2.21.

The vascular supply of the brainstem has been worked out by Foix,[39–41] Stopford,[42] Gillilan,[43] and Duvernoy[44] and is illustrated in Figure 2.22. Large paramedian arteries and smaller, short circumferential arteries penetrate through the basal portions of the brainstem into the tegmentum. Long circumferential arteries course around the brainstem giving off branches to the lateral tegmentum. The PCAs give off penetrating arteries to the midbrain and thalamus, course around the cerebral peduncles, and then supply the occipital lobes and inferior surface of the temporal lobes (Figure 2.23). The circle of Willis allows for connections between the anterior circulations of each side, through the anterior communicating artery, and between the posterior and anterior circulations of each side through the posterior communicating artery (Figure 2.24).

The blood supply of the spinal cord will be covered in Chapter 16, which deals with spinal cord strokes.

Composition of cervico-cranial artery walls

The walls of the extracranial arteries consist of three well developed layers; intima, media, and adventitia[45,46] (see Figure 2.2A). The intima is composed of a single row of endothelial cells that forms a continuous barrier between the arterial wall and the circulating blood. The endothelium sits on a basal membrane that is separated from the internal elastic lamina and the media by a space that contains an acellular matrix containing collagen, elastin, and glycoproteins. The internal elastic lamina is a thick fenestrated layer of elastin that separates the intima from the media. The media is the thickest component of the arterial wall and is composed of smooth muscle, elastic fibers, and an extracellular matrix. The external elastic lamina separates the media and adventitia. The outermost layer of the arterial wall, the adventitia, is composed of loose connective tissue and adipose cells. Nerves and vessels (so-called *vasa vasorum*) penetrate the adventitia and may extend into the media.

Intracranial arteries are morphologically different from extracranial arteries. Intracranial arteries have no external elastic membrane and have a thinner intimal layer. The media and adventitia are relatively poor in elastic fibers when compared to extracranial arteries of comparable size.[45,46]

Venous and dural sinus anatomy

The veins within the cranium contain approximately 70% of the cerebral blood volume. The cerebral blood volume, largely sustained by the veins, plays a critical role in both arterial and

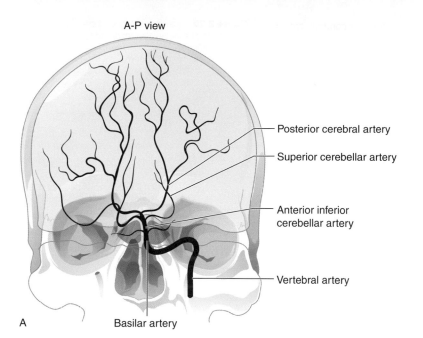

A-P view

Posterior cerebral artery

Superior cerebellar artery

Anterior inferior
cerebellar artery

Vertebral artery

Basilar artery

A

Figure 2.21 Large intracranial posterior circulation arteries as they appear on arteriograms. Anteroposterior (A-P) view (A) and lateral projection (B).

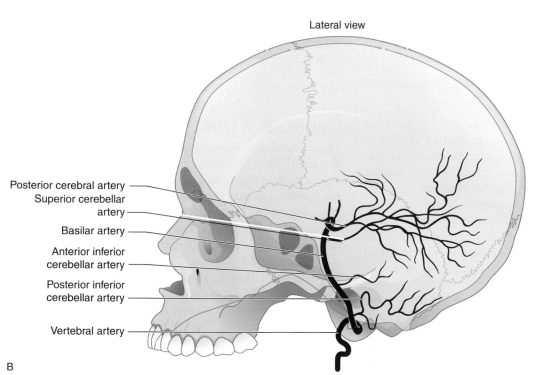

Lateral view

Posterior cerebral artery
Superior cerebellar
artery
Basilar artery
Anterior inferior
cerebellar artery
Posterior inferior
cerebellar artery

Vertebral artery

B

venous stroke syndromes. The venous blood pool is an important factor in the balance of intracranial pressure dynamics. The intracranial venous circulation is usually divided into the superficial and deep venous drainage systems.[33,44,47] Most descriptions focus on the larger dural sinuses and veins, as there is marked variability and redundancy in smaller venous channels. Although variations exist, the superficial venous drainage of the brain is typically on the right side with deep venous drainage developed from the left side. During development, these lateral systems often fuse in the midline, similar to the pairing of arterial structures.

The dural venous sinuses are trabeculated, endothelial-lined channels whose fibrous walls are formed by the inner and outer layers of the dura mater. The sinuses are situated at the junctions and edges of the falx cerebri and the tentorium cerebelli. The intracranial veins drain into the dural sinuses, which in turn empty into the neck veins to drain into the superior vena cava. A system of venous lakes within the skull also drains into the dural sinuses. Venous blood flow distribution is often described as drainage, but pooling or retention of blood volume occurs due to valves and the capacitance that distinguish the veins from arteries in the brain.

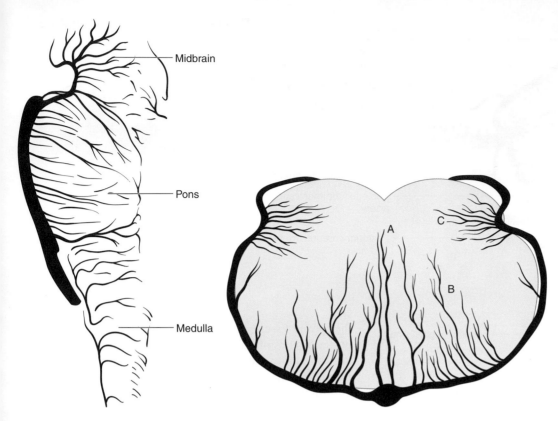

Figure 2.22 Drawings of the penetrating arteries to the pons showing the pattern of arterial supply. A, Midline large median arteries; B, paramedian penetrators; C, penetrating arteries into the lateral tegmentum of the pons.

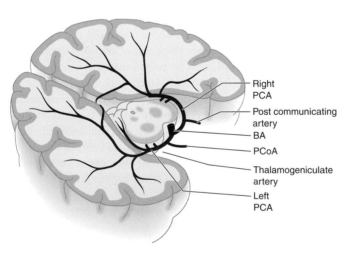

Figure 2.23 Drawing showing the course and branching of the PCAs as they course around the midbrain, and branches to the temporal and parieto-occipital lobes. BA, basilar artery; PCA, posterior cerebral artery; PCoA, posterior communicating artery.

The paired cavernous sinuses are located on the lateral surface of the body of the sphenoid bone and are connected to each other by the anterior and posterior intercavernous sinuses (Figure 2.25). The cavernous sinuses reach the superior orbital fissure anteriorly and posteriorly extend to the petrous apices. The ophthalmic and facial veins drain into the cavernous sinuses. The ICAs lie within the medial walls of the cavernous sinuses.

The superior sagittal sinus courses in an arc from anteriorly to far posteriorly in the superior margin of the falx cerebri and ends at the internal occipital protuberance by draining into the confluens of the sinuses (torcular Herophili) (Figure 2.26). The superior sagittal sinuses drain most of the blood from the cerebral hemispheres. The posterior portion of the superior sagittal sinus is better developed than the anterior portion. The inferior sagittal sinus is smaller and shorter than the superior sagittal sinus and runs in the inferior margin of the falx until it joins with the great cerebral vein of Galen to form the straight sinus.

The paired transverse sinuses originate at the torcular and course anterolaterally along the skull between the attachments of the tentorium cerebelli. At the petrous portion of the temporal bones, the transverse sinuses empty into the sigmoid sinuses, which course medially and inferiorly to reach the jugular foramina where they become the jugular veins. Figure 2.27 is a normal MR venogram that shows the major dural sinus structures. One of the transverse sinuses (most often the left) is sometimes hypoplastic or absent as it typically arises from the deep system as described above. The superior and inferior petrosal sinuses begin at the cavernous sinuses and drain into the sigmoid sinuses and the jugular veins. The majority of the venous blood flow within the cranium flows posteriorly and drains into the sigmoid sinuses into the jugular veins and from there into the superior vena cava. These drainage patterns, however, are dependent on head position as the jugular drainage usually collapses in the upright position.

The superior group of cerebral veins drains most of the medial surface, the superior parts of the lateral surfaces, and the anterior portions of the ventral surfaces of the cerebral hemispheres. The veins empty into the frontal and parietal

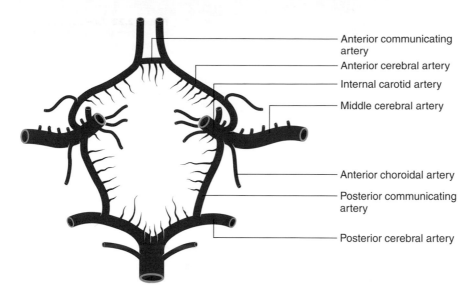

Figure 2.24 Drawing of the arterial "circle" of Willis.

- Anterior communicating artery
- Anterior cerebral artery
- Internal carotid artery
- Middle cerebral artery
- Anterior choroidal artery
- Posterior communicating artery
- Posterior cerebral artery

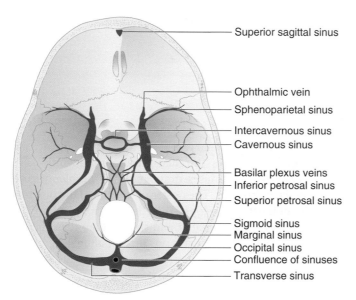

- Superior sagittal sinus
- Ophthalmic vein
- Sphenoparietal sinus
- Intercavernous sinus
- Cavernous sinus
- Basilar plexus veins
- Inferior petrosal sinus
- Superior petrosal sinus
- Sigmoid sinus
- Marginal sinus
- Occipital sinus
- Confluence of sinuses
- Transverse sinus

Figure 2.25 Drawing of the base of the skull with the brain removed showing the various dural sinuses.

regions of the superior sagittal sinus. The middle cerebral veins consist of a superficial and a deep vein. The superficial middle cerebral veins drain the sylvian fissures and the opercula and empty into the cavernous sinuses. The deep middle cerebral veins form on the insular surfaces and drain into the basal veins of Rosenthal. The basal veins arise on the ventral surface of the brain lateral to the optic chiasm and course posteriorly to the cerebral peduncles where the interpeduncular vein connects the two basal veins. The basal veins then course around the cerebral peduncles next to the PCAs and empty into the great cerebral vein of Galen. The inferior cerebral veins drain from the inferior and lateral surfaces of the temporal and occipital lobes into the transverse sinuses.

Some large veins are often readily identified on cerebral angiography. The superficial middle cerebral veins course in the sylvian fissure. The veins of Trolard anastamose with the posterior ends of the middle cerebral veins and course superiorly to empty into the superior sagittal sinus. The veins of Labbé anastamose with the middle cerebral veins and empty into the transverse sinuses. Figure 2.28 shows the major veins on the lateral surface of the cerebral hemispheres. The veins of Trolard and Labbé are quite variable in size and location, balancing the relative sizes of the adjacent venous structures. Figure 2.7 is a magnetic resonance imaging (MRI) scan that shows a hemorrhage caused by occlusion of the vein of Labbé.

The deep venous system veins drain into structures at or near the midsagittal plane. The paired internal cerebral veins originate behind the foramina of Monro and course posteriorly side by side near the midline. The thalamostriate veins course with the stria terminalis between the caudate nucleus and the thalamus on each side to drain into the internal cerebral veins. The two internal cerebral veins and the basal veins of Rosenthal join below or behind the splenium of the corpus callosum to form the great cerebral vein of Galen. Figure 2.29 shows the deep venous drainage system.

The veins that drain the brainstem and cerebellum are divided into three groups. The superior group drains the superior portions of the cerebellum and the rostral and dorsal brainstem. They empty into the vein of Galen, the basal veins of Rosenthal, or the petrosal veins, which drain into the petrosal sinuses. One of the superior veins, the precentral vein, is an important anatomical landmark because it separates the pons, which lies below the vein, from the midbrain, which lies above the vein. The petrosal group of veins drains the ventral surface of the brainstem, the superior and inferior surfaces of the cerebellar hemispheres, and the lateral recesses of the IVth ventricle. They drain into the superior petrosal sinuses or their tributaries. The tentorial group of veins is posteriorly located and drains the inferior vermis and the medial portions of the cerebellar hemispheres. They drain into the straight sinus or lateral sinuses near the torcular.[33,44] Figure 2.30 shows the major posterior fossa venous structures.

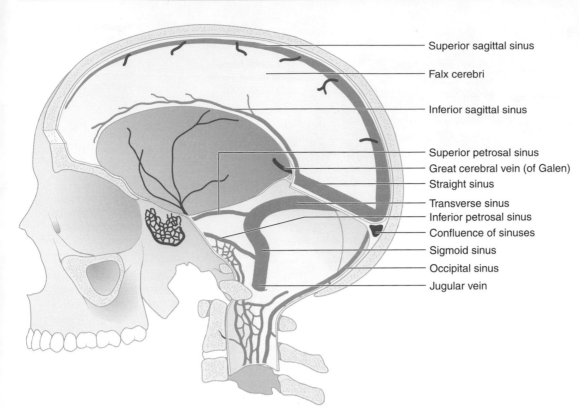

Superior sagittal sinus

Falx cerebri

Inferior sagittal sinus

Superior petrosal sinus
Great cerebral vein (of Galen)
Straight sinus
Transverse sinus
Inferior petrosal sinus
Confluence of sinuses
Sigmoid sinus
Occipital sinus
Jugular vein

Figure 2.26 Drawing of a midsagittal view of the skull showing the major large veins and dural sinuses.

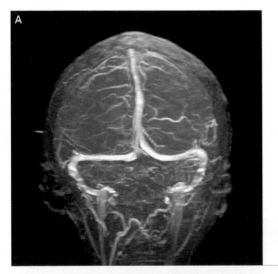
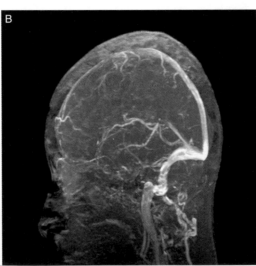

Figure 2.27 (A,B) Magnetic resonance venogram showing the superior and inferior sagittal sinuses, the lateral and sigmoid sinuses, and the jugular veins.

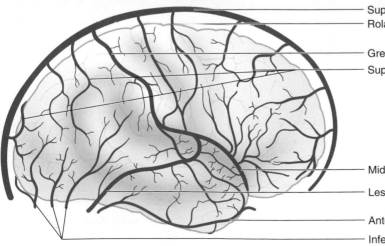

Superior sagittal sinus
Rolandic vein

Greater anastomotic vein (Trolard)
Superior cerebral veins

Middle cerebral vein (Sylvian)

Lesser anastomotic vein (Labbé)

Anterior temporal cerebral vein

Inferior cerebral veins

Figure 2.28 Drawing of major superficial veins seen on lateral surface of the left cerebral hemisphere.

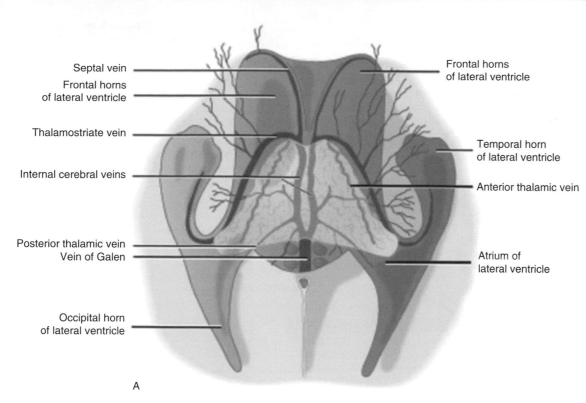

Septal vein

Frontal horns
of lateral ventricle

Thalamostriate vein

Internal cerebral veins

Posterior thalamic vein
Vein of Galen

Occipital horn
of lateral ventricle

Frontal horns
of lateral ventricle

Temporal horn
of lateral ventricle

Anterior thalamic vein

Atrium of
lateral ventricle

A

Figure 2.29 Drawing of the deep venous drainage system: (A) axial section showing the veins and their relations to the lateral ventricles; (B) sagittal section.

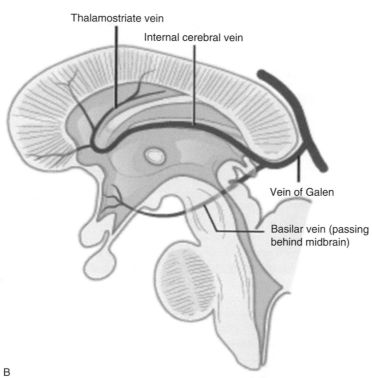

Thalamostriate vein

Internal cerebral vein

Vein of Galen

Basilar vein (passing behind midbrain)

B

Distribution of vascular pathology

Thrombosis

Atherosclerotic narrowing most often occurs at the origins of the ICAs in the neck. The remaining nuchal ICAs are seldom affected, but the carotid siphon is a frequent site for atheromas. This predilection for atherosclerotic narrowing of specific carotid segments is likely determined by flow patterns, as variation in hemodynamics such as shear stress strongly influences atherosclerosis and vascular remodeling. The supraclinoid carotid arteries and the mainstem MCAs and ACAs are affected less often than the ICAs in the neck and the siphon in the general population,[6,48,49] although in black and Asian patients, MCA disease is more common than disease of the ICAs.[50–54]

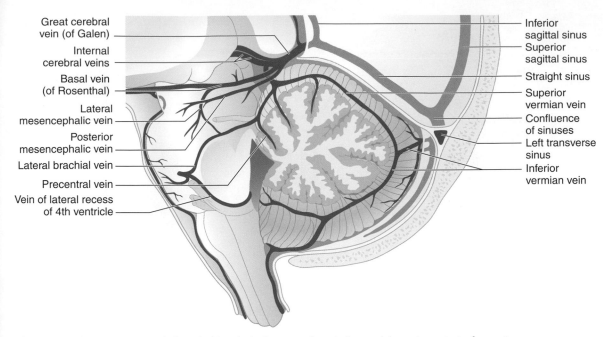

Figure 2.30 Drawing in a sagittal plane showing the brainstem and cerebellum and the major posterior fossa veins.

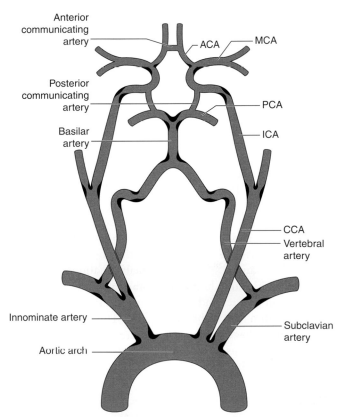

Figure 2.31 Drawing showing sites of predilection for atherosclerotic narrowing; black areas represent plaques. ACA, anterior cerebral artery; CCA, common carotid artery; ICA, internal carotid artery; MCA, middle cerebral artery; PCA, posterior cerebral artery.

Sites of predilection for atherosclerotic narrowing in the posterior circulation include the proximal origins of the VAs and the subclavian arteries, the proximal and distal ends of the intracranial VAs, the basilar artery, and the origins of the PCAs.[6,38] Figure 2.31 shows the most frequent locations of

atherosclerosis. Atherosclerotic narrowing rarely affects the distal superficial branches of the cerebral (ACA, MCA, PCA) or cerebellar (PICA, AICA, SCA) arteries.

Lipohyalinosis and medial hypertrophy secondary to hypertension affect mainly: (1) penetrating lenticulostriate branches of the MCAs (see Figure 2.14); (2) anterior perforating artery branches of the ACA, often referred to as the recurrent artery of Heubner (Figure 2.32; see also Figure 2.13); (3) penetrating arteries originating from the AChAs (see Figures 2.15 and 2.18); (4) thalamoperforating and thalamogeniculate penetrators from the PCAs (see Figure 2.32); and (5) paramedian perforating vessels to the pons, midbrain, and thalamus from the basilar artery (Figure 2.22).[7,55]

At times, atheromatous plaques within parent arteries or microatheromas within the orifices of branches cause blockage of penetrating arteries[56] (Figure 2.33). The distribution of atheromatous branch disease is the same as that of lipohyalinosis except that atheromatous branch disease may also obstruct larger branches (e.g., the AChA branches of the ICAs and the thalamogeniculate pedicles from the PCAs).

Arterial dissection – traumatic or spontaneous tearing of a vessel wall with intramural bleeding – usually involves the pharyngeal portion of the carotid arteries and the VAs between their origin and penetration into the intravertebral foramina and in their third portion as they wind around the rostral cervical vertebrae before penetrating the dura mater to enter the skull.[12,38,57,58] In these regions, the neck arteries are mobile and not anchored to other arteries or bony structures. Tearing of neck arteries is most often due to sudden stretching of the arteries or direct trauma. Less common are dissections of the intracranial ICAs, MCAs, VAs, and basilar arteries.[38,59,60] Temporal arteritis characteristically affects the ICAs and VAs just before they pierce the dura to enter the cranial cavity, as

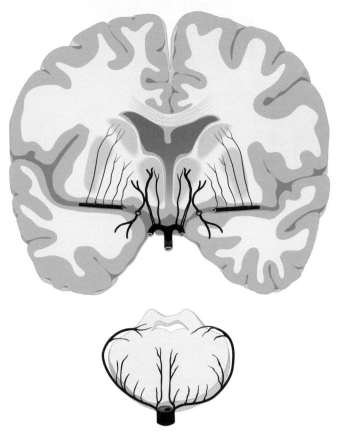

Figure 2.32 Drawing showing penetrating arteries that supply the basal ganglia and thalamus.

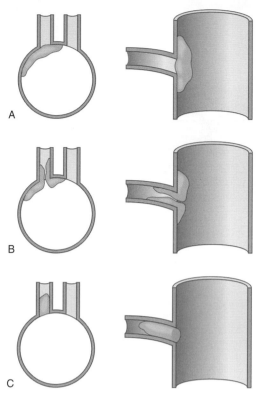

Figure 2.33 Drawing showing the arterial pathology in atheromatous branch disease: (A) plaque in the parent artery obstructing a branch, (B) a junctional plaque extending into the branch, (C) a microatheroma formed at the orifice of a branch.

well as the branches of the ophthalmic arteries before they pierce the globe.[11,61]

Embolism

Emboli can block any artery depending on the size and nature of the embolic material.[62] Large emboli, often clots formed within the heart, can block even large extracranial arteries, such as the innominate, subclavian, carotid, and vertebral arteries in the neck. More often, smaller thrombi formed in the heart or the proximal arteries embolize to block intracranial arteries, such as the ICAs, ACAs, VAs, basilar arteries, PCAs, and especially the MCAs and their superior and inferior trunks.[62] Within the anterior circulation, there is a strong predilection for emboli to go to the MCAs and their specific branches. Small balloons released into the ICAs in experimental animals consistently follow flow patterns to travel to MCA branches.[63] Within the posterior circulation, emboli preferentially block the intracranial VA, the distal basilar artery, and the PCAs.[38] Smaller fragments, such as tiny or fragmented thrombi, platelet–fibrin clumps, cholesterol crystals or other fragments from atheromatous plaques, and calcified fragments from heart valves and arterial surfaces, tend to embolize to superficial small branches of the cerebral and cerebellar arteries and the ophthalmic and retinal arteries.

Intracerebral hemorrhage

Intracerebral hemorrhage is most often caused by hypertension and has the same vascular distribution as lipohyalinosis (Figure 2.34).[28,29] In 1872, Charcot and Bouchard originally described microaneurysms, which they believed had ruptured, causing intracerebral hemorrhage.[26,27] Sudden increases in blood pressure and blood flow can also cause these same penetrating arteries to break, even in the absence of chronic hypertensive changes.[28,29] Vascular malformations can occur anywhere within the brain. Cerebral amyloid angiopathy involves small arteries and arterioles within the subarachnoid space and within the cerebral cortex.[64,65] The pattern or location of hemorrhage in the brain, predominantly cortical or subcortical, helps distinguish amyloid angiopathy from hypertensive bleeds.

Subarachnoid hemorrhage

Aneurysms most often affect junctional regions of the larger arteries of the circle of Willis, although any branch point, such as the origin of the PICAs from the VA may also be affected. The ICA–posterior communicating artery junction, anterior communicating artery–ACA junction, and the MCA trifurcations are the most common sites. The supraclinoid ICAs, pericallosal arteries, vertebral–PICA junctions, and apex of the basilar artery are also frequent sites (Figure 2.35).[23,46,66,67] Arteriovenous malformations that cause the syndrome of

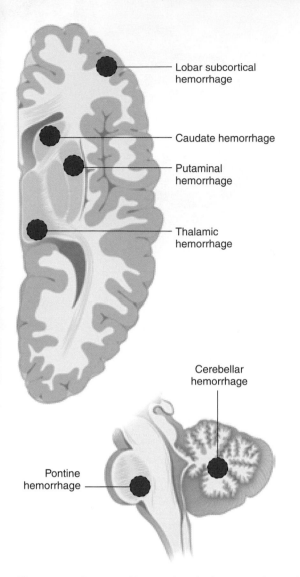

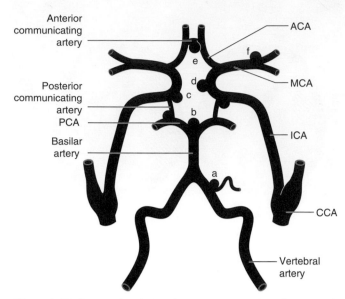

Figure 2.35 Drawing that depicts the most common sites of intracranial aneurysms; (a) posterior inferior cerebellar artery (PICA), (b) basilar artery, (c) posterior communicating artery, (d) internal carotid artery (ICA), (e) anterior communicating artery, and (f) bifurcation of the middle cerebral artery (MCA). ACA, anterior cerebral artery; CCA, common carotid artery; PCA, posterior cerebral artery.

Figure 2.34 Drawings of horizontal cerebral section and sagittal brainstem section, showing most common sites of intracerebral hemorrhage.

subarachnoid hemorrhage are either located in the brain, abutting on pial or ventricular surfaces, or situated within the ventricular system or the subarachnoid space. Some large malformations are located entirely within the subarachnoid cerebrospinal fluid compartment.

Distribution of brain pathology

Ischemia

The distribution of brain lesions caused by thrombosis is not easily distinguished from that owing to embolism, because in many patients thrombosis of an artery can lead to distal artery-to-artery embolism. Usually, the region of ischemia tends to lie in the center of the supply of the occluded artery. The extent and size of the infarct depends on the location of the occlusion, rate of development of the occlusion, adequacy of collateral circulation, and resistance of brain structures to ischemia. In patients with angiographically documented occlusion of the

ICA in the neck, Ringelstein and colleagues separated those patients with an intra-arterial embolus to the MCA and its branches ("occlusio supra occlusionem") from those who had cortical and subcortical infarcts that were considered related to diminished blood flow secondary to the ICA occlusion.[68] Figure 2.36 shows common patterns of infarction in patients with ICA occlusions. In a separate study, Ringelstein and colleagues studied the distribution of lesions in the brain in patients with cardiogenic cerebral embolism. Figure 2.37 illustrates various patterns of infarction associated with brain embolism based on this report.[69]

In patients who have systemic hypoperfusion, in contrast, the regions most vulnerable to ischemia are located in the borderzones between major arterial supply zones (see Figure 2.6A). The situation has been likened to a watering system for a field.[20,70] If a hose is blocked and the pressure of water in the pump remains constant, the portion of the field least well supplied is at the center of the blocked hose (see Figure 2.6B). More water flows through the open or collateral hoses to supply the edges of territory supplied by the blocked hose. However, if pump pressure is reduced, water trickles out of each hose, and only the center of supply of each hose receives water (see Figure 2.6C). Low pressure reduces flow to the borderzone regions or watersheds between hoses. Some borderzones are cortical or cortical–subcortical while others are deep; the latter are usually referred to as internal borderzones. Another way to consider the distribution of damage in patients with low flow is the concept of distal fields.[20] The regions that receive the least blood are those farthest from the center of the longest vessels. These distal fields are situated at the edges of the major vessel distributions and most often are located in the posterior portions of

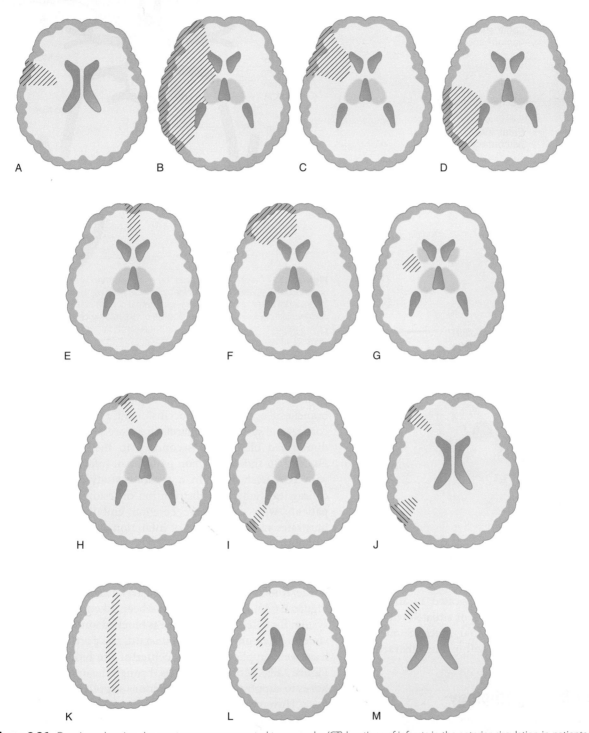

Figure 2.36 Drawings showing the most common computed tomography (CT) locations of infarcts in the anterior circulation in patients with ICA occlusions; infarcts are shown by hatched gray: (A) wedge-shaped MCA infarct; (B) entire MCA territory; (C) superior division MCA; (D) inferior division MCA; (E) ACA; (F) ACA and MCA; (G) striatocapsular infarct; (H) wedge-shaped, anterior watershed infarct; (I) wedge-shaped, posterior watershed infarct; (J) anterior and posterior watershed infarcts; (K) linear internal watershed infarct; (L) oval-shaped, deep watershed infarct; (M) small white matter watershed infarct.

the cerebral hemispheres. The common borderzone infarct regions are shown in Figure 2.36H–M. Any vascular territory has potential collateral vessels that can provide blood flow from adjacent regions. Immediately after the blockage or occlusion of a vessel, the diminished downstream pressure in the vessel segments allows higher pressure blood flow from collaterals to fill. Such collateral flow patterns can actually be shown as reverse flow in the main arterial tree if the upstream artery is completely or severely blocked.

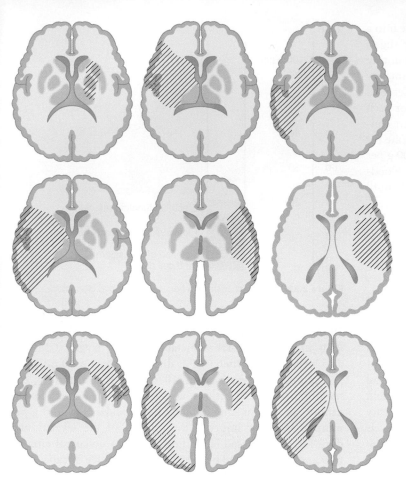

Figure 2.37 Drawings of computed tomography (CT) scans that show the most common infarct patterns in patients with embolic strokes. Adapted from Ringelstein EB, Koschorke S, Holling A, et al. *Computed tomographic pattern of proven embolic brain infarctions. Ann Neurol* 1989;26:759–765.

Intracerebral hemorrhage

The most common brain locations for hypertensive intracerebral hemorrhages are as follows: lateral ganglionic (putaminal or pallidal) and capsular (40%), thalamus (12%), lobar white matter (15–20%), caudate nucleus (8%), pons (8%), and cerebellum (8%)[29,71] (see Figure 2.34). Such bleeding sites are often supplied by perforatoring arteries that have become frail due to chronic hypertension. Bleeding does not usually conform to territories supplied by larger arteries since hemorrhages often dissect across arterial boundary territories. Hemorrhages owing to vascular malformations have no special predilection sites but are most often either subcortical or near the brain surface. Hemorrhages caused by amyloid angiopathy are usually lobar, often occipital, and seldom affect the basal ganglia or posterior fossa structures.[65,72]

Hemorrhages related to illicit drug use, especially cocaine and amphetamines, have the same general distribution as hypertensive hemorrhages, probably because the mechanism of bleeding is an acute increase in blood pressure. Patients who develop intracranial hemorrhages after using cocaine have a much higher frequency of aneurysms and vascular malformations than hemorrhages that develop after amphetamine use.[73] Hemorrhages in patients who are being treated with anticoagulants preferentially involve the cerebral white matter and the cerebellum.[74,75]

Physiology and pathophysiology of brain ischemia and hemorrhage

Ischemia

Normal metabolism and blood flow

The brain is a metabolically very active organ. Despite its relatively small size, the brain uses about one-quarter of the body's energy supply. Brain cells depend mainly on oxygen and sugar to survive. Unlike other body organs, the brain uses glucose as its sole substrate for energy metabolism. Glucose is oxidized to carbon dioxide (CO_2) and water (H_2O). Glucose metabolism leads to conversion of adenosine diphosphate (ADP) into adenosine triphosphate (ATP). A constant supply of ATP is needed to maintain neuronal integrity and to keep the major extracellular cations Ca^{2+} (calcium ions) and Na^+ (sodium ions) outside the cells and the intracellular cation K^+ (potassium ions) within the cells. Production of ATP is much more efficient in the presence of oxygen. Although in the absence of oxygen anaerobic glycolysis leads to formation of ATP and lactate, the energy yield is relatively small, and lactic acid accumulates within and outside of cells.[76] The brain requires and uses approximately 500 ml of oxygen and 75–100 mg of glucose each minute, a total of 125 g of glucose each day.[77]

41

These requirements for oxygen and glucose translate into a need for lots of oxygenated blood containing adequate sugar. Even though the brain is a relatively small organ, accounting for only 2% of adult body weight, the brain uses approximately 20% of the cardiac output when the body is resting.[76] Cerebral blood flow (CBF) is normally approximately 50 ml for each 100 g of brain tissue per minute, and cerebral oxygen consumption, usually measured as the cerebral metabolic rate for oxygen ($CMRO_2$), is normally approximately 3.5 ml/100 g per minute.[78] By increasing oxygen extraction from the bloodstream, compensation can be made to maintain $CMRO_2$ until CBF is reduced to a level of 20–25 ml/100 g per minute.[76] Positron emission tomography (PET) can measure CBF, $CMRO_2$, and oxygen extraction fraction (OEF) and the cerebral metabolic rate for glucose ($CMRg_1$) in various brain regions of interest.[78,79] PET scanning is discussed in more detail in Chapter 4.

Brain energy use and blood flow depend on the degree of neuronal activity. In 1890, Roy and Sherrington first demonstrated the ability of the brain to increase local blood flow in response to regional changes in neuronal activity.[80,81] PET and functional MRI show that using the right hand increases metabolism and CBF in the left motor cortex. Clearly, it is critical for survival of brain tissue that there are systems to maintain CBF despite changes in systemic blood pressure. The capacity of the cerebral circulation to maintain relatively constant levels of CBF despite changing blood pressure has traditionally been termed *autoregulation*. CBF remains relatively constant when mean arterial blood pressures are between 50 and 150 mmHg.[76] When blood pressure is chronically raised, both the upper and lower levels of autoregulation are raised, indicating a higher tolerance to hypertension but also increased sensitivity to hypotension.[82]

Mean blood flow velocities as measured by transcranial Doppler (TCD) within the intracranial arteries range from 35 to 75 cm per second but vary considerably with age, sex, blood pressure, hematocrit, and blood vessel location.[83] When CBF increases or an artery narrows, the velocity in that segment of artery increases. At first glance, increased velocity in response to a reduction in luminal diameter seems paradoxical. One must try, however, to visualize a simple everyday example of velocity of liquid flow – an ordinary garden hose. When using a hose to wash off a pavement or a patio, to generate a high pressure jet of water, the nozzle is turned to reduce the luminal diameter. The narrower the nozzle lumen, the more pressure in the stream until the lumen is nearly effaced, at which time water dribbles out, and velocity becomes greatly reduced. This analogy will be useful to recall in Chapter 4, when we discuss transcranial Doppler measurements of blood flow velocities in proximal segments of the intracranial arteries.

Local brain effects of ischemia

When blood flow to a brain region is reduced, survival of the at-risk tissue depends on the intensity and duration of the ischemia and the availability of collateral blood flow. Animal experiments provide estimates of thresholds of brain ischemia (Figure 2.38).[76] At blood flow levels of approximately

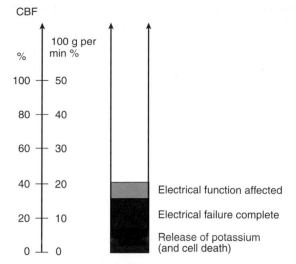

Figure 2.38 Thresholds of brain ischemia. CBF, cerebral blood flow.

20 ml/100 g per minute, electroencephalographic (EEG) activity is affected. The cerebral metabolic rate of oxygen ($CMRO_2$) also begins to fall when CBF is diminished below 20 ml/100 g per minute. At levels below 10 ml/100 g per minute, cell membranes and functions are severely affected. Neurons cannot survive for long at blood flows below 5 ml/100 g per minute. Ischemic injury is the product of the severity and duration of decreased blood flow, offset by collateral circulation and also modified by the ischemic tolerance or capacity of specific brain tissue to sustain injury.

When neurons become ischemic, a number of biochemical changes potentiate and enhance cell death: K^+ moves across the cell membrane into the extracellular space, and Ca^{2+} moves into the cell, where it greatly compromises the ability of intracellular membranes to control subsequent ion fluxes and causes mitochondrial failure;[78] normally, there is a 10-fold gradient difference between extracellular and intracellular (cytosolic) Ca^{2+}. Decreased oxygen availability leads to production of oxygen molecules with unpaired electrons, termed *oxygen-free radicals*. These free radicals cause peroxidation of fatty acids in cell organelles and plasma membranes, causing severe cell dysfunction.[84,85] With decreased oxygen availability, anaerobic glycolysis leads to an accumulation of lactic acid and a decrease in pH. The resulting acidosis also greatly impairs cell metabolic functions.

The activity of neurotransmitters, often referred to as *excitatory neurotransmitters* (glutamate, aspartate, and kainic acid), is significantly increased in regions of brain ischemia.[85–88] Hypoxia, hypoglycemia, and ischemia all contribute to cause energy depletion and an increase in glutamate release but a decrease in glutamate uptake. This increased availability of glutamate causes vulnerable neurons to receive toxic exposure to glutamate, thereby increasing the likelihood of cell death. Glutamate entry opens membranes and increases Na^+ and Ca^{2+} influx into cells. Large influxes of Na^+ are followed by entry of chloride ions and water, causing cell swelling and edema. Glutamate is an agonist at both *N*-methyl-D-aspartate (NMDA) and

non-NMDA (kainate and quisqualate) receptor types, but only NMDA receptors are linked to membrane channels with high calcium permeability.[87] Knowledge of these changes in the neuronal and extracellular spaces is important to recall when treatment of acute stroke patients is discussed in Chapter 6.

These aforementioned local metabolic changes cause a self-perpetuating cycle of changes that lead to increasing neuronal damage and cell death. Changes in ionic concentrations of Na^+, K^+, and Ca^{2+}; release of oxygen-free radicals; acidosis; and release of excitatory neurotransmitters further damage cells, leading to more local biochemical changes, which in turn cause more neuronal damage.[87,88] At some point, the process of ischemia becomes irreversible, despite reperfusion of tissues with adequate oxygen and glucose-rich blood. At times, although the severity of ischemia is insufficient to cause neuronal necrosis, ischemia may nevertheless set in motion a process of programmed cell death referred to as *apoptosis*.[89]

The degree of ischemia caused by blockage of an artery varies in different zones supplied by that artery. In the center of the zone, blood flow is lowest and ischemic damage is most severe. This region of the most severe damage is often referred to as the *core* of the infarct. On the periphery of the affected vascular territory, collateral blood flow allows continued delivery of blood. The capacity of collateral circulation also markedly varies across individuals. Referring to Figure 2.38, metabolism at the center of blood supply may be reduced sufficiently to cause cell necrosis (0–10 ml/100 g/minute), whereas at the periphery, supplies of 10–20 ml/100 g per minute might stun the brain, causing electrical failure but not permanent cell damage. The zone of dysfunctional, but not dead, brain surrounding the center of infarction has traditionally been referred to as the *ischemic penumbra* (Figure 2.39). Garcia and Anderson eloquently describe this region as follows: "Penumbral neurons are thought to be paralyzed in a shadowy state between life and death, merely awaiting the restoration of either adequate blood flow or other as yet unknown conditions before resuming full life."[85] Some neurons are thought to be more vulnerable to hypoxia and decreased fuel supply than other neurons, termed *selective vulnerability*.[86] Recent advanced imaging approaches to stroke with multimodal computed tomography (CT) and MRI often refer to these penumbral zones as regions at-risk of ischemic infarction as it remains difficult to standardize penumbral definitions across various imaging modalities and measures.

Arterial occlusion and reaction to the occlusive process

Brain ischemia should not be viewed as a static anatomic–pathological process. It is usually an incredibly dynamic, often unstable, condition. Brain tissue, in imminent danger of irreversible death, nevertheless often recovers remarkably well, leaving no trace of its previous precarious situation. To treat patients optimally, physicians must understand the various factors that affect outcome. The discussion of pathophysiology has so far centered on the function and metabolism of local regions of brain tissue. To understand the variety of factors affecting outcome, we now turn to a more macroscopic view of both the process of arterial occlusion and the way in which occlusive changes are handled by the body.

Vascular occlusion most often begins with formation of atherosclerotic plaques within extracranial and large intracranial arteries. These plaques contain a mixture of lipid, smooth muscle, fibrous and collagen tissues, macrophages, and inflammatory cells. Plaques may enlarge quickly when hemorrhages occur within the plaques. When a critical plaque size and significant encroachment on the lumen develop, the atherosclerotic process often accelerates. Reduced luminal area and the bulk of the protruding plaque alter the physical and mechanical properties of blood flow and create regions of local turbulence and stasis. Platelets often adhere to irregular plaque surfaces. Secretion of chemical mediators within platelets and within the underlying vascular endothelium causes aggregation and further adherence of platelets to the endothelium. ADP, epinephrine, and collagen can all increase platelet aggregation.[90] Activated platelets release ADP and arachidonic acid. In the presence of the enzyme cyclooxygenase, arachidonic acid is metabolized to prostaglandin endoperoxides, which can be converted by thromboxane synthetase to thromboxane A_2, a potent vasoconstrictor and inducer of further platelet aggregation and secretion.[3] At the same time, the vascular endothelium may secrete prostacyclin, a potent vasodilator and inhibitor of platelet aggregation.[91] Both vascular patency and the formation of platelet–fibrin clots are influenced by the balance between thromboxane A_2, prostacyclin, and other factors. Platelets begin to stick together and adhere to the endothelial lining of the plaque. A "white clot" composed of platelets and fibrin develops (Figure 2.40; see also Figure 2.2C).

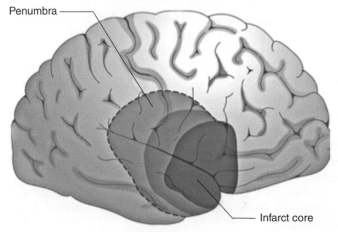

Figure 2.39 Cartoon showing the core and penumbra of a brain infarct. The darkest region represents the core – tissue already infarcted. The surrounding gray zones represent areas with decreased blood flow but capable of recovery if the blood supply improves. In the most peripheral gray zone, the blood supply decrement is least severe.

Penumbra

Infarct core

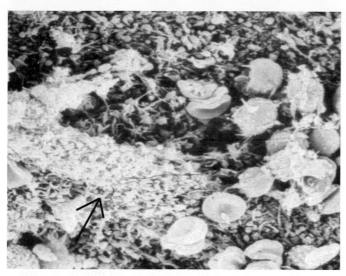

Figure 2.40 Phase microscope image of a white fibrin–platelet thrombus (black arrow) formed in a high flow system. Courtesy of S H Hanson and C H Kessler, Emory University, Division of Hematology.

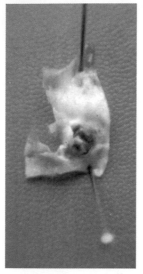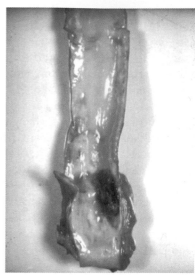

Figure 2.41 Ulcerated internal carotid artery (ICA) plaques in specimens of arteries removed at surgery. A black and white version of this figure will appear in some formats. For the color version, please refer to the plate section.

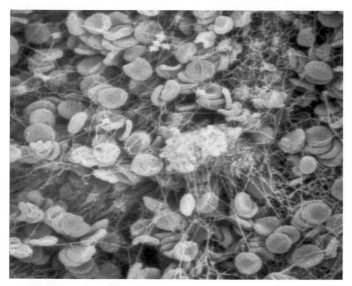

Figure 2.42 Phase microscope image of a red thrombus, composed of fibrin and erythrocytes, formed in a thrombogenic system, in a vessel with a low flow rate. Courtesy of S H Hanson and C H Kessler, Emory University, Division of Hematology.

Plaques often interrupt the endothelial lining of arteries and ulcerate. Figure 2.41 shows ulcerated irregular plaques within specimens of carotid arteries removed at surgery. Breaches in the endothelium allow cracks and fissures to form, allowing contact of the constituents of the plaque with the blood within the lumen. Tissue factor, an important stimulator of the body's coagulation system, is released. The coagulation cascade is activated by this contact and a "red thrombus" composed of erythrocytes and fibrin forms within the lumen (Figure 2.42; see also Figure 2.2C). Platelet secretion can also activate the serine proteases that form the body's coagulation system and also promotes the formation of red clots. When white or red thrombi first form, they are poorly organized and only loosely adherent. They often propagate and embolize. Figure 2.4 shows an occluded carotid artery found at

necropsy. The specimen contains a large mobile red thrombus, a part of which had embolized to the brain. Within a period of 1–2 weeks, thrombi organize and become more adherent and fragments are less likely to break off and embolize. A variety of different materials – cholesterol crystals, calcified plaque fragments, white clots, and red thrombi – can form the substance of intra-arterial emboli. Recent analyses of retrieved thrombi have shown mixtures of red and white thrombi, likely due to associated conditions and the hemodynamic milieu as well as sampling variation in such specimens.

Atherosclerotic plaques and vascular stenosis cause brain ischemia in a variety of ways. Progressive intimal thickening leads to stenosis or occlusion of the artery, resulting in reduced distal blood flow. Stasis of blood flow enhances the formation of thrombi that often embolize. Physical factors are clearly important in the formation, lysis, clearance, and washout of thromboemboli. Blood flow at arterial bifurcations is complex even in normal non-stenotic arteries. Eddies, turbulence, flow separation, and vortices are common and vary with location along the arteries.[92] As an artery narrows, blood flow velocity increases within the center of the artery and flow separation becomes more prominent.[92] Flow is reduced in some parts of the artery, especially on the outer perimeter of the residual lumen. When subtotal or complete occlusion of an artery develops, the blood-stream flow diminishes because of reduced volume of flow, and blood flow velocity also is decreased.[92–94] Antegrade perfusion becomes less effective. This reduced perfusion and pressure decreases washout and throughput of emboli, especially in remote borderzone portions of the brain circulation.[95–97] Hypoperfusion and embolism interact and complement each other to promote and enhance brain infarction.[93,94]

Thrombus formation

Thrombi form in situ when the body's coagulation system has been activated and the blood is hypercoagulable. In some

patients with hypercoagulability, red thrombi form simultaneously or sequentially in multiple, systemic extracranial and intracranial arteries and veins. In other patients with arterial lesions (e.g., arterial atherosclerotic plaques or dissections), the process of occlusive thrombosis is accelerated at sites of vascular disease. Hypercoagulability can be a lifelong hereditary problem. Systemic diseases, such as cancer, regional enteritis, and thrombocytosis, can cause increased clotting. The process of atherothrombosis (e.g., in the coronary or cerebrovascular systems) can also activate serological coagulation factors that promote further thrombosis.[98–102]

Much of the treatment of patients with thromboembolic stroke concerns attempts to affect or reverse the coagulation process or to facilitate clot lysis or removal. Clinicians treating patients with ischemia should be familiar with the general features of blood coagulation to effectively choose and monitor antithrombotic and thrombolytic therapies.

The final step in the coagulation cascade is the conversion of the soluble protein fibrinogen into insoluble polymers termed *fibrin*. These strands of fibrin form a network of fibers that entangle formed blood elements (i.e., platelets and erythrocytes) into a clot. Fibrin is quite adhesive and has the capability of contracting. The fibrinogen-to-fibrin reaction occurs when factor II, prothrombin, is converted to thrombin. The amounts of circulating fibrinogen and prothrombin are important in these reactions.

Prothrombin can be activated in two different ways: In the so-called extrinsic system of coagulation, a tissue or endothelial injury releases thromboplastic substances, known as tissue factors, which in turn cause both platelet activation and activation of some of the blood serine protease coagulation factors, especially factors V and VII. Tissue factor forms a complex with factor VIIa; the tissue factor-VIIa complex converts factor X to Xa. Factor Xa activates a prothrombinase complex composed of activated factor V, Ca^{2+}, and phospholipids, which in turn with factor Xa catalyzes the reaction of prothrombin to thrombin. Activation of platelets causes them to agglutinate, to adhere to the injured vessel wall, and to release various intracellular substances, which in turn activate the coagulation system.[98–100]

The complementary intrinsic coagulation system refers to blood-coagulation factors that circulate in inactive forms (factors V, VIII [antihemophilic globulin], IX, X, XI, XII) and are intrinsic to the blood. Activation of factor XII from an inert precursor form to an activated form triggers a series of reactions, described as the *coagulation cascade* in which the various blood-clotting factors are sequentially converted to their active enzymatic forms. Ultimately, these reactions lead to activation of factor X, which catalyzes the prothrombin → thrombin reaction.[100–102] Figure 2.43 is a simplified diagram of the coagulation reactions. Thrombin, in turn, in addition to converting fibrinogen to fibrin, has an important influence on blood platelets, causing them to swell, aggregate, and release substances that affect vascular tone and blood coagulability.

Also important are various natural inhibitors of coagulation: antithrombin III, protein C, and protein S. Deficiencies in any of these serum proteins can cause increased coagulability.

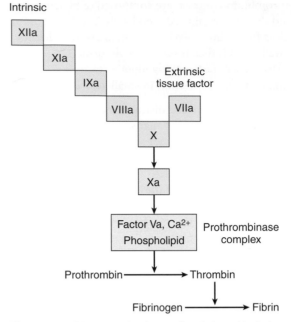

Figure 2.43 Diagrammatic scheme of extrinsic and intrinsic coagulation systems.

Genetically transmitted disorders can also lead to hypercoagulability. One common inherited disorder leads to functional resistance to the anticoagulant effects of activated protein C.[103] This genetic defect is termed the *factor V Leiden mutation* and is caused by a point mutation in factor V.[104] Another genetic disorder that predisposes to thrombosis is caused by a mutation in the prothrombin gene.[105] These mutations in the prothrombin and factor V genes are common in patients who develop cerebral venous thrombosis and phlebothromboses, especially if they also take oral contraceptives.[106]

Key components in the coagulation system are factor Xa, prothrombin, and thrombin. Factor Xa is especially important since it is the focal point at the intersection of both the intrinsic and extrinsic portions of the coagulation cascade. Heparins cause a conformational change in antithrombin III, which increases its ability to inactivate factor Xa. Warfarins inhibit the action of vitamin K necessary for the biosynthesis of prothrombin and factor X. Researchers and clinicians are now exploring the potential for using agents that inactivate factor Xa or directly inhibit thrombin generation and function.

Naturally occurring factors also exist that act to lyse clots once they are formed. Tissue plasminogen activator and other substances activate plasminogen to form plasmin, a potent fibrinolytic enzyme. Plasminogen is also activated by various coagulation factors, such as factor XII, so that the process of coagulation itself activates the thrombolytic system. Various plasmin inhibitors ("antiplasmins") are also present.[102,107]

Pathologists and hematologists recognize and describe three types of thrombi[101]:

1. Red thrombi are composed mostly of red blood cells and fibrin; they form in areas of slowed blood flow. Their formation does not require an abnormal vessel wall or tissue thromboplastin (see Figure 2.42).

2. White thrombi, in contrast, are composed of platelets and fibrin and do not contain red blood cells (see Figure 2.40). White clots form almost exclusively in areas in which the arterial wall or endothelial surface is abnormal, characteristically in fast-moving bloodstreams.
3. Disseminated fibrin deposition in small vessels.

These types of thrombi are distinct and are affected by different therapeutic agents. In many cases, the thrombus begins as a white platelet–fibrin clot and then a red thrombus is laid down as a cap over the initial platelet mass.[101]

When a major artery occludes, a crisis ensues. Pressure drops distal to the occlusion, and the brain region supplied by that vessel is acutely deprived of blood. Diminished blood flow in turn activates protective mechanisms that help restore needed blood flow to the ischemic region. Low pressure helps to draw blood from higher pressure regions. Collateral circulation is allowed to enter the downstream territory from adjacent vascular territories. Ischemic cell damage causes release of lactic acid and other metabolites. The resulting local tissue acidosis leads to vasodilation, augmenting regional CBF.[108] If brain tissue is deprived of blood and needed nourishment for too long, it dies. At times, there are varying grades of ischemia, ranging from irreversible cell death in the most deprived zone to a reversible situation of diminished electrical activity but normal or only slightly elevated extracellular potassium concentration in the threatened ischemic penumbral zone.[71,85,86,108,109] The severity of the ischemic crisis depends on the rate of vascular occlusion. A vessel that gradually occludes may already have stimulated abundant collateral circulation so that final occlusion produces less stress on the system.

Factors that affect tissue survival

The survival of the brain regions at risk depends on a number of factors: (1) the adequacy of collateral circulation; (2) the state of the systemic circulation; (3) serological factors; (4) changes within the obstructing vascular lesion; and (5) resistance within the microcirculatory bed; (6) brain edema and increased intracranial pressure.

Adequacy of the collateral circulation

Variation in collateral circulation due to vascular capacity or patterns at the circle of Willis and in leptomeningeal or pial vessels can radically alter the outcome of ischemic stroke. Although persistent fetal patterns are often described at the circle of Willis, serial imaging studies show dynamic changes in vascular segments of this structure during adult life due to changes in blood flow. The specific determinants of collateral grade or capacity remain an area of focused research due to their importance in stroke outcomes. Hypertension or diabetes diminishes blood flow in smaller arteries and arterioles and so reduces the potential of the vascular system to supply blood flow to the needy region.

State of the systemic circulation

Cardiac pump failure, hypovolemia, and increased blood viscosity all reduce CBF. The two most important determinants of blood viscosity are the hematocrit and the fibrinogen levels.[110–112] In patients with hematocrits in the range of 47–53%, lowering of the hematocrit by phlebotomy to below 40% can increase CBF by as much as 50%.[112] Blood pressure is also very important. Elevation of blood pressure except at malignant ranges increases CBF. Surgeons take advantage of this fact by injecting catecholamines to raise blood pressure and flow during the clamping phase of carotid endarterectomy. Low blood pressure significantly reduces cerebral blood flow. In some patients, the balance is so tenuous that simply sitting in bed or standing lowers collateral pressure enough to induce symptoms.[113,114] Low blood and fluid volume also limit available blood flow in collateral channels. Many older individuals limit their fluid intake, especially in the evening, to avoid getting up at night to urinate. After the stroke, there may not have been any fluid intake because of swallowing difficulty or lack of feeding during the trip to the hospital and the initial hospital encounters.

Serological factors

The blood functions as a carrier of needed oxygen and other nutrients. Hypoxia is clearly detrimental because each milliliter of blood delivers a less-than-normal oxygen supply.[115] Low blood sugar similarly increases the risk of cell death. Higher-than-normal blood sugar also can be detrimental to the ischemic brain.[116,117] Elevated serum calcium levels[118,119] and high blood-alcohol content[120] are also potential important detrimental variables. These factors are also discussed in Chapter 6 on treatment.

Changes within the obstructing vascular lesion

Embolic occlusive thrombi do not adhere to the vessel wall of the recipient artery and frequently move on. The moving embolus can block a more distal intracranial artery, causing added or new ischemia, or it may fragment and pass through the vascular bed. Clot formation activates an endogenous thrombolytic system that includes tissue plasminogen activator (tPA).[102,107] Inhibitors of tPA are also present. Sudden obstruction of a vascular lumen can cause reactive vasoconstriction (spasm), which in turn causes further luminal compromise. Thrombolysis, passage of clots, and reversal of vasoconstriction all promote reperfusion of the ischemic zone. If reperfusion occurs quickly enough, the stunned, reversibly ischemic brain may recover quickly. The occlusive clot may propagate further proximally or distally along the vessel, blocking potential collateral channels. The distal end of the thrombus can also break loose and embolize to an intracranial receptive site. Hypercoagulable states promote such extension of thrombi.

Resistance within the microcirculatory bed

The vast majority of CBF does not occur in the large macroscopic arteries at the base of the brain or along the surface. Most flow occurs through microscopic-sized vessels: the arterioles, capillaries, and venules.[102] Resistance to flow in these small vessels is affected by prior diseases, such as hypertension and diabetes, which often cause thickening of arterial and arteriolar walls. Experimental animals and patients that have

been hypertensive before a vascular occlusion fare worse than individuals previously normotensive, presumably because of these microcirculatory changes. Both hyperviscosity and diffuse thromboses within the capillaries and microvessel bed greatly reduce flow through the microcirculation. Ischemic insults may produce biochemical changes that lead to platelet activation, clumping of erythrocytes, and plugging of the microcirculation. Ames referred to these changes as causing a "no reflow" state in the microvascular bed, even when large arteries are reperfused.[121] In general, studies of CBF are sensitive to changes in resistance in the microcirculatory bed. Remember that flow is inversely proportional to resistance in the vascular bed, the majority of which is microcirculatory.

Brain edema and increased intracranial pressure

Edema and pressure changes within the brain and cranial cavity also influence survival of brain tissue and patient recovery after vascular occlusions. There are two types of brain edema: (1) water accumulation inside cells, termed *cytotoxic edema*; and (2) fluid within the extracellular space, often termed *vasogenic edema*.[122] Extracellular edema is also often referred to as *wet edema* because in such cases, the cut surface of the brain oozes edema fluid, whereas intracellular (cytotoxic) edema is termed *dry edema*.[122] Cytotoxic edema is caused by energy failure, with movement of ions and water across the cell membranes into cells. Extracellular edema is influenced by hydrostatic pressure factors, especially increased blood pressure and blood flow, and by osmotic factors. When proteins and other macromolecules enter the brain extracellular space because of breakdown of the blood–brain barrier, they exert an osmotic gradient pulling water into the extracellular space. This vasogenic edema accumulates more in the cerebral and cerebellar white matter because of the difference in compliance between gray and white matter.

Brain swelling caused by cytotoxic edema means a large volume of dead or dying brain cells, which implies a bad outcome. On the other hand, edema within the extracellular space does not necessarily imply neuronal injury, and fluid in the extracellular compartment can potentially be mobilized and removed. Severe edema may cause gross swelling of the brain; shifts in position of brain tissue, with potential pressure damage; and herniation of brain contents from one compartment to another.

Intracranial pressure may also be increased, leading to increased morbidity and decreased CBF. When intracranial pressure is increased, the pressure in the venous sinuses and draining veins must also increase if blood is to be drained normally from the cranium. There must be a gradient between venous pressure and intracranial pressure for drainage to occur. Also, for tissue perfusion to occur, arterial pressure must exceed venous pressure. Blood flow is compromised in the presence of arterial and venous occlusions. When the intracranial venous system contains occlusions, venous pressure is increased. The limited drainage often causes fluid to back up into the brain, causing vasogenic edema. Increased intracranial pressure places an additional stress on the system, forcing even higher the flow values required for tissue survival.

Brain edema and increased intracranial pressure also cause headache, decreased consciousness, and vomiting.[123] Pressure shifts and herniation cause pressure-related damage to adjacent tissues and signs of dysfunction of the compressed structures.[32,123,124] Because pressure shifts and herniations are more common after intracerebral hemorrhage, due to the additional presence in the brain of an extra mass of tissue (hematoma), we discuss herniations further in the discussion of intracerebral hemorrhage.

Events during the first three weeks after vascular occlusion

Experience shows that the tenuous balance created by occlusion of a major artery is temporary and usually resolves in 2–3 weeks at most. During this period, any systemic changes, such as decrease in fluid volume or positional or pharmacologically mediated drops in blood pressure, can cause worsening of symptoms. By 3 weeks, either the brain tissue has died, causing a brain infarct, or collateral sources of blood flow develop that adequately supply the region at risk. By 2–3 weeks, collateral circulation stabilizes, and the patient is less vulnerable to positional or circulatory changes. In addition to causing ischemia through low perfusion, the occlusive thrombus, which at first loosely adheres to the vessel wall, can propagate distally or can fragment and embolize to a distal artery. By 2–3 weeks, the clot has become more adherent and has much less tendency to embolize. Most studies of patients with anterior[125,126] and posterior circulation ischemia[38,127–131] show a low frequency of progression of acute ischemic deficits after 2 weeks.

During the hours, days, and early weeks after a vascular occlusion, the question of death or survival of at-risk brain tissue can be viewed as a clash between factors acting to worsen ischemia and natural body responses that prevent or limit ischemia. Table 2.1 summarizes these "good guys" versus "bad guys" responses, which are useful to keep in mind when treatment is discussed. Clinicians hope to build on the body's natural defenses and counteract the factors that promote ischemia.

Table 2.1 Balancing of factors after vascular occlusion

Factors promoting ischemia	Responses limiting ischemia
Decreased blood flow due to occlusion	Opening of collateral vascular channels
Embolization of clot	Passing and fragmentation of emboli
Activation of coagulation factors and inhibitors of thrombolysis	Activation of thrombolytic factors
Propagation of clot	Lysis of clot
Decreased blood flow due to hypotension, hypovolemia, low cardiac output	Improvement in general medical condition, especially after correction of abnormalities

This process of shifting vulnerability translates clinically into fluctuating variable symptoms and signs during the early period after a vascular occlusion. Acute blockage of an artery often translates into the sudden onset of symptoms. After vascular occlusion, a weighing of the balance of positive and adverse factors toward the adverse side causes transient deficits or causes fluctuating, stepwise, or gradual worsening of neurological symptoms and signs. Sudden worsening is often related to distal embolization.

Intracerebral hemorrhage

Hemorrhage into the brain parenchyma is often preceded by hypertensive damage to small cerebral penetrating arteries and arterioles. Small aneurysmal dilatations, first hypothesized by Charcot and Bouchard in the 1870s, pepper the penetrating vascular territories of hypertensive patients[26,27] and in some patients represent weak points that rupture under increased arterial tension. In most patients, abrupt elevation in blood pressure causes rupture of small penetrating arteries that had no prior vascular damage.[28,29] Leakage from these small vessels produces a sudden but local pressure effect on surrounding capillaries and arterioles, causing them in turn to break.[132] An avalanche-type effect ensues, in which vessels at the circumference break, adding volume to the gradually enlarging hemorrhage (Figure 2.44). The accumulation of blood along the circumference of the hematoma is like a snowball rolling downhill, gathering volume along its outer surfaces as it descends. High blood pressure and this avalanche effect enlarge the hemorrhage, while mounting local tissue pressure acts as a tamponade to the bleeding.

Trauma, bleeding disorders, and degenerative changes in congenitally abnormal blood vessels within vascular malformations also may initiate intracerebral bleeding, which then progresses in a manner similar to hypertensive intracerebral hemorrhage. The gradual increase in size of the hematoma translates clinically into gradual worsening of symptoms and signs until the hematoma attains its final size. Hematomas can stop enlarging and may drain themselves by emptying into the ventricular system or the cerebrospinal fluid (CSF) at the pial surface.

If the hemorrhage becomes sizable, the increase in intracranial volume must increase intracranial pressure. When intracranial pressure rises, the venous pressure in the draining dural sinuses increases pari passu. To perfuse the brain, the arterial pressure must rise to produce an effective arteriovenous difference. The patient with intracerebral hemorrhage may have a markedly elevated blood pressure because of the hemorrhage, not necessarily reflecting the true level of premorbid blood pressure. Although lowering this pressure does help to stop bleeding, caution must be exercised because the elevated pressure also serves to perfuse the areas of the brain not damaged by the hemorrhage.

Patients with intracerebral hemorrhage often worsen during the first 24–48 hours after their initial symptoms. This worsening can be explained by continued bleeding but most often is related to the development of edema around the

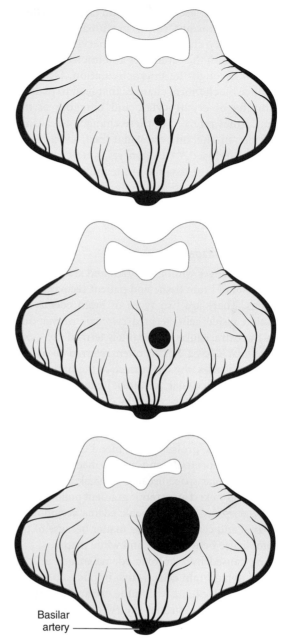

Figure 2.44 Drawing illustrating avalanche-type effect in pontine hemorrhage, showing gradual development of hemorrhage due to rupture of small vessels on the periphery of the hemorrhage.

lesion,[132,133] to the effects of the lesion on blood flow and metabolism, and, in large hemorrhages, to shifts in brain contents and herniations. Effects caused by masses in patients with hematomas are more common than in patients with ischemia because an extra volume of substance has been added (blood in the hematoma) in addition to the surrounding edema. Most often, pressure effects in hemispheral hematomas result in a shift of the midline without herniation of brain contents. The brain is compartmentalized by bony fortresses (anterior, middle, and posterior fossas) and by dural structures (falx cerebri and tentorium cerebelli), which, under normal circumstances, contain their usual contents. When mass

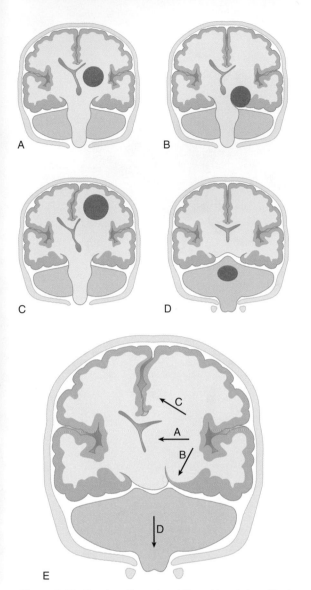

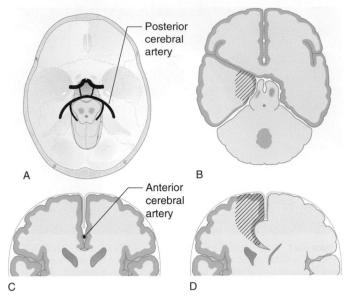

Figure 2.46 Drawing illustrating infarcts due to compression of arteries: (A) Normal anatomy showing posterior carotid artery (PCA) crossing up and over the edge of the tentorium; (B) infarction of medial temporal lobe due to compression of PCA between herniated uncus and tentorium; (C) anatomy showing anterior carotid artery (ACA) in relation to falx; (D) infarction of medial frontal lobe, due to compression of ACA against the falx cerebri.

Figure 2.45 Drawings illustrating shifts and herniations. Displacement of brain tissues due to mass-producing strokes is illustrated by patients with hematomas. (A) Basal ganglionic hematoma causes compression of the ipsilateral ventricle and shift of the midline to the opposite side. (B) Deep hematoma causes uncal herniation. The medial temporal lobe exerts pressure on the upper brainstem. (C) Frontal hematoma causes herniations of the cingulum under the falx cerebri. (D) Cerebellum hematoma causes increased posterior fossa pressure with herniation of the cerebellum (E) through the foramen magnum. These patterns are also illustrated in E.

effects are severe, brain tissue bulges or spills out of its usual abode into a different compartment – a process called *herniation*.[30–32,124]

Brain shifts and herniations and their effects are shown in Figure 2.45. The most common are: (1) herniation of the temporal lobe through the tentorial notch, to compress the midbrain (see Figure 2.45A); (2) symmetric, downward pressure by the swollen cerebral hemispheres on the rostral brainstem, causing elongation (see Figure 2.45B); (3) herniation of the anterior medial frontal lobe, usually of the cingulate gyrus, under the falx cerebri (see Figure 2.45C); (4) herniation of the cerebellum upward through the tentorial notch, to

compress the brainstem (see Figure 2.45D); and (5) downward herniation of the cerebellar tonsils through the foramen magnum, compressing the medulla and upper cervical spinal cord (see D in Figure 2.45E).

Shifts in brain contents can also lead to compression or stretch of arteries and infarction in areas of supply and secondary hemorrhages. The most common loci of secondary vascular changes leading to infarction involve the PCAs where they pass between the tentorium and the medial temporal lobe and the ACAs adjacent to the falx (Figure 2.46). Distortion of the upper brainstem at the tentorial opening often leads to secondary hemorrhages in the brainstem. These usually involve the midline and paramedian vessels and are called *Düret hemorrhages*, after the French clinician and researcher who first described them.[134] A necropsy specimen of a Düret hemorrhage is shown in Figure 2.47 and a drawing of another Düret hemmorhage is shown in Figure 2.48B.

The ventricular system may also be compressed at variable sites. Hematomas in the putamen or cerebral lobes may distort the foramen of Monro, causing dilatation of the contralateral lateral ventricle. Thalamic hematomas often obstruct and compress the IIIrd ventricle, leading to hydrocephalus of both lateral ventricles. Cerebellar hemorrhages can compress the IVth ventricle or cerebral aqueduct, leading to obstructive hydrocephalus of the third and lateral ventricles. Shifts in brain contents, herniations, and secondary infarctions, as well as Düret hemorrhages and hydrocephalus, all cause clinical worsening of signs and symptoms. Intracerebral hemorrhages are discussed in detail in Chapter 14.

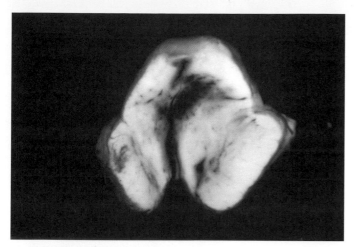

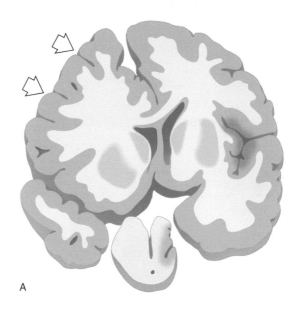

Figure 2.47 A necropsy specimen of a Düret midbrain hemorrhage. A left subdural hematoma was present on the lateral surface of the cerebral hemisphere. A black and white version of this figure will appear in some formats. For the color version, please refer to the plate section.

A

Subarachnoid hemorrhage

Subarachnoid bleeding nearly always abruptly increases intracranial pressure (ICP). Systemic blood pressure and volume must be maintained or augmented to preserve brain perfusion in the face of the increased ICP. After the initial bleeding, three major risks affect subsequent events: rebleeding, vasoconstriction, and hydrocephalus. Once the outer wall of abnormal blood vessels, most often aneurysms and vascular malformations, has been breached, the vessels are vulnerable to rebleeding. Clearly, a second or third bleed poses substantial threats for survival because each bleed increases ICP and the amount of blood in the CSF. Arteries bathed in bloody CSF often become constricted.[135,136] Vasoconstriction can be local or more diffuse and frequently leads to ischemia, brain edema, and infarction.[136–138] Blood within the CSF can clog the absorptive membranes, leading to communicating hydrocephalus and dilation of all of the ventricular system. At times, the initial bleed or subsequent bleeds are into the brain, as well as on its surface. In these patients, the discussion of intracerebral hemorrhage also applies because they have both intracerebral and subarachnoid hemorrhages.

Having presented the basic building blocks for understanding the mechanisms of stroke, we proceed directly to clinical diagnosis at the bedside and then laboratory diagnosis in the following chapters. Subarachnoid hemorrhage, aneurysms, and vascular malformations are discussed in Chapter 13.

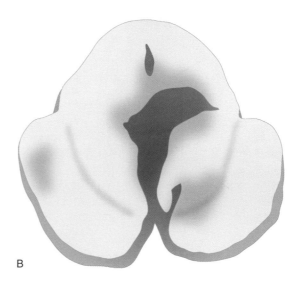

B

Figure 2.48 Drawings of autopsy findings in patients who died of lesions that increased intracranial pressure. (A) A subdural hematoma was present in the region shown by the open arrows. The underlying brain is flattened and compressed in contrast to the opposite cerebral hemisphere. The extrinsic pressure on the brain has caused compression of the ipsilateral lateral ventricle and a shift in midline structures. The increased pressure forced the midbrain against the contralateral tentorium, causing injury to the contralateral cerebral peduncle – "Kernohan's notch." (B) A Düret hemorrhage in the midbrain that developed in a patient with a large intracerebral hemorrhage.

References

1. Wagner KR, Xi G, Hua Y, et al: Early metabolic alterations in edematous perihematomal brain regions following experimental intracerebral hemorrhage. *J Neurosurg* 1998;**88**:1058–1065.

2. Bullock R, Brock-Utne J, van Dellen J, Blake G: Intracerebral hemorrhage in a primate model: effect on regional cerebral blood flow. *Surg Neurol* 1988;**29**:101–107.

3. Weiss H: Platelet physiology and abnormalities of platelet function. *N Engl J Med* 1975;**293**:531–540,580–588.

4. Ashby B, Daniel JL, Smith JB: Mechanisms of platelet activation and inhibition. *Hematol Oncol Clin North Am* 1990;**4**:1–26.

5. Baker A, Iannone A: Cerebrovascular disease. I. The large arteries of the circle of Willis. *Neurology* 1959;**9**:321–332.

6. Fisher CM, Gore I, Okabe N, et al: Atherosclerosis of the carotid and vertebral arteries–extracranial and

intracranial. *J Neuropathol Exp Neurol* 1965;**24**:455–476.

7. Fisher CM: Lacunes: Small deep cerebral infarcts. *Neurology* 1965;**15**:774–784.

8. Fisher CM: The arterial lesions underlying lacunes. *Acta Neuropathol* 1969;**12**:1–15.

9. Luscher TF, Lie JT, Stanson AW, et al: Arterial fibromuscular dysplasia. *Mayo Clin Proc* 1987;**62**:931–952.

10. Shinohara Y: Takayasu disease. In Bogousslavsky J, Caplan LR (eds): *Uncommon Causes of Stroke*. Cambridge: Cambridge University Press, 2001, pp 37–42.

11. Davis SM: Temporal arteritis. In Bogousslavsky J, Caplan LR (eds): *Uncommon Causes of Stroke*. Cambridge: Cambridge University Press, 2001, pp 10–17.

12. Mokri B: Cervicocephalic arterial dissections. In Bogousslavsky J, Caplan LR (eds): *Uncommon Causes of Stroke*. Cambridge: Cambridge University Press, 2001, pp 211–229.

13. Imparato A, Riles T, Mintzer R, et al: The importance of hemorrhage in the relationship between gross morphologic characteristics and cerebral symptoms in 376 carotid artery plaques. *Ann Surg* 1983;**197**:195–203.

14. DeGeorgia M, Belden J, Pao L, et al: Thrombus in vertebrobasilar dolichoectatic artery treated with intravenous urokinase. *Cerebrovasc Dis* 1999;**9**:28–33.

15. Caplan LR, Manning W: Cardiac sources of embolism: The usual suspects. In Caplan LR, Manning WJ (eds): *Brain Embolism*. New York: Informa Healthcare, 2006, pp 129–159.

16. Caplan LR: Arterial sources of embolism. In Caplan LR, Manning WJ (eds): *Brain Embolism*. New York: Informa Healthcare, 2006, pp 203–222.

17. Gautier JC, Durr A, Koussa S, et al: Paradoxical cerebral embolism with a patent foramen ovale. A report of 29 patients. *Cerebrovasc Dis* 1991;**1**:193–202.

18. Caplan LR: Embolic particles. In Caplan LR, Manning WJ (eds): *Brain Embolism*. New York: Informa Healthcare, 2006, pp 259–275.

19. Caplan LR: Cardiac arrest and other hypoxic-ischemic insults. In Caplan LR, Hurst JW, Chimowitz M (eds): *Clinical Neurocardiology*. New York: Marcel Dekker, 1999, pp 1–34.

20. Mohr J: Neurological complications of cardiac valvular disease and cardiac surgery including systemic hypotension. In Vinken P, Bruyn G (eds): *Handbook of Clinical Neurology*, vol **38**. Amsterdam: North Holland, 1979, pp 143–171.

21. Romanul F, Abramowicz A: Changes in brain and pial vessels in arterial boundary zones. *Arch Neurol* 1964;**11**:40–65.

22. Fisher CM, Adams RD: Observations on brain embolism with special reference to hemorrhagic infarction. In Furlan A (ed): *The Heart and Stroke*. London: Springer-Verlag, 1987, pp 17–36.

23. Weir B: *Aneurysms Affecting the Nervous System*. Baltimore: Williams & Wilkins, 1987.

24. Chicoine MR, Dacey RG: Clinical aspects of subarachnoid hemorrhage. In Welch KMA, Caplan LR, Reis DJ, et al. (eds): *Primer on Cardiovascular Diseases*. San Diego: Academic Press, 1997, pp 425–432.

25. Kaufman HH (ed): *Intracerebral Hematomas*. New York: Raven Press, 1992.

26. Cole F, Yates P: Intracerebral microaneurysms and small cerebrovascular lesions. *Brain* 1967;**90**:759–768.

27. Rosenblum W: Miliary aneurysms and "fibrinoid" degeneration of cerebral blood vessels. *Hum Pathol* 1977;**8**:133–139.

28. Caplan LR: Intracerebral hemorrhage revisited. *Neurology* 1988;**38**:624–627.

29. Caplan LR: Hypertensive intracerebral hemorrhage. In Kase C, Caplan LR (eds): *Intracerebral Hemorrhage*. Boston: Butterworth–Heinemann, 1993, pp 99–116.

30. Finney L, Walker A: *Transtentorial Herniation*. Springfield, Ill: Thomas, 1962.

31. Fisher CM: Observations concerning brain herniation. *Ann Neurol* 1983;**14**:110.

32. Ropper AH: Lateral displacement of brain and level of consciousness in patients with acute hemispheral mass. *N Engl J Med* 1986;**314**:953–958.

33. Stephens R, Stilwell D: *Arteries and Veins of the Human Brain*. Springfield, IL: Charles C Thomas Publisher, 1969.

34. de Oliveira E, Tedeschi H, Rhoton Jr AL, Peace DA: Microsurgical anatomy of the internal carotid artery: Intrapetrous, intracavernous, and clinoidal segments. In Carter LP, Spetzler RF, Hamilton MG (eds): *Neurovascular Surgery*. New York: McGraw-Hill, 1995, pp 3–10.

35. Helgason C, Caplan LR, Goodwin J, Hedges T: Anterior choroidal artery – territory infarction. *Arch Neurol* 1986;**43**:681–686.

36. Tatu L, Moulin T, Bogousslavsky J, Duvernoy H: Arterial territories of the human brain: Cerebral hemispheres. *Neurology* 1998;**50**:1699–1708.

37. Lie T: Congenital malformations of the carotid and vertebral arterial systems, including the persistent anastomoses. In Vinken P, Bruyn G (eds): *Handbook of Clinical Neurology*, vol **12**. Amsterdam: North Holland, 1972, pp 289–339.

38. Caplan LR: *Posterior Circulation Disease: Clinical Findings, Diagnosis, and Management*. Boston: Blackwell, 1996.

39. Foix C, Hillemand P: Contributions a l'etude des ramolissements protuberentiels. *Rev Med* 1926;**43**:287–305.

40. Foix C, Hillemand P: Les Arteres de l'axe encephalique jusqu'a diencephale inclusivement. *Rev Neurol* 1925;**32**:705–739.

41. Caplan LR: Charles Foix – The first modern stroke neurologist. *Stroke* 1990;**21**:348–356.

42. Stopford J: The arteries of the pons and medulla oblongata. *J Anat Physiol* 1915,1916;**50**:131–164,255–280.

43. Gillilan L: Anatomy and embryology of the arterial system of the brainstem and cerebellum. In Vinken P, Bruyn G (eds): *Handbook of Clinical Neurology*, vol **11**. Amsterdam: North Holland, 1972, 24–44.

44. Duvernoy HM: *Human Brainstem Vessels*. Berlin: Springer-Verlag, 1978.

45. Capron L: Extra-and intracranial atherosclerosis. In Toole JF (ed): *Vascular Diseases*, Part 1, vol **53**, Bruyn G, Klawans HL (eds): *Handbook of Clinical Neurology*. Amsterdam: Elsevier Science, 1988, pp 91–106.

46. Stehbens WE: *Pathology of the Cerebral Blood Vessels*. St Louis: Mosby, 1972.

47. Taveras JM, Wood EH: *Diagnostic Neuroradiology*. Baltimore: Williams & Wilkins, 1964.

48. Moosy J: Morphology, sites, and epidemiology of cerebral

atherosclerosis in research publications. *Assoc Res Nerv Ment Dis* 1966;**51**:1–22.

49. Caplan LR: Cerebrovascular disease: Large artery occlusive disease. In Appel S (ed): *Current Neurology*, vol **8**. Chicago: Yearbook Medical, 1988, pp 179–226.

50. Gorelick PB, Caplan LR, Hier DB, et al: Racial differences in the distribution of anterior circulation occlusive cerebrovascular disease. *Neurology* 1984;**34**:54–59.

51. Caplan LR, Gorelick PB, Hier DB: Race, sex, and occlusive cerebrovascular disease: A review. *Stroke* 1986;**17**:648–655.

52. Caplan LR: Cerebral ischemia and infarction in blacks. Clinical, autopsy, and angiographic studies. In Gillum RF, Gorelick PB, Cooper ES (eds): *Stroke in Blacks*. Basel: Karger, 1999, pp 7–18.

53. Kieffer S, Takeya Y, Resch J, et al: Racial differences in cerebrovascular disease: Angiographic evaluation of Japanese and American populations. *AJR Am J Roentgenol* 1967;**101**:94–99.

54. Feldmann E, Daneault N, Kwan E, et al: Chinese–white differences in the distribution of occlusive cerebrovascular disease. *Neurology* 1990;**40**:1541–1545.

55. Mohr JP: Lacunes. *Stroke* 1982;**13**:3–11.

56. Caplan LR: Intracranial branch atheromatous disease. *Neurology* 1989;**39**:1246–1250.

57. Caplan LR, Zarins C, Hemmatti M: Spontaneous dissection of the extracranial vertebral artery. *Stroke* 1985;**16**:1030–1038.

58. O'Connell BF, Towfighi J, Brennan RW, et al: Dissecting aneurysms of head and neck. *Neurology* 1985;**35**:993–997.

59. Caplan LR, Baquis GD, Pessin MS, et al: Dissection of the intracranial vertebral artery. *Neurology* 1988;**38**:868–877.

60. Chaves C, Estol C, Esnaola M, et al: Spontaneous intracranial internal carotid artery dissection. *Arch Neurol* 2002;**59**:977–981.

61. Wilkinson I, Russell R: Arteries of the head and neck in giant cell arteritis. *Arch Neurol* 1972;**27**:378–391.

62. Caplan LR: Recipient artery: Anatomy and pathology. In Caplan LR, Manning WJ (eds): *Brain Embolism*. New York: Informa Healthcare, 2006, pp 31–59.

63. Gacs G, Merei FT, Bodosi M: Balloon catheter as a model of cerebral emboli in humans. *Stroke* 1982;**13**:39–42.

64. Vinters HV, Gilbert JJ: Cerebral amyloid angiopathy: Incidence and complications in the aging brain. II. The distribution of amyloid vascular changes. *Stroke* 1983;**14**:924–928.

65. Kase CS: Cerebral amyloid angiopathy. In Kase C, Caplan LR (eds): *Intracerebral Hemorrhage*. Boston: Butterworth–Heinemann, 1993, pp 179–200.

66. Bull J: Contribution of radiology to the study of intracranial aneurysms. *BMJ* 1922;**2**:1701–1708.

67. Alpers B: Aneurysms of the circle of Willis. In Fields WS (ed): *Intracranial Aneurysms and Subarachnoid Hemorrhage*. Springfield, IL: Charles C Thomas Publisher, 1965, pp. 5–24.

68. Ringelstein E, Zeumer H, Angelou D: The pathogenesis of strokes from internal carotid artery occlusion. *Stroke* 1983;**14**:867–875.

69. Ringelstein EB, Koschorke S, Holling A, et al: Computed tomographic pattern of proven embolic brain infarctions. *Ann Neurol* 1989;**26**:759–765.

70. Zulch K, Behrends R: The pathogenesis and topography of anoxia, hypoxia, and ischemia of the brain in man. In Meyer J, Gastant H (eds): *Cerebral Anoxia and the EEG*. Springfield, IL: Charles C Thomas Publisher, 1961, 144–163.

71. Caplan LR: Clinical features at different sites. In Kase C, Caplan LR (eds): *Intracerebral Hemorrhage*. Boston: Butterworth–Heinemann, 1993, pp 305–308.

72. Smith EE, Eichler F: Cerebral amyloid angiopathy and lobar intracerebral hemorrhage. *Arch Neurol* 2006;**63**:148–151.

73. Caplan LR: Drugs. In Kase C, Caplan LR (eds): *Intracerebral Hemorrhage*. Boston: Butterworth–Heinemann, 1993, pp 201–220.

74. Kase CS: Bleeding disorders. In Kase C, Caplan LR (eds): *Intracerebral Hemorrhage*. Boston: Butterworth–Heinemann, 1993, pp 117–152.

75. Kase C, Robinson K, Stein R, et al: Anticoagulant-related intracerebral hemorrhage. *Neurology* 1985;**35**:943–948.

76. Jafar JJ, Crowell RM: Focal ischemic thresholds. In Wood JH (ed): *Cerebral Blood Flow*. New York: McGraw-Hill, 1987, pp 449–457.

77. Toole JF: *Cerebrovascular Disorders*, 4th ed. New York: Raven Press, 1990.

78. Frackowiak R, Lenzi G, Jones T, et al: Quantitative measurements of regional cerebral blood flow and oxygen metabolism in man using 150 and positron emission tomography: Therapy, procedure, and normal values. *J Comput Assist Tomogr* 1980;**4**:722–736.

79. Baron J-C: Positron emission tomography. In Babikian VL, Wechsler LR, Higashida RT (eds): *Imaging Cerebrovascular Disease*. Philadelphia: Butterworth–Heinemann, 2003, pp 115–130.

80. Roy CS, Sherrington CS: On the regulation of the blood-supply of the brain. *J Physiol (London)* 1890;**11**:85–108.

81. Friedland RP, Iadecola C: Roy and Sherrington (1890): A centennial reexamination of "On the regulation of the blood-supply of the brain". *Neurology* 1991;**41**:10–14.

82. Symon L: Pathological regulation in cerebral ischemia. In Wood JH (ed): *Cerebral Blood Flow*. New York: McGraw-Hill, 1987, pp 413–424.

83. Tong DC, Albers GW: Normal values. In Babikian VL, Wechsler LR (eds): *Transcranial Doppler Ultrasonography*, 2nd ed. Boston: Butterworth–Heinemann, 1999, pp 33–46.

84. Kontos HA: Oxygen radicals in cerebral ischemia: The 2001 Willis Lecture. *Stroke* 2001;**32**:2712–2716.

85. Garcia JH, Anderson ML: Pathophysiology of cerebral ischemia. *Crit Rev Neurobiol* 1989;**4**:303–324.

86. Collins RC, Dobkin BH, Choi DW: Selective vulnerability of the brain: New insights into the pathophysiology of stroke. *Ann Intern Med* 1989;**110**:992–1000.

87. Choi DW: Excitotoxicity and stroke. In Caplan LR (ed): *Brain Ischemia: Basic Concepts and Clinical Relevance*. London: Springer, 1995, pp 29–36.

88. Garcia JH: Mechanisms of cell death in ischemia. In Caplan LR (ed): *Brain Ischemia: Basic Concepts and Clinical Relevance*. London: Springer, 1995, pp 7–18.

89. Mattson MP, Barger SW: Programmed cell life: Neuroprotective signal transduction and ischemic brain injury. In Caplan LR (ed): *Cerebrovascular Diseases, Nineteenth Princeton Stroke Conference, Moskowitz, MA*. Boston: Butterworth–Heinemann, 1995, pp 271–290.

90. Nurden AT, Duperat V-G, Nurden P: Platelet function and pharmacology of antiplatelet drugs. *Cerebrovasc Dis* 1997(suppl 6):2–9.

91. Moncada S, Higgs E, Vane J: Human arterial and venous tissues generate prostacyclin (prostaglandin 4) a potent inhibitor of platelet aggregation. *Lancet* 1977;**1**:18–20.

92. Schmid-Schonbein H, Perktold K: Physical factors in the pathogenesis of atheroma formation. In Caplan LR (ed): *Brain Ischemia: Basic Concepts and Clinical Relevance*. London: Springer, 1995, pp 185–213.

93. Caplan LR, Hennerici M: Impaired clearance of emboli (washout) is an important link between hypoperfusion, embolism, and ischemic stroke. *Arch Neurol* 1998;**55**:1475–1482.

94. Caplan LR, Wong KS, Gao S, Hennerici MG: Is hypoperfusion an important cause of strokes? If so, how? *Cerebrovasc Dis* 2006;**21**:145–153.

95. Masuda J, Yutani C, Ogata J, et al: Atheromatous embolism in the brain: A clinicopathologic analysis of 15 autopsy cases. *Neurology* 1994;**44**:1231–1237.

96. McKibbin DW, Bulkley BH, Green WR, et al: Fatal cerebral atheromatous embolization after cardiac bypass. *J Thorac Cardiovasc Surg* 1976;**71**:741–745.

97. Pollanen MS, Deck JHN: The mechanism of embolic watershed infarction: Experimental studies. *Can J Neurol Sci* 1990;**17**:395–398.

98. Fisher M, Francis R: Altered coagulation in cerebral ischemia. *Arch Neurol* 1990;**47**:1075–1079.

99. Tohgi H, Kawashima M, Tamura K, et al: Coagulation-fibrinolysis abnormalities in acute and chronic phases of cerebral thrombosis and embolism. *Stroke* 1990;**21**:1663–1667.

100. Feinberg WM: Coagulation. In Caplan LR (ed): *Brain Ischemia: Basic Concepts and Clinical Relevance*. London: Springer, 1995, pp 85–96.

101. Deykin D: Thrombogenesis. *N Engl J Med* 1967;**276**:622–628.

102. del Zoppo GJ: Vascular hemostasis and brain embolism. In Caplan LR, Manning WJ (eds): *Brain Embolism*. New York: Informa Healthcare, 2006, pp 243–258.

103. Svensson PJ, Dahlback B: Resistance to activated protein C as a basis for

venous thrombosis. *N Engl J Med* 1994;**330**:517–522.

104. Bertina RM, Koelman BPC, Rosendall FR, et al: Mutation in the blood coagulation factor V associated with resistance to activated protein C. *Nature* 1994;**369**:64–67.

105. Poort SR, Rosendaal FR, Reitsma PH, Bertina RM: A common genetic variation in the 3' untranslated region of the prothrombin gene is associated with elevated plasma prothrombin levels and an increase in venous thrombosis. *Blood* 1996;**88**:3698–3703.

106. Martinelli I, Sacchi E, Landi G, et al: High risk of cerebral vein thrombosis in carriers of a prothrombin-gene mutation and in users of oral contraceptives. *N Engl J Med* 1998;**338**:1793–1797.

107. Sloan M: Thrombolysis and stroke. *Arch Neurol* 1987;**44**:748–768.

108. Raichle M: The pathophysiology of brain ischemia. *Ann Neurol* 1983;**13**:2–10.

109. Astrup J, Siesjo B, Simon L: Thresholds in cerebral ischemia: The ischemic penumbra. *Stroke* 1981;**12**:723–725.

110. Thomas D, du Boulay G, Marshall J, et al: Effect of hematocrit on cerebral blood flow in man. *Lancet* 1977;**2**:941–943.

111. Thomas D, Marshall J, Russell RW, et al: Cerebral blood flow in polycythemia. *Lancet* 1977;**2**:161–163.

112. Tohgi H, Yasmanouchi H, Murakami M, et al: Importance of the hematocrit as a risk factor in cerebral infarction. *Stroke* 1978;**9**:369–374.

113. Caplan LR, Sergay S: Positional cerebral ischemia. *J Neurol Neurosurg Psychiatry* 1976;**39**:385–391.

114. Toole J: Effects of change of head, limb, and body position on cephalic circulation. *N Engl J Med* 1968;**279**:307–311.

115. Kim HY, Singhal AB, Lo EH: Normobaric hyperoxia extends the reperfusion window in focal cerebral ischemia. *Ann Neurol* 2005;**57**:571–575.

116. Ginsberg M, Welsh F, Budd W: Deleterious effect of glucose pretreatment on recovery from diffuse cerebral ischemia in the cat. *Stroke* 1980;**11**:347–354.

117. Plum F: What causes infarction in ischemic brain? *Neurology* 1983;**33**:222–233.

118. Siesjo BK, Kristian T, Katsura K: The role of calcium in delayed postischemic brain damage. In Caplan LR (ed): *Cerebrovascular Diseases, the Nineteenth Princeton Stroke Conference, Moskowitz MA*. Boston: Butterworth–Heinemann, 1995, pp 353–370.

119. Gorelick PB, Caplan LR: Calcium, hypercalcemia and stroke. *Curr Concepts Cerebrovasc Dis (Stroke)* 1985;**20**:13–17.

120. Hillbom M, Kaste M: Ethanol intoxication: A risk factor for ischemic brain infarction in adolescents and young adults. *Stroke* 1981;**12**:422–425.

121. Ames III A, Wright RL, Kouada M, et al: Cerebral ischemia. II. The no-reflow phenomenon. *Am J Pathol* 1968;**52**:437–453.

122. O'Brien MD: Ischemic cerebral edema. In Caplan LR (ed): *Brain Ischemia: Basic Concepts and Clinical Relevance*. London: Springer, 1995, pp 43–50.

123. Ropper AH: Brain edema after stroke, clinical syndrome and intracranial pressure. *Arch Neurol* 1984;**41**:26–29.

124. Ropper AH: A preliminary MRI study of the geometry of brain displacement and level of consciousness with acute intracranial masses. *Neurology* 1989;**39**:622–627.

125. Barnett H: Delayed cerebral ischemic episodes distal to occlusion of major cerebral arteries. *Neurology* 1978;**28**:769–774.

126. Fisher CM: Occlusion of the internal carotid artery. *Arch Neurol Psychiatry* 1951;**65**:346–377.

127. Caplan LR: Occlusion of the vertebral or basilar artery. *Stroke* 1979;**10**:277–282.

128. Glass TA, Hennessey PM, Pazdera L, et al: Outcome at 30 days in the New England Medical Center Posterior Circulation Registry. *Arch Neurol* 2002;**59**(3):369–376.

129. Caplan LR, Wityk RJ, Glass TA, et al: New England Medical Center Posterior Circulation Registry. *Ann Neurol* 2004;**56**:389–398.

130. Savitz SI, Caplan LR: Current concepts: Vertebrobasilar disease. *N Engl J Med* 2005;**352**:2618–2626.

131. Jones H, Millikan C, Sandok B: Temporal profile of acute vertebrobasilar system infarction. *Stroke* 1980;**11**:173–177.

132. Fisher CM: Pathological observations in hypertensive cerebral hemorrhage. *J Neuropathol Exp Neurol* 1971;**30**:536–550.

133. Herbstein D, Schaumberg H: Hypertensive intracerebral hematoma: An investigation of the initial hemorrhage and rebleeding using Cr 51 labeled erythrocytes. *Arch Neurol* 1974;**30**:412–414.

134. Duret H: *Traumatismes Cranio-Cerebaux*. Paris: Librarie Felix Alcan, 1919.

135. Fisher CM, Kistler JP, Davis JM: Relation of cerebral vasospasm to subarachnoid hemorrhage visualized by computerized tomographic scanning. *Neurosurgery* 1980;**6**:1–9.

136. MacDonald RL: Cerebral vasospasm. In Welch KMA, Reis DJ, Caplan LR, et al. (eds): *Primer on Cerebrovascular Diseases*. San Diego: Academic Press, 1997, pp 490–497.

137. Hijdra A, van Gijn J, Nagelkerke NJD, et al: Prediction of delayed cerebral ischemia, rebleeding, and outcome after aneurysmal subarachnoid hemorrhage. *Stroke* 1988;**19**:1250–1256.

138. Aygun N, Perl II J: Subarachnoid hemorrhage. In Babikian VL, Wechsler LR, Higashida RT (eds): *Imaging Cerebrovascular Disease*. Philadelphia: Butterworth–Heinemann, 2003, pp 241–269.

Chapter 3

Diagnosis and the clinical encounter

Louis R Caplan and Fernando Barinagarrementeria

A 36-year-old man, JH, became confused at work. His wife was called and she came to the workplace and brought him to the hospital. On arrival about 4 hours after symptom onset, it is obvious that his left limbs are weak. He is very sleepy and at times barely arousable. The nurse in the emergency ward at the hospital calls you, his physician, and relates that your patient is having a stroke.

Information used for stroke diagnosis

The preceding brief patient vignette describes a seriously ill man, presumably an acute stroke patient. The clinician's first task is to decide what is the matter with him. This chapter follows the process of diagnosis by a stepwise consideration of the facts in his case. Before proceeding with the specific case example, however, we will review the general process of stroke diagnosis. Clinical diagnosis is often difficult, but the process becomes easier and more logical if approached systematically. We routinely follow several steps and rules and urge each individual clinician to become familiar with the diagnostic methods that he or she uses. Routines and thoroughness prevent errors made by snap guesses or impulsive diagnoses. We have elaborated elsewhere in much more detail on the subject of clinical neurological diagnosis[1,2] and only summarize briefly the main points here.

First, the clinician must decide on the key questions to be asked. Answers are difficult unless the questions are clearly framed. The most general questions should be asked first, followed by more specific queries. In neurology, two diagnostic questions always require an answer: (1) *What* is the disease mechanism – the pathology and pathophysiology? And (2) *Where* is the lesion(s) – the anatomy of the disorder? In regard to the stroke patient, the "what" question concerns which of the five stroke mechanisms (hemorrhage – subarachnoid or intracerebral; ischemia – thrombotic, embolic, or decreased global perfusion) is present. Of course, before distinguishing among stroke mechanisms, clinicians should first ask whether the findings could be caused by a non-vascular process, such as a brain tumor, metabolic abnormality, infection, intoxication, seizure disorder, or traumatic injury that mimics stroke. The *where* question concerns the anatomical location of the condition, both in the brain and in the vascular system that supplies and drains the brain.

Different data are used to answer these two quite different questions. In determining stroke mechanism – the *What* question – the following clinical bedside data are most helpful:

1. Ecology – the past and present personal and family illnesses.
2. Presence and nature of past strokes or transient ischemic attacks (TIAs).
3. Activity at the onset of the stroke, such as physical effort.
4. Temporal course and progression of the findings. (Was the stroke onset sudden with the deficit maximal at onset? Did the deficit improve, worsen, or remain the same after onset? If it worsened, did this occur in a stepwise, remitting or gradually progressive fashion? Were there fluctuations between normal and abnormal?)
5. Accompanying symptoms such as headache, vomiting, seizures, and decreased level of consciousness.

Information about these items can all be gleaned from a thorough and thoughtful history from the patient, a review of physicians' and medical records, and data collected from observers, family members, and friends. These data are primarily historical and require little sophisticated knowledge of neurology. The general physical examination, which uncovers disorders not known from the history, adds to the data used for diagnosing the stroke mechanism. Elevated blood pressure, cardiac enlargement, murmurs or arrythmia, and vascular bruits are examples of physical findings that influence identification of the stroke mechanism.

Diagnosis of stroke location – the *Where* question – is made using very different information:

1. Analysis of the neurological symptoms and their distribution.
2. Findings on neurological examination.
3. Findings from brain and vascular imaging.

The history and knowledge of general systemic diseases tells the clinician *what* is wrong; the neurological examination tells more *where* the disease process is located.

Mechanism and anatomical diagnoses are not absolute. More realistic are estimates of probabilities. In one patient, intracerebral hemorrhage (ICH) may be by far the most likely diagnosis, but embolism and thrombosis are also possible and should not be eliminated from consideration. In another patient, there might be an apparent toss-up between thrombosis and embolism.

The process of diagnosis involves two basic techniques: (1) hypothesis generation and testing; and (2) pattern matching.

The inductive method – sequential hypothesis generation and testing

Hypothesis generation should begin as soon as the first information about the patient becomes available. This may come from a call to the doctor, for example by an emergency room nurse – as in the vignette at the beginning of the chapter, or when the patient is first seen. As the patient or another individual, relates the history, the clinician should be thinking of possible diagnoses. It is best to first let the patient (or other historian) give an overview of the events while the doctor listens without interrupting. The information conveyed should generate hypotheses and queries. Ask the patient and available others questions whose answers should help confirm or refute the hypotheses about the two questions that should be answered, "What" and "Where." For example, an elderly patient with known coronary and peripheral limb atherosclerosis has a left hemiparesis noted on awakening. In such a case, considering the patient's risk factors and time of onset, we would first think of thrombosis because that would be a common stroke mechanism. We would then ask whether there had been prior transient episodes of left limb symptoms. Their presence would strongly favor thrombosis.

Anatomical hypotheses are also generated. A left hemiparesis raises the possibility of a right cerebral or brainstem lesion, so we ask about accompanying visual, sensory, or brain stem symptoms that would help generate a more specific anatomical localization. The process of anatomical diagnosis is much like locating a missing person. First, the clinician must determine whether the person is in the United States before limiting the whereabouts to Massachusetts, then the Boston vicinity, then to a specific street in the Brookline neighborhood. Similarly, regarding the diagnosis of mechanism, the physician must decide on ischemia versus hemorrhage before hypothesizing about subtypes of those mechanisms. The physician must identify thrombosis versus embolism versus global hypoperfusion before distinguishing subtypes of thrombosis, such as lacunar (small penetrating artery disease) or large artery, anterior or posterior circulation. Thus, the clinician proceeds systematically from the more general to the more specific. Clearly, the amount of available data may limit reasonable hypotheses to the most general inferences. In some patients, few historical data are available. In patient JH it would have been particularly helpful to know if he had had right monocular visual symptoms which would localize the vascular lesion to the right internal carotid artery. On admission he was too drowsy to reliably obtain that information.

Pattern matching

The other technique used by most clinicians is pattern matching. For example, we recognize the person we call "Jim" by comparing the individual in front of us with a mental image of Jim that we conjure up in our minds' eye. We do not ordinarily list individual features (e.g., height, glasses, hair style). Similarly, clinicians try to identify a constellation of findings that match their mental images of patterns of stroke mechanisms and pathology and anatomy. For example, the diagnosis of Parkinsonism may become readily obvious to you even as you walk with a new patient into your office because of the resemblance of the patient's facial expression, posture, gait, and tremor to other Parkinsonian patients that have been seen in the past.

Although the diagnostic thinking analysis should be pursued sequentially, accumulating information that would answer the *What* and *Where* questions should proceed concurrently. While obtaining the patient's history, have the patient describe information that will allow prediction of the probability of various stroke mechanisms and locations. At the end of the history, be prepared to list these and to assign rough probability estimates. Next, think about and plan the examination. In this patient, what additional findings are important and help to confirm or refute the preliminary diagnoses? What data will allow more specificity? In the patient with left hemiparesis, the presence of a left visual field deficit or left visual neglect would localize the lesion to the right cerebral hemisphere. Nystagmus or a gaze palsy to the right or an internuclear ophthalmoplegia would favor a brainstem site in the pons or midbrain. A right carotid bruit or a cholesterol crystal found on examining the retina of the right eye would favor a right carotid artery site. After the general and neurological examinations, re-examine the original hypotheses and their probabilities. New or unexpected findings from the examinations might stimulate new hypotheses or might confirm or refute prior hypotheses. A blood pressure of 260/140 mmHg would clearly increase the likelihood of hemorrhage. The absence of a pulse or presence of papilledema on examination would change prior estimated probabilities. The presence of a cardiac murmur and fever suggests a systemic condition such as infectious endocarditis.

Next, proceed to ask what imaging laboratory testing might help refine the hypotheses generated at the end of the history and the examinations. Also, initial test results help determine the need for other tests. Laboratory tests should also be planned, reviewed, and ordered sequentially (this topic is elaborated in Chapter 4). Overall, the process of diagnosis should be logical, systematic, and sequential.

Procedure for diagnosis of stroke mechanism and brain localization

Mimicking a computer

Computers have taught clinicians to be more aware of the process and mechanics of diagnosis. In an individual patient, how would a computer estimate the most likely stroke mechanism diagnosis? Physicians can emulate the logic and methodology of the computer process for a more systematic diagnostic strategy. One technique of computer diagnosis is the use of Bayes' theorem.[3,4] Information needed for this methodology are knowledge of: (1) the incidence of each illness (in this case,

stroke mechanism) in the population studied; and (2) the incidence of a given finding in each illness (stroke mechanism). Armed with this information and the findings in the individual patient, the computer calculates the probability of a given stroke mechanism in that patient. The use of probabilities mimics the way clinicians usually approach a diagnostic problem. Seldom is a single diagnosis absolutely certain (100%). More often, a given diagnosis (e.g., brain embolism) is considered most likely (perhaps 70% probable); but thrombotic occlusion also should be considered (perhaps 20%); and ICH, although unlikely (10%), still enters into the differential diagnosis.

Knowing the frequencies of the various stroke mechanisms provides what is often called a priori odds. Data from large stroke studies and registries[5–23] yields much information about the relative frequencies of various stroke subtypes. Table 3.1 shows data from some of these analyses that show that approximately 80% of all strokes are ischemic and 20% are hemorrhagic. Therefore, if no other specific information were available about a stroke patient, the diagnosis of ischemic stroke would be correct 4 out of 5 times, but subarachnoid hemorrhage (SAH) would be correct for only about 1 patient in 10. The remainder of the computer prediction uses individual factors (e.g., headache preceding stroke, presence of TIAs, activity at onset, prior evidence of atherosclerosis etc) to predict the likely stroke mechanism. For example, Table 3.2 shows the relative frequency of headache during the days or weeks preceding stroke.[7] Relatively few patients had headaches preceding stroke, but the finding was slightly more common in patients with thrombotic stroke and ICH and less common in patients with either SAH or brain embolism. In this example, the difference in frequency is small. Some causes of stroke that present after preceding headache such as arterial dissections and cerebral venous thrombosis were not tabulated in the Harvard Stroke Registry. In contrast, headache at or near the onset of stroke (Table 3.3) invariably occurred in patients with SAH, but was less often present in patients with other mechanisms of stroke.

These data can also be presented in graphic form; Figure 3.1 from a study of patients seen on the stroke service at the Michael Reese Hospital and the University of Illinois,[24] shows the frequency-by-stroke subtype of headache preceding stroke (often called sentinel headache) and headache at onset. The computer and the alert physician sum the individual data items, factor in the a priori odds, and arrive at a total probability for a given stroke mechanism in each stroke patient. During the discussion of individual topics in the remainder of this chapter, we include important data results selected from stroke-registry experience.

Ecology

Included within ecology are prior medical diseases and demographic data that might predispose the patient to have one or more of the various stroke mechanisms. When called to see a patient with stroke, the physician usually has available some background information from the family, another physician, or the clinician's own experience with the patient. For example, a call from the hospital emergency room might describe a "65-year-old man with angina pectoris, two prior heart attacks, diabetes, and hypertension who arrived here today with ..." This information leads the physician to consider the probability of particular stroke mechanisms in the patient who is about to be seen. In this example, the presence of diabetes and coronary artery disease strongly favors a diagnosis of associated atherosclerosis of the extracranial cervical arteries and a thrombotic (or artery-to-artery embolus) mechanism of stroke. The presence of prior heart disease raises the possibility of arrhythmia, mural thrombosis, ventricular aneurysm, and valvular heart disease – all potential sources of brain embolism. The presence of hypertension increases the probability of ICH, especially if the hypertension is severe, a determination that can be made quickly when the patient is seen. An alert physician would also be sure to inquire whether the patient was being treated with anticoagulants for his cardiac disease, a factor that would greatly increase the chance of ICH. Neck and/or face pain in young physically active individuals raises the possibility of arterial dissection. A stroke that develops rapidly in a young person while defecating or during sex raises the possibility of a patent foramen ovale or other cardiac shunt causing a brain embolus.

The clinician uses the presence of individual risk factors to alter the likelihood that an individual patient has a particular stroke mechanism. Perhaps another example will help clarify this statement – on average, 60% of strokes are considered thrombotic, 20% are embolic, 12% are ICH, and 8% are due to SAH. The presence of severe hypertension (e.g., 220/130 mmHg) would certainly make hemorrhage, especially ICH, much more likely. This factor would significantly shift the odds toward ICH and slightly to SAH. If another factor, such as age, is then added (e.g., if the severely hypertensive patient were a 23-year-old woman, this would make the major alternative diagnosis, thrombotic stroke, much less likely and would further increase the likelihood of a hemorrhagic mechanism. This shift of probabilities can be described as "loading on" or "detracting from" a specific diagnosis: For example, severe hypertension loads heavily on ICH (+ + + +); youthfulness detracts from thrombosis. Data from prior experience, such as those found in registries, can help determine quantitatively the relative shift of odds.

Table 3.4 lists the frequencies of diabetes, hypertension, and coronary artery disease in the various subtypes of stroke in the Harvard Stroke Registry (HSR)[7] and the frequencies of other similar variables in the Michael Reese Stroke Registry (MRSR).[10] Note that hypertension was more common in all groups in the MRSR and atherosclerosis more prominent in the HSR. The populations in these two registries were quite different: the HSR included a predominantly white, middle- and upper-class population with a high incidence of atherosclerosis, whereas the MRSR had more young, black, hypertensive individuals with a lower prevalence of atherosclerosis. Black, Chinese, and Japanese populations have a higher incidence of ICH and intracranial occlusive disease than white populations.[25–34] Table 3.5 lists estimated loading

Table 3.1 Frequency and types of stroke in various studies

Study	Year	N	T	LA	Lac	ICU	Emb	ICH	SAH	Isc Total	Hem Total
Aring and Merritt[5]	1935	407	81	–	–	–	3	–	–	84	15
Whisnant et al.[8]	1971	548	75	–	–	–	3	10	5	78	15
Matsumoto et al.[9]	1973	993	71	–	–	–	8	10	6	79	16
Harvard Stroke Registry[7]	1978	694	53	34	19	–	31	10	6	84	16
Michael Reese Stroke Registry[10]	1983	472	31	18	13	30	17	14	8	78	22
Austin Hospital[11]	1983	700	68	45	23	18	8	6	Excl	94	6
South Alabama[17]	1984	160	19	6	13	40	26	8	6	85	14
Lausanne Stroke Registry[13]	1988	1000	56	43	13	8	20	11	Excl	89	11
Stroke Data Bank[12]	1988	1805	25	6	19	32	14	13	13	71	26
Lehigh Valley Stroke Registry[21]	1989	2639	60	–	9	–	20	9	Excl	91	9
Oxfordshire Community Stroke Project[19]	1990	675	–	–	–	–	–	10	5	81	15
Taiwan Stroke Registry[22]	1997	676	46	17	29	20	29	Excl	Excl	100	Excl
Community Hospital Stroke Program[23]	1990	4129	32	–	–	–	11	5	2	60	10

Emb, embolism; Excl, excluded from study; Hem, hemorrhage; ICH, intracerebral hemorrhage; ICU, infarct cause unknown; Isc, ischemia; LA, large artery; Lac, lacune; SAH, subarachnoid hemorrhage; T, thrombosis (sum of large artery and lacune).

Table 3.2 Headache preceding stroke (from the Harvard Stroke Registry[7])

	Thrombosis	Embolism	ICH	SAH
Yes	27 (8.2%)	8 (4%)	6 (8%)	1 (3%)
No	291 (89%)	177 (87%)	61 (77%)	27 (87%)
No information	9 (2%)	18 (9%)	12 (15%)	3 (10%
Totals	**327**	**203**	**79**	**31**

ICH, intracerebral hemorrhage; SAH, subarachnoid hemorrhage.

Table 3.3 Headache at onset of stroke

Registry	Thrombosis (%)	Lacune (%)	Embolism (%)	SAH (%)	ICH (%)	ICU (%)
HSR	12	3	9	78	33	–
MRSR	29	16	17	98	80	13

HSR, Harvard Stroke Registry; ICU, infarct cause unknown; ICH, intracerebral hemorrhage; MRSR, Michael Reese Stroke Registry; SAH, subarachnoid hemorrhage.

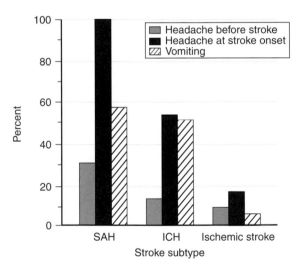

Figure 3.1 Graph showing frequency of headache patterns and vomiting in patients with ischemic strokes and hemorrhages in the Michael Reese and University of Illinois stroke registries. From Gorelick PB, Hier DB, Caplan LR, et al. Headache in acute cerebrovascular disease. *Neurology* 1986;36:1445–1450 with permission.

weights that could be assigned to various risk factors. At times, the effect of a condition is indirect; for example, the presence of diabetes increases the chance of myocardial infarction, which in turn increases the likelihood of a cardiac-origin embolism.

We now return to the patient JH discussed at the beginning of this chapter. We continue to discuss his case and its analysis during the remainder of the discussion of clinical diagnosis.

After the call from the emergency room, before leaving for the hospital, the doctor asked her secretary to pull JH's office chart. He had last been seen 1 year ago, at age 35 years, because of bronchitis. Notes indicate that he smoked three packs of cigarettes a day, had always had normal blood pressures, and had no history of cardiac or neurological symptoms. He had described, however, a high incidence of heart attacks in his family. He had been overweight, and his blood cholesterol level last year was 295. He was advised to pursue a weight-reduction program, to reduce his intake of fats and cholesterol-containing foods, to stop smoking, and to return for a recheck. He had not returned.

When leaving for the hospital, think about the information known, based on the emergency room nurse's call and on JH's records. The illness was said to have begun rather suddenly, and the brain lesion must be focal because he has an obvious left limb paralysis. Abrupt-onset focal brain lesions are most often strokes, but his youth serves as a reminder to be certain to consider focal brain lesions other than stroke. Brain tumors, abscesses, trauma, and encephalitis can cause focal findings, and without other information, it is not yet clear how abruptly the symptoms began and progressed. Subacute and chronic subdural hematomas can present with focal signs appearing "acutely." If the process is a stroke, as would be statistically most likely, review the background information regarding risks for the different stroke mechanisms. His past smoking, family history of cardiac disease, and high blood cholesterol level suggest to you the possibility of premature atherosclerosis, with large artery occlusive disease as the mechanism of the stroke. An unusual type of cardiac disease with brain embolism is another mechanism that is suggested by the family history of cardiac disease. ICH could also cause left-sided paralysis and sleepiness, but the absence of past hypertension makes this less likely, unless he had recently developed hypertension. Make a mental note to quickly check his blood pressure and seek signs of organ damage due to hypertension on examination. The first hypothesis regarding preliminary stroke mechanism is large artery atherosclerosis with embolism; cardiac-origin embolism and ICH are also to be seriously considered. Systemic hypoperfusion and SAH seldom cause severe hemiplegia at outset.

Table 3.4 Incidence of various risk factors in each type of stroke

	Thrombosis (%)	Lacune (%)	Embolus (%)	ICH (%)	SAH (%)
HSR					
Atherosclerosis*	56	37	34	11	5
Diabetes	26	28	13	15	2
Past hypertension	55	75	40	72	19
MRSR					
Angina pectoris	13	8	20	5	0
Past MI	23	16	40	12	0
Recent MI	7	12	12	3	0
Past hypertension	75	55	55	68	44

HSR, Harvard Stroke Registry; ICH, intracerebral hemorrhage; MI, myocardial infarction; MRSR, Michael Reese Stroke Registry; SAH, subarachnoid hemorrhage.
* Includes peripheral vascular disease, coronary artery disease, neck bruit.

Table 3.5 Weighting of ecological factors

	Thrombosis	Lacune	Embolus	ICH	SAH
Hypertension	++	+++		++	+
Hypertension +++		+		++++	++
Coronary disease	+++		++		
Claudication	+++		+		
Atrial fibrillation			++++		
Sick sinus syndrome			++		
Valvular heart disease			+++		
Diabetes	+++	+	+		
Bleeding diathesis				++++	+
Smoking	+++		+		+
Cancer	++		++		
Old age	+++	+	+	+	
Black or Asian origin	+	+		++	

ICH, intracerebral hemorrhage; SAH, subarachnoid hemorrhage.
Hypertension +++ = severe hypertension.

So far, little detail about neurological symptoms are available that could help localize the lesion. The patient is said to have a left-sided paralysis, and so the right cerebral hemisphere and right pons are the most likely sites of pathology. The report of confusion at work favors a cerebral hemispheric lesion. Plan to ask questions that will promote more precise localization.

Having used the ecological data to shift the usual stroke mechanism probabilities, carry these probabilities into an investigation of the next data items, such as prior cerebrovascular symptoms, course of illness, accompanying symptoms, and so on-each of which then further modifies the probabilities.

When you arrive at the emergency room, the nurse says that JH's pulse and blood pressure are normal. The patient is awake but cannot give any account of his illness. He seems unaware that his left limbs are paralyzed. The coworker who was with him when he became ill says that he suddenly seemed dazed and quickly became hemiplegic, falling to the ground. His wife says that he did not follow previous dietary advice and was still smoking heavily. She said he had not been ill, but a week before he told her that for 10 minutes one morning, his left arm and face had temporarily felt numb, symptoms he attributed to a draft from an air conditioner in the office.

Prior cerebrovascular symptoms especially TIAs

Although not especially common, prior cerebrovascular events so heavily load probabilities that they should be given considerable importance. Recent TIAs in the same vascular territory are frequent precursors of thrombotic stroke, so their presence, especially when multiple, is virtually diagnostic of that stroke mechanism. If a patient presenting to the hospital with aphasia and right limb weakness had had an attack of transient right-handed weakness three weeks earlier and an attack of right face and right hand numbness and weakness one week earlier, the clinician could be relatively certain that the stroke was a result of thrombotic occlusive disease within the left anterior circulation. If, in addition, that same individual had also had a black shade descending over the left eye, causing temporary blindness, the location could be further refined, and it would seem certain that the occlusive lesion involved the internal carotid artery before its ophthalmic artery branch. The presence, nature, and duration of TIAs are important. Information about the presence of TIAs must be vigorously and repeatedly sought.

Many patients are quite naive about the functions of the body, especially the nervous system. Some stroke patients attribute their weakness, lack of feeling, and visual deficits to the local limbs or to the eyes; they often do not understand that the central nervous system (CNS) control of these functions has been damaged. They often wonder why the head is being studied and imaged rather than the arm or leg, where surely the trouble resides. Patients usually do not volunteer information they think is unrelated to their present trouble. A woman with visual difficulty will not tell her eye doctor about a vaginal discharge, considering the latter problem in the province of her gynecologist. Similarly, a patient with hand weakness might not tell the physician about prior leg weakness, not realizing that the conditions are related. The same individual will surely not tell the doctor about temporary visual dysfunction, considering the eye problem to belong to the ophthalmologist. Patients often attribute their temporary symptoms to banal causes in the environment (e.g., an air conditioner draft, as in the case of JH). Symptoms of TIA must be elicited specifically: "Have you ever had temporary weakness of your right hand, your right leg, your face? Have you had difficulty speaking, seeing, and so forth?" On entry to the hospital, or during the early physician encounters, patients are often not at their optimum performance levels. They may be sick, frightened, tired, or worried and therefore suboptimal observers and witnesses. Many patients have told me on the third or even sixth day of stroke about prior TIAs, having denied their presence when queried on admission.

Physicians should acquire as much detail as possible about the TIAs. Some features of TIAs are helpful in diagnosing a subtype of brain ischemia, as will be discussed below. When there were multiple attacks, when was the first and when was the last? Are they getting more frequent or is the interval between attacks becoming longer? Are the episodes stereotyped and nearly identical in all attacks? How long do the TIAs last? What is the shortest, longest, and average duration? Are attacks becoming longer or shorter?

Are TIAs provoked by standing or activity? Are they positional? Neck positioning can occasionally temporarily occlude stenotic vertebral arteries producing symptoms of brainstem or cerebellar dysfunction.

Some patients cannot provide information about a TIA because of aphasia, altered level of consciousness, amnesia, and so on. Some patients with right hemisphere dysfunction do not realize when things go wrong. Other observers, such as family, hospital visitors, and friends, should be queried because the patient may have told them about prior symptoms, or these individuals may have observed altered function in the patient. Caution must be exercised in exploring symptoms at the patient's work site, because knowledge about a patient's neurological problem might adversely affect job status. Clearly, permission should be sought before approaching employers or coworkers for health information. In this case, the coworker and wife were present and could provide useful data when the patient could not.

Many studies in varied populations have shown that TIAs carry a very substantial risk of imminent brain infarction and should be handled emergently.[35–41] Johnston and colleagues analyzed outcomes among 1707 patients with TIAs that presented to emergency departments in 16 hospitals in the San Francisco Bay area in California.[35] During the 90 days after emergency-room presentation, 180 patients (10.5%) returned with a stroke, occurring in half the patients within the first 2 days.[35] Kleindorfer et al. performed a population-based study of TIAs occurring in the Cincinnati–northern Kentucky region during one year.[37] During the year 1023 TIA events occurred among 927 patients. Within 6 months of the index TIA, 144 patients had an ischemic stroke and 77 died. The median time for stroke to develop was 12 days.[37] Rothwell and Warlow used a different approach.[39] They retrospectively reviewed data from 2146 stroke admissions in the UK. A preceding TIA was present in 23%; 17% of TIAs occurred on the day of the stroke, 9% on the preceding day, and 43% during the preceding week.[39]

Prognostic scores have been developed in order to identify patients who have a high risk of developing a stroke soon after one or more TIAs. The tabulations used in the most common score (the ABCD2 score)[42,43] are shown in Table 3.6. This score has prognostic features but in our opinion should never be used to exclude from admission or further investigations those patients whose scores are low. Every patient with a TIA requires urgent clinical and laboratory evaluations including brain and vascular imaging and blood tests.

The designation TIA should mean what it says. *Transient* implies temporary, although not stating how temporary – at least not permanent; *ischemic* identifies the cause – lack of blood flow; and "attack" implies a suddenness and limited time duration of a discrete event, although again not stating the duration of the attack or the rapidity of onset. The two key words are "ischemic" conveying an etiology, and "transient" meaning not permanent, not causing irreversible cell death, infarction. The old definition created by the Committee on Cerebrovascular Disease in 1975 " transient ischemic attack is defined as a cerebral dysfunction of ischemic nature lasting no

Table 3.6 The ABCD2 score

Risk factor	Points
Age ≥60 years	1 point
Systolic **B**lood pressure ≥140 mmHg or diastolic ≥90 mmHg	1 point
Clinical manifestation Unilateral weakness with or without speech impairment OR Speech impairment without unilateral weakness	2 points 1 point
Duration TIA duration ≥60 min TIA duration 10–59 min	2 points 1 point
Diabetes	1 point
Total ABCD2 Score	0–7 points
ABCD2 Score	2-day stroke risk Score of 0–3 gives a 1% stroke risk

Table 3.7 Transient ischemic attacks (TIAs) in patients with severe carotid artery occlusive disease (from the Harvard Stroke Registry[7])

Time	First TIA N = 59	Last TIA N = 56*
<1 day	2	16
1 day–1 week	9	25
1 week–1 month	14	7
>1 month	34	8

* In three patients the timing of the last TIA was unknown.

longer than 24 hours with a tendency to recur"[44] is outdated and should no longer be used. The 24-hour duration was arbitrarily chosen without data. Studies have shown that, in fact, most TIAs last only a few minutes and the great majority last less than an hour. Those lasting longer than an hour are often associated with brain infarction on modern brain imaging that includes magnetic resonance imaging (MRI) with diffusion-weighted images (DWIs).[45] The new definition which we strongly favor is "a TIA is a brief episode of neurological dysfunction caused by focal brain or retinal ischemia, with clinical symptoms typically lasting less than an hour, and without evidence of acute infarction."[45] The neurological deficit should not be related to convulsive activity.

Although the term TIA designates ischemia, it does not differentiate between an embolic and a thrombotic mechanism, or between a small artery and a large artery site. Brain embolism can produce a transient disorder that would qualify as a TIA. Some evidence supports the notion that embolism is more likely to produce less frequent but longer attacks, whereas low flow states produce briefer but more frequent attacks. The term embolism denotes that material (usually thrombus) originates in one site and then travels to a distant site. The main components are the donor source where the material originates, the material (thrombus, calcium, bacteria, fat, air, etc.), and the recipient site where the embolus comes to rest. The donor source of the embolus varies and includes the heart, aorta, proximal cervico-cranial arteries, and systemic veins in the case of paradoxical embolism. Embolism is not synonymous with cardiac-source cardioembolism. Shotgun-like repeated episodes of ischemia in the same vascular territory virtually always indicate a critical degree of vessel narrowing with hemodynamic failure. Single but longer attacks are more often associated with an ulcerated plaque or another embolic source (artery-to-artery embolism). Bilateral and non-simultaneous TIAs and brain infarcts are highly suggestive of a cardiac or aortic donor source of emboli.

In patients with penetrating artery disease (lacunar infarction), TIAs occur but are less common. In the HSR, TIAs occurred in 23% of patients with lacunar disease, compared with 50% of patients with large artery arteriosclerosis.[7] When present, TIAs in patients with lacunar disease are more likely to be stereotyped (e.g., weakness of face, arm, and leg in each attack) and are usually limited to a period of days. In 1993 Donnan et al. coined the term "warning capsular syndrome" when they described recurrent crescendo TIAs affecting face, arm, and leg due to ischemia in the region of internal capsule[46] and Saposnik et al. described the "pontine warning syndrome" with fluctuating symptoms such as dysarthria, ataxic-hemiparesis and gaze palsies.[47] In contrast, patients with occlusion of larger arteries, such as the internal carotid artery (ICA) in the neck, may have TIAs during a period of weeks or months. It takes longer for a large vessel (8–15 mm in diameter) to occlude than for a small artery (several hundred microns in diameter) to do so. In large artery disease, TIAs may be less stereotyped, with weakness of a hand in one attack and aphasia and facial numbness in another. The larger the vascular territory, the more opportunity there is for variety of symptoms. Note, in Table 3.7, which includes data from the HSR, that in patients who had carotid artery occlusion, the initial TIA most often occurred months before the stroke, whereas the last TIA often preceded the stroke by less than a week. As an artery occludes, TIAs may become more frequent. A TIA occurring yesterday is much more ominous than a single TIA that occurred 3 months ago; the recent TIA would demand more urgent evaluation and treatment.

The nature of the symptoms and their posited localization are also important in making a diagnosis. Occasionally, a patient gives a history of transient deficits in different vascular territories. Such a patient was DB, who awakened one night with numbness of his left arm and leg, symptoms that were gone by morning when he told his wife about the occurrence. Two nights later, while on his way to the bathroom, he noted weakness and numbness of his right limbs. In the morning, his physician could still document slight weakness of the right hand but noted no other abnormalities on examination. Had this patient confused his left and right sides and mislocalized

the initial night symptoms? A week later, the same patient suddenly developed a cold, painful right leg, and investigations confirmed bacterial endocarditis as the source of his multiple embolizations. The clinical key in this patient was the bilateral sequential TIAs in different vascular territories, suggesting a central source of embolism.

In the patient, JH, the single TIA provided an important clue in predicting the most probable stroke mechanism. The symptoms involved the left arm and face, making it unlikely that the cause was a local disturbance in these parts of the body. This must have been a transient brain event and one localized to the same side of the brain, probably the same vascular territory as the stroke since the same side of the body was involved in the TIA and the later stroke. A thrombotic event seems the most likely mechanism. TIAs do not usually precede ICH. If the mechanism was cardiac-origin embolism, emboli would have had to have hit the same general target twice in a row, an unusual occurrence. It would help if he were alert enough to tell whether there had been more transient attacks because many attacks in the same territory make cardiac-origin embolism quite unlikely. Knowledge about eye involvement would also have been helpful in localizing the occlusive process along the right carotid artery system.

A history of past strokes also helps the alert clinician pinpoint a stroke mechanism. A patient with three prior strokes during the past year involving the vertebrobasilar, left carotid, and right carotid artery systems has a high probability of brain embolism probably from a cardiac or aortic source or a hypercoagulable state. A normotensive patient with several prior ICHs in different loci has a high probability of having a bleeding diathesis or cerebral amyloid angiopathy as the cause of a propensity for ICH. JH had no history of a prior stroke.

Activity at onset

Traditional teaching states that most thrombotic strokes occur when the circulation is least active and most sluggish (e.g., during the night or during a nap, with the deficit usually noticed on arising). Embolism and hemorrhage, in contrast, would be more likely to occur when the circulation is more active or when blood pressure rises. New data show that most ischemic[48] and hemorrhagic strokes[49] actually occur during the morning hours, especially between 10 AM and noon after the patient has awakened and begun daily activities. Table 3.8 contains data from the MRSR on the frequencies of the various stroke mechanisms in relationship to activity at onset.[10]

A significant number of hemorrhages do occur at night, and thrombotic deficits can occur during activity. It is, however, unusual for a thrombotic stroke or a lacune to develop during vigorous physical activity or during sex. A particularly common time for embolism to occur is on arising at night to urinate, the so-called matudinal (morning) embolus. The onset in JH was during relatively sedentary activities at work.

Certain physical activities and situations are related to particular stroke subtypes. A valsalva maneuver immediately before stroke symptoms should suggest paradoxical embolism related to an increase in right atrial pressure in patients with a patent foramen ovale (PFO).[50] Coughing or a vigorous sneeze can also shake loose an embolic particle, resulting in brain embolism. Physical efforts that involve neck trauma or sudden neck movements and stroke after neck manipulations should raise suspicion of arterial dissection. Arterial dissections have also been described after labor and during the postpartum period[51] or after weight lifting.

Early course of development of the deficit

Table 3.9 contains data from the HSR,[7] the MRSR,[10] and the Lausanne Stroke Registry[13] concerning the temporal course of the neurological deficits. Often, the early course gives important information about the stroke mechanism. We encourage clinicians to construct "course of illness" graphs that show the temporal pattern of the findings.[1,52] A few examples may serve to illustrate.

> WC, a previously hypertensive man, suddenly became aphasic and hemiplegic while eating lunch with his family. When initially examined in the emergency room, he was mute and had a severe right hemiplegia. Two hours later, he was much improved and could lift his right leg and say a few words. Four hours after the symptoms began, he had returned to normal except for minor weakness of the right hand and arm.

Figure 3.2 illustrates the course of illness in patient WC. The improvement shortly after onset of the deficit argues strongly against an ICH. The deficit, which was maximal at onset and was unassociated with headache, is most compatible with an embolic mechanism. Cardiac rhythm monitoring in this patient later showed intermittent atrial fibrillation. The next patient illustrates a different scenario.

> RP was admitted to the hospital, and the intern called the attending physician to report that RP had developed a gradually progressive hemiplegia throughout the day. On closer

Table 3.8 Activity at onset in subtypes of stroke (from the Michael Reese Stroke Registry[10])

Activity at onset	Thromb (%)	Emb (%)	Lacune (%)	ICU (%)	ICH (%)	SAH (%)
On arising	40	17	50	31	13	15
Stress	1	5	1	5	10	15
ADL	54	68	47	50	64	64
Unknown	5	10	2	14	13	6

ADL, activities of daily living; Thromb, thrombosis; Emb, embolus; ICU, infarct cause unknown; ICH, intracerebral hemorrhage; SAH, subarachnoid hemorrhage.

Table 3.9 Early course of deficit in various registries (%)

| | T | | | Lac | | | Emb | | | ICH | | | SAH | |
	HSR	MRSR	LSR	HSR	MRSR	LSR	HSR	MRSR	LSR	HSR	MRSR	LSR	HSR	MRSR
Maximal at onset	40	45	66	38	40	54	79	89	82	34	38	44	80	64
Stepwise/stutter	34	30	27	32	28	40	11	10	13	3	9		3	14
Gradual, smooth	13	14		20	24		5	1		63	51	52	14	18
Fluctuating	13	11	7	10	8	5	5	0	5	0	2	4	3	4

Emb, embolism; HSR, Harvard Stroke Registry; ICH, intracerebral hemorrhage; Lac, lacune; LSR, Lausanne Stroke Registry; MRSR, Michael Reese Stroke Registry; SAH, subarachnoid hemorrhage; T, thrombosis.

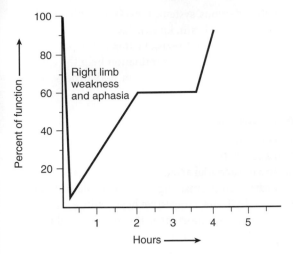

Figure 3.2 Course of illness for patient WC.

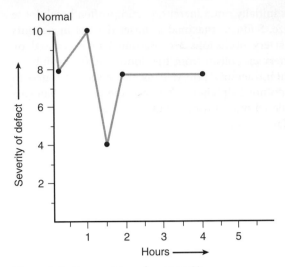

Figure 3.3 Course of illness for patient RP.

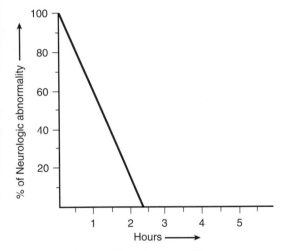

Figure 3.4 Course of illness for patient BK.

We call the process of eliciting the historical details from RP "walking through" the course of illness with the patient. Most patients have difficulty quantifying their deficits and estimating the course of their illness. When patients are asked to describe their activities, an alert observer can often better gauge the course of development of the deficit. Inspection of these course of illness graphs (Figures 3.2 and 3.3) helps experienced physicians predict stroke mechanism. Such a graph (Figure 3.4) would also aid diagnosis in the following case.

> BK was admitted to the hospital with a note that said that she had the sudden onset of left hemiplegia while shopping. A review of the events with her sister who accompanied her and a call to the shopkeeper revealed a different story. While the patient was trying on a hat in a store, the shopkeeper had noted a droop of the face and had called for an ambulance, against the patient's wishes. The shopkeeper recalled the patient walking to the next room and gesturing with both hands. When the ambulance arrived 10 minutes later, the patient could walk to the ambulance but had a limp and less swing of the left arm. On arrival at the hospital 30 minutes after onset, she had a severe left hemiplegia, eyes and head were deviated to the right, and she vomited and reported a headache. During the next 2 hours she continued to worsen and became comatose.

The gradual development of a progressive focal deficit, accompanied by gradually developing symptoms of increased ICP suggested ICH, a diagnosis confirmed by computed tomography (CT). In this case, a more detailed account of the early course of illness helped to suggest the correct diagnosis.

In patient JH, the onset was abrupt and presumably maximal at onset because he fell with a hemiplegia. Among the two stroke mechanisms with the highest probability so far – atherosclerosis with thrombosis and later embolism and cardiac-origin embolism – each has a tendency to begin abruptly and to have maximal deficit at or near onset. Recall from the discussion in Chapter 2 that when atherosclerotic large artery lesions critically reduce the size of the residual lumen, an occlusive thrombus often develops. Because the

questioning by the attending physician, RP related the following account: At 9:30 AM, while eating breakfast, her left hand became clumsy, and she dropped a piece of bread. When she climbed the stairs to go to her room, she noticed a slight limp in her left foot. Worried about her problem, she rested for an hour and was comforted when, on rising, she could walk down the stairs without any difficulty and clear the table without a trace of left hand awkwardness. Thirty minutes later while sitting on the couch, her left limbs became weak and she could lift neither her left arm nor leg. Twenty minutes or so after this worsening, her left limb function improved and remained the same until her arrival in the hospital about 3 hours after the first onset of symptoms. When she was seen at the hospital 3 hours after onset, the left limbs were slightly weak.

This course of illness in RP (Figure 3.3) was typical of a stuttering onset, with improvement in the deficit, followed by worsening and a second improvement. Again, this course would be difficult to understand if the initial deficit had been caused by ICH; the tempo was most compatible with a thrombotic process, most likely due to penetrating artery disease since the deficit was solely motor.

thrombus is initially not adherent, portions often break loose and embolize. Sudden, maximal-at-onset deficits in patients with large artery occlusions are presumed to be caused by artery-to-artery embolism from the donor site of thrombosis to a recipient intracranial artery. Thus, the onset and course to date of JH do not help choose between the two mechanisms being considered most strongly, but the preceding TIA in the same vascular territory favors artery-to-artery embolism over cardiac-origin embolism.

Accompanying symptoms

Headache, particularly if it is sudden and severe at onset, is an invariable symptom of SAH. Sudden release of blood into the subarachnoid space increases ICP and usually leads to severe headache, vomiting, and a decrease in the level of consciousness. In ICH, the focal deficit usually develops progressively, and only later, when there has been enlargement of the hematoma, do headache, vomiting, and decreased consciousness develop. Loss of consciousness is common in SAH and is rare in ischemic stroke unless the ischemia involves the brain stem bilaterally. Occasionally, very transient loss of consciousness occurs in patients with ischemic strokes particularly those due to embolism. Seizures are rare in the early period after stroke onset; their presence argues for embolic stroke or ICH. Table 3.10 lists the frequency of accompanying features by stroke mechanism.

Combining two pieces of information often adds greatly to the accuracy of the probabilities. An example of this is seen in Table 3.11, which analyzes information about the presence of vomiting among patients in the HSR for each stroke mechanism in relation to the location of the stroke in the anterior or posterior circulation. Vomiting is common in both ischemic and hemorrhagic posterior circulation strokes, presumably because of involvement of the so-called vomiting center in the floor of the IVth ventricle. Vomiting is rare in ischemic strokes in the anterior circulation, however, whether thrombotic or embolic. In the anterior circulation, ICH was accompanied by vomiting, presumably because of the associated increase in ICP. Thus, vomiting and anterior circulation location usually equals ICH. A patient with a right hemiparesis and aphasia who vomits early during the stroke has a high likelihood of harboring an ICH.

Patient JH denied headache but did have lethargy, qualifying as some decrease in level of consciousness. Decrease in level of consciousness is very rare in lacunar infarction, one subtype of thrombotic stroke. He had not vomited. These features do not, in his case, help differentiate between thrombosis with embolism and cardiogenic embolism.

Localization and detection of the vascular lesion

Having pursued the history as thoroughly as possible, the clinician should be ready to perform a general and neurological examination. While proceeding, the principal aims should be kept in mind. They are: (1) to detect vascular and cardiac abnormalities that aid in determining stroke mechanism and localization of vascular lesions; and (2) to localize the process within the central nervous system. Once the clinician knows where the lesion is in the brain, knowledge about the anatomy of the vascular supply, about the risk factors in the patient, and about the results of the vascular examination help the clinician predict the most likely vascular location and process in the patient.

Findings from examination of the heart

The diagnosis of cardiogenic embolism is important because its evaluation and treatment differ from intrinsic disease of the extracranial and intracranial arteries. A careful detailed history of possible cardiac symptoms, angina, myocardial infarction, palpitations or arrhythmia, congestive heart failure, and rheumatic heart disease is as important as the neurological history. The heart should be examined thoroughly, taking time to estimate size, character, and quality of heart sounds and gallops; listening for murmurs is not enough.

Findings from examination of the vascular system

Examination of the available systemic and extracranial arteries may give clues to the presence of atherosclerosis or diminished flow not detectable by history. Note the pulse for at least a minute, seeking any irregularities. Feel the radial pulses simultaneously, looking for a significant difference in the strength of the pulses or a delay on one side. In all reported examples of subclavian steal, the diminished blood flow to the arm related to subclavian artery occlusive disease produced a definite pulse alteration;[53,54] the radial pulse is smaller and delayed on the ischemic side. If the pulses are equal and synchronous, it is not necessary to check the blood pressures in each arm. Feel the femoral and foot pulses and listen to the femoral region for an arterial bruit. Remember that some patients with a hyperdynamic circulation (e.g., fever, anemia, or hyperthyroidism) have bruits over many peripheral vessels. When a femoral bruit is present, listen over the antecubital and supraclavicular fossas to determine whether bruits are a generalized phenomenon and do not necessarily indicate focal disease.

Next, gently palpate the carotid artery in the neck. Recall that you are feeling the common carotid artery (CCA) until you reach the bifurcation high in the neck. The ICA then proceeds posteriorly and usually cannot be felt; the external carotid artery (ECA) projects slightly forward and laterally and can be traced. The left carotid artery is positioned more posteriorly and deeper, so that the carotid pulses rarely feel equal. Feeling a carotid pulse in the neck tells the examiner that the CCA is patent; it gives no information about the ICA. Even if the proximal ICA is occluded, a pulse can often be seen and felt along the ICA because of propagation of the pulse wave from the CCA. All too often, a bounding carotid pulse is falsely considered evidence against an ICA occlusion. Listening to the carotid artery beginning low in the neck and progressing cranially is important.

The stethoscope used to listen over arteries should have a relatively small diameter bell. Most newer stethoscopes (Littman types) have too large flat bells and diaphragms and are not very suitable for listening to arteries or examining blood vessels in children. The bell of an old-fashioned

Table 3.10 Frequency of accompanying symptoms at or near onset by stroke subtype (%)

| | Thrombosis | | | Lacune | | | Embolus | | | ICH | | | SAH | |
	HSR	LSR	SDB	HSR	LSR	SDB	HSR	LSR	SDB	HSR	LSR	SDB	HSR	SDB
Decreased consciousnes	15	13	14	20	12	29	3	3	2	39	50	57	68	48
Vomiting	11	–	8	6	–	5	3	–	1	46	–	29	48	45
Seizures	0.3	1	3	4	0	3	0	0	1	7	7	9	7	7
Headache	12	17	11	9	18	10	3	7	5	33	40	41	78	87

HSR, Harvard Stroke Registry; ICH, intracerebral hemorrhage; LSR, Lausanne Stroke Registry; SAH, subarachnoid hemorrhage; SDB, Stroke Data Bank.

Table 3.11 Vomiting and location and type of stroke (from the Harvard Stroke Registry[7])

Intracerebral hemorrhage	
Anterior circulation	19/29 (65.5%)
Posterior circulation	8/12 (67%)
Thrombosis	
Anterior circulation	3/141 (2%)
Posterior circulation	24/83 (29%)
Embolism	
Anterior circulation	4/198 (2%)
Posterior circulation	6/21 (29%)

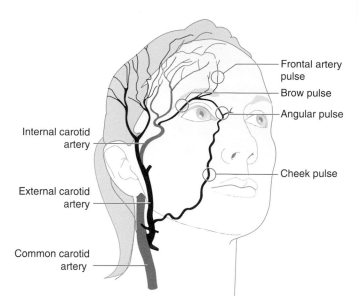

Figure 3.5 Lateral view showing internal (ICA) and external (ECA) carotid arteries. ECA branches supply collateral circulation after ICA occlusion. Palpation points for angular, brow, cheek, and frontal pulses are shown.

stethoscope is usually superior to the diaphragm or flat bell of the newer stethoscopes for bruit detection and analysis.

Recall that many non-stenosing processes can cause carotid bruits. The most common of these are transmitted cardiac murmurs, especially aortic stenosis, tortuous vessels, dilated aortas, anemia, chronic kidney disease, and hyperdynamic circulatory states. Transmitted heart and aortic murmurs and hyperdynamic states produce bruits usually heard over the entire artery, often loudest at the base of the neck. These bruits are usually low-pitched, relatively short, and are invariably heard best over the supraclavicular fossa, perhaps because of the presence of lung tissue just beneath this region, which better transmits the sound. The auscultatory features of a focal vascular constriction can be compared with that of mitral stenosis because each impedes flow and creates a pressure differential beyond the area of blockage. The bruit caused by local constriction of a carotid or vertebral artery is usually:

1. Focal in location – often loudest at the bifurcation high in the neck and not audible at the base – Osler said that the murmur of mitral stenosis is often limited to the region of a dime; the same explanation is valid for the focality of a localized region of carotid artery stenosis.
2. Long – It takes longer for blood to course across a constricted vessel; the diastolic murmur of tight mitral stenosis is also long.
3. High-pitched – The blood flow velocity is often increased in regions of arterial stenosis. The increased velocity is associated with a high-pitched sound.

At times, stenosis at the origin of the ECA produces a bruit that can be confused with an ICA-origin lesion. When the lesion is in the ECA, the bruit can sometimes be traced forward toward the area of the facial artery. Also, blockage of the major ECA branches by finger pressure reduces or obliterates an ECA bruit but does not alter a bruit of ICA origin[55]

After examining the carotid arteries, listen over the supraclavicular fossa and then follow the course of each vertebral artery (VA), first within the posterior cervical triangle and then up the sternocleidomastoid muscle to the mastoid region. Sometimes, a unilateral vertebral artery bruit is a reflection of augmented flow to compensate for a contralateral VA occlusion; the bruit is then on the "wrong side" for the symptoms.

Clues to the patency of the carotid system arteries can also be obtained by careful palpation of the ECA branches on the face. The most readily palpable arteries in normal individuals are the facial artery along the edge of the lower jaw; the preauricular artery just anterior to the ear; and the superficial temporal artery in the temple region. It is important to feel both sides simultaneously to detect a delay or asymmetry of the pulses. When the ECA or CCA on one side is occluded or severely stenosed, the facial, preauricular, and superficial temporal pulses are diminished on that side, and the regions of supply may feel cool to the touch. When the ICA is occluded before its ophthalmic artery branch, the ECA may supply critical collateral vessels, usually about the orbit.

The augmented flow can often be felt as brisk increased pulsation at the cheek, brow, or inner angle of the eye. Fisher designated these pulses ABC (angular, brow, cheek) for easy recall (Figure 3.5).[56] At times, the superficial temporal artery provides collateral supply to the supraorbital and supratrochlear branches of the ophthalmic artery feeding the low pressure ophthalmic–carotid system.[56] In the normal situation, blood flows from the ICA to the ophthalmic artery to the supraorbital (frontal artery) and supratrochlear branches cephalad from the eye brow toward the hair line. In the normal situation, obliteration of these arteries at the brow blocks the distal pulse above it. When there is low pressure in the ophthalmic system, flow goes down these vessels from superficial temporal artery collaterals into the orbit. In that circumstance, obliteration of the brow pulse does not block the forehead pulses, but a finger on the forehead pulses stops the pulsation in the brow, a reversal of the usual normal pattern of flow (Figure 3.6). This finding is called the frontal artery sign.[57]

Remember that there is alternative rich collateral circulation at the circle of Willis, especially through the anterior

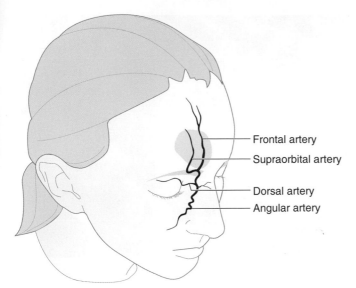

Figure 3.6 Drawing shows the major arterial branches about the eye. The shaded region is supplied by the frontal and supraorbital branches of the ophthalmic artery.

- Frontal artery
- Supraorbital artery
- Dorsal artery
- Angular artery

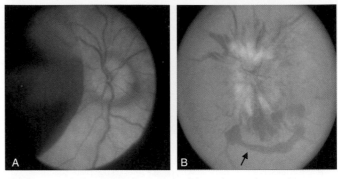

Figure 3.7 (A) This retinal photograph of the right eye shows a large subhyaloid hemorrhage. (B) Papilledema and multiple retinal flame-shaped hemorrhages are present (black arrow) in the retina of the left eye. Photographs kindly submitted by Kathleen Digre, MD, University of Utah. A black and white version of this figure will appear in some formats. For the color version, please refer to the plate section.

communicating and posterior communicating arteries, which bring collaterals from the opposite cerebral hemisphere and posterior circulation, respectively. The absence of augmented facial collateral vessels does not mean that the ICA system is not obstructed. On the other hand, the presence of collateral flow through the orbit is diagnostic of a low pressure ophthalmic–carotid artery system and so is important clinically. The technique for detecting this is easy to master at the bedside.

Also feel for the occipital artery behind the mastoid process. This branch of the ECA often provides collateral circulation to the distal extracranial VA in the neck when the VA is occluded at its origin. A bounding occipital artery pulse on one side provides some evidence of VA occlusive disease.

In temporal arteritis, the superficial temporal and occipital arteries are often tender, nodular, and pulseless. Compression of these arteries in patients who have temporal arteritis often reveals firm arterial walls in contrast to the normal situation. Unless a clinician gains experience by routinely palpating these arteries, they will not be able to recognize pathological changes when they occur.

Be sure to feel the femoral and pedal pulses and to inspect the fingers and toes. Claudication and peripheral vascular occlusive disease highly correlate with atherostenosis of the carotid and vertebral arteries in the neck.[7] Cyanosis, coldness, or frank gangrene of digits usually means either embolism from the heart or the aorto-iliac region blocking the distal digital arteries, or in-situ thrombosis of digital arteries owing to a coagulopathy or severe occlusive peripheral vascular disease. Endocarditis is often associated with tender small nodules in the pulp of the fingers and toes.

JH had a normal-sized heart and rhythm. There were no cardiac murmurs. Blood pressure was 130/70 mmHg. All pulses were palpable, and there were no vascular bruits. The facial pulses were normal and symmetric.

The results of the cardiac and vascular examinations provided no new clues in JH. The absence of a carotid artery bruit and the presence of normal facial pulses did not exclude severe carotid artery disease in the neck but offered no positive evidence for its occurrence.

Findings from examination of the eyes

The eyes provide a window into the body's vascular system and can yield clues concerning stroke mechanism. Subhyaloid hemorrhages (Figure 3.7), large round hemorrhages with a fluid level, represent sudden bleeding below the retina and almost always reflect a sudden change in ICP. They are often seen in patients with SAH and also occur in acutely developing large ICHs.

The severity of hypertensive retinopathy and arteriosclerotic changes is important to note. In long-standing stenosis of the ICA, the reduced pressure in the ophthalmic artery tributaries may minimize hypertensive changes ipsilateral to the stenosis. The same phenomenon is well known as the Goldblatt phenomenon in experimental renal artery stenosis. The kidney arteries on the side of the ligature are spared the systemic hypertensive effects, whereas the opposite renal arteries and arterioles and systemic arteries show advanced hypertension.

Examination of the retina can also yield signs of embolism, most often from the carotid artery but sometimes from the heart and its valves or the aorta. Some patients with retinal embolism have had attacks of transient monocular blindness but some give no history of transient or persistent visual loss. The most important and common ophthalmoscopic finding in patients with transient monocular blindness is the presence of embolic particles within retinal arteries. The commonest particles that are seen are cholesterol crystals (Hollenhorst plaques), which are white but may appear bright, often glinting, and yellow–orange in color (Figure 3.8). These crystals are usually small (10–250 μm). They most often lodge at bifurcations of retinal arteries and do not ordinarily block distal blood flow. They can move or disappear rapidly, but may injure the vascular wall leading to sheathing of the artery. Compressing the orbit may cause crystals to move, flip over, or "flash,"

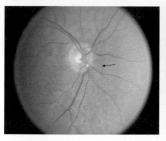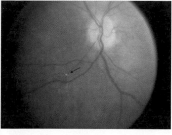

Figure 3.8 Retinal photographs showing cholesterol crystal emboli (black arrows point to the emboli). A black and white version of this figure will appear in some formats. For the color version, please refer to the plate section.

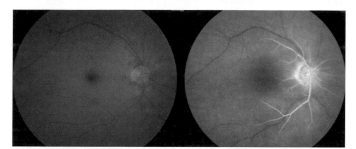

Figure 3.10 Retinal photographs showing acute central retinal artery occlusion in the right eye. (left) The arteries are very attenuated and the ischemic retina appears pale and edematous. The fovea remains red because it receives its blood supply from the choroid (so-called cherry red spot). (right) Retinal fluorescein angiogram 30 seconds after injection of fluorescein showing delayed filling of all retinal vessels which appear dark. Photograph kindly submitted by Dr Valerie Biousse, Emory University. A black and white version of this figure will appear in some formats. For the color version, please refer to the plate section.

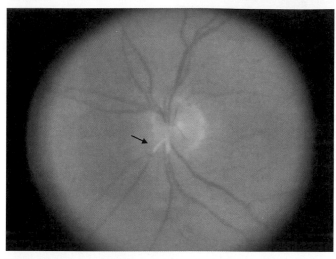

Figure 3.9 Retinal photograph showing a long white platelet–fibin plug (black arrow) impacted in two arterial branches. A black and white version of this figure will appear in some formats. For the color version, please refer to the plate section.

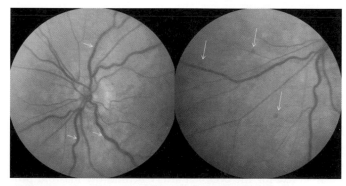

Figure 3.11 Venous stasis retinopathy in the left eye in a patient with a left internal carotid artery occlusion. (left) The posterior pole of the eye appears normal, but the veins are dilated and tortuous (arrows). (right) There are numerous dot-blot hemorrhages (arrows) in the mid-periphery of the retina, beyond the vascular arcades. The right eye is normal. Photograph kindly submitted by Dr Valerie Biousse, Emory University. A black and white version of this figure will appear in some formats. For the color version, please refer to the plate section.

making them more visible with the ophthalmoscope. Platelet–fibrin emboli ("white clots") are longer gray–white columns that gradually progress through small retinal arteries with distal fragments breaking off as the column moves (Figure 3.9).[58,59] Other embolic materials occasionally seen on ophthalmoscopy are calcium fragments that appear chalky white and usually remain in one location obstructing blood flow, and talc, cornstarch, and other foreign body emboli in patients who inject intravenously mashed-up pills intended for oral use after dissolving the tablets in water.[60]

In some patients, ophthalmoscopy will show retinal artery occlusions (Figure 3.10) or branch retinal artery occlusions. Retinal infarcts and focal cotton-wool spots called cytoid bodies that represent retinal microinfarcts are often seen. Patients with carotid artery occlusions sometimes develop a condition of chronic ocular ischemia that has been called venous stasis retinopathy.[61,62] The diagnosis of venous stasis retinopathy is made on the basis of small blot and dot hemorrhages (especially at the mid-periphery of the retina), darkening and dilatation of retinal veins, disc edema, and retinal edema (Figure 3.11). These findings provide evidence of low pressure in the ophthalmic–ICA system. In chronic ocular ischemia the optic disc may be revascularized and the retina show cotton-wool spot infarcts (Figure 3.12). The iris is also supplied by tributaries of the ophthalmic artery and can reveal ischemic damage in patients with ICA disease.[63] In occasional patients the pupil on the side of chronic severe ICA disease can be dilated in relation to iris ischemia.[64] Venous stasis

retinopathy develops in about one-third of patients with symptomatic carotid artery occlusion.

Occlusion of the central retinal vein often produces very dramatic abnormalities on ophthalmoscopy. There are often florid hemorrhages in the peripapillary region and the retinal veins become dilated and tortuous. Central retinal vein occlusion is often a clue to the presence of a coagulopathy.[65,66]

Neuro-ophthalmologists at Emory University in Atlanta, Georgia recently showed that the ocular fundus can be reliably photographed using an iPhone without first instilling mydriatic agents or administering sedatives.[67,68] Emergency room physicians, accustomed to reading other images, can be trained to accurately interpret findings from these photographs.[68,69] Most present day recently trained (non-ophthalmologist) physicians are not skilled or experienced in viewing the ocular fundus. Introduction of these easily acquired photographs of the retina could greatly improve the use of eye findings as a guide to cardiovascular diagnosis.

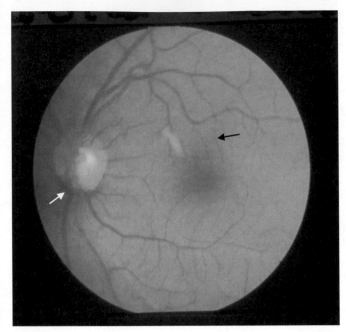

Figure 3.12 Retinal photograph showing neovascularization of the optic disc (white arrow) and retina and a cotton-wool spot retinal infarct (black arrow). Photograph kindly submitted by Kathleen Digre, MD, University of Utah. A black and white version of this figure will appear in some formats. For the color version, please refer to the plate section.

Stroke localization

Findings from the neurological examination

Clinical localization of the brain lesion is primarily from the patient's description of their neurological symptoms and the findings on neurological examination.[1,70] It would be impossible and probably unprofitable to review here the full details of the neurological examination. Many non-neurologists feel uncomfortable when confronted with a stroke patient because they feel ill-equipped to detect neurological signs and to explain them in anatomical detail. Actually, the neurological findings do not have much impact on the diagnosis of stroke mechanism, although the findings do help with the anatomical location of the lesion. Useful anatomical data for practical diagnosis can be summarized rather briefly. Rather than systematically reviewing the examination, we comment here only on important, practical, useful features. More detailed discussions of the neurological examination are published elsewhere.[1,66]

We have been impressed that the most important and most frequently missed signs of brain dysfunction involve abnormalities of: (1) higher cortical function; (2) level of alertness; (3) the visual and oculomotor systems; and (4) gait. These are parts of the examination most often overlooked by non-neurologists, which provide key clues to anatomical localization.

Bedside tests of high-level cortical function

Cognitive function testing should always include examination of language function, especially if the patient has symptoms or signs referable to the right limbs or the right visual field. A good screening test is the writing of a brief paragraph describing the stroke or TIA. Alternatively ask the patient to write a few lines about the town where they live. Asking the patient to read a paragraph from a newspaper or a magazine is also helpful. Ask the patient to name objects in the environment and to repeat spoken language. Remember that there is a large difference between dysarthria (an abnormality of speech articulation and pronunciation) and aphasia (altered content, expression, and understanding of language). If patients are mute and do not write, it is often difficult to be sure whether they are aphasic unless they follow commands or select objects or words from choices in a clearly erroneous manner.

When symptoms or signs of dysfunction are present in the left limbs or visual field, it is especially important to test visual spatial functions and to look for neglect of the left side of space.[1,70–72] Ask the patient to draw a clock or a house and to copy a single two-dimensional figure. Patients with right hemispheric cortical lesions will often omit the left side of their figures and their drawings often contain abnormal angles and proportions. Ask the patient to read a brief paragraph or headline or to look at a picture with the examiner. Left neglect is manifested by omitting words, phrases, or people on the left side of the page. Also notice how the patient responds to environmental stimuli on the right and left sides.

Memory can also be affected by a focal CNS lesion, usually involving the posterior cerebral artery (PCA) territories. The clinician can test memory by asking patients to recall the material contained in the paragraph they read, a picture they were shown, or what they wrote in the paragraph that they wrote earlier. Alternatively, patients may be asked to recall three or more items or a story that they were given to recall later.

Level of alertness

Decreased level of consciousness is an important sign of increased ICP or lesions of the brain stem reticular activating system or bilateral cerebral hemispheres.[2,73–76] Nonetheless, often there is no comment in the record regarding whether the patient was bright and alert or drowsy or delirious. Does the patient require frequent prodding to stay alert? Often, the nurses on the floor or the family who are with the patient for much of the day can best answer this question. They should always be interrogated about the patient's alertness and the appropriateness of mental performance or deviations from behavior before the stroke.

Visual and oculomotor function

Much of the mammalian brain is concerned with visual interpretation and exploration, looking and seeing. Large lesions of the posterior portions of the cerebral hemispheres may produce only visual dysfunction and may leave speech, movement, and other sensations unscathed. Not to test the visual fields in a stroke patient is a cardinal sin, similar to failing to palpate the abdomen in a patient with unexplained shock. Test the visual fields by presenting a visual stimulus, usually a finger or pin in the peripheral portion of each visual field in each eye, and determine on confrontation when the patient sees it. Also ask the patient to look at something – a picture, a paragraph, or the

scene outside the window. Is there consistent omission of objects on one side? Is the individual scanning the materials presented and visual environment normally?

Probably the most common eye movement abnormality in patients with stroke is a conjugate-gaze paralysis. The eyes may be deviated to one side, usually the side of the hemispheric lesion, and both eyes fail to look toward the opposite side. This abnormality usually means a frontal or deep hemispheric lesion in the hemisphere opposite to the gaze palsy[73,76,77] or a lesion in the pontine tegmentum on the same side as the gaze palsy. Nystagmus, a rhythmic oscillation of the eyes on horizontal or vertical gaze, is usually diagnostic of a vertebrobasilar location of the stroke, as are dysconjugate palsies or paralysis of movement of one eye or one eye muscle.

Gait

Some patients with cerebellar lesions have a normal examination when recumbent or seated but cannot walk. These patients are too often discharged from the emergency room only to return later, desperately ill from cerebellar hemorrhage or infarction. Observation of gait also gives a great deal of information about motor function and its symmetry. Is there dragging of one foot, delay in hip flexion on one side, or less arm swing on one side? Are tremors or odd posturing of a limb seen as the patient walks?

Aspects of motor function

Having covered the usual omissions, we now turn to an evaluation of the motor system. Be sure to test each limb proximally and distally. In central lesions, the most important weakness is usually in the shoulder abductors, arm extensors, finger extensors and abductors, thigh flexors, leg flexors, and foot and toe dorsiflexors and everters. Check for drift of the outstretched hands. Try to estimate the relative motor strength in face, arms, hands, and legs. In hemiparetic patients, are any of these regions disproportionately affected or preserved? Test coordination of each limb by the finger-nose, toe-object maneuvers. Deep tendon reflexes are of little importance in central lesions during the acute stroke, but it is informative to elicit the Babinski responses.

Somatosensory functions

In patients with cerebral lesions, higher sensory functions – such as position sense, object recognition, and extinction – are more often affected than elementary pin or touch perception. A useful single screening test is: (1) have the patient close the eyes; (2) touch a specific spot on the patient's fingers, hand, or foot; and then (3) direct the patient to touch precisely the same spot with the opposite hand. This test requires no equipment and is an excellent measure of point-position localization, a good reflection of higher sensory tactile function. Of course, at the same time, you are also testing fine touch because if patients cannot feel the touch, they fail the test. Also, with the patient's eyes still closed, touch both arms, both hands, and then both legs simultaneously, to see whether the patient fails to recognize the touch consistently on one side of the

body. Again, try to assess the relative sensory involvement in face, arms, hands, and legs for disproportionately severe involvement or sparing.

When you have tabulated in your mind the neurological abnormalities, step back from the bedside and *think*. Where is the lesion likely to be? If there is more than one possible or probable location, you may think of further bedside testing that could distinguish among these possibilities. Do not leave the bedside before you feel confident in your clinical localization.

Common localization patterns

Neurological signs most often fall into recognizable patterns that predict the likely anatomical localization of the brain lesion. The neurological symptoms and signs can usually be placed in one of seven general categories. The process is simply one of pattern recognition – that is, matching the patient's clinical deficit with that of patients with known lesions in one of the following regions. Also, are there expected findings that are absent or unexpected added findings beyond those described among these patterns?

1. Left hemisphere lesion (in the anterior hemisphere in the territory of the ICA and its middle cerebral artery (MCA) and anterior cerebral artery (ACA) tributaries) – Aphasia, right limb weakness, right limb sensory loss, right visual field defect, reduced right conjugate gaze, difficulty reading, writing, and calculating.

2. Right hemisphere lesion (in ICA–ACA–MCA distribution) – Neglect of the left visual space, difficulty drawing and copying, left visual field defect, left limb motor weakness, left limb sensory loss, reduced left conjugate gaze, extinction of the left stimulus of two simultaneously given visual or tactile stimuli.

3. Left PCA lesion – Right visual field defect, difficulty reading with retained writing ability, difficulty naming colors and objects presented visually, normal repetition of spoken language, numbness and sensory loss in the right limbs.

4. Right PCA lesion – Left visual field defect, often with neglect, left limb numbness and sensory loss.

5. Vertebrobasilar territory infarction[78] – Spinning dizziness, diplopia, weakness or numbness of all four limbs or bilateral regions, crossed motor or sensory findings (e.g., numbness or weakness of one side of the face and the opposite side of the body), ataxia, vomiting, headache in the occiput, mastoid, or neck, bilateral blindness or dim vision; on examination, nystagmus or dysconjugate gaze, gait or limb ataxia out of proportion to weakness, bilateral recently acquired weakness or numbness (i.e., one side not due to an old stroke or other defect), crossed signs, bilateral visual-field defects, amnesia.

Acute isolated vertigo is most often explained by a peripheral origin in the ear structures. There are some caveats worth remembering: (1) Transient isolated vertigo in some patients is due to vertebrobasilar territory ischemia. In these patients, vertigo usually lasts more than an hour; (2) hearing loss is usually an inner-

ear symptom but when it appears acutely it often has a vascular origin. (Remember that the internal auditory artery is a branch of the anterior inferior cerebellar artery (AICA). Deafness and/or vertigo can herald AICA territory brainstem infarction.)

Newman-Toker, Kattah, and colleagues use a three-part test entitled HINTS (Head–Impulse–Nystagmus–Test of Skew) to separate patients with brainstem and cerebellar ischemia from those with vestibular neuritis or other peripheral causes of vertigo.[79,80] These tests apply to patients who have continuous feelings of vertigo or dizziness but is not useful in patients with momentary position-related transient vertigo (often benign positional vertigo) or those with TIAs who are not dizzy when examined. The head impulse test (also called head thrust) is performed by the clinician sitting face to face with the patient holding the patient's head from the front. The patient is directed to keep their gaze fixed on a target (e.g., usually the examiner's nose) and the head is moved gently about 20 degrees to the side and then quickly thrust back to the midline. This maneuver is performed first on one side and then from the other side while watching the eyes for the presence or absence of any corrective movements. The patient is able to maintain eye fixation in brainstem and cerebellar lesions while in patients with peripheral lesions there is often a refixation saccade on impulse to one side.[79,80] This manifestation of the oculo-vestibular reflex is preserved in central lesions (except when VIIIth-nerve nuclei fascicles are affected in the lateral pons) and is abnormal when the VIIIth nerve or peripheral labyrinth are affected. Peripheral vestibular lesions often are accompanied by nystagmus that is always in the same direction while nystagmus in patients with brainstem and cerebellar lesions often changes direction when looking to one side and then the other. Brainstem and cerebellar lesions sometimes cause a slight skew deviation. The Test for Skew involves covering one eye and seeing if there is a vertical shift in the eye when uncovered. The formula that suggests a brainstem or cerebellar lesion on HINTS testing is: a bilaterally normal head impulse test; or direction changing nystagmus; or vertical displacements on the cover/uncover testing for skew.[79,80] A peripheral lesion is characterized by unilaterally abnormal head impulse test with unidirectional nystagmus beating horizontally (and towards the opposite side from the abnormal impulse), and normal vertical eye alignment.

6. Pure motor stroke (internal capsule or basis pontis) or ataxic hemiparesis – Weakness of face, arm, and leg on one side of the body, without abnormalities of higher cortical function, sensory or visual dysfunction, or reduced alertness. Included in this category are patients with mixed weakness and incoordination or ataxia on the same side of the body.

7. Pure sensory stroke (Thalamus) – Numbness or decreased sensibility of face, arm, and leg on one side of the body, without weakness, incoordination, visual or higher cortical function abnormalities.

In some patients, the findings are quite limited and do not represent the full clinical syndrome. For example, the abnormality may be limited to aphasia, yet this is sufficient to place the patient in the category of left hemisphere anterior circulation disease because no other pattern includes aphasia. Similarly, nystagmus and ataxia are diagnostic of a brainstem or cerebellar process in the category of vertebrobasilar disease. In other patients, the findings are not sufficient to allow definite localization but suggest a number of possibilities. Acute decrease in activity level and motivation are found in patients with caudate nucleus,[81–89] thalamic,[84–86] and frontal lobe infarction.[84,87,88] Weakness limited to a single limb could fit into a number of these categories depending on other neurological signs (numbers 1–6 in the preceding list).

The neurological findings also may help predict the stroke mechanism. An example would be a hypertensive patient with pure motor stroke on the right. This lesion is invariably due to a small lacunar infarct in the internal capsule or pons or a small hemorrhage in these areas. A patient with sudden onset of Wernicke-type fluent aphasia without accompanying weakness or motor signs has a left temporal embolus or a small posterior putaminal hemorrhage undercutting the left temporal lobe. We now return to the patient JH who had a different presentation.

> JH was very sleepy. He could not cooperate for tests of drawing or copying. He was not aware of his left limb paralysis. He did not notice visual stimuli to his left. His eyes were deviated to the right but moved fully to the left with passive head rotation. There was severe paralysis of the left face, arm, and leg, with virtually no movement to pinch or other stimulation. He did not feel touch on his left limbs and could not reliably tell whether his fingers and toes were moved up or down. Pin and pinch were felt as a general discomfort which he could not localize. Deep tendon reflexes were reduced on the left, and the left plantar response was extensor.

The neurological findings in JH clearly localize the process to the right cerebral hemisphere (category 2 above). The severe motor, somatosensory, and vision loss and lack of awareness of the deficit point to a large lesion involving the frontal and paracentral regions. The decreased level of alertness and the involvement of multiple systems (motor, somatosensory, visual) suggest a large area of brain abnormality or a deep lesion involving subcortical structures and the internal capsule. Conjugate eye deviation is especially common in deep lesions.

We now review our hypotheses about stroke mechanisms and localization in JH. The site of brain dysfunction is surely the frontal and central portions of the right cerebral hemisphere. The vascular pathway supplying this region involves blood coming from the heart to the aorta to the right innominate, internal carotid, and middle cerebral arteries. Vascular examination has offered no evidence for disease at any of these locations. The ecology suggests the possibility of large artery occlusive disease, which would be statistically most commonly located at the origin of the ICA in the neck. Atherostenosis of the ICA within the siphon and within the proximal MCA are less likely but possible sites of occlusive disease.

Table 3.12 Diagnosis in patients with and without Wernicke's aphasia (from the Harvard Stroke Registry[7])

	Thrombosis	Embolism	ICH	SAH	Total
With Wernicke's aphasia	8 (15%)	35 (65%)	8 (15%)	3 (6%)	54
Without Wernicke's aphasia	222 (53%)	124 (30%)	39 (9%)	30 (7%)	415

ICH, intracerebral hemorrhage; SAH, subarachnoid hemorrhage.

Table 3.13 Diagnosis: No motor weakness with and without Wernicke's aphasia (from the Harvard Stroke Registry[7])

	Thrombosis	Embolism	ICH	SAH	Total
With Wernicke's aphasia	0 (0%)	12 (75%)	3 (19%)	1 (6%)	16
Without Wernicke's aphasia	56 (58%)	24 (25%)	2 (2%)	14 (15%)	96

ICH, intracerebral hemorrhage; SAH, subarachnoid hemorrhage.

Probable stroke mechanisms can be listed, in order of likelihood, as: (1) premature atherosclerotic occlusive disease with thrombosis and distal intra-arterial embolization of clot; (2) cardiogenic embolism; and (3) ICH. The clinical findings on neurological examination exclude the possibility of lacunar infarction. The focality of findings and absence of headache exclude SAH. ICH is possible, given the reduction in alertness and the likelihood of a large deep cerebral hemispheral lesion, but the absence of risk factors (e.g., hypertension, bleeding abnormality, anticoagulation, and drug use) and the presence of a preceding TIA argue strongly against ICH. The absence of any history of cardiac disease and the normal cardiac findings place cardiogenic embolism below thrombosis as a probable stroke mechanism. We are now ready to test and refine these hypotheses by laboratory and imaging investigations, which are discussed in the next chapter.

Using information from a stroke registry or data bank

Early in the discussion of clinical diagnosis, we introduced the computer, emphasizing the utility of the clinician emulating computer logic. We now return to the computer. Suppose that data were available from detailed analyses of patients with stroke. The registry could be the clinician's own data, collected from patients seen at a single institution, or it could be data gleaned by others or pooled from many registries. We have cited information from such databases and registries throughout this chapter.[5–23] Ideally, these registries should include information from each of the categories discussed so far (i.e., demography, risk factors, past TIAs and strokes, onset and course of the deficit, accompanying symptoms, cardiac and vascular abnormalities on examination, and localization from the clinical and imaging tests). The clinician could then search the registry data for patients with characteristics matching his or her patients. The final diagnosis in these matching cases would help the clinician to estimate more accurately the probability of particular stroke mechanisms and causative vascular lesions in his or her own patients.

We now illustrate the use of such registry data. First let's explore computer driven searches in a patient who is agitated and has Wernicke's aphasia as the only abnormality on neurological examination. Tables 3.12 through 3.14[7] show the results of searches using data from the HSR.[7] From among all testable patients with information about aphasia (469 patients), 54 had Wernicke's aphasia. The distribution of diagnoses in patients with and without Wernicke's aphasia is shown in Table 3.12. The Wernicke's aphasia group differs from patients without Wernicke's aphasia because they include more patients with emboli and ICH and fewer examples of thrombosis. However, there are significant numbers of patients showing all stroke mechanisms, so that this information only suggests general probabilities. Next, we think of a way to make the groups more specifically like our patient: This patient had no motor weakness. We search again the group with Wernicke's aphasia but now stipulate the absence of motor weakness, so the findings might be more useful. We then search the database for patients with Wernicke's aphasia with no motor weakness, comparing patients who have Wernicke's aphasia but no weakness with patients who have no Wernicke's aphasia and no weakness (Table 3.13). Now the figures are more impressive because the registry does not contain a single example of thrombosis with Wernicke's aphasia and no weakness. There are, however, a significant number of patients with ICH. From these data, the major differential diagnosis using the past experience of the HSR would be embolus versus ICH.

We now think harder and ask whether there is any other factor that could be added that would differentiate these two conditions: This patient had no history of hypertension and was not hypertensive in the hospital. Hypertension is, of course, common in ICH. If no hypertension is added to the list of search criteria (Table 3.14), only five patients remain who have Wernicke's aphasia, no weakness, and no hypertension, and all had brain embolism. Using the past experience of the HSR, this patient probably has had a brain embolus. Of course, the odds would be much higher if the number of

Table 3.14 Diagnosis: No motor weakness and no hypertension with and without Wernicke's aphasia (from the Harvard Stroke Registry[7])

	Thrombosis	Embolism	ICH	SAH	Total
With Wernicke's aphasia	0 (0%)	5 (100%)	0 (0%)	0 (0%)	5
Without Wernicke's aphasia	16 (41%)	15 (38%)	1 (3%)	7 (18%)	39

ICH, intracerebral hemorrhage; SAH, subarachnoid hemorrhage.

patients with Wernicke's aphasia, no weakness, and no hypertension were 100 rather than 5, but the computer has allowed quick and precise comparison of this patient with the experience of the registry. Large databases provide clinicians with an opportunity to explore in detail the findings in large groups of stroke patients.

References

1. Caplan LR, Hollander J. *The Effective Clinical Neurologist*, 3rd edn. Shelton, CT: People's Medical Publishing House – USA, 2011.

2. Caplan LR, Kelly JJ. *Consultations in Neurology*. Toronto: BC Decker, 1988.

3. Bayes T. An essay towards solving a problem in the doctrine of chances. *Philos Trans R Soc Lond* 1763;**53**:270–418. Reprinted in *Biometrika* 1935;**45**:296–315.

4. Winkler RL. *Introduction to Bayesian Inference and Decision*. New York: Holt, Rinehart & Winston, 1972.

5. Aring C, Merritt H. Differential diagnosis between cerebral hemorrhage and cerebral thrombosis. *Arch Intern Med* 1935;**56**:435–456.

6. Dalsgaard-Nielsen T. Survey of 1000 cases of apoplexia cerebri. *Acta Psychiatr Neurol Scand* 1955;**30**:169–185.

7. Mohr JP, Caplan LR, Melski JW, et al. The Harvard Cooperative Stroke Registry: A prospective registry. *Neurology* 1978;**28**:754–762.

8. Whisnant J, Fitzgibbons J, Kurland L, et al. Natural history of stroke in Rochester, Minnesota, 1945–1954. *Stroke* 1971;**2**:11–22.

9. Matsumoto N, Whisnant J, Kurland L, et al. Natural history of stroke in Rochester, Minnesota, 1955–1969. *Stroke* 1973;**4**:20–29.

10. Caplan LR, Hier DB, D'Cruz I. Cerebral embolism in the Michael Reese Stroke Registry. *Stroke* 1983;**14**:530–536.

11. Chambers BR, Donnan GA, Bladin PF. Patterns of stroke: An analysis of the first 700 consecutive admissions to the Austin Hospital Stroke Unit. *Aust N Z J Med* 1983;**13**:57–64.

12. Foulkes MA, Wolf PA, Price TR, et al. The Stroke Data Bank: Design, methods, and baseline characteristics. *Stroke* 1988;**19**:547–554.

13. Bogousslavsky J, Mille GV, Regli F. The Lausanne Stroke Registry: An analysis of 1,000 consecutive patients with first stroke. *Stroke* 1988;**19**:1083–1092.

14. Moulin T, Tatu L, Crepin-Leblond T, Chavot D, Berges S, Rumbach T. The Besancon Stroke Registry: An acute stroke registry of 2,500 consecutive patients. *Eur Neurol* 1997;**38**(1):10–20.

15. Heuschmann PU, Kolominsky-Rabas PL, Misselwitz B, et al. German Stroke Registers Study Group. Predictors of in-hospital mortality and attributable risks of death after ischemic stroke: The German Stroke Registers Study Group. *Arch Intern Med* 2004;**164**:1761–1768.

16. Vemmos KN, Takis CE, Georgilis K, et al. The Athens Stroke Registry: Results of a five-year hospital-based study. *Cerebrovasc Dis* 2000; **10**:133–141.

17. Gross CR, Kase CS, Mohr JP, et al. Stroke in south Alabama: incidence and diagnostic features – a population based study. *Stroke* 1984;**15**:249–255.

18. Oxfordshire Community Stroke Project. Incidence of stroke in Oxfordshire: First year's experience of a community stroke registry. *BMJ* 1983;**287**:713–717.

19. Bamford J, Sandercock P, Dennis M, et al. A prospective study of acute cerebrovascular disease in the community: the Oxfordshire Community Stroke Project: 1981–1986. *J Neurol Neurosurg Psychiatry* 1990;**53**:16–22.

20. Alter M, Sobel E, McCoy RC, et al. Stroke in the Lehigh Valley: Incidence based on a community-wide hospital registry. *Neuroepidemiology* 1985;**4**:1–15.

21. Friday G, Lai SM, Alter M, et al. Stroke in the Lehigh Valley: Racial/ethnic difference. *Neurology* 1989;**39**:1165–1168.

22. Yip P-K, Jeng JS, Lee T-K, et al. Subtypes of ischemic stroke in hospital-based stroke registry in Taiwan. *Stroke* 1997;**28**:2507–2512.

23. Coull BM, Brockschmidt JK, Howard G, et al. Community hospital-based stroke programs in North Carolina, Oregon and New York: IV. Stroke diagnosis and its relation to demographics, risk factors, and clinical status after stroke. *Stroke* 1990;**21**:867–873.

24. Gorelick PB, Hier DB, Caplan LR, et al. Headache in acute cerebrovascular disease. *Neurology* 1986;**36**:1445–1450.

25. Gorelick PB, Caplan LR, Hier DB, et al. Racial differences in the distribution of anterior circulation occlusive disease. *Neurology* 1984;**34**:54–59.

26. Kieffer S, Takeya Y, Resch J, et al. Racial differences in cerebrovascular disease: angiographic evaluation of Japanese and American populations. *AJR Am J Roentgenol* 1967;**101**:94–99.

27. Heyman A, Fields WS, Keating RD. Joint study of extracranial arterial occlusion: VI. Racial differences in hospitalized patients with ischemic stroke. *JAMA* 1972;**222**:285–289.

28. Russo LS. Carotid system transient ischemic attacks, clinical, racial, and angiographic correlations. *Stroke* 1981;**12**:470–473.

29. Heyden S, Heyman A, Goree J. Nonembolic occlusion of the middle cerebral and carotid arteries: a comparison of predisposing factors. *Stroke* 1970;**1**:363–369.

30. Barnett HJM. The international collaborative study of superficial temporal artery – middle cerebral

artery anastomosis. In FC Rose (ed), *Advances in Stroke Therapy*. New York: Raven Press, 1982, pp 179–182.

31. Huang CY, Chan FL, Yu YL, et al. Cerebrovascular disease in Hong Kong Chinese. *Stroke* 1990;**21**:230–235.

32. Feldmann E, Daneault N, Kwan E, et al. Chinese–white differences in the distribution of occlusive cerebrovascular disease. *Neurology* 1990;**40**:1541–1545.

33. Caplan LR, Gorelick PB, Hier DB. Race, sex, and occlusive vascular disease: A review. *Stroke* 1986;**17**:648–655.

34. Caplan LR. Cerebral ischemia and infarction in blacks. Clinical, autopsy, and angiographic studies. In RF Gillum, PB Gorelick, ES Cooper (eds), *Stroke in Blacks*. Basel: Karger, 1999, pp 7–18.

35. Johnston SC, Gress DR, Browner WS, Sidney S. Short-term prognosis after emergency department diagnosis of TIA. *JAMA* 2000;**284**:2901–2906.

36. Daffertshofer M, Mielke O, Pullwitt A. Felsenstein M, Hennerici M. Transient ischemic attacks are more than "ministrokes." *Stroke* 2004;**35**:2453–2458.

37. Kleindorfer D, Pangos P, Pancoli A, et al. Incidence and short-term prognosis of transient ischemic attack in a population-based study. *Stroke* 2005;**36**:720–724.

38. Hill MD, Yiannakoulias N, Jeerakathil T, Tu JV, Svenson LW, Swchopflocher DP. The high risk of stroke immediately after transient ischemic attack. A population-based study. *Neurology* 2004;**62**:2015–2020.

39. Rothwell PM, Warlow CP. Timing of TIAs preceding stroke. Time window for prevention is very short. *Neurology* 2005;**64**;817–820.

40. Touze E, Varenne O, Chatellier G, Peyrard S, Rothwell PM, Mas J-L. Risk of myocardial infarction and vascular death after transient ischemic attack and ischemic stroke. *Stroke* 2005;**36**:2748–2755.

41. Nguyen-Huynh MN, Johnston SC. Transient ischemic attack: A neurologic emergency. *Curr Neurol Neurosci Rep* 2005;**5**:13–20.

42. Rothwell PM, Giles MF, Flossmann E, et al. A simple score (ABCD) to identify individuals at high early risk of stroke after transient ischemic attack. *Lancet* 2005;**366**:29–36.

43. Johnston SC, Rothwell PM, Nguyen-Huynh MN, et al. Validation and refinement of scores to predict very early stroke after transient ischemic attack. *Lancet* 2007;**369**:283–292.

44. Advisory Council for the National Institute of Neurological Diseases and Blindness. A classification and outline of cerebrovascular diseases: a report by an ad hoc committee established by the Advisory Council for the National Institute of Neurological Diseases and Blindness, Public Health Service. *Neurology* 1958;**8**:395–434.

45. Albers GW, Caplan LR, Easton JD et al. Transient ischemic attack – proposal for a new definition. *N Engl J Med* 2002;**347**:1713–1716.

46. Donnan GA, Melley HM, Quang L, Hurley S, Bladin PF. The capsular warning syndrome: Pathogenesis and clinical features. *Neurology* 1993;**43**:957–962.

47. Saposnik G. Noel de Tilly L, Caplan LR. Pontine warning syndrome. *Arch Neurol* 2008;**65**:1375–1377.

48. Marler J, Price TR, Clark GL, et al. Morning increase in onset of ischemic stroke. *Stroke* 1989;**20**:473–476.

49. Sloan M, Price TR, Foukes MA, et al. Circadian rhythmicity of stroke onset: intracerebral and subarachnoid hemorrhage. *Ann Neurol* 1990;**28**:226–227.

50. Caplan LR. Clinical diagnosis of brain embolism. *Cerebrovasc Dis* 1995;**5**:79–88

51. Baffour FI, Kirchoff-Torres KF, Einstein FH, Karakash S, Miller TS. Bilateral internal carotid artery dissection in the postpartum period. *Obstet Gynecol* 2012;**119**:489–492.

52. Caplan, LR. Course-of-illness graphs. *Hosp Pract* 1985;**20**:125–136.

53. Baker R, Rosenbaum A, Caplan LR. Subclavian steal syndrome. *Contemp Surg* 1974;**4**:96–104.

54. Caplan LR. *Posterior Circulation Disease*. Boston, Blackwell Science 1996.

55. Reed C, Toole J. Clinical technique for identification of external carotid bruits. *Neurology* 1981;**31**:744–746.

56. Fisher CM. Facial pulses in internal carotid artery occlusion. *Neurology* 1970;**20**:476–478.

57. Caplan LR. The frontal artery sign:A bedside indicator of internal carotid occlusive disease. *N Engl J Med* 1973;**288**:1008–1009.

58. Caplan LR. Transient ischemia and brain and ocular infarction. In DM Albert, FA Jakobiec (eds), *Principles and Practice of Ophthalmology*, vol **4** JF Rizzo, S Lessell (eds) *Neuroophthalmology*. Philadelphia: W B Saunders, 1994, pp 2653–2669.

59. Wray SH. Visual aspects of extracranial internal carotid artery disease. In EF Bernstein (ed), *Amaurosis Fugax*. New York: Springer-Verlag, 1988, pp 72–80.

60. Atlee W. Talc and cornstarch emboli in the eyes of drug abusers. *JAMA* 1972;**219**:49–51.

61. Fisher CM. Observations of the fundus oculi in transient monocular blindness. *Neurology* 1959;**9**:333–347.

62. Kearns T, Hollenhorst R. Venous stasis retinopathy of occlusive disease of the carotid artery. *Mayo Clin Proc* 1963;**38**:304–312.

63. Carter JE. Chronic ocular ischemia and carotid vascular disease. In EF Bernstein (ed), *Amaurosis Fugax*. New York: Springer-Verlag, 1988, pp 118–134.

64. Fisher CM. Dilated pupil in carotid occlusion. *Trans Am Neurol Assoc* 1966;**91**:230–231.

65. Prisco D, Marcucci R. Retinal vein thrombosis: Risk factors, pathogenesis and therapeutic approach. *Pathophysiol Haemost Thromb* 2002;**32**:308–311.

66. Lahey JM, Kearney JJ, Tunc M. Hypercoagulable states and central retinal vein occlusion. *Curr Opin Pulm Med* 2003;**9**:385–392.

67. Lamirel C, Bruce BB, Wright DW, Newman NJ, Biousse V. Non-mydriatic digital ocular fundus photography on the iPhone 3G: The PHOTO-ED study. *Arch Opthalmol* 2012;**130**(7):939–940.

68. Bidot S, Bruce BB, Newman NJ, Biousse V. Nonmydriatic retinal photography in the evaluation of acute neurological conditions. *Neurol Clin Pract* 2013;**1**:527–531.

69. Bruce BB, Thulasi P, Fraser CL, et al. Diagnostic accuracy and use of nonmydriatic ocular fundus photography by emergency physicians: phase II of the PHOTO-ED study. *Ann Emerg Med* 2013;**62**(1):28–33.

70. Caplan LR. The neurological examination. In M Fisher, J Bogousslavsky (eds), *Textbook of Neurology*. Boston: Butterworth–Heinemann, 1998, pp 3–18.

71. Heir D, Mondlock J, Caplan LR. Behavioral deficits after right hemisphere stroke. *Neurology* 1983;**33**:337–344.

72. Caplan LR, Bogousslavsky J. Abnormalities of the right cerebral hemisphere. In J Bogousslavsky, LR Caplan (eds), *Stroke Syndromes*. Cambridge: Cambridge University Press, 1995, pp 162–168.

73. Caplan LR. The patient with reduced consciousness or coma. In J Skillman (ed), *Intensive Care*. Boston: Little, Brown, 1975, pp 559–567.

74. Posner J, Saper CB, Schiff N, Plum F. *Plum and Posner's Diagnosis of Stupor and Coma.* New York: Oxford University Press, 2007.

75. Young GB, Ropper AH, Bolton CFB. *Coma and Impaired Consciousness: A Clinical Perspective.* New York: McGraw-Hill, 1998.

76. Fisher CM. The neurologic examination of the comatose patient. *Acta Neurol Scand* 1969;**45**(suppl 36):1–56.

77. Mohr J, Rubinstein L, Kase C, et al. Gaze palsy in hemispheral stroke: the NINCDS Stroke Data Bank. *Neurology* 1984;**34**:199.

78. Savitz S, Caplan LR. Current concepts: Vertebrobasilar disease. *N Engl J Med* 2005;**352**:2618–2626.

79. Newman-Toker DE, Katah JC, Alvernia JE, Wang DZ. Normal head impulse test differentiates acute cerebellar strokes from vestibular neuritis. *Neurology* 2008;**70**:2378–2385.

80. Kattah JC, Talkad AV, Wang DZ, Hsieh YH, Newman-Toker DE. Hints to diagnose stroke in the acute vestibular syndrome: Three-step bedside oculomotor examination more sensitive than early MRI diffusion-weighted imaging. *Stroke.* 2009;**40**(11):3504–3510.

81. Caplan LR, Schmahmann JD, Kase CS, et al. Caudate infarcts. *Arch Neurol* 1990;**47**:133–143.

82. Mendez MF, Adams NL, Skoog-Lewandowski K. Neurobehavioral changes associated with caudate lesions. *Neurology* 1989;**39**:349–354.

83. Caplan LR. Caudate infarct. In G Donnan, B Norrving, J Bamford, J Bogousslavsky (eds), *Subcortical Stroke*, 2nd edn. Oxford: Oxford University Press, 2002, pp 209–223.

84. Ghoshal S, Gokhale S, Rebovich G, Caplan LR. The neurology of decreased activity: Abulia. *Rev Neurol Dis* 2011;**8**:e55–67.

85. Graff-Radford NR, Eslinger PJ, Damasio AR, et al. Nonhemorrhage infarction of the thalamus: Behavioral, anatomic and physiologic correlates. *Neurology* 1984;**34**:14–23.

86. Bogousslavsky J, Regli F, Uske A. Thalamic infarcts: Clinical syndromes, etiology, and prognosis. *Neurology* 1988;**38**:837–848.

87. Barth A, Bogousslavsky J, Caplan LR. Thalamic infarcts and hemorrhages. In J Bogousslavsky, LR Caplan (eds), *Stroke Syndromes*, 2nd edn. Cambridge: Cambridge University Press, 2001, pp 461–468.

88. Eslinger PJ, Reichwein RK. Frontal lobe stroke syndromes. In J Bogousslavsky, LR Caplan (eds), *Stroke Syndromes*, 2nd edn. Cambridge: Cambridge University Press, 2001, pp 232–241.

89. Fisher CM. Honored guest presentation: Abulia minor vs. agitated behavior. *Clin Neurosurg* 1983;**31**:9–31.

Chapter

4

Imaging and laboratory diagnosis

Louis R Caplan, Bruce Campbell, and Stephen Davis

Having reviewed the basic elements on which diagosis is based and the preliminary diagnostic impressions from the clinical encounter, we now turn to imaging and laboratory testing. These investigations should be planned to test, confirm, and elaborate on the hypotheses of stroke mechanism and anatomical localization generated from the clinical encounter. A shotgun approach to testing is discouraged. Instead, an individualized and eclectic program of tests should be tailored to the individual patient's problems. Whenever possible, tests should be selected and interpreted sequentially. Results of the initial investigations should be used to help determine the next steps in testing.

In this chapter, we consider various tests in relation to the following series of questions that clinicians should ask sequentially:

1. Is the brain lesion(s) caused by ischemia or hemorrhage, or is it related to a non-vascular stroke mimic?
2. Where is the brain lesion(s)? What is its size, shape, and extent?
3. What are the nature, site, and severity of the vascular lesion(s), and how do the vascular lesion(s) and brain perfusion abnormalities relate to the brain lesion(s)?
4. Are abnormalities of blood constituents causing or contributing to brain ischemia or hemorrhage?
5. Is the patient with stroke or transient neurological deficits having seizures?

6. Are there genetic abnormalities that might clarify the etiology of the cerebrovascular disease and potentially guide treatment of the patient and prevention or management of relatives?

With these questions in mind, we continue to follow JH, the 36-year-old patient with left hemiparesis introduced in Chapter 3, as he proceeds through the diagnostic laboratory tests.

Question 1: Is the brain lesion(s) caused by ischemia or hemorrhage, or is it related to a non-vascular stroke mimic?

Computed tomography

In JH, the most likely stroke mechanism diagnoses after the clinical encounter are large-artery occlusive disease and cardiogenic brain embolism, with infarction of the frontal and central regions of the right cerebral hemisphere. Hemorrhage from an unusual cause and even non-stroke etiologies are much less likely but possible causes. The next step is a brain-imaging procedure that allows the clinician to distinguish among these possibilities. A computed tomography (CT) scan in this patient (Figure 4.1A) shows a large, hypodense lesion in the right cerebral hemisphere. This clearly identifies the process as ischemic. A non-vascular lesion such as a brain tumor or abscess large enough to

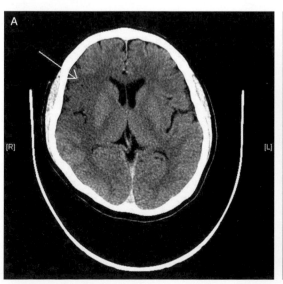 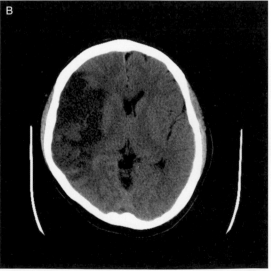

Figure 4.1 CT non-enhanced scans. (A) Recent large infarct (white arrow) involving the right MCA territory of the cerebral cortex and underlying white matter. (B) Very well-demarcated infarct shown on CT scan taken 36 hours after onset. There is edema surrounding the infarct and mass effect on the ipsilateral lateral ventricle.

Caplan's Stroke: A Clinical Approach, 5th Edition, ed. Louis R Caplan. Published by Cambridge University Press. © Cambridge University Press, 2016.

Table 4.1 CT abnormalities in patients with acute brain ischemia

Loss of distinction between gray and white matter (indicating irreversible injury)
- Obscuring of basal ganglia density
- Loss of definition of the insular cortex

Sulcal effacement/early swelling (reversible)

Hypodensity within the infarcted zone

Hyperdense arteries indicating thrombosis

Calcific emboli within arteries

cause a hemiplegia would usually be visible on CT. The lesion shown conforms well to the middle cerebral artery (MCA) territory and involves the surface and depth in a triangular configuration quite typical for infarction. CT scans taken at a later time after brain infarction show more clearly demarcated hypodensity and surrounding edema and mass effect if the infarcts are large (Figure 4.1B).

CT is readily available in most hospitals and can reliably show intracerebral hemorrhage (ICH). Immediately after the onset of bleeding, intracerebral hematomas are seen on CT as well-circumscribed areas of high density with smooth borders.[1] Sequential scans in some patients have shown continued bleeding with enlargement of the hematomas in later scans. Occasionally, a blood-fluid level is seen within acute hematomas. Edema develops within the first days and is seen as a dark rim around the white hematoma. As absorption of blood proceeds, the white image becomes more irregular and hypodense, and edema subsides. Ring enhancement of the outer dark zone may occur and may remain evident for weeks after the bleeding. In patients with low hematocrits, or those scanned initially weeks after stroke onset, hematomas can appear as solely hypodense lesions.

When the mechanism is ischemic, CT may show infarction as a low-density lesion or may initially remain normal. The early ischemic changes on CT scans can be quite subtle in the first few hours of the onset of symptoms.[1-3] Table 4.1 lists the key diagnostic signs. Newer-generation helical CT scanners yield images in a very short time and provide clearer images and are better able to show these early signs than older generation scanners. Viewing the images on a computer with the ability to vary the contrast also helps identify subtle abnormalities and asymmetries.

Subarachnoid hemorrhage (SAH) is not as reliably diagnosed by CT, especially if the bleeding is minor or has occurred days previously. Increased density is in the cerebrospinal fluid (CSF) adjacent to bone. Visualization depends more on the hematocrit (Hct) in the CSF than on the iron content.[4] Because contrast infusions make this meningeal area bright on CT, SAH is particularly difficult to diagnose if there has not been an unenhanced scan. In those circumstances when SAH is suspected from the clinical findings of headache and restlessness, lumbar puncture (LP) with spectrophotometry for xanthochromia is needed to confirm or exclude SAH.[5,6]

Magnetic resonance imaging

MRI shows tomographic sections in multiple planes of proton distribution modified by spin-lattice (T1) and spin-spin (T2) relaxation time.[7,8] Ischemia alters water content in the affected region, prolonging the T1 and T2 relaxation constants and appears as a dark, hypointense region on T1-weighted sequences and as a bright, hyperintense lesion on T2-weighted images.[7,8] T1-weighted MRI images performed during the first day show infarcts as a loss of gray–white contrast and decreased image intensity (darkness). T2-weighted sequences show hyperintense bright foci of ischemia. During the next days, lesions become darker on T1-weighted and brighter on T2-weighted images.

Increased signal on T2-weighted images due to gliosis may be evident years after the stroke. T2 fluid-attenuated inversion recovery (FLAIR) images, which remove bright signal from CSF, improve the visual conspicuity of many cerebral lesions including stroke.[9]

MRI is far more sensitive than CT in detecting early ischemic changes. Diffusion-weighted imaging (DWI) is especially sensitive for detection of acute brain infarcts as it detects the extracellular-to-intracellular shift of water that occurs in cytotoxic edema, within minutes of stroke onset.[10-13] Infarcted areas are shown as bright on DWI and dark on apparent diffusion coefficient (ADC) images. DWI is diagnostically effective in both the anterior and posterior circulations.[10-14] Acute, small dot-like white matter, basal ganglionic, and cerebral cortical and cerebellar infarcts are readily shown on DWI images that are not detected on CT scans. The location, pattern, and multiplicity of DWI ischemic lesions can help in suggesting the causative stroke mechanism.[14-16] For example, a patient who presents with a left MCA infarct but also has a small DWI lesion in the contralateral hemisphere is likely to have a central embolic source, such as atrial fibrillation, which requires investigation. DWI positivity wanes during the first 7–10 days after stroke onset. Lesions seen on DWI images (and confirmed by ADC) usually correspond to areas of infarction but can also be seen in cerebral abscess, some hypercellular tumors and demyelinated plaques. If DWI is repeated soon after reperfusion of the stroke there can be a temporary "reversal" of the lesion which later reappears. True permanent reversal of ischemic diffusion lesions is rare.[17-19] T2-weighted scans show established infarcts as bright. Since DWI images contain some T2 weighting, infarcts that appear bright on T2-weighted images also look bright on DWI images. Care must be taken that the lesions on DWI do not represent the same lesions seen on T2-weighted scans – so-called T2 shine-through. In that circumstance, ADC images do not show a dark region concordant with the DWI + area and the clinician can conclude that the lesions are not hyperacute.

MRI can also accurately show ICH. The most sensitive technique is susceptibility-weighted imaging (SWI), which demonstrates blood products as hypointense.[20-24] The T2*-weighted (gradient recalled echo) sequence can also show thrombi within intracranial arteries and dural sinuses and veins[25] and cerebral microbleeds. Microbleeds can be due to

Table 4.2 Imaging findings in patients with ICH at various stages

Stage	CT	T2*	T1	T2
Hyperacute	Bright	Dark	If detectable, dark	If detectable, bright with dark rim
Acute	Bright	Dark	Isodense	Dark
Subacute	Isodense	Dark	Bright	Dark (early); bright (late)
Chronic	Dark	Dark	Dark	Dark

Note: Dark refers to low signal, and bright to high signal.
Adapted from Bui JD, Caplan LR. Magnetic resonance imaging in intracerebral hemorrhage. *Semin Cerebrovasc Dis Stroke* 2005;5:172–177.

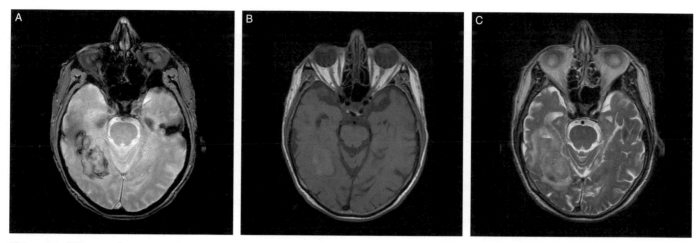

Figure 4.2 MRI scans of a patient with an acute right temporal lobe hemorrhage. (A) Gradient-recalled echo (T2*-weighted) scan, (B) T1-weighted scan, and (C) T2-weighted scan.

hypertensive injury, amyloid angiopathy or trauma and are also common in patents with infective endocarditis. The pattern of microbleeds can provide a clue to the etiology of ICH as discussed below. The appearances of ICH on other MR sequences depends on the duration of time since the bleed, and the choice of MRI technique.[7,8,20–24,26]

Hemoglobin derivatives have paramagnetic effects. The imaging appearance depends on the nature of the compound, oxyhemoglobin, methemoglobin, hemosiderin, or ferritin. The appearance on MRI is also dependent on whether the hemoglobin-derived substances are present inside cells or in the interstitial extracellular spaces. During the first 12 hours after intracerebral bleeding, hematomas contain mostly oxyhemoglobin, which is not paramagnetic. The hematoma appearance during that time reflects mostly protein and water content. On T1-weighted images, the acute hematoma appears as isointense or slightly hypointense (dark), with a surrounding hypointense darker rim. T2-weighted images are often hyperintense (bright), reflecting water content. Between 12 and 48 hours after the onset of hemorrhage, deoxyhemoglobin is formed within extravascular red blood cells (RBCs), especially within the depth of the hematoma.

Figure 4.2 shows various MRI sequences of an acute ICH. During the next week, oxidation to methemoglobin occurs, beginning at the periphery of the lesion. By day 5 or 6, T1-weighted images show a central area of bright signal due to short T1, and a darker signal around the hematoma due to edema. On T2-weighted images, the center often becomes dark and is surrounded by bright images. Chronic bleeds contain hemosiderin within macrophages and tissues and show as dark, hypointense areas on T2-weighted images.[26] Table 4.2 reviews the MRI findings in patients with hematomas at various times after bleeding. Figure 4.3 shows a left thalamic hematoma imaged by CT and MRI.

Patients with aneurysmal SAH are not easy to study by MRI. Restless, ill patients often have difficulty holding still for the time required to produce high-quality images. The relaxation times of blood admixed with CSF approximate the signal from normal brain parenchyma, especially in T1-weighted images. T2 images often do show a bright signal. T2 FLAIR images are highly sensitive to SAH as a bright signal adjacent to the nulled, low-signal-intensity CSF.[23,27]

Computed tomography versus magnetic resonance imaging

Brain imaging has become an absolutely integral part of the evaluation of all patients with cerebrovascular disease. Stroke is such a potentially devastating disease that clinicians need all of the objective data available to prognosticate, diagnose, and treat individual stroke patients. CT and MRI are non-invasive and safe, and new-generation scanners produce an enormous

amount of clinically useful information. For urgent diagnosis, CT is far more readily available in most emergency departments. However, MRI has advantages in sensitivity to small infarcts and in elucidating underlying pathology. Either a CT or an MRI scan should be performed as an emergency investigation in all stroke patients. In many centers, an emergent CT scan will be followed by an MRI in the next few days to provide additional diagnostic information. Table 4.3 lists the advantages of CT scanning while Table 4.4 lists the disadvantages.

CT and MRI results depend on the time of the scan in relation to the clinical event. In patients with ischemia, early CT scans are often normal or contain only subtle abnormalities. Careful windowing to maximize gray–white contrast and a systematic approach in reviewing scans (e.g., using the Alberta Stroke Program Early CT Score – ASPECTS[28]) can improve sensitivity. However, agreement between different clinicians on the presence and extent of these changes is at best modest. Fortunately, subtle loss of gray–white differentiation is not a contraindication to thrombolysis. During the first days after stroke onset, infarcts are usually round or oval and have poorly defined margins. Later, infarcts become more hypodense and dark, and are more wedge-like and circumscribed. Contrast enhancement of infarcts can occur and sometimes makes differentiation from tumor difficult if presentation is delayed. Some infarcts that had been hypodense become isodense during Weeks 2 and 3 after stroke onset. This so-called fogging effect may obscure the lesion for some time.[1,29] Later, infarcts become hypodense again. Edema also begins to develop within the first days in patients with large infarcts. Edema is manifested by low density surrounding the lesion and mass effect with displacement of adjacent structures.

MRI is the investigation of choice for patients with transient ischemic attacks (TIAs). The earliest imaging abnormality in ischemia is detected by diffusion-weighted MRI, followed some hours later by T2 FLAIR hyperintensity. Despite the fact that a patient clinically has had a TIA and has no residual symptoms or signs at the time of brain imaging, scans often show a brain infarct. These lesions are now regarded as small strokes, despite rapid resolution of symptoms within 24 hours. Nicolaides and colleagues studied 149 patients with hemispheral TIAs and found that 48% had an infarct on CT, most often in the symptomatic hemisphere.[30] MRI is clearly more sensitive than CT in detecting infarcts in patients with clinical "TIAs." Inatomi and colleagues studied 129 consecutive TIA patients.[31] The mean time from TIA to MRI was 4.7 ± 2.6 days. Fifty-seven patients (44%) had DWI lesions appropriate to the TIA symptoms. TIA duration of more than 30 minutes and a higher cortical function abnormality during the TIA

Table 4.3 Advantages of CT scanning in stroke patients

At present, CT is more readily available. It is generally easier to obtain an acute CT scan in most hospitals than an urgent MRI

CT is less expensive than MRI

CT imaging and its interpretation are much less dependent than MRI on selection of technique and filming planes. More experience with CT interpretation makes these scans easier to read by most clinicians who are not stroke neurologists or neuroradiologists

CT scans of ICH are easier to interpret than MRI scans and, in most circumstances, yield adequate data for clinical decision making without the need for MRI scanning

CT images subarachnoid blood as well as MRI, and the shorter scanning time of CT is important in restless patients whom you do not want to heavily sedate

Table 4.4 Disadvantages of CT scanning in stroke patients

CT is not as sensitive as MRI in detecting and imaging acute brain infarcts

CT is not accurate in delineating lesions adjacent to bony surfaces (e.g., in the orbital, frontal poles, and temporal lobes). CT is quite inferior to MRI in imaging brainstem and cerebellar infarcts

CT is not useful in detecting and delineating spinal cord infarcts

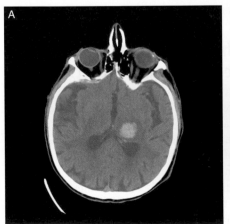
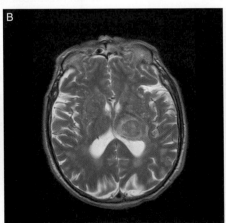
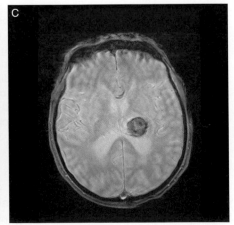

Figure 4.3 Acute left thalamic ICH imaged by (A) CT scan, (B) T2-weighted MRI scan, and (C) T2* (GRE) MRI scan.

predicted the presence of DWI lesions.[31] Winbeck et al. analyzed signal intensity on DWI and hypodensity on ADC maps to separate TIAs that showed positivity on DWI and strokes.[32] Stroke patients had an increased signal on b-1000 DWI images and a reduced intensity on ADC maps compared with DWI-positive TIA patients.[32]

Lamy and colleagues analyzed how often DWI abnormalities found in TIA patients resolved, and how often they represented brain infarction.[33] They showed that 76% of 59 brain ischemic lesions identified in patients who had clinical TIAs represented regions of brain infarction.[33] They confirmed that the TIA-related ADC decrease was moderate when compared to stroke patients, and that ADC values measured in the core of the lesion were quite predictive of long-term brain tissue outcome.[33]

When brain infarcts in an appropriate location to explain symptoms are found on DWI in patients who have clinical TIAs, the frequency of recurrent brain ischemia is higher than if no infarcts are shown.[34-38] Infarcts on DWI of different ages are particularly indicative of a high risk of recurrent brain ischemia.[37,38] If the infarcts are in different vascular territories then brain embolism from a central (cardiac or aortic) source is the likely mechanism. When various infarcts of different ages are in the same vascular territory, a proximal large-artery occlusive lesion is likely.

Two other considerations heavily affect the choice of CT versus MR brain imaging – whether the patient is a candidate for thrombolysis, and whether vascular imaging will also be performed acutely. If the patient is a potential candidate for thrombolysis, time is crucial. The availability of emergent CT or MRI will decide which to choose. In the great majority of stroke patients, a study that shows the cervico-cranial arteries should be performed concurrent with brain imaging. The need, availability, and feasibility of vascular imaging should also guide the choice of CT versus MRI. Magnetic resonance angiography (MRA) images are readily obtainable at the same time as MRI brain imaging. Time-of-flight MRA does not require contrast infusion. Computed tomography angiography (CTA) requires intravenous contrast that can be a problem in patients with allergy to the contrast and in those with severely reduced kidney function.

In JH, by the time that the patient was seen, 5 hours had elapsed since symptom onset, outside the current 4.5-hour time window for thrombolysis. MR scanning was not readily available and there were no contraindications to CTA. CT showed the infarct quite well and had indicated without a doubt that the lesion was ischemic. The established hypodensity within the stroke and the time that had already elapsed indicted that he was not a candidate for thrombolysis.

Lumbar puncture

Lumbar puncture (LP), introduced into clinical medicine by Quincke in 1891, is still an important diagnostic test. LP is especially important in the diagnosis and management of patients with SAH, and in patients in whom an infectious cause of stroke is suspected. CT and MRI are not particularly sensitive tests for the detection of SAH, especially if bleeding is minor in degree and occurred days before scanning. The accuracy of CT in documenting subarachnoid blood diminishes after 24 hours.[6,39] Large SAHs are often preceded by small warning leaks that are easily overlooked by CT but readily diagnosed by LP. By definition, subarachnoid blood rapidly disseminates and is present in the lumbar theca within minutes. The absence of blood on LP excludes the diagnosis of SAH. When blood is present, the quantity of blood and the pressure of CSF can also be measured and followed by later spinal taps.

Counting the number of erythrocytes in the first and third or fourth tubes of CSF, measurement of the CSF Hct, and spectrophotometric analysis of the CSF give an accurate quantitative database. When RBCs lyse, oxyhemoglobin is released into the CSF, reaches a maximum level in approximately 36 hours, and gradually disappears between days 7 and 10.[40-43] Bilirubin is first detectable approximately 10 hours after SAH, reaches a maximum at 48 hours, and persists for approximately 2–4 weeks after large hemorrhages. Oxyhemoglobin and methemoglobin are detected at maximal light-absorption peaks at 415 μm on spectrophotometry. The bilirubin peak is approximately 460 μm.[42,43] Sequential LPs with measurement of CSF pressure, the quantity of blood, and the relative quantities of oxyhemoglobin and bilirubin help to determine the time since the last bleeding and can show evidence of fresh bleeding.

The presence of visible xanthochromia in the CSF can also be helpful, although formal spectrophotometry is far more sensitive and should be routinely performed.[42] The CSF collected in a test tube should be spun down quickly in a centrifuge and the supernatant held up against a white piece of paper for comparison to determine if there is a yellowish tint to the fluid. It takes a few hours for the CSF to become xanthochromic after a bleed. A very high CSF protein level can also render the CSF xanthochromic. In the absence of a very high protein content, the presence of xanthochromia indicates that there is a substantial number of RBCs within the subarachnoid space – either due to a SAH or a traumatic spinal tap.

Question 2: Where is the brain lesion(s)? What is its size, shape, and extent?

The next important questions that the clinician must ask concern the characteristics of the brain lesion found. Where is the lesion? How large is it? What is its extent? What is the effect of the lesion on intracranial structures? Does the location and characteristics of this lesion correlate well with the clinical findings and explain the patient's symptoms and signs? Are there other lesions, and if so, do they have similar or different characteristics from the symptomatic lesion?

Having differentiated ischemia from hemorrhage and from stroke mimics, the clinician needs to know more about the

lesion to predict the most likely stroke mechanism, localize the underlying vessels involved, prognosticate the probable future course, and select optimal treatment. The laboratory answers to the delineation of the morphology of the brain process usually come from neuroimaging with CT or MRI or both. Diffusion-weighted MRI scans are especially helpful when patients are tested soon after stroke onset.

Perfusion CT or MR can be helpful in localization of the fundamental abnormality in the brain in some patients in whom the results of standard CT and MRI scans are normal or incompletely explain the clinical presentation. Clinicians are fortunate to have available clinical data from the neurological examination before brain imaging. Having already made hypotheses about lesion localization, clinicians can match these hypotheses with the imaging results. Does the location of the lesion(s) on CT or MRI explain the clinical signs? Could the lesion(s) be asymptomatic, incidental findings not related to the recent event? Are the clinical signs more severe than would be expected from the imaging studies? A discrepancy might indicate that some tissue, although not morphologically damaged enough to show on scans, is not functioning normally. Davalos and colleagues have dubbed this discrepancy a clinical–imaging mismatch.[44]

What if the lesion is an infarct?

Brain ischemia occurs in 80% of stroke patients. In these patients, CT or MRI does not show a hematoma. Hemorrhagic stippling (hemorrhagic infarction) may be present. Analysis of the neuroimaging findings should allow useful information about the lesion location and morphology. In JH, the lesion shown on CT scan was clearly a brain infarct (see Figure 4.1).

What vascular territory is involved?

Identification of the arteries and or veins supplying an area of symptomatic infarction is the first step toward identifying the causative vascular lesion. Ultrasound and vascular imaging tests can then be planned to show the vascular structures involved. Once a plumber has pinpointed a blocked sink, the plumber can examine the water tank, the pump, and the pipes that lead to that blocked region, knowing that mischief must be located within the water delivery system. In 36-year-old JH with left hemiparesis, CT has shown an infarct that involves the deep and superficial territory of the right MCA. Infarction is present above and below the sylvian fissure. The responsible vascular lesion must involve the vascular tree proximal to the origin of the lenticulostriate arteries, which supply the deep territory that is infarcted. These vessels branch from the mainstem of the MCA. The vascular process probably involves the proximal right MCA. Possibilities from viewing only the imaging data include: (1) in-situ occlusive disease of the right MCA; (2) cardiogenic embolism to the MCA; (3) an intra-arterial embolus from the aorta, right common carotid artery, or right internal carotid artery (ICA); and (4) propagation of clot or embolism from the intracranial portion of the right ICA.

Suppose that the infarct had involved the paramedian frontal lobe cortex in the supply region of the anterior cerebral artery (ACA), in addition to the MCA territory. Clearly, the vascular process would then have had to originate proximal to the ICA intracranial bifurcation into the ACA and MCA. Similarly, within the posterior circulation, the location of infarction yields important clues to the location of the vascular process. In a patient with quadriparesis, MRI shows an infarct in the paramedian basis pontis bilaterally. Careful scrutiny of the films also shows a small infarct in the right cerebellum in the territory of the anterior inferior cerebellar artery (AICA), which originates from the lower to midportion of the basilar artery. The lesion must involve the basilar artery proximal to the AICA branches. The vascular process could be an insitu occlusive lesion within the basilar artery or an embolus to this region arising from the heart, the aorta, the innominate or subclavian arteries, or the cervical or intracranial portion of one of the vertebral arteries. If the cerebellar lesion had involved the posterior inferior cerebellar artery territory, the clinician would know that the vascular lesion must have affected the intracranial vertebral artery from which the posterior inferior cerebellar artery branches.

Knowledge of vascular distribution and supply is essential to localizing the vascular abnormality. Chapter 2 includes diagrams and descriptions of the vascular territories and examples of anterior circulation infarct distributions (see Figures 2.11–2.17, 2.35, 2.36).

How large is the infarct?

The size of the lesion is helpful in prognosis. Although the severity of the clinical deficit is not always directly proportional to infarct size, large lesions in the same anatomical area cause more severe deficits than small lesions in the same location. The infarct size, as shown on CT or MRI, should be matched in the clinician's mind with the size of the vascular territory involved. The non-infarcted tissue (entire vascular territory minus the infarct) represents the tissue at risk for further ischemia. To determine the at-risk tissue, the vascular lesion must be known. For example, a small infarct in the territorial supply of a lenticulostriate branch might represent the entire supply of that small penetrating branch. If the vascular lesion were in the MCA proximal to that lenticulostriate branch, a large area of brain tissue would still be at risk for spread of the ischemic damage. Diffusion-weighted and perfusion MRI studies and perfusion CT scanning can give more direct information about the brain tissue at risk for infarction by a given vascular lesion. When the perfusion defect is larger than the diffusion-weighted zone of infarction, the remainder of the brain showing the perfusion deficit is at imminent risk if blood flow to that zone is not improved.

Large lesions often exert mass effect and displace normal intracranial contents, especially if edema develops. Large lesions are also more often accompanied by a reduced level of alertness. Mass effect and stupor often dictate treatment strategies aimed at these problems. Large infarcts also represent a relative contraindication for anticoagulant treatment because brain hemorrhages develop much more often in large infarcts than in small ones.

Does the location and extent of the infarct correlate with the clinical findings? Are other ischemic lesions present?

Clinicians should decide if the lesion found on brain imaging is appropriate to the patient's clinical symptoms and signs. In JH, the right cerebral hemisphere lesion explains quite well his left hemiplegia. A lesion in the left cerebral hemisphere or cerebellum would not have correlated with the clinical findings. In the case of JH, the clinicians could be quite confident that the symptomatic lesion was identified. In some other patients – especially those with TIAs or minor clinical symptoms and signs, and those patients with minor or equivocal brain-imaging findings – it may be more difficult to determine if a brain-imaging lesion relates to the clinical findings. It is also useful to match the extent of the infarct with the severity of the neurological deficit. When the clinical findings outweigh the brain-imaging lesion, there may be considerable brain tissue that is not functioning normally but is not yet infarcted. This "stunned" brain often retains the ability to return to normal when reperfused.

Many patients have brain infarcts that do not relate to their symptoms. These so-called "silent infarcts" are common;[45] in these patients, clinical manifestations were absent, minor, or forgotten. The presence of silent and symptomatic infarcts can yield clues as to the mechanism of the present symptomatic infarction. Guilt by association – identification by the company it keeps – is an important, but by no means an infallible, strategy. For example, suppose that a patient is admitted with a pure motor hemiparesis involving his left limbs. CT and MRI do not show a lesion involving the right descending corticospinal system, but five small lacunes in other regions are noted. The likelihood is high that the symptomatic vascular process is also lacunar infarction. Data from the Lausanne Stroke Registry indicates that 62% of recurrent strokes have the same stroke mechanism as the first stroke.[46] If CT or MRI shows multiple scattered cortical infarcts in different vascular territories, then cardiogenic embolism, multiple large-artery occlusive disease, and a hypercoagulable state are the most likely stroke mechanisms.

Are edema or mass effect present?

Edema can develop around infarcts and may even be potentiated by reperfusion of a blocked artery.[47] Sometimes the zone of actual infarction is quite small, but the surrounding edema zone is large. In young patients, edema may be more threatening than in older patients in whom brain atrophy might allow room for brain expansion. Displacement of midline structures,[48,49] effacement of gyri, encroachment on cisternal spaces, and brainstem displacement can often be judged well on diagnostic-quality CT and MRI scans.

What is the age of the infarct?

There are some general rules for identifying the age of an ischemic lesion. In the beginning of this chapter, we noted some sequential changes that occur in brain infarcts. On CT, well-defined borders, severe hypodensity, and shrinkage of the infarcted brain region all suggest a chronic infarct that is months old. Poor definition from the surrounding brain, edema, mass effect, and contrast enhancement all suggest an acute process. In practice, however, these rules are not often as helpful as clinicians would like them to be. Diffusion-weighted images usually only show bright signal in infarcts that are less than 1-week old. The age of brain infarcts can be estimated by analyzing the lesion characteristics using DWI, ADC, and FLAIR MRI sequences.[37,50]

Usually, the history gives the clinician a relatively accurate time of reference. Surprisingly, some acute lesions quickly become well delineated and defined and appear on brain images to be older than they actually are. Also, lesions that are months old are not appreciably different on imaging than those that are years old.

What if the imaging lesion represents an intracerebral hemorrhage?

Does the location provide a clue as to etiology of the hemorrhage?

Chapter 2 described and illustrated (Figure 2.34) the usual locations of hypertensive brain hemorrhages. These are usually deep and are most often located in the lateral ganglionic region, subcortex, thalamus, caudate nucleus, pons, and cerebellum. In a hypertensive patient with a hematoma confined to one of these regions, the likelihood of an etiology other than hypertension is relatively low. Angiography in patients with hypertension and deep hematomas has a low yield for showing aneurysms, arteriovenous malformations (AVMs), or other vascular lesions. However, CTA is non-invasive and has a relevant yield up to 15% in some studies.[51,52] An MRI performed 6–8 weeks after onset is often helpful to exclude underlying vascular or neoplastic lesions once the initial hematoma has substantially resolved. MRI susceptibility-weighted imaging can also provide clues to etiology as hypertensive bleeds are often associated with a predominance of microbleeds in the basal ganglia whereas amyloid angiopathy leads to a predominance of microbleeds in lobar regions close to the cerebral cortex.

Hematomas resulting from aneurysms, so-called meningocerebral bleeds, are invariably contiguous to the aneurysms at the brain base or surface. In amyloid angiopathy, hemorrhages are lobar, often multiple, and can be accompanied by small infarcts.[53,54] Anticoagulant-related ICHs are most often lobar or cerebellar, evolve gradually, and enlarge.[55,56] AVMs may be located anywhere in the brain, especially in subependymal locations. Calcifications and heterogeneity within the hematoma raise suspicion of an underlying AVM.

How large is the hematoma?

Is there mass effect? By definition, a hematoma represents an extra volume of material in the cranium. Mass effect is more common and more serious in hematomas than in brain infarction. Large size (e.g., >60 ml) correlates with poor outcome in hematomas at any location and the volume can be readily calculated by clinicians using the ABC/2 method.[57] In this method, a representative slice at the center of the hematoma

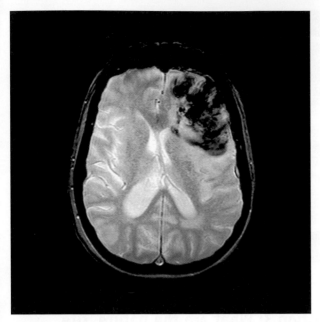

Figure 4.4 T2* (GRE) MRI scan showing a large left frontal hemorrhage with surrounding edema and mass effect.

is first selected. The maximum linear length (A) in centimeters is multiplied by the maximum width (B) in centimeters and the maximum depth (C) in centimeters. The depth (C) is determined by multiplying the number of slices in which the hematoma is seen by the slice thickness listed on the CT scan. To obtain the volume in cubic centimeters (cm³) the volume is divided by two.[57] Both mass effect and displacement of adjacent structures are readily analyzed on CT and MRI images. Figure 4.4 is an MRI scan that shows a large ICH with mass effect.

Is there a spot sign?

ICH is a dynamic process. Most patients show some degree of hematoma expansion, if studied acutely (within 3 h of symptom onset) and then again at 24 hours. Significant hematoma enlargement (defined as >6 ml or more than 1/3 of the original volume) is an independent risk factor for mortality and poor functional outcome. Density heterogeneity on non-contrast CT has also been associated with hematoma expansion. A major recent imaging finding was the recognition of the "spot sign," shown on CTA.[58] The spot sign is a unifocal or multifocal region of contrast enhancement within an acute primary ICH that is visible on CTA source images and discontinuous from adjacent normal or abnormal blood vessels. It should not be present on pre-contrast images. It corresponds to sites of active, dynamic hemorrhage and is a signature of active bleeding in ICH. Patients with the spot sign have a far greater risk of hematoma expansion.[59] The finding of the spot sign may indicate a potential role for intravenous hemostatic therapy.

Does the hematoma drain into the cerebrospinal fluid?

Is the hemorrhage causing hydrocephalus? Hematomas decompress themselves by draining into the CSF on the surface of the brain and into the ventricular system. Intraventricular hemorrhage is an adverse prognostic factor, together with hematoma volume, age, decreased level of consciousness, and location of the hematoma. Infratentorial ICH has a worse prognosis than supratentorial bleeds.

The mass effect produced by the hematoma and blood within the ventricular system can obstruct the flow of CSF. Blockage of the ventricular system is most common at the foramen of Munro (putaminal bleeds) and at the level of the IIIrd (thalamic hemorrhage) and IVth ventricle (cerebellar hemorrhage). Dilatation of the ventricular system (hydrocephalus) augments the mass effect of the hematoma and is often amenable to surgical decompression by temporary drainage or permanent shunting of CSF.

What if imaging studies show subarachnoid hemorrhage?

Where is the blood?

Where is the blood located? Blood may accumulate around a bleeding aneurysm or in the adjacent subarachnoid spaces and cisterns, thus yielding a clue as to the site of bleeding. Blood in the suprasellar cisterns and frontal interhemispheric fissure predicts an anterior communicating artery aneurysm.[60,61] Blood localized predominantly in one sylvian fissure suggests an MCA bifurcation aneurysm on that side.[60,61] Thick blood in the pontine and cerebellopontine angle cisterns predicts a posterior fossa aneurysm. Since the early 1980s, van Gijn and colleagues have identified a pattern of perimesencephalic hemorrhage that does not seem to reflect aneurysmal rupture and has a benign prognosis.[62–64] Focal "convexal" SAH is an interesting entity that deserves mention. In elderly patients convexal subarachnoid bleeding is most often a manifestation of amyloid angiopathy and usually presents with "TIA"-like symptoms in the absence of headache.[65] A detailed thorough history will often reveal a migratory quality to the symptoms and there are recurrent stereotyped events. Their significance lies in the high risk of subsequent amyloid-related ICH and the need to avoid antiplatelet agents that would otherwise be given for a TIA patient. Convexal SAH, particularly in younger patients, can be a manifestation of cortical vein thrombosis or reversible cerebral vasoconstriction syndrome.[65] Recognition of convexal SAH in an elderly patient generally obviates the need for catheter angiography, essential in all other patients with SAH.

How much bleeding has occurred generally or locally?

The thickness of blood on CT or MRI correlates roughly with the degree of bleeding. Figure 4.5A shows a CT scan with thick blood in the subarachnoid cisterns. Figure 4.5B is a CT scan that shows more focal subarachnoid bleeding after trauma. Large subarachnoid bleeds are more often complicated by hydrocephalus and delayed cerebral infarction owing to vasoconstriction than are smaller leaks. Vertical layers of blood clot more than 1 mm thick, or local clots larger than 5 mm in size are often associated with angiographically documented vasoconstriction and secondary ischemic

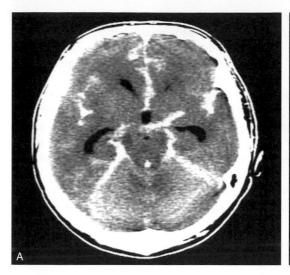
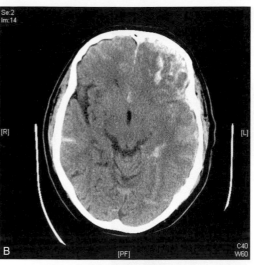

Figure 4.5 CT scans showing subarachnoid blood: (A) Diffuse white staining of the cisterns and subarachnoid space in a patient with SAH from a ruptured aneurysm, and (B) a left frontal contusion after trauma with prominent subarachnoid spread of blood especially seen in the left sulci.

complications.[66,67] Repeated LPs, washing away of the blood at the time of aneurysm surgery, and installation of thrombolytic agents such as recombinant tissue plasminogen activator (rt-PA), are strategies that have been used to deal with large subarachnoid bleeds.

In addition to the bleeding, do regions of infarction exist?

SAH is often complicated by vasoconstriction and delayed ischemic brain damage. Infarction is most often localized to the territory supplied by the artery harboring the aneurysm, but can be located elsewhere. The presence of acute ischemia clearly suggests that vasoconstriction is present. Widespread vasoconstriction can also produce a pattern of generalized brain ischemia without focal infarction. In brain imaging, this often has the appearance of diffuse brain edema.

Is hydrocephalus present?

Blood within the subarachnoid space can diminish the absorptive capability of the arachnoid granulations. Communicating hydrocephalus develops because CSF production exceeds absorption. In Figure 4.5A, the temporal horns of the lateral ventricles are dilated indicating early hydrocephalus. This complication can be managed by temporary or permanent CSF drainage or shunting.

What if CT and MRI show no acute brain lesions?

Normal neuroimaging is common in patients with transient ischemia. Although highly sensitive, even diffusion MRI may not detect some small infarcts, especially in the brainstem.[10–14,36,50] Transient reversal of DWI lesions can occur immediately following reperfusion. In patients who have only transient ischemia, or persistent ischemia without infarction, the clinical symptoms and signs provide clues as to localization. Detection of a potentially causative vascular lesion or perfusion abnormality that corresponds to the clinical localization is very strong evidence that the process is ischemic.

Question 3: What are the nature, site, and severity of the vascular lesion(s), and how do the vascular lesion(s) and brain perfusion abnormalities relate to the brain lesion(s)?

Having localized, characterized, and quantified the process in the brain, the clinician is now ready to identify the vascular lesion(s). The clinical findings and brain imaging results have usually narrowed down the vascular region of interest in the individual stroke patient. In patient JH, it is known that the vascular process must be within the right carotid artery system or lie more proximally in the heart, aorta, or innominate artery.

What if the stroke mechanism is ischemia?

Ultrasound

Although Christian Doppler discovered the principal idea that underlies ultrasound in 1842, the first clinically applicable devices used to study blood flow were not introduced until the early 1960s. During the 1970s, amplitude modulation and brightness-modulation (B-mode) pulse echo ultrasound were introduced into clinical examinations of the extracranial arteries to detect atherosclerotic changes. The duplex scanner that produced a B-mode image of the extracranial artery being insonated, combined with a pulsed Doppler spectrum analysis, was first introduced in 1979. During the 1980s, duplex scanning became widely used in clinics throughout the world as a means of detecting and quantifying disease of the carotid arteries. Since the early 1980s, major advances in computer technology and electronics have made ultrasound an important tool for identifying occlusive vascular lesions within the neck and basal intracranial cerebral arteries. Ultrasound energy is used to detect interfaces among structures of different densities and to detect moving targets such as RBCs. The ultrasonic

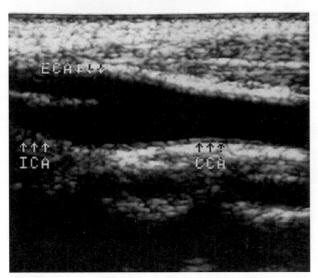

Figure 4.6 B-mode ultrasound of carotid artery bifurcation region. On the left is a small plaque near the origin of the ICA (white arrows). There is also a thin plaque in the common carotid artery (black arrows). CCA, common carotid artery; ECA, external carotid artery; ICA, internal carotid artery.

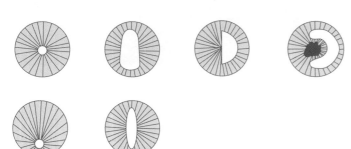

Figure 4.8 Transverse sections through various types of plaques. The plaque on the upper right has had an intramural hemorrhage. From Hennerici M, Steinke W. *Durchblutungsstorungen des Gehirns – Neue Diagnostische Moglichkeiten*. Gütersloh: Verlag Bertelsmann Stiftung, 1987 with permission.

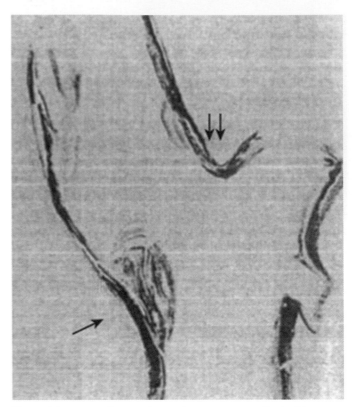

Figure 4.7 Picture of a stained carotid artery specimen: The double arrows point to the flow divider between the ICA on the left and the external carotid artery on the right. The single arrow points to a plaque in the characteristic location along the posterior wall of the ICA opposite the flow divider. From Hennerici M, Steinke W. *Durchblutungsstorungen des Gehirns – Neue Diagnostische Moglichkeiten*. Gütersloh: Verlag Bertelsmann Stiftung, 1987 with permission.

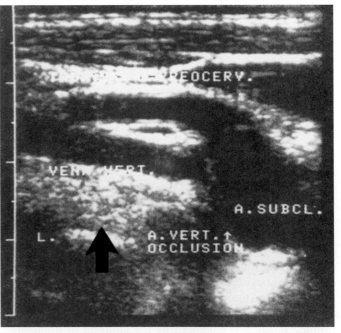

Figure 4.9 B-mode ultrasound figure that shows the subclavian artery on the right and the origin and proximal portion of the right VA that courses from right to left on the figure. The left VA is occluded (black arrow). The vascular structures above the occluded artery are the vertebral vein and the thyrocervical artery. From Caplan LR. *Posterior Circulation Disease: Clinical Findings, Diagnosis, and Management*. New York: Blackwell Science, 1996 with permission of Blackwell Publishing Ltd.

information is received through a probe or transducer held over the artery being studied, and the information is converted into electrical energy, either for developing an image or for generating Doppler curves of blood-flow velocity.

Brightness-modulation (B-mode) imaging

High-resolution B-mode ultrasound scanning of the neck provides images in several planes of the neck arteries. Figure 4.6 is a B-mode image of a carotid artery plaque. Figure 4.7 shows the usual location of atherosclerotic plaques that develop at the carotid bifurcation in the neck. Figure 4.8 shows a cartoon of transverse sections through various types of carotid artery plaques.

Advances in technology can show these lesions in different planes and allow three-dimensional reconstruction of the arterial lesions (see Figure 4.7). B-mode scanning is quite accurate at the carotid bifurcation in the neck and at the origin of the vertebral artery (VA) from the subclavian artery. Lesions higher in the neck and more proximally located are technically harder to image well. Figure 4.9 shows a B-mode image of an occluded VA.

B-mode is quite accurate in assessing the degree of luminal narrowing, in the identification of ulcerations and intraplaque

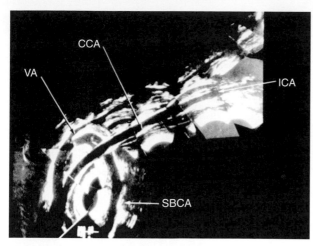

Figure 4.10 Composite B-mode ultrasound image shows the innominate artery and its subclavian, carotid, and VA branches in the neck. Courtesy of Burt Eikelboom, MD, and Rob Ackerstaf,f MD. CCA, common carotid artery; ICA, internal carotid artery; SBCA, subclavian artery; VA, vertebral artery. From Caplan LR. *Posterior Circulation Disease: Clinical Findings, Diagnosis, and Management.* New York: Blackwell Science, 1996 with permission of Blackwell Publishing Ltd.

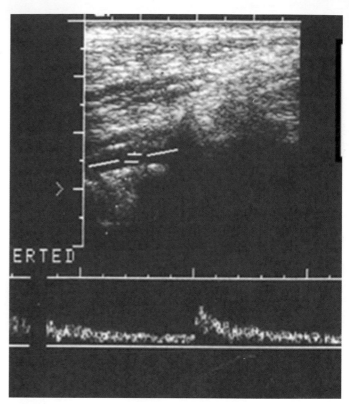

Figure 4.11 Duplex scan of a normal VA. Top panel shows a brightness modulation of the VA (white lines mark the lumen). Bottom panel shows the Doppler spectrum from this artery.

hemorrhages, and for delineating the gross surface-wall characteristics of the carotid arteries.[68,69] When compared with angiography and pathological study of the arteries at endarterectomy, B-mode generally has good sensitivity and specificity (80%) for detection of significant occlusive lesions.[70–73] Figure 4.10 is a composite B-mode ultrasound image that shows the great potential of the technique for imaging all of the major proximal cervical arteries. However, B-mode performed by itself has limitations. The large size of the ultrasound probe and sharp angulation of the arteries sometimes prevents adequate display of the vessels, especially at the VA origin. Calcifications and clots are not imaged. Soft, irregular, ulcerated plaques and firm, fibrous, or calcified plaques can often be characterized well. Echolucent plaques are usually rich in cholesterol[74] and are susceptible to reduction in size as well as progression. Calcified, hard echodense plaques in contrast usually do not change much with time.[74] Echolucent plaques with an irregular surface are more likely than echogenic plaques to progress and cause brain infarction.[71,73,75]

Thrombi within the arterial lumen can usually be detected using a combination of the Doppler flow spectra and B-mode ultrasound images. B-mode is quite accurate at separating normal arteries and those with minor plaques from those arteries with severe stenosing lesions (≥70% narrowed). More difficult is separation of arteries with severe preocclusive stenosis from those in whom the artery is occluded. Analysis of B-mode images also requires experience and familiarity with the vascular anatomy. Arteries can be misidentified, especially from analyzing only one view. Experience has shown that B-mode imaging is enhanced by the addition of multigated, pulsed-Doppler apparatus. The combined B-mode and Doppler diagnostic systems are called duplex systems. The pulsed-Doppler in this duplex system helps identify the arteries and orientation of B-mode images. The analysis of flow-velocity patterns by Doppler, recorded from different positions within

the arterial lumen, provides qualitative and quantitative information about hemodynamic changes. The B-mode images help show the location of the velocity changes. The duplex system offers advantages over either B-mode scanning or Doppler analysis alone. Figure 4.11 shows a duplex scan of a normal VA.

B-mode ultrasound can also be effective in measuring the diameters of the various components of the arterial wall. The intima-media thickness (IMT) can be accurately quantified and followed during sequential ultrasound examinations.[71,73] Thickening of the wall of the carotid artery has been shown to be a marker for systemic atherosclerosis.[71,73,76–78] Finding an increased IMT diameter might stimulate measures to better control atherosclerotic risk factors such as hypertension, smoking, diabetes, and hypercholesterolemia. B-mode imaging can also be performed by using a special probe applied to the posterior pharyngeal wall.[79,80] This transoral approach is useful in showing the pharyngeal carotid artery and diagnosing and monitoring carotid artery dissections.[79,80]

Doppler sonography systems

Continuous-wave and pulsed-Doppler systems

There are two main Doppler systems: continuous-wave (CW) Doppler measures an average velocity for blood moving through an artery or vein beneath the probe; pulsed-Doppler is range gated to measure the velocity of blood in small volumes at specific selected sites within the vessel lumen.[71,73] The CW Doppler device can readily determine mean-flow

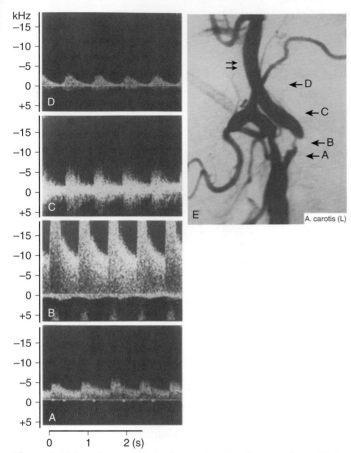

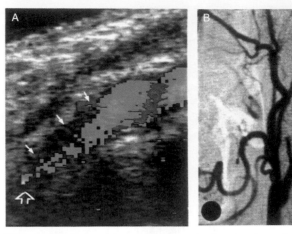

Figure 4.13 An image is shown from a color-flow Dopplar study of an ICA. (A) Blood flows from right-to-left. Blood flow in the image is red. The lumen is severely narrowed and flow is diminished (white open arrows) by an extensive atherosclerotic plaque (dark zone above the region of diminished flow to which small white arrows point). The image in (B) is a cerebral angiogram in the same patient that seems to show a complete occlusion of the artery (open arrow). A black and white version of this figure will appear in some formats. For the color version, please refer to the plate section.

Figure 4.12 Doppler spectra taken from various sites from a patient with the arteriogram shown on the right (E). At (A), the maximal systolic frequency is reduced to 5 kHz; at (B), there is increased velocity at the region of stenosis to a maximum of 20 kHz, with an end-diastolic velocity of 10 kHz; (C) and (D) show velocities within the distal artery. The spectra are broadened and show decreased antegrade velocities. From von Reutern G, Budingen HJ. *Ultraschalldiagnostik der Hirnversorgenden Arterien.* Stuttgart: Georg Thieme Verlag, 1989 with permission.

velocities of the periorbital arteries, the carotid arteries in the neck, and the VAs at their origins and at the cervical region near the skull base (C1 and C2). Moving the Doppler probe along the course of the carotid and vertebral arteries allows identification of the bifurcation of the carotid arteries and major changes in audible blood-flow signals. Doppler curves can be analyzed using fast Fourier transform spectral analysis to detect peak frequencies and broadening of the spectrum.[71,81,82]

Figure 4.12 shows Doppler spectra in a patient with carotid artery stenosis in the neck. The severity of stenosis is estimated by the increase in peak systolic frequency, the presence and severity of poststenotic turbulence, and an increase in diastolic blood-flow velocity. Most readers are familiar with the task of washing off a pavement by using a hose. Turning the adjustable end of the hose changes the diameter of the lumen of the nozzle. When the nozzle is tightened, the jet stream of the water is under higher velocity and is more effective in washing the surface. If the nozzle is tightened too much, however, the stream dribbles out or stops altogether. Similarly, in regions of luminal narrowing, blood velocity increases in an inverse proportion to the size of the lumen until a critical reduction in lumen size severely limits flow.

In patients with suspected occlusive disease of the subclavian and innominate arteries, a variety of non-invasive tests can measure blood flow in the arm. The relative velocity of pulsed-wave propagation in the two arms then can be compared. Forearm blood flow can also be studied by oscillography and venous occlusive plethysmography.

Color Doppler flow imaging, power Doppler, and compounded imaging

Color Doppler flow imaging (CDFI) improves analysis of arterial plaque surface and configuration. In this technique, the spatial and temporal distribution of color-coded Doppler signals are visualized in real time and displayed as color images superimposed on gray-scale images of the surrounding tissues.[71,81-85] Figure 4.13 shows a CDFI in a patient with near occlusion of an ICA. This technique is especially good for showing changes in blood-flow patterns near small plaques. This technique has an extremely high sensitivity and accuracy for detecting minor, moderate, and severe degrees of carotid artery stenosis.[82-85] CDFI improves evaluation of the extent of carotid artery plaques by the simultaneous two-dimensional display of tissue structure and flow-velocity profile. Real-time images are easier to see and interpret than are curves of velocity. The technology also helps differentiate smooth from irregular surfaces and from ulcerative niches. Severe stenosis cannot always be differentiated from complete occlusion by CDFI.[84] This technique also helps visualization of VA lesions in the neck.

Power Doppler is a system based on the display of the integrated power of the Doppler signal obtained from an insonated artery.[71,86,87] This technique is able to remove some of the artifacts and improve some limitations of CDFI. The color display on power Doppler imaging is independent of the angle of insonation. The intravascular surface is better shown using power Doppler. Calcification within plaques can also be visualized with this system. Power Doppler improves

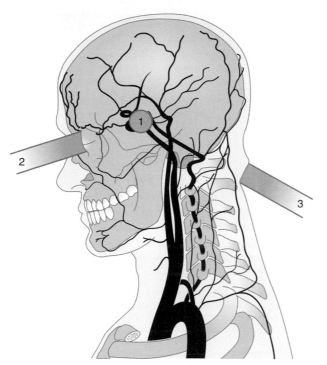

Figure 4.14 Diagram shows locations for TCD probes: (1) temporal window, (2) orbital window, (3) suboccipital foramen magnum window. Redrawn from von Reutern G, Budingen HJ. *Ultraschalldiagnostik der Hirnversorgenden Arterien.* Stuttgart: Georg Thieme Verlag, 1989 with permission.

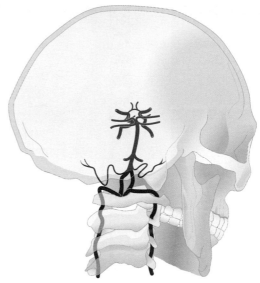

Figure 4.15 The suboccipital window is shown along with the location of the distal vertebral arteries in the neck and the intracranial vertebral and basilar arteries. Adapted from von Reutern G, Budingen HJ. *Ultraschalldiagnostik der Hirnversorgenden Arterien.* Stuttgart: Georg Thieme Verlag, 1989.

the assessment of the severity of carotid artery stenosis and plaque morphology compared with CDFI.[86]

Real-time compounded imaging is a technique that can enhance visualization and characterization of arterial plaques. The technique uses ultrasound beams that are steered off-axis from the orthogonal beams used in conventional B-mode ultrasound.[68,71] The frames acquired from different angles are then averaged to reduce speckle and improve tissue differentiation. Compound B-mode imaging can suppress edge shadowing and provides better contrast resolution than standard B-mode imaging.[68,71] Plaque motion can also be studied using compound imaging techniques.[88] Plaque movement in relation to the arterial wall can result in potential "hammering" of the plaque promoting plaque rupture and fissuring and increasing the likelihood of an arterial stenotic lesion becoming symptomatic.[88]

Transcranial Doppler ultrasound

One of the major advances in the field of analysis of vascular lesions was the introduction of the transcranial Doppler (TCD) system, which permits study of the intracranial arteries. Extracranial ultrasound examinations use pulse frequencies ranging from 2 to 10 MHz. These ultrasound frequencies cannot penetrate bone sufficiently to reflect signals from the intracranial arteries. Aaslid and colleagues showed that signals could be obtained from the MCA and ACA, using a 2-MHz probe directed intracranially from the temporal bone just above the zygomatic arch.[89] Three separate windows are customarily used for probe placement, taking advantage of natural skull foramina or soft-tissue regions.[89–91] The temporal

window is used for insonating the MCA and its major branches, the proximal ACA, and the ICA bifurcation as well as the posterior cerebral arteries. A transorbital probe is placed near the eye and is used for studying blood velocities in the ICA siphon and ophthalmic arteries. A suboccipital window through the foramen magnum allows recording of frequencies from the intracranial VAs and the proximal portion of the basilar artery.[92,93] Figure 4.14 shows these ultrasonic windows. From the suboccipital window imaging of the distal VA in the neck and the intracranial VA can be performed (Figure 4.15).

Early studies using TCD confirmed normal values and techniques and showed that the technology was useful in detecting severe stenosis or occlusion of basal cerebral arteries, and for yielding information about the impact of extracranial occlusive disease on flow in intracranial arteries.[92–99] A microprocessor-controlled, directional pulsed-wave adjustable probe is placed at one of the windows and moved until maximal signals are obtained; velocities are then recorded at different depths along the arteries. The introduction of three-dimensional display vascular maps helps orient the insonation to the location of the artery being studied. Specially designed helmets and headbands can be used to hold the probes in place, facilitating monitoring of arteries over time. These improvements allowed the introduction of duplex scanning of intracranial arteries. Power Doppler technology has also been applied to transcranial duplex scanning.[87,100,101] B-mode images of the intracranial arteries can be produced and color-coded scans can be obtained from intracranial arteries during transcranial sonography.[83,100,101] Solutions that contain microbubbles can be injected intravenously to obtain contrast-enhancement of the transcranial ultrasound signals. In European countries, the commonest ultrasound contrast agent used is the galactose-palmitic, acid-based agent called "levovist."[100] Contrast enhancement improves the diagnostic

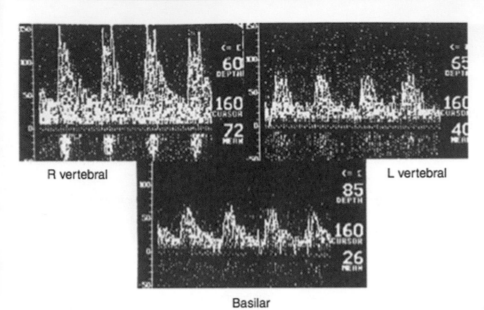

Figure 4.16 TCD spectra: The velocities in the right intracranial VA are much higher than in the left VA and the basilar artery. Arteriography showed a region of severe stenosis in the intracranial right VA.

R vertebral

L vertebral

Basilar

capability of transcranial ultrasound scans.[100–104] Newer ultrasonic contrast-enhancing agents are being investigated.[105] Unfortunately, until now microbubble contrast enhancers have not been approved for use in the United States. Interpretation of the results of TCD depends on integrating information from extracranial and transcranial ultrasound and from study of all of the major intracranial arteries at various depths.

TCD has improved the ability of clinicians to study stroke patients at the bedside.[106] TCD can accurately detect important atherostenotic lesions within the major basal cerebral arteries – the intracranial ICAs, MCAs, intracranial vertebral arteries, and the proximal and middle portions of the basilar artery.[90–92,96–99,106–108] TCD is also helpful in showing the hemodynamic effects of extracranial occlusive lesions on velocities in the intracranial branches. The combination of CW Doppler, color-flow Doppler, and TCD is effective in screening for major occlusive lesions within the extracranial and intracranial arteries within the posterior circulation as well as in the anterior circulation.[83,109,110] Vascular narrowing due to vasoconstriction and augmented flow through collateral channels and through AVMs all increase blood-flow velocity. TCD can be used to monitor vasoconstriction in patients with SAH.[81,100,111,112] Figure 4.16 shows TCD velocity curves in a patient with an intracranial VA stenosis.

TCD is also useful in studying collateral circulation in patients with large-artery occlusive lesions. In patients with carotid artery territory occlusions, blood flow to the ischemic hemisphere through the posterior communicating artery from the vertebrobasilar arterial system and from the contralateral cerebral hemisphere through the anterior communicating artery can be analyzed and quantified.[113–115] Reserve capacity for augmenting blood flow in patients with arterial occlusions can also be studied using TCD and vasodilator stimuli.[116–118] The most common techniques involve either injection of acetazolamide or inhalation of a gas mixture containing carbon dioxide (CO_2). These promote vasodilatation in normal arteries. Blood flow velocities are monitored using TCD. In normal patients and those with good "vasomotor reactivity," cerebral blood flow (CBF) increases. When collateral vessels are already maximally dilated, they fail to further augment flow when acetazolamide is injected or when their pCO_2 level is increased. Reduced cerebrovascular reserve capability has been correlated with an increased stroke risk in patients with severe occlusive carotid artery disease.[119] The reduced blood flow reserve capacity reflects a tenuous circulation which is at risk if further vascular stenosis or occlusion develops.

Embolus detection and monitoring using transcranial Doppler

So far we have discussed the ability of TCD techniques to analyze the presence of arterial occlusions and the effect of occlusions on blood flow. The other very important capability of TCD relates to its use in patients suspected of having brain embolism. Emboli of all kinds can be detected as sudden alterations in flow, with characteristic sound signals.[91,106,120–126] In this technique TCD probes are positioned over brain arteries, most often the middle and posterior cerebral arteries on each side. When particles pass through the arteries being monitored, they produce an audible chirping noise and high-intensity transient signals (HITS) visible on an oscilloscope. Figure 4.17 shows a microembolic signal (HIT).

The signal characteristics depend on the nature of the particles (gas, thrombus, calcium, cholesterol crystal, etc.), particle size, and particle transit time. Monitoring probes can be placed on the neck and brain arteries. Emboli that arise from the heart or aorta should go equally to each side, proportionately to the anterior and posterior circulation arteries, and the signals should appear in the neck before appearing intracranially. In contrast, emboli that originate in a neck artery should go only to the intracranial arterial branches on the side of the donor artery and embolic signals do not appear in the neck. For example, emboli from the left ICA generate embolic signals detectable in the left MCA and not in the neck, posterior cerebral or right-sided arteries. This technique now allows

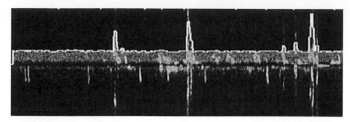

Figure 4.17 TCD ultrasound monitoring of a MCA showing high intensity transient signals (sharp spikes) representing a microemboli.

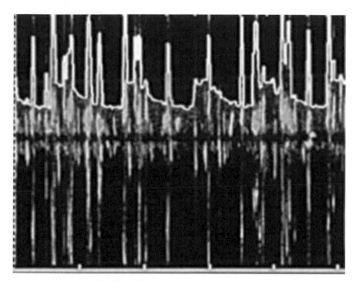

Figure 4.18 TCD ultrasound monitoring of a MCA after intravenous installation of air in a patient with a patent foramen ovale.

better identification of the nature of embolic materials and their sources and also allows some quantification of the emboli load and a means of monitoring the effect of various therapies on lessening that load.

Emboli monitoring can serve several functions. In patients with TIAs or acute strokes, monitoring can suggest the source of emboli and the quantity of microembolic signals. Monitoring is also useful in patients with known sources of emboli in the heart, aorta, or large arteries. The presence of microemboli in patients with known cardiac lesions may help predict the risk of embolic stroke and also be useful in assessing the effectiveness of various prophylactic regimens in reducing the microembolic load.[123] Monitoring is also helpful in patients with carotid artery disease in the neck.[127,128] Microemboli in patients with severe carotid occlusive disease are often detected after TIAs and minor strokes. The microembolus load decreases soon after carotid occlusion. TCD embolus detection is also useful in patients with known intracranial arterial occlusive disease.[129–131] Long-term ambulatory monitoring is also possible.[132] TCD monitoring has also been used during procedures such as cardiac surgery, carotid artery surgery, and carotid artery stenting. Emboli monitoring is discussed again in the chapter on brain embolism.

TCD can also be used to detect potential right-to-left circulatory system shunts and paradoxical embolism.[91,133–139]

Table 4.5 Protocol for TCD detection and reporting of right-to-left circulatory shunts

Performance

1. The patient is in supine position, and an 18-gauge needle is inserted into a cubital vein

2. A three-way stop-cock connector with two 10-ml syringes is connected to intravenous access

3. 9 ml of isotonic (preferably bacteriostatic) saline is forcefully mixed with 1 ml of air

4. <1 ml of patient blood may be suctioned into syringe for better bubble formation with agitation

5. At least one MCA is monitored with TCD

6. The first bolus injection of agitated saline is made with the patient breathing normally

7. A second bolus injection of similarly prepared agitated saline is made with 10 s Valsalva maneuver initiated 5 s after beginning of saline injection

8. If negative, TCD monitoring is extended up to 1 min in order to detect potentially late-arriving bubbles suggesting a pulmonary arteriovenous shunt

Interpretation

1. At times, a so-called curtain of almost continuous signals develops. A four-level categorization is proposed by the International Consensus Criteria[126]

2. No MES detected (negative "bubble" test)

3. 1–10 MES detected (positive "bubble" test)

4. >10 MES detected with no curtain

5. A curtain indicates the presence of a large and functional shunt

MCA, middle cerebral artery; MES, microembolic signals; TCD, transcranial Doppler.
From Molina CA, Alexandrov AV. Transcranial Doppler ultrasound. In Caplan LR, Manning WJ (eds), *Brain Embolism*. New York: Informa Healthcare, 2006, pp 113–128 with permission.

Bubbles are injected into an arm vein while the TCD probe is held over a temporal window. In patients without cardiac shunts, no change is noted over the probe. In the presence of cardiac defects with shunting or pulmonary arteriovenous shunts, air emboli are heard and can be recorded. Figure 4.18 shows air microembolic signals in an MCA during testing for a venous to arterial circulatory shunt. Table 4.5 includes the suggested protocol and reporting.

In patient JH, ultrasound examinations were quite helpful. Duplex scanning of the ICAs in the neck suggested an occlusion of the right ICA at its origin. The left ICA had only minor disease. TCD showed an inability to detect blood flow in the right MCA. Collateral flow was detected through the right ACA and posterior communicating-cerebral artery (PCA). There was also some damping of flow in the ICA siphon, presumably due to the proximal ICA obstruction in the neck. The left MCA showed normal velocities.

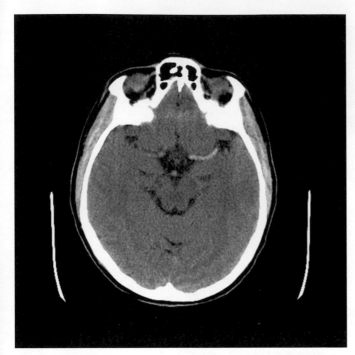

Figure 4.19 CT scan showing a very prominent hyperdense left MCA. A cerebral angiogram showed a completely occluded MCA and a long thrombus was later extracted from this vessel.

Transcranial Doppler of cranial venous structures

TCD technology has also occasionally been used to study cerebral veins and dural sinuses.[140–144] The major problem is visualizing the location of the veins. Some venous structures such as the superior sagittal sinus are far away from the usual insonating windows. Power-based and color-coded duplex sonography have been most effective in showing the major veins and dural sinuses especially after bubble ultrasound contrast injections.[140] In normal individuals, the deep cerebral veins especially the basal vein of Rosenthal and the vein of Galen can usually be visualized.[141] The dural sinuses are more difficult to image. The straight sinus and transverse sinus can be imaged in more than 50% of individuals but sagittal sinus visualization is poor. Dural sinus occlusion can be suspected by failure to visualize a sinus,[142] by reversal of normal flow direction in a draining vein, and by increased blood flow velocities in the venous structures.[140–144] The patency of the jugular veins can also be assessed. To date, Doppler sonography is probably not an effective screening technique for diagnosis of cerebral venous thrombosis, but may prove useful as a bedside non-invasive method of following changes in the venous system in patients with venous thrombosis identified by MR venography, CT venography, or catheter cerebral angiography.

Computed tomography and magnetic resonance imaging

Some information about the neck and intracranial vessels can often be gleaned from careful scrutiny of CT and MRI scans, especially after contrast enhancement. On plain CT, an acutely thrombosed artery can sometimes be seen as a hyperdense image that has the shape and distribution of an artery or vein.[145] Sensitivity for acute thrombus is greatly improved by the use of thin slice reformats (e.g., 1 mm), which can be obtained using the same image dataset (no extra time or radiation required).[146] The MCA is the most frequently involved artery.[145,147,148] Sometimes the intracranial ICA and both the anterior cerebral and MCA branches are hyperdense, indicating a top-of-the-carotid-artery occlusion. The hyperdense MCA sign (Figure 4.19) is virtually diagnostic of the presence of a clot within the MCA and is associated with a worse prognosis, particularly with larger proximal hyperdense signs, related to the large arterial territory involved and lower probability of recanalization with tPA. Careful scrutiny may show distal dots (dot sign) in the Sylvian region, indicating distal thrombi. Occasionally, the basilar artery and the PCAs can show similar hyperdensity on unenhanced scans indicating thromboembolic occlusion of these arteries. Calcific particle emboli arising from calcific material in heart valves or a calcified atherostenotic plaque can also sometimes be identified within brain arteries on plain CT scans. Figure 4.20 shows a calcific embolus in an intracranial ICA shown on a CT scan.

Occasionally an intracranial artery can image as a dark linear hypodense structure indicating fat embolism to that artery.[149] Contrast enhancement can show large berry aneurysms and dolichoectatic fusiform aneurysms; absence of opacification of an artery can indicate the high probability of occlusion of that vessel. CT can also suggest dural sinus thrombosis by showing thrombosed serpiginous cortical veins, the superior sagittal, or other sinuses as high-density clots on plain CT scans. After contrast enhancement, CT venograms may show a filling defect, representing a clot within the sagittal sinus, the so-called empty delta sign. Serial cross-sectional CT images of the neck after contrast infusion can also yield information about carotid artery plaques, occlusions, and plaque hemorrhages. High-resolution spiral CT scanning can also show plaque characteristics in patients with atherosclerotic lesions in neck arteries[150] and can also show spontaneous and traumatic arterial dissections.

High-resolution MRI is now being used in some centers to characterize atherosclerotic plaques in neck arteries. First used in the heart to show vulnerable coronary artery plaques,[151] the technology has now been explored in imaging atherosclerotic carotid arteries in the neck.[152–158] Using a surface coil, and high-resolution 1.5-tesla MR scanners, the fibrous caps of atherosclerotic plaques image as a low signal band just outside of the lumen. Rupture of a region within the fibrous cap can also sometimes be imaged. Intraplaque hemorrhages show high signal intensities indicating the presence of a complicated plaque. Researchers are exploring the use of fibrin-specific contrast agents for imaging thrombi within neck arteries; this technique has already been applied to the coronary arteries with success.[159,160] Cross-section views of cervical arterial dissections often show intramural hematomas and luminal encroachment. Fat-saturated images show dissections best. The characteristic finding is a dark small circular or elliptical-shaped flow void representing the compressed lumen surrounded by a bright hyperintense crescent or donut-shaped zone that represents bleeding within the wall of the artery. Figure 4.21 shows a VA dissection confirmed by MRI.

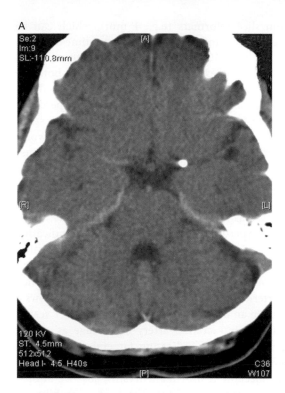

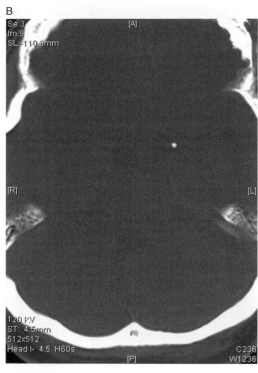

Figure 4.20 (A) CT scan with contrast shows a bright white calcium particle in the right ICA. (B) A bone density film showing that the particle has the same density as bone. Courtesy of Steven Tanabe, MD, New England Medical Center, Boston.

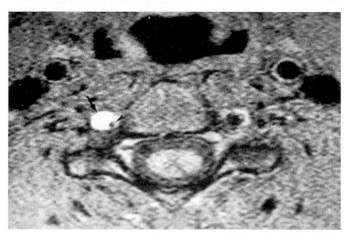

Figure 4.21 MRI with fat-saturation technique showing a dissection within the VA on the left of the picture (black arrows). The black flow voids in the contralateral VA and the carotid arteries are well seen in contrast to the tiny flow void in the dissected artery.

Flow within intracranial arteries can also be studied with MRI. Vessels with high-velocity flow appear black (signal void) on T2 MRI images, whereas arteries with slower flow (e.g., leptomeningeal collateral vessels) may show as linear hyperintensities best seen on T2 FLAIR. Occlusions can be inferred when a flow void is not seen on images that show cross-section views of arteries. Aneurysms and dissections can also frequently be identified and followed by MRI scanning. High-resolution MRI scanning is also used to characterize intracranial arterial plaques. MRI performed using a 1.5-tesla scanner, 8-channel brain array coils, and a multicontrast imaging technique can show plaques within intracranial arteries.[161] Plaques within the basilar[162] and MCAs[163,164] have been imaged using this technique. Figure 4.22 shows a

cross-section image of a stenosing plaque in a MCA obtained by this MRI technique.

T2*-weighted (also called susceptibility) images can show thrombi within intracranial arteries and veins. Gradient echo images that contain dark hypointense regions that take the shape of intracranial arteries are the MR equivalent of the hyperdense MCA sign seen on CT brain imaging.[165–170] This finding is most common after cardiac and intra-arterial embolic stroke but also may occur in thrombosis engrafted upon intrinsic atherostenotic intracranial lesions. Diffusion-weighted MR images can also show thrombi within veins as hyperintense regions.[171,172]

Enhancement of arteries can be seen after intravenous injection of gadopentetate dimeglumine-diethylenetriaminepentaacetic acid in patients with brain ischemia and infarction.[173,174] Fluid-attenuated inversion recovery (FLAIR) images after gadolinium may show delayed enhancement of CSF spaces especially on the side of brain infarction. This finding indicates breakdown in the blood–brain barrier and was termed hyperintense acute reperfusion marker (HARM) by Warach and colleagues.[175–177] HARM indicates a high risk of hemorrhagic transformation, increased brain edema, and poor outcome after reperfusion. Another MRI technique, referred to as T2*-permeability imaging can also be used to predict the likelihood of hemorrhagic complications after brain infarction especially after thrombolysis.[178] However, both these approaches work best following reperfusion. The risk of post-reperfusion hemorrhage relates to the severity and duration of ischemia which can be assessed prior to reperfusion by examining cerebral blood volume maps for regions of very low CBV or T_{MAX} maps for very delayed flow.[179–182]

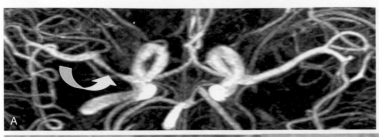

Right MCA
stenosis

Figure 4.22 The top image shows a stenosis in the MCA on the left of the picture (arrow). The images below are cross-sections through the normal MCA (B, D, F) and the stenosed MCA (C, E, G). Courtesy of Isabelle Klein, MD, Phillippa Lavallee, MD, and Pierre Amarenco, MD, Bichat Hospital, Paris, France.

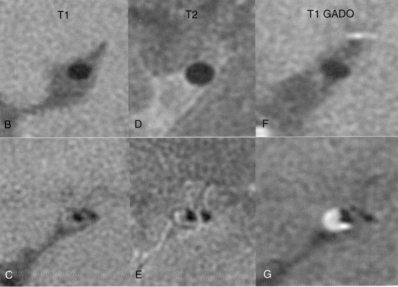

Left MCA

Right MCA

Magnetic resonance angiography

MRA offers many advantages over other non-invasive methods of vascular imaging and is a standard component of MRI ischemia protocols.[183–186] Time-of-flight (TOF) MRA uses a T1-weighted sequence to capture information about the flow of blood without the need for contrast. Contrast-enhanced MRA can also be used and is generally preferred for accurate characterization of stenoses as the TOF technique tends to overestimate severity of stenosis.[187–189] Another technique used less frequently nowadays is phase-contrast MRA. This provides lower resolution images but does give information on direction of flow. Knowledge of the likely location of the vascular lesions helps the examiner focus on particular regions, improving the yield of the examination. Veins can also be studied; the imaging of veins is referred to as MR venography.

TOF MRA is a functional process that creates an image of flow in blood vessels. Unlike standard contrast injection angiograms, the images do not show anatomy. When flow is reduced in an artery, the vessel may appear narrowed or absent even when the artery is normal by contrast angiography; for example, when both intracranial vertebral arteries are severely stenosed or occluded, the basilar artery may not opacify and yet be widely patent. In some patients with severe dolichoectasia, TOF MRA may fail to image the artery because to and fro flow cancel each other and there is insufficient antegrade flow to provide opacity in the artery.

Within the anterior circulation, the ICA origins are usually well visualized, but at times TOF MRA overestimates the severity of luminal narrowing.[190,191] TOF MRA is quite accurate in patients with complete ICA occlusions and has similar sensitivity and specificity to duplex ultrasound in screening for the presence of severe ICA stenotic lesions.[190] The changing angles and curvature of the ICA in the siphon often makes interpretation of this region more difficult than the straight portions of the artery. The intracranial anterior circulation large arteries are well seen but distal branch arteries are not well imaged.[192–194] The horizontal segment of the MCA and the proximal portions of the superior and inferior divisions of the MCA are usually well shown.

TOF MRA of the VA origins from the subclavian arteries is often suboptimal because of the overlapping of arteries. Superimposition of arteries sometimes makes images difficult to interpret with multiplanar reformats required to see the origins of the VAs. The second portion of the VA within the intervertebral foramina is well shown on TOF MRA. The third portion of the VA, that section of the artery that curves around the rostral cervical vertebrae, is often not well seen on TOF MRA because of the sharp angulation and curvature of the artery. The intracranial vertebral arteries and the basilar artery are usually well shown on intracranial TOF MRA, especially the rostral bifurcation of the basilar artery into the PCAs. All of the above-mentioned limitations of TOF-MRA can be reduced or avoided through the use of gadolinium contrast-enhanced MRA, provided the patient has acceptable kidney function. Note that this would require a separate injection of contrast in addition to any perfusion imaging sequence.

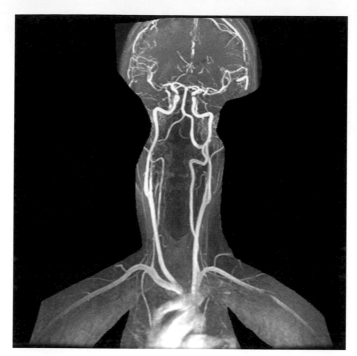

Figure 4.23 MRA of the head and neck after gadolinium infusion.

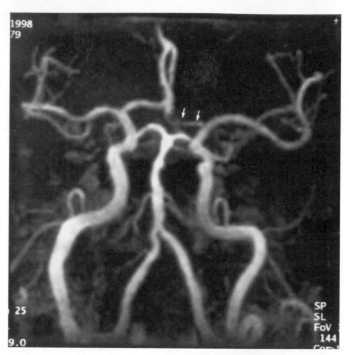

Figure 4.24 Intracranial MRA. The carotid arteries and their intracranial branches and the vertebral and basilar arteries are well seen. The left A1 segment of the ICA is hypoplastic (white arrows). The basilar artery has irregularities due to plaques but there are no important stenosing lesions.

Qureshi and colleagues evaluated the ability of TOF MRA to detect significant occlusive lesions among 118 patients with brain infarcts.[185] Among the 176 large arteries visualized by both MRA and conventional angiography, angiography confirmed 9 out of 10 (90%) extracranial and 32 out of 40 (80%) intracranial abnormalities shown by MRA. There were few false-negative or false-positive abnormalities.[185] MRA has proven to be an excellent screening technique for occlusive disease. CT or catheter contrast angiography may still be needed in some patients to better delineate the vascular lesions. In some patients who are studied with TOF MRA images of the neck, the jugular vein is also shown. This means that there is reversed flow in the vein, suggesting a proximal stenosis or occlusion of the innominate vein on that side.[195]

Quantitative magnetic resonance angiography (QMRA) is a newer technology that can quantify regional cerebral blood flow. This technique has been used to study blood flow in the vertebrobasilar system providing hemodynamic information.[196] Flow in stenotic posterior circulation arteries correlates with residual diameter, but flow decreases significantly when there are tandem stenotic lesions. Distal flow blood flow, incorporating collateral capacity, is not well predicted by the severity or location of the disease, but is improved using QMRA.[196]

Figure 4.23 shows a normal MRA taken after gadolinium infusion. Figure 4.24 shows an intracranial MRA in a patient with an irregular basilar artery. In patient JH, MRA confirmed a right ICA occlusion in the neck. Intracranial views also showed occlusion of the proximal MCA.

Computed tomography angiography

Development of rapid spiral (helical) CT scanners has enabled the development of CTA.[197] This technique involves intravenous injection of a bolus of dye followed by helical scanning. Volumetric data acquisition and improved computerized image manipulation have improved the CTA image display into three-dimensional reformats. CTA is based on anatomical imaging, and when blood flow is severely reduced, CTA has theoretical advantages over MRA, which is a functional imaging technique. The ICAs are well shown in the neck and the results of CTA for quantification of carotid stenosis are comparable to those obtained with MRA.[197–201] Figure 4.25 shows a CTA of a normal extracranial VA. Figure 4.26 shows lesions in a carotid artery (Figure 4.26A) and in the neck in a VA (Figure 4.26B). Compared with conventional angiography there are few false-positive and false-negative results.[197–200]

CTA also provides useful images of intracranial arteries and can show regions of intracranial stenosis, dolichoectasia, and aneurysms.[192,197,202–205] Figure 4.27 shows reconstruction images of CTAs that show intracranial MCA lesions. Bash and colleagues compared CTA, MRA, and digital subtraction catheter angiography in 28 patients who had 115 diseased intracranial vascular segments.[192] CTA had a higher sensitivity for intracranial artery stenosis than MRA (98% vs. 70%) and for occlusion (100% vs. 87%). CTA was superior to MRA especially in patients with low flow states in the posterior circulation.[192] CTA reliably detects aneurysms larger than 3 mm in size,[204] and is often used as the initial screen for cerebral aneurysms, although catheter angiography remains the definitive diagnostic technique.[206] A caveat in the interpretation of CTA is that an arterial occlusion (e.g., terminal ICA) may prevent contrast entry into the entire artery, at least during the time taken to acquire the CTA, as there is insufficient outflow rostrally. The length of the occluded segment

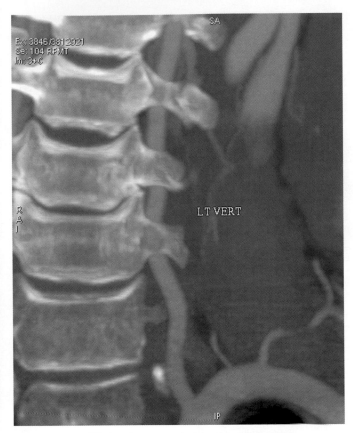

Figure 4.25 A CTA showing a normal origin of the left VA in the neck. The artery can be seen to enter the intervertebral foramina and course rostrally.

may, therefore, not be accurately represented on CTA. This will become clear if the patient proceeds to catheter angiogram but can sometimes be predicted by careful examination of the non-contrast CT for the extent of hyperdense thrombus.

CTA has also been used to predict enlargement and progression of ICHs.[207] Hematoma growth is a strong predictor of poor outcome.[208] Tiny enhancing foci within hematomas ("spot sign") shown by CTA indicates active bleeding and correlates with hematoma progression.[207] Clearly the development of a spot sign is a dynamic process. The prevalence of a spot sign is greater with later (e.g., venous-phase) CTA and even higher in post-contrast CT. However, the association with hemorrhage growth is strongest in patients with spot signs detected in the early arterial phase.[209]

Imaging cerebral venous sinus thrombosis

Both CT venography (CTV) and MR venography (MRV) can show lack of flow in the major cerebral veins with excellent sensitivity. As mentioned above, the thrombus may be evident as a hyperdensity on non-contrast CT. Both time-of-flight and contrast-enhanced techniques can be used for MRV. MRI has the advantage of multiple confirmatory sequences to differentiate an occluded sinus from congenital hypoplasia and better delineates parenchymal abnormalities as a consequence of the thrombosis.

Perfusion imaging

CT or MRI can be used to image the dynamic passage of a contrast bolus through the cerebral circulation – so-called perfusion imaging. CT perfusion involves injection of iodinated contrast and repeated imaging of the brain every 1–3 seconds, sometimes with table movement to increase brain coverage. MR perfusion involves rapid acquisitions with a repetition time of approximately 1.5 seconds after Gd-DTPA injection. These dynamic images of the passage of contrast generate a concentration-time curve in each image voxel that can be mathematically manipulated to calculate parametric maps. Some parameters can be calculated directly from the concentration-time curve such as regional cerebral blood volume (rCBV – area under curve) and time to peak (TTP – delay to peak contrast intensity). Others are calculated via a process of "deconvolution" which uses the concentration-time curve in a normal vessel (the "arterial input function" AIF) to estimate the concentration-time curve in tissue that would have occurred after a theoretical "instantaneous" contrast bolus arrival. Deconvolution allows the calculation of regional cerebral blood flow (rCBF), mean transit time (MTT – calculated as CBV/CBF), and time to maximum perfusion (T_{max}).[210–219]

When MRI is used, the diffusion lesion is used to define the irreversibly injured ischemic core.[219–221] However, with CT perfusion, reduced cerebral blood volume or severely reduced CBF can provide an estimate of the ischemic core.[222–225] Regions supplied by leptomeningeal collateral flow have delayed contrast arrival (the TTP, or deconvoluted equivalent "T_{max}" is increased) as well as dispersion, which prolongs the MTT. A thresholded T_{max} greater than 6 seconds has been proposed as a way to separate ischemic penumbra (at risk of infarction without reperfusion) from "benign oligemia" (hypoperfused tissue that will not proceed to infarction regardless of reperfusion).[226,227] A "mismatch" between a small ischemic core and larger perfusion lesion has been used as a surrogate for the presence of ischemic penumbra and identifies a patient population whose outcome clearly diverges based on whether reperfusion is achieved.[228–230] In some patients perfusion in an area that correlates with the clinical symptoms and signs suggests the possibility that the symptoms are related to a seizure rather than brain ischemia.

Multimodal imaging of brain, blood vessels, and brain perfusion using magnetic resonance imaging and computed tomography in acute ischemic stroke

The advent of thrombolysis in 1996 made it important for medical centers evaluating patients with acute brain ischemia to obtain anatomical and functional information quickly and safely. Major ongoing efforts attempt to streamline treatment and reduce delays to thrombolysis and efficient imaging is a key component. New technology and improvements in older techniques now provide clinicians with a menu of different strategies for brain and vascular studies in patients with ischemia. At the simplest level, tPA trials were based on the use of non-contrast CT to exclude hemorrhage and established infarction. In clinically straightforward cases this remains

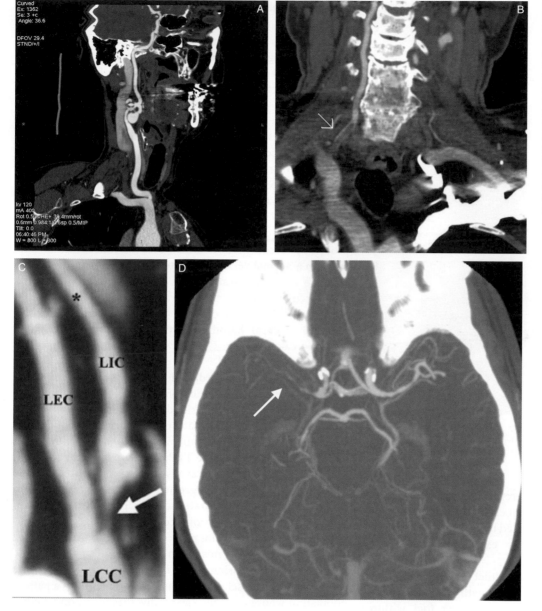

Figure 4.26 Neck and intracranial CTAs. (A) An aneurysm is arising from the ICA. (B) A thrombus is seen within the proximal portion of a VA (white arrow). (C) Close up of a CT angiogram showing a severe stenosis at the origin of the left ICA (white arrow). An asterix in the distal left ICA identifies partial collapse and narrowing of the artery distal to the stenosis. Kindly submitted by Dr Robert Ackerman. LCC, left common carotid; LEC, left external carotid; LIC, left internal carotid. (D) Intracranial view showing a region of severe stenosis involving a long segment of the mainstem MCA (white arrow). Calcifications are seen in the bilateral intracranial carotid arteries.

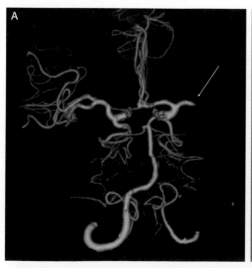

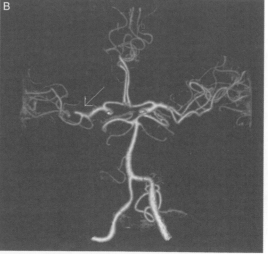

Figure 4.27 Intracranial CTAs – maximal intensity projections (MIPS). (A) Abrupt occlusion of the left mainstem MCA (white arrow). (B) Occlusion of the superior division of the right MCA (white arrow).

sufficient information to deliver thrombolysis with minimum delay. However, in less certain cases, treating clinicians may wish to confirm the diagnosis of ischemic stroke by showing a perfusion abnormality or vessel occlusion. They may also want to know how much brain is already irreversibly injured (termed the "ischemic core"), whether large brain-supplying arteries are occluded as a target for endovascular therapy or a risk for clinical deterioration. In addition, the location and volume of the brain that may be contributing to the clinical deficit but remains salvageable with rapid reperfusion (ie the ischemic penumbra) may help guide therapy. Although a condensed stroke protocol MRI (DWI, FLAIR, MRA, SWI, and perfusion) can be performed within a few minutes, access to the scanner and magnet safety clearance would now cause unacceptable delays in many health systems. As a result, CT remains the workhorse in acute stroke at most centers. A sequential approach with thrombolysis initiated on the CT table as soon as sufficient information is available, be that after the non-contrast CT or after CT perfusion has lead to the fastest "door-to-needle" times.[231,232] Extracranial and transcranial ultrasound can be used as the diagnostic vascular tests in patients who have only had brain imaging or can be used to corroborate and quantify the blood-flow effects of vascular lesions found by CTA and MRA. Ultrasound is also used effectively to monitor the progression and regression of vascular occlusive lesions once they are identified.

Magnetic resonance imaging multimodal protocols

Modern acute stroke MRI protocols include diffusion and perfusion imaging along with T2 and T2*-weighted images and MRA. Brain perfusion can be imaged using dynamic susceptibility (contrast-enhanced) MR scans.[219–215]

If MRI is to be used prior to reperfusion therapies, time is of the essence. Perfusion imaging must be processed and interpreted immediately. The availability of automated software packages for this purpose has greatly improved the practical relevance of perfusion imaging. In the presence of large vessel occlusion, similar information to the perfusion–diffusion mismatch can be gleaned from the diffusion-weighted scan and the MRA since in most patients, prediction of the hypoperfused region can be estimated by the severity and location of the occluded artery and the clinical neurological signs (clinical–imaging mismatch.)[44]

Researchers and clinicians are now exploring imaging perfusion without the need for contrast infusion. The technique is referred to as arterial spin labeling.[233–236] A radiofrequency pulse is given to the arterial blood column in the neck giving the blood a magnetic label. Continuous arterial spin labeling perfusion magnetic resonance imaging (CASL-pMRI) uses magnetically labeled arterial blood water as a tracer to obtain quantifiable measurements of CBF.[233–236] Current ASL sequences are limited in resolution and their ability to resolve the degree of hypoperfusion within the brain ischemic region as the vascular tagging signal decays too rapidly in regions of delayed collateral flow. Another potential capability of ASL is to show vascular occlusions. Arteries harboring thrombi can appear bright on MRI ASL. These bright vessels correlate well

with MRA and the appearance on T2*-weighted susceptibility signs.[237]

Comparison of the region of probable infarction on diffusion-weighted scans with the region of reduced perfusion (either from perfusion-weighted scans or estimated by the MRA results) gives an indication of the part of the brain that is underperfused but not yet infarcted (the presumed ischemic penumbra).[214,215] When the region of reduced perfusion matches the zone of infarction, progression of infarction and progression of neurological signs are rare. When this information is supplemented by vascular imaging, usually MRA that is acquired at the same time as the diffusion-weighted and perfusion MRI scans, the treating physician has all the useful information needed to assess brain perfusion and to allow a logical decision about the likely utility of acute reperfusion therapies. Figure 4.28 illustrates the components of a multimodal MRI examination emphasizing perfusion–diffusion mismatch. The information gained from the MRI protocols is often used to evaluate acute stroke patients. A patient with an occluded MCA shown by MRA who has a large zone of reduced perfusion within the MCA territory shown by perfusion MRI, and a relatively small region of infarction shown by diffusion-weighted MRI represents the ideal candidate for reperfusion. On the other hand, a large zone of infarction on diffusion-weighted MRI, open ICA and MCA on MRA, and perfusion

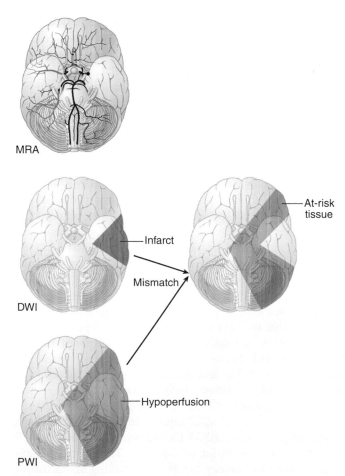

MRA

DWI

PWI

Infarct

Mismatch

At-risk tissue

Hypoperfusion

Figure 4.28 A multimodal MRI protocol emphasizing a perfusion–diffusion mismatch.

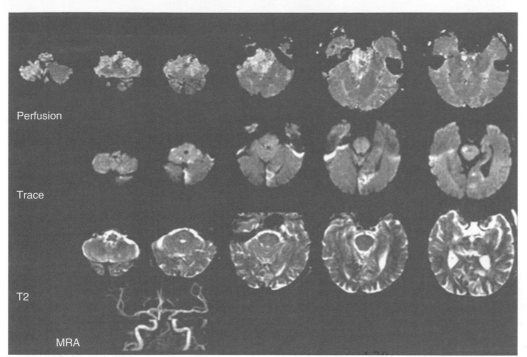

Figure 4.29 Multimodal MRI protocol of patients with severe posterior circulation occlusive disease. A patient with bilateral occlusive lesions involving the intracranial vertebral arteries. The perfusion images at the top of the figure show marked reduction in perfusion in the medulla and pons and the right cerebellum. The diffusion images (labeled Trace) show a small infarct in the right pons and left occipital lobe. The T2-weighted images show no definite infarction. The MRA shows very poor opacification of the intracranial vertebral arteries. The midbasilar artery is faintly shown because of reduced intracranial VA flow. The perfusion abnormality far exceeds the diffusion abnormality in this patient.

deficits that match or are less than the zone of infarction on diffusion-weighted scans are characteristics of candidates in whom reperfusion has little likely utility. In patients who show a large perfusion–diffusion mismatch in whom MRA shows that the artery supplying the ischemia zone is occluded, the infarct generally enlarges if the artery is not opened quickly.[184] When MRA shows patency of the intracranial artery leading to an ischemic zone, usually no added infarction occurs.[217] The presence of a large-artery occlusion is the main predictor of subsequent acute vascular events in patients with TIAs[238] and strokes, so that vascular imaging is crucial in patients with cerebrovascular ischemia.

Guidelines for thrombolysis emphasize time; a 4.5-hour window is usually cited. Modern multimodal MR imaging, however, often shows that important diffusion–perfusion mismatch can still be present long after the 4.5-hour window. One study showed that among 42 patients in whom MR imaging was performed more than 48 hours after neurological symptom onset, 15 (36%) still showed a mismatch pattern indicating brain still at risk for further infarction.[239] Figure 4.29 shows results of acute MRI stroke protocols in patients with posterior circulation occlusive disease.[240] These findings have led to the hypothesis that the time window for effective reperfusion strategies might be individualized, based on advanced imaging information and hence the basis of current trials.[241,242] Although most studies and literature emphasize the utility of multimodal MRI in patients with anterior circulation strokes, the technique can be just as useful in the posterior circulation.[240]

Figure 4.30 shows MRI studies before and after tissue plasminogen activator (tPA) thrombolysis in a patient with an acute embolic occlusion of the MCA. The use of MRI and other imaging technology for decision making about thrombolysis and other potential therapies will be discussed further in Chapter 6.

Computed tomography perfusion and computed tomography protocols

Brain perfusion can also be studied using contrast-enhanced CT techniques.[243–248] Within the ischemic core both rCBF and rCBV are reduced; within penumbral zones vascular dilatation usually leads to an increase in rCBV so that rCBF is decreased but rCBV is preserved or increased.[244] These measurements are theoretically more quantitative than perfusion MRI but have much lower contrast-to-noise ratio.[247]

When perfusion CT is combined with CT angiography and non-contrast CT scans, comparable information to MRI protocols can be obtained.[237–247] Figure 4.31 shows studies of a patient with a MCA occlusion studied by a multimodal CT protocol. The major difference between acute CT and MRI protocols are that CT does not show the acute area of infarction as well as diffusion-weighted MRI. In the past, CT often had incomplete brain coverage so that some underperfused regions were not shown. Figure 4.32 shows another patient with an acute MCA occlusion studied using a multimodal CT protocol before and after mechanical thrombectomy. This is no longer an issue with current generation scanners. Although cerebellar perfusion lesions can be identified using CTP, posterior circulation thromboembolism is less well suited to CT protocols.

Another method using CT and dye infusion has become popular in Korea and in Calgary, Canada. Injection of contrast followed by sequential imaging at specific time intervals ("triphasic perfusion computed tomography") using helical CT can yield rapid information about regions of brain ischemia and blockage of intracranial arteries.[249–252] The technique involves giving a bolus injection using a power injector of contrast into an antecubital vein after a non-contrast CT has been performed. Early, middle, and late phase images are obtained 18, 30, and 80 seconds after the contrast has been injected.

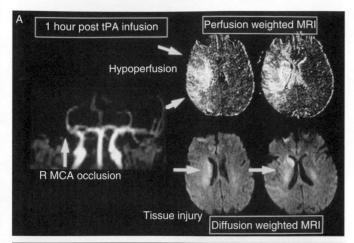

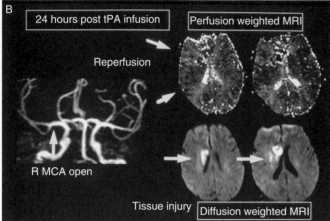

Figure 4.30 MRI protocols in relation to thrombolysis. (A) The MRI images were taken 1 hour after tPA infusion was begun. The right MCA is occluded on the MRA image (white arrow). The perfusion-weighted images show markedly reduced perfusion in the entire right-MCA territory. The diffusion-weighted images show an area of reduced diffusion adjacent to the right lateral ventricle. (B) The same MRI protocol taken 24 hours after tPA infusion. The right MCA has now reopened (white arrow). The perfusion has returned to normal and the diffusion-weighted images show only a minimal increase in the area of reduced diffusion compared to the prior DWI images in A.

Occlusion of the MCA or its main branches can be detected from the images even without reformation, allowing rapid decision about thrombolysis. Figure 4.33 is an example of a triphasic CT perfusion study in a patient with a right MCA occlusion. The original method had limited brain coverage but whole brain acquisitions are now possible and have been used to grade collateral flow quality.[253]

Multimodal techniques using MRI or CT that include brain, vascular and perfusion imaging are effective in studying patients with acute ischemic stroke for the feasibility of reperfusion.[254,255] CT has the advantage of ready accessibility but MRI using DWI and ADC imaging more accurately and effectively shows regions of acute ischemia that will go on to infarction than CT techniques.[255]

Other techniques for studying perfusion and vascular disease

A number of other metabolic and perfusion techniques have been used, predominantly in the context of research.

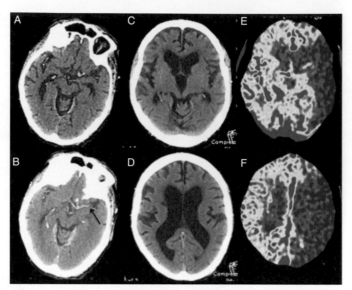

Figure 4.31 Multimodal CT protocol in a patient taken 90 minutes after the onset of dysphasia and right hemiparesis. (A) Thin slice non-contrast CT showing hyperdense thrombus in the intracranial left ICA. (B) Maximum intensity projection image showing full extent of the hyperdense thrombus in the carotid T and the MCA (black arrow). (C&D) Non-contrast CT showing minimal evidence of ischemia at this early stage. (E&F) CT perfusion showing severely reduced cerebral blood volume due to very poor collateral flow indicating a large irreversibly injured ischemic core. A black and white version of this figure will appear in some formats. For the color version, please refer to the plate section.

Inhalation of xenon, an inert gas that is not metabolized, has been used for decades to study CBF. The development of xenon inhalation combined with CT scanning (XeCT) has allowed imaging of rCBF changes on sequential standard CT slices.[256–258] Xenon enhances or modifies the images, allowing visualization of relative rCBF in regions of interest. This technique facilitates comparison of the zone of infarction on CT with regions of reduced CBF.

Single-photon-emission computed tomography (SPECT) uses ordinary radionuclear camera equipment and does not require a cyclotron to generate radionuclides. The most common radioisotopes used now are technetium-99M-labeled hexamethylpropylene amineoxime (HMPAO) and technetium-99m-labeled ethyl cysteinate dimer (Tc ECD).[259–263] Regional radiotracer uptake can be imaged in three planes. The isotopes measure rCBF rather than metabolic activity. SPECT and XeCT contain no important metabolic information.

A major advantage of SPECT scanning is that imaging does not have to be performed immediately after injection of the radionuclide. The findings on SPECT imaging represent those that were present at the time of injection. Acute treatment could be instituted immediately after injection even before the scans are performed. SPECT does not show the region of infarction but can be used with CT and can be helpful in the diagnosis and management of stroke patients, when the proper questions are asked.[260] Wintermark and colleagues compared perfusion imaging using MRI, CT, XeCT, and SPECT.[264] Despite these studies, XeCT and SPECT have little role in current clinical practice.

In the past, positron-emission tomography (PET) scanning was used extensively in research centers to quantify

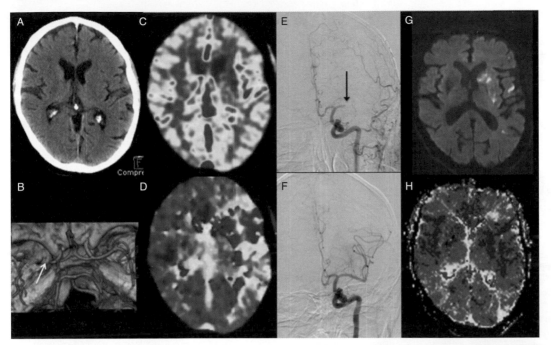

Figure 4.32 Multimodal CT protocol in a patient with the acute onset of a MCA occlusion who had good collateral blood flow. (A). Non-contrast CT brain – subtle loss of gray–white differentiation in the left caudate and putamen. (B) CT angiogram showing proximal left MCA occlusion (white arrow). (C) CT perfusion scan showing reduced cerebral blood volume in the left caudate and putamen confirming the suspicion on non-contrast CT of an ischemic core. (D) CT perfusion showing delayed flow (increased time to peak) in the MCA territory indicating the region supplied by collateral flow which is contributing to the severe clinical deficit but is potentially salvageable with rapid reperfusion. (E) Digital subtraction angiogram with left carotid injection showing persistent MCA occlusion (black arrow) 1 hour after a tPA infusion was begun. (F) Repeat angiogram after mechanical thrombectomy showing recanalization of the MCA. (G) MRI diffusion imaging 24 hours later showing the expected left striatal infarct but salvage of most of the MCA territory. (H) MRI perfusion 24 hours after treatment showing normalization of flow in the left MCA (time to peak map). A black and white version of this figure will appear in some formats. For the color version, please refer to the plate section.

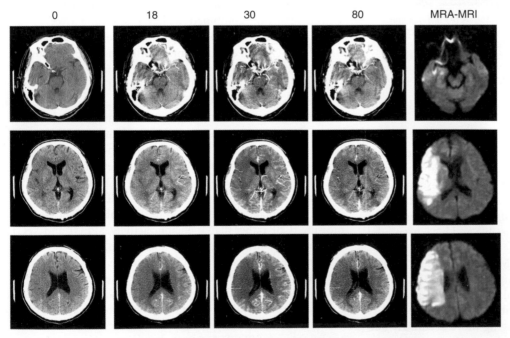

Figure 4.33 Triphasic CT perfusion. The columns show CT scans taken at various sections through the cerebral hemispheres before and 18, 30, and 80 seconds after a contrast infusion. In the upper row, the MCA on the left of the figures is occluded. The MCA territory on the side of the occlusion has much less blood vessel and tissue opacification indicating infarction. The comparable MRA-MRI figures are shown in the far right column. Courtesy of S J Lee, MD, Samsung Medical Center, Seoul, Korea.

cerebral blood flow and metabolism. But PET uses rapidly metabolized radioisotopes and proved to be not practical in the management of patients with acute stroke. MRI has virtually replaced PET in clinical practice, but PET is still used for research.

PET is a functional imaging technique that makes it possible to measure in vivo chemical reactions in body organs. Only a small number of suitable positron-emitting radionuclides are available that are integral to most organic biological compounds. These radionuclides have short half-lives, and so a dedicated medical cyclotron is required on site for synthesis, thereby making the equipment and its maintenance quite expensive. Research physicists and chemists are also often needed.

The positron-emitting radionuclides are tagged to physiologically active compounds and given to the patient at acceptably low radiation doses. CT or MRI studies of the distribution of these radionuclides allow for images of brain physiology and metabolism during life. PET scanning allows for quantification and imaging of CBF, the metabolic rate of oxygen, the metabolic rate of glucose, and the oxygen extraction function. These measurements give useful information about blood flow, the metabolic activity, and avidity for oxygen in the local regions studied.[265–269] Reduced rCBF in the range of 10–20 ml/100 g per minute can lead to brain stunning (not functioning normally but not irreversibly damaged), a state characterized by decreased electrical activity and reduced cerebral metabolism but increased extraction of oxygen.

In the normal situation, blood flow and metabolism are coupled; however, flow and metabolism are often different in the core of infarcts, when compared with the peripheral zone (penumbra). When oxygen metabolism is markedly depressed, either in association with low rCBF or out of proportion to rCBF, the likelihood of useful return of function in the tissue is small. If oxygen metabolism is preserved and there is a relatively high oxygen extraction function (OEF), then the outlook for recovery is better. Baron dubbed this situation of avidity of the local tissue for oxygen in the presence of poor perfusion the misery perfusion syndrome, the hallmark being the elevated OEF.[267,269] In chronic infarcts, CT regions of hypodensity and PET images of rCBF and the metabolic rate of oxygen are essentially congruous, showing dead tissue with little flow and little metabolism. During some phases of a stroke, rCBF may be increased relative to metabolism, a phenomenon dubbed luxury perfusion. Figure 4.34 illustrates the data generated from PET examinations in a patient with a MCA territory infarct.

Metabolic depression can also occur at sites distant from the zones of infarction. This finding has sometimes been called diaschisis. For example, metabolic depression may be evident in the cerebellum contralateral to hemispheric infarction, termed crossed cerebellar diaschisis. The recognized regions of reduced metabolism distant from brain infarcts and hemorrhages are noted in Table 4.6. These regions that show distant effects provide insight into brain pathways and help guide physiological approaches to rehabilitation. They also

Table 4.6 Regions of diaschisis (reduced metabolism) distant from brain infarcts and hemorrhages

Thalamus ipsilateral to a cerebral infarct
Cerebral cortex ipsilateral to thalamic lesion
Cerebral hemisphere contralateral to supratentorial infarct of the opposite hemisphere
Cerebellar hemisphere contralateral to cerebral lesion
Cerebellar hemisphere ipsilateral to pontine infarct

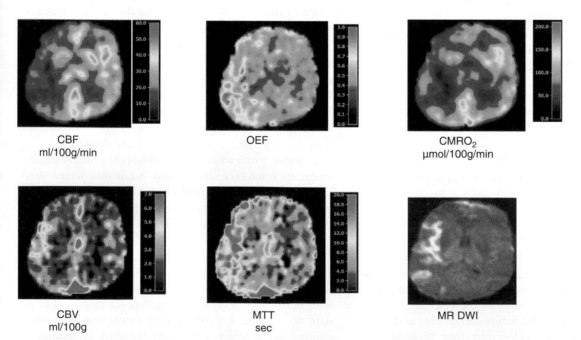

CBF
ml/100g/min

OEF

CMRO$_2$
µmol/100g/min

CBV
ml/100g

MTT
sec

MR DWI

Figure 4.34 PET parametric maps of cerebral blood flow (CBF), oxygen extraction fraction (OEF), oxygen consumption (CMRO$_2$), cerebral blood volume (CBV) and mean transit time (MTT), as well as the diffusion-weighted (DWI) scan, obtained in a 51-year-old man, 7–9 hours after acute-onset right-sided hemiparesis, homonymous hemianopia and neglect, and global dysphasia. One axial plane is shown for illustration. Images are shown in neurological orientation (i.e., right is shown on the right side). Quantitative gray–white intensity scales are shown to the right of each PET image for interpretation. There is extensive hypoperfusion over the entire left MCA territory, with CBF below the penumbra threshold of 20 ml/100 g/min in large parts of the affected cortex. The CMRO$_2$ is also reduced in the entire MCA territory, but less so than predicted by the CBF with massively increased OEF ("misery perfusion"). The CMRO$_2$ lies above the threshold for irreversible damage (around 39 µmol/100 g/min) throughout except around the posterior insula and surrounding white matter. The CBV and the MTT are also increased throughout, indicating overridden autoregulation from low perfusion pressure. The DWI lesion is heterogeneous and extensive but smaller than the area of hypoperfusion ("mismatch"); although it is partly congruent with the areas of very low CMRO$_2$ indicating irreversible damage, it also straddles areas of penumbra, characterized by CBF <20 ml/100 g/min, high OEF, and CMRO$_2$ above the irreversibility threshold. Courtesy of J-C Baron, J V Guadagno, M Takasawa, E A Warburton, et al., University of Cambridge, UK. A black and white version of this figure will appear in some formats. For the color version, please refer to the plate section.

help in understanding previously confusing rCBF results associated with xenon inhalation.

PET can also be used to study changes in flow and metabolism after various types of stimulation. Visual stimuli augment activity in the lateral geniculate body and striate regions. Auditory stimuli activate the medial geniculate body and various temporal and parietal regions, depending on whether music, language, or other auditory stimuli are used and the content of the sound. Speaking and right-limb movement activate parasylvian and frontal regions, predominantly in the left cerebral hemisphere. These studies give important insights into how the brain functions. Also, in some circumstances, rCBF and metabolism might be adequate for baseline function but may not be able to augment satisfactorily after stimulation. These functional studies also have the potential of telling how the damaged brain functions with sensory stimuli and how patterns of metabolism and flow change with recovery. Insight into reparative and adaptive mechanisms could ensue.

Without question, PET has opened up large vistas with potential insights into brain function. The expense of the equipment, the length of time required for testing, and the importance of ancillary physicists and chemists limit the applicability of the PET technique to large research centers funded for their studies. Functional MRI (fMRI) studies have begun to develop the capability of demonstrating brain function and activity without the need for a cyclotron. Furthermore, fMRI can be performed on the same equipment used for brain and vascular imaging.

Recently PET has been used to diagnose cerebral amyloid angiopathy and Alzheimer's disease.[270,271] Radionuclides with an affinity for amyloid (Pittsburgh compound B and fluoroethyl methyl amino-2-naphthyl ethylidene malonitrile) are used during PET scanning (PiB-PET) to show the quantity and distribution of amyloid within the brain and within brain blood vessels.[270,271]

Catheter digital subtraction angiography

MRA and CTA have the advantage of being able to be performed at the same time as brain imaging and are non-invasive. The advent of high-quality CTA, MRA, and cervical and transcranial ultrasonography have led to a marked decrease in the indications for catheter contrast angiography. Catheter angiography is now performed using a digital subtraction technique that allows for less dye injection than was used in the past. Digital subtraction cerebral angiography is indicated when the preliminary testing does not satisfactorily clarify the nature of the vascular lesions and when treatment depends on the nature and severity of those vascular lesions. For example, angiography may be used in patients in whom dissection or stenosis has been inadequately demonstrated by non-invasive testing. Angiography is often required to better define cerebral aneurysms and vascular malformations. Catheter angiography is used as a prelude to intravascular interventions such as intra-arterial thrombolysis and mechanical thrombectomy and angioplasty and stenting because the treatment is given directly within the artery. In experienced hands, angiography gives valuable information and has a

Table 4.7 Factors related to complications of cerebral angiography

Equipment, dye, and catheters used
Method, quantity, and rate of dye infusion
Number of injections
Training and experience of angiographer
Whether a large volume of contrast is injected into aortic arch
General medical and psychological state of the patient
Adequacy of hydration
Kidney function
Nature and severity of the occlusive cervico-cranial vascular disease

relatively low incidence of serious complications. The commonest factors that relate to complications are noted in Table 4.7.

Angiography should be tailored to the clinical question and therapeutic alternatives. Brain and non-invasive vascular imaging (CT or MRI) or ultrasonography, or both, usually should precede angiography. These tests help the angiographer focus on the particular regions of interest. Screening of other arterial regions by non-invasive techniques allows the angiographer to limit the angiographic procedure, thus helping reduce morbidity, time, and expense. The clinician and the angiographer should decide together on the important data clinically needed, considering the clinical context of the study.

The following critical angiography "rules" are useful:[272]

1. Tailor angiography to the patient and the individual problem. Avoid extra injections, catheterization, and dye because they increase the risk of the procedure.

2. Follow Sutton's law. Sutton robbed banks because that is where the money is – go after the highest-yield information first. Angiographers, after a catheter had flipped unexpectedly into a vessel that was not the primary focus of attention, often take several films "while they were there," believing that the films might be necessary anyway. Too often, a complication or other unforeseen exigency curtails the procedure before the important data are obtained. First things first.

3. The clinician responsible for the patient and the angiographer should plan and discuss the procedure together. Ideally, the procedure should be performed with both present, choosing together the next shot as the data accumulate. Because of time constraints and other commitments, this is not always possible. Telephone contact at critical decision points often is an acceptable substitute. If a clinician cannot be reached during the procedure, discussion of the plan of attack and treatment choices with the angiographer is a minimum requirement. In some circumstances, the relationship between angiographer and clinician is so well oiled by shared past experiences that the angiographer learns how the clinician approaches most common situations.

In that case, consultation during the procedure would occur only if unexpected or unusual findings were uncovered. Ideally, if the responsible clinician is not the surgeon who will perform an operative procedure, the surgeon also should be contacted when findings are uncovered that would dictate an operation. Surgeons may have their own demands for studies before surgery, and this is best accomplished during the angiography. Communication between clinicians and neuroradiologists is also important for the performance and interpretation of MRA and CTA protocols, because neuroradiologists should monitor the studies as they are performed to be sure that the information derived answers the queries raised by the clinicians caring for the patient.

4. Avoid an aortic arch injection whenever possible. The yield of arch opacification studies is low. Akers and colleagues reviewed the results of 1000 consecutive patients who had arch angiography, followed by selective catheterization of both carotid and vertebral arteries.[273] Only 6 (0.6%) had intrathoracic vascular pathology that was hemodynamically important, including 4 lesions at the common carotid artery origin and 2 at the innominate artery origin. Three of these lesions (two common carotid arteries and one innominate) would have been discovered if only selective catheterization were performed. Inability to selectively catheterize these arteries and fluoroscopy identify most cases requiring arch injection. The absence of a significant lesion in the head or neck should alert the angiographer to opacify the origin of the artery on the way out. Arch injections usually require 40–50 ml of contrast material injected under pressure, so cardiac overload and renal toxicity do occur. A large bolus of dye used for filming the arch limits the amount of dye that should be used during selective catheterization. Arch films are also not easy to read because of overlapping of vessels. In my opinion, there is no reason to perform routine arch angiography. Only the major arteries of interest should be studied using the Seldinger technique of selective catheterization. In addition, intra-arterial digital subtraction filming techniques allow use of less dye while retaining high-quality films.

5. Use the least amount of dye and injections to arrive at a therapeutic decision. Often, the initial opacification provides enough information so that other injections are not needed.

6. Talk to and examine the patient at least briefly after each dye injection, to detect any complication that might dictate stopping the procedure. The neurological examination depends on the vessels studied. For example, after posterior circulation opacification, check vision and memory; after carotid artery injection, check speech and arm movement.

In JH, LRC did not perform contrast angiography. The concordance of the MRA, ultrasound data, and the unlikelihood of a treatable lesion persuaded LRC not to pursue angiography. His clinical deficit was also severe and not reversible.

Cardiac evaluation

Cardioembolic mechanisms of ischemic stroke are common. The proportion of ischemic strokes generally considered to have originated from cardioembolic sources has increased dramatically with the development of sophisticated technology that has the capability of defining cardiac and vascular lesions. A wide variety of different cardiac lesions are now known to be potential sources of embolism, while in the remote past, only acute myocardial infarction and rheumatic mitral stenosis with atrial fibrillation were generally accepted cardiac sources.

Cardiac emboli arise from a varied assortment of diseases that affect the heart valves, heart rhythm, endocardial surface, and myocardium.[274] Of these, non-valvular atrial fibrillation is the commonest pathology. Pump failure can cause general cerebral hypoperfusion. In addition, many patients with brain ischemia caused by neck and intracranial atherosclerosis have coexisting coronary artery atherosclerosis. Late deaths in series of patients with ischemic stroke are most often caused by coronary artery disease and myocardial infarction rather than by cerebrovascular disease. These facts should direct the physician's attention to the stroke patient's heart, as well as to the brain and its vascular supply.

The question is not whether to look at the heart but how thoroughly to do so. What is the yield of intensive cardiac investigation? Is it worth the cost? Most clinicians agree that it is important to take a careful cardiac history, particularly seeking symptoms of arrhythmia, congestive heart failure, angina pectoris, and prior myocardial infarctions. The heart should be carefully examined, noting heart size, quality of sounds, rhythm, and presence of gallops, in addition to seeking and characterizing murmurs. An electrocardiogram and chest x-ray should also be obtained routinely because of their high screening value, safety, and low cost.

Table 4.8 lists the demographic features and history features in ischemic stroke patients that indicate the need for echocardiography. Table 4.9 lists the situations recognizable after the preliminary investigations in which echocardiography has a high yield. In these circumstances, intensive cardiac testing is essential. Transthoracic echocardiography (TTE) is often performed first, and the results may be definitive, and, thus, transesophageal echocardiography (TEE) would not be required. Because the left atrium is directly anterior to the

Table 4.8 Situations in which echocardiography has a high yield in ischemic stroke patients

Known prior heart disease

Clinical course suggestive of brain embolism – that is, sudden onset of neurological deficit, while active, without prior TIAs

A history of peripheral embolism in the limbs or abdominal viscera

Young age with no atherosclerotic risk factors. (Young patients who have no known risk factors for atherosclerosis often harbor unexpected cardiac sources, such as cardiac tumors, intra-atrial defects, or cardiomyopathy)

Table 4.9 Preliminary investigation results leading to important yield of echocardiography in ischemic stroke patients

Absence of extracranial and intracranial vascular disease on non-invasive testing

Superficial infarct on CT or MRI in the distribution of a peripheral branch of the MCA or PCA or cerebellar arteries

Hemorrhagic transformation of a brain infarct in one vascular territory

CT or MRI showing infarcts in multiple vascular territories

Normal CTA, MRA, or contrast arteriography in a patient whose clinical deficit and brain imaging are not compatible with lacunar infarction

Angiography (CTA, MRA, or standard catheter) that shows distal cut-off of a brain artery branch or a luminal filling defect without severe proximal arterial stenosis

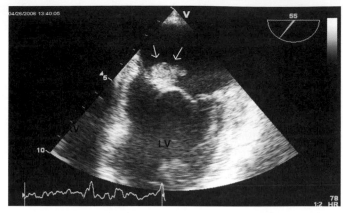

Figure 4.35 Transesophageal image of large vegetation (white arrows) on the anterior mitral valve leaflet. Courtesy of Susan Yeon, MD, Beth Israel Deaconess Medical Center and Harvard Medical School, Boston, MA.

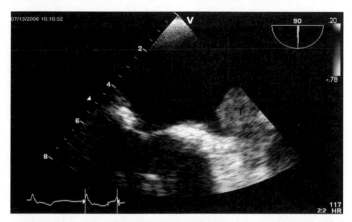

Figure 4.36 TEE image at the midesophageal level at 90-degree transducer orientations. A large thrombus (T) is seen along the lateral wall of the left atrium (LA) and filling the left atrial appendage. Courtesy of Warren Manning, MD, Beth Israel Deaconess Medical Center and Harvard Medical School, Boston, MA.

esophagus, atrial lesions, occult valvular disorders, and ulcerative lesions of the proximal aorta, often missed by transthoracic echocardiography, are detected by the TEE approach. TEE shows many abnormalities not revealed by TTE. The use of TEE in patients with strokes and TIAs has been extensively reviewed.[274–279] TEE is more accurate than TTE in showing atrial and ventricular thrombi, in detecting and quantifying intracardiac shunts, and more often shows spontaneous echo contrast than TTE. The significance of finding a patent foramen ovale (present in 25% of the general population but over-represented in "cryptogenic" stroke) is debated. There are certainly instances where paradoxical embolism via the patent foramen ovale (PFO) have caused strokes but in many cases it may be an innocent bystander. Some features such as the presence of an atrial septal aneurysm and large volume shunts have been associated with a higher risk of stroke recurrence. However, whether device closure of the PFO reduces the risk of recurrent stroke has not been established in large randomized trials, and this remains a controversial area.[280,281] Figure 4.35 shows a vegetation on the mitral valve. Figure 4.36 shows an

atrial thrombus identified on echocardiography in patients with cardiogenic brain embolism.

TEE may not be able to identify a potential cardiac source of emboli. Some thromboemboli are too small to be detected. An embolus that is 1 or 2 mm in size can produce a devastating neurological deficit, and this size particle is often beyond the resolution of echocardiography.[274,282,283] The other major reason for failure of echocardiography to show a thrombus is that thrombosis and embolism are dynamic processes. When a thrombus leaves the heart to go to the brain, echocardiography may not show a residual thrombus within the heart if performed soon after the clinical event.[282,283] The thrombus may re-form later.

TEE also yields important information about the proximal aorta, a region not imaged by TTE.[284] Figure 4.37 shows different types of aortic plaques detected by TEE. It has been established that substantial aortic arch atheroma, indicated by plaque thickness of greater than 4 mm or a mobile plaque are independent risk factors for recurrent stroke.[284] The optimal therapy for major arch atheroma has not been clarified.[285] TEE is important in all patients in whom TTE suggests, but does not adequately define, the cardiac pathology, and in all patients in whom other studies (cerebrovascular, hematological, and other cardiac investigations) do not satisfactorily show the cause of brain embolism and brain ischemia.[277,282] Radionuclide testing, including gated blood pool imaging (multigated acquisition scans), also may be helpful in selected patients as might other cardiac imaging techniques.[286]

The aorta is an important potential source of embolism, especially during angiography and cardiac surgery.[284,287] Presently, TEE is the most common method of imaging the aorta for plaques and thrombi. The ascending aorta can also be insonated using a duplex ultrasound probe placed in the right supraclavicular fossa. The arch and proximal descending thoracic aorta can be imaged using a left supraclavicular probe.[288] The results so far are preliminary but promising. Most plaques are located in the curvature of the arch from the distal ascending aorta to the proximal descending aorta, regions shown by B-mode ultrasound.[288]

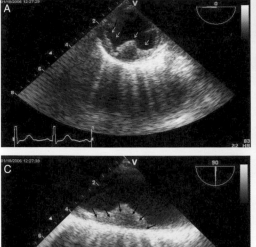

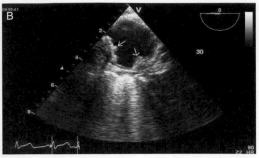

Figure 4.37 (A) Transesophageal long-axis (90 degrees) view of thoracic aorta with complex plaque (white arrows). (B) TEE image at the mid-esophageal level in the horizontal (0 degree) transducer orientation. Two atherosclerotic plaques (white arrows) are visible and invaginate into the aortic lumen. (C) Transesophageal long-axis (90 degrees) view of thoracic aorta with complex plaque (black arrows). Courtesy of Susan Yeon, MD, and Warren Manning, MD, Beth Israel Deaconess Medical Center and Harvard Medical School, Boston, MA.

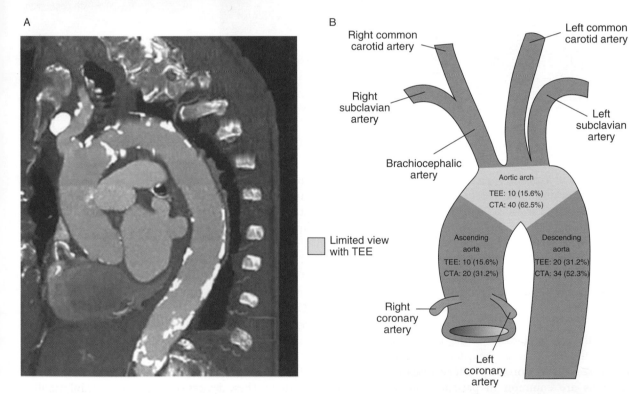

Figure 4.38 (A) CTA, lateral view of the aorta showing calcified plaques within the ascending, arch, and descending aorta. (B) Drawing showing location and frequency of plaques within portions of the aorta detected by CTA versus TEE. From Chatzikonstantinou A, Krissak R, Flüchter S. CT angiography of the aorta is superior to transesophageal echocardiography for determining stroke subtypes in patients with cryptogenic ischemic stroke. *Cerebrovasc Dis* 2012;33:322–328 with permission.

TEE is fairly invasive and is not always well tolerated by patients. The distal part of the ascending aorta and the proximal right portion of the aortic arch are often poorly visualized in TEE due to the location of the trachea and the right main stem bronchus between the esophagus and the aorta. CTA has increasingly been used to define and localize aortic arch plaques.[289] Figure 4.38A shows a CTA of the

aorta and Figure 4.38B shows the location of aortic plaques shown by CTA as compared to the frequency detected by TEE in one study.[289] The majority of plaques are found by CTA in the aortic arch and a significant number are also found in the proximal thoracic portion of the descending aorta. Studies of blood flow in the aorta show that particles discharged from the descending aorta can flow retrograde

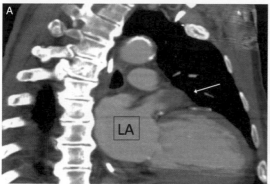

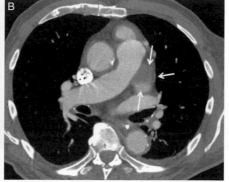

Figure 4.39 Contrast-enhanced chest CT. (A) Oblique reformatted image that shows a thrombus within the left atrial appendage. (B) Axial reformatted image showing a left atrial appendage filling defect that represents a thrombus. Courtesy of Susan Yeon, MD, and Warren Manning, MD, Beth Israel Deaconess Medical Center and Harvard Medical School, Boston, MA.

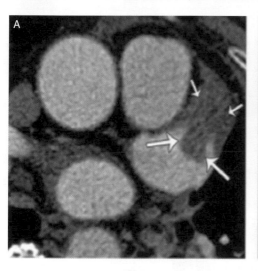

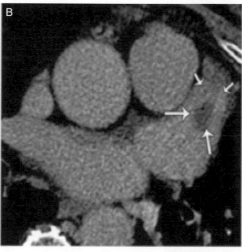

Figure 4.40 Early and late phase cardiac CTA images showing (A) an oval-shape filling defect in the left atrial appendage (white arrows) with circulatory stasis just distal to the thrombus, and (B) the filling defect distal to the thrombus caused by circulatory stasis disappears on late-phase imaging. From Hur J, Kim Y J, Lee H-J, et al., Cardiac computed tomographic angiography for detection of cardiac sources of embolism in stroke patients. *Stroke* 2009;40:2073–2078 with permission.

into the aortic arch and so potentially embolize to the brain.[290]

When clinical suspicion of a cardiac source embolism is high and echocardiography is not diagnostic, chest CT with contrast enhancement (Figure 4.39A,B), cardiac CTA (Figure 4.40), and cardiac MRI all have the capability of showing thrombi within cardiac chambers.[291] Documentation of a potential cardioembolic source – such as mitral valve prolapse, patent foramen ovale, mitral annulus calcification, or akinetic zones – does not mean per se that the patient has had brain embolism. Coexistent atherosclerotic disease may be the cause and these pathologies often coexist.

Many patients with atherosclerosis of the carotid and vertebral arteries in the neck have coexistent peripheral vascular occlusive disease and coronary artery disease.[292] Myocardial infarctions are common in patients who had first presented with strokes.[293] Stroke patients, especially those with carotid artery disease, show a high prevalence of coexistent coronary artery disease. Because coronary artery disease, even when silent, can be life-threatening, screening of these patients for silent myocardial ischemia and for the presence of coronary artery disease is important, especially if surgery is considered. Coronary artery CTA[294], CT scanning of the heart for calcification of the coronary arteries[295] and coronary MRA[296] are techniques now being investigated for non-invasive recognition of coronary artery disease. Calcification within coronary arteries does correlate

with coronary artery stenosis and the risk of myocardial infarction.[297] If severe coronary artery disease is suggested by screening tests, coronary angiography may be needed to localize and quantify the coronary artery disease to guide treatment.

The importance of ambulatory monitoring for cardiac rhythm disturbances is increasingly recognized. In patients suspected of brain embolism, the yield is probably high enough to dictate the use of heart rhythm monitoring. Monitoring can involve simply continuous electrocardiogram (ECG) while hospitalized or short term (24–48 h) or longer term ambulatory cardiac rhythm monitoring after the hospitalization.[298–301] Ambulatory rhythm monitors can be worn for 30 days. More recently "loop" recorders can be implanted under the skin of the chest to record the heart's electrical activity. These devices continuously store information in their circular memory (the "loop") as ECGs. Arrhythmias are recorded by "freezing" a segment of the memory for later review. Typically, up to three episodes of abnormal activity can be stored with the most recent episode replacing the oldest. The devices can effectively monitor heart rhythms for a year or more. Some patients have single or multiple very brief episodes of atrial fibrillation. Uncertainty still surrounds the significance of these very short instances of arrhythmia. Long-term monitoring studies have detected significant episodes of atrial fibrillation in 10–15% of stroke patients labeled "cryptogenic" stroke after standard investigations.[301]

In patients with lacunar infarcts and those with a well-defined atherosclerotic extracranial vascular cause for their stroke, the yield is probably low. Cardiac rhythm monitoring should probably be done in any patient whose initial EEG suggests a cardiac rhythm abnormality. More recently biomarker testing has been studied to identify those patients likely to have or develop atrial fibrillation. A high level of brain natriuretic peptide (BNP), especially its metabolite N-terminal pro-B-type natriuretic peptide seems to be useful in detecting the presence or risk of atrial fibrillation.[302,303] Cardiologists are exploring other means of predicting the development of atrial fibrillation and the risk of associated brain embolism. In some patients who have normal sinus rhythm on ECG, pulsed-wave Doppler interrogation of the left atrial appendage shows an atrial fibrillation phenotype.[304] The morphology of the left atrial appendage may also help predict the presence of intermittent atrial fibrillation and so stimulate monitoring.

Other investigations

A wide variety of other tests have been used in the past to study arterial flow in the brain vessels. Most of these investigations have been superseded by newer ultrasound technology and neuroimaging techniques. These include oculoplethysmography and ophthalmodynamometry, techniques that were described in the first two editions of this book but have now been superseded by TCD. A new ultrasound technology, color Doppler imaging of the vessels that supply the eye, has become available and can accurately image and define vascular lesions that involve the ophthalmic and central retinal arteries.[305,306]

The tests described so far help localize and quantify morphological structural abnormalities in the brain and the brain-supplying arteries. Two other advances, MR spectroscopy (MRS) and fMRI, have added new dimensions to the study of stroke and brain ischemia. During MRS, regions of interest as identified by MRI can be analyzed for the relative volumes and localization of various chemical constituents such as choline, creatine, N-acetyl aspartate, lactate, and glutamate.[307–309] Elevated lactate is found soon after infarction; decreased N-acetyl aspartate, creatine, and choline are characteristic of the MRS spectrum in the region of brain infarction. MRS analysis may be useful in the future in distinguishing tissue that is destined to become infarcted from tissue that is reversibly ischemic. MRS may also prove useful in studying patients with various stroke-related metabolic problems, such as mitochondrial disorders that alter brain metabolism.[308]

When certain MRI techniques are used during perceptual, cognitive, and motor tasks, small changes in signal intensity show alterations in local blood flow related to increased brain activity and function during these tasks.[310–312] fMRI can yield insights into which parts of the brain are being used to perform various brain functions. This information is probably most relevant to the study of recovery from stroke and may give important insights into spontaneous recovery and the potential of various rehabilitative therapies. Figures 4.41, 4.42, and 4.43 show fMRI scans in some patients with strokes.

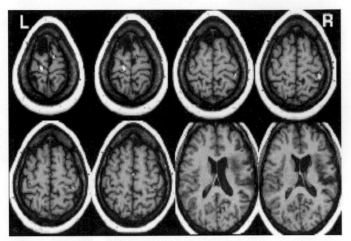

Figure 4.41 fMRI scans of a patient with a right cerebral infarct (best seen on the image at the bottom right). When he is asked to try and move his left hand, both the right and left motor regions are activated as shown by spots. Courtesy of Gottfried Schlaug, MD, Beth Israel Deaconess Medical Center and Harvard Medical School, Boston, MA.

What if brain imaging shows an intracerebral hemorrhage?

The most common cause of ICH is hypertension, either acute or chronic. When the blood pressure is high and CT or MRI shows a hematoma in a typical location for hypertensive ICH (putamen, caudate nucleus, thalamus, pons, cerebellum), a search for AVMs or aneurysms has a very low yield but a CT angiogram is probably worthwhile. In young patients with no hypertension or with intraventricular or lobar hematomas, however, studies of the intracerebral arteries often show vascular lesions. Patients with ICH after using cocaine, especially the hydrochloride form, have a relatively high incidence of underlying vascular malformations.[313,314]

MRI can show AVMs and cavernous angiomas well. Vascular channels, serpiginous arteries, mixed-density heterogeneous signals, and the presence of old bleeds containing hemosiderin are clues to the presence of vascular malformations. Contrast-enhanced CT and MRI, plain or enhanced with gadolinium, can show large aneurysms if they are in the plane of the sections taken. CTA and MRA effectively show AVMs and aneurysms. In some patients, digital subtraction angiography with opacification of the arteries supplying the ICH, is needed for definitive exclusion of small AVMs and aneurysms larger than 3 mm. Cavernous and venous angiomas are usually not detected by cerebral angiography. Repeating the MRI after 6–8 weeks when the hematoma has at least partially resolved may increase the yield for underlying vascular and neoplastic lesions.

What if brain imaging or lumbar puncture show subarachnoid hemorrhage?

Cerebral angiography is still often required for the study of patients with SAH not explainable by trauma or a known bleeding diathesis. Aneurysmal re-rupture is such a potentially lethal event that clinicians must be sure an aneurysm is not present in patients with SAH. CTA has achieved sufficient

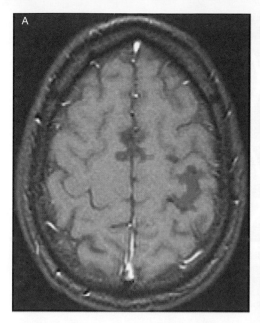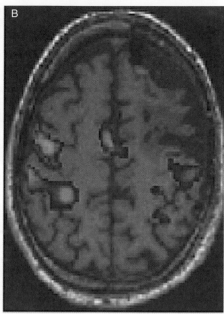

Figure 4.42 fMRI scans. (A) Scan after a normal patient is asked to move the left hand. The gray regions in the right frontal convexal and paramedian areas represent activation. (B) A patient with a right cerebral infarct is asked to move the left hand. The activation in this patient (white regions in the left cerebral hemisphere and black regions in the right cerebral hemisphere) is bilateral but mostly in the non-affected hemisphere. Courtesy of Alvaro Pascual-Leone, MD, Beth Israel Deaconess Medical Center and Harvard Medical School, Boston, MA.

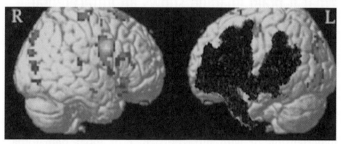

Figure 4.43 fMRI scans in a patient with a large left cerebral infarct that rendered him aphasic. The infarct is shaded black on the figure at the right. Activation is predominantly in the right cerebral hemisphere contralateral to the infarct in the figure on the left that is a lateral view of the right cerebral hemisphere. Courtesy of Alvaro Pascual-Leone, MD, Beth Israel Deaconess Medical Center and Harvard Medical School, Boston, MA.

resolution that it is often possible to determine endovascular versus surgical management on the basis of this non-invasive test.[204,315] However, lesions of the floor of the anterior cranial fossa and pial lesions (e.g., dural arteriovenous fistulas) are generally better shown using digital catheter angiography. MRI may also be helpful in detecting small vascular malformations near the ependymal and pial surfaces. MRA and CTA may be useful in following patients after surgical or endovascular treatment of aneurysms and AVMs, and in following unruptured aneurysms and AVMs not treated surgically. TCD is helpful in following patients with aneurysmal SAH in detecting and monitoring vasoconstriction in the basal intracranial arteries.[81,316,317]

Question 4: Are abnormalities in the blood causing or contributing to brain ischemia or hemorrhage?

Once the clinician has determined the nature, site, and severity of the vascular lesion, it is important to find out whether abnormalities of blood constituents are causing or contributing to brain ischemia or hemorrhage. Clinicians must not forget the blood. Abnormalities of the clotting system can lead to hypercoagulability and thrombosis. Even in patients with lesions known to predispose to thromboembolism and brain ischemia, the acute event is often precipitated by a change in the blood and its coagulability. Infections, cancer, and inflammatory bowel disease are examples of conditions that are associated with release of acute-phase reactants that may alter coagulability sufficiently to promote thromboembolism – especially if there is a pre-existing lesion that affects an endothelial surface. Bleeding diatheses often cause intracranial bleeding. Abnormalities of the viscosity of blood can alter blood flow, especially in small arterioles and capillaries of the brain, and in patients with occlusive lesions. Increased viscosity can cause or contribute to regional decreases in CBF and potentiate ischemia. Autoimmunity, which can be detected and monitored by blood tests, can lead to occlusive cerebrovascular disease.

What if the problem is ischemia?

The formed cellular elements of the blood – erythrocytes, leukocytes, and platelets – should always be studied. Screening tests of coagulation functions should also be a part of the routine evaluation of patients with brain ischemia. In addition, other blood components may be analyzed, such as serum proteins, coagulation factors, antiphospholipid antibodies, and blood viscosity.

Erythrocytes

Quantitative and qualitative RBC abnormalities can affect blood flow and clotting. The level of the Hct clearly affects whole blood viscosity and the rheological properties of blood. Physicians have long been aware that high Hct levels, such as 60% or more, can cause clotting in normal young adults. In

older patients with pre-existing atherosclerosis and small-vessel disease, high Hcts that are still within the normal range can compound the vascular disease and limit perfusion. Studies in animals[318] and humans[319–321] confirm that the Hct level can affect blood flow and prognosis even when Hct levels are not frankly polycythemic. The Hct level also has a heavy impact on blood viscosity.[322,323] Lowering the Hct from 45 to 32 results in doubling of CBF.[324] High Hct levels are a factor in reducing reperfusion of ischemic brain and are associated with larger brain infarcts.[325] These studies have led to the concept that acute hemodilution with reduction of Hct and increased cerebral blood flow could be effective in acute ischemic stroke, but clinical trials have been uniformly negative.

Sickle cell disease and other hemoglobinopathies can lead to altered flow and hypercoagulability. Sickle cell disease and spherocytosis are associated with multifocal brain infarcts. TCD documents abnormalities of flow velocities even in young patients with sickle cell disease. These abnormalities correlate well with regions of arterial narrowing and with the occurrence of strokes[326–328] and help select patients for prophylactic blood transfusions.[329,330]

Hemoglobin and Hct certainly should be measured in every patient with stroke. Lowering of relatively high Hct levels by blood donations has been advocated as a measure to prophylactically reduce the risk of stroke in stroke-prone individuals. Hemoglobin electrophoresis is important in those with racial and genetic predispositions to hemoglobinopathies, especially if anemia is present. Careful examination of a stained blood smear for the morphology of RBCs can suggest the possibility of a hemoglobinopathy. Severe anemia promotes hypercoagulability and also can compound brain ischemia, but low Hct levels are not common in stroke patients.

Leukocytes

The white blood cell (WBC) count is often elevated in patients with myocardial infarction and is also often slightly elevated in patients with brain infarcts. Some have correlated a high WBC count with the severity of carotid atherosclerosis[331] and carotid[332] and aortic arch plaque[333] thickness but interpretation of this finding is clouded by the fact that cigarette smoking is one cause of a high WBC count. Patients with elevated WBC counts also seem to have reduced endothelial reactivity.[334] A relatively elevated WBC is also a marker predicting the likelihood of developing a first stroke.[335] A high WBC count is also a marker of inflammatory activity in the body and inflammation is an important cause of blood vessel damage.[336]

Leukemia with high WBC counts can cause packing of capillaries and small arterioles with aggregates of large WBCs, causing multiple small infarcts and hemorrhages. This is suggested by a high leukocrit in the capillary tube used to measure Hct. Measurement of WBC count is usually a routine part of a complete blood cell count, which should be ordered on each stroke patient.

Platelets

Platelets are critical structures active in the initiation of blood coagulation. Evidence of the central importance of platelets in cerebrovascular disease is the enthusiasm clinicians have had for platelet inhibition as a major treatment for patients who have or are at risk of developing brain ischemia. Quantitative and qualitative platelet abnormalities can cause hypercoagulability and bleeding.[337–339] Thrombocytosis, especially with platelet counts greater than 1 million, can cause hypercoagulability and vascular occlusion and brain infarction.[340,341] Platelet counts should be a routine part of the initial evaluation of patients with ischemic stroke because thrombocytosis can potentiate thrombosis. Low platelet counts can suggest the presence of other disorders, such as the antiphospholipid antibody syndrome, heparin-induced thrombocytopenia, consumptive coagulopathies, systemic lupus erythematosus, and thrombotic thrombocytopenic purpura – all of which are often complicated by brain ischemia. Platelet counts can fall during the course of illness (e.g., heparin-induced thrombocytopenia),[342,343] so that a baseline count before treatment is useful for later comparison.

Some patients with platelet counts in the normal range have increased platelet aggregation and secretion, or qualitative abnormalities of platelet morphology and function. In-vitro platelet function tests are usually performed in hematological research laboratories, and even experts disagree on their applicability to the in-vivo state. Studies to date have not confirmed any clinical value of using platelet function testing and hence routine testing is not recommended. Platelet aggregation is usually measured after the addition of various agents known to increase aggregation, such as arachidonic acid, adenosine diphosphate, epinephrine, and collagen.[338,344] The extent of platelet activation can also be studied by measuring the levels of beta-thromboglobulin in the blood.[338,344–346] Beta-thromboglobulin is secreted during platelet-release reactions, and, when optimal venipuncture technique is used, the levels are good markers of in vivo platelet activation and secretion. Simultaneous measurement of platelet factor 4, which has a short half-life, can help control in-vitro platelet changes.[347,348] Heparin-induced thrombocytopenia is characterized by elevated antiheparin/platelet factor 4 antibody titers and these can be measured in patients on heparin.[344,348]

Platelet production of thromboxane B_2 can be performed by radioimmunoassays and von Willebrand factor antigen can also be quantified.[349–351] Polymorphisms in the platelet glycoprotein II/III fibrinogen receptor have been described; these may also predispose to hypercoagulability and brain and myocardial ischemia.[352]

Fibrinogen, albumin and globulins, blood viscosity, and lipids

Fibrinogen is an important part of the coagulation system because fibrinogen is converted to fibrin monomers by the action of thrombin. Fibrin is an essential component of red and white thrombi. Fibrinogen also contributes to blood viscosity because high levels of fibrinogen can increase blood viscosity. Under ordinary circumstances, the Hct and fibrinogen levels are the two most important single predictors of whole-blood viscosity.[320,321]

Normal fibrinogen levels usually range from 250 to 400 mg/dl. High levels of fibrinogen have been shown to be risk factors for stroke in many studies.[353–359] Fibrinogen levels can also rise as acute-phase reactants in the early period after stroke. Ancrod (a defibrogenating enzyme of Malayan pit-viper venom), has been used to lower fibrinogen levels and to decrease fibrin formation, potentially lyse thrombi, and increase blood flow.[360,361] However, clinical trials have been negative. High fibrinogen levels decrease the likelihood of effective reperfusion after thrombolysis.[362] Omega 3 fish oil preparations containing eicosapentaenoic acid may also act to decrease fibrinogen content.[363]

Patients with a predisposition to stroke recurrence have a slightly lower serum albumin level and albumin–globulin ratio than those without recurrence.[355] Abnormally high levels of immunoglobulin (Ig) A, IgG, and IgM can indicate autoimmune disease and can be a clue to diagnosis in patients with unexplained brain ischemia. Macroglobulins found in Waenström's macroglobulinemia and multiple myeloma also can increase blood viscosity and cause or potentiate multiple loci of ischemia. Immunoglobulin measurements are now not a part of the routine evaluation of stroke patients because of their low yield. In selected patients with clinical and ophthalmoscopic suggestions of hyperviscosity, and in those with a high serum globulin level, serum immunoelectrophoresis can be helpful. Another unusual cause of hyperviscosity is a very high titer of lipoproteins. High levels of triglycerides, chylomicra, low-density and very-low-density lipoprotein cholesterol fractions can increase whole blood viscosity.[364,365] Measurement of blood lipids should be performed in every patient with brain ischemia and those with a family history of hyperlipidemia.

Studies have also shown that elevated levels of lipoprotein (a) [Lp(a)] are an independent risk factor for stroke and other important cardiovascular conditions.[366–368] In a large study among 5888 community-dwelling individuals aged more than 65 years, men in the highest quintile of Lp(a) had three times the risk of stroke and three times the risk of vascular disease-related death compared to the lowest quintile.[367] High Lp(a) levels also have been correlated with the extent of symptomatic intracranial atherosclerosis.[368]

Studies of coagulation factors and coagulation

The prothrombin time (PT) or the international normalized ratio (INR) and the activated partial thromboplastin time (aPTT) are excellent screening tests of coagulation function and are routinely available in nearly all hospital laboratories. Measurement of the PT (or INR) and the aPTT should usually be part of stroke evaluation. Indications for sometimes ordering other tests of coagulation are noted in Table 4.10.

Some serum proteins – such as antithrombin, protein C, and protein S – are natural inhibitors of coagulation. A decrease in the level of these substances because of a familial inherited condition or an acquired disease can cause hypercoagulability. An inherited coagulation deficit, usually referred to as resistance to activated protein C, has been described by Dutch investigators from Leiden.[369–372] In most instances, resistance to

Table 4.10 Potential reasons to order coagulation testing for ischemic stroke patients

Hypercoagulable state is suspected by acceleration of PT or aPTT
Multiple vascular occlusions are present and no cardiac source of embolism has been detected
Occlusion of veins in the upper or lower extremities and the presence of an ischemic stroke
Dural sinus and/or cerebral venous occlusion
A past history of recurrent thrombophlebitis or miscarriages
Known neoplastic, collagen, vascular, rheumatological, or inflammatory diseases are present

activated protein C is caused by a point mutation in the gene that encodes for coagulation factor V.[370] The presence of this mutation, called factor V Leiden, is accompanied by a threefold to fivefold increase in the frequency of venous thromboembolism in the lower extremities[372] and an increased frequency of cerebral venous thrombosis. Factor V Leiden is the most common recognized genetic disorder that leads to hypercoagulability but its relevance for arterial thromboembolism has not yet been unequivocally established. The second most common genetic mutation that leads to a prothrombotic state is a mutation in the gene encoding prothrombin.[371,373] This mutation involves a transition from guanine to adenine at position 20210 in the sequence of the 3' untranslated region of the prothrombin gene.[373] The frequency of cerebral and peripheral venous thrombosis is greatly increased in carriers of the prothrombin gene mutation, especially if they also take oral contraceptive pills.[374] Genetic analysis is warranted in patients with unexplained hypercoagulability, especially those with cerebral venous thrombosis and recurrent peripheral venous thromboembolism.

The level of coagulation factors VII, VIII, IX, and X can be measured in most hematological laboratories but have not been well studied in large groups of stroke patients. Abnormal levels of factor VIII can cause hypercoagulability and recurrent strokes.[375–377] Factor VIII elevation can be chronic, precede and predispose to stroke, increase as an acute-phase reactant in systemic illnesses such as ulcerative colitis, and can increase secondary to thrombosis. In the latter case, it is a marker and not the cause of the thrombosis.[375–377] High levels of factor VIII activity have been correlated with carotid and coronary atherosclerosis.[378] In a study performed in India of patients with non-puerperal, non-infectious cerebral venous thrombosis, factor VIII levels were nearly twice as high as controls (235.4 vs. 121.2 IU/dL).[379] In this study the patients' fibrinogen levels were not increased indicating that the elevated factor VIII levels likely preceded and contributed to the venous occlusion rather than reflected elevation as an acute phase reactant.[379] Levels of other factors have been explored and may be utilized more in the future. High levels of plasma von Willebrand factor increase the risk of stroke and other vascular events in patients with atrial fibrillation,[380] and is a risk factor for first ischemic strokes.[381]

Hemostatic markers of coagulation activity have been used to detect and monitor hypercoagulability.[382,383] Thrombin acts as a catalyst of the proteolysis of fibrinogen to fibrin. During this reaction, fibrinopeptide A is generated. The level of fibrin D-dimer is an index of fibrin generation. The level of the prothrombin activation fragment F1.2 is a measure of in vivo thrombin generation.[383] Increasing intensity of anticoagulation is accompanied by decreasing thrombin generation as measured by the F1.2 levels.[384,385] Fibrinolysis involves the dissolution of fibrin by endogenous fibrinolytic mechanisms. Fibrinolytic activity can be estimated by the levels of fibrinopeptide B-beta 1–42 and of tissue plasminogen activator and its inhibitor. Thrombosis is favored when thrombin proteolysis of fibrinogen (increased fibrinopeptide A and D-dimer levels) exceeds plasmin proteolysis (increased fibrinopeptide B-beta 1–42 and tissue plasminogen activator to its inhibitor ratio).[346,385–387] Several studies have monitored the levels of these substances in acute stroke patients and during follow-up.[346,383,387] D-dimer testing has been used to monitor the continued need for anticoagulation in patients with venous thromboembolism.[322,388]

Antiphospholipid antibodies

Antiphospholipid antibodies (APLAs) are usually IgG or IgM antibodies that bind to negatively charged phospholipids. Phospholipids are important constituents of vascular endothelium, heart proteins, platelets, and other cells.[389–391] Laboratory studies show that sera from patients with APLAs have increased immunoglobulin binding to cerebral endothelium.[392] The two most commonly measured APLAs are anticardiolipin antibody and the so-called lupus anticoagulant (LA). LAs are acquired immunoglobulins that are associated clinically with thrombosis, not bleeding; most patients with LA do not have systemic lupus erythematosus. The laboratory hallmark of LA is a prolonged aPTT that does not correct when normal plasma is added. This indicates the presence of an inhibitor of clotting rather than a deficiency of a necessary coagulation factor.

LA can be sought using a sensitive phospholipid reagent, the kaolin clotting time, or the Russell viper venom time.[390,391] Anticardiolipin antibodies of the IgG or IgM types can be measured as well as more specific antibodies to beta-2-glycoprotein 1. IgG antibody levels, especially those greater than 40 GPL (IgG phospholipid) units, correlate with a relatively high risk of stroke and recurrent stroke.[393] Antiphospholipid antibodies are actually antibodies to a protein, most often beta-2-glycoprotein 1, that is usually bound to a phospholipid.[394] Measurement of beta-2-glycoprotein 1 antibodies is often useful in defining autoimmune activity. Two other antibodies, antiphosphatidyl serine[395] and antiphosphatylinositol,[396] show a high correlation with ischemic stroke especially in the young and in those without another determined cause.[397] The screening tests for syphilis – the VDRL and Reiter protein reaction – depend on the activity of APLAs. False-positive serological tests for syphilis are often found in patients with APLAs, and thrombocytopenia is present in a third of APLA-positive patients.

Table 4.11 Suggested hypercoagulability screening battery

Genetic test for factor V Leiden mutation or coagulation assay for activated protein C resistance (if abnormal confirm genetically)
Genetic test for prothrombin *G20210A* mutation
Functional assay of antithrombin
Functional assay of protein C
Functional assay of protein S and measurements of total and free protein S antigen
Homocysteine
Factor VIII level
Lupus anticoagulant, cardiolipin antibodies, beta-2 glycoprotein 1 antibodies

Note: Ken Bauer, MD, Hematology-Coagulation Department, Harvard Medical School, Cambridge, MA, assisted with the preparation of this table.

The clinical APLA syndrome consists of frequent venous and arterial thrombotic events, such as thrombophlebitis, pulmonary embolism, TIAs, strokes, myocardial infarctions, and recurrent fetal loss in women.[388,390] It is likely that the mechanism of recurrent brain ischemia is excessive clotting. APLAs may be directed against the endothelium or platelet membranes and may alter coagulability and vascular functions. APLAs should be measured in situations in which the usual risk factors for ischemic stroke are not present, and certainly in patients with livedo reticularis and strokes (Sneddon's syndrome), and those patients with clinical features matching the primary APLA syndrome.[388,389,391,398] Table 4.11 suggests a screening battery in patients suspected of having ischemic strokes related to hypercoagulability.

Other blood measurements

After the demonstration that sugar administration could worsen experimentally induced brain ischemia,[399,400] Plum and colleagues noted a poorer prognosis in stroke patients with elevated blood sugar levels.[401,402] Blood sugar elevation can be triggered by tissue damage with release of catecholamines and mobilization of sugar. Large infarcts and hemorrhages are often associated with elevations in the blood sugar level. Because blood sugar is a critical metabolite for the brain, abnormally low levels can be deleterious to patients with stroke. Elevated levels of blood sugar are also often associated with an increased risk of brain damage in patients with brain ischemia and hemorrhage, perhaps linked to increased lactate production. Although most patients with post-stroke hyperglycemia have recognized or newly diagnosed diabetes, stress hyperglycemia can occur in nondiabetics and also predicts a higher mortality and worse outcome after ischemic or hemorrhagic stroke. Although guidelines emphasize good glycemic control, intravenous insulin infusions have not been associated with better outcomes; hypoglycemia is a significant risk of aggressive insulin administration and this approach is not recommended.[403]

Patients with hypercalcemia due to hyperparathyroidism also have a higher frequency of stroke, probably due to the vascular and platelet effects of calcium.[404–407] Low serum magnesium can have a similar effect to hypercalcemia. Dehydration diminishes blood volume, thus potentially decreasing blood flow. Measurements of blood urea nitrogen and electrolytes are useful in determining the presence and degree of dehydration and would show important electrolyte imbalance. Blood lipids, including total cholesterol and fractionation into high-density lipoprotein and low-density lipoprotein components, should be measured in each patient with brain ischemia. Markedly increased levels of triglycerides, low-density lipoproteins, and chylomicra can increase blood viscosity. These levels are useful to analyze in patients with known familial hyperlipidemia, premature atherosclerosis, and patients who have clinical hyperviscosity syndromes. A clue to the presence of chylomicra is the presence of milky, lipemic serum, especially after a meal.

> Patient JH had an Hct of 41 and normal WBC and platelet counts. The PT and aPTT were also normal. Renal function and electrolytes were normal. Blood sugar on admission was 145, but levels returned to normal after a few days. HDL cholesterol level was 40 and LDL cholesterol 185.

Other blood testing that reflects risk factors

Some measurements are useful in assessing risk factors for stroke and other cardiovascular diseases especially in patients seen in an outpatient setting. In some patients primary stroke prevention is considered, others have already had one or more strokes and secondary prevention of another stroke is the consideration. Prevention has been shown to be most effective when patients are studied in the hospital and preventive measures are begun at discharge.[408,409] We find it useful to measure these risk factors in the hospital, recognizing that sometimes some elevations may represent acute-phase reactions and not persist later. In that case the measurements should be repeated when the patients are seen as ambulatory patients in follow-up.

An elevated erythrocyte sedimentation rate can be an important clue to the presence of a systemic inflammatory disease or unsuspected vasculitis. It should be ordered in patients with suspected temporal arteritis and in young and elderly patients with unexplained strokes. Studies also show that elevated C-reactive protein (CRP) and fibrinogen levels as well as homocysteine are risk factors for coronary heart disease, peripheral arterial disease, and stroke.

Elevated homocysteine levels have convincingly been shown to correlate with the risk of ischemic stroke and with large-artery atherosclerosis.[410–415] Homocysteine is a sulfur containing amino acid derived from the metabolism of methionine that circulates bound to plasma proteins. Folic acid, pyridoxine, and B_{12} intake and metabolism are important determinants of homocysteine blood levels. A deficiency in methylenetetrahydrofolate reductase (MTHFR) caused by a polymorphism in the *A677V MTHFR* gene is a common and important cause of a high homocysteine level.[414] Vegetarians

and those with low serum vitamin levels are especially likely to have high serum homocysteine levels. Homocysteine has been associated with hypercoagulability – especially dural sinus thrombosis[416] and with endothelial injury. LRC has seen a number of patients with very high serum homocysteine levels (>40 µmol/l) who had multiple lacunar-like infarcts in the absence of other risk factors. Homocysteine serum levels are worth measuring, but large trials of vitamin treatment have not been shown to have any clinical benefits in secondary stroke prevention, except in patients with very low B_{12} levels.

Studies now show convincingly that elevated high-sensitivity CRP levels correlate with a risk of stroke, cardiovascular disease, and carotid and intracranial large-artery atherosclerosis.[408,417–421] CRP is an acute-phase protein discovered in the 1930s that was named for its reaction with the C-polysaccharide cell wall of *Streptococcus pneumoniae*. It is produced in the liver and is a final common pathway of cytokine activation and is produced in response to a variety of infectious and inflammatory stimuli. Some patients with significant atherosclerotic lesions have normal lipids, but high CRP levels, indicating the likely importance of inflammation in contributing to their vascular disease. C-reactive protein levels are also an important measure of activity in patients with temporal arteritis and Takayasu's arteritis.[422]

Measurement of the ESR, fibrinogen level, HDL and LDL cholesterol, high-sensitivity CRP, and homocysteine are useful in suggesting and quantifying the risk of vascular disease and hopefully contributing to preventive measures. We believe they are important to study in patients suspected of having cerebrovascular disease. Table 4.12 notes our suggestions for laboratory testing in patients with ischemic strokes, TIAs, and known cervico-cranial arterial lesions.

Table 4.12 Suggestions for blood testing in all patients with ischemic stroke or TIA

Hemoglobin
Hematocrit
WBC count (and differential if abnormally high or low)
Platelet count
aPTT
PT–INR
Serum fibrinogen level
Blood sugar
Serum calcium
Total cholesterol and HDL and LDL cholesterol
Blood urea nitrogen
Electrolytes (sodium, chloride, potassium, and carbon dioxide)
Homocysteine
C-reactive protein
ESR

What if the patient has intracerebral hemorrhage or subarachnoid hemorrhage?

Bleeding diatheses are important causes of intracranial bleeding. Probably the most common bleeding disorders are now iatrogenic, including the use of anticoagulants (heparins, vitamin K and direct thrombin and factor Xa inhibitors), rt-PA and other fibrinolytic compounds, and more marginally the use of aspirin and other antiplatelet substances. Stroke clinicians will be particularly familiar with ICH associated with warfarin and increasingly with the newer direct acting oral anticoagulants (DOACs), although these prothombin and Xa inhibitors are generally safer. Usually, these clinical situations are known and are not diagnostic dilemmas. Hereditary bleeding disorders such as hemophilia are usually well known to both patients and physicians and most patients have had prior systemic hemorrhages before intracranial bleeding events. Thrombocytopenia is another important cause of intracranial bleeding. More recently attention has been focused on an acquired hemorrhagic condition dubbed "hemophilia A," a severe autoimmune bleeding disorder resulting from the presence of autoantibodies directed against clotting factor VIII.[423,424]

A history of prior bleeding episodes (vaginal, dental, postoperative, and so forth) and the presence of systemic purpura or active gum, urine, or bowel bleeding are the best clues to the presence of a bleeding diathesis.

Measurement of PT and INR and partial thromboplastin time (PTT) are usually sufficient to screen for these disorders. Platelet counts detect thrombocytopenia, and the bleeding time is a useful screening procedure measuring platelet function, among other conditions. Hemophilia and other lifelong bleeding diatheses are usually known before the intracranial bleed occurs. Measurement of antihemophilic globulin, antibodies to factor VIII, and other coagulation factors is helpful in patients with previously uncharacterized bleeding disorders.

Question 5: Is the patient with stroke or transient neurological deficits having seizures?

Electrical tests of brain function

Electroencephalography (EEG) is the oldest available non-invasive test of brain function. Experience has shown that the use of EEG in stroke diagnosis and management is very limited. There are, however, occasional circumstances in which EEG is quite helpful. Seizures and postictal neurological signs can mimic TIAs. In some patients with stroke or other central nervous system lesions, worsening of a neurological deficit is caused by clinically unapparent or subtle seizure activity, which is usually dramatically captured by EEG. Some patients with recent-onset strokes, especially those caused by subcortical ICHs or brain embolism, have seizures. Patients with acute pontine ischemia or hemorrhage can have unusual limb movements that are easily confused with seizures by those inexperienced with brainstem strokes.[425,426]

In patients in whom the differential diagnosis is between seizures and other transient neurological conditions, EEG can document seizure discharges or show an EEG suggestive of a seizure disorder. In patients with strokes and known seizures or in less than fully alert patients in whom seizures are a potential cause of decreased alertness, sequential EEGs or EEG monitoring can document and quantify seizure discharges and thereby guide anticonvulsant management. EEG monitoring of acute stroke patients shows a previously unexpected frequency of seizure activity.[427] Seizures are also quite common in the days, months, and few years after stroke and EEGs can be quite helpful in these patients.[428]

EEGs can also be recorded during somatosensory, visual, and auditory stimuli, and while the patient is performing various cognitive tasks. Computers then subtract the baseline electrical activity and generate a printout of that part of the electrical activity directly attributable to the stimulus and the task-related evoked potentials. Evoked potentials can also be studied via topographic mapping techniques to better localize the abnormalities. These techniques are particularly useful in unresponsive patients, especially after cardiac arrest, when it is impossible to clinically assess cognitive and sensory functions, and in patients under anesthesia.[429-431] In patients with brainstem disease, electrophysiological diagnostic testing of reflex functions including brainstem auditory evoked responses and quantified testing of the blink and masseter reflexes can help localize the functional abnormality to particular portions of the brainstem.[432]

These electrical and electrophysiological tests are most helpful in answering the following questions: Is the patient having seizures? How much residual electrical activity is present in this comatose patient's cerebrum, and what is the prognosis for long-term outcome? Is this anesthetized patient now having cerebrovascular surgery undergoing damage during the procedure? Are there functional changes in the brain or brainstem not shown by brain-imaging techniques?

In JH, functional imaging or electrical testing was not performed. His clinical deficit was severe, and morphological studies (CT) had shown an extensive infarct. Moreover, his vascular lesion was not treatable. Newer MR technologies were not available at the time he was treated.

Question 6: Are there genetic abnormalities that might clarify the etiology of the cerebrovascular disease and potentially guide treatment of the patient and prevention or management of relatives?

During the last quarter-century, there has been a revolution in molecular biology and genetics. Genetic influences clearly play a large influence in determining who will develop strokes and which subtypes of stroke.[433-440] Genetic analyses

will undoubtedly become even more important in the future. For this reason, we have added a full chapter (Chapter 5) on stroke genetics in this fifth edition. We also discuss some genetically mediated conditions in Chapter 12 on nonatherosclerotic causes of stroke.

A stimulus to further genetic research was the finding by deCODE genetics that polymorphisms of the phosphodiesterase 4D, camp-specific (*PDE4D*) gene were prevalent in patients with stroke.[441,442] Genetic analysis of mutations has become instrumental in the diagnosis and understanding of some specific and genetic and mitochondrial diseases. A number of genetic disorders have been shown to cause abnormal bleeding and hypercoagulability. Further advances are likely in coming years. The availability of high-density microarrays that allow rapid screening of genome-wide sets that range from 100 000 to more than a million single-nucleotide polymorphisms (SNPs), shows promise of revealing important genetic associations with stroke and stroke risk factors.[439] Identifying the genetic etiology and influences on cerebrovascular disease can help the patient's relatives and progeny as well as the patient.

References

1. Eckert B, Zeumer H: Brain computed tomography. In Ginsberg MD, Bogousslavsky J (eds): *Cerebrovascular Disease: Pathophysiology, Diagnosis, and Management*, vol 2. Boston: Blackwell Science, 1998, pp 1241–1264.

2. von Kummer R, Nolte PN, Schnittger H, et al: Detectability of cerebral hemisphere ischaemic infarcts by CT within 6 hours of stroke. *Neuroradiology* 1996;38:31–33.

3. Moulin T, Cattin F, Crepin-Leblond T, et al: Early CT signs in acute middle cerebral artery infarction: Predictive value for subsequent infarct location and outcome. *Neurology* 1996;47:366–375.

4. Norman D, Price D, Boyd D, et al: Quantitative aspects of computed tomography of the blood and cerebrospinal fluid. *Radiology* 1977;7:223–228.

5. Caplan LR, Flamm ES, Mohr JP, et al: Lumbar puncture and stroke: A statement for physicians by a committee of the Stroke Council of the American Heart Association. *Stroke* 1987;18:540A–544A.

6. Edlow JA, Caplan LR: Primary care: Avoiding pitfalls in the diagnosis of subarachnoid hemorrhage. *N Engl J Med* 2000;341:29–36.

7. Beauchamp NJ, Bryan RN: Neuroimaging of stroke. In Welch KMA, Caplan LR, Reis DJ, Siesjo BK, Weir B (eds): *Primer on Cerebrovascular Diseases*. San Diego: Academic Press, 1997, pp 599–611.

8. Baird AE, Warach S: Magnetic resonance imaging of acute stroke. *J Cereb Blood Flow Metab* 1998;18:583–609.

9. Brant-Zawadski M, Atkinson D, Detrick M, et al: Fluid-attenuated inversion recovery (FLAIR) for assessment of cerebral infarction: Initial clinical experience in 50 patients. *Stroke* 1996;27:1187–1191.

10. Warach S, Chien D, Li W, et al: Fast magnetic resonance diffusion-weighted imaging of acute human stroke. *Neurology* 1992;42:1717–1723.

11. Warach S, Gaa J, Siewert B, et al: Acute human stroke studied by whole brain echo planar diffusion-weighted magnetic resonance imaging. *Ann Neurol* 1995;37:231–241.

12. Lansberg MG, Norbash AM, Marks MP, et al: Advantages of adding diffusion-weighted magnetic resonance imaging to conventional imaging for evaluating acute stroke. *Arch Neurol* 2000;57:1311–1316.

13. Engelter ST, Wetzel SG, Radue EW, et al: The clinical significance of diffusion-weighted imaging in infratentorial strokes. *Neurology* 2004;62:574–580.

14. Kang DW, Chalela JA, Ezzeddline MA, Warach S: Association of ischemic lesion patterns on early diffusion-weighted imaging with TOAST stroke subtypes. *Arch Neurol* 2003;60:1730–1734.

15. Bonati LH, Lyrer PA, Wetzel SG, et al: Diffusion-weighted imaging, apparent diffusion coefficient maps and stroke etiology. *J Neurol* 2005;252:1387–1393.

16. Bonati LH, Kessel-Schaefer A, Linka AZ, et al: Diffusion-weighted imaging in stroke attributable to patent foramen ovale. *Stroke* 2006;37:2030–2034.

17. Kidwell CS, Saver JL, Mattiello J, et al: Thrombolytic reversal of acute human cerebral ischemic injury shown by diffusion/perfusion magnetic resonance imaging. *Ann Neurol* 2000;47:462–469.

18. Chemmanam T, Campbell BCV, Christensen S, et al: Ischemic diffusion lesion reversal is uncommon and rarely alters perfusion–diffusion mismatch. *Neurology* 2010;75:1040–1047.

19. Campbell BCV, Purushotham A, Christensen S, et al: The infarct core is well represented by the acute diffusion lesion: sustained reversal is infrequent. *J Cereb Blood Flow Metab* 2012; 32:50–56.

20. Patel MR, Edelman RR, Warach S: Detection of hyperacute primary intraparenchymal hemorrhage by magnetic resonance imaging. *Stroke* 1996;27:2321–2324.

21. Linfante I, Llinas RH, Caplan LR, Warach S: MRI features of intracerebral hemorrhage within 2 hours from symptom onset. *Stroke* 2002;30:2263–2267.

22. Chalela JA, Latour LL, Jeffries N, et al: Hemorrhage and early MRI evaluation from the emergency room (HEME-ER): A prospective single center comparison of MRI to CT for the emergency diagnosis of intracranial hemorrhage in patients with suspected acute cerebrovascular disease. *Stroke* 2003;34:239–240.

23. Schellinger PD, Fiebach JB, Mohr A, et al: The role of stroke MRI in intracranial and subarachnoid hemorrhage. *Nervenarzt* 2001;72:907–917.

24. Schellinger PD, Jansen O, Fiebach JB, et al: A standardized MRI protocol comparison with CT in hyperacute intracerebral hemorrhage. *Stroke* 1999;30:765–768.

25. Assouline E, Benziane K, Reizine D, et al: Intra-arterial thrombus visualized on T2 gradient echo imaging in acute ischemic stroke. *Cerebrovasc Dis* 2005;20:6–11.

26. Dul K, Drayer BP: CT and MR imaging of intracerebral hemorrhage. In Kase CS, Caplan LR (eds): *Intracerebral Hemorrhage*. Boston: Butterworth–Heinemann, 1994, pp 73–93.

27. Rumboldt Z, Kalousek M, Castillo M: Hyperacute subarachnoid hemorrhage on T2-weighted MR images. *AJNR Am J Neuroradiol* 2003;24:472–475.

28. Pexman JHW, Barber PA, Hill MD, et al.: Use of the Alberta Stroke

Program Early CT Score (ASPECTS) for Assessing CT Scans in Patients with Acute Stroke. *AJNR Am J Neuroradiol* 2001;**22**:1534–1542.

29. Becker H, Desch H, Hacker H, et al: CT fogging effect with ischemic cerebral infarcts. *Neuroradiol* 1978;**18**:185–192.

30. Nicolaides AN, Kalodiki E, Ramaswami G, et al: The significance of cerebral infarcts on CT scans in patients with transient ischemic attacks. In Bernstein EF, Callow AD, Nicolaides AN, Shifrin EG (eds): *Cerebral Revascularisation.* London, Med-Orion, 1993, pp 159–178.

31. Inatomi Y, Kimura K, Yonehara T, et al: DWI abnormalities and clinical characteristics in TIA patients. *Neurology* 2004;**62**:376–380.

32. Winbeck K, Bruckmaier K, Etgen T, et al: Transient ischemic attack and stroke can be differentiated by analyzing early diffusion-weighted imaging signal intensity changes. *Stroke* 2004;**35**:1095–1099.

33. Lamy C, Oppenheim C, Calvet D, et al: Diffusion-weighted MR imaging in transient ischaemic attacks. *Eur Radiol* 2006;**16**:1090–1095.

34. Bykowski J, Latour LL, Warach S: More accurate identification of reversible ischemic injury in human stroke by cerebrospinal fluid suppressed diffusion-weighted imaging. *Stroke* 2004;**35**:1100–1106.

35. Prabhakaran S, Chong JY, Sacco RL: Impact of abnormal diffusion-weighted imaging results on short-term outcome following transient ischemic attack. *Arch Neurol* 2007;**64**:1105–1109.

36. Redgrave JNE, Coutts SB, Schulz UG, et al: Systematic review of associations between the presence of acute ischemic lesions on diffusion-weighted imaging and clinical predictors of early stroke risk after transient ischemic attack. *Stroke* 2007;**38**:1482–1488.

37. Sylaja PN, Coutts SB, Subramaniam S, et al: Acute ischemic lesions of varying ages predict risk of ischemic events in stroke/TIA patients. *Neurology* 2007;**68**:415–419.

38. Caplan LR: Transient ischemic attack with abnormal diffusion-weighted imaging results. What's in a name? *Arch Neurol* 2007; **64**:1080–1082.

39. Adams Jr HP, Kassell NF, Turner JC, et al: CT and clinical correlations in recent aneurysmal subarachnoid hemorrhage: A preliminary report of the Cooperative Aneurysm Study. *Neurology* 1983;**33**:981–988.

40. Fishman RA: Cerebrospinal fluid in cerebrovascular disorders. In Barnett HJM, Mohr JP, Stein BM, Yatsu FJ (eds): *Stroke: Pathophysiology, Diagnosis, and Management.* New York: Churchill Livingstone, 1986, pp 109–117.

41. Schluep M, Bogousslavsky J: Cerebrospinal fluid in cerebrovascular disease. In Ginsberg MD, Bogousslavsky J (eds): *Cerebrovascular Disease: Pathophysiology, Diagnosis, and Management,* vol **2**. Boston: Blackwell Science, 1998, pp 1221–1226.

42. Van der Meulen JP: Cerebrospinal fluid xanthrochromia: An objective index. *Neurology* 1966;**16**:170–178.

43. Soderstrom CE: Diagnostic significance of CSF spectrophotometry and computer tomography in cerebrovascular disease: A comparative study in 231 cases. *Stroke* 1977;**8**:606–612.

44. Davalos A, Blanco M, Pedraza S, et al: The clinical-DWI mismatch: A new diagnostic approach to the brain tissue at risk of infarction. *Neurology.* 2004;**62**:2187–2192.

45. Caplan LR: Significance of unexpected (silent) brain infarcts. In Caplan LR, Shifrin EG, Nicolaides AN, Moore WS (eds): *Cerebrovascular Ischaemia: Investigation and Management.* London: Med-Orion, 1996, pp 423–433.

46. Yamamoto H, Bogousslavsky J: Mechanisms of second and further strokes. *J Neurol Neurosurg Psychiatry* 1998;**64**:771–776.

47. Caplan LR: Reperfusion of ischemic brain: Why and why not? In Hacke W, del Zoppo G, Hirschberg M (eds): *Thrombolytic Therapy in Acute Stroke.* Berlin: Springer, 1991, pp 36–45.

48. Ropper AH: Lateral displacement of the brain and level of consciousness in patients with an acute hemispheral mass. *N Engl J Med* 1986;**314**:953–958.

49. Ropper AH: A preliminary MRI study of the geometry of brain displacement and level of consciousness with acute intracranial masses. *Neurology* 1989;**39**:622–627.

50. Lansberg MG, Thijs VN, O'Brien MW, et al: Evolution of apparent diffusion coefficient, diffusion-weighted, and T2-weighted signal intensity of acute stroke. *AJNR Am J Neuroradiol* 2001;**22**:637–644.

51. Weisberg LA, Stazio A, Shamsnia M, et al: Nontraumatic parenchymal brain hemorrhages. *Medicine (Baltimore)* 1990;**69**:277–295.

52. Delgado Almandoz JE, Schaefer PW, Forero NP, et al: Diagnostic accuracy and yield of multidetector CT angiography in the evaluation of spontaneous intraparenchymal cerebral hemorrhage. *AJNR Am J Neuroradiol* 2009;**30**:1213–1221.

53. Kase CS: Cerebral amyloid angiopathy. In Kase CS, Caplan LR (eds): *Intracerebral Hemorrhage.* Boston: Butterworth–Heinemann, 1994, pp 179–200.

54. Hauw J-J, Seilhean D, Duyckaerts CH: Cerebral amyloid angiopathy. In Ginsberg MD, Bogousslavsky J (eds): *Cerebrovascular Disease: Pathophysiology, Diagnosis, and Management.* Boston: Blackwell, 1998, pp 1772–1794.

55. Kase C, Robinson R, Stein R, et al: Anticoagulant-related intracerebral hemorrhages. *Neurology* 1985;**35**:943–948.

56. Kase CS: Bleeding disorders. In Kase CS, Caplan LR (eds): *Intracerebral Hemorrhage.* Boston: Butterworth–Heinemann, 1994, pp 117–151.

57. Broderick JP, Brott TG, Duldner JE, Tomsick T, Huster G. Volume of intracerebral hemorrhage: a powerful and easy-to-use predictor of 30-day mortality. *Stroke* 1993;**24**:987–993.

58. Wada R, Aviv RI, Fox A, et al: CT angiography "spot sign" predicts hematoma expansion in acute intracerebral hemorrhage. *Stroke* 2007;**38**:1257–1262.

59. Demchuk AM, Dowlatshahi D, Rodriguez-Luna D, et al; and PREDICT Group: Prediction of haematoma growth and outcome in patients with intracerebral haemorrhage using the CT-angiography spot sign (PREDICT): A prospective observational study. *Lancet Neurol* 2012;**11**:307–314.

60. Weisberg L: Computed tomography in aneurysmal subarachnoid hemorrhage. *Neurology* 1979;**29**:802–808.

61. Adams H, Kassell N, Torner J, et al: CT and clinical correlations in recent aneurysmal subarachnoid hemorrhage: A preliminary report of the cooperative aneurysm study. *Neurology* 1983;**33**:981–988.

62. van Gijn J, van Dongen K: Computerized tomography in subarachnoid hemorrhage: Difference between patients with and without an aneurysm on angiography. *Neurology* 1980;**30**:538–539.

63. van Gijn J, van Dongen KJ, Vermeulen M, et al: Perimesencephalic hemorrhage: A non-aneurysmal and benign form of subarachnoid hemorrhage. *Neurology* 1985;**35**:493–497.

64. Rinkel GJ, Wijdicks EF, Vermeulen M, et al: Outcome in perimesencephalic (non-aneurysmal) subarachnoid hemorrhage: A follow-up study in 37 patients. *Neurology* 1990;**40**:1130–1132.

65. Kumar S, Goddeau Jr RP, Selim MH, et al: Atraumatic convexal subarachnoid hemorrhage: clinical presentation, imaging patterns, and etiologies. *Neurology* 2010;**74**:893–899.

66. Kistler JP, Crowell R, Davis K, et al: The relation of cerebral vasospasm to the extent and location of subarachnoid blood visualized by CT scan: A prospective study. *Neurology* 1983;**33**:424–437.

67. Mohsen F, Pominis S, Illingworth R: Prediction of delayed cerebral ischemia after subarachnoid hemorrhage by computed tomography. *J Neurol Neurosurg Psychiatry* 1984;**47**:1197–1202.

68. Kern R, Szabo K, Hennerici M, Meairs S: Characterization of carotid artery plaques using real-time compound B-mode ultrasound. *Stroke* 2004;**35**:870–875.

69. Landry A, Spence JD, Fenster A: Measurement of carotid plaque volume by 3-dimensional ultrasound. *Stroke* 2004;**35**:864–869.

70. O'Donnell TF, Erdoes L, Mackey W, et al: Correlation of B-mode ultrasound imaging and arteriography with pathologic findings at carotid endarterectomy. *Arch Surg* 1985;**120**:443–449.

71. Hennerici M, Baezner H, Daffertshofer M: Ultrasound of cervical arteries. In Caplan LR, Manning WJ (eds): *Brain Embolism*. New York: Informa Healthcare, 2006, pp 223–242.

72. Schenk EA, Bond G, Aretz T, et al: Multicenter validation study of real-time ultrasonography, arteriography and pathology: Pathologic evaluation of carotid endarterectomy specimens. *Stroke* 1988;**19**:289–296.

73. Hennerici M, Meairs S: Imaging arterial wall disease. *Cerebrovasc Dis* 2000;**10**(Suppl 5):9–20.

74. Gronholdt M-LM, Nordestgaard BG, Nielsen TG, Sillesen H: Echolucent carotid artery plaques are associated with elevated levels of fasting and postprandial triglyceride-rich lipoproteins. *Stroke* 1996;**27**:2166–2172.

75. Geroulakos G, Hobson RW, Nicolaides AW: Ultrasonic carotid plaque morphology. In Caplan LR, Shifrin EG, Nicolaides AN, Moore WS (eds): *Cerebrovascular Ischaemia: Investigation and Management*. London: Med-Orion, 1996, pp 25–32.

76. O'Leary DH, Polka JF, Kronmal RA, et al: Thickening of the carotid wall: A marker for atherosclerosis in the elderly? *Stroke* 1996;**27**:224–231.

77. Bots ML, Hoes AW, Koudstaal PJ, et al: Common carotid intima-media thickness and risk of stroke and myocardial infarction: The Rotterdam Study. *Circulation* 1997;**96**:1432–1437.

78. O'Leary DH, Polak JF, Kronmal RA, et al: Carotid artery intima and media thickness as a risk factor for myocardial infarction and stroke risk in older adults. *N Engl J Med* 1999;**340**:14–22.

79. Yakushiji Y, Yasaka M, Takada T, Minematsu K: Serial transoral carotid ultrasonographic findings in extracranial internal carotid artery dissection. *J Ultrasound Med* 2005;**24**:877–880.

80. Yakushijji Y, Takase Y, Kosugi M, et al: Transoral carotid ultrasonography is useful for detection and follow-up of extracranial internal carotid artery dissecting aneurysm. *Cerebrovasc Dis* 2007;**24**:144–146.

81. Forteza A, Krejza J, Koch S, Babikian V: Ultrasound imaging of cerebrovascular disease. In Babikian VL, Wechsler LR, Higashida RT (eds): *Imaging Cerebrovascular Disease*. Philadelphia: Butterworth–Heinemann, 2003, pp 3–35.

82. von Reutern GM, von Budingen HJ: *Ultrasound Diagnosis of Cerebrovascular Disease*. New York: Georg Thieme, 1993.

83. Bartels E: *Color-Coded Duplex Ultrasonography of the Cerebral Vessels*. Stuttgart: Schattauer, 1998.

84. Steinke W, Kloetzsch C, Hennerici M: Carotid artery disease assessed by color Doppler flow imaging: correlation with standard Doppler sonography and angiography. *AJNR Am J Neuroradiol* 1990;**11**:259–266.

85. Steinke W, Hennerici M, Rautenberg W, Mohr JP: Symptomatic and asymptomatic high-grade carotid stenosis in Doppler color-flow imaging. *Neurology* 1992;**42**;131–138.

86. Steinke W, Ries S, Artemis N, et al: Power Doppler imaging of carotid artery stenosis. Comparison with color Doppler flow imaging and angiography. *Stroke* 1997;**28**:1981–1987.

87. Griewing B, Doherty C, Kessler CH: Power Doppler ultrasound examination of the intracerebral and extracerebral vasculature. *J Neuroimaging* 1996;**6**:32–35.

88. Lenzi GL, Vicenzini E: The ruler is dead: An analysis of carotid plaque motion. *Cerebrovasc Dis* 2007;**23**:121–125.

89. Aaslid R: *Transcranial Doppler Sonography*. New York: Springer, 1986.

90. Alexandrov AV (ed): *Cerebrovascular Ultrasound in Stroke Prevention and Treatment*. New York: Futura Blackwell Publishing, 2003.

91. Molina CA, Alexandrov AV: Transcranial Doppler ultrasound. In Caplan LR, Manning WJ (eds): *Brain Embolism*. New York: Informa Healthcare, 2006, pp 113–128.

92. Babikian VL, Wechsler LR (eds): *Transcranial Doppler Ultrasonography*, 2nd ed. Boston: Butterworth–Heinemann, 1999.

93. Otis SM, Ringelstein EB: The transcranial Doppler examination: Principles and applications of transcranial Doppler sonography. In Tegeler CH, Babikian VL, Gomez CR (eds): *Neurosonology*. St Louis: Mosby, 1996, pp 113–128.

94. Gomez CR, Brass LM, Tegeler CH, et al: The trans-cranial Doppler standardization project. Phase 1 results. The TCD Study Group, American Society of Neuroimaging. *J Neuroimaging* 1993;**3**:190–192.

95. Caplan LR, Brass LM, DeWitt LD, et al: Transcranial Doppler ultrasound: Present status. *Neurology* 1990;**40**:696–700.

96. Hennerici M, Rautenberg W, Sitzer G, et al: Transcranial Doppler ultrasound for the assessment of intracranial arterial flow velocity. *Surg Neurol* 1987;**27**:439–448.

97. Hennerici M, Rautenberg W, Schwartz A: Transcranial Doppler ultrasound for the assessment of intracranial arterial flow velocity. II. Evaluation of intracranial arterial disease. *Surg Neurol* 1987;**27**:523–532.

98. Demchuk A, Christou I, Wein T, et al: Accuracy and criteria for localizing arterial occlusion with transcranial Doppler. *J Neuroimaging* 2000;**10**:1–12.

99. Demchuk AM, Christou I, Wein T, et al: Specific transcranial Doppler flow findings related to the presence and site of arterial occlusion. *Stroke* 2000;**31**:140–146.

100. Baumgartner RW: Transcranial color duplex sonography in cerebrovascular disease: A systematic review. *Cerebrovasc Dis* 2003;**16**:4–13.

101. Krejza J, Baumagartner RW: Clinical applications of transcranial color-coded duplex sonography. *J Neuroimaging* 2004;**14**:215–225.

102. Burns PN: Overview of echo-enhanced vascular ultrasound imaging for clinical diagnosis in neurosonology. *J Neuroimaging* 1997;7(Suppl 1):S2–S14.

103. Bogdahn U, Becker G, Schlief R, et al: Contrast-enhanced transcranial color-coded real-time sonography. *Stroke* 1993;**24**:676–684.

104. Delcker A, Turowski B: Diagnostic value of three-dimensional transcranial contrast duplex sonography. *J Neuroimaging* 1997;**7**:139–144.

105. Stolz E, Kaps M: New techniques in ultrasound. In Babikian VL, Wechsler LR, Higashida RT (eds): *Imaging Cerebrovascular Disease*. Philadelphia: Butterworth–Heinemann, 2003, pp 383–401.

106. Sharma VK, Tsivgoulis G, Lao AY, Alexandrov AV: Role of transcranial Doppler ultrasonography in evaluation of patients with cerebrovascular disease. *Curr Neurol Neurosci Rep* 2007;**7**:8–20.

107. Tsivgoulis G, Sharma VK, Lao AY, et al: Validation of transcranial Doppler with computed tomography angiography in acute cerebral ischemia. *Stroke* 2007;**38**:1245–1249.

108. Sharma VK, Tsivgoulis G, Lao AY, et al: Noninvasive detection of diffuse intracranaial disease. *Stroke* 2007;**38**:3175–3181.

109. Caplan LR: *Posterior Circulation Disease: Clinical Findings, Diagnosis, and Management*. Boston: Blackwell, 1996.

110. Sliwka U, Rautenberg W: Multimodal ultrasound versus angiography for imaging the vertebrobasilar circulation. *J Neuroimaging* 1998;**8**:182.

111. Seiler RW, Grolimund P, Asaslid R, et al: Cerebral vasospasm evaluated by transcranial ultrasound correlated with clinical grade and CT-visualized subarachnoid hemorrhage. *J Neurosurg* 1986;**64**:594–600.

112. Becker G, Greiner K, Kaune B, et al: Diagnosis and monitoring of subarachnoid hemorrhage by transcranial color-coded real time sonography. *Neurosurgery* 1991;**28**:814–820.

113. Chaudhuri R, Padayachee TS, Lewis RR, et al: Non-invasive assessment of the circle of Willis using transcranial pulsed Doppler ultrasound with angiographic correlation. *Clin Radiol* 1992;**46**:193–197.

114. Anzola GP, Gasparotti R, Magoni M, Prandini F: Transcranial Doppler sonography and magnetic resonance angiography in the assessment of collateral hemispheric flow in patients with carotid artery disease. *Stroke* 1995;**26**:214–217.

115. Klotzsch C, Popescu O, Berlit P: Assessment of the posterior communicating artery by transcranial color-coded duplex sonography. *Stroke* 1996;**27**:486–489.

116. Piepgras A, Schmiedek P, Leinsinger G, et al: A simple test to assess cerebrovascular reserve capacity using transcranial Doppler sonography and acetazolamide. *Stroke* 1990;**21**:1306–1311.

117 Dahl A, Russell D, Rootwelt K, et al: Cerebral vasoreactivity assessed with transcranial Doppler and regional cerebral blood flow measurements. Dose, concentration, and time of the response to acetazolamide. *Stroke* 1995;**26**:2302–2306.

118. Valdueza JM, Draganski B, Hoffman O, et al: Analysis of CO_2 vasomotor reactivity and vessel diameter changes by simultaneous venous and arterial Doppler recordings. *Stroke* 1999;**30**:81–86.

119. Yonas H, Smith HA, Durham SR, et al: Increased stroke risk predicted by compromised cerebral blood flow reactivity. *J Neurosurg* 1993;**79**:483–489.

120. Markus HS: Transcranial Doppler detection of circulating cerebral emboli: A review. *Stroke* 1993;**24**:1246–1250.

121. Markus HS, Harrison MJ: Microembolic signal detection using ultrasound. *Stroke* 1995;**26**:1517–1519.

122. Tong DC, Albers GW: Transcranial Doppler-detected microemboli in patients with acute stroke. *Stroke* 1995;**26**:1588–1592.

123. Sliwka U, Job F-P, Wissuwa D, et al: Occurrence of transcranial Doppler high-intensity transient signals in patients with potential cardiac sources of embolism: A prospective study. *Stroke* 1995;**26**:2067–2070.

124. Daffertshofer M, Ries S, Schminke U, Hennerici M: High-intensity transient signals in patients with cerebral ischemia. *Stroke* 1996;**27**:1844–1849.

125. Sliwka U, Lingnau A, Stohlmann W-D, et al: Prevalence and time course of microembolic signals in patients with acute strokes: A prospective study. *Stroke* 1997;**28**:358–363.

126. Ringelstein EB, Droste DW, Babikian VL, et al: Consensus on microembolus detection by TCD. International Consensus Group on Microembolus Detection. *Stroke* 1998;**29**:725–729.

127. Siebler M, Nachtmann A, Sitzer M, et al: Cerebral microembolism and the risk of ischemia in asymptomatic high-grade internal carotid artery stenosis. *Stroke* 1995;**26**:2184–2186.

128. Molloy J, Markus HS: Asymptomatic embolization predicts stroke and TIA risk in patients with carotid artery stenosis. *Stroke* 1999;**30**:1440–1443.

129. Segura T, Serena J, Molins A, Davalos A: Clusters of microembolic signals: A new form of cerebral microembolism presentation in a patient with middle cerebral artery stenosis. *Stroke* 1998;**29**:722–724.

130. Wong KS, Li H, Chan YL, et al: Use of trans-cranial Doppler to predict outcome in patients with intracranial large-artery occlusive disease. *Stroke* 2003;**31**:2641–2647.

131. Gao S, Wong KS, Hansberg T, et al: Microembolic signal predicts recurrent cerebral ischemic events in acute stroke patients with middle cerebral artery stenosis. *Stroke* 2004;**35**:2832–2836.

132. Mackinnon AD, Aaslid R, Markus HS: Long-term ambulatory monitoring for cerebral emboli using transcranial Doppler ultrasound. *Stroke* 2004;**35**:73–78.

133. Teague SM, Sharma MK: Detection of paradoxical cerebral echo contrast embolization by transcranial Doppler ultrasound. *Stroke* 1991;**22**:740–745.

134. Chimowitz MI, Nemec JJ, Marwick TH, et al: Transcranial Doppler ultrasound identifies patients with right-to-left cardiac or pulmonary shunts. *Neurology* 1991;**41**:1902–1904.

135. Albert A, Muller HR, Hetzel A: Optimized transcranial Doppler

technique for the diagnosis of cardiac right-to-left shunts. *J Neuroimaging* 1997;**7**:159–163.

136. Di Tullio M, Sacco RL, Venketasubramanian N, et al: Comparison of diagnostic techniques for the detection of a patent foramen ovale in stroke patients. *Stroke* 1993;**24**:1020–1024.

137. Klotzsch C, Janzen G, Berlit P: Transesophageal echocardiography and contrast-TCD in the detection of a patent foramen ovale. Experiences with 111 patients. *Neurology* 1994;**44**:1603–1606.

138. Jauss M, Zanette E: Detection of right-to-left shunt with ultrasound contrast agent and trans-cranial Doppler sonography. *Cerebrovasc Dis* 2000;**10**:490–496.

139. Sastry S, Daly K, Chengodu T, McCollum C: Is transcranial Doppler for the detection of venous-to-arterial circulation shunts reproducible? *Cerebrovasc Dis* 2007;**23**:424–429.

140. Baumgartner RW, Gonner F, Arnold M, Muri R: Transtemporal power- and frequency-based color-coded duplex sonography of cerebral veins and sinuses. *AJNR Am J Neuroradiol* 1997;**18**:1771–1781.

141. Stolz E, Kaps M, Dorndorf W: Assessment of intracranial venous hemodynamics in normal individuals and patients with cerebral venous thrombosis. *Stroke* 1999;**30**:70–75.

142. Ries S, Steinke W, Neff KW, Hennerici M: Echocontrast enhanced transcranial color-coded sonography for the diagnosis of transverse sinus thrombosis. *Stroke* 1997;**28**:696–700.

143. Valdueza JM, Hoffmann O, Weih M, et al: Monitoring of venous hemodynamics in patients with cerebral venous thrombosis by transcranial Doppler ultrasound. *Arch Neurol* 1999;**56**:229–234.

144. Becker G, Bogdahn U, Gehlberg C, et al: Transcranial color-coded real-time sonography of intracranial veins. *J Neuroimaging* 1995;**5**:87–94.

145. Pressman BD, Tourje EJ, Thompson JR: An early sign of ischemic infarction: Increased density in a cerebral artery. *AJNR Am J Neuroradiol* 1987;**8**:645–648.

146. Riedel CH, Zoubie J, Ulmer S, Gierthmuehlen J, Jansen O: Thin-slice reconstructions of nonenhanced CT images allow for detection of thrombus in acute stroke. *Stroke* 2012;**43**:2319–2323.

147. Lays D, Pruvo JP, Godefroy O, et al: Prevalence and significance of hyperdense middle cerebral artery in acute stroke. *Stroke* 1992;**23**:317–324.

148. Tomsick T, Brott T, Barsan W, et al: Prognostic value of the hyperdense middle cerebral artery sign and stroke scale score before ultraearly thrombolytic therapy. *AJNR Am J Neuroradiol* 1996;**17**:79–85.

149. Lee TC, Bartlett E, Fox AJ, Symons SP: The hypodense artery sign. *AJNR Am J Neuroradiol* 2005;**26**:2027–2029.

150. Grunholdt ML: B-mode ultrasound and spiral CT for the assessment of carotid atherosclerosis. *Neuroimaging Clin N Am* 2002;**12**:421–435.

151. Frank H: Characterization of atherosclerotic plaque by magnetic resonance imaging. *Am Heart J* 2001;**141**(Suppl 2):S45–S48.

152. Yuan C, Mitsumori LM, Beach KW, Maravilla KR: Carotid atherosclerotic plaque: Noninvasive MR characterization and identification of vulnerable lesions. *Radiology* 2001;**221**:285–299.

153. Adams GJ, Greene J, Vick 3rd GW, et al: Tracking regression and progression of atherosclerosis in human carotid arteries using high-resolution magnetic resonance imaging. *Magn Reson Imaging* 2004;**22**:1249–1258.

154. Honda M, Kitagawa N, Tsutsumi K, et al: High-resolution magnetic resonance imaging for detection of carotid plaques. *Neurosurgery* 2006;**58**:338–346.

155. Hatsukami TS, Ross R, Polissar NL, Yuan C: Visualization of fibrous cap thickness and rupture in human atherosclerotic carotid plaque in vivo with high-resolution magnetic resonance imaging. *Circulation* 2000;**102**:959–964.

156. Moody AR, Murphy RE, Morgan PS, et al: Characterization of complicated carotid plaque with magnetic resonance direct thrombus imaging in patients with cerebral ischemia. *Circulation* 2003;**107**:3047–3052.

157. Saloner D, Acevedo-Bolton G, Wintermark M, Rapp JH: MRI of geometric and compositional features of vulnerable carotid plaque. *Stroke* 2007;**38**(2):637–641.

158. Touzé E, Toussaint J-F, Coste J, et al; for the High-Resolution Magnetic Resonanace Imaging in Atherosclerotic Stenosis of the Carotid Artery (HIRISC) Study Group: Reproducibility of high-resolution MRI for the identification and the quantification of carotid atherosclerotic plaque components. *Stroke* 2007;**38**:1812–1819.

159. Yuan C, Mitsumori LM, Ferguson MS, et al: In vivo accuracy of multispectral magnetic resonance imaging for identifying lipid-rich necrotic cores and intraplaque hemorrhage in advanced human carotid plaques. *Circulation* 2001;**104**:2051–2056.

160. Botnar RM, Buecker A, Wiethoff AJ, et al: In vivo magnetic resonance imaging of coronary thrombosis using a fibrin-binding molecular magnetic resonance contrast agent. *Circulation* 2004;**110**:1463–1466.

161. Sirol M, Fuster V, Badimon JJ, et al: Chronic thrombus detection with in vivo magnetic resonance imaging and a fibrin-targeted contrast agent. *Circulation* 2005;**112**:1594–1600.

162. Klein IF, Lavallee PC, Schouman-Claeys E, Amaraenco P: High-resolution MRI identifies basilar artery plaques in paramedian pontine infarct. *Neurology* 2005;**64**:551–552.

163. Klein IF, Lavallee PC, Touboul P-J, et al: In vivo middle cerebral artery plaque imaging by high-resolution MRI. *Neurology* 2006;**67**:327–329.

164. Lam WW, Wong KS, So NM, et al: Plaque volume measurement by magnetic resonance imaging as an index of remodeling of middle cerebral artery: Correlation with transcranial color Doppler and magnetic resonance angiography. *Cerebrovasc Dis* 2004;**17**:166–169.

165. Chalela JA, Haaymore JB, Ezzeddine MA, et al: The hypointense MCA sign. *Neurology* 2002;**58**:1470.

166. Cho K-H, Kim JS, Kwon SU, et al: Significance of susceptibility vessel sign on T2*-weighted gradient echo imaging for identification of stroke subtypes. *Stroke* 2005;**36**:2379–2383.

167. Hermier M, Nighoghossian N: Contribution of susceptibility-weighted imaging to acute stroke assessment. *Stroke* 2004;**35**:1989–1994.

168. Assouline E, Benziane K, Reizine D, et al: Intra-arterial thrombus visualized on T2* gradient echo imaging in acute ischemic stroke. *Cerebrovasc Dis* 2005;**20**:6–11.

169. Idbaih A, Boukobza M, Crassard I, et al: MRI of clot in cerebral venous thrombosis: high diagnostic value of susceptibility-weighted images. *Stroke* 2006;**37**:991–995.

170. Selim M, Fink J, Linfante I, et al: Diagnosis of cerebral venous thrombosis with echo-planar T2*-weighted magnetic resonance imaging. *Arch Neurol* 2002;**59**:1021–1026.

171. Lovblad KO, Bassetti C, Schneider J, et al: Diffusion-weighted MR in cerebral venous thrombosis. *Cerebrovasc Dis* 2001;**11**:169–176.

172. Favrole P, Guichard JP, Crassard I, et al: Diffusion-weighted imaging of intravascular clots in cerebral venous thrombosis. *Stroke* 2004;**35**:99–103.

173. Essig M, von Kummer R, Egelhof T, et al: Vascular MR contrast enhancement in cerebrovascular disease. *AJNR Am J Neuroradiol* 1996;**17**:887–894.

174. Lazar EB, Russell EJ, Cohen BA, et al: Contrast-enhanced MR of cerebral arteritis: Intravascular enhancement related to flow stasis within areas of focal arterial ectasia. *AJNR Am J Neuroradiol* 1992;**13**:271–276.

175. Warach S, Latour LI: Evidence of reperfusion injury, exacerbated by thrombolytic therapy, in human focal brain ischemia using a novel imaging marker of early blood–brain barrier disruption. *Stroke* 2004;**35**(Suppl 1):2659–2661.

176. Latour LL, Kang DW, Ezzeddine MA, et al: Early blood–brain barrier disruption in human focal brain ischemia. *Ann Neurol* 2004;**56**:468–477.

177. Schellinger PD, Chalela JA, Kang DW, et al: Diagnostic and prognostic value of early MR Imaging vessel signs in hyperacute stroke patients imaged <3 hours and treated with recombinant tissue plasminogen activator. *AJNR Am J Neuroradiol* 2005;**26**:618–624.

178. Bang OY, Buck BH, Saver JL, et al: Prediction of hemorrhagic transformation after recanalization therapy using T2*-permeability magnetic resonance imaging. *Ann Neurol* 2007;**62**:170–176.

179. Singer OC, Humpich MC, Fiehler J, et al: Risk for symptomatic intracerebral hemorrhage after thrombolysis assessed by diffusion-weighted magnetic resonance imaging. *Ann Neurol* 2008;**63**:52–60.

180. Campbell BCV, Christensen S, Butcher KS, et al: Regional very low cerebral blood volume predicts hemorrhagic transformation better than diffusion-weighted imaging volume and thresholded apparent diffusion coefficient in acute ischemic stroke. *Stroke* 2010;**41**:82–88.

181. Kim JH, Bang OY, Liebeskind DS, et al: Impact of baseline tissue status (diffusion-weighted imaging lesion) versus perfusion status (severity of hypoperfusion) on hemorrhagic transformation. *Stroke* 2010;**41**: e135–e142.

182. Campbell BCV, Christensen S, Parsons MW, et al: Advanced imaging improves prediction of hemorrhage after stroke thrombolysis. *Ann Neurol* 2013;**73**:510–519.

183. Edelman RR, Mattle HP, Atkinson DJ, et al: MR angiography. *AJR Am J Roentgenol* 1990;**154**:937–946.

184. Bradley WG: Magnetic resonance angiography. In Babikian VL, Wechsler LR, Higashida RT (eds): *Imaging Cerebrovascular Disease.* Philadelphia: Butterworth–Heinemann, 2003, pp 37–50.

185. Qureshi A, Isa A, Cinnamon J, et al: Magnetic resonance angiography in patients with brain infarction. *J Neuroimaging* 1998;**8**:65–70.

186. Gillard JH, Oliverio PJ, Barker PB, et al: MR angiography in acute cerebral ischemia of the anterior circulation: A preliminary report. *AJNR Am J Neuroradiol* 1997;**18**:343–350.

187. Yano T, Kodama T, Suzuki Y, Watanabe K: Gadolinium-enhanced 3D time-of-flight MR angiography. *Acta Radiol* 1997;**38**:47–54.

188. Leclerc X, Martinat P, Godefroy O, et al: Contrast-enhanced three-dimensional fast imaging with steady-state precession (FISP) MR angiography of supraaortic vessels: Preliminary results. *AJNR Am J Neuroradiol* 1998;**19**:1405–1413.

189. U-King-Im J, Trivedi R, Graves M, et al: Contrast-enhanced MR angiography for carotid disease: Diagnostic and potential clinical impact. *Neurology* 2004;**62**:1282–1290.

190. Mitti RL, Broderick M, Carpenter JP, et al: Blinded-reader comparison of magnetic resonance angiography and Duplex ultrasonography for carotid artery bifurcation stenosis. *Stroke* 1994;**25**:4–10.

191. Levi CR, Mitchell A, Fitt G, Donnan GA: The accuracy of magnetic resonance angiography in the assessment of extracranial carotid artery occlusive disease. *Cerebrovasc Dis* 1996;**6**:231–236.

192. Bash S, Villablanca JP, Duckwiler G, et al: Intracranial vascular stenosis and occlusive disease. Evaluation with CT angiography, MR angiography, and digital subtraction angiography. *AJNR Am J Neuroradiol* 2005;**26**:1012–1021.

193. Uehara T, Mori E, Tabuchi M, et al: Detection of occlusive lesions in intracranial arteries by three-dimensional time-of-flight magnetic resonance angiography. *Cerebrovasc Dis* 1994;**4**:365–370.

194. Johnson BA, Heiserman JE, Drayer BP, Keller PJ: Intracranial MR angiography: Its role in the integrated approach to brain infarction. *AJNR Am J Neuroradiol* 1994;**15**:901–908.

195. Ko SB, Kim D-E, Kim SH, Roh J-K: Visualization of venous system by time-of-flight magnetic resonance angiography. *J Neuroimaging* 2006;**16**:353–356.

196. Amin-Hanjani S, Du X, Rose-Finnell L, et al; on behalf of the VERiTAS Study Group: Hemodynamic features of symptomatic vertebrobasilar disease. *Stroke* 2015;**46**:1850–1856.

197. Roberts HC, Lee TJ, Dillon WP: Computed tomography angiography. In Babikian VL, Wechsler LR, Higashida RT (eds): *Imaging Cerebrovascular Disease.* Philadelphia: Butterworth–Heinemann, 2003, pp 51–71.

198. Leclerc X, Godefroy O, Pruvo JP, Leys D: Computed tomographic angiography for the evaluation of carotid artery stenosis. *Stroke* 1995;**26**:1577–1581.

199. Josephson S, Bryant S, Mak H, et al: Evaluation of carotid stenosis using CT angiography in the initial evaluation of stroke and TIA. *Neurology* 2004;**63**:457–460.

200. Feasby T, Findlay J: CT angiography for the assessment of carotid stenosis. *Neurology* 2004;**63**:412–413.

201. Bartlett ES, Walters TD, Symons SP, Fox AJ: Carotid stenosis index revisited with direct CT angiography measurement of carotid arteries to quantify carotid stenosis. *Stroke* 2007;**38**:286–291.

202. Wong KS, Liang EY, Lam WWM, et al: Spiral computed tomography angiography in the assessment of middle cerebral artery occlusive disease. *J Neurol Neurosurg Psychiatry* 1995;**59**:537–539.

203. Skutta B, Furst G, Eilers J, et al: Intracranial stenoocclusive disease: Double detector helical CTA versus digital subtraction angiography. *AJNR Am J Neuroradiol* 1999;**20**:791–799.

204. Brisman J, Song JK, Newell DW: Cerebral aneurysms. *N Engl J Med* 2006;**355**:928–939.

205. Nguyen-Huynh MN, Wintermark M, English J, et al: How accurate is CT angiography in evaluating intracranial atherosclerotic disease? *Stroke* 2008;**39**:1184–1188.

206. Nijjar S, Patel B, McGinn G, West M: Computed tomographic angiography as the primary diagnostic study in spontaneous subarachnoid hemorrhage. *J Neuroimaging* 2007;**17**:295–299.

207. Wada R, Aviv RI, Fox AJ, et al: CT angiography "spot sign" predicts hematoma expansion in acute intracerebral hemorrhage. *Stroke* 2007;**38**:1257–1262.

208. Davis SM, Broderick J, Hennerici M, et al: Hematoma growth is a determinant of mortality and poor outcome after intracerebral hemorrhage. *Neurology* 2006;**66**:1175–1181.

209. Rodriguez-Luna D, Dowlatshahi D, Aviv RI, et al; and the PRSICS Group: Venous phase of computed tomography angiography increases spot sign detection, but intracerebral hemorrhage expansion is greater in spot signs detected in arterial phase. *Stroke* 2014;**45**:734–739.

210. Warach S, Li W, Ronthal M, Edelman R: Acute cerebral ischemia: evaluation with dynamic contrast-enhanced MR imaging and MR angiography. *Radiology* 1992;**182**:41–47.

211. Fisher M, Prichard JW, Warach S. New magnetic resonance techniques for acute ischemic stroke. *JAMA* 1995;**274**:908–911.

212. Rother J, Guckel F, Neff W, et al: Assessment of regional cerebral blood flow volume in acute human stroke by use of a single-slice dynamic susceptibility contrast-enhanced magnetic resonance imaging. *Stroke* 1996;**27**:1088–1093.

213. Sorensen AG, Buonanno F, Gonzalez RG, et al: Hyperacute stroke: evaluation with combined multisection diffusion-weighted and hemodynamically weighted echo-planar MR imaging. *Radiology* 1996;**199**:391–401.

214. Schlaug G, Benfield A, Baird AE, et al: The ischemic penumbra operationally defined by diffusion and perfusion MRI. *Neurology* 1999;**53**:1528–1537.

215. Schellinger PD, Fiebach JB, Jansen O, et al: Stroke magnetic resonance imaging within 6 hours after onset of hyperacute cerebral ischemia. *Ann Neurol* 2001;**49**:460–469.

216. Chaves C, Silver B, Staroselskaya I, et al: Relation of perfusion-weighted magnetic resonance imaging (MRI) and clinical outcome in patients with ischemic stroke. *Cerebrovasc Dis* 1999;**9**(Suppl 1):56.

217. Staroselskaya I, Chaves C, Silver B, et al: Relationship between magnetic resonance arterial patency and perfusion–diffusion mismatch in acute ischemic stroke and its potential clinical use. *Arch Neurol* 2001;**58**:1069–1074.

218. Neumann-Haefelin T, Moseley ME, Albers GW: New magnetic resonance imaging methods for cerebrovascular disease: emerging clinical applications. *Ann Neurol* 2000;**47**:559–570.

219. Ostergaard L, Sorensen AG, Chesler DA, et al: Combined diffusion-weighted and perfusion-weighted flow heterogeneity magnetic resonance imaging in acute stroke. *Stroke* 2000;**31**:1097–1103.

220. Chaves CJ, Staroselskaya I, Linfante I, Llinas R, et al: Patterns of perfusion-weighted imaging in patients with carotid artery occlusive disease. *Arch Neurol* 2003;**60**:237–242.

221. Kane I, Carpenter T, Chappell F, et al: Comparison of 10 different magnetic resonance perfusion imaging processing methods in acute ischemic stroke. *Stroke* 2007;**38**:3158–3164.

222. Wintermark M, Flanders AE, Velthuis B, et al: Perfusion-CT assessment of infarct core and penumbra: receiver operating characteristic curve analysis in 130 patients suspected of acute hemispheric stroke. *Stroke* 2006;**37**:979–985.

223. Bivard A, McElduff P, Spratt N, Levi C, Parsons M: Defining the extent of irreversible brain ischemia using perfusion computed tomography. *Cerebrovasc Dis* 2011;**31**:238–245.

224. Campbell BC, Christensen VS, Levi CR, et al: Cerebral blood flow is the optimal CT perfusion parameter for assessing infarct core. *Stroke* 2011;**42**:3435–3440.

225. Kamalian S, Maas MB, Goldmacher GV, et al: CT cerebral blood flow maps optimally correlate with admission diffusion-weighted imaging in acute stroke but thresholds vary by postprocessing platform. *Stroke* 2011;**42**:1923–1928.

226. Olivot JM, Mlynash M, Thijs VN, et al: Optimal T_{max} threshold for predicting penumbral tissue in acute stroke. *Stroke* 2009;**40**:469–475.

227. Zaro-Weber O, Moeller-Hartmann W, Heiss WD, Sobesky J: Maps of time to maximum and time to peak for mismatch definition in clinical stroke studies validated with positron emission tomography. *Stroke* 2010;**41**:2817–2821.

228. Albers GW, Thijs VN, Wechsler L, et al: Magnetic resonance imaging profiles predict clinical response to early reperfusion: the diffusion and perfusion imaging evaluation for understanding stroke evolution (DEFUSE) study. *Ann Neurol* 2006;**60**:508–517.

229. Lansberg MG, Straka M, Kemp S, et al: MRI profile and response to endovascular reperfusion after stroke (DEFUSE 2): A prospective cohort study. *Lancet Neurol* 2012;**11**:860–867.

230. Davis SM, Donnan GA, Parsons MW, et al: Effects of alteplase beyond 3 h after stroke in the Echoplanar Imaging Thrombolytic Evaluation Trial (EPITHET): A placebo-controlled randomised trial. *Lancet Neurol* 2008;**7**:299–309.

231. Meretoja AD, Strbian D, Mustanoja S, et al: Reducing in-hospital delay to 20 minutes in stroke thrombolysis. *Neurology* 2012;**79**:306–313.

232. Meretoja A, Weir L, Ugalde M, et al: Helsinki model cut stroke thrombolysis delays to 25 minutes in Melbourne in only 4 months. *Neurology* 2013;**81**:1071–1076.

233. Wong EC: Quantifying CBF with pulsed ASL: Technical and pulse sequence factors. *J Magn Reson Imaging* 2005;**22**:727–731.

234. Wang Z, Wang J, Connick TJ, et al: Continuous ASL (CASL) perfusion MRI with an array coil and parallel imaging at 3T. *Magn Reson Med* 2005;**54**:732–737.

235. Fernandez-Seara MA, Wang Z, Wang J, et al: Continuous arterial spin labeling perfusion measurements using single shot 3D GRASE at 3 T. *Magn Reson Med* 2005;**54**:1241–1247.

236. Ances BM, McGarvey ML, Abrahams JM, et al: Continuous arterial spin labeled perfusion magnetic resonance imaging in patients before and after carotid endarterectomy. *J Neuroimaging* 2004;**14**:133–138.

237. Yoo R-E, Yun TJ, Rhim JH, et al: Bright vessel appearance on arterial spin labeling MRI for localizing arterial occlusion in acute ischemic stroke. *Stroke* 2015;**46**:564–567.

238. Park K-Y, Youn YC, Chung C-S, et al: Large-artery stenosis predicts subsequent vascular events in patients with transient ischemic attack. *J Clin Neurol* 2007;**3**:169–174.

239. Perez A, Restepo L, Kleinman J, et al: Patients with diffusion–perfusion mismatch on magnetic resonance imaging 48 hours or more after stroke symptom onset: Clinical and imaging features. *J Neuroimaging* 2006;**16**:329–333.

240. Linfante I, Llinas RH, Schlaug G, et al: Diffusion-weighted imaging and National Institutes of Health Stroke Scale in the acute phase of posterior-circulation stroke. *Arch Neurol* 2001;**58**:621–628.

241. Ma H, Parsons MW, Christensen S, et al: A multicentre, randomized, double blinded, placebo controlled phase 3 study to investigate EXtending the time for Thrombolysis in Emergency Neurological Deficits (EXTEND). *Int J Stroke* 2012;**7**:74–80.

242. Campbell BC, Mitchell PJ, Yan B, et al; and E-I investigators: A multicenter, randomized, controlled study to investigate EXtending the time for Thrombolysis in Emergency Neurological Deficits with Intra-Arterial therapy (EXTEND-IA). *Int J Stroke* 2014;**9**:126–132.

243. von Kummer R, Weber J: Brain and vascular imaging in acute ischemic stroke: The potential of computed tomography. *Neurology* 1997;**49**(Suppl 4):S52–S55.

244. Nabavi DG, Kloska SP, Nam E-M, et al: MOSAIC: Multimodal stroke assessment using computed tomography. Novel diagnostic approach for the prediction of infarction size and clinical outcome. *Stroke* 2002;**33**:2819–2826.

245. Koroshetz W: Contrast computed tomography scan in acute stroke: "You can't always get what you want but . . . you get what you need." *Ann Neurol* 2002;**51**:415–416.

246. Wintermark M, Reichhart M, Thiran J-P, et al: Prognostic accuracy of cerebral blood flow measurement by perfusion computed tomography, at the time of emergency room admission, in acute stroke patients. *Ann Neurol* 2002;**51**:417–432.

247. Wintermark M, Reichart M, Cuisenaire O, et al: Comparison of admission perfusion computed tomography and qualitative diffusion- and perfusion-weighted magnetic resonance imaging in acute stroke patients. *Stroke* 2002;**33**:2025–2031.

248. Parsons MW, Pepper EM, Bateman GA, et al: Identification of the penumbra and infarct core on hyperacute noncontrast and perfusion CT. *Neurology* 2007;**68**:730–736.

249. Na DG, Byun HS, Lee KH, et al: Acute occlusion of the middle cerebral artery: Early evaluation with triphasic helical CT – Preliminary results. *Radiology* 1998;**207**:113–122.

250. Lee KH, Cho S-J, Byun HS, et al: Triphasic perfusion computed tomography in acute middle cerebral artery stroke. *Arch Neurol* 2000;**57**:990–999.

251. Lee KH, Lee S-J, Cho S-J, et al: Usefulness of triphasic perfusion computed tomography for intravenous thrombolysis with tissue-type plasminogen activator in acute ischemic stroke. *Arch Neurol* 2000;**57**:1000–1008.

252. Kohrmann M, Juttler E, Huttner HB, et al: Acute stroke imaging for thrombolytic therapy – an update. *Cerebrovasc Dis* 2007;**24**:161–169.

253. Menon BK, Smith EE, Modi J, et al: Regional leptomeningeal score on CT angiography predicts clinical and imaging outcomes in patients with acute anterior circulation occlusions. *AJNR Am J Neuroradiol* 2011;**32**:1640–1645.

254. Wintermark M, Meuli R, Browaeys P, et al: Comparison of CT perfusion and angiography and MRI in selecting stroke patients for acute treatment. *Neurology* 2007;**68**:694–697.

255. Chalela JA, Kidwell CS, Nentwich LM, et al: Magnetic resonance imaging and computed tomography in emergency assessment of patients with suspected acute stroke: A prospective comparison. *Lancet* 2007;**369**:293–298.

256. Yonas H, Wolfson SK, Gur D, et al: Clinical experience with the use of xenon-enhanced CT blood flow mapping in cerebral vascular disease. *Stroke* 1984;**15**:443–450.

257. Yonas H, Darby JM, Marks EC, et al: CBF measured by Xe-CT: Approach to analysis and normal values. *J Cereb Blood Flow Metab* 1991;**11**:716–725.

258. Hilman J, Sturnegk P, Yonas H, et al: Bedside monitoring of CBF with xenon-CT and a mobile scanner: A novel method in neurointensive care. *Br J Neurosurg* 2005;**19**:395–401.

259. Fayad P, Brass LM: Single photon emission computed tomography in cerebrovascular disease. *Stroke* 1991;**22**:950–954.

260. Caplan LR: Question-driven technology assessment: SPECT as an example. *Neurology* 1991;**41**:187–191.

261. Masdeu JC, Brass LM: SPECT imaging of stroke. *J Neuroimaging* 1995;**5**:514–522.

262. Therapeutics and Technology Subcommittee of the American Academy of Neurology: Assessment of Brain SPECT. *Neurology* 1996;**46**:278–285.

263. Masdeu JC: Imaging of stroke with single-photon emission computed tomography. In Babikian VL, Wechsler LR, Higashida RT (eds): *Imaging Cerebrovascular Disease*. Philadelphia: Butterworth–Heinemann, 2003, pp 131–143.

264. Wintermark M, Sesay M, Barbier E, et al: Comparative overview of brain perfusion imaging techniques. *JNR J Neuroradiol* 2005;**32**:294–314.

265. Frackowiak R: PET CBF investigations of stroke. In Welch KMA, Caplan LR, Reis DJ, Siesjo B, Weir B (eds): *Primer on Cerebrovascular Diseases*. San Diego: Academic Press, 1997, pp 636–640.

266. Phelps M, Mazziotta J, Huang S: Study of cerebral function with positron computed tomography. *J Cereb Blood Flow Metab* 1982;**2**:113–162.

267. Baron JC, Bousser M-G, Rey A, et al: Reversal of focal misery-perfusion syndrome by extra-intracranial arterial bypass in hemodynamic cerebral ischemia. *Stroke* 1981;**12**:454–459.

268. Marchal G, Furlong M, Beaudouin V, et al: Early spontaneous hyperperfusion after stroke: A marker of favorable tissue outcome. *Brain* 1996;**119**:409–419.

269. Baron J-C: Positron emission tomography. In Babikian VL, Wechsler LR, Higashida RT (eds): *Imaging Cerebrovascular Disease*. Philadelphia: Butterworth–Heinemann, 2003, pp 115–130.

270. Johnson KA, Gregas M, Becker JA, et al: Imaging of amyloid burden and distribution in cerebral amyloid angiopathy. *Ann Neurol* 2007;**62**:229–234.

271. Vinters HV: Imaging cerebral microvascular amyloid. *Ann Neurol* 2007;**62**:209–212.

272. Caplan LR, Wolpert SM: Angiography in patients with occlusive cerebrovascular disease: A stroke neurologist and neuroradiologist's views. *AJNR Am J Neuroradiol* 1991;**12**:593–601.

273. Akers DL, Markowitz IA, Kerstein MD: The value of aortic arch study in the evaluation of cerebrovascular insufficiency. *Am J Surg* 1987;**154**:230–232.

274. Caplan LR, Manning WJ: Cardiac sources of embolism: The usual suspects. In Caplan LR, Manning WJ (eds): *Brain Embolism*. New York: Informa Healthcare, 2006, pp 129–159.

275. DeRook FA, Comess KA, Albers GW, Popp RL: Transesophageal echocardiography in the evaluation of stroke. *Ann Intern Med* 1992;**117**:922–932.

276. Grullon C, Alam M, Rosman HS, et al: Transesophageal echocardiography in unselected patients with focal cerebral ischemia: When is it useful? *Cerebrovasc Dis* 1994;**4**:139–145.

277. Daniel WG, Mugge A: Transesophageal echocardiography. *N Engl J Med* 1995;**332**:1268–1279.

278. Horowitz DR, Tuhrim S, Weinberger J, et al: Transesophageal echocardiography: Diagnostic and clinical applications in the evaluation of the stroke patient. *J Stroke Cerebrovasc Dis* 1997;**6**:332–336.

279. Manning WJ: Cardiac sources of embolism: Pathophysiology and identification. In Caplan LR, Manning WJ (eds): *Brain Embolism*. New York: Informa Healthcare, 2006, pp 161–186.

280. Furlan AJ, Reisman M, Massaro J, et al; and CI Investigators: Closure or medical therapy for cryptogenic stroke with patent foramen ovale. *N Engl J Med* 2012;**366**:991–999.

281. Carroll JD, Saver JL, Thaler DE, et al; and R Investigators: Closure of patent foramen ovale versus medical therapy after cryptogenic stroke. *N Engl J Med* 2013;**368**:1092–1100.

282. Caplan LR: Of birds and nests and cerebral emboli. *Rev Neurol* 1991;**147**:265–273.

283. Caplan LR: Brain embolism. In Caplan LR, Chimowitz M, Hurst JW (eds): *Practical Clinical Neurocardiology*. New York: Marcel Dekker, 1999, pp 35–185.

284. Caplan LR: The aorta as a donor source of brain embolism. In Caplan LR, Manning WJ (eds): *Brain Embolism*. New York: Informa Healthcare, 2006, pp 187–201.

285. Amarenco P, Davis S, Jones EF, et al; for The Aortic Arch Related Cerebral Hazard Trial Investigators: Clopidogrel plus aspirin versus warfarin in patients with stroke and aortic arch plaques. *Stroke* 2014;**45**:1248–1257.

286. Johnson LL, Pohost GM: Nuclear cardiology. In Schlant RC, Alexander RW (eds): *Hurst's The Heart*, 8th ed. New York: McGraw-Hill, 1994, pp 2281–2323.

287. Caplan LR. Translating what is known about neurological complications of coronary artery bypass grafting into action. *Arch Neurol* 2009;**66**:1063–1064.

288. Weinberger J, Azhar S, Danisi F, et al: A new noninvasive technique for imaging atherosclerotic plaque in the aortic arch of stroke patients by transcutaneous real-time B-mode ultrasonography. *Stroke* 1998;**29**:673–676.

289. Chatzikonstantinou A, Krissak R, Flüchter S: CT angiography of the aorta is superior to transesophageal echocardiography for determining stroke subtypes in patients with cryptogenic ischemic stroke. *Cerebrovasc Dis* 2012;**33**:322–328.

290. Svedlund S, Wetterholm R, Volkmann R, Caidahl K: Retrograde blood flow in the aortic arch determined by transesophageal Doppler ultrasound. *Cerebrovasc Dis* 2009;**27**:22–28.

291. Hur J, Kim YJ, Lee H-J, et al: Cardiac computed tomographic angiography for detection of cardiac sources of embolism in stroke patients. *Stroke* 2009;**40**:2073–2078.

292. Rokey R, Rolak LA, Harati Y, et al: Coronary artery disease in patients with cerebrovascular disease: A prospective study. *Ann Neurol* 1985;**16**:50–53.

293. Dhamoon MS, Tai W, Boden-Albala B, et al: Risk of myocardial infarction or vascular death after first ischemic stroke. The Northern Manhattan Study. *Stroke* 2007;**38**:1752–1758.

294. Calvet D, Touzé E, Varenne O, et al: Prevalence of asymptomatic coronary artery disease in ischemic stroke patients: The PRECORIS study. *Circulation* 2010;**121**:1623–1629.

295. Yoo J, Yang JH, Choi BW, et al: The frequency and risk of preclinical coronary artery disease detected using multichannel cardiac computed tomography in patients with ischemic stroke. *Cerebrovasc Dis* 2012;**33**:286–294.

296. Kim WY, Danias PG, Stuber M, et al: Coronary magnetic resonance angiography for the detection of coronary stenoses. *N Engl J Med* 2001;**345**:1863–1869.

297. Budoff MJ, Shaw LJ, Liu ST, et al: Long-term prognosis associated with coronary calcification: Observations from a registry of 25,253 patients. *J Am Coll Cardiol* 2007;**49**:1860–1870.

298. Liao J, Khalid Z, Scallan C, et al: Noninvasive cardiac monitoring for detecting paroxysmal atrial fibrillation or flutter after acute ischemic stroke: A systematic review. *Stroke* 2007;**38**:2935–2940.

299. Rizos T, Güntner J, Jenetsky E, et al: Continuous stroke unit electrocardiographic monitoring versus 24-hour holter electrocardiography for detection of paroxysmal atrial fibrillation after stroke. *Stroke* 2012;**43**:2689–2694.

300. Rabinstein A: Prolonged cardiac monitoring for detection of paroxysmal atrial fibrillation after cerebral ischemia. *Stroke* 2014;**45**:1208–1214.

301. Kishore A, Vail A, Majid A, et al: Detection of atrial fibrillation after ischemic stroke or transient ischemic attack: a systematic review and meta-analysis. *Stroke* 2014;**45**:520–526.

302. Patton KK, Ellinor PT, Hecklert SR, et al: N-terminal pro-B-type natriuretic peptide is a major

predictor of the development of atrial fibrillation. *Circulation* 2009;**120**:1768–1777.

303. Hijazi Z, Wallentin L, Siegbahn A, et al: N-terminal pro–B-type natriuretic peptide for risk assessment in patients with atrial fibrillation. *J Am Coll Cardiol* 2013;**61**:2274–2284.

304. Warraich HJ, Gandhavadi M, Manning WJ: Mechanical discordance of the left atrium and appendage. A novel mechanism of stroke in paroxysmal atrial fibrillation. *Stroke* 2014;**45**:1481–1484.

305. Lieb WE, Flaharty PM, Sergott RC, et al: Color Doppler imaging provides accurate assessment of orbital blood flow in occlusive carotid artery disease. *Ophthalmology* 1991;**98**:548–552.

306. Hedges TR. Ocular ischemia. In Caplan LR (ed): *Brain Ischemia: Basic Concepts and Clinical Relevance*. London: Springer, 1995, pp 61–73.

307. Castillo M, Kwock L, Mukherji SK: Clinical applications of proton MR spectroscopy. *AJNR Am J Neuroradiol* 1996;**17**:1–15.

308. Pavlakis SG, Kingsley PB, Kaplan GP, et al: Magnetic resonance spectroscopy: Use in monitoring MELAS treatment. *Arch Neurol* 1998;**55**:849–852.

309. Koroshetz WJ: New techniques in computed tomography, magnetic resonance imaging, and optical imaging in cerebrovascular disease. In Babikian VL, Wechsler LR, Higashida RT (eds): *Imaging Cerebrovascular Disease*. Philadelphia: Butterworth–Heinemann, 2003, pp 403–412.

310. Cramer SC, Nelles G, Benson RR, et al: A functional MRI study of subjects recovered from hemiparetic stroke. *Stroke* 1997;**28**:2518–2527.

311. Ward NS, Brown MM, Thompson AJ, Frackowiak RSJ: Neural correlates of motor recovery after stroke: a longitudinal fMRI study. *Brain* 2003;**126**:2476–2496.

312. Love T, Haist F, Nicol J, Swinney D: A functional neuroimaging investigation of the roles of structural complexity and task-demand during auditory sentence processing. *Cortex* 2006;**42**:577–590.

313. Levine SR, Brust JCM, Futrell N, et al: A comparative study of the cerebrovascular complications of

cocaine-alkaloidal versus hydrochloride – a review. *Neurology* 1991;**41**:1173–1177.

314. Caplan LR: Drugs. In Kase CS, Caplan LR (eds): *Intracerebral Hemorrhage*. Boston: Butterworth–Heinemann, 1994, pp 201–220.

315. Alberico RA, Patel M, Casey S, et al: Evaluation of the circle of Willis with three-dimensional CT angiography in patients with suspected intracranial aneurysms. *AJNR Am J Neuroradiol* 1995;**16**:1571–1578.

316. Sekhar L, Wechsler L, Yonas H, et al: Value of transcranial Doppler examination in the diagnosis of cerebral vasospasm after subarachnoid hemorrhage. *Neurosurgery* 1988;**22**:813–821.

317. Sloan MA, Haley EC, Kassell NF, et al: Sensitivity and specificity of transcranial Doppler ultrasonography in the diagnosis of vasospasm following subarachnoid hemorrhage. *Neurology* 1989;**39**:1514–1518.

318. Pollock S, Tsitsopoulas P, Harrison M: The effect of hematocrit on cerebral perfusion and clinical status following occlusion in the gerbil. *Stroke* 1982;**13**:167–170.

319. Harrison M, Pollock S, Kindoll B, et al: Effect of hematocrit on carotid stenosis and cerebral infarction. *Lancet* 1981;**2**:114–115.

320. Thomas D, duBoulay G, Marshall J, et al: Effect of hematocrit on cerebral blood flow in man. *Lancet* 1977;**2**:941–943.

321. Tohgi H, Yamanouchi H, Murakami M, et al: Importance of the hematocrit as a risk factor in cerebral infarction. *Stroke* 1978;**9**:369–374.

322. Grotta J, Ackerman R, Correia J, et al: Whole-blood viscosity parameters and cerebral blood flow. *Stroke* 1982;**13**:296–298.

323. Thomas D: Whole blood viscosity and cerebral blood flow. *Stroke* 1982;**13**:285–287.

324. Kee Jr DB, Wood JH: Influence of blood rheology on cerebral circulation. In Wood JH (ed): *Cerebral Blood Flow: Physiological and Clinical Aspects*. New York: McGraw-Hill, 1987, pp 173–185.

325. Allport LE, Parsons MW, Butcher KS, et al: Elevated hematocrit is associated with reduced reperfusion and tissue survival in acute stroke. *Neurology* 2005;**65**:1382–1387.

326. Adams RJ, Nichols FT, Figueroa R, et al: Transcranial Doppler correlation with cerebral angiography in sickle cell disease. *Stroke* 1992;**23**:1073–1077.

327. Switzer JA, Hess DC, Nichols FT, Adams RJ: Pathophysiology and treatment of stroke in sickle-cell disease: Present and future. *Lancet Neurol* 2006;**5**:501–512.

328. Adams RJ: TCD in sickle cell disease: An important and useful test. *Pediatr Radiol* 2005;**35**:229–234.

329. Adams RJ, McKie VC, Hsu L, et al: Prevention of a first stroke by transfusions in children with sickle cell anemia and abnormal results on transcranial Doppler ultrasonography. *N Engl J Med* 1998;**339**:5–11.

330. Adams RJ, Brambilla D: Optimizing Primary Stroke Prevention in Sickle Cell Anemia (STOP 2) Trial Investigators: Discontinuing prophylactic transfusions used to prevent stroke in sickle cell disease. *N Engl J Med* 2005;**353**:2769–2778.

331. Mercuri M, Bond MG, Evans G, et al: Leukocyte count and carotid atherosclerosis. *Stroke* 1991;**22**:134.

332. Elkind MS, Cheng I, Boden-Albala B, et al: Elevated white blood cell count and carotid plaque thickness: The Northern Manhattan Stroke Study. *Stroke* 2001;**32**:842–849.

333. Elkind MS, Sciacca R, Boden-Albala B, et al: Leukocyte count is associated with aortic arch plaque thickness. *Stroke* 2002;**33**:2587–2592.

334. Elkind MS, Sciacca RR, Boden-Albala B, et al: Leukocyte count is associated with reduced endothelial reactivity. *Atherosclerosis* 2005;**181**:329–338.

335. Elkind MS, Sciacca RR, Boden-Albala B, et al: Relative elevation in baseline leukocyte count predicts first cerebral infarction. *Neurology* 2005;**64**:2121–2125.

336. Elkind MS: Inflammation, atherosclerosis, and stroke. *Neurologist* 2006;**12**:140–148.

337. Bennett JS, Kolodziej MA: Disorders of platelet function. *Dis Month* 1992;**38**:557–563.

338. Anderson IR, Feinberg WM: Primary platelet disorders. In Welch KMA, Caplan LR, Reis DJ, Siesjo BK, Weir B (eds): *Primer on Cerebrovascular Diseases*. San Diego, Academic Press, 1997, pp 401–405.

339. Wu K: Platelet hyperaggregability and thrombosis in patients with thrombocythemia. *Ann Intern Med* 1978;**88**:7–11.

340. Arboix A, Besses C, Acin P, et al: Ischemic stroke as first manifestation of essential thrombocythemia: Report of six cases. *Stroke* 1995;**26**:1463–1466.

341. Ogata J, Yonemura K, Kimura K, et al: Cerebral infarction associated with essential thrombocythemia: An autopsy case study. *Cerebrovasc Dis* 2005;**19**:201–205.

342. Atkinson JLD, Sundt TM, Kazmier FJ, et al: Heparin-induced thrombocytopenia and thrombosis in ischemic stroke. *Mayo Clin Proc* 1988;**63**:353–361.

343. Arepally GM, Ortel TL: Clinical practice. Heparin-induced thrombocytopenia. *N Engl J Med* 2006;**355**:809–817.

344. Uchyama S, Takeuchi M, Osawa M, et al: Platelet function tests in thrombotic cerebrovascular disorders. *Stroke* 1983;**14**:511–517.

345. Ludlam CA: Evidence for the platelet specificity of beta-thromboglobulin and studies on its plasma concentration in healthy individuals. *Br J Haematol* 1979;**41**:271–278.

346. Fisher M, Francis R: Altered coagulation in cerebral ischemia: Platelet, thrombin, and plasmin activity. *Arch Neurol* 1990;**47**:1075–1079.

347. Helgason CH, Bolin KM, Hoff JA, et al: Development of aspirin resistance in persons with previous ischemic stroke. *Stroke* 1994;**25**:2331–2336.

348. Yeh RW, Everett BM, Foo SY, et al: Predictors for the development of elevated anti-heparin/platelet factor 4 antibody titers in patients undergoing cardiac catheterization. *Am J Cardiol* 2006;**98**:419–421.

349. Qizilbash N, Duffy S, Prentice CRM, et al: von Willebrand factor and risk of ischemic stroke. *Neurology* 1997;**49**:1552–1556.

350. Blann AD: Plasma von Willebrand factor, thrombosis, and the endothelium: The first 30 years. *Thromb Haemost* 2006;**95**:49–55.

351. Bowen DJ, Collins PW: Insights into von Willebrand factor proteolysis: Clinical implications. *Br J Haematol* 2006;**133**:457–467.

352. Weiss EJ, Bray PF, Tayback M, et al: A polymorphism of a platelet glycoprotein receptor as an inherited risk factor for coronary thrombosis. *N Engl J Med* 1996;**334**:1090–1094.

353. Kannel WB, Wolf PA, Castelli WP, et al: Fibrinogen and risk of cardiovascular disease. *JAMA* 1987;**258**:1183–1186.

354. Coull BM, Beamer NB, deGarmo PL, et al: Chronic blood hyperviscosity in subjects with acute stroke, transient ischemic attack, and risk factors for stroke. *Stroke* 1991;**22**:162–168.

355. Beamer N, Coull BM, Sexton G, et al: Fibrinogen and the albumin-globulin ratio in recurrent stroke. *Stroke* 1993;**24**:1133–1139.

356. Ernst E, Resch KL: Fibrinogen as a cardiovascular risk factor: A meta-analysis and review of the literature. *Ann Intern Med* 1993;**118**:956–963.

357. Danesh J, Lewington S, Thompson SG, et al: Plasma fibrinogen level and the risk of major cardiovascular diseases and nonvascular mortality: An individual participant meta-analysis. *JAMA* 2005;**294**:1799–1809.

358. Rothwell PM, Howard SC, Power DA, et al: Fibrinogen concentration and risk of ischemic stroke and acute coronary events in 5113 patients with transient ischemic attack and minor ischemic stroke. *Stroke* 2004;**35**:2300–2305.

359. Mora S, Rifai N, Buring JE, Ridker PM: Additive value of immunoassay-measured fibrinogen and high-sensitivity C-reactive protein levels for predicting incident cardiovascular events. *Circulation* 2006;**114**:381–387.

360. The Ancrod Stroke Study Investigators: Ancrod for the treatment of acute ischemic brain infarction. *Stroke* 1994;**25**:1755–1759.

361. Atkinson RP: Ancrod in the treatment of acute ischemic stroke. a review of clinical data. *Cerebrovasc Dis* 1998;**8**(Suppl 1):23–28.

362. Gonzales-Conejero R, Fernandez-Cadenas I, Iniesta JA, et al: Role of fibrinogen levels and factor XIII V34L polymorphism in thrombolytic therapy in stroke patients. *Stroke* 2006;**37**:2288–2293.

363. Radack K, Deck C, Huster G: Dietary supplementation with low-dose fish oils lowers fibrinogen levels: A randomized double-blind controlled study. *Ann Intern Med* 1989;**111**:757–758.

364. Dashe J: Hyperviscosity and stroke. In Bogousslavsky J, Caplan LR (eds): *Uncommon Causes of Stroke*. Cambridge: Cambridge University Press, 2001, pp 100–109.

365. Rosenson RS, Lowe GD: Effects of lipids and lipoproteins on thrombosis and rheology. *Atherosclerosis* 1998;**140**:271–280.

366. Ariyo A, Thach C, Tracy R; for the Cardiovascular Health Study Investigators: Lp (a) lipoprotein, vascular disease, and mortality in the elderly. *N Engl J Med* 2003;**349**:2108–2115.

367. Ohira T, Schreiner P, Morrisett JD, et al: Lipoprotein (a) and incident ischemic stroke. The Atherosclerosis Risk in Communities (ARIC) Study. *Stroke* 2006;**37**:1407–1412.

368. Arenillas JF, Molina CA, Chacon P, et al: High lipoprotein (a), diabetes, and the extent of symptomatic intracranial atherosclerosis. *Neurology* 2004;**63**:27–32.

369. Dahlback B, Carlsson M, Svensson PJ: Familial thrombophilia due to a previously unrecognized mechanism characterized by poor anticoagulant response to activated protein C: Prediction of a cofactor to activated protein C. *Proc Natl Acad Sci U S A* 1993;**90**:1004–1008.

370. Zoller B, Dahlback B: Linkage between inherited resistance to activated protein C and factor V gene mutation in venous thrombosis. *Lancet* 1994;**343**:1536–1538.

371. Coull BM, Skaff PT: Disorders of coagulation. In Bogousslavsky J, Caplan LR (eds): *Uncommon Causes of Stroke*. Cambridge: Cambridge University Press, 2001, pp 86–95.

372. Ridker PM, Miletich JP, Stampfer MJ, et al: Factor V Leiden and risks of recurrent idiopathic venous thromboembolism. *Circulation* 1997;**95**:1777–1782.

373. Poort SR, Rosendaal FR, Reitsma PH, et al: A common genetic variation in the 3' untranslated region of the prothrombin gene is associated with elevated prothrombin levels and an increase in venous thrombosis. *Blood* 1996;**88**:3698–3703.

374. Martinelli I, Sacchi E, Landi G, et al: High risk of cerebral-vein thrombosis in carriers of a prothrombin-gene mutation and in users of oral contraceptives. *N Engl J Med* 1998;**338**:1793–1797.

375. Kosik KS, Furie B: Thrombotic stroke associated with elevated plasma factor VIII. *Arch Neurol* 1980;**8**:435–437.

376. Bhopale GM, Nanda RK: Blood coagulation factor VIII: An overview. *J Biosci* 2003;**28**:783–789.

377. Estol C, Pessin MS, DeWitt LD, et al: Stroke and increased factor VIII activity. *Neurology* 1989;**39**:225.

378. Pan W-H, Bai C-H, Chen J-R, Chiu H-C: Associations between carotid atherosclerosis and high factor VIII activity, dyslipidemia, and hypertension. *Stroke* 1997;**28**:88–94.

379. Anadure RK, Nagaraja D, Christopher R: Plasma factor VIII in non-puerperal cerebral venous thrombosis: a prospective case-control study. *J Neurol Sci* 2014;**339**:140–143.

380. Lip GYH, Lane D, Van Walraven C, Hart RG: Additive role of plasma von Willebrand factor levels to clinical factors for risk stratification of patients with atrial fibrillation. *Stroke* 2006;**37**:2294–2300.

381. Bongers TN, de Maat MP, van Goor ML, et al: High von Willebrand factor levels increase the risk of first ischemic stroke: Influence of ADAMTS 13, inflammation, and genetic variability. *Stroke* 2006;**37**:2672–2677.

382. Markus HS, Hambley H: Neurology and the blood: haematological abnormalities in ischaemic stroke. *J Neurol Neurosurg Psychiatry* 1998;**64**:150–159.

383. Feinberg WM, Bruck DC, Ring ME, et al: Hemostatic markers in acute stroke. *Stroke* 1989;**20**:592–597.

384. Feinberg WM, Cornell ES, Nightingale SD, et al: Relationship between prothrombin activation fragment F1.2 and international normalized ratio in patients with atrial fibrillation. *Stroke* 1997;**28**:1101–1106.

385. Toghi H, Kawashima M, Tamura K, et al: Coagulation–fibrinolysis abnormalities in acute and chronic phases of cerebral thrombosis and embolism. *Stroke* 1990;**21**:1663–1667.

386. Jeppeson LL, Jorgensen HS, Nakayama H, et al: Tissue plasminogen activator is elevated in women with ischemic stroke. *J Stroke Cerebrovasc Dis* 1998;**7**:187–191.

387. Feinberg WM: Coagulation. In Caplan LR (ed): *Brain Ischemia: Basic Concepts and Clinical Relevance.* London: Springer, 1995, pp 85–96.

388. Palareti G, Cosmi B, Legnani C, et al: D-dimer testing to determine the duration of anticoagulant therapy. *N Engl J Med* 2006;**355**:1780–1789.

389. Stallworth C, Brey R: Antiphospholipid antibody syndrome. In Bogousslavsky J, Caplan LR (eds): *Uncommon Causes of Stroke.* Cambridge: Cambridge University Press, 2001, pp 63–77.

390. Coull BM, Goodnight SH: Antiphospholipid antibodies, prothrombotic states, and stroke. *Stroke* 1990;**21**:1370–1374.

391. Levine SR, Welch KMA: The spectrum of neurologic disease associated with antiphospholipid antibodies: Lupus anticoagulants, and anticardiolipin antibodies. *Arch Neurol* 1987;**44**:876–883.

392. Hess DC, Sheppard S, Adams RJ: Increased immunoglobulin binding to cerebral endothelium in patients with antiphospholipid antibodies. *Stroke* 1993;**24**:994–999.

393. Levine SR, Salowich-Palm L, Sawaya K, et al: IgG anticardiolipin antibody titer ϒ40GPL and the risk of subsequent thrombo-occlusive events and death. A prospective cohort study. *Stroke* 1997;**28**:1660–1665.

394. Ortel TL: The antiphospholipid syndrome: What are we really measuring? How do we measure it? And how do we treat it? *J Thromb Thrombolysis* 2006;**21**:79–83.

395. Tuhrim S, Rand JH, Horowitz DR, et al: Antiphosphatidyl serine antibodies are independently associated with ischemic stroke. *Neurology* 1999;**53**:1523–1527.

396. Toschi V, Motta A, Castelli C, et al: High prevalence of antiphosphatidylinositol antibodies in young patients with cerebral ischemia of undetermined cause. *Stroke* 1998;**29**:1759–1764.

397. Tanne D, Triplett D, Levine SR: Antiphospholipid-protein antibodies and ischemic stroke: Not just cardiolipin anymore. *Stroke* 1998;**29**:1755–1758.

398. Francès C, Papo T, Wechsler B, et al: Sneddon syndrome with or without antiphospholipid antibodies. A comparative study in 46 patients. *Medicine* 1999;**78**:209–219.

399. Myers R, Yamaguchi S: Nervous system effects of cardiac arrest in monkeys. *Arch Neurol* 1977;**34**:65–74.

400. Pulsinelli W, Waldman S, Rawlinson D, et al: Hyperglycemia converts ischemic neuronal damage into brain infarction. *Neurology* 1982;**32**:1239–1246.

401. Plum F: What causes infarction in ischemic brain? *Neurology* 1983;**33**:222–233.

402. Pulsinelli W, Levy D, Sigsbel B, et al: Increased damage after ischemic stroke in patients with hyperglycemia with or without established diabetes mellitus. *Am J Med* 1983;**74**:540–544.

403. Bellolio MF, Gilmore RM, Stead LG: Insulin for glycaemic control in acute ischaemic stroke. *Cochrane Database Syst Rev* 2011 Sep 7;(9):CD005346. doi:10.1002/14651858.CD005346.pub3.

404. Walker G, Williamson P, Ravich R, et al: Hypercalcemia associated with cerebral vasospasm causing infarction. *J Neurol Neurosurg Psychiatry* 1980;**43**:464–467.

405. Gorelick PB, Caplan LR: Calcium, hypercalcemia, and stroke. Current concepts of cerebrovascular disease. *Stroke* 1985;**20**:13–17.

406. Siesjo B, Kristian T: Cell calcium homeostasis and calcium-related ischemic damage. In Welch KMA, Caplan LR, Reis DJ, et al. (eds): *Primer on Cerebrovascular Diseases.* San Diego: Academic Press, 1997, pp 172–178.

407. Henderson GV, Caplan LR: Calcium, hypercalcemia, magnesium, and brain ischemia. In Bogousslavsky J, Caplan LR (eds): *Uncommon Causes of Stroke.* Cambridge: Cambridge University Press, 2001, pp 110–113.

408. Ovbiagele B, Saver J, Fredieu A, et al: In-hospital initiation of secondary stroke prevention therapies yields high rates of adherence at follow-up. *Stroke* 2004;**35**:2879–2883.

409. Ovbiagele B, Saver J, Fredieu A, et al: PROTECT. A coordinated stroke treatment program to prevent recurrent thromboembolic events. *Neurology* 2004;**63**:1217–1222.

410. Ridker PM, Stampfer MJ, Rifai N: Novel risk factors for systemic atherosclerosis: A comparison of C-reactive protein, fibrinogen, homcysteine, lipoprotein (a), and standard cholesterol screening as predictors of peripheral arterial disease. *JAMA* 2001;**285**:2481–2485.

411. Sacco RL, Anand K, Lee H-S, et al: Homocysteine and the risk of ischemic stroke in a triethnic cohort. The Northern Manhattan Study. *Stroke* 2004;**35**:2263–2269.

412. Tanne D, Haim M, Goldbourt U, et al: Prospective study of serum homocysteine and risk of ischemic stroke among patients with preexisting coronary heart disease. *Stroke* 2003;**34**:632–636.

413. Eikelboom JW, Hankey GJ, Anand SS, et al: Association between high homocyst(e)ine and ischemic stroke due to large and small-artery disease but not other etiologic subtypes of ischemic stroke. *Stroke* 2000;**31**:1069–1075.

414. Bova I, Chapman J, Sylantiev C, et al: The A677V methylenetetrahydrofolate reductase gene polymorphism and carotid atherosclerosis. *Stroke* 1999;**30**:2180–2182.

415. Selhub J, Jacques PF, Rosenberg IH, et al: Serum total homocysteine concentrations in the Third National Health and Nutrition Examination Survey (1991–1994): Population reference ranges and contribution of vitamin status to high serum concentrations. *Ann Intern Med* 1999;**331**–339.

416. den Heijer, Rosendaal FR, Blom HJ, Gerrits WB, Bos GM: Hyperhomocysteinemia and venous thrombosis: a meta-analysis. *Thromb Haemost* 1998;**80**:874–877.

417. Ridker PM, Rifai N, Rose L, et al: Comparison of C-reactive protein and low-density lipoprotein cholesterol levels in the prediction of first cardiovascular events. *N Engl J Med* 2002;**347**:1557–1565.

418. Eikelboom JW, Hankey GJ, Baker RI, et al: C-reactive protein in ischemic stroke and its etiologic subtypes. *J Stroke Cerebrovasc Dis* 2003;**12**:74–81.

419. Arenillas JF, Alvarez-Sabin J, Molina CA, et al: C-reactive protein predicts further ischemic events in first-ever transient ischemic attack or stroke patients with intracranial large-artery occlusive disease. *Stroke* 2003;**34**:2463–2470.

420. Wakugawa Y, Kiyohara Y, Tanizaki Y, et al: C-reactive protein and risk of first-ever ischemic and hemorrhagic stroke in general Japanese population. The Hisayama Study. *Stroke* 2006;**37**:27–32.

421. Schlager O, Exner M, Miekusch W, et al: C-reactive protein predicts future cardiovascular events in patients with carotid stenosis. *Stroke* 2007;**38**:1263–1268.

422. Salvarani C, Canini F, Boiardi L, Hunder GG: Laboratory investigations useful in giant cell arteritis and Takayasu's arteritis. *Clin Exp Rheumatol* 2003;**21**(Suppl 32):523–528.

423. Lavigne-Lissalde G, Schved JF, Granier C, Villard S: Anti-factor VIII antibodies: A 2005 update. *Thromb Haemost* 2005;**94**:760–769.

424. Franchini M: Acquired hemophilia A. *Hematology* 2006;**11**:119–125.

425. Saposnik G, Caplan LR: Convulsive-like movements in brainstem stroke. *Arch Neurol* 2001;**54**:654–657.

426. Ropper AH: "Convulsions" in basilar artery occlusions. *Neurology* 1988;**38**:1500–1501.

427. Carrera E, Michel P, Despland PA, et al: Continuous assessment of electrical epileptic activity in acute stroke. *Neurology* 2006 **11**;67:99–104.

428. Bladin CF, Alexandrov A, Bellavance A, et al: Seizures after stroke: A prospective multicenter study. *Arch Neurol* 2000;**57**:1617–1622.

429. Wilber DJ, Garan H, Finkelstein D, et al: Out-of-hospital cardiac arrest: Use of electrophysiologic testing in the prediction of long-term outcome. *N Engl J Med* 1988;**318**:19–24.

430. Madl C, Kramer L, Domanovits H, et al: Improved outcome prediction in unconscious cardiac arrest survivors with sensory evoked potentials compared with clinical assessment. *Crit Care Med* 2000;**28**:721–726.

431. Wijdicks EF, Hijdra A, Young GB, et al; For the Quality Standards Subcommittee of the American Academy of Neurology Practice Parameter: Prediction of outcome in comatose survivors after cardiopulmonary resuscitation (an evidence-based review). Report of the Quality Standards Subcommittee of the American Academy of Neurology. *Neurology* 2006;**67**:203–210.

432. Marx J, Thoömke F, Urban PP, Bense S, Dieterich M: Electrophysiologic diagnostics. In Urban PP, Caplan LR (eds): *Brainstem Disorders*, Berlin: Springer-Verlag, 2011, pp 61–101.

433. Alberts MJ: Genetics of cerebrovascular disease. *Stroke* 2004;**35**:342–344.

434. Meschia JF, Worrall BB: New advances in identifying genetic anomalies in stroke-prone probands. *Curr Neurol Neurosci Rep* 2004;**4**:420–426.

435. Dichgans M, Hegele RA: Update on the genetics of stroke and cerebrovascular disease – 2006. *Stroke* 2007;**38**:216–218.

436. Dichgans M: Genetics of ischaemic stroke. *Lancet Neurol* 2007;**6**:149–161.

437. Sims KB, Alberts MJ, Caplan LR. *New Insights into the Diagnosis of Single-gene Disorders Associated with Cryptogenic Ischemic Stroke*. CME Monograph. Lexington, KY: University of Kentucky College of Medicine and CE Health Sciences Inc, 2010.

438. Debette S, Bis JC, Fornage M, et al: Genome-wide association studies of MRI-defined brain infarcts: Meta-analysis from the CHARGE Consortium. *Stroke* 2010;**41**:210–217.

439. Caplan LR, Arenillas J, Cramer SC, et al: Stroke-related translational research (review). *Arch Neurol* 2011;**68**:1110–1123.

440. Falcone GJ, Malik R, Dichgans M, Rosand J: Current concepts and clinical applications of stroke genetics. *Lancet Neurol* 2014;**13**:405–418.

441. Gretarsdottir S, Thorleifsson G, Reynisdottir ST, et al: The gene encoding phosphodiesterase 4D confers risk of ischemic stroke. *Nat Genet* 2003;**35**:131–138.

442. Yee RYL, Brophy VH, Cheng S, et al: Polymorphisms of the phosphodiesterase 4D, camp-specific (*PDE4D*) gene and risk of ischemic stroke: A prospective, nested case-control evaluation. *Stroke* 2006;**37**:2012–2017.

Genetics of stroke

Stéphanie Debette and Louis R Caplan

Introduction

Stroke is one of the most common neurological diseases, with a lifetime risk of 1 in 5 for middle-aged women and 1 in 6 for middle-aged men.[1] Besides being the first cause of acquired disability in adults and the second cause of death,[2] stroke is also a major contributor to cognitive decline and dementia.[3–5]

Although a number of important risk factors for stroke are known and actionable, a substantial proportion of stroke risk remains unexplained. Converging evidence suggests that genetic risk factors likely contribute to this residual risk. In rare instances stroke can be directly caused by single gene disorders. In most patients genetic risk factors contribute to the risk of stroke as part of a multifactorial predisposition, with each genetic variation being responsible only for modest increases in risk. The advent of high throughput genotyping and sequencing technologies in the past decade has led to important progress in the discovery of genes underlying complex forms of stroke.[6] The main application expected from these discoveries is to improve understanding of the biological pathways and mechanisms of the various subtypes of stroke and by doing so improve prevention.[7] While improved risk prediction also remains a long-term goal, its implementation is complex given the small effect size of genetic risk variants and their paucity to date compared to other complex phenotypes. A major challenge in the identification of genetic determinants of stroke, which requires very large samples, is the complexity of the phenotype. In contrast to other common vascular and neurological conditions such as myocardial infarction and Alzheimer's disease, stroke is not a single disease but a syndrome that can be caused by multiple, extremely diverse etiologies.

In this chapter, we will first describe the main single-gene disorders causing stroke. Second, we will present a summary of genetic-risk variants identified as contributing to stroke risk and the implications of these discoveries. In both cases ischemic stroke and intracerebral hemorrhage will be discussed separately, although some monogenic diseases or genetic-risk variants can be associated with both presentations. We will not discuss the genetics of subarachnoid hemorrhage, which is mentioned in Chapter 13.

Rare monogenic causes of stroke

Single-gene (monogenic) disorders are responsible for a very small proportion of strokes, probably less than 1%.[8] The mechanisms by which these monogenic disorders result in stroke are varied. Features that should prompt investigations towards identifying an underlying monogenic disorder in stroke patients are summarized in Table 5.1. If genetic testing is being performed, appropriate genetic counseling by a specialized team needs to be proposed. The monogenic disorders presented below are those for which stroke is one of the main clinical manifestations. Inherited cardiopathies (e.g., familial atrial fibrillation) or vascular malformations (e.g., familial cavernomas) that can cause stroke are not discussed in this chapter. Cavernous malformations are discussed in Chapter 13.

Ischemic stroke

Monogenic disorders causing small artery occlusion (lacunar) ischemic stroke

Cerebral autosomal dominant arteriopathy with subcortical infarcts and leukoencephalopathy

Cerebral autosomal dominant arteriopathy with subcortical infarcts and leukoencephalopathy (CADASIL) is a rare autosomal dominant disease (one mutated allele is sufficient to cause the disease) affecting cerebral small arteries, due to mutations in the NOTCH3 gene on chromosome 19p13.2–p13.1.[9,10] It is the most common inherited cerebral small artery disease. NOTCH3 encodes a cell-surface receptor involved in vascular smooth muscle cell survival and vascular remodeling.

Table 5.1 Stroke characteristics that should lead to genetic investigation

Young age
Family history (highly suggestive, but not necessarily present in monogenic forms, as penetrance can be variable and mutations can occur de novo)
Absence of defined etiology and conventional vascular risk factors (hypertension, diabetes, dyslipidemia, obesity, smoking, alcohol consumption)
Some magnetic resonance imaging (MRI) features: • Multiple old infarcts or intracerebral hemorrhages • Presence of extensive white matter hyperintensities on brain MRI, especially in the absence of hypertension • Multiple microbleeds, in the absence of known etiology

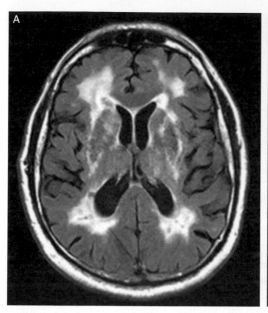 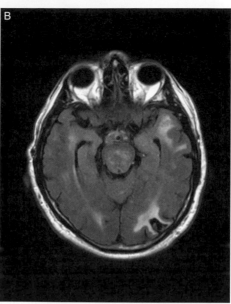

Figure 5.1 MRI FLAIR images from a 45-year-old CADASIL patient. (A) Extensive white matter hyperintensities in the external and internal capsules, basal ganglia and frontal white matter. Kindly submitted by Dr Joshua Klein of the Brigham and Womans Hospital, Boston. (B) The left temporal and occipital lobes are involved. The pontine white matter also is hyperintense.

The underlying vascular lesion is a non-arteriosclerotic, amyloid-negative angiopathy involving small arteries and capillaries.[11] The prevalence of this disorder has been estimated at about 1 in 24 000, which is probably an underestimate.[12] CADASIL has been reported to account for 2% of cases of lacunar stroke with white matter lesions in patients under age 65 and for 11% in those under age 50.[13]

CADASIL patients have recurrent lacunar strokes, the most common manifestation of the condition (60–85%), occurring at a mean age of 49 years, often in the absence of conventional stroke risk factors.[9] The phenotype also includes progressive cognitive impairment (the second most common manifestation, initially mostly detectable with tests of executive function and processing speed), migraine with aura (20–40% of patients, usually the first symptom when it is present), and psychiatric disturbances (20%, especially mood disturbances, including severe depression). Magnetic resonance imaging (MRI) abnormalities appear before the onset of clinical symptoms, at a mean age of 30 years.[9] The earliest and most common abnormalities are white matter hyperintensities (WMH) on T2-weighted or fluid-attenuated inversion recovery (FLAIR) MRI. These are located in the periventricular and deep white matter, but also in the basal ganglia and thalamus, the external capsule and the anterior temporal lobe, the latter location being highly suggestive of CADASIL.[14] Figure 5.1 from a CADASIL patient shows these white matter lesions. The brainstem and corpus callosum are also occasionally affected. WMH are initially punctate but evolve towards diffuse, confluent lesions over time. Lacunar infarcts can been seen on T1-weighted images as areas of decreased signal intensity; they tend to occur later in life than WMH.[15] Sometimes multiple simultaneous acute infarcts are seen on diffusion-weighted imaging (DWI).[16] Other MRI features include dilated perivascular spaces (Virchow–Robin spaces), in the basal ganglia but typically also in the temporal lobes and subinsular areas.[17]

Although the clinical expression of CADASIL is mostly due to ischemic lesions, microbleeds are also often seen on gradient echo images (T2*). The definitive diagnostic test is the molecular genetic analysis of the *NOTCH3* gene. Skin biopsy can show characteristic granular osmiophilic material within the vascular basal lamina on electron microscopy.[18] Only symptomatic treatments are available. Stroke risk fators when present should be optimized. Antiplatelet agents are sometimes used to prevent ischemic events. A randomized controlled trial testing the effect of donepezil on cognitive decline in CADASIL patients failed to show a benefit for the primary end-point (progression on the cognitive subscale of the vascular Alzheimer's disease assessment scale), with improvements seen on secondary end-points of executive function.[19]

Cerebral autosomal recessive arteriopathy with subcortical infarcts and leukoencephalopathy

Cerebral autosomal recessive arteriopathy with subcortical infarcts and leukoencephalopathy (CARASIL) is a rare autosomal recessive disease (two mutated alleles are required to cause the disease) affecting cerebral small arteries, due to mutations in the *HTRA1* gene on chromosome 10q25.[20] *HTRA1* encodes a serine protease that is thought to repress signaling by transforming growth factor-beta (TGF-beta) family members. The exact prevalence of CARASIL is unknown, as only few patients have been described. Most of them were diagnosed in Japan, with a few additional cases reported in Chinese, Turkish, Spanish, and Romanian patients.[21–25] In addition to lacunar stroke, CARASIL patients present with early-onset dementia, gait disturbance, alopecia, and low back pain.[26] Lacunar strokes have been reported in a quarter to half of CARASIL patients, mainly in the basal ganglia or brainstem.[26,27] Alopecia, confined to the head, is usually the first clinical symptom, present in 75–90% of patients during adolescence. Early-onset dementia, starting in the thirties, is another common clinical feature, often accompanied by gait and mood changes (apathy and irritability).[26,27] Severe acute mid and lower

back pain can occur, beginning in the twenties.[28] Most patients become bedridden within 10 years from onset. By age 20, T2-weighted or FLAIR brain MRI shows diffuse and symmetrical WMH, more often in the periventricular and deep white matter, but also in basal ganglia, thalami, brainstem, cerebellum, temporal lobes and external capsules, usually at a less early stage than in CADASIL for the latter two locations.[26,27] Multiple lacunar infarcts are observed. There is no known effective treatment. The effectiveness of antiplatelet agents in preventing ischemic stroke recurrences is unclear.[27]

Retinal vasculopathy and cerebral leukodystrophy

Retinal vasculopathy and cerebral leukodystrophy (RVCL) is a group of inherited small vessel diseases comprised of cerebro-retinal vasculopathy (CRV), hereditary vascular retinopathy (HVR), and hereditary endotheliopathy with retinopathy, nephropathy and stroke (HERNS), due to mutations in the TREX1 gene on chromosome 3p21.1–21.3.[29–32] The mode of inheritance is autosomal dominant. The prevalence is unknown as only a few cases and families have been described (<1/1 million, www.orpha.net). All types of RVCL are characterized by progressive loss of visual acuity secondary to retinal vasculopathy (telangiectasias, microaneurysms and retinal capillary obliteration starting in the macula) and variable neurological findings. Visual loss, stroke, and dementia begin in middle age, and death occurs in most families 5–10 years later.[32] In a subset of affected individuals, systemic vascular involvement is present, with Raynaud's phenomenon and slight liver and kidney dysfunction.[32] The commonly observed neurological manifestations are transient ischemic attacks and lacunar ischemic strokes, seizures, cognitive dysfunction, headaches, personality disorders, depression, and anxiety. Cerebral MRI findings usually consist of multiple subcortical lacunar infarcts, WMH involving the periventricular and deep white matter, as well as contrast enhancing lesions in the white matter of the cerebrum and cerebellum.[32] No specific treatment is available.

Collagen 4A1 (COL4A1) syndrome

This condition is described in detail in the Intracerebral hemorrhage section in Chapter 5, as cerebrovascular complications are predominantly hemorrhagic.

Monogenic disorders causing large artery atherosclerosis and small artery occlusion (lacunar) ischemic stroke

Sickle cell disease

Sickle cell disease is an autosomal recessive disorder that can be due to either a homozygous state for hemoglobin S (HbS) or to the combined heterozygous state with other hemoglobinopathies such as hemoglobin C (HbC) or mild β-thalassemia.[33] HbS results from a mutation on the HBB (hemoglobin beta) gene on chromosome 11.[33] Populations predominantly affected by sickle cell disease are those of sub-Saharan origin and also Indian, Arab, and some Mediterranean populations.[34] The prevalence of sickle cell disease is highest in sub-Saharan

Africa (over 0.74% of births), due to selection for carriers through their survival advantage in malaria-endemic regions.[35]

Stroke affects up to 25% of patients by age 45, and includes large-artery and lacunar ischemic stroke (with a peak incidence in early childhood), as well as hemorrhagic stroke (mainly in adults).[36] Most overt strokes are due to large artery vasculopathy affecting the intracranial internal carotid arteries and proximal middle and anterior cerebral arteries, associated with intimal thickening, fibroblast and smooth muscle cell proliferation, and thrombus formation.[11,33] "Silent" or covert brain infarcts are also common in sickle cell disease patients (22–35%),[37] and are mostly secondary to small artery occlusion (lacunar brain infarcts), probably caused by sludging and intravascular sickling in smaller vessels. These covert brain infarcts are associated with cognitive deficits.[38]

Intracranial bleeding is less common but can occur, mostly between ages 20 and 30, typically in association with a moyamoya-like syndrome or brain aneurysms.[35,39] Other clinical features include vaso-occlusive or painful crises, retinopathy, chronic leg ulcers, increased susceptibility to infections, and anemia.[33] The treatment of sickle cell disease is beyond the scope of this chapter, but it is important to note that transfusion therapy can reduce the risk of stroke in patients with increased transcranial Doppler blood flow velocities.[40,41] After a first stroke, the risk of recurrence is very high (>60%), but substantially reduced by starting a transfusion program.[42]

Homocystinuria

Homocystinuria includes several heritable, mainly autosomal recessive, diseases causing elevated plasma concentrations of homocysteine, and homocystinuria. The most frequent cause is a mutation in the CBS (cystathionine beta-synthase) gene on chromosome 21q22.3. Based on data from newborn screening the rate of occurrence of homocystinuria is approximately 1 in 344 000 (www.orpha.net), but prevalence rates of up to 1 in 20 500 have been described in some European countries.[43] Thromboembolism is a key clinical feature, affecting large and small arteries, and veins. The chances of having a thromboembolic event were estimated at 25% by age 16 and 50% by age 29, over half of these events being venous, and 32% cerebrovascular.[44] Ischemic stroke in homocystinuria has been primarily attributed to accelerated atherosclerosis.[45] Some pathological studies suggest that arterial damage in homocystinuria differs from atherosclerosis, most notably by a lack of lipid deposition.[46] Other mechanisms could include endothelium-mediated thrombosis through direct toxicity of homocysteine on the endothelium.[46]

Isolated instances of cervical artery dissection have also been reported,[47] but whether these are mere coincidence or reflect a true association is unclear. Other clinical features include mental retardation, ectopia lentis, and skeletal abnormalities ("marfanoid," with excessive height and length of the limbs, and osteoporosis). Mental retardation is the most frequent central nervous system complication of homocystinuria due to CBS deficiency, and often the presenting feature.

Decreased cognitive abilities usually becomes obvious in middle childhood. CBS-deficient patients not treated from infancy are also at risk of seizures. Treatments to lower plasma homocysteine levels and stroke risk include pyridoxine, methionine-restricted diet, folate and vitamin B_{12} supplementation, and betaine.

Fabry's disease

Fabry's disease is an X-linked disease caused by a mutation in the *GLA* gene (chromosome Xq21.3-q22), encoding the α-galactosidase A gene, which belongs to the group of lysosomal storage disorders. Women heterozygous for the mutation can also be symptomatic, but are usually less severely affected than men. Fabry's disease can affect all ethnic groups. Reported incidences range from 1 in 476 000 to 1 in 117 000 in the general population, but newborn screening initiatives have found a prevalence as high as 1 in 3100 newborns in Italy and 1 in 1500 in Taiwan.[48] In a large survey of 721 young patients with cryptogenic ischemic stroke, 4.9% of men and 2.4% of women carried a mutation in *GLA*.[49] This high percentage was not confirmed in subsequent studies of cryptogenic ischemic stroke, although numbers were smaller and diagnostic methods partly differed.[50–52] In a very large study on 5023 patients aged 18–55 years with a diagnosis of ischemic stroke (3396, not only cryptogenic), hemorrhagic stroke (271), or transient ischemic attack (1071) from 15 European countries, definite Fabry's disease occurred in 0.5% and probable Fabry's disease in further 0.4% of young stroke patients.[53] An analysis of a large cohort of 2446 patients in the Fabry Registry (www.Fabryregistry.com) reported a stroke in 6.9% of men and 4.3% of women with Fabry's disease, with 87% of first strokes being ischemic and 13% hemorrhagic.[54] Most Fabry patients had their first stroke between the age of 20 and 50 years, and in 50% of men and 38% of women, Fabry's disease had not yet been diagnosed when the stroke occurred.[54] Ischemic stroke can be due to both small artery occlusion and large artery vasculopathy, with a predominance in the vertebro-basilar circulation.[49] The pathophysiology of cerebrovascular events in Fabry's disease is complex and incompletely understood, probably resulting from a combination of abnormalities in blood vessel walls, altered blood components, and altered blood flow.[55] Deposition of globotriaosylceramide in the vascular wall and dolichectasia of the basilar and vertebral arteries have been described.[11] Ischemic stroke in Fabry's disease can also be cardioembolic, resulting from arrhythmia caused by cardiomyopathy.[55] Seldom, hemorrhagic stroke has been reported in patients with Fabry's disease, likely resulting from cerebral small artery disease.[56]

On brain MRI Fabry's disease patients often have non-specific WMH (symmetrical, in the periventricular, deep and subcortical white matter), reported to be present in all patients by age 54.[57] A significantly enlarged basilar artery diameter has been reported in patients with Fabry's disease compared with the general population.[58] Other early clinical features of Fabry's disease, often beginning in childhood or adolescence, include acroparesthesia (sometimes burning pain in the extremities), hypohidrosis (decreased ability to sweat), and

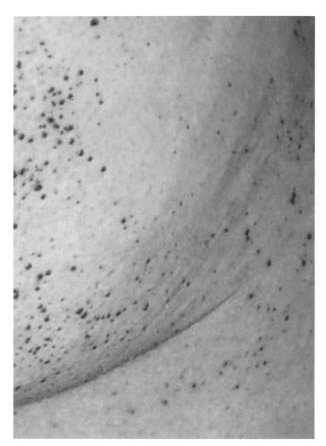

Figure 5.2 Angiokeratomas on the buttocks region in a patient with Fabry's disease. A black and white version of this figure will appear in some formats. For the color version, please refer to the plate section.

angiokeratomas (small, raised, dark-red spots typically found on the lower back, buttocks, groin, flanks, and upper thighs (Figure 5.2)). Later, systemic complications occur, which worsen with increasing age, including chronic kidney disease (beginning with microalbuminuria and proteinuria in the second or third decade of life) and cardiomyopathy (left ventricular hypertrophy, arrhythmia, myocardial ischemia, and heart failure).[48] Deafness, often of sudden onset, is also common.

Although measuring α-galactosidase A activity in male patients is a practical screening tool, all suspected cases of Fabry's disease in both genders must be confirmed using the gold standard mutation analysis.[59] Enzyme-replacement therapy was recently shown to improve some symptoms, but the effect on stroke prevention remains unclear.[60] Prophylactic treatment with antiplatelet agents are often given. Anticoagulants are prescribed in the presence of cardiac arrhythmia.[48]

Pseudoxanthoma elasticum

Pseudoxanthoma elasticum (PXE) is a rare autosomal recessive disorder caused by mutations in the *ATP-binding Cassette C6* (*ABCC6*) gene on chromosome 16p13.1. *ABCC6* encodes an ATP-dependent transmembrane transporter, the biological substrate of which is unknown but is believed to be important for connective tissue homeostasis.[61] The prevalence is

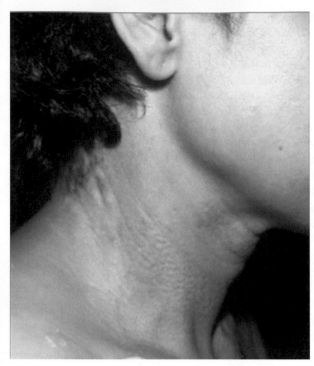

Figure 5.3 Neck skin redundancy in a patient with pseudoxanthoma elasticum. Kindly submitted by Dr Graeme Hankey, Perth, Australia. A black and white version of this figure will appear in some formats. For the color version, please refer to the plate section.

estimated at 1 in 75 000.[61] PXE is characterized by progressive calcification and fragmentation of elastic fibers in the skin, retina, and arterial walls (www.orpha.net). Increased rates of brain ischemia, mostly transient ischemic attacks, compared to the general population have been reported in patients with PXE (7–15%),[61–63] but published data is extremely limited. The etiology of ischemic stroke in PXE patients is believed to be either accelerated large vessel atherosclerosis or small artery disease, but further studies on large PXE series are needed to explore the underlying mechanisms.[63–67] Hypertension is a confounding feature since penetrating artery disease can be attributed to the blood pressure elevations. Other clinical manifestations include: skin lesions (mainly papular *peau d'orange* lesions and increased laxity and redundancy of skin (Figure 5.3) appearing initially in flexural areas); ocular complications (especially angioid streaks, hemorrhage, and progressive loss of visual acuity); cardiovascular manifestations with an increased prevalence of hypertension, peripheral artery disease, coronary artery disease; gastrointestinal bleeding due to rupture of vessels in the gastric and intestinal mucosa has also been described.[61,68–70]

Monogenic disorders causing ischemic stroke of other etiologies

Vascular Ehlers–Danlos syndrome

Vascular Ehlers–Danlos syndrome (vEDS) is a rare autosomal dominant disease, due to a mutation in the *COL3A1* gene on chromosome 2q31. The prevalence is estimated at 0.2–1.0 per 100 000.[71] The diagnosis is suggested clinically by the presence of at least two out of four major clinical criteria:[72] easy bruising, thin skin with visible veins, characteristic facial features, and rupture of arteries, the uterus or intestines. In addition, the diagnosis must be confirmed by the demonstration of either an abnormal type III procollagen synthesis or a mutation in the *COL3A1* gene. Phenotypic features can be subtle and most patients are unaware of the diagnosis at the time of their first major complication.[73] The latter usually occurs at a young age, before age 40 in 80% of patients.[73] Among the vascular complications of vEDS, about one-quarter involve head and neck vessels.[73] In a study of 202 well-characterized vEDS patients whose records were reviewed for central nervous system complications, 19 patients (9.4%) had at least one cerebrovascular complication,[74] which included carotid-cavernous fistula, cervical artery dissection (CeAD), intracranial aneurysms, and arterial rupture (this percentage may be higher in a prospective setting with systematic screening for cerebrovascular complications). The mean age at occurrence of the first cerebrovascular complication was 28 years (range: 17–48 years).[74]

Ischemic stroke can occur in vEDS as a complication of cervical artery dissection. In the two largest, partly overlapping, series of biologically confirmed vEDS patients, 2% of the patients had a history of CeAD.[73,74] The reported frequency of vEDS cases in large published series of consecutive CeAD patients is very low, around 0.5–2.0%.[75–79] In the general population about three-quarters of CeAD patients have transient or permanent cerebral or retinal ischemia (transient ischemic attack, transient monocular blindness, or ischemic stroke);[80–82] whether this frequency is similar among vEDS patients is unknown. Due to the vulnerability of the arterial wall, conventional angiography is contra-indicated in vEDS patients, given the high risk of iatrogenic arterial dissection and rupture. Magnetic resonance (MR) or computed tomography angiography (CTA) should be used to confirm the diagnosis.[82] In the general population, antiplatelet agents or anticoagulants are recommended at the acute phase of CeAD to prevent primary or recurrent ischemic events, but their efficacy has never been assessed and compared in a randomized trial.[79,82,83] In vEDS patients, antiplatelet agents might be the preferred treatment, as fatal bleeding may occur under anticoagulants.[71] While long-term prevention of cerebral ischemia with antiplatelet agents is often proposed in CeAD patients with residual stenosis, occlusion, or aneurysmal dilation, in vEDS patients the risk–benefit ratio of long-term antiplatelet therapy should be carefully weighed.[84] Prophylactic treatment with celiprolol is now recommended to prevent recurrences of dissection or arterial rupture.[85]

Marfan's syndrome

Marfan's syndrome (MFS) is an autosomal dominant condition due to a mutation in the *fibrillin-1* (*FBN1*) gene on chromosome 15q21.1. The prevalence is estimated at 1 in 5000 individuals.[86] The clinical signs in MFS are mainly musculoskeletal, ocular, and cardiac, with aortic and mitral valve anomalies, aortic aneurysms, and dissections mainly affecting the outcome. While an early review suggested that ischemic events of the brain or spinal cord occur in

10–20% of patients with MFS,[87] a later retrospective analysis of neurovascular complications among 513 MFS patients identified only 15 patients (2.9%) with an ischemic event, among whom 11 had a transient ischemic attack, 2 an ischemic stroke, and 2 a spinal cord infarct.[88] A cardioembolic source was identified in 12 of the 13 patients with a transient ischemic attack or ischemic stroke, including prosthetic cardiac valves ($N = 9$), atrial fibrillation ($N = 4$), and mitral valve prolapse ($N = 2$).[88] MFS patients have a high prevalence of mitral valve prolapse, sometimes requiring valve repair or replacement, and are at increased risk of aortic regurgitation and atrial fibrillation.[89] The most severe cardiovascular complication is aortic dissection, usually starting in the ascending aorta.[89] CeAD occasionally occurs as an extension of a proximal aortic dissection into the brachiocephalic arteries.[90–92] CeAD occasionally occurs in MFS patients independent of aortic lesions.[75,93–95] In a retrospective series of 513 MFS patients none was reported to have CeAD.[88] In large cohorts of CeAD patients, a few isolated instances of MFS are mentioned (<1%),[75,76,79,80] but information about the criteria used for the diagnosis of MFS is often lacking.

The clinical characteristics of ischemic stroke in MFS patients do not differ from those of ischemic stroke in the general population and current recommendations for the management of ischemic stroke during the acute phase and secondary prevention also apply to MFS patients. In the retrospective series of 513 MFS patients, 3 patients (0.6%) had a hemorrhagic event: of these two were subdural hematomas, one was in a patient on chronic anticoagulation; and one was a spinal subarachnoid hemorrhage followed by a cerebral subarachnoid hemorrhage in a patient on anticoagulation in whom autopsy revealed vertebral dolichoectasia with suspected rupture of a vertebral artery.[88] The clinical diagnostic criteria of MFS were revised in 2010 and are based on a combination of family history, presence of aortic root dilatation at sinuses of Valsalva or aortic root dissection, ectopia lentis, and a systemic score that combines signs such as Marfonoid habitus (e.g., reduced upper–lower segment ratio and increased arm span–height ratio, pectus carinatum), dural ectasia, and pneumothorax.[96] FBN1 genetic testing is not a formal requirement, depending on the clinical criteria that are present. Treatment with beta-blockers for the prevention of aortic complications is now recommended in all MFS patients. The use of angiotensin-converting enzyme receptor agonists is being investigated. Lifestyle recommendations include avoiding contact sports and exercising to exhaustion and isometric activities with Valsalva maneuver.[96] Prophylactic aortic surgery is considered when the diameter at Valsalva sinuses reaches 5 cm.[96]

Monogenic mitochondrial disorders

Mitochondrial myopathy, encephalopathy, lactic acidosis and stroke-like episodes

Mitochondrial myopathy, encephalopathy, lactic acidosis and stroke-like episodes (MELAS) is a progressive neurodegenerative disorder characterized by acute neurological episodes resembling brain ischemia associated with hyperlactatemia and mitochondrial myopathy. It is the most prevalent inherited mitochondrial disorder. The disease is caused by mitochondrial DNA mutations, with 80% of MELAS patients being due to the 3243A>G mutation in the leucine transfer RNA gene (tRNA Leu). Mitochondrial DNA mutations are transmitted according to maternal inheritance (an affected man cannot transmit the disease). The exact prevalence of MELAS is unknown, but the estimated prevalence of the 3243A>G mutation ranges from 5 to 16 per 100 000 in the white population.[97,98] Identification of the causal mutation needs to take into account heteroplasmy; i.e., the coexistence of mutated mitochondrial DNA with a residual population of wild-type mitochondrial DNA. Mutation proportions can differ considerably between tissues. MELAS is a multi-system disorder with onset typically in childhood between the ages of 2 and 10 years, with some persons having delayed onset between the ages of 10 and 40 years (www.orpha.net). The most common initial symptoms are seizures, recurrent headaches, anorexia, recurrent vomiting, and myopathy with exercise intolerance or proximal limb weakness. Additional features include short stature, hearing loss and visual impairment, migraine, abdominal pain, obstipation, cognitive deficits (but early development is normal), diabetes, and cardiomyopathy.

Stroke-like episodes are the clinical disease hallmark. They are usually characterized by aphasia, cortical blindness, hemianopia, or hemiparesis, which are at least partially reversible, sometimes with impaired consciousness. Eventually there is a progressive accumulation of neurological deficits and cognitive and behavioral abnormalities.[99] The term "stroke-like episodes" was coined to stress the non-ischemic origin of these events, but the exact underlying mechanisms are incompletely understood. During stroke-like episodes, affected areas on brain imaging do not correspond to classical vascular distributions. Lesions typically present in an asymmetric pattern affecting predominantly the temporal, parietal, and occipital lobes and are often restricted to the cortex, with relative sparing of the deep white matter.[99] Figure 5.4 is an MRI that shows scattered regions of abnormality in the predominantly temporal lobe cortex and white matter in a MELAS patient. Deep gray matter such as the thalamus may be involved and lesions may migrate over time. There is contradictory data in the literature on the presence of an increased apparent diffusion coefficient on diffusion-weighted MRI, higher ADC (apparent diffusion coefficient) value being possibly related to a longer interval.[100,101] These episodes likely represent energy failure.

The diagnostic evaluation includes a combination of clinical and radiological findings and laboratory and genetic testing. Lactate levels, pyruvate levels, and lactate–pyruvate ratio are typically elevated in serum and cerebrospinal fluid of MELAS patients, and on skeletal muscle biopsy, ragged red fibers are found.[102] No specific treatment for MELAS exists.

The administration of coenzyme Q10 (CoQ10) (50–100 mg 3×/day) and L-carnitine (1000 mg 3×/day) has been of some benefit to some individuals and in small randomized trials.[103] Idebenone, an analog of CoQ10 that crosses the blood–brain

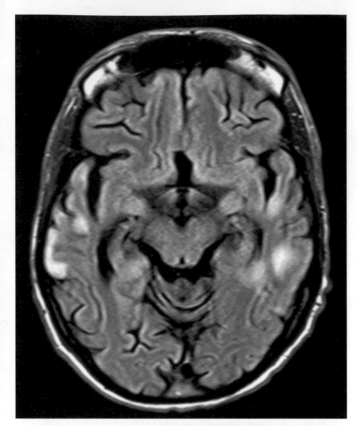

Figure 5.4 MRI FLAIR image showing scattered acute hyperintensity cortical and subcortical lesions in a 44-year-old patient with MELAS.

barrier more efficiently, has also been reported as beneficial in anecdotal reports.[104] L-arginine showed promise in treating stroke-like episodes.[105] Because febrile illnesses may trigger acute exacerbations, individuals with MELAS should receive appropriate vaccinations, including flu and pneumococcal vaccine. Mitochondrial toxins such as aminoglycoside antibiotics, linezolid, cigarettes, and alcohol should also be avoided.

Intracerebral hemorrhage

Familial cerebral amyloid angiopathy

Cerebral amyloid angiopathy (CAA) is a heterogeneous group of biochemically and genetically diverse central nervous system disorders, all sharing the presence of amyloid fibrils in the walls of small to medium-sized arteries, sometimes also in the capillaries of central nervous system parenchyma and leptomeninges.[106] While CAA mostly occurs sporadically in older adults, we focus here on rare familial forms of CAA occurring in younger patients (often <55 years). These forms usually have a more severe course. We limit the discussion to one form of familial CAA, namely hereditary cerebral hemorrhage with amyloidosis (HCHWA), as other forms of familial CAA are not often associated with intracerebral hemorrhage. HCHWA is comprised of various subtypes that all have an autosomal dominant pattern of inheritance, but are caused by different types of mutation: in the *APP* gene chromosome 21q21.2 for most (Dutch, Italian, Flemish, Iowa, and Piedmont

types), and in the *CST3* gene on chromosome 20p11.2 (encoding Cystatin C) for another (Icelandic type).[107–109] The accumulating peptide in the arterial walls is Aβ for the first five types and ACys for the Icelandic type.[106] The prevalence is unknown, about 400 patients have been described. Typically, patients can present with hemorrhagic stroke and/or dementia (either slowly progressive, of the Alzheimer type, or progressing in a stepwise fashion). Transient neurological symptoms and seizures also occur.

Patients carrying the same mutation may have different clinical phenotypes, predominantly intracerebral hemorrhage in some and dementia in others.[110] Definitive diagnosis of CAA requires pathological examination. According to the Boston Criteria, a probable diagnosis of CAA can be made in sporadic CAA, in the absence of pathological examination, in the presence of multiple strictly lobar cortical or cortico–subcortical intracerebral hemorrhages (including cerebellar and microbleeds) detected by gradient echo (T2*) MRI sequences, in the absence of another definite cause of intracerebral hemorrhage, in patients aged 55 years or older.[111–113] In the presence of otherwise unexplained multiple lobar hemorrhages and a typical family history, the finding of a causative mutation is considered sufficient for a definite diagnosis of HCHWA in vivo (www.orpha.net). No specific treatment is available for HCHWA. Careful blood pressure control is recommended in case of hypertension, but its efficacy on CAA progression is not evidence-based.

Collagen 4A1 (COL4A1) syndrome

Mutations in the *COL4A1* gene have been recently identified as a cause of autosomal dominant hereditary cerebrovascular disease, due to mutations in the *COL4A1* gene on chromosome 13q34 that lead to reduced stability and basement membrane defects. COL4A1-related disorders cover a spectrum of overlapping phenotypes characterized by cerebral small vessel disease of varying severity, associated at varying degrees with eye abnormalities and systemic findings, mainly in kidney and muscles. COL4A1-related disorders include the following entities, now considered as part of a continuum with overlapping features: (1) autosomal dominant type 1 porencephaly;[114] (2) brain small vessel disease with hemorrhage;[115] (3) brain small vessel disease with Axenfeld–Rieger anomaly;[116] and (4) hereditary angiopathy with nephropathy, aneurysms, and muscle cramps (HANAC) syndrome.[117] The prevalence is unknown as only few families have been described. Given its recent identification and variable clinical expression, COL4A1-related disorders are probably largely underestimated.

There is an important diversity in the clinical expression of the disease, even within the same family.[118,119] Cerebrovascular manifestations include perinatal intracerebral hemorrhage and porencephaly, adult or childhood-onset intracerebral hemorrhage (in all locations), and less often lacunar ischemic strokes. Of note, intracerebral hemorrhage can be seen in adults in the absence of any perinatal or childhood events.[120] In a systematic review of published studies describing patients with *COL4A1* mutations, stroke often occurred as

the first presentation of the disease, with a mean age of onset of 36 years.[120] Other neurological manifestations can be associated, including migraine, with or without aura, seizures, intellectual disability, and dementia.[121]

On brain MRI old intracranial hemorrhages can be seen, mostly located in the basal ganglia, centrum semiovale and pons.[118] Patients with COL4A1-related disorders also have diffuse WMH (63.5%), microbleeds (52.9%), dilated perivascular spaces (19.2%), and lacunar infarcts (16.5%), reflecting an underlying cerebral small artery disease.[120] WMH are usually bilateral and symmetrical, mainly in supratentorial regions with a pattern that seems predominant in the frontal and parietal lobes, the periventricular regions and the centrum semiovale; brainstem, especially pons, and cerebellar deep white matter may also be affected.[118] Asymptomatic intracranial aneurysms are common in patients with *COL4A1* mutations (44.4% of 18 patients with angiography),[120] particularly in the HANAC phenotype; they are usually small, on the carotid siphon (extra- or intradural), and may be multiple.[118]

Extraneurological symptoms of COL4A1-related disorders include: (1) retinal signs, especially retinal arteriolar tortuosities, retinal hemorrhage, but also congenital or juvenile cataract, Axenfeld–Rieger syndrome; (2) renal manifestations with chronic hematuria, bilateral renal cysts, mild renal failure; (3) muscular symptoms with muscle cramps and elevated serum creatine phosphokinase levels.[118] There is no specific treatment for COL4A1 syndrome. Head trauma, intensive exercise, and use of anticoagulants increase the risk of intracerebral haemorrhage and should be avoided. Classical vascular risk factors, especially hypertension, should be treated and closely monitored. Cesarean delivery is recommended for pregnancies in which the fetus is at risk for a COL4A1-related disorder to prevent hemorrhagic stroke secondary to birth trauma in newborns.[121]

Osteogenesis imprfecta

Osteogenesis imperfecta is a group of heritable disorders caused by various mutations in the *COL1A1* or *COL1A2* gene on chromosome 17q21.33 and chromosome 7q22.1, encoding the alpha 1 and alpha 2 chains of type I collagen, respectively. Different types of osteogenesis imperfecta are known, mostly with an autosomal dominant inheritance pattern, although there are also some recessive forms.[122,123] Incidence rates from 1 in 10 000 to 1 in 20 000 live births are reported. Clinically, the condition is characterized by varying degrees of skeletal fragility leading to fractures and bone deformities, ligamentous laxity, and easy bruising. Collagen mutations in osteogenesis imperfecta lead to platelet dysfunction and vascular wall fragility, which account for easy bruising and hemorrhages due to trivial trauma. Some patients have blue scleras. Isolated case reports and small case series suggest an association of osteogenesis imperfecta with intracranial bleeding, aneurysms and cervical artery dissection.[124–126] Figure 5.5 is a CT scan that shows a midbrain hemorrhage in a woman who has osteogenesis imperfecta.

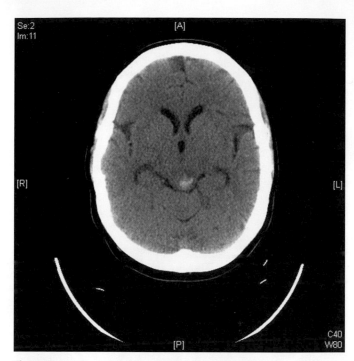

Figure 5.5 CT scan showing a midbrain hemorrhage in a woman with osteogenesis imperfecta.

Genetic contributions to common multifactorial stroke

Importance of genetic factors in common multifactorial stroke

Analyses of twin studies,[127] and reviews of the frequencies of a family history of stroke[128–134] convincingly show that genetic factors substantially contribute to stroke susceptibility. There are important heterogeneity of heritability estimates. Many studies combine ischemic and hemorrhagic stroke, and only a few studies consider ischemic stroke subtypes.[131] In four hospital-based series in which ischemic stroke patients were compared to healthy controls, a family history of stroke was found to be independently associated with an increased risk of large artery ischemic stroke (odds ratio (OR) = 1.88 (95% clearance interval (CI) 1.02–3.44) to 2.24 (1.49–3.36)) and small artery occlusion ischemic stroke (OR = 1.79 (95%CI 1.13–2.84) to 2.76 (95% CI 1.55–4.91)); the association with cardioembolic ischemic stroke was weaker.[125,127–129] The advent of genome-wide genotyping (i.e., genotyping of hundreds of thousands or millions of genetic variants distributed across the chromosomes), has stimulated novel approaches to estimate the pseudo-heritability of diseases in the absence of familial information, based solely on genome-wide genotypes.[135] This pseudo-heritability corresponds to the proportion of phenotypic variance explained by genome-wide genotypes. Recently, the pseudo-heritability of stroke has been estimated based on data from large genome-wide association studies, confirming a substantial heritability,[136,137] but also important differences according to stroke subtypes. Pseudo-heritability estimates were: 40.3% for large artery ischemic stroke, 32.6% for cardioembolic ischemic stroke,

16.1% for small artery occlusion ischemic stroke, 73% for lobar intracerebral hemorrhage, and 34% for deep intracerebral hemorrhage.[136,137]

Genetic variants predisposing to stroke could act at various levels; for example, by increasing the risk of and susceptibility to "conventional" stroke risk factors such as hypertension and diabetes, by influencing specific mechanisms underlying stroke, such as the occurrence and progression of atherosclerosis or lipohyalinosis, by predisposing to arterial thrombosis or bleeding, or by modifying tolerance to brain ischemia or more largely brain injury.[138] The underlying genetic model is considered multifactorial, involving several genetic polymorphisms that each confer small increases in risk.[139,140]

Recently, large collaborative efforts have identified a number of common genetic risk variants associated with an increased risk of stroke, both ischemic and hemorrhagic stroke.[141–147] Earlier studies had consisted of testing the association of stroke with a few genetic variants in one or few candidate genes, selected based on a priori hypothesis on the mechanisms underlying the disease, leading to disappointing results, as most associations that were identified could not be confirmed in independent samples.[148] Most robust genetic associations with stroke were identified through genome-wide association studies, an approach that consists of genotyping a very large number of genetic variants across the genome and testing their association with a phenotype, without any a priori hypothesis on the underlying biology.[139,149,150] This

approach has led to the identification of a very large number of genetic associations with various traits and diseases that have been convincingly replicated in independent samples, mostly near previously unsuspected genes, providing new hypotheses on the underlying biology.[7] For stroke most genome-wide significant associations were identified for specific ischemic or hemorrhagic subtypes,[141–144,151] suggesting that the genetic contributions to stroke risk are largely subtype specific. Some risk loci for all ischemic strokes have also been reported.[146,147] An elaborate analysis of shared genetic variation also showed a high genetic correlation between the large-artery atherosclerosis and small artery disease subtypes of ischemic stroke.[152] These discoveries have required large collaborative efforts which were made possible through the creation of international consortia, especially the International Stroke Genetics Consortium (ISGC, www.strokegenetics.org), and also the Cohorts of Heart and Aging Research in Genomic Epidemiology (CHARGE) consortium.[153–155]

Ischemic stroke

Genome-wide significant associations with ischemic stroke (i.e., yielding a P-value $<5 \times 10^{-8}$, to account for approximately one million of independent statistical tests performed at the genome-wide level) are summarized in Table 5.2.

Most ischemic stroke genetic risk loci to date were identified for subtypes of ischemic stroke. All genetic loci that were

Table 5.2 Genome-wide risk loci for complex forms of ischemic and hemorrhagic stroke

SNP	Chr	Gene	Phenotype	Risk allele	Risk allele frequency	N*	OR	P
Ischemic stroke[†]								
rs10744777	12	ALDH2	All IS	T	66%	17970/ 70764	1.10	7.1×10^{-11}
rs11833579	12	NINJ2	All IS	A	23%	1164/18058	1.41	2.3×10^{-10}
rs6843082	4	PITX2	CE-IS	G	21%	2365/12389	1.36	7.8×10^{-16}
rs879324	16	ZFHX3	CE-IS	A	19%	2365/12389	1.25	2.3×10^{-8}
rs556621	6	CDC5L	LAA-IS	A	33%	400/1172	1.62	3.9×10^{-8}
rs2107595	7	HDAC9	LAA-IS	A	16%	2167/12389	1.39	2.0×10^{-16}
rs660599	11	MMP12	LAA-IS	A	19%	3197/62912	1.18	2.6×10^{-8}
Intracerebral hemorrhage[†]								
rs429358/ rs7412	19	APOE	Lobar ICH	ε2	7%	931/3744	1.82	6.6×10^{-10}
rs429358/ rs7412	19	APOE	Lobar ICH	ε4	12%	931/3744	2.20	2.4×10^{-11}
rs2984613	1	PMF1/ SLC25A44	Deep ICH	C	32%	881/1481	1.33	2.2×10^{-10}

CE, cardioembolic; ICH, intracerebral hemorrhage; IS, ischemic stroke; LAA, large artery atherosclerosis.
*N cases/N controls
†[136–142]

found to be associated with cardioembolic ischemic stroke were already known risk loci for atrial fibrillation (*PITX2*, *ZFHX3*), which is not surprising, as atrial fibrillation is the most common source of cardioembolic events.[156–158] Recent experimental data showed that murine *Pitx2*–/– mutants had reduced and discontinuous smooth muscle actin staining of cerebral vessels and increased cerebral vessel density, and imaging studies in large population-based samples found *PITX2* variants to be associated with increased white matter hyperintensity burden, suggesting that *PITX2* could perhaps also contribute to stroke risk independently of atrial fibrillation.[154] Evidence for this in stroke genetic association studies is lacking to date.[142]

Genetic variants showing genome-wide association with large artery ischemic stroke (*HDAC9*, *MMP12*, *CDC5L*) were all in previously unsuspected loci.[141,142,145] The *HDAC9* locus was later also identified as a risk locus for coronary artery disease.[159] Risk allele carriers of the main *HDAC9* susceptibility variant for large artery ischemic stroke (rs2107595) were found to be associated with increased mRNA levels of *HDAC9*.[160] Compared with *Hdac9*+/+*Apoe*–/– mice, *Hdac9*–/–*Apoe*–/– mice had markedly reduced atherosclerotic lesion size throughout the aorta,[160] suggesting that HDAC9 may be a plausible drug target candidate for atherosclerosis prevention. The *MMP12* locus was identified by implementing an age-at-onset informed genome-wide association analysis (i.e., a regression analysis conditioning on age-at-onset).[141] This analysis was driven by the assumption that early-onset stroke may have increased genetic liability.[161] In addition to these genome-wide significant findings, a few candidate gene based associations (requiring a less stringent threshold for significance) have been robustly replicated in large independent studies, such as the chr9p21 locus (rs2383207) or the *ABO* locus (rs505922) on chromosome 9 with large artery ischemic stroke.[142,162,163] The *ABO* locus also showed association with cardioembolic ischemic stroke.[163]

So far no common genetic risk variant for the small artery disease subtype of ischemic stroke has been consistently identified.[142] Pseudo-heritability estimates were also smaller for this subtype (16% vs. 40%, and 33% for large artery and cardioembolic ischemic stroke).[136] While this could reflect a lesser contribution of genetic factors to this ischemic stroke subtype, it could also mirror the heterogeneity and imprecision in the phenotype definition of small artery disease according to the most commonly used TOAST subtyping algorithm.[164] Genetic liability to small artery occlusion may also differ according to ethnic origin. This subtype is much more prevalent in Asian populations and a significant association of a variant in the *PRKCH* gene (chromosome 14) with small artery occlusion ischemic stroke was described in Japanese and Chinese populations. The corresponding risk variant is monomorphic in European populations and no convincing association was shown between nearby variants in *PRKCH* and small artery occlusion ischemic stroke in Europeans.[142,165–167]

Two novel genetic risk loci (chr12p13 and chr12q24.12) were found to be associated with all ischemic stroke at a genome-wide significant level. The association with the chr12p13 locus, near the *NINJ2* gene, was subject to controversy. This locus had shown genome-wide significant association with incident stroke (all stroke and ischemic stroke); i.e., stroke occurring during follow-up of prospective population-based cohort studies participating in the CHARGE consortium,[147] but was not replicated in a large hospital-based cross-sectional study comparing stroke patients to healthy controls.[168] A potential explanation for these discrepant results is that the chr12p13 locus may be associated with stroke severity and mortality more than with stroke risk. For hospital-based cross-sectional studies, given high early mortality rates of stroke, death might occur very early before hospitalization or before samples can be taken. In prospective cohort studies severe strokes leading to early death are included, as blood samples were taken at recruitment in the study, often years before the onset of stroke; incident stroke ascertainment also comprises strokes that do not lead to hospitalization. Recent data emerging from targeted sequencing around the *NINJ2* region suggests that allelic heterogeneity at this locus, caused by multiple rare, low frequency, and common variants with disparate effects on risk, may also explain the difficulties in replicating the original genome-wide association studies' results.[169]

The second genetic risk locus for all ischemic stroke (chr12q24.12) was identified in a very large case-control dataset with over 17 000 ischemic stroke patients, and found to be equally associated with all subtypes of ischemic stroke. The single nucleotide polymorphism (SNP) showing the most significant association is in linkage disequilibrium with a nonsynonymous variant in *SH2B3* and is associated with gene expression of *ALDH2*, pointing to a potential role of these two genes in the association.[146] Given the very large sample size this case-control study also found genome-wide association of the *PITX2* and *ZFHX3* loci with all ischemic stroke, but there was no indication of an association between these loci and ischemic stroke subtypes other than cardioembolic.[146]

Novel genetic risk loci have also recently been discovered for other well characterized ischemic stroke etiologies, such as cervical artery dissections, which despite being uncommon at the general population level is a major cause of ischemic stroke in young adults.[170] This large collaborative study from the CADISP consortium (www.cadisp.com) found a common variant at *PHACTR1* to be associated with a lower risk of cervical artery dissection. The same variant was independently shown to be associated with a lower risk of migraine (especially without aura) and with an increased risk of myocardial infarction,[159,170,171] suggesting that this locus may play a pivotal role in vascular biology. The function of *PHACTR1* is poorly understood. Experimental studies revealed a pivotal role in vascular tube formation and actin polymerization, suggesting a possible role in angiogenic processes.[40,41] Up-regulation of *PHACTR1* by TGFβ has been described in breast cancer cell lines,[42] potentially pointing to a connection with the TGFβ signaling pathway.

Brain hemorrhage

A highly significant and robust association with intracerebral hemorrhage was shown for the *APOE* locus in a large candidate gene association study on 2189 cases and 4041 controls.[150] Both *APOEε2* and *APOEε4* alleles were associated with lobar intracerebral hemorrhage at a "genome-wide significance level," with ORs of 1.82 ($P = 6.6 \times 10^{-10}$) and 2.20 ($P = 2.4 \times 10^{-11}$) respectively. Associations were even stronger when restricting the analysis to patients with definite or probable underlying CAA. The *APOEε4* was also associated with an increased risk for deep intracerebral hemorrhage, at a lower significance level (OR = 1.21, $P = 2.6 \times 10^{-4}$), suggesting that mechanisms linking *APOEε4* to intracerebral hemorrhage may expand beyond CAA-mediated effects.[151,172] In a later analysis, the authors also showed a strong association of the *APOE* locus with hemorrhage size and growth.[173] For patients with lobar intracerebral hemorrhage, carriers of the *APOEε2* allele had larger hemorrhage volumes than did non-carriers in the discovery phase at a very high level of significance ($P = 3.2 \times 10^{-8}$).[173]

Another candidate gene study was based on the assumption that *COL4A1* and *COL4A2*, which harbor mutations for Mendelian diseases causing intracerebral hemorrhage, could also be involved in common, complex forms of intracerebral hemorrhage. Common variants in *COL4A2*, but not *COL4A1* were associated with an increased risk of deep intracerebral hemorrhage ($P = 0.00003$), and also showed suggestive associations with small artery occlusion and white matter hyperintensity burden, possibly via increased liability to cerebral small vessel disease.[174] Another study found that rare variants in *COL4A1* were associated with an increased risk of intracerebral hemorrhage.[175]

The first genome-wide association analysis of intracerebral hemorrhage was published in 2014 by the International Stroke Genetics Consortium, based on 1545 patients with intracerebral hemorrhage (664 lobar and 881 non-lobar) and 1481 controls.[143] This study identified one novel genome-wide significant locus on chromosome 1q22 associated specifically with an increased risk of non-lobar (deep) intracerebral hemorrhage, with replication in an independent sample.[143] This locus was also recently found to be associated at a genome-wide level with increasing white matter hyperintensity burden, the most plausible pathophysiological link between both associations being an increased liability to cerebral small artery disease.[176,177] The identified genetic risk variants are located in a region that contains *PMF1* and *SLC25A44*, and they are associated with expression levels of a nearby gene, *SEMA4A*.[143] The results of this study also emphasize the biological heterogeneity across ICH subtypes, as this association was found exclusively for non-lobar ICH.

Implications, limitations, and perspectives

Overall, the discovery of common genetic variants associated with stroke and its subtypes has substantially broadened knowledge of the underlying pathophysiology. Recent findings have also emphasized the need to carefully consider ischemic and hemorrhagic stroke not as single entities, but as composite entities comprised of various underlying conditions, some of which may share common mechanisms. This heterogeneity, combined with difficulties to collect very large samples given the severity of this acute disease, is probably the main explanation for the fact that, despite important discoveries, the search for genetic determinants of stroke has been less successful than for a number of other complex phenotypes, including other neurological or vascular phenotypes, for which many more loci have been revealed.[159,178] Understanding of stroke genetics may be enriched by exploring MRI-based endophenotypes for specific stroke subtypes, such as white matter hyperintensity burden, a marker of cerebral small vessel disease, which is strongly correlated with small artery occlusion ischemic stroke. Five genome-wide significant risk loci for white matter hyperintensity burden have been identified (chr17q25, chr10q24, chr2p21, chr1q22, and chr2p16).[176]

So far most studies on complex stroke genetics have focused on common single-nucleotide polymorphisms, and, as in other complex diseases, these identified common risk variants explain only a small proportion of the disease heritability.[179] Other types of variation, such as low frequency (1–5%) or rare (<1%) single nucleotide variants, or structural variation such as copy number variants, have been insufficiently explored. New genome-wide genotyping arrays now also partly cover lower frequency variants and more importantly the advent of next generation sequencing technologies has made sequencing of large samples more accessible and opened new avenues for studying unexplored rare variants as well as structural variation.[180,181] So far no major results have emerged yet for stroke, but there are encouraging preliminary findings.

One important discovery of genome-wide association studies is the amount of pleiotropy or shared genetic variation between stroke and other complex phenotypes, which also tells us more about disease mechanisms.[182] For example, substantial overlap was observed between the genetic risk of ischemic stroke, and particularly the large artery subtype, with coronary artery disease, contributing to a better understanding of common underlying biological pathways.[183]

As part of the International Stroke Genetics Consortium, the METASTROKE collaboration, the US National Institutes of Health (NIH)-funded SiGN initiative and the CHARGE consortium, efforts are ongoing to perform genome-wide association studies of stroke in much larger samples of patients, in order to increase the power to detect genetic association with stroke and its subtypes. These projects take advantage of the most recent 1000 genomes reference panel (www.1000genomes.org) that enables more reliable imputation (statistical inference) of genotypes for millions of genetic variants that have not been genotyped. Efforts are also being made to expand genetic studies to non-European ethnic groups. Data on rare variants is also being obtained through exome chip genotyping, whole exome and whole genome sequencing is being accrued. In addition to uncovering new

risk loci, sequencing will likely help fine-map genetic risk loci discovered by genome-wide association studies and facilitate the identification of the underlying causal variant and gene.

Understanding of the genetic underpinnings of stroke will be further enriched by combining genomic information with trancriptomic, epigenomic, and metabolomic data.

References

1. Seshadri S, Wolf PA. Lifetime risk of stroke and dementia: Current concepts, and estimates from the Framingham Study. *Lancet Neurol* 2007;**6**:1106–1114.

2. Johnston SC, Mendis S, Mathers CD. Global variation in stroke burden and mortality: Estimates from monitoring, surveillance, and modelling. *Lancet Neurol* 2009;**8**:345–354.

3. Gorelick PB, Scuteri A, Black SE, et al. Vascular contributions to cognitive impairment and dementia: A statement for healthcare professionals from the American Heart Association/American Stroke Association. *Stroke* 2011;**42**:2672–2713.

4. Viswanathan A, Rocca WA, Tzourio C. Vascular risk factors and dementia: How to move forward? *Neurology* 2009;**72**:368–374.

5. Pendlebury ST, Rothwell PM. Prevalence, incidence, and factors associated with pre-stroke and post-stroke dementia: A systematic review and meta-analysis. *Lancet Neurol* 2009;**8**:1006–1018.

6. Falcone GJ, Malik R, Dichgans M, Rosand J. Current concepts and clinical applications of stroke genetics. *Lancet Neurol* 2014;**13**:405–418.

7. Manolio TA. Bringing genome-wide association findings into clinical use. *Nat Rev Genet* 2013;**14**:549–558.

8. Leys D, Bandu L, Henon H, et al. Clinical outcome in 287 consecutive young adults (15 to 45 years) with ischemic stroke. *Neurology* 2002;**59**:26–33.

9. Chabriat H, Joutel A, Dichgans M, Tournier-Lasserve E, Bousser M-G. Cadasil. *Lancet Neurol* 2009;**8**:643–653.

10. Joutel A, Corpechot C, Ducros A, et al. Notch 3 mutations in CADASIL, a hereditary adult-onset condition causing stroke and dementia. *Nature* 1996;**383**:707–710.

11. Dichgans M. Monogenic causes of ischemic stroke. In *Stroke Genetics*, H Markus (ed). Oxford: Oxford University Press, 2003.

12. Razvi SS, Davidson R, Bone I, Muir KW. The prevalence of cerebral autosomal dominant arteriopathy with subcortical infarcts and

leucoencephalopathy (CADASIL) in the west of Scotland. *J Neurol Neurosurg Psychiatry* 2005;**76**:739–741.

13. Dong Y, Hassan A, Zhang Z, Huber D, Dalageorgou C, Markus HS. Yield of screening for CADASIL mutations in lacunar stroke and leukoaraiosis. *Stroke* 2003;**34**:203–205.

14. O'Sullivan M, Jarosz JM, Martin RJ, Deasy N, Powell JF, Markus HS. MRI hyperintensities of the temporal lobe and external capsule in patients with CADASIL. *Neurology* 2001;**56**:628–634.

15. Chabriat H, Levy C, Taillia H, et al. Patterns of MRI lesions in CADASIL. *Neurology* 1998;**51**:452–457.

16. Gobron C, Viswanathan A, Bousser M-G, Chabriat H. Multiple simultaneous cerebral infarctions in cerebral autosomal dominant arteriopathy with subcortical infarcts and leukoencephalopathy. *Cerebrovasc Dis* 2006;**22**:445–446.

17. Yao M, Herve D, Jouvent E, et al. Dilated perivascular spaces in small-vessel disease: A study in CADASIL. *Cerebrovasc Dis* 2014;**37**:155–163.

18. Ruchoux MM, Chabriat H, Bousser M-G, Baudrimont M, Tournier-Lasserve E. Presence of ultrastructural arterial lesions in muscle and skin vessels of patients with CADASIL. *Stroke* 1994;**25**:2291–2292.

19. Dichgans M, Markus HS, Salloway S, et al. Donepezil in patients with subcortical vascular cognitive impairment: A randomised double-blind trial in CADASIL. *Lancet Neurol* 2008;**7**:310–318.

20. Hara K, Shiga A, Fukutake T, et al. Association of *HTRA1* mutations and familial ischemic cerebral small-vessel disease. *N Engl J Med* 2009;**360**:1729–1739.

21. Bayrakli F, Balaban H, Gurelik M, Hizmetli S, Topaktas S. Mutation in the *HTRA1* gene in a patient with degenerated spine as a component of CARASIL syndrome. *Turk Neurosurg* 2014;**24**:67–69.

22. Zheng DM, Xu FF, Gao Y, Zhang H, Han SC, Bi GR. A Chinese pedigree of cerebral autosomal recessive arteriopathy with subcortical infarcts and leukoencephalopathy (CARASIL):

Clinical and radiological features. *J Clin Neurosci* 2009;**16**:847–849.

23. Mendioroz M, Fernandez-Cadenas I, Del Rio-Espinola A, et al. A missense *HTRA1* mutation expands CARASIL syndrome to the Caucasian population. *Neurology* 2010;**75**:2033–2035.

24. Yanagawa S, Ito N, Arima K, Ikeda S. Cerebral autosomal recessive arteriopathy with subcortical infarcts and leukoencephalopathy. *Neurology* 2002;**58**:817–820.

25. Bianchi S, Di Palma C, Gallus GN, et al. Two novel *HTRA1* mutations in a European CARASIL patient. *Neurology* 2014;**82**:898–900.

26. Nozaki H, Nishizawa M, Onodera O. Features of cerebral autosomal recessive arteriopathy with subcortical infarcts and leukoencephalopathy. *Stroke* 2014;**45**:3447–3453.

27. Fukutake T. Cerebral autosomal recessive arteriopathy with subcortical infarcts and leukoencephalopathy (CARASIL): From discovery to gene identification. *J Stroke Cerebrovasc Dis* 2011;**20**:85–93.

28. Fukutake T, Hirayama K. Familial young-adult-onset arteriosclerotic leukoencephalopathy with alopecia and lumbago without arterial hypertension. *Eur Neurol* 1995;**35**:69–79.

29. Terwindt GM, Haan J, Ophoff RA, et al. Clinical and genetic analysis of a large Dutch family with autosomal dominant vascular retinopathy, migraine and Raynaud's phenomenon. *Brain* 1998;**121**(Pt 2):303–316.

30. Grand MG, Kaine J, Fulling K, et al. Cerebroretinal vasculopathy. A new hereditary syndrome. *Ophthalmology* 1988;**95**:649–659.

31. Jen J, Cohen AH, Yue Q, et al. Hereditary endotheliopathy with retinopathy, nephropathy, and stroke (HERNS). *Neurology* 1997;**49**:1322–1330.

32. Richards A, van den Maagdenberg AM, Jen JC, et al. C-terminal truncations in human 3'-5' DNA exonuclease TREX1 cause autosomal dominant retinal vasculopathy with cerebral leukodystrophy. *Nat Genet* 2007;**39**:1068–1070.

33. Stuart MJ, Nagel RL. Sickle-cell disease. *Lancet* 2004;**364**:1343–1360.

34. Howard J, Davies SC. Sickle cell disease in North Europe. *Scand J Clin Lab Invest* 2007;**67**:27–38.

35. Rees DC, Williams TN, Gladwin MT. Sickle-cell disease. *Lancet* 2010;**376**:2018–2031.

36. Ohene-Frempong K, Weiner SJ, Sleeper LA, et al. Cerebrovascular accidents in sickle cell disease: Rates and risk factors. *Blood* 1998;**91**:288–294.

37. Bernaudin F, Verlhac S, Arnaud C, et al. Impact of early transcranial Doppler screening and intensive therapy on cerebral vasculopathy outcome in a newborn sickle cell anemia cohort. *Blood* 2011;**117**:1130–1140.

38. Switzer JA, Hess DC, Nichols FT, Adams RJ. Pathophysiology and treatment of stroke in sickle-cell disease: Present and future. *Lancet Neurol* 2006;**5**:501–512.

39. Kossorotoff M, Brousse V, Grevent D, et al. Cerebral haemorrhagic risk in children with sickle-cell disease. *Dev Med Child Neurol* 2015;**57**:187–193.

40. Fullerton HJ, Adams RJ, Zhao S, Johnston SC. Declining stroke rates in Californian children with sickle cell disease. *Blood* 2004;**104**:336–339.

41. Adams RJ, McKie VC, Hsu L, et al. Prevention of a first stroke by transfusions in children with sickle cell anemia and abnormal results on transcranial Doppler ultrasonography. *N Engl J Med* 1998;**339**:5–11.

42. Verduzco LA, Nathan DG. Sickle cell disease and stroke. *Blood* 2009;**114**:5117–5125.

43. Gaustadnes M, Ingerslev J, Rutiger N. Prevalence of congenital homocystinuria in Denmark. *N Engl J Med* 1999;**340**:1513.

44. Mudd SH, Skovby F, Levy HL, et al. The natural history of homocystinuria due to cystathionine beta-synthase deficiency. *Am J Hum Genet* 1985;**37**:1–31.

45. Welch GN, Loscalzo J. Homocysteine and atherothrombosis. *N Engl J Med* 1998;**338**:1042–1050.

46. Bellamy MF, McDowell IF. Putative mechanisms for vascular damage by homocysteine. *J Inherit Metab Dis* 1997;**20**:307–315.

47. Kelly PJ, Furie KL, Kistler JP, et al. Stroke in young patients with hyperhomocysteinemia due to cystathionine beta-synthase deficiency. *Neurology* 2003;**60**:275–279.

48. Germain DP. Fabry disease. *Orphanet J Rare Dis* 2010;**5**:30.

49. Rolfs A, Bottcher T, Zschiesche M, et al. Prevalence of Fabry disease in patients with cryptogenic stroke: A prospective study. *Lancet* 2005;**366**:1794–1796.

50. Sarikaya H, Yilmaz M, Michael N, Miserez AR, Steinmann B, Baumgartner RW. Zurich Fabry study – prevalence of Fabry disease in young patients with first cryptogenic ischaemic stroke or TIA. *Eur J Neurol* 2012;**19**:1421–1426.

51. Wozniak MA, Kittner SJ, Tuhrim S, et al. Frequency of unrecognized Fabry disease among young European-American and African-American men with first ischemic stroke. *Stroke* 2010;**41**:78–81.

52. Brouns R, Sheorajpanday R, Braxel E, et al. Middelheim Fabry Study (MiFaS): A retrospective Belgian study on the prevalence of Fabry disease in young patients with cryptogenic stroke. *Clin Neurol Neurosurg* 2007;**109**:479–484.

53. Rolfs A, Fazekas F, Grittner U, et al. Acute cerebrovascular disease in the young: The Stroke in Young Fabry Patients Study. *Stroke* 2013;**44**:340–349.

54. Sims K, Politei J, Banikazemi M, Lee P. Stroke in Fabry disease frequently occurs before diagnosis and in the absence of other clinical events: Natural history data from the Fabry Registry. *Stroke* 2009;**40**:788–794.

55. Kolodny E, Fellgiebel A, Hilz MJ, et al. Cerebrovascular involvement in Fabry disease: Current status of knowledge. *Stroke* 2015;**46**:302–313.

56. Nakamura K, Sekijima Y, Hattori K, et al. Cerebral hemorrhage in Fabry's disease. *J Hum Genet* 2010;**55**:259–261.

57. Crutchfield KE, Patronas NJ, Dambrosia JM, et al. Quantitative analysis of cerebral vasculopathy in patients with Fabry disease. *Neurology* 1998;**50**:1746–1749.

58. Fellgiebel A, Keller I, Martus P, et al. Basilar artery diameter is a potential screening tool for Fabry disease in young stroke patients. *Cerebrovasc Dis* 2011;**31**:294–299.

59. Zarate YA, Hopkin RJ. Fabry's disease. *Lancet* 2008;**372**:1427–1435.

60. Schiffmann R, Kopp JB, Austin HA, 3rd, et al. Enzyme replacement therapy in Fabry disease: A randomized controlled trial. *JAMA* 2001;**285**:2743–2749.

61. Vanakker OM, Leroy BP, Coucke P, et al. Novel clinico-molecular insights in pseudoxanthoma elasticum provide an efficient molecular screening method and a comprehensive diagnostic flowchart. *Hum Mutat* 2008;**29**:205.

62. Debette S, Germain DP. Neurologic manifestations of inherited disorders of connective tissue. *Handb Clin Neurol* 2014;**119**:565–576.

63. van den Berg JS, Hennekam RC, Cruysberg JR, et al. Prevalence of symptomatic intracranial aneurysm and ischaemic stroke in pseudoxanthoma elasticum. *Cerebrovasc Dis* 2000;**10**:315–319.

64. Germain DP, Boutouyrie P, Laloux B, Laurent S. Arterial remodeling and stiffness in patients with pseudoxanthoma elasticum. *Arterioscler Thromb Vasc Biol* 2003;**23**:836–841.

65. Dalloz MA, Debs R, Bensa C, Alamowitch S. [White matter lesions leading to the diagnosis of pseudoxanthoma elasticum]. *Rev Neurol (Paris)*;**166**:844–848.

66. Renard D, Castelnovo G, Jeanjean L, Perrochia H, Brunel H, Labauge P. Teaching neuroimage: Microangiopathic complications in pseudoxanthoma elasticum. *Neurology* 2008;**71**:e69.

67. Pavlovic AM, Zidverc-Trajkovic J, Milovic MM, et al. Cerebral small vessel disease in pseudoxanthoma elasticum: Three cases. *Can J Neurol Sci* 2005;**32**:115–118.

68. Neldner KH. Pseudoxanthoma elasticum. *Clin Dermatol* 1988;**6**:1–159.

69. De Paepe A, Viljoen D, Matton M, et al. Pseudoxanthoma elasticum: Similar autosomal recessive subtype in Belgian and Afrikaner families. *Am J Med Genet* 1991;**38**:16–20.

70. Uitto J, Li Q, Jiang Q. Pseudoxanthoma elasticum: Molecular genetics and putative pathomechanisms. *J Invest Dermatol*;**130**:661–670.

71. Germain DP. Ehlers–Danlos syndrome type IV. *Orphanet J Rare Dis* 2007;**2**:32.

72. Beighton P, De Paepe A, Steinmann B, Tsipouras P, Wenstrup RJ. Ehlers–Danlos syndromes: Revised nosology, Villefranche, 1997. Ehlers–Danlos National Foundation (USA) and Ehlers–Danlos Support Group (UK). *Am J Med Genet* 1998;**77**:31–37.

73. Pepin M, Schwarze U, Superti-Furga A, Byers PH. Clinical and genetic features of Ehlers–Danlos syndrome type IV, the vascular type. *N Engl J Med* 2000;**342**:673–680.

74. North KN, Whiteman DA, Pepin MG, Byers PH. Cerebrovascular complications in Ehlers–Danlos syndrome type IV. *Ann Neurol* 1995;**38**:960–964.

75. Debette S, Goeggel Simonetti B, Schilling S, et al. Familial occurrence and heritable connective tissue disorders in cervical artery dissection. *Neurology* 2014;**83**:2023–2031.

76. Arnold M, Bousser M-G, Fahrni G, et al. Vertebral artery dissection: Presenting findings and predictors of outcome. *Stroke* 2006;**37**:2499–2503.

77. Leys D, Moulin T, Stojkovic T, Begey S, Chavot D, DONALD Investigators. Follow-up of patients with history of cervical artery dissection. *Cerebrovasc Dis* 1995;**5**:43–49.

78. Schievink WI, Mokri B, O'Fallon WM. Recurrent spontaneous cervical-artery dissection. *N Engl J Med* 1994;**330**:393–397.

79. Beletsky V, Nadareishvili Z, Lynch J, Shuaib A, Woolfenden A, Norris JW. Cervical arterial dissection: Time for a therapeutic trial? *Stroke* 2003;**34**:2856–2860.

80. Touze E, Gauvrit JY, Moulin T, Meder JF, Bracard S, Mas JL. Risk of stroke and recurrent dissection after a cervical artery dissection: A multicenter study. *Neurology* 2003;**61**:1347–1351.

81. Arnold M, Kappeler L, Georgiadis D, et al. Gender differences in spontaneous cervical artery dissection. *Neurology* 2006;**67**:1050–1052.

82. Debette S, Leys D. Cervical-artery dissections: Predisposing factors, diagnosis, and outcome. *Lancet Neurol* 2009;**8**:668–678.

83. Engelter ST, Brandt T, Debette S, et al. Antiplatelets versus anticoagulation in cervical artery dissection. *Stroke* 2007;**38**:2605–2611.

84. Schievink WI, Limburg M, Oorthuys JW, Fleury P, Pope FM. Cerebrovascular disease in Ehlers–Danlos syndrome type IV. *Stroke* 1990;**21**:626–632.

85. Ong KT, Perdu J, De Backer J, et al. Effect of celiprolol on prevention of cardiovascular events in vascular Ehlers–Danlos syndrome: A prospective randomised, open, blinded-endpoints trial. *Lancet* 2010;**376**:1476–1484.

86. Gray JR, Bridges AB, West RR, et al. Life expectancy in British Marfan syndrome populations. *Clin Genet* 1998;**54**:124–128.

87. Schievink WI, Michels VV, Piepgras DG. Neurovascular manifestations of heritable connective tissue disorders. A review. *Stroke* 1994;**25**:889–903.

88. Wityk RJ, Zanferrari C, Oppenheimer S. Neurovascular complications of Marfan syndrome: A retrospective, hospital-based study. *Stroke* 2002;**33**:680–684.

89. Ho NC, Tran JR, Bektas A. Marfan's syndrome. *Lancet* 2005;**366**:1978–1981.

90. Lynch DR, Dawson TM, Raps EC, Galetta SL. Risk factors for the neurologic complications associated with aortic aneurysms. *Arch Neurol* 1992;**49**:284–288.

91. Spittell PC, Spittell JA, Jr., Joyce JW, et al. Clinical features and differential diagnosis of aortic dissection: Experience with 236 cases (1980 through 1990). *Mayo Clin Proc* 1993;**68**:642–651.

92. Bonnin P, Giannesini C, Amah G, Kevorkian JP, Woimant F, Levy BI. Doppler sonograpy with dynamic testing in a case of aortic dissection extending to the innominate and right common carotid arteries. *Neuroradiology* 2003;**45**:472–475.

93. Youl BD, Coutellier A, Dubois B, Leger JM, Bousser M-G. Three cases of spontaneous extracranial vertebral artery dissection. *Stroke* 1990;**21**:618–625.

94. Schievink WI, Bjornsson J, Piepgras DG. Coexistence of fibromuscular dysplasia and cystic medial necrosis in a patient with Marfan's syndrome and bilateral carotid artery dissections. *Stroke* 1994;**25**:2492–2496.

95. Harrer JU, Sasse A, Klotzsch C. Intimal flap in a common carotid artery in a patient with Marfan's syndrome. *Ultraschall Med* 2006;**27**:487–488.

96. Loeys BL, Dietz HC, Braverman AC, et al. The revised Ghent nosology for the Marfan syndrome. *J Med Genet* 2010;**47**:476–485.

97. Majamaa K, Moilanen JS, Uimonen S, et al. Epidemiology of *A3243G*, the mutation for mitochondrial encephalomyopathy, lactic acidosis, and stroke-like episodes: Prevalence of the mutation in an adult population. *Am J Hum Genet* 1998;**63**:447–454.

98. Testai FD, Gorelick PB. Inherited metabolic disorders and stroke part 1: Fabry disease and mitochondrial myopathy, encephalopathy, lactic acidosis, and strokelike episodes. *Arch Neurol* 2010;**67**:19–24.

99. Sproule DM, Kaufmann P. Mitochondrial encephalopathy, lactic acidosis, and stroke-like episodes: Basic concepts, clinical phenotype, and therapeutic management of MELAS syndrome. *Ann N Y Acad Sci* 2008;**1142**:133–158.

100. Ito H, Mori K, Kagami S. Neuroimaging of stroke-like episodes in MELAS. *Brain Dev* 2011;**33**:283–288.

101. Yoneda M, Maeda M, Kimura H, Fujii A, Katayama K, Kuriyama M. Vasogenic edema on MELAS: A serial study with diffusion-weighted MR imaging. *Neurology* 1999;**53**:2182–2184.

102. Thambisetty M, Newman NJ, Glass JD, Frankel MR. A practical approach to the diagnosis and management of MELAS: Case report and review. *Neurologist* 2002;**8**:302–312.

103. Rodriguez MC, MacDonald JR, Mahoney DJ, Parise G, Beal MF, Tarnopolsky MA. Beneficial effects of creatine, CoQ10, and lipoic acid in mitochondrial disorders. *Muscle Nerve* 2007;**35**:235–242.

104. Napolitano A, Salvetti S, Vista M, Lombardi V, Siciliano G, Giraldi C. Long-term treatment with idebenone and riboflavin in a patient with MELAS. *Neurol Sci* 2000;**21**:S981–982.

105. Koga Y, Povalko N, Nishioka J, Katayama K, Kakimoto N, Matsuishi T. MELAS and L-arginine therapy: Pathophysiology of stroke-like episodes. *Ann N Y Acad Sci* 2010;**1201**:104–110.

106. Biffi A, Greenberg SM. Cerebral amyloid angiopathy: A systematic review. *J Clin Neurol* 2011;**7**:1–9.

107. De Jonghe C, Zehr C, Yager D, et al. Flemish and Dutch mutations in amyloid beta precursor protein have different effects on amyloid beta secretion. *Neurobiol Dis* 1998;**5**:281–286.

108. Bornebroek M, De Jonghe C, Haan J, et al. Hereditary cerebral hemorrhage with amyloidosis Dutch type (AbetaPP 693): Decreased plasma amyloid-beta 42 concentration. *Neurobiol Dis* 2003;**14**:619–623.

109. Palsdottir A, Snorradottir AO, Thorsteinsson L. Hereditary cystatin C amyloid angiopathy: Genetic, clinical, and pathological aspects. *Brain Pathol* 2006;**16**:55–59.

110. Van Nostrand WE, Melchor JP, Cho HS, Greenberg SM, Rebeck GW. Pathogenic effects of D23N Iowa mutant amyloid beta-protein. *J Biol Chem* 2001;**276**:32860–32866.

111. Viswanathan A, Greenberg SM. Cerebral amyloid angiopathy in the elderly. *Ann Neurol* 2011;**70**:871–880.

112. Greenberg SM, O'Donnell HC, Schaefer PW, Kraft E. MRI detection of new hemorrhages: Potential marker of

progression in cerebral amyloid angiopathy. *Neurology* 1999;53:1135–1138.

113. Knudsen KA, Rosand J, Karluk D, Greenberg SM. Clinical diagnosis of cerebral amyloid angiopathy: Validation of the Boston criteria. *Neurology* 2001;**56**:537–539.

114. Gould DB, Phalan FC, Breedveld GJ, et al. Mutations in *COL4A1* cause perinatal cerebral hemorrhage and porencephaly. *Science* 2005;**308**:1167–1171.

115. Vahedi K, Massin P, Guichard JP, et al. Hereditary infantile hemiparesis, retinal arteriolar tortuosity, and leukoencephalopathy. *Neurology* 2003;**60**:57–63.

116. Sibon I, Coupry I, Menegon P, et al. *COL4A1* mutation in Axenfeld–Rieger anomaly with leukoencephalopathy and stroke. *Ann Neurol* 2007;**62**:177–184.

117. Plaisier E, Alamowitch S, Gribouval O, et al. Autosomal-dominant familial hematuria with retinal arteriolar tortuosity and contractures: A novel syndrome. *Kidney Int* 2005;**67**:2354–2360.

118. Vahedi K, Alamowitch S. Clinical spectrum of type IV collagen (*COL4A1*) mutations: A novel genetic multisystem disease. *Curr Opin Neurol* 2011;**24**:63–68.

119. Vahedi K, Boukobza M, Massin P, Gould DB, Tournier-Lasserve E, Bousser M-G. Clinical and brain MRI follow-up study of a family with *COL4A1* mutation. *Neurology* 2007;**69**:1564–1568.

120. Lanfranconi S, Markus HS. *COL4A1* mutations as a monogenic cause of cerebral small vessel disease: A systematic review. *Stroke* 2010;**41**: e513–518.

121. Gould DB, Phalan FC, van Mil SE, et al. Role of *COL4A1* in small-vessel disease and hemorrhagic stroke. *N Engl J Med* 2006;**354**:1489–1496.

122. Rauch F, Glorieux FH. Osteogenesis imperfecta. *Lancet* 2004;**363**:1377–1385.

123. Prockop DJ, Kivirikko KI. Heritable diseases of collagen. *N Engl J Med* 1984;**311**:376–386.

124. Goddeau RP Jr, Caplan LR, Alhazzani AA. Intraparenchymal hemorrhage in a patient with osteogenesis imperfecta and plasminogen activator inhibitor-1 deficiency. *Arch Neurol* 2010;**67**:236–238.

125. Martin JJ, Hausser I, Lyrer P, et al. Familial cervical artery dissections: Clinical, morphologic, and genetic studies. *Stroke* 2006;**37**:2924–2929.

126. Caplan LR, Gonzales G, Buonanno FS. Case 18 – A 35-year old man with neck pain, hoarseness and dysphagia. *N Engl J Med* 2012;**366**:2306–2313.

127. Bak S, Gaist D, Sindrup SH, Skytthe A, Christensen K. Genetic liability in stroke: A long-term follow-up study of Danish twins. *Stroke* 2002;**33**:769–774.

128. Kiely DK, Wolf PA, Cupples LA, Beiser AS, Myers RH. Familial aggregation of stroke. The Framingham Study. *Stroke* 1993;**24**:1366–1371.

129. Liao D, Myers R, Hunt S, et al. Familial history of stroke and stroke risk. The Family Heart Study. *Stroke* 1997;**28**:1908–1912.

130. Jood K, Ladenvall C, Rosengren A, Blomstrand C, Jern C. Family history in ischemic stroke before 70 years of age: The Sahlgrenska Academy Study on Ischemic Stroke. *Stroke* 2005;**36**:1383–1387.

131. Flossmann E, Schulz UG, Rothwell PM. Systematic review of methods and results of studies of the genetic epidemiology of ischemic stroke. *Stroke* 2004;**35**:212–227.

132. Jerrard-Dunne P, Cloud G, Hassan A, Markus HS. Evaluating the genetic component of ischemic stroke subtypes: A family history study. *Stroke* 2003;**34**:1364–1369.

133. Polychronopoulos P, Gioldasis G, Ellul J, et al. Family history of stroke in stroke types and subtypes. *J Neurol Sci* 2002;**195**:117–122.

134. Lee TH, Hsu WC, Chen CJ, Chen ST. Etiologic study of young ischemic stroke in Taiwan. *Stroke* 2002;**33**:1950–1955.

135. Yang J, Benyamin B, McEvoy BP, et al. Common SNPs explain a large proportion of the heritability for human height. *Nat Genet* 2010;**42**:565–569.

136. Bevan S, Traylor M, Adib-Samii P, et al. Genetic heritability of ischemic stroke and the contribution of previously reported candidate gene and genomewide associations. *Stroke* 2012;**43**:3161–3167.

137. Devan WJ, Falcone GJ, Anderson CD, et al. Heritability estimates identify a substantial genetic contribution to risk and outcome of intracerebral hemorrhage. *Stroke* 2013;**44**:1578–1583.

138. Hassan A, Markus HS. Genetics and ischaemic stroke. *Brain* 2000;**123**(Pt 9):1784–1812.

139. Zondervan KT, Cardon LR. Designing candidate gene and genome-wide case-control association studies. *Nat Protoc* 2007;**2**:2492–2501.

140. Zeggini E, Scott LJ, Saxena R, et al. Meta-analysis of genome-wide association data and large-scale replication identifies additional susceptibility loci for type 2 diabetes. *Nat Genet* 2008;**40**:638–645.

141. Traylor M, Makela KM, Kilarski LL, et al. A novel MMP12 locus is associated with large artery atherosclerotic stroke using a genome-wide age-at-onset informed approach. *PLoS Genet* 2014;**10**:e1004469.

142. Traylor M, Farrall M, Holliday EG, et al. Genetic risk factors for ischaemic stroke and its subtypes (the METASTROKE Collaboration): A meta-analysis of genome-wide association studies. *Lancet Neurol* 2012;**11**:951–962.

143. Woo D, Falcone GJ, Devan WJ, et al. Meta-analysis of genome-wide association studies identifies 1q22 as a susceptibility locus for intracerebral hemorrhage. *Am J Hum Genet* 2014;**94**:511–521.

144. Bellenguez C, Bevan S, Gschwendtner A, et al. Genome-wide association study identifies a variant in HDAC9 associated with large vessel ischemic stroke. *Nat Genet* 2012;**44**:328–333.

145. Holliday EG, Maguire JM, Evans TJ, et al. Common variants at 6p21.1 are associated with large artery atherosclerotic stroke. *Nat Genet* 2012;**44**:1147–1151.

146. Kilarski LL, Achterberg S, Devan WJ, et al. Meta-analysis in more than 17,900 cases of ischemic stroke reveals a novel association at 12q24.12. *Neurology* 2014;**83**:678–685.

147. Ikram MA, Seshadri S, Bis JC, et al. Genomewide association studies of stroke. *N Engl J Med* 2009;**360**:1718–1728.

148. Hirschhorn JN, Lohmueller K, Byrne E, Hirschhorn K. A comprehensive review of genetic association studies. *Genet Med* 2002;**4**:45–61.

149. Feero WG, Guttmacher AE, Collins FS. Genomic medicine – An updated primer. *N Engl J Med* 2010;**362**:2001–2011.

150. McCarthy MI, Abecasis GR, Cardon LR, et al. Genome-wide association studies for complex traits: Consensus, uncertainty and challenges. *Nat Rev Genet* 2008;**9**:356–369.

151. Biffi A, Sonni A, Anderson CD, et al. Variants at APOE influence risk of deep and lobar intracerebral hemorrhage. *Ann Neurol* 2010;**68**:934–943.

152. Holliday EG, Traylor M, Malik R, et al. Genetic overlap between diagnostic subtypes of ischemic stroke. *Stroke* 2015;**46**:615–619.

153. Battey TW, Valant V, Kassis SB, et al. Recommendations from the International Stroke Genetics Consortium, part 2: Biological sample collection and storage. *Stroke* 2015;**46**:285–290.

154. Majersik JJ, Cole JW, Golledge J, et al. Recommendations from the International Stroke Genetics Consortium, part 1: Standardized phenotypic data collection. *Stroke* 2015;**46**:279–284.

155. Psaty BM, O'Donnell CJ, Gudnason V, et al. Cohorts for Heart and Aging Research in Genomic Epidemiology (CHARGE) Consortium: Design of prospective meta-analyses of genome-wide association studies from 5 cohorts. *Circ Cardiovasc Genet* 2009;**2**:273–280.

156. Gretarsdottir S, Thorleifsson G, Manolescu A, et al. Risk variants for atrial fibrillation on chromosome 4q25 associate with ischemic stroke. *Ann Neurol* 2008;**64**:402–409.

157. Lemmens R, Buysschaert I, Geelen V, et al. The association of the 4q25 susceptibility variant for atrial fibrillation with stroke is limited to stroke of cardioembolic etiology. *Stroke* 2010;**41**:1850–1857.

158. Gudbjartsson DF, Holm H, Gretarsdottir S, et al. A sequence variant in ZFHX3 on 16q22 associates with atrial fibrillation and ischemic stroke. *Nat Genet* 2009;**41**:876–878.

159. Deloukas P, Kanoni S, Willenborg C, et al. Large-scale association analysis identifies new risk loci for coronary artery disease. *Nat Genet* 2013;**45**:25–33.

160. Azghandi S, Prell C, van der Laan SW, et al. Deficiency of the stroke relevant HDAC9 gene attenuates atherosclerosis in accord with allele-specific effects at 7p21.1. *Stroke* 2015;**46**:197–202.

161. Cheng YC, Cole JW, Kittner SJ, Mitchell BD. Genetics of ischemic stroke in young adults. *Circ Cardiovasc Genet* 2014;**7**:383–392.

162. Gschwendtner A, Bevan S, Cole JW, et al. Sequence variants on chromosome 9p21.3 confer risk for atherosclerotic stroke. *Ann Neurol* 2009;**65**:531–539.

163. Williams FM, Carter AM, Hysi PG, et al. Ischemic stroke is associated with the ABO locus: The EuroCLOT study. *Ann Neurol* 2013;**73**:16–31.

164. McArdle PF, Kittner SJ, Ay H, et al. Agreement between TOAST and CCS ischemic stroke classification: The NINDS SiGN study. *Neurology* 2014;**83**:1653–1660.

165. Wu L, Shen Y, Liu X, et al. The 1425G/A SNP in PRKCH is associated with ischemic stroke and cerebral hemorrhage in a Chinese population. *Stroke* 2009;**40**:2973–2976.

166. Serizawa M, Nabika T, Ochiai Y, et al. Association between PRKCH gene polymorphisms and subcortical silent brain infarction. *Atherosclerosis* 2008;**199**:340–345.

167. Kubo M, Hata J, Ninomiya T, et al. A nonsynonymous SNP in PRKCH (protein kinase Ceta) increases the risk of cerebral infarction. *Nat Genet* 2007;**39**:212–217.

168. International Stroke Genetics Consortium, Wellcome Trust Case-Control Consortium 2. Failure to validate association between 12p13 variants and ischemic stroke. *N Engl J Med* 2010;**362**:1547–1550.

169. Bis JC, DeStefano A, Liu X, et al. Associations of NINJ2 sequence variants with incident ischemic stroke in the Cohorts for Heart and Aging in Genomic Epidemiology (CHARGE) consortium. *PLoS One* 2014;**9**:e99798.

170. Debette S, Kamatani Y, Metso TM, et al. Common variation in PHACTR1 is associated with susceptibility to cervical artery dissection. *Nat Genet* 2015;**47**:78–83.

171. Anttila V, Winsvold BS, Gormley P, et al. Genome-wide meta-analysis identifies new susceptibility loci for migraine. *Nat Genet* 2013;**45**:912–917.

172. Rannikmae K, Kalaria RN, Greenberg SM, et al. APOE associations with severe CAA-associated vasculopathic changes: Collaborative meta-analysis. *J Neurol Neurosurg Psychiatry* 2014;**85**:300–305.

173. Biffi A, Anderson CD, Jagiella JM, et al. APOE genotype and extent of bleeding and outcome in lobar intracerebral haemorrhage: A genetic association study. *Lancet Neurol* 2011;**10**:702–709.

174. Rannikmae K, Davies G, Thomson PA, et al. Common variation in COL4A1/COL4A2 is associated with sporadic cerebral small vessel disease. *Neurology* 2015;**84**:918–926.

175. Weng YC, Sonni A, Labelle-Dumais C, et al. COL4A1 mutations in patients with sporadic late-onset intracerebral hemorrhage. *Ann Neurol* 2012;**71**:470–477.

176. Verhaaren BF, Debette S, Bis JC, et al. Multiethnic genome-wide association study of cerebral white matter hyperintensities on MRI. *Circ Cardiovasc Genet* 2015;**8**:398–409.

177. Fornage M, Debette S, Bis JC, et al. Genome-wide association studies of cerebral white matter lesion burden: The CHARGE consortium. *Ann Neurol* 2011;**69**:928–939.

178. Lambert JC, Ibrahim-Verbaas CA, Harold D, et al. Meta-analysis of 74,046 individuals identifies 11 new susceptibility loci for Alzheimer's disease. *Nat Genet* 2013;**45**:1452–1458.

179. Eichler EE, Flint J, Gibson G, et al. Missing heritability and strategies for finding the underlying causes of complex disease. *Nat Rev Genet* 2010;**11**:446–450.

180. Panoutsopoulou K, Tachmazidou I, Zeggini E. In search of low-frequency and rare variants affecting complex traits. *Hum Mol Genet* 2013;**22**: R16–21.

181. Kiezun A, Garimella K, Do R, et al. Exome sequencing and the genetic basis of complex traits. *Nat Genet* 2012;**44**:623–630.

182. Sivakumaran S, Agakov F, Theodoratou E, et al. Abundant pleiotropy in human complex diseases and traits. *Am J Hum Genet* 2011;**89**:607–618.

183. Dichgans M, Malik R, Konig IR, et al. Shared genetic susceptibility to ischemic stroke and coronary artery disease: A genome-wide analysis of common variants. *Stroke* 2014;**45**:24–36.

Treatment

Louis R Caplan and Jeffrey Saver

Some men see things as they are and say "Why?" I dream things that never were and say "Why not?"
George Bernard Shaw

Introduction

The last quarter of the twentieth century and first decades of the twenty-first can be legitimately considered a time when neurological and stroke therapeutics reached center stage. Advances in diagnostic technology made it possible to quickly and safely determine the cause of most strokes. The methodology of randomized therapeutic trials progressed as researchers and physicians began to systematically study various treatments. In this chapter, we introduce the general underlying principles of treatment of patients who have acute strokes and outline the types of therapy available. We will devote the most space to neurothrombectomy and thrombolysis since these treatments have expanded dramatically since the fourth edition of this monograph. Prophylactic treatments and stroke prevention strategies will be discussed in Chapter 18, avoidance and management of complications in Chapter 19, and strategies to enhance recovery and rehabilitation in Chapter 20.

Factors that influence treatment and various therapeutical strategies are also discussed. The emphasis of all treatments is on the anatomy, pathology, and pathophysiology of the cerebrovascular process and on the patient in all of their socio-psycho-economic-environmental complexity. Clinicians must use all information available to make difficult treatment decisions for individual patient situations. Specific treatments for patients with individual vascular pathologies and mechanisms (e.g., stenosis of an internal carotid artery (ICA), cardiac-origin embolism, and cerebral venous sinus thrombosis) are considered in Part II of this book.

Randomized trials and so called evidence-based medicine

Randomized trials are important but have limitations.[1] Trials are expensive, time-consuming, and require enormous resources. To provide statistically valid results, randomized trials must contain large numbers of patients with enough end-points to analyze. Sufficient end-points must be reached in a relatively short period. Many cerebrovascular conditions are unsuitable for trials. The issue of numbers versus specificity limits trials. For randomized trials to yield statistically valid results, many patients must be included in the study. If the results are to be useful, the data must be specifically applicable to individual patients. To achieve an adequate number of patients, the condition studied must be common and a "lumping" strategy must predominate over "splitting." Patients who are too ill, too old, too young, and are women of childbearing age are often excluded from trials. Those incapable of giving informed consent, or who have too complex or multiple illnesses are also frequently left out of trials. These exclusions are just the type of stroke patients that doctors care for every day.

The results of many randomized trials cannot be applied directly to individual patients. The term *evidence-based* must be used cautiously when applied to a particular circumstance if that circumstance has not been specifically studied. Information from trials must be weighed according to the context of specific treatment decisions. Conducting trials is different from caring for sick patients. In trials, the same treatments are given to all eligible patients depending only on randomization. Departure from the specified treatment makes the results difficult to interpret. In the clinic, doctors treat individual patients. George Thibault said it well:[2]

> We then need to decide which approach in our large therapeutic armamentarium will be most appropriate in a particular patient, with a particular stage of disease and particular coexisting conditions, and at a particular age. Even when randomized clinical trials have been performed (which is true for only a small number of clinical problems), they will often not answer this question specifically for the patient sitting in front of us in the office or lying in the hospital bed.

First, find out what is wrong with each patient in as much detail as possible. This includes the anatomy, pathology, and pathophysiology of the brain and vascular lesions. The methodology of diagnosis has been considered in Chapters 3 and 4. If there is clear therapeutic guidance from randomized trials that apply to the patient at hand then follow those guidelines. If not, use all information from what you know about the condition, what you know about the person, what has been written from published observations, case series and reports, and what is known about potential treatments to make rational considered treatment decisions.

What factors should the clinician consider when planning treatment for the individual stroke patient?

Socioeconomic and psychological factors

Socioeconomic and psychological factors may influence treatment for some patients and their families. A previously unreliable and non-compliant patient cannot be depended on to take anticoagulants. Some patients do not have the economic resources for particular therapies. In other cases, lack of caring family members or friends limits subsequent follow-up and treatment. One person might be disabled by fear of impending disability when informed of the presence of carotid artery disease and a threat of stroke whereas another individual with a similar condition may weigh the alternatives more dispassionately.

Other medical conditions

The presence of pre-existent and coexistent medical problems and conditions affects and often limits available treatments. Physicians are more conservative when suggesting surgery for stroke patients who have severe heart disease or advanced cancer. Particular concurrent conditions contraindicate some treatments. An active peptic ulcer or severe uncontrolled arterial hypertension makes anticoagulation unwise. Other conditions, such as severe heart or lung disease, increase the risks of anesthesia and surgery.

The patient's premorbid function and intellect are also critical. A hopelessly demented nursing home resident with a new stroke should be treated humanely but certainly not aggressively. An older widow, depressed and lonely for many years after the passing of her husband and friends, would be managed differently from a happy and pleasant but slightly demented grandmother who draws joy from her family and surroundings. Age is never an absolute contraindication to stroke treatment. Elderly patients cannot tolerate medical and surgical treatments as well as younger patients, nor do they share the same ability to rebound from strokes. The elderly should be handled cautiously. The same diagnostic and therapeutic strategies that apply to younger individuals, however, should be considered for geriatric patients.

Nature of the stroke

Vascular lesion

Stroke is a *cerebrovascular disease*. The nature of the causative cerebrovascular process is certainly one of the very most important determinants of potential treatments. Management of ICA occlusion is different from severe ICA stenosis or carotid plaque disease without stenosis. These extracranial large artery lesions differ greatly from lipohyalinosis of intracranial penetrating arteries caused by hypertension. These intrinsic vascular lesions differ from cardiogenic embolism and hypercoagulability as causes of vascular occlusion. Venous and dural sinus occlusions present very different issues from arterial occlusive disease.

The nature, location, and severity of the vascular lesions are key factors in selecting possible and optimal therapeutic strategies.

The blood

Does the patient have a high hematocrit (Hct) or platelet count? What is the blood viscosity? Are the platelets activated or sticky? Is there a bleeding diathesis? Abnormalities of blood constituents and coagulation functions might suggest some therapeutic strategies and contraindicate other treatments.

In a small number of patients, the hematological disorder is the primary condition that leads to vascular thrombosis or hemorrhage. In many patients, the coagulation disorder contributes to vascular occlusion. Many acute medical conditions, including infections, systemic vascular occlusions (e.g., myocardial infarction), cancers, and inflammatory diseases such as regional enteritis and ulcerative colitis, are accompanied by platelet activation and an increase in acute phase reactants that increase blood coagulability. In patients with pre-existing cardiac and vascular lesions (e.g., atrial fibrillation, congestive heart failure, and arterial stenosis or ulceration), the increase in coagulability and platelet activation incites the formation of white thrombi, red thrombi, or both at the site of the pre-existing condition.

Mechanisms and pathophysiology of stroke

Was the ischemia caused by local vascular thrombosis, embolism, or circulatory failure? (For example, was the brain ischemia caused by reduced perfusion, or artery-to-artery embolism, or a combination of hypoperfusion and embolism in a patient with severe ICA stenosis?)

Nature, location, extent, and reversibility of the brain lesions

If the entire middle cerebral artery (MCA) territory is destroyed, there is little point in reperfusing the MCA territory because only dead brain would be irrigated. Reperfusion might even be harmful.[3,4] In the Diffusion and perfusion imaging Evaluation For Understanding Stroke Evolution (DEFUSE) trial, reperfusion of patients with large infarcts worsened outcomes.[5] If, however, the MCA territory ischemia is reversible and the neurons are stunned and dysfunctional but not yet infarcted, the argument for augmenting MCA blood flow is substantially greater. Imaging using modern CT or MR can define the state of the brain as discussed in Chapter 4. Imaging results can show if feeding arteries are still occluded and the potential reversibility of the ischemia.

The cause of the ischemia and the severity and location of the cardio-cerebrovascular lesion is also important in determining the risk for further ischemia. Even if the entire MCA territory in one cerebral hemisphere is irreversibly damaged by cardiac-origin embolism, the opposite cerebral hemisphere and the territory supplied by the posterior circulation is still at risk for further damage.

The size of the lesion, severity of the neurological deficit, and length of time since the last worsening have traditionally

been used to decide if a stroke is "completed."[6] The term completed stroke is variously defined and applied and should be discarded. Short of an infallible crystal ball or direct guidance from a deity, doctors cannot predict the future. The fact that a patient is stable today does not tell whether he or she will worsen tomorrow. Patients with so-called completed stroke have as high a frequency of further brain ischemia as those with a transient ischemic attack (TIA) or reversible ischemic neurological deficit (RIND).[6] If, however, the vascular mechanism and pathology are known, the tissue at risk can be estimated. In a patient with penetrating artery disease, a 5 mm basal-ganglionic lacune may represent infarction of the entire territory of that artery. If the same patient with a small basal-ganglia infarct had severe stenosis of the MCA causing reduced flow in the lenticulostriate territory, the potential for further extensive damage is much greater.

"Stroke in evolution" is a non-specific term. Almost 30% of stroke patients worsen after entry into the hospital. These worsening deficits are related to numerous factors listed in Box 6.1. Knowledge that a patient is worsening should stimulate action. The nature of the therapeutic action, however, depends on the pathophysiology of the patient's particular problem that is causing the worsening.

Pace of the stroke

We have already emphasized that tempo of the illness should not be used as the only criterion for treatment. This does not mean, however, that it should not be considered at all. In fact, the pace of progression dictates the urgency and speed of evaluation and treatment. A patient with a TIA this morning has a greater probability of stroke tomorrow than a patient with a single TIA 3 months ago. The patient with a single TIA a week ago differs from the patient with a flurry of 5–10 TIAs yesterday and today. Patients worsening under immediate supervision require more urgent management than patients stable for the past week. An improving patient makes the physician pause before deciding to tamper with natural forces that seem to be at least temporarily succeeding.

Box 6.1 Explanations for worsening among acute stroke patients

- Failure of collateral circulation
- Systemic hypotension
- Hypovolemia
- Cardiac arrhythmias
- Embolization or propagation of thrombus
- Progressive occlusion of the arterial lumen
- Hemorrhagic transformation or hemorrhage expansion
- Brain edema
- Intercurrent infections, especially pneumonia and urinary tract infection
- Seizures
- Pulmonary embolism
- Depression

The goal of treatment is to prevent brain damage whenever possible. The major determinant of treatment is the nature of the causative cardio-cerebrovascular lesion.[7] Ideally, treatments indicated because of the nature of that lesion should begin before the patient develops any neurological worsening.

Personnel and technology available for a given treatment or evaluation

Complications and success rates vary widely between different hospitals and even within the same medical center depending on the personnel involved. There is striking variability in morbidity and mortality for the same surgical procedure – carotid endarterectomy.[8,9] The risk–benefit ratio of carotid endarterectomy when the complication rate is 2% is quite different from the situation when it is 10%. The use and complication rate for diagnostic tests, such as cerebral angiography, also vary with the skill, training, and experience of the angiographer and the equipment available. Especially in this era of limited resources, not all medical centers are economically able to specialize equally in all fields. Physicians owe patients the best available care. Responsibility to the patient must exceed loyalty to one's colleagues and institution if physicians are to continue to deserve the respect of the community. If a physician or hospital has limited training, experience, interest and capability in stroke management and the patient's condition and socioeconomic status make it feasible for the patient to go elsewhere, then the physician should send the patient to where the best care is available. The Golden Rule – do unto others what you would want for yourself – is the most important guide to treatment.

Some therapeutic strategies are general and apply to all stroke patients whereas other strategies depend on the specific problems in the individual patient. Examples of specific problems include: (1) focal brain ischemia caused by low flow in a patient with a documented occlusive vascular lesion; (2) increased (ICP) caused by the mass effect of a hematoma and its surrounding brain edema; (3) a threatened second embolism in a patient with a known cardiac source of embolism; and (4) a threatened recurrence of subarachnoid hemorrhage (SAH) in a patient with a cerebral aneurysm. The key treatment strategies are listed in Box 6.2.

Box 6.2 General strategies of stroke treatment

1. Control stroke risk factors to prevent further strokes and vascular disease
2. Prevent stroke complications (e.g., decubitus ulcers, urinary infections, phlebothrombosis, and pulmonary embolism)
3. Treat specific pathologies and pathophysiologies (e.g., draining a brain hematoma, reperfusion of an occlusive vascular lesion, managing increased intracranial pressure, reducing coagulability to prevent thrombus formation in patients with atrial fibrillation)
4. Facilitate recovery
5. Improve neurological function

General care

Important general care goals for physicians are to limit suffering, give comfort, and prevent complications. Patients deserve excellent nursing and general care even when no specific therapy seems warranted because of the severity of the deficit, type of stroke, or severe comorbidities. Stroke patients are often at least partially immobilized and may not be able to care for their bodily needs. Key goals are: (1) maintenance of adequate nutrition; (2) prevention of contractures or painful, stiff, or frozen joints; (3) prevention of decubiti and of pressure-related peripheral nerve palsies; and (4) prevention of thromboembolic, pulmonary, genitourinary, and skin complications. Table 6.1 lists some stroke complications and general types of

Table 6.1 General problems and treatments in patients with stroke

Problems	Treatments
Nutritional maintenance (especially if dysphagia is present)	Balanced diet that conforms to suggested calories and content (e.g., low cholesterol and low salt), vitamins when indicated, intravenous feeding, nasogastric tubes, gastrostomy
Pulmonary complications (aspiration, pneumonia atelectasis, pulmonary emboli)	Care or avoidance in oral feeding; in dysphagics, study of swallowing before oral feeding; respiratory therapy; early antibiotic treatment of infection; no smoking; anticoagulants (low-dose heparin, low-molecular-weight heparin, or synthetic pentasaccharide); use of intermittent pneumatic compression boots to prevent phlebothrombosis
Immobility (body or one or more limbs)	Frequent full range-of-motion exercises, frequent turning, prevention of pressure palsies and joint dislocations by slings, and careful limb positioning
Urinary-tract complications (bladder distension, urinary retention, infection)	Catheterization using sterile technique when needed; avoidance when possible of indwelling catheters; early antibiotic treatment; urinary acidification
Skin (decubiti)	Careful, frequent turning; pillows and pads to protect pressure areas; water beds; skin surveillance
Psychological (apathy and depression)	Positive outlook; entire medical care personnel functioning as a team; antidepressants

Modified from Caplan LR. A general therapeutic perspective on stroke treatment. In Dunkel R, Schmidley J (eds), *Stroke in the Elderly: New Issues in Diagnosis; Treatment and Rehabilitation*. New York: Springer Publishing, 1987, pp 60–69 with permission.

treatment for their prevention. Complications are discussed in detail in Chapter 19. Perhaps just as important as these physical problems is maintenance of a positive but realistic outlook for patients, their families, and significant others. Depression is common after stroke, so measures should be instituted early to prevent discouragement.[10,11] Depression should be recognized and treated when it occurs.

Patients' visits to doctors' gives physicians important opportunities to view the whole person and his or her environment. In the hurry to diagnose and treat acute stroke problems, preventive measures are often overlooked. The stroke patient of today, irrespective of cause, is at risk for future strokes and vascular disease in other important organs. Prevention strategies should begin as early as possible. Patients receive wrong messages when some factors are neglected (e.g., food trays rich in red meats, cheese, and ice cream tell the patient with hypercholesterolemia that diet is not important). Nurses or aides who help the patient smoke also convey approbation. While the specific stroke mechanism is investigated and treated, explore general health practices and stroke risk factors and deal with them early in the course. Box 6.3 lists some of these risk factors. These are explored in more detail in Chapter 18 on stroke prevention.

While exploring diagnosis and treatment of acute stroke, begin to develop rehabilitation strategies. Restorative or rehabilitation therapy depends on the type of handicap and disability, not on the stroke etiology or mechanism. Limb weakness, gait abnormalities, language disturbances, dysphagia, neglect of the left side of space, and hemianopia are different problems that require different rehabilitation and therapy strategies. To be maximally effective, rehabilitation should focus on the individual patient, taking past capabilities, activities, and future needs into consideration. Recovery and rehabilitation are discussed at more length in Chapter 20.

Rehabilitation involves two complementary processes. The first is activity-dependent plasticity. The brain's substantial capacity for neural repair and reorganization is driven by engagement in tasks and activities. The second is an educational process, training patients and their caregivers to understand their residual handicaps, and devising strategies to overcome them. Recall that the word doctor is derived from

---

Box 6.3 Risk factors and potentially unhealthy practices

Smoking
Heart disease
Hypertension
Illicit drug use (especially cocaine and amphetamines)
Prescription drugs and their overuse
Overuse of alcohol
Abnormal blood lipids
Oral contraceptives
Sedentary lifestyle, lack of regular exercise
Diabetes
Highly stressful work and home situations
Being overweight
Low fluid intake

the Latin word *docere*, which means "to teach" or "to lead." Sometimes well-learned routine tasks, such as walking, eating, or getting on and off a toilet seat, must be performed in different ways. Patients must be instructed and trained to use new approaches. To be successful, the rehabilitation and education process must be shared with the family and others who live with and help the patient. They must carry on and amplify the gains made in the hospital after the patient returns home. If friends and family know the nature of the patient's disabilities, they understand when the patient cannot perform particular tasks and, thus, modify the patient's environment to make things easier. A kind, understanding, and unhurried approach by all personnel involved is needed. Rehabilitation, like prevention, should start early during the acute stroke period. Passive range-of-movement exercises, speech therapy, and explanation of the neurological dysfunction can begin during the first days after the stroke.

In many medical centers and physician practices, the locations and personnel involved in stroke prevention, acute treatment, and rehabilitation are different. Primary care physicians have the most opportunity to encourage stroke prevention practices when they see patients in their offices. Neurologists, hospitalists, and other acute-care specialists treat acute strokes in acute-care facilities, sometimes in special stroke or intensive care units (ICUs). Neurologists do not usually see patients until they already have had a stroke or other cerebrovascular event. Other specialists, such as physiatrists, often manage the patient during the recuperative period in rehabilitation hospitals. All phases of care should be a continuum. Ideally, the three types of practitioners should be involved during the acute-care phase. Rehabilitation personnel must be aware of the preventive and acute treatment strategies used during rehabilitation. After being urged to refrain from smoking and watch their diet in the acute-care hospital, what message do patients receive if they are allowed to smoke and eat as they please in the rehabilitation hospital?

Stroke units and stroke centers

One of the most important therapeutic advances during the last decades of the twentieth and the first decade of the twenty-first century in the treatment of patients with acute stroke was the development of stroke services, stroke nurses, stroke specialists, stroke units, and stroke centers. Technological advances in diagnosis and treatment of stroke patients and the complexity of stroke prevention, acute care, and rehabilitation led to the development of specialized stroke services and units in many academic hospitals in the United States, Europe, and Australasia. The advent of thrombolysis and potentially effective care of acute stroke patients gave a boost to this movement and made it clear that efficient rapid throughput of stroke patients by experienced physicians and nurses was essential and it was advantageous to route patients to designated stroke center hospitals and therein segregate stroke patients in ICUs and specialized stroke units.

These stroke center hospitals established policies for rapid, multidisciplinary care of acute stroke patients in the emergency department, imaging and interventional suites,

and inpatient wards.[12–14] These stroke units include nurses with experience and training in stroke, internists, and stroke neurologists. They are able to deliver: specialized nursing care; attention to management of blood pressure, fluid volumes, and other physiological and biochemical factors; protocols and practices to facilitate rapid and thorough evaluation and treatment, monitor treatment, carry out randomized therapeutic trials, and prevent complications, and educate patients and their families and caregivers about stroke and its prevention and treatment.[15–20] Stroke units also promote an up-beat optimistic view of stroke recovery in contrast to the situation previously present on medical wards where stroke patients were often considered undesirable patients with hopeless outcomes.

Once these centers and units began to proliferate, it became clear that they were a very important major advance. Dedicated stroke center hospitals and inpatient stroke units have been convincingly shown to decrease mortality, limit stroke morbidity, and allow more patients to retain their independence and to return home after stroke.[15–19,21–24] The milieu and patient care in dedicated stroke units leads to better outcomes. Mortality is reduced. More patients return home and less are transferred to chronic hospitals and nursing homes. Short-term and long-term functional outcomes are also improved. There is no longer any doubt that stroke units work.

Ischemic stroke

Although mechanisms of ischemia vary, particular themes are applicable to all patients with brain ischemia. Ischemia means inadequate delivery of blood containing required nutrients. The major nutrients that the brain needs are oxygen and glucose. Maximizing blood flow to ischemic zones is clearly important. Can areas of vascular blockage in large arteries be opened or circumvented by medical or surgical treatments? Can local perfusion through the microcirculation supplying the ischemic zone be improved? Occlusive thrombosis and thromboembolism are important in most patients with ischemic stroke. Can the coagulation system be altered to diminish the development of white platelet–fibrin clots and red thrombin-dependent clots? Metabolic changes within the ischemic zone are important in causing cell death. Can the brain be made more resistant to ischemia by manipulating its chemical environment? Edema and raised intracranial pressure (ICP) can promote nerve cell damage. Can they be controlled? We discuss these different issues separately.

Maximizing blood flow

Different medical and surgical strategies are available to try to improve circulation to an ischemic region distal to a vascular occlusive lesion.

Controlling position and activity

In some patients, sitting, standing, and even elevating the head of the bed increase ischemic symptoms.[25,26] The minor reduction in cephalad flow accompanying postural change decreases

blood flow through the stenotic vessel or collateral channels just enough to decompensate a fragile equilibrium. Ischemic stroke patients may improve when they are treated in a supine or head down position.[27,28] Physicians should note if patients are sensitive to postural changes. Initially after the acute stroke, patients should be observed when first sitting or standing, to ensure that blood pressure does not drop excessively or postural symptoms appear. Patients with progressive symptoms caused by ischemia should be nursed supine, sometimes with the feet slightly or moderately elevated.

Managing blood pressure, blood volume, and cardiac output

Cerebral blood flow (CBF) increases with rising blood pressure until the pressure becomes high, approaching the malignant range. For this reason, surgeons often administer intravenous (IV) agents, such as phenylephrine, to raise blood pressure just before clamping the ICA during an endarterectomy. During the first 24 hours of ischemic stroke, it is unwise to lower the systemic pressure unless it is extremely high (e.g., >200/120 mmHg). In some Emergency Rooms or ICUs, however, exposing physicians to an elevated blood pressure is like waving a red flag before a bull; they want to move all of the patient's numbers into the normal range, including blood pressure. Remember that physicians treat patients not numbers. The patient's symptoms, signs, and neurological function are better guides to the appropriateness of a treatment than the measured blood pressure.

In some patients with arterial occlusive lesions, giving medications such as phenylephrine to raise the blood pressure can lead to improved neurological function.[29-32] Improvement in function is especially likely when there is an arterial occlusion and MRI studies show a diffusion–perfusion mismatch indicating the presence of considerable viable brain tissue.

Blood volume also affects perfusion pressure and blood flow. Some patients who are not able to eat normally become dehydrated and relatively hemoconcentrated. Other factors (i.e., vomiting, eating restrictions because of concern for aspiration, or simply the rush of diagnostic testing occupying patients at mealtimes) contribute to reduced fluid intake during the early hours and days after stroke onset. In general, it is wise to keep blood volume, especially plasma volume, high. Fluids must often be given intravenously or by nasogastric tube. Care, however, must be taken to avoid fluid overload and the complications of cardiac failure and brain edema. Careful monitoring of cardiac and brain function should accompany any therapeutic attempt to augment fluid volume.

Some patients have anoxic-ischemic brain damage caused by cardiac malfunction; in others, a strong pump helps maximize CBF. Attention to cardiac rhythm and pump function is important, especially during the acute, fragile period of brain ischemia. Cardiac output can sometimes be improved by: (1) use of inotropic agents, vasodilators, pacemakers, or medications to treat slow rhythms and heart block; (2) adjustment of already prescribed drugs such as digitalis and diuretics;

Box 6.4 Strategies used to effect reperfusion of ischemic brain regions

1. Direct arterial surgery – endarterectomy
2. Angioplasty
3. Stenting
4. Thrombolysis
5. Mechanical clot retrieval or clot aspiration
6. Vasodilator treatment of vasoconstriction
7. Surgically bypassing an obstructed artery
8. Augmenting collateral circulation

---

(3) correction of abnormal serum K^+ and Ca^{2+} levels; and (4) control of tachyrhythmias. Cardiac-ejection fractions and output can be monitored non-invasively by echocardiography.

Reperfusion strategies

Box 6.4 lists the various strategies that can be used to effect reperfusion of ischemic zones. Often more than one strategy can be used.

Surgical endarterectomy or local reconstruction

Endarterectomy has been the most common method of unblocking a vessel by direct surgery. This strategy differs from other techniques that augment flow through collateral vessels because endarterectomy of a tightly stenotic vessel produces a suddenly large increase in flow. Capillaries, small arterioles, and neurons are often damaged during ischemia. When flooded with blood under high pressure, these abnormal vessels can then bleed. The carotid sinus is also damaged during endarterectomy, leading to failure of the carotid sinus reflex and accelerated hypertension in the hours and days after carotid endarterectomy.[33-35] Elevated blood pressure and flooding of damaged vessels can lead to brain edema and ICH after carotid endarterectomy.[35-37] Care must be taken in the timing of endarterectomy. The blood pressures of patients undergoing carotid endarterectomy must be carefully monitored during the postoperative period. Usually, completely occluded arteries do not lend themselves to direct repair because clots form and propagate distally beyond the site of surgical access in the presence of low flow.

Carotid endarterectomy has been shown to be clearly more effective than medical therapy in patients with neurologically symptomatic, severe (70–99% luminal narrowing) carotid artery stenosis.[38-40] Endarterectomy not only removes the obstructing lesion dramatically augmenting flow but also removes the source of intra-arterial emboli. Endarterectomy has also been shown to be somewhat effective in selected patients with luminal stenosis in the 50–69% range.[41,42] However, patients must be carefully chosen because neurological and cardiac morbidity and mortality are significant risks.

Vertebral artery surgery can also be performed successfully with low morbidity and mortality when performed by surgeons with extensive experience with the procedure.[43-45] The most common method of vertebral artery reconstruction is to anastamose the vertebral artery to the carotid artery. Vertebral artery endarterectomy can also be performed.

Several randomized trials showed that carotid endarterectomy in carefully selected patients who had severe carotid artery stenosis but no recent symptoms considered related to the carotid disease was more effective than medical treatment in preventing strokes.[46,47] The selected patients had no symptoms of retinal or brain ischemia, severe cardiac disease, or other serious comorbidities and were operated on by selected surgeons who had low surgical complication rates. Women and those over 65 years of age in the European Asymptomatic Carotid Surgery trial (ACST) did not fare as well as men and younger individuals.[47] We rarely suggest carotid endarterectomy or stenting in asymptomatic patients.

Endarterectomy has also occasionally been performed successfully in stenosing lesions of the intracranial vertebral arteries.[48,49] Insufficient cases have been studied to determine the indications and effectiveness of surgery versus medical therapy in patients with vertebral artery lesions. Emboli have also been removed directly from the MCA during craniotomy but the procedure did not lessen stroke severity.[50]

Angioplasty and stenting

Since the 1980s, catheter-based neurointerventional techniques have become an important therapeutic alternative for many cerebrovascular conditions. At first, interventional techniques using coils, catheters, balloons, glues, and other devices were applied mostly to treatment of patients with intracranial aneurysms and vascular malformations. Transluminal angioplasty, sometimes with insertion of vascular stents, first developed for coronary artery and peripheral vascular occlusive disease of the limbs, also became an important option for cervical and cerebral arteries, both for atherosclerosis and for fibromuscular dysplasia.

Angioplasty/stenting of neck arteries

Although coronary artery angioplasty began much earlier, Kerber et al. published the first report of endovascular treatment of carotid artery disease with balloon angioplasty

in 1980.[51–53] By 1995, a review of worldwide experience among 523 patients claimed favorable results: 96.2% technical success, 2.1% morbidity, 6.3% transient minor complications, and no deaths.[52,53] Operator experience was important in determining the technical success and treatment outcomes: centers with limited experience (<50 cases) reported nearly twice the rate of complications (5.9% vs. 2.6%) than those with more substantial experience.[53–55]

The development of stenting in conjunction with balloon angioplasty for carotid stenosis was based on reports that showed improved outcomes during coronary interventions when stents were used. These coronary artery studies reported greater event-free survival at one year with a lower rate of repeat angioplasty for recurrent stenosis after stenting as compared with angioplasty alone. Stents seemed to reduce the risk of plaque dislodgement, significant intimal dissection, elastic recoil of the vessel wall, and both early and late restenosis. Figure 6.1 is an example of stenting of a very stenotic ICA.

Increasing experience showed that angioplasty, with or without stenting, to treat atherosclerotic disease generated embolic debris composed of atheromatous plaque, cholesterol crystals, thrombus, and platelet aggregates.[56–59] An important further technical advance was the development of embolus protection devices. Most often these were "distal" protection devices that consist of baskets or umbrellas placed above the target atherosclerotic lesion to trap debris dislodged by angioplasty before it reached the brain. Less often interventionalists deploy "proximal" protection approaches, such as flow reversal through the target stenosis by balloon occlusion at the level of the common carotid artery.[60] Protection devices appeared to reduce the frequency of embolic stroke occurring during angioplasty procedures.

Hoffman and colleagues reviewed the risk scores for peri-interventional complications of carotid artery stenting derived from a prospective registry of 606 consecutive patients treated at a "secondary care hospital" in Austria.[61] The acute stroke rate was 3% (including 13 minor and 5 major periprocedural

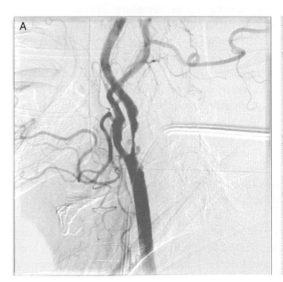
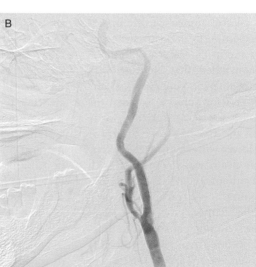

Figure 6.1 Carotid artery lesion treated with stent placement. (A) Catheter contrast angiogram lateral view showing a long very irregular atherosclerotic lesion that begins in the distal common carotid artery and extends several centimeters into the ICA. (B) Angiographic film after successful placement of a stent across the lesion. Kindly submitted by Dr Ajith Thomas, Neurosurgery, Beth Israel Deaconess Medical Center, Boston, MA.

non-fatal strokes) and 1.3% deaths including 4 fatal strokes. Patients treated with distal protection devices fared better than those who did not have protection devices.[61]

Potential problems may arise in some patients in deploying protection devices. When stenotic lesions are very severe, expansion of the lumen by balloon stretching was needed in order to advance the device past the stenotic area. This can add risk to the procedure. The protective devices can also irritate or denude the intima above the ultimate stent placement making it a potential nidus for thrombus formation in the hours and days after the procedure.[53]

Several multicenter studies clarified the evolving usefulness of carotid angioplasty and stenting compared to carotid endarterectomy. Early carotid angioplasty techniques showed promise but also problems in the Carotid and Vertebral Transluminal Angioplasty Study (CAVATAS), a large, prospective, randomized, multicenter, trial that compared carotid endarterectomy to carotid angioplasty. Five hundred and four patients with a symptomatic stenosis (70–99% stenosis) were randomized to angioplasty or surgery during 5 years.[62–64] Among the catheter-treated patients, angioplasty alone was used in three-quarters and stents in one-quarter, so CAVATAS was primarily a pre-stent era trial. No significant difference in the risk of stroke or death related to either carotid endarterectomy or carotid angioplasty was found. The rate of any stroke lasting greater than 7 days, or death within 30 days of first treatment, was approximately 10–12% in both the surgical and angioplasty groups, and the rate of disabling stroke or death within 30 days of first treatment was 6% in both groups. Long-term follow-up showed no difference in the rate of ipsilateral stroke or any disabling stroke in patients up to 8 years after randomization.[65] However, the rate of restenosis in the endovascular group was three times higher in the surgical cohort, 31% versus 11%, respectively.[63–66]

The Stenting and Angioplasty with Protection in Patients at High Risk for Endarterectomy (SAPPHIRE) study compared carotid stenting using an embolic protection device to endarterectomy in surgically "high-risk" patients with specific comorbidities.[67] Overall, 747 patients with 50–99% symptomatic stenosis, or with 80–99% asymptomatic stenosis, were enrolled; all enrollees were distinctive in that they had conditions that placed them at high risk for surgical carotid operations. Primary end-points were a composite of death, stroke, or myocardial infarction at 30 days and ipsilateral stroke or death within 1 year. The authors concluded that stenting with distal embolic protection was not inferior to endarterectomy ($P = 0.004$). Among these high risk for surgery patients, the results narrowly missed the mark for statistical superiority of stenting ($P = 0.053$). Overall the risk of stroke, death or myocardial infarction was 39% lower with stenting at 30 days. The risk of ipsilateral stroke or death was 7.9% lower with stenting at 1 year. Fewer stented patients required re-operation than those who had endarterectomy.[67]

Three randomized trials in the stent era compared carotid stenting to carotid endarterectomy among patients not at distinctively high risk for surgery. While these trials uniformly used stents in the catheter intervention arms, the use of protection devices, which were still evolving, was variable. The SPACE trial included 1183 German, Austrian, and Swiss patients with symptomatic eye or brain ischemia and severe (50–99% luminal narrowing by NASCET criteria) ipsilateral carotid artery stenosis who were allocated to carotid surgery (599) or carotid artery stenting (584).[68] Choice of protection devices, predilatation, balloon size, and stents was left up to the interventionalists. Only 27% of stented patients had protection devices, but there were no differences in end-points among those treated with and without protective devices. The rate of death or ipsilateral ischemic stroke at 30 days was 6.34% with surgery and 6.84% with stenting, an insignificant difference. Older patients and women tended to do worse with either treatment.[68] In a French trial of carotid endarterectomy versus stenting (EVA-3S), the rates of stroke and death were higher in the stent group than the surgical group.[69] The frequency of stroke or death at 30 days was 3.9% in the endarterectomy group and 9.6% in the stented group.[69] Five different stents and 7 different protection devices were used; in about 20% of instances (mostly at the beginning of the trial) protection devices were not deployed. The requirements for prior experience of the interventionalists who performed the stenting was less restrictive than in other trials.[70]

The largest study to date is the CREST trial, which enrolled 2502 patients with either symptomatic carotid disease and 50–99% stenosis or asymptomatic carotid disease and 60–99% stenosis.[71] In the angioplasty arm, all patients had stenting and distal protection whenever technically possible. The primary end-point was stroke, myocardial infarction, or death from any cause in the periprocedure period or any stroke on the side of the carotid intervention thereafter. Overall, there was no difference between the two groups, 7.2% in the stenting patients and 6.8% in the endarterectomy patients at 4 years.[71] The type of periprocedural complications differed between the two treatments, with more strokes occurring with stenting and more myocardial infarctions occurring with endarterectomy. Patient age emerged as an important modifier of treatment effect. Younger patients (<70 years) fared better with stenting, while older patients (≥70 years) had better outcomes with endarterectomy.[72] In older patients, greater vessel tortuosity appears to make stenting technically more difficult. Crossing the aorta in order to deploy the stent likely led to more emboli in older patients than those who were younger. A retrospective analysis of hospital data regarding treatment of asymptomatic carotid artery stenosis showed that among 17 716 patients who had carotid endarterectomies and 3962 who had carotid artery stenting, the postoperative stroke or in-hospital death rate was higher among those stented (4.0% vs. 1.5%, $P < 0.001$).[73]

The collective results of the major trials suggest that it is naïve to conclude that one of the two treatments would always be superior. Patients with long lesions, smooth lesions, and very high bifurcations, especially those with coronary artery disease might better be treated using catheter-based techniques. Patients with focal irregular ulcerated lesions and older patients with tortuous arteries making catheter access difficult might better be treated surgically. Surgeons are learning both direct surgical and interventional techniques so that they could

fit the preferred technique in the individual case to the lesion and the patient.

Angioplasty and stenting has also been used to treat occlusive lesions in other neck arteries. Studies of balloon angioplasty and/or stenting for treatment of subclavian stenosis report excellent patency rates and more favorable results than surgery with amelioration of presenting symptoms in 72–100%, technical success in 90–100%, periprocedural complications in 0–10%, with stroke and death in 0–4%.[74–76] Henry et al. reported on 113 patients treated for subclavian stenosis or occlusion with either angioplasty alone ($N = 57$) or angioplasty/stenting ($N = 46$) with 91% technical success and 2.6% complication rate.[77] Procedural failures occurred mostly in occluded vessels. During 4.3 years of average follow-up, restenosis occurred in 16%, the majority of which had been treated with angioplasty only.[77] Schillinger et al. reported a higher rate of initial technical success in 115 patients treated for subclavian stenosis with stents: 95% of stented vessels remained patent at 1 year versus 76% treated with angioplasty; however, by 4 years, only 59% of stented vessels remained patent compared with 68% for angioplasty alone.[78]

There is relatively little data on the results of stenting for vertebral artery stenosis near the origin of the artery.[79–82] The vertebral artery is smaller in diameter than the carotid artery and takes off at an almost 90-degree angle from the subclavian artery making stenting more difficult than in the carotid artery. Although a restenosis rate of 43% at 6 months follow-up was reported in the Stenting of Symptomatic Atherosclerotic Lesions in the Vertebral or Intracranial Arteries (SSYLVIA) trial,[82] a more recent multicenter registry enrolling 148 patients found a lower restenosis rate of 16%.[83]

Angioplasty/stenting of intracranial arteries

The first balloon angioplasties for intracranial occlusive disease were reported in the mid 1980s.[53,84,85] Introduction of improved micro-balloon catheters and smaller balloon-expandable stents led to a dramatic increase in intracranial interventions. Several case series showed good technical success, but the complication rate was substantial.[85–87] Connors and Wojack noted that their continued experience led to a change in technique during a 9-year period during which they had treated 70 patients with intracranial occlusive disease.[88] They had learned to use slow-inflation of an undersized balloon and aimed at moderate reduction of the luminal stenosis rather than normalization. They, Takis et al.,[89] and others reported complications that included: arterial dissections; arterial thrombi that required thrombolysis; and procedural-related brain infarcts.

Following the experience in the coronary and carotid arteries, intracranial stents began to be used.[90–92] Long-term results were reported by Marks et al. among 37 intracranial angioplasties[93] and by Wojak et al. among their 84 procedures (62 angioplasties and 22 stents).[94] There were two periprocedural deaths and one minor stroke in the series of Marks et al.[93] The average stenosis decreased from 84% to 43%. The annual stroke rate in the territory of the treated lesions was 3.4% but

was 4.5% in patients with greater than 50% residual stenosis.[93] In the Wojak et al. series, the periprocedural stroke or death rate was 4.8%.[94] During a mean of 4.6 months, angiographic restenosis developed in 23 patients, 13 of whom were retreated without recognized complications.[94]

Several non-randomized, multicenter studies also suggested potential benefit of intracranial stenting for symptomatic intracranial atherosclerosis. The SSYLVIA trial was a multicenter, non-randomized, prospective feasibility study that evaluated the Neurolink intracranial stent system for treatment of patients with single target vertebral or intracranial artery stenosis greater than 50%.[82] Among 61 patients enrolled, 43 (70.5%) had an intracranial stenosis, and 18 (29.5%) had an extracranial vertebral artery stenosis. During the first 30 days, 6.6% of patients had strokes but no deaths. Successful stent placement was achieved in 58 of 61 (95%) procedures. Although restenosis occurred in 35% of patients, 61% were asymptomatic.[82] Revascularization using the WingSpan stent was performed in a prospective multicenter study among 45 patients, enrolled from 12 European sites, with symptomatic intracranial atherosclerosis (>50% stenosis).[95,96] Among these patients, 95% had strokes, and 29% had had TIAs. Technical success was achieved in 98% (44/45) of patients. The composite 30-day death or ipsilateral stroke rate was 4.5% (2/44), the 6-month death or ipsilateral stroke rate was 7.1% (3/42), and the all cause stroke rate was 9.5% (4/42).[96] One report described the results of WingSpan stent deployment among US centers in 78 patients with 82 intracranial atherostenotic lesions.[97] Two-thirds of the lesions had greater than 70% stenosis. All but one of the lesions was successfully stented during the first procedure session. There were 5 (6.1%) major procedural neurological complications, 4 of which proved fatal within 30 days after the procedure.[97]

Figure 6.2 is an example of a lesion in the proximal portion of the left MCA in a patient with acute left hemisphere brain ischemia treated with angioplasty and a neuroform stent. The patient's clinical symptoms and left hemisphere brain perfusion, as studied by CT perfusion, normalized after the stent was placed.

Based on these encouraging studies, two randomized trials of intracranial stenting for symptomatic intracranial atherosclerosis were performed. Both failed to show a benefit of stenting, in part due to a better than expected outcome in the medical therapy control arms. In the Stenting versus Aggressive Medical Therapy for Intracranial Arterial Stenosis (SAMMPRIS) trial, 451 patients with recent ischemic stroke or TIA due to 70–99% atherosclerotic stenosis of a major intracranial artery were randomized to aggressive medical therapy alone or aggressive medical therapy plus stenting with the WingSpan system.[98] There was a high early complication rate in the stented patients, with 14.7% rate of stroke or death in the first month after stenting.[98] Beyond the first month, both the medical and stent arm patients had the same rate of stroke within the territory of the target artery. At 2 years after randomization the stent group had higher rates of any stroke, 21.9% versus 14.9%.[99] A unique aspect of

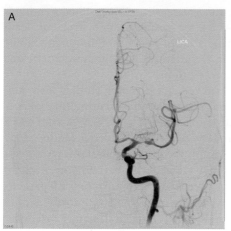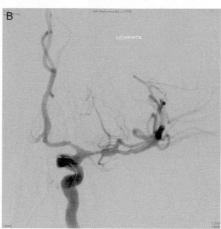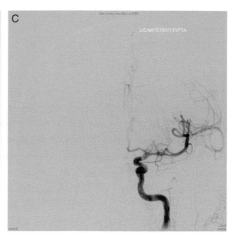

Figure 6.2 Intracranial lesion treated with stent placement. Left carotid angiograms in a patient with acute left cerebral ischemia. (A) The first angiogram shows severe stenosis of the left MCA beginning near the origin of the artery. There is post-stenotic dilatation. (B) Angiogram after angioplasty before stent placement. (C) Angiogram after placement of a neuroform stent. Kindly submitted by Dr Ajith Thomas, Neurosurgery, Beth Israel Deaconess Medical Center, Boston, MA.

the SAMMPRIS trial was mandated lifestyle modifications in nutritional intake, weight, and exercise monitored by assigned coaches. The intensive medical therapy used in SAMMPRIS also included high potency statins, aggressive control of blood pressure with frequent monitoring of results, and double antiplatelet therapy (combined aspirin and clopidogrel). This intensive and closely monitored medical therapy protocol yielded better outcomes in the medical arm than prior medically treated cohorts. In prior trials of surgical or interventional versus medical therapy, "best medical therapy" was not systematically described and the effectiveness of the medical therapy in modifying risk factors was not closely monitored. In SAMMPRIS, post-procedural complications were most common when the basilar artery was stented, and many infarcts were located within territory supplied by penetrating arterial branches of the stented arteries.

Results similar to SAMMPRIS were preliminarily reported in the VISSIT trial. Among 112 patients with symptomatic intracranial stenosis, more patients randomized to intracranial stenting with the Vitesse stent had stroke at 1 year than patients randomized to medical therapy, 36.2% versus 15.1%.[100]

The results of these two randomized trials indicate that aggressive medical therapy remains the best first treatment strategy for patients with symptomatic intracranial stenting. Patients who fail aggressive medical therapy might be considered for stenting, especially if they have evidence of poor collaterals,[101] but stenting carries too high an immediate stroke risk to use as a first-line treatment.

Drug-eluting stents have been used in the coronary circulation to attempt to reduce restenosis rates. These stents may require longer-term more aggressive antiplatelet therapy to reduce the risk of white-platelet thrombi formation on the stents than on bare stents. Drug-eluting stents are now also being used to treat both extracranial and intracranial arterial stenoses but their relative long-term safety and efficacy are as yet uncertain.[102–105] Further studies are needed to tell if drug-elution provides an important benefit.

Thrombolysis

Rationale and early studies

Clots can also be lysed chemically. In the body, thrombus formation stimulates an endogenous fibrinolytic mechanism for thrombolysis. Factor XII, the release of tissue plasminogen activator, and other substances promote conversion of plasminogen to plasmin, the active fibrinolytic enzyme.[106–108] Plasmin activity is concentrated at the sites of fibrin deposition. Fibrinolytic drugs degrade the fibrin network mesh of red erythrocyte–fibrin clots. They do not lyse white platelet–fibrin thrombi but instead may activate platelets.[108] Endogenous formation of plasmin is probably responsible for some examples of spontaneous recanalization of thrombosed arteries. The ideal thrombolytic agent would adhere specifically to fibrin in clots and would not cause systemic fibrinogenolysis. Lowering fibrinogen levels excessively can promote bleeding.

Physicians began to explore the use of thrombolytic agents during the 1950s for a variety of systemic thromboembolic conditions. Early attempts used bovine or human thrombolysins or streptokinase. During the early 1960s, Meyer and colleagues randomized 73 patients with worsening strokes to receive streptokinase IV and/or concomitant anticoagulants within 3 days of stroke onset.[109,110] Clot lysis was successful in some patients, but 10 patients died, and some had brain hemorrhages. After these studies, use of streptokinase for systemic and cardiac thromboembolism was considered contraindicated in the presence of brain lesions or past strokes.

Observational studies of intravenous and intra-arterial thrombolysis in patients with known arterial lesions before the National Institute of Neurological Disorders and Stroke (NINDS) study

During the 1980s, stimulated by success in treating coronary artery thrombosis, clinicians turned again to "clot busters" to treat cerebrovascular thromboembolism. Caplan, Pessin, and

colleagues at the New England Medical Center in Boston were involved in some of the early studies with American, German, and Japanese colleagues. Streptokinase, urokinase, and recombinant tissue plasminogen activator (rt-PA) were the most common agents used. In these early studies, acute stroke patients were screened clinically and by computed tomography (CT), and then angiography was performed. If an intracranial arterial occlusion was shown, thrombolytic drugs were given either intra-arterially (IA) into the clots, or intravenously (IV). Follow-up angiography was performed after treatment to assess recanalization. Both anterior and posterior circulation thromboembolism were treated. These studies were observational only, since controls were seldom used and patients were not randomized, but successive patients meeting protocol requirements were treated.

In all of these early angiographic studies, and in angiographically controlled trials since release of rt-PA, recanalization heavily correlated with outcome. As far as is known, thrombolytic agents act beneficially only by lysing clots. If arteries are not opened the drugs do not facilitate recovery. Knowing the recanalization rate of agents given IV and IA in patients with various occlusive arterial lesions is extremely helpful in choosing appropriate therapy.

Among patients treated using IA thrombolytic agents under angiographic control, the agents were given within 24 hours.[109–112] The presence and extent of reperfusion depended mostly on the location of the occluded artery and the mechanism of the stroke. Among 449 patients treated in 17 studies, 64% had effective recanalization after therapy. Mainstem and divisional MCA occlusions responded best, while ICA occlusions responded poorly. Distal MCA branch occlusions did not respond as well as more proximal MCA lesions, probably because the blockage was beyond the reach of interventional catheters. Basilar artery occlusions were recanalized in 69% of patients. Thrombolysis of occlusions of the ICA bifurcation (the carotid "T" portion) was almost invariably unsuccessful. Embolic occlusions were more successfully recanalized than thrombosis engrafted upon in-situ atherosclerosis. Reocclusions did occur and transluminal angioplasty was sometimes used after thrombolysis to keep occluded arteries open. Recanalization was helped by mechanical clot disruption. Intracranial hemorrhagic complications occurred in 18.5% of patients and 42% of treated patients had good outcomes as judged by the authors of the reports.[111–114]

In other clinical studies, the vascular lesions were defined by angiography but thrombolytic drugs were given IV.[111–114] Only two of these studies had control patients that were not given a thrombolytic drug. In 6 series, rt-PA was given within 6 hours, and one study had an 8-hour window. Among 370 patients treated with IV rt-PA, one-third of the arteries treated showed significant recanalization compared to only 5% of 58 control arteries. MCA branch occlusions recanalized best followed by occlusions of the superior and inferior divisions of the MCA. Mainstem MCA occlusions recanalized less often than branch and division MCA lesions. ICA occlusions recanalized seldom and there were no recanalizations when both the ICA and MCA were occluded. Very few patients with

documented basilar artery occlusions were given IV rt-PA, and only one-sixth recanalized.[115] Embolic occlusions recanalized more often than in-situ thrombosis of atherostenotic arteries. Recanalization was better when there was angiographic evidence of good collateral circulation prior to administration of rt-PA. Both hemorrhagic infarction and hematomas were more common with IV than with IA treatment possibly because of the larger dose used in IV treatment.[111–114]

Randomized trials of intravenous and intra-arterial therapy

Intravenous thrombolytic therapy

Based on the encouraging results of observational studies, several randomized trials of IV and IA thrombolysis were performed during the past two decades. By 2014, at least 27 randomized trials enrolling over 10 000 patients had been reported.[116,117] Few of the IV randomized trials recommended or reported vascular testing before treatment; they used clinical findings and CT as entry requirements. The randomized trials of IA treatment required catheter or non-invasive angiography before treatment.

The first reported large multicenter randomized trial of IV thrombolysis was the European Cooperative Acute Stroke Study (ECASS) which included 620 patients with acute hemispheral strokes among 75 hospitals in 14 European countries.[118,119] A total of 313 patients were randomized to receive rt-PA (1.1 mg/kg) and 307 patients were randomized to placebo. Treatment was given within 6 hours of the onset of symptoms of brain ischemia. Patients who had major early infarct signs (diffuse hemispheral swelling, parenchymal hypodensity, effacement of cerebral sulci in >1/3 of the MCA territory) and hemorrhage on initial CT scans, which were read at the local site, were excluded. An independent blinded CT scan reading panel later retrospectively reviewed the CT scans and determined protocol violations of the CT scan entry criteria. Many patients (109 – including 66 patients in the rt-PA group and 43 in the placebo-treated group) were judged to have protocol deviations, mostly because of failure at local centers to recognize CT abnormalities that should have excluded patients. Considering the whole group of patients treated, the study was considered negative. There was a bimodal result – more patients treated with rt-PA had good outcomes but more patients did poorly and more patients died.[118,119]

In ECASS I, among rt-PA treated patients in the target population (those patients who had no protocol violations) there was a significantly better outcome and hospital stay was significantly shorter. Intracerebral hemorrhages and death were more common in rt-PA treated patients but these differences were not statistically significant. Large parenchymal hematomas were more often found in rt-PA treated patients. Patients treated with rt-PA within 3 hours did better than controls and those treated with rt-PA between 3 and 6 hours.[120]

The ECASS I study showed that treatment of patients with early infarct signs on CT scan could be hazardous. Reading of

the CT scans at the local hospitals was often unreliable. Some hemorrhages and many early infarcts were missed by local physicians. The mortality and brain hemorrhage rate among patients with protocol violations treated with rt-PA was extremely high, 33.3% and 40% respectively. Among 52 patients included in the study despite major early infarct signs, 40% died.[118-120]

The next two trials were reported together as the NINDS study.[121] The major study differences compared to ECASS were: lower rt-PA dose; earlier treatment (302 patients were treated within 90 min and 322 between 90 and 180 min); and no exclusion of patients because of brain ischemia on entry CT scans. Patients who received IV rt-PA were at least 30% more likely to have minor or no disability at 3 months. Symptomatic intracerebral hemorrhages were more common in the rt-PA treated patients (6.4% vs. 0.6%) and more often developed in patients who had more severe neurological deficits at entry and in patients 75 years or older. The mortality at 3 months was 17% in the rt-PA group versus 21% in the placebo group.[121] The benefit of lytic therapy seemed to be equal across the groups with varying etiologies, but the quick entry and absence of vascular and cardiac imaging made the clinical diagnosis of stroke etiology and mechanism tentative at best. A committee that reviewed the NINDS results reported that the stroke subtype results were not valid.[122]

Subsequent trials confirmed that IV rt-PA is beneficial in acute ischemic stroke, but also showed that its benefits are highly time dependent.[123-125] IV lytic therapy confers substantial benefit when started within the first 1.5 hours after onset (improving final outcome in 26/100 treated patients), solid benefit in the 1.5–3.0-hour window, and modest benefit in the 3.0–4.5-hour window. But the therapeutic yield steadily diminishes. Table 6.2 shows the odds ratio at 3 months of a favorable outcome using pooled data from the NINDS, ECASS, and Alteplase Thrombolysis for Acute Noninterventional Therapy in Ischemic Stroke (ATLANTIS) trials.

Between 1.0 and 4.5 hours after stroke onset, with every 10 minute delay in the start of rt-PA infusion, 1 fewer patient out of 100 has an improved disability outcome.[126] Beyond 4.5 hours of onset, treating unselected patients actually causes more harm than good.[127-130] Streptokinase use was associated with an unacceptable rate of bleeding.[131]

Intra-arterial thrombolysis

The first large, multicenter randomized trials of direct catheter delivery of pharmacological lytic agents to target cerebral clots were the Prolyse in Acute Cerebral Thromboembolism (PROACT) trials, which studied the effectiveness of IA administered pro-urokinase (r-proUK) in patients who had angiographically documented MCA occlusions.[132-134] PROACT I compared the recanalization rate of locally injected, IA r-proUK versus heparin within 6 hours of onset in patients with a radiographically proven MCA occlusion.[132] The interventionalist was not permitted to mechanically disturb the clot (contrary to the usual practice in the community) and was to inject r-proUK at the proximal end of the thrombus. There was successful recanalization in 15 out of 26 (58%) patients treated with r-proUK while 2 out of 14 patients (14%) recanalized with heparin alone.

PROACT II was more extensive.[133] Although it was an open-label study, the follow-up was blinded to medication versus placebo. About one-fifth of patients thought clinically by their doctors to have MCA occlusions had no occlusive arterial lesions at angiography. Forty percent of patients in the treatment group had slight or no neurological disability at day 90 compared with 25% of the control group ($P = 0.04$). The mortality rates were similar: 25% in the treatment group versus 27% in the placebo group. The symptomatic hemorrhage rate was 10% in the treatment group versus 2% in the placebo group ($P = 0.04$). The study showed favorable recanalization rates in the treatment group (66%) versus 18% in the control group ($P < 0.001$).[133] Patients overall benefited from IA thrombolysis despite the excess hemorrhage rate and there was no excess mortality.[133,134] Although IA thrombolytic treatment was effective and met the pre-trial guidelines discussed with the US Food and Drug Administration (FDA), the drug was not approved.

A randomized trial of IA urokinase in patients with angiographically confirmed occlusions of the M1 or M2 portions of one of the MCAs was performed in Japan.[135,136] IV heparin was given and angiograms performed. In patients with MCA occlusions IA urokinase was given and disruption of clot by guide-wire was allowed. Patients (57 in the urokinase group and 57 controls) were treated within 6 hours. Favorable outcome (Rankin score 0–2 at 90 days) was present in 49% of the urokinase group and 39% of the control group, and excellent

Table 6.2 Pooled analysis of the NINDS, ECASS, and ATLANTIS trials odds ratio for favorable outcome at 3 months after brain infarct

Time range	Odds ratio	Confidence interval	rt-PA treated	Placebo
0–90 min	2.81	1.75–4.5	161	150
91–180 min	1.55	1.12–2.15	302	315
181–270 min	1.40	1.05–1.85	390	411
270–360 min	1.15	0.90–1.47	538	508

From Lees KR, Bluhmki E, von Kummer R, et al. Time to treatment with intravenous alteplase and outcome in stroke: An updated pooled analysis of ECASS, ATLANTIS, NINDS, and EPITHET trials. *Lancet* 2010;375:1695–1703 with permission.

outcome (Rankin score 0–1 at 90 days) occurred in 42% of the urokinase group and 23% of controls.[135] Intracerebral hemorrhage during the first day occurred in 9% after IA urokinase and in 2% of controls. The death rate was 5% in the fibrinolytic group and 3.5% in the control group. The study was prematurely stopped when IV rt-PA was approved in Japan. Although the results did not show a statistically significant advantage of IA urokinase, the results looked promising if a sufficient number of patients had been enrolled.[136]

Results of thrombolytic drug use after FDA approval of rt-PA in the United States

Release of the results of the NINDS trial gave momentum to a movement in the United States to quickly (perhaps too quickly in our opinion) introduce IV thrombolysis widely into the community. During the summer of 1996, about half a year after the publication of the NINDS trial, the FDA approved the use of rt-PA for the treatment of stroke patients when the drug was given within the first 3 hours. Committees of the American Heart Association[137] and the American Academy of Neurology[138] published treatment recommendations that exactly followed the inclusion and exclusions and the treatment protocols of the NINDS trial. The recommendations suggest that a CT scan done before thrombolysis should not show major infarction, mass effect, edema, or hemorrhage. The guidelines do not require or suggest magnetic resonance imaging (MRI) or vascular tests before treatment. The most recent American Heart Association/American Stroke Association Guidelines published in 2013 concerning early management of adults with ischemic stroke provide some degree of additional sophistication concerning IV tPA administration.[139,140]

The post-marketing experience with IV rt-PA is an instructive example of the slow but increasing adoption of a novel treatment advance in conservative medical practice. Finally there was a drug that all agreed was an effective stroke treatment. Before tPA therapeutic nihilism prevailed. Approval of tPA was a wake-up call. *Stroke can and should be treated.* Stroke patients must be hustled quickly into medical centers, and doctors and hospitals must become prepared and able to treat them. Doctors and the media, politicians, and authorities called the attention of the public and of doctors to stroke.

But, unfortunately, doctors and medical centers were initially slow to heed the call. As a profoundly time-urgent treatment, thrombolytic therapy with IV rt-PA was a disruptive medical innovation that when first introduced could not easily be incorporated into existing patterns of care. Neurologists resisted the changes in practice that lytic therapy required, including the need to respond emergently to the emergency department.[141] Radiologists resisted reading CT or MR scans emergently, rather than the following morning during routine reading sessions.[142] Emergency physicians resisted having to give a therapy with risks as well as benefits, for a complex brain disease, if they were not supported by neurologist, radiologist, and institutional backing.[143] Delivering fibrinolytic therapy effectively required multiple system changes in acute stroke, including: cultural and generational change among neurologists to develop a critical mass of stroke specialists schooled in emergent response;[144,145] cultural and generational change among emergency physicians to develop a critical mass of emergency specialists ready to participate as vital members of stroke response teams;[146] hospital-level commitments to create stroke units and stroke centers;[12] development of regional and national certifying authorities to designate and regulate stroke centers;[147] changes in reimbursement to defray the added up-front costs of delivering fibrinolytic therapy (more than recouped at the system level by reduced long-term nursing home costs from implementation of an efficacious treatment);[148] supportive data confirming benefit from additional controlled trials and large-scale practice registries indicating safety and benefit in community as well as academic hospitals;[116,124,149–151] and studies indicating safety and benefit across race–ethnic groups with distinctive stroke etiologies and hemorrhage propensities (including Asians and blacks).[152–154]

Development of competent medical centers and stroke patients delivery to those centers

Not all hospitals are equally suited to manage acute brain ischemia patients. An important accomplishment was developing regional Comprehensive Stroke Centers with advanced capabilities in stroke management.[13] Many large US and European cities now have such centers. Also needed were community Primary Stroke Centers that were widely distributed and had adequate personnel and technology to efficiently and safely administer thrombolytics and supportive medical treatments.[155] Since many self-designated centers are not adequately equipped, criteria and evaluation strategies had to be developed for accrediting competent centers. Listed in Box 6.5 are alternatives for hospitals that receive acute stroke patients. Telemedicine has been used effectively for stroke in diverse locations throughout the world.[156–160] This allows doctors at stroke centers to help with the acute care of stroke patients at distant sites. The use of telemedicine has increased the frequency and appropriateness of stroke thrombolysis at rural hospitals and other facilities that do not have locally available neurologist expertise.[158,161]

Box 6.5 Alternatives for hospitals that receive acute stroke patients

1. If your medical center intends to treat acute stroke patients, develop systems and protocols for rapid delivery, efficient evaluation, and rapid throughput of patients with suspected acute strokes and TIAs. Be sure that physicians managing the patients are experienced in stroke care and the technology available is adequate
2. Choose not to accept patients suspected of having acute stroke and divert them to a nearby stroke center if such is available
3. Upgrade the facility to meet standards and then accept patients
4. If it is not feasible to divert to a nearby facility consider connecting with such a facility by telemedicine or consultative arrangements to facilitate care

---

Over the past decade, throughout the developed world, regional systems of acute care were built to route patients preferentially to thrombolysis-capable hospitals, increasing the frequency of treatment delivery.[162–165] In countries and regions with more advanced networks, IV fibrinolytic use within the first 3 hours of onset has increased from 1–2% to 5–20% of all ischemic stroke patients.[166–169]

Within established stroke centers, further improvements in outcome from IV rt-PA have been achieved by systematic efforts to reduce the time interval from patient arrival to start of drug infusion – the "door to needle (DTN) time." Because of the importance of rapid treatment, treatment guidelines recommend that hospitals complete the clinical and imaging evaluation of acute ischemic stroke patients and initiate IV tPA therapy within 60 minutes of patient arrival in those without contraindications.[139,170,171] Key best practice strategies that are associated with achieving faster DTN times in acute ischemic stroke include: (1) Emergency Medical Service pre-arrival-notification, allowing activation of the stroke team and readying of the CT scanner before patient arrival; (2) activating all stroke team members with a single group alert; (3) rapid acquisition and interpretation of brain imaging, pre-mixing rt-PA, rapid data feedback, and paramedic delivery of patients directly to CT scanners.[172,173] Implementation of these approaches reduced DTN times nationwide in the United States, with resulting reduced stroke mortality and improved functional outcomes.[174–183]

Clearly also important are the earliest steps: Educating patients and the public about calling 911 in the United States in case of suspected stroke; training those who answer the calls to recognize an acute neurological problem and to dispatch an ambulance as an emergency that is appropriately equipped with experienced personnel and technology; and training ambulance personnel in recognition of strokes and in their emergency management.

IA delivery of thrombolytic drugs was also pursued in the community and in academic centers after PROACT II.[135,184–186] However, in recent years, with the rise of mechanical catheter-based approaches to reperfusion (discussed later in this chapter), IA delivery of lytic drugs has become a secondary therapy, used to treat more distal occlusions in smaller intracranial arteries that mechanical devices cannot easily access.[135,184–188]

A look ahead – recent technology and therapeutic developments

Earlier treatment

Spurred by the availability of a proven treatment for acute ischemic stroke, researchers and clinicians have explored a number of new strategies for rapid treatment and reperfusion.[189] We list in Box 6.6 the most important new strategies.

The most expeditious way to begin treatment of patients is to begin treatment in the field when the ambulance personnel arrive. Physicians are exploring the feasibility of pre-hospital administration of drugs, especially

---

Box 6.6 New thrombolytic strategies

1. Faster treatment – even before the hospital. Use of mobile stroke units equipped with CT scanners
2. Lengthening the time window for treatment and improving selection of candidates by using more advanced CT, MRI, and ultrasound technologies including vascular imaging
3. Telemedicine communications with stroke centers
4. Newer thrombolytics
5. Bridging strategies – IV and then selective IA thrombolysis
6. Enhancing thrombolysis by using transcranial Doppler-related techniques
7. Multiple reperfusion and neuroprotection combinations
8. Mechanical recanalization as an assist to thrombolysis

---

neuroprotective agents.[190–192] Theoretically increasing the brain's resistance to ischemia would provide a longer time window for thrombolysis. Several neuroprotective agents have been tested in initial trials, including magnesium sulfate, nitroglycerin, and remote ischemic conditioning.[192–195] With this approach treatment can be initiated within the first 60 minutes after onset, the "golden hour" when the great preponderance of threatened brain tissue is still salvageable.[193] The Field Administration of Stroke Therapy–Magnesium (FAST-MAG) trial was a large innovative study carried out in southern California between 2005 and 2013.[192] It involved collaboration between 315 ambulances, 40 emergency medical service agencies, 60 receiving hospitals, and 2988 paramedics. The study showed that 74% of the 1700 study patients in Los Angeles and Orange counties were treated within the first hour, with the magnesium administered within a median time of 45 minutes.[192] Unfortunately, the administration of magnesium at the ambulance site was not shown to be effective. The study did demonstrate the feasibility of treating acute stroke patients rapidly and in the field.

Better clinical and technological diagnosis in the field would also accelerate early treatment. An intriguing approach to accelerate the start of IV rt-PA is to deploy a specialized stroke ambulance that is equipped with a mobile CT scanner, a mobile blood laboratory, and a neurologist on board, in person or via telemedicine. This strategy "brings the hospital to the patient, rather than the patient to the hospital," allowing the brain to be imaged and rt-PA to be started at the scene.[196,197] In the Prehospital Acute Neurological Treatment and Optimization of Medical care in Stroke Study (PHANTOM-S) randomized trial in Germany, a mobile CT ambulance was deployed in intervention weeks and compared with standard ambulance transport in 6182 code stroke transports. Patients treated in the specialized stroke ambulance received IV rt-PA 25 minutes faster than patients treated after transport to hospital in a standard ambulance.[198] Further studies are needed to determine if the stroke-mobile approach is cost-effective and can be made feasible in diverse geographical settings.[199]

Selection of candidates for thrombolysis using modern up-to-date technology

When the ECASS and NINDS studies were planned, available technology was limited. Since then there has been a dramatic up-grade in MRI, CT, and ultrasound technology. The capability of this technology to yield information about the presence, location, and amount of infarcted brain and arterial and venous occlusions has been discussed in detail in Chapter 4. Most authorities agree that thrombolysis can be effective if given up to 4.5 hours following present guidelines, but are the present guidelines optimal? Could thrombolytic treatment be improved? Are there patients now excluded such as those who awaken with neurological symptoms, those who have minor deficits or have improved substantially, and those treatable only after 4.5 hours that could respond to treatment? Are there some patients now treated under the guidelines who should not be treated because of little likelihood of success and high risk of hemorrhage or edema?

Knowledge gained from modern brain and vascular imaging can help select for IV thrombolysis treatment some patients now included and excluded under present guidelines. The present guidelines are: Use a firm 4.5-hour window; do not incorporate vascular imaging in decision-making; exclude patients who awaken with deficits; and exclude patients who have mild or improving signs.

1. Some patients have brain that is at risk for further ischemia hours after the present 4.5 hour deadline. Early and recent studies document many instances of improvement and recanalization after the 4.5-hour window when the volume of irreversibly infarcted tissue is still small and volume of threatened tissue is still large.[112,114,115,200–205]

2. Patients who awaken with neurological symptoms often have brain and vascular imaging that shows treatable vascular occlusion patterns and no or small infarcts and are excellent candidates for thrombolysis.[206,207]

3. Many patients who enter with slight deficits or improving signs later develop severe strokes. Improving or slight deficits are one of the most common reasons patients are now excluded from thrombolysis. Several series show that a substantial number of patients who later deteriorate have occlusive vascular lesions that are amenable to thrombolytic treatment.[208–211]

4. Many patients already have large infarcts and little recoverable brain when brain imaging is performed within 3 hours. These patients can be harmed by thrombolysis.[5,118]

5. Seizures at or near onset do occur in some acute ischemic stroke patients, especially those with embolic strokes.[212] The occurrence of a seizure should not exclude an otherwise appropriate candidate for thrombolysis from being treated.

Knowing whether there is an arterial occlusion and its location and the extent of infarction already present might lead clinicians to choose no thrombolysis, IV treatment, or to consider catheter-based treatment, or combined IV then catheter-based treatment. The site of arterial occlusion and the size of the clot ("clot burden") clearly strongly effects the likelihood of reperfusion after IV thrombolysis.[112,114,200,201,212,213] The more one knows about the patient, the more logically the clinician can choose acute and more chronic treatment. The present guidelines would benefit from futher revision to account for information gained since the original NINDS trials about tailoring thrombolytic therapy to each individual's stroke process.

Modern MRI and CT protocols along with clinical data are now being used to attempt to better select patients likely to benefit from thrombolysis and those at most risk of hemorrhage and other complications.[214–230] A selection system based on pathology and pathophysiology is preferred over selection by a clock. Trials (the Echoplanar Imaging Thrombolytic Evaluation Trial (EPITHET),[205] the Desmoteplase in Acute Ischemic Stroke Trial (DIAS),[231] and the Diffusion and Perfusion Imaging Evaluation for Understanding Stroke Evolution trial (DEFUSE)[5]) and extensive experience[225] have established the feasibility of using modern brain and vascular imaging to optimally choose patients for thrombolysis.

Three trials (DEDAS, DIAS 1, and DIAS 2) have tested using brain and vascular imaging to select patients beyond 3 hours of onset for IV thrombolysis with desmoteplase.[223,232,233] Desmoteplase is derived from vampire bat saliva and is a plasminogen activator fibrinolytic enzyme with high fibrin selectivity and a long-terminal half-life.[234] Fibrin-selectivity is important since the agent tends to bind at the site of the thrombus and not cause systemic fibrinogenolysis. In the 3 demoteplase trials patients were selected for fibrinolysis if they had core infarcts smaller than at risk penumbral regions on MRI and CT within a 3–9-hour window. When the more reliable MRI selection method was employed, patients treated with desmoteplase had a higher rate of reperfusion and better clinical outcomes than placebo-treated controls.[231]

The DEFUSE trial studied whether MRI criteria helped determine responders to IV tPA in patients treated between 3 and 6 hours after stroke symptom onset.[5] A perfusion–diffusion mismatch occurred in 54% of patients with interpretable perfusion scans and, in this group, early reperfusion was associated with a favorable response in 56% of patients compared to only 19% of patients with no mismatch. In addition, those with large diffusion-weighted imaging (DWI) lesions fared worse with a very low rate of good clinical response and a high rate of hemorrhage when reperfusion occurred.[5] Magnetic resonance angiograms (MRA) showed that 44 of 68 (65%) patients had a symptomatic arterial occlusion before treatment. Complete early recanalization occurred in 27% and partial recanalization in 16% as determined by follow-up MRA. Patients with early recanalization had a 74% reduction in perfusion-weighted imaging (PWI) volume compared with 16% with no recanalization.[5] Symptomatic intracerebral bleeding occurred in 9.5% of patients, especially in those with a large DWI volume infarct before thrombolysis.[225]

The EPITHET randomized patients with a favorable MRI profile 3–6 hours after stroke onset to IV rt-PA or placebo.[205] Among the 101 enrolled patients, reperfusion was more

common with rt-PA than with placebo and was associated with less infarct growth, better neurological outcome, and better functional outcome than was no reperfusion. The investigators posited that 200–300 MRI-selected late patients would need to be enrolled to definitively confirm benefit in a successor trial.[205]

EPITHET, DEFUSE, and the desmoteplase trials strongly suggest that MRI and MRA could be used effectively to select patients for thrombolysis even within the 4.5–9.0-hour window. Modern CT profiles that include CTA and perfusion CT should also be able to select patients with arterial occlusions with no or small infarcts and larger perfusion defects that would be amenable to thrombolysis irrespective of time.[215,216,235–237]

Box 6.7 lists the data needed for optimal treatment of patients with acute brain ischemia.

Improving intravenous thrombolysis

Stroke physicians recognize that IV rt-PA is often ineffective. The success in chemically digesting the clot and achieving recanalization varies with the volume of the target thrombus – the clot burden. In smaller, distal arteries, like the M2 branches of the MCA, rt-PA achieves early reperfusion 60–70% of the time. In the larger M1 stem segment of the MCA, early reperfusion rates are only 40–50%. And in the very large terminal ICA, IV rt-PA yields early reperfusion only 5–15% of the time.[197] Strategies to improve IV recanalization rates include testing newer generation thrombolytic drugs,[238] combining rt-PA with other modalities such as ultrasound,[239,240] and drugs to enhance its effectiveness, giving IV tPA first and then pursuing intra-arterial tPA or catheter mechanical thrombectomy treatment if large arteries remain occluded.[240–247]

Thrombolytics other than rt-PA

Streptokinase

Streptokinase has been used widely in patients with coronary ischemia, although patients with past strokes were excluded from most streptokinase cardiac trials. There were three randomized trials of IV streptokinase in patients with acute ischemic strokes; all were stopped prematurely because of a high rate of brain hemorrhages in patients treated with

streptokinase.[131] No vascular studies were reported and inclusion depended on CT scan results. Researchers and clinicians speculated that the dose of streptokinase may have been excessive in these trials and the drug could be effective at lower doses,[244] but no streptokinase trials have been launched.

Urokinases

IV and IA urokinase was used often in early pre-NINDS observational studies and continues to be given in some medical centers.[249–253] r-ProUK was used in the successful PROACT trials,[132–134] but has not been approved to be marketed and is not presently available.[250] IA urokinase was used in the Middle Cerebral Artery Embolism Local Fibrinolytic Intervention Trial (MELT) in Japan, and showed promise.[135]

Ancrod

Ancrod, a purified venom extract from the Malaysian pit viper induces rapid systemic defibrinogenation.[254–256] It has been used in Canada and Europe since the 1970s in patients with peripheral limb vascular disease, deep vein thrombosis, and central retinal artery thrombosis to induce reperfusion.[256] Two preliminary studies in the 1980s involving respectively 20 and 30 ischemic stroke patients indicated that ancrod was possibly safe and effective.[257,258]

A randomized, placebo-controlled trial was performed in the United States of ancrod in ischemic stroke patients ($N = 132$) treated within 6 hours of symptom onset.[254] Neurological function as measured by the Scandinavian Stroke Scale was significantly better in the ancrod-treated patients ($P = 0.04$) and there were no recognized symptomatic intracranial hemorrhages. No vascular studies were reported so that the mechanism of improvement was not clear. Did the lowering of fibrinogen lyse occlusive clots? Did lowering of fibrinogen effectively reduce blood viscosity so that blood flow was increased in collateral vessels?

A second study, The Stroke Treatment with Ancrod Trial (STAT), was performed in the United States and Canada.[255] A total of 500 patients with acute or progressing ischemic deficits were treated with a continuous 72 hour infusion of ancrod ($N = 248$) or placebo ($N = 252$) followed by 1 hour infusions at 96 and 120 hours. The aim was to reduce fibrinogen levels to below 200. More patients treated with ancrod achieved favorable functional status than those treated with placebo (42.2% vs. 34.4%, $P = 0.04$). There were more symptomatic and asymptomatic intracranial hemorrhages in the ancrod treated group. No data about vascular lesions was included in the report of the trial.[255] The European Stroke Treatment with Ancrod trial (ESTAT) was performed and enrolled 1222 patients.[259] Patients were treated within 6 hours in contrast to the 3-hour window in the STAT trial. Functional outcome at 3 months was the same in the ancrod and placebo-treated groups. There were more hemorrhages and more deaths in the ancrod-treated group.[259] No further trials of ancrod are being pursued or planned, as far as we know.

Tenecteplase

Tenecteplase (TNK) is a biogenetic variant of wild-type rt-PA that may be given as a single bolus injection.[254] It is posited to have an eightfold higher affinity for fibrin and a longer halflife than rt-PA. In a trial of 17 000 patients with myocardial infarction, TNK was compared with rt-PA in reference to bleeding; fewer patients treated with TNK had major systemic bleeding but intracranial bleeding and mortality were similar.[260] For stroke patients, a preliminary dose-finding trial found too high a rate of hemorrhage at a dose of 0.4 mg/kg, but lower doses of 0.1 and 0.25 mg/kg appeared promising when compared with IV rt-PA in under 3 hour patients.[261] An Australian trial compared two doses of TNK (0.1 and 2.5 mg/kg) versus IV rt-PA in patients selected by CT imaging to have known occlusions in medium-sized arteries (middle, anterior, or posterior cerebral artery) and perfusion-core mismatch.[262] The TNK groups had more frequent reperfusion, 79% versus 55%, and more frequent final good recovery, 72% versus 44%.[262] Given these promising findings, TNK is currently being studied in larger trials.

Desmoteplase

As noted earlier when discussing imaging selection, desmoteplase is derived from vampire bat saliva and is a plasminogen activator fibrinolytic enzyme with high fibrin selectivity and a long-terminal half-life.[234] Desmoteplase's signals of potential benefit in the Desmoteplase in Acute Ischemic Stroke (DIAS)[233] and Dose Escalation of Desmoteplase for Acute Ischemic Stroke (DEDAS)[232] trials are now being followed up with larger, definitive international trials.

Reperfusion using mechanical techniques

Catheter-based mechanical thrombectomy techniques to reopen acutely occluded arteries have made rapid technical advances over the past decade. Endovascular mechanical therapies offer several distinct advantages over both IV and IA delivery of thrombolytic drugs.[263] Catheter-based mechanical therapies typically work more rapidly, achieving recanalization within a few minutes, rather than the up to 120 minutes required with lytic drug administration. Mechanical techniques may have lower intracerebral and systemic hemorrhage risk, due to the avoidance of pharmacological lysis. Catheter-based mechanical therapies are more effective removing large clot burdens in proximal vessels, such as carotid T occlusions, where the sheer volume of clot to be digested retards pharmacological lysis. And the most recently developed catheter-based mechanical thrombectomy devices are more effective at achieving substantial reperfusion than pharmacological approaches.[263,264] At times, papaverine is infused IA during mechanical thrombectomy to reduce the vasoconstriction that can follow mechanical perturbation of the endothelium.[265]

The variety of target vascular lesions in acute ischemic stroke has fostered development of a range of mechanical treatment options. In many patients, the intracranial occlusion is an embolus that has arisen from the heart or an arterial source, such as the aorta or the cervical carotid artery, and landed in a relatively normal recipient brain artery. Such target thrombi respond well to devices that fish the clot out (retrieval devices) or suck the clot out (aspiration devices). In other patients, the occlusive lesion is comprised largely of a local atherosclerotic plaque with small thrombus on top of it. Retrieval and aspiration devices may be able to remove the small thrombus component of these blockages, but not the atherosclerotic plaque. However, the plaque can respond well to angioplasty and stenting, which mechanically crack open the underlying atherosclerotic lesions.

The currently widely employed endovascular mechanical interventions can be classified into three categories: angioplasty/stent devices; suction thrombectomy devices; and thrombus retrieval devices.

Angioplasty and/or stenting

Angioplasty and/or stenting are highly effective at reopening blocked brain arteries when target occlusions are local atherosclerotic plaques with superimposed occlusive thrombi,[266–268] but there are risks associated with the angioplasty and/or stenting strategy. Compared with heart arteries, intracranial arteries are more prone to vessel dissection and to a "snow plow" effect in which plaque displaced by the stent piles up and blocks the opening of small perforating branches exiting the parent artery. As a result, acute angioplasty and stenting is currently used as a fallback strategy, when other approaches have not been successful.

Suction thrombectomy

Suction thrombectomy devices use vacuum aspiration to suck the occlusive clot out of the blocked artery. The first successful suction device was the Penumbra system. Progress in developing aspiration devices required a technical solution to the problem of clogging of aspiration tips, a common occurrence when applyiing suction through the small catheter tubes that could be maneuvered to intracranial arteries. The Penumbra system overcame this obstacle by adding a separator wire with a bulbous tip inside the suction tube. A physician continually advances and retracts the separator wire while the vacuum is turned on, keeping the tip of the catheter tube clear and also pulling in thrombus ahead of the catheter. In a multicenter study, the Penumbra System was tested in 125 patients within 8 hours of onset who were ineligible for rt-PA or who had received rt-PA but failed to recanalize.[269] The average National Institutes of Health Stroke Scale (NIHSS) score was 18. The system was able to be technically deployed in the vast preponderance of patients. Symptomatic intracranial hemorrhage occurred in 11.2% of patients and independent final outcomes tended to be more frequent among patients in whom recanalization was achieved, 29% versus 9%.[269] In subsequent large single series, rates of substantial reperfusion with the Penumbra system have been 50–75%.[270,271]

A recent innovation in suction thrombectomy has been the development of larger bore catheters that are flexible and steerable enough to be maneuvered to target clots in intracranial arteries. With these larger devices, clogging of the tip during direct aspiration without a separator wire is not a problem, and substantial vacuum power can be generated

simply by having the physician pull back strongly with a syringe. In large series of acute stroke patients treated with direct aspiration, immediate substantial reperfusion rates have been 50–75%, improving to 85–95% when retrieval devices were used in cases that did not open with direct aspiration alone.[272,273]

Clot retrieval devices

Clot retrieval devices were first developed to capture coils and other foreign bodies that had embolized within the brain circulation during endovascular procedures. A natural next step was to apply these devices to capture and remove naturally arising thromboemboli. These devices ensnare a thrombus and then withdraw it out of the body. The first approved family of retrieval devices were the Merci retrievers. These devices look like corkscrews, and pull the clot out of the artery like a corkscrew removing a cork from a wine bottle. The Mechanical Embolus Removal in Cerebral Ischemia (MERCI) study evaluated the safety and efficacy of this mechanical embolectomy device. The prospective, non-randomized, multicenter trial enrolled 151 patients who were ineligible for IV tPA.[274] Substantial recanalization was achieved in 48% (68/141) of patients in whom the device was deployed. Clinically important procedural complications occurred in 10 (7.1%) patients. Symptomatic intracranial hemorrhages developed in 11 of 141 (7.8%) patients. Good neurological outcomes (modified Rankin score (mRS) ≤2) were more frequent at 90 days in patients with successful recanalization compared with patients with unsuccessful recanalization (46% vs. 10%; and mortality was less (32% vs. 54%, $P = 0.01$)).[274] As a result of this trial the MERCI retriever in 2004 became the first device approved by the US FDA for use in patients with acute intracranial occlusions.

The Multi-MERCI then evaluated the Merci Retrievers in a broader group of patients within 8 hours of symptom onset, including patients who had received IV tPA but did not recanalize.[275] The primary outcomes were vascular recanalization and safety. Among 164 patients in whom the thrombectomy procedure was performed, 48 (29%) had received IV tPA before intervention. Treatment with the retriever alone resulted in substantial recanalization in 90 (55%) patients and 112 (68%) after adjunctive therapy (IA tPA or other mechanical manipulation). Symptomatic intracranial hemorrhage occurred in 16 (9.8%) patients, 5 of 48 (10.4%) in patients pretreated with IV tPA, and 11 of 116 (9.5%) in those without. Clinically significant procedural complications occurred in 9 (5.5%) patients, including groin hemorrhages and emboli to previously uninvolved territories.[276]

The most recent and most successful family of thrombectomy devices to be developed are the stent retrievers.[277,278] These are mesh columns that are expanded inside the target clot, pushing it aside and entangling it within the crossing struts of the stent. The stent is then withdrawn in its unfolded state, bringing out with it the enmeshed thrombus. Stent retrievers have two major advantages over the Merci corkscrew retriever and other retrieval devices: (1) restoration of flow immediately upon deployment within the target artery, rather than only upon successful clot extraction; and (2) substantially higher successful recanalization rates than other embolectomy devices.

The stent retrievers were tested against corkscrew retrievers in two randomized trials. The first was the Solitaire With the Intention For Thrombectomy (SWIFT) trial, a multicenter, prospective, randomized trial.[279] SWIFT was designed to enroll 200 patients undergoing neurothrombectomy, randomizing them to treatment with the Solitaire stent retriever or the Merci corkscrew retriever as the first deployed device. However, the trial was stopped early by the Data Safety and Monitoring Board, after only 113 patients were enrolled, due to overwhelming demonstration of superiority of the Solitaire device at an interim analysis. Substantial recanalization was achieved more often with the stent retriever. When the stent retriever was the first device deployed, substantial recanalization was achieved with the device in 37 of 54 patients (69%) and after additional adjunctive therapy (IA tPA or other mechanical) in 48 of 54 (89%). When the corkscrew retriever was the first device used, substantial recanalization was attained with the device in 16 of 53 patients (30%) and after adjunctive therapy in 37 of 55 (67%). The better recanalization rates translated into better clinical outcomes. Good neurological outcome at 3 months was achieved in 32 of 55 (58%) patients treated with the stent retriever versus 16 of 48 patients (33%) treated with the corkscrew retriever. The rates of symptomatic intracranial hemorrhage were markedly lower in stent retriever than corkscrew retriever patients, 1.7%, versus 10.9%. Death by 3 months after stroke was reduced in the stent retriever arm, 17.2% versus 38.2%.[279]

Similar results were found for a different stent retriever, the Trevo device, in the Thrombectomy REvascularization of large Vessel Occlusions in acute ischemic stroke (TREVO) 2 trial.[280] The multicenter study randomized 178 patients to initial treatment with the Trevo stent retriever or the Merci corkscrew retriever. Better vessel reopening occurred with the stent retriever, with minimal or greater recanalization with the first device type used in 86% of stent retriever patients versus 60% of corkscrew retriever patients. Better functional outcome resulted, with independence at 3 months in 40% of stent retriever patients versus 22% of corkscrew retriever patients. However, unlike with the Solitaire stent retriever in the SWIFT trial, hemorrhage rates were not reduced with the Trevo stent retriever and death by 3 months tended to be increased compared with the corkscrew retriever, 34.1% versus 24.1%.[280]

A challenge in medical research, particularly when studying rapidly evolving device therapies, is that technologies may evolve so quickly that treatments being studied in a multi-year clinical trial may already be outmoded by the time the study is concluded. This phenomenon occurred with catheter-based reperfusion therapies for acute ischemic stroke.[193] Before the stent retrievers were developed, three randomized trials were started to evaluate first generation catheter-based approaches. The SYNTHESIS expansion (362 patients), Interventional Management of Stroke III (IMS-III) (656 patients), and the Mechanical Retrieval and Recanilization of Stroke Clots Using Embolectomy (MR RESCUE)

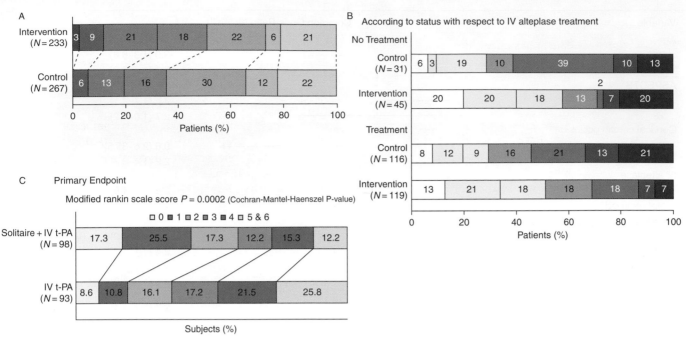

Figure 6.3 Modified Rankin scale outcomes in the (A) MR CLEAN, (B) ESCAPE, and (C) SWIFT PRIME trials.

(118 patients) tested primarily combinations of IA thrombolysis and corkscrew retrievers.[281–283] All three trials had disappointing results, failing to show an added benefit of first-generation catheter-based treatments above that of IV tPA or supportive medical care alone. However, just as these trials were being completed, the stent retrievers appeared and were shown to be far superior to first-generation catheter therapies.

The results of the SWIFT and TREVO trials suggested a potential new era in reperfusion therapy for acute cerebral ischemia. For the first time, stroke physicians can offer patients a highly effective recanalization intervention, achieving substantial reperfusion in 80–95% of patients. During the first few months of 2015, 3 trials showed that intra-arterial therapy of selected patients with acute occlusions of large intracranial anterior circulation arteries was more effective than standard treatment including IV tPA. The Multicenter Randomized Clinical Trial of Endovascular Treatment for Acute Ischemic Stroke in the Netherlands (MR CLEAN) trial was a phase 3 multicenter clinical trial performed in the Netherlands characterized by randomized treatment-group assignments, open-label treatment, and blinded end-point evaluation.[284] Patients with a NIHSS score of 2 or higher who could be treated IA within 6 hours were included if acute vascular imaging (computed tomography angiography (CTA), magnetic resonance angiography (MRA), or digital subtraction angiography (DSA)) showed occlusion of the intracranial ICA, MCA (M1 or M2) or anterior cerebral artery (ACA). IV tPA was given to 445 patients (89%) before randomization. Among the 500 acute ischemic stroke patients, 233 were assigned to intra-arterial treatment and 267 to usual care alone. Intra-arterial treatment consisted of retrievable stents in 190 of the 233 patients (81.5%) assigned to intra-arterial treatment. The median NIHSS score before treatment was 17 in the intra-arterial

group and 18 in the control usual care group. The results showed a shift in the distribution of the primary-outcome scores in favor of intra-arterial treatment. The adjusted common odds ratio (OR) was 1.67 (95% confidence interval (CI), 1.21–2.30).[284] The mRS at 90 days are shown in Figure 6.3A in this trial. The shift toward better outcomes in favor of the intervention was consistent for all categories of the mRS, except death. The absolute between-group difference in the proportion of patients who were functionally independent (mRS 0–2) was 13.5 percentage points (95% CI, 5.9–21.2) in favor of intra-arterial treatment (32.6% vs. 19.1%), with an adjusted OR of 2.16 (95% CI, 1.39–3.38). There were no significant differences in mortality or the occurrence of symptomatic intracerebral hemorrhage.[284]

The Endovascular Treatment for Small Core and Anterior Circulation Proximal Occlusion with Emphasis on Minimizing CT to Recanalization Times (ESCAPE) trial, with headquarters in Calgary, Canada, randomly assigned 118 patients with acute ischemic stroke to receive standard care (the control group) and 118 to receive standard care and endovascular treatment using a thrombectomy device.[285] Patients with a proximal intracranial occlusion (ICA or MCA, M1 or M2) in the anterior circulation shown by CTA who had small infarct cores, and good collateral circulation were included when treated up to 12 hours after symptom onset. IV tPA was given to 238 patients (120 in the intervention group and 118 in the control group). Patients were investigated and treated very quickly in this study. In the intervention group, the median time from CT to first reperfusion was 84 minutes. Modern stent retrievers were used and clot retrieval was performed sooner than in preceding trials. The trial was stopped early for efficacy. The rate of functional independence (90 day mRS 0–2) was (53.0%, vs. 29.3% in the control group; P < 0.001) (Figure 6.3B). This primary outcome favored the intervention (common OR, 2.6;

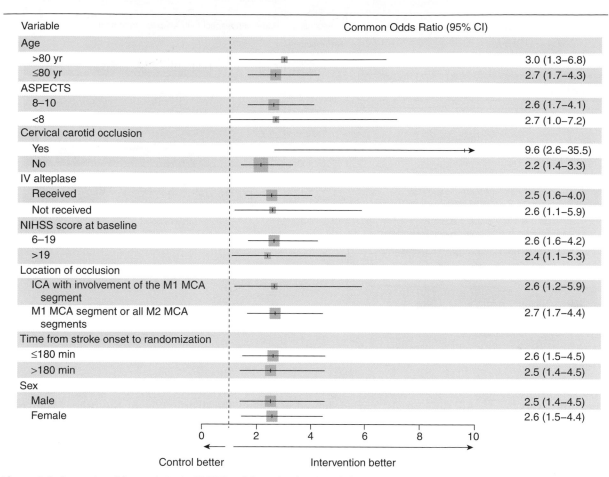

Variable	Common Odds Ratio (95% CI)	
Age		
>80 yr		3.0 (1.3–6.8)
≤80 yr		2.7 (1.7–4.3)
ASPECTS		
8–10		2.6 (1.7–4.1)
<8		2.7 (1.0–7.2)
Cervical carotid occlusion		
Yes		9.6 (2.6–35.5)
No		2.2 (1.4–3.3)
IV alteplase		
Received		2.5 (1.6–4.0)
Not received		2.6 (1.1–5.9)
NIHSS score at baseline		
6–19		2.6 (1.6–4.2)
>19		2.4 (1.1–5.3)
Location of occlusion		
ICA with involvement of the M1 MCA segment		2.6 (1.2–5.9)
M1 MCA segment or all M2 MCA segments		2.7 (1.7–4.4)
Time from stroke onset to randomization		
≤180 min		2.6 (1.5–4.5)
>180 min		2.5 (1.4–4.5)
Sex		
Male		2.5 (1.4–4.5)
Female		2.6 (1.5–4.4)

Control better — Intervention better

Figure 6.4 Forest plot of the results in the ESCAPE trial. From Goyal M, Demchuk AM, Menon BK et al. for the ESCAPE Trial Investigators. Randomized assessment of rapid endovascular treatment if ischemic stroke. *N Engl J Med* 2015;371:1019–1030 with permission.

95% CI, 1.7–3.8; $P < 0.001$), and the intervention was associated with reduced mortality (10.4%, vs. 19.0% in the control group, $P = 0.04$). Symptomatic intracerebral hemorrhage occurred in 3.6% in the intervention group and 2.7% of participants in the control group ($P = 0.75$).[285] The forest plot showing the results of this trial is shown in Figure 6.4.

The Solitaire With the Intention For Thrombectomy as PRIMary Endovascular treatment (SWIFT PRIME) trial was also stopped because of efficacy after 98 patients each were randomized to an IV tPA group or an interventional group that was treated with IV tPA and clot retrieval using a Solitaire stent retriever.[286] Inclusions were: IV tPA given within 4.5 hours and stent retriever able to be applied within 6 hours after stroke onset; CTA confirmation of an intracranial ICA occlusion or an M1 occlusion; infarct core less than one-third MCA territory or less than 100 ml. IV tPA was given within 2 hours in each group. The results showed an increase in good functional outcomes and a decrease in death and severe disability. Functional independence (mRS 0–2 at 90 days) was attained by 60% of patients treated with IV tPA plus Solitaire thrombus retrieval compared to 36% of patients treated with IV tPA alone.[286] (Figure 6.3C).

The Extending the Time for Thrombolysis in Emergency Neurological Deficits–Intra-Arterial (Extend IA) trial was an investigator-initiated trial performed in Australia and New Zealand.[287] The protocol was similar to the trials above. The goal was to assess whether treatment using IV tPa followed by intervention using an intra-arterial stent retriever (Solitaire) had better outcomes than treatment with IV tPA alone. Patients needed to be eligible to receive IV tPA within 4.5 hours. Inclusion criteria included an intracranial ICA or M1 or M2 occlusion, infarct volume less than 70 ml, and a mismatch as determined on a rapid evaluation (Stanford) multimodal CT imaging protocol. Groin puncture must be made before 6 hours for patients to be included. The study was stopped after 70 patients were treated for efficacy. Early recovery occurred in 37% of the IV tPA group versus 80% in the interventional group, and 9 patients died in the interventional group versus 20 in the IV tPA-alone group.[287] The number needed to treat (NNT) with interventional treatment was similar to that found in the other trials.

These trials showed that rapid interventional treatment using stent retrievers in carefully selected acute ischemic stroke patients was very effective. Patients should be evaluated using modern CT and/or MRI protocols. Patients selected for interventional treatment should have: intracranial large artery occlusions, no or small infarct cores, and good potential collateral vessels. These selected patients should be treated at

advanced stroke centers by interventionalists who have training and experience and good track records.

Multiple neuroprotective and thrombolytic combinations –– The history of acute stroke treatment reflects the limited effectiveness of any single treatment. Reperfusion of occluded arteries is considered by all to be the single most important goal of treatment. Reperfusion is strongly associated with improved clinical outcome.[266] The faster that arteries are opened, the better the outcome.[124,151,288,289]. Even late reperfusion is associated with better outcomes than failure to reperfuse.[290,291] Unfortunately, thrombolysis is underutilized often because appropriate candidates for thrombolysis do not reach stroke centers equipped to manage them in sufficient time to be treated effectively.

Even in patients who are treated "in time," IV recanalizes the occluded artery 40% of the time. Researchers and clinicians have begun to explore multiple sequential or concurrent treatments – a "cocktail' approach.[292] The three most commonly used strategies are: (1) giving a neuroprotective drug before thrombolysis in an attempt to lengthen the time window available for thrombolysis. Increasing the brain's resistance to ischemia could lengthen the time that reperfusion might save neurons; (2) augmenting the effect of the presently used thrombolytic agents by using antiplatelet or anticoagulant drugs concurrently or after thrombolysis to open arteries and to keep arteries open; and (3) using mechanical thrombectomy or IA lysis as a second recanalization intervention when IV tPA alone has not reopened a target artery.

Clinicians continue to search for effective neuroprotective agents. Unfortunately the search has been mostly unsuccessful. We discuss neuroprotection in some detail later in this chapter. Combining neuroprotection with thrombolysis has several potential advantages. Ambulance delivery of neuroprotective agents could stabilize threatened tissues, so that more salvageable brain is present when IV tPA is given after hospital arrival. Although magnesium sulfate delivered in the ambulance was not found to be beneficial in the FAST-MAG trial, early trials have suggested potential benefits from ambulance administration of nitroglycerin, which alters brain nitric oxide signaling, and of remote ischemic conditioning, which induces brain resistant to hypoxia by briefly inflating blood pressure cuffs on the arms to make them temporarily ischemic.[194,195]

Physicians are exploring the potential for hypothermia to be used in combination with thrombolysis.[293–295] Hypothermia is an extremely powerful neuroprotective intervention in animal models. Theoretically the concurrent use of a safe and an effective neuroprotectant might help resuscitate ischemic neurons, protect against reperfusion injury, as well as lengthen the time window for reperfusion.[295]

In many patients IV thrombolytic agents are ineffective in lysing clots and in effecting important reperfusion. In other patients thrombolysis is initially effective but the artery reoccludes.[296] Alexandrov and Grotta found that reocclusion after initial recanalization developed in about one-third of their patients who had initially recanalized after IV rt-PA.[296] Clinicians have explored the use of glycoprotein (Gp) IIb/IIIa inhibitors and direct thrombin inhibitors as an adjunct to thrombolysis and other reperfusion strategies. The Gp

IIb/IIIa inhibitors abciximab,[297,298] tirofiban,[299–301] and eptifibatide,[302,303] have all been administered in preliminary studies along with thrombolytics. Hemorrhage was a major concern in the Abciximab in Emergent Stroke Treatment Trial (AbESTT), a trial of abciximab for acute ischemic stroke,[298,304] and was a problem when abciximab was combined with neurointerventional procedures and thrombolysis.[297] Tirofiban has been used: with heparin before IA urokinase and mechanical devices;[93] concurrent with IV rt-PA;[94] and after IV rt-PA.[95] The dose of thrombolytics was usually reduced. Preliminary results were suggestive of an added effect and hemorrhage was not a major problem in these preliminary explorations with tirofiban. Eptifibatide was used in combination with a reduced dose (0.6 mg/kg) of IV tPA in two multicenter trials.[302,303] In the most recent trial, among 126 randomized subjects, 101 were assigned to the combined treatment arm.[304] Patients in the combined treatment group tended to have a lower symptomatic hemorrhage rate (2% vs. 12%) and a higher rate of final excellent outcome (50% vs. 36%).[304] The Argatroban tPA Stroke Study explored the safety and efficacy of giving argatroban after IV rt-PA.[305,306] Among the 65 enrolled patients treated with combination therapy, the rate of symptomatic hemorrhage was 4.6% and early recanalization assessed by transcranial Doppler (TCD) occurred in 61%, suggesting safety and potential greater efficacy than IV tPA alone.[305,306]

Standard anticoagulants and antiplatelet agents have also been used as adjuncts to thrombolytic drugs.[307] Heparin has been variously used immediately after IV and IA thrombolysis although its use was prohibited for 24 hours in the 2 NINDS and the 2 PROACT trials. In one study the use of heparin just after thrombolysis did not increase the rate of symptomatic hemorrhagic complications.[308] In another study, among 300 consecutive acute stroke patients treated with IV rt-PA, 92 were pre-treated with aspirin (100–500 mg) and with low-dose (N = 122) or high-dose (N = 153) heparin.[309] The authors concluded that pre-treatment with aspirin in this group of patients did not increase the rate of symptomatic hemorrhage even in those also given heparin.[309] Addition of aspirin to IV tPA was subsequently found to be harmful in a randomized trial. In the Antiplatelet therapy in combination with Rt-PA Thrombolysis in Ischemic Stroke (ARTIS) study, 642 patients receiving IV tPA were randomized to also receive aspirin 300 mg or no immediate antiplatelet therapy.[310] The trial was stopped early because symptomatic hemorrhage occurred more often in the combined therapy group, 4.3% versus 1.6%.[310]

Use of ultrasound to enhance reperfusion

Transcranial Doppler ultrasound (TCD) has been used effectively to diagnose and localize intracranial arterial occlusions and to monitor whether spontaneous or treatment-related recanalization has occurred.[296,311] Preliminary small studies suggested that continuous monitoring of the MCA using TCD ultrasound during thrombolysis might augment the lytic effect of the thrombolytic agent.[312,313] Ultrasound waves increase the transport of rt-PA into the thrombus, promote the opening and cleaving of the fibrin polymers, and improve the

binding of tPA to fibrin.[314] In a randomized trial, combined lysis of thrombus in brain ischemia using transcranial ultrasound and systemic tPA (CLOTBUST), patients were randomly assigned to receive continuous 2 MHz TCD (the target group, N = 63) or placebo (the control group, N = 63).[315] The primary combined end-point was complete recanalization as assessed by TCD or dramatic clinical recovery. Symptomatic intracerebral hemorrhage occurred in three patients in the target group and in three in the control group. Complete recanalization or dramatic clinical recovery within 2 hours after the administration of a tPA bolus occurred in 31 patients in the target group (49%), compared with 19 patients in the control group (30%, $P = 0.03$). Twenty-four hours after treatment, 24 patients in the target group (44%) and 21 in the control group (40%) had a dramatic clinical recovery ($P = 0.7$). At 3 months, 22 of 53 (42%) patients in the target group and 14 of 49 in the control group (29%) had favorable outcomes (as indicated by mRS 0–1) ($P = 0.20$).[315] Using standard TCD ultrasound to enhance thrombolysis has a substantial practical drawback – the pulse wave Doppler technique requires the immediate availability of a skilled ultrasound technician to position the ultrasound window on the target clot. A novel, continuous wave Doppler device that can be placed by any health professional has recently been developed.[240] This more practical technique for ultrasound enhancement of brain thrombolysis is now being testing in a large trial.

The clot disrupting effects of ultrasound energy can be further increased by adding gaseous microsphere ultrasound contrast agents, which resonate, expand, oscillate, and detonate near and within the thrombus when subjected to externally applied ultrasound. Combining rt-PA not only with ultrasound, but also with microbubbles that will be popped at the clot by the ultrasound, may further increase recanalization rates.[316]

Ultrasound alone, without thrombolytic drug, has the potential to physically loosen fibrin bridges within red blood clots, allowing erythrocytes to escape and the clot to dissolve.[317] In a preliminary study 15 patients who were ineligible for thrombolysis were randomized to have or not have continuous TCD monitoring.[318] The group that had TCD monitoring more often recanalized and showed more neurological improvement than those patients not monitored but the numbers were very small.[318] In another preliminary study, TCD monitoring of thrombolysis was compared with no monitoring, and with monitoring combined with 3 doses of 2.5 g (400 mg/ml) of a galactose-based microbubble solution.[319] There was a suggestion that the microbubble infusion potentiated and accelerated the effect of ultrasound on thrombolysis.[319] There are many reasons to recommend TCD monitoring during and shortly after thrombolysis in centers that have the capability.

Thrombolytic treatment has brought much excitement and enthusiasm to the care of patients with acute ischemic stroke. As one can readily see from the length and complexity of this review, the field is ever changing and new agents, devices, and means of evaluation are being explored and studied in observation studies and trials. Box 6.8 lists our present recommendations for thrombolysis. Key to these decisions are:

Box 6.8 Our present recommendations for thrombolysis at stroke centers that have experienced stroke clinicians and modern technology

1. If the patient is seen within 4.5 hours and the cause is clear clinically (e.g., atrial fibrillation) and the CT does not show a large region of hypodensity, it is reasonable to give IV tPA using the guidelines without further study
2. If the cause is not obvious and/or the patient does not meet the present guidelines (stroke on awakening, uncertain onset time, >4.5 hours of symptoms, minor or improving deficit) then further brain and vascular imaging are suggested. This could be MRI with T2*, DWI, MRA or CT with CTA, or CT or MR with neck and TCD
3. TCD monitoring before, during, and shortly after thrombolysis is optimal if available. This allows recognition of recanalization and reocclusions

After brain and vascular evaluation

Situations in which we do not recommend thrombolysis:

a. Large infarct already present and little at-risk tissue
b. Spontaneous recanalization has already occurred

Situations in which we recommend IV thrombolysis (followed by IA and or mechanical clot retrieval if recanalization does not occur):

a. Occluded intracranial artery (e.g., carotid T occlusion, M1 or M2 MCA, vertebral artery, or basilar artery), especially if the mechanism is embolic and no or small infarct and considerable at-risk tissue
b. Occluded ICA in the neck seen within 3 hours (although treatment is often unsuccessful)

Situations in which we usually recommend angiography with consideration of endovascular recanalization therapy:

a. Basilar artery occlusions
b. Bilateral vertebral artery occlusive disease
c. >4.5 hours after symptom onset
d. Some patients with ICA neck occlusions
e. Some patients whose clinical picture (demography and recurrent TIAs) suggest in-situ atherothrombotic intracranial occlusive disease especially after IV treatment does not produce effective recanalization

knowledge of the presence, location, size, and nature of an arterial occlusion, time since symptom onset if known, presence and amount of infarction and threatened brain, availability of other potentially effective treatments, and the wishes of patients informed about the risks and benefits of the recommendations.

Surgically bypassing regions of blockage

A surgical bypass can be created connecting one vessel to another beyond an obstruction in the neck (e.g., a common carotid artery to vertebral artery connection) or intracranially creating an artificial conduit between extracranial branches and intracranial arteries. This is performed by connecting one artery directly to another or by interposing a venous or artificial conduit. When the vessel to be bypassed is stenotic but still patent, creation of a high pressure distal shunt has been shown to further reduce flow through the region of stenosis and promote thrombotic occlusion of the previously stenotic artery.[320,321] Clots that form at the site of occlusion might embolize distally, causing new ischemic damage.

Many anecdotal reports noted the effectiveness of high flow extracranial-to-intracranial (EC-IC) bypass using the superficial temporal artery as the donor artery and an MCA branch as the recipient artery. A large, randomized study of the effectiveness of such EC-IC bypasses, however, proved beyond reasonable doubt that the surgery as it was customarily performed at the time had no benefit.[322] In some circumstances, operated patients fared worse than patients treated medically.[322] The patients in this series had surgery approximately 6 weeks or more after the last symptomatic episode of brain ischemia or stroke to prevent reperfusion hemorrhage in regions where the capillaries and arterioles might be ischemic and vulnerable to leakage. Following the report of this study, surgeons, and stroke clinicians wondered:[323] (1) Would bypass procedures earlier in the course (although more risky) be more effective? (2) Would a larger recipient artery (e.g., intracranial ICA, mainstem MCA or a large conduit such as an interposed vein or larger artery) improve results? (3) Might there be some small well-selected groups of patients (e.g., those with severe persistent hypoperfusion confirmed by modern technology) who could benefit?[324–328]

Subsequent studies showed that using brain imaging to identify ICA occlusion patients with poor collateral flow and reduced cerebrovascular reserve identified a subpopulation at particularly increased risk of stroke.[329–333] The Carotid Occlusion Study showed that ipsilateral increased O_2 extraction fraction (OEF), as measured by positron emission tomography (PET), was a powerful independent risk factor for subsequent strokes in patients with symptomatic complete ICA occlusion.[332,333] The ipsilateral ischemic stroke rate at 2 years was 5.3% in 42 patients with normal OEF and 26.5% in 39 patients with increased OEF ($P = 0.004$).[332,333]

These studies gave impetus to a second trial of the EC-IC bypass; the Carotid Occlusion Surgery Study (COSS) enrolled 195 patients with recently symptomatic ICA occlusion and increased ipsilateral OEF.[334–336] There were no differences in outcome in the surgical and medical arm at 2 years.

Perioperative stroke and death or later ipsilateral stroke occurred in 21% of the surgical group versus 23% for the medical group. Although the surgical group had lower rates of stroke once they were more than 30 days out from their surgery, this advantage was negated by a high rate of stroke during the first 30 days, 14.3% in the surgical group versus 2.0% in the non-surgical group.[335]

Bypass surgery needs to be made substantially safer if it is to provide an advantage over medical therapy. One recent innovation is to perform indirect, rather than direct, surgical bypass.[337] This approach avoids connecting the new, supplying artery directly to a recipient brain artery with resulting high pressure flow into a chronically stressed brain vascular bed. Instead, the supplying artery is simply placed on the cortical surface, and small collateral channels grow from the artery into the brain substance slowly over the next several weeks and months. This approach is modeled on the procedure used in patients with moyamoya syndrome. In children with moyamoya syndrome, a variety of different structures have been placed over the ischemic brain including omentum, gracilis muscle, temporalis muscle with its blood supply, superficial temporal artery with attached galea, and a vascular portion of the dura mater and arachnoid.[338] These procedures are often considered effective in children with moyamoya, although they have not been studied definitively in randomized trials.[339] Superficial temporal artery to middle cerebral artery anastamoses have also been performed, but in young individuals the arteries are rather small. Adult patients with moyamoya often present with hemorrhages from deep penetrating arteries that are overloaded in attempting to deliver adequate collateral blood supply. A multicenter, prospective randomized trial (Japan Adult Moyamoya Trial) found that rebleeding was reduced in patients who underwent bilateral EC-IC bypass.[340] A study is under way in Japan to determine if EC–IC bypass will be useful in patients with moyamoya who present with brain hemorrhage.[341] Treatment of moyamoya will also be discussed in Chapter 12.

Bypass operations have also been performed in the past for vertebro-basilar ischemia. These procedures have now been almost entirely superceded by intracranial angioplasty and stenting.

Increasing blood flow in the collateral circulation and perfusion in the ischemic-zone capillary bed

Vasodilating agents have long been prescribed to increase blood flow. Carbon dioxide (CO_2) is the oldest known vasodilator. Physicians have attempted to dilate brain arteries by asking patients to breathe air with high CO_2 content. Other agents include cyclandelate, isoxsuprine, hydergine, papaverine, phosphodiesterase inhibitors, and nicotinic acid. A woeful lack of information exists regarding the effect and use of vasodilating agents on CBF in patients with TIAs or ischemic strokes.[342] Abnormal or even paradoxical responses of the cerebral circulation in stroke patients might theoretically render vasodilator treatment

ineffective or even harmful.[342] Cerebral arteries have relatively few elastic fibers in the media and are less responsive than systemic vessels to vasodilator stimuli. Vasodilator agents produce more systemic than cerebral vasodilation and could, thus, lead to hypotension or globally decreased CBF. Arteries within non-ischemic regions should retain the ability to vasodilate, whereas arteries within ischemic zones could be sufficiently damaged by ischemia and so lose their ability to dilate. In that circumstance, vasodilating drugs could result in an increased flow into non-ischemic areas creating a type of "steal away" from the ischemic areas.

Some pharmaceutical agents have vasoconstrictive effects in some arteries and vasodilator effects in others. Even individual drugs sometimes have different effects on the same circulation depending on dose and other factors. Serotonin has been shown to dilate normal coronary arteries but constrict coronary arteries when the endothelium is diseased.[343] None of the available agents have been thoroughly studied in individuals with cerebrovascular disease. Technology to study regional cerebral blood flow (rCBF) and flow in the brain arteries is now available allowing more definitve analysis of the effect of various agents on blood flow, symptoms, and outcomes.

In situations such as SAH or migraine, in which there is known vasoconstriction, agents that decrease vasoconstriction may have beneficial effects. Acetazolamide (Diamox) has been used as a provocative agent to acutely dilate brain arteries to test the brain's vascular reserve capability to further augment blood flow. Flow is measured in basal intracranial arteries by TCD or perfusion CT before and after acetazolamide is given IV.[344,345] In one study of patients with occlusive disease of intracranial or extracranial arteries, IV acetazolamide increased rCBF but mostly on the non-obstructed side.[346] Acetazolamide is taken orally and could be administered to outpatients with occlusive disease in an attempt to augment blood flow but this strategy has not been extensively studied as a treatment in ischemic stroke patients.

Calcium-channel blocking agents have been tested since 1987 to determine if they improve function in patients with ischemic stroke and SAH. Calcium has a number of actions that can influence the outcome of ischemia.[347] These include: promoting vasoconstriction by effects on vascular smooth muscle; altering coagulation (some of the coagulation reactions require Ca^{2+}); killing cells when extracellular Ca^{2+} passes through cell membranes into the intracellular compartment; and lowering systemic blood pressure.[347,348] A preliminary study of nimodipine in patients with SAH suggested some beneficial effects on cerebral vasospasm.[349] Later studies also showed some beneficial effects on morbidity, mortality, and on prevention of delayed ischemic infarction in patients with SAH. It was not clear in these studies whether or not nimodipine successfully increased blood flow or decreased the arterial vasoconstriction.[350–352] Trials of the effectiveness of nimodipine in patients with ischemic stroke have had disappointing results,[353] although nimodipine may help in the most severe cases if given early enough.[354] Therapeutic benefits probably result more from blockage of extracellular-to-intracellular movement of Ca^{2+} than from reversal of vasoconstriction.

Systemic injection of calcium-channel blockers results in low agent concentrations in target arteries. Super-selective injection by catheter directly into brain arteries yields higher concentrations and better physiological results. Intra-arterial injections of calcium-channel blockers have been shown to reverse vasospasm, both after SAH and in the reversible cerebral vasoconstriction syndrome.[355,356]

Volume expansion is another method used to attempt to augment CBF and increase perfusion within the microcirculation of the brain. Physicians have attempted to increase blood volume by simply increasing fluid intake or by using various volume expanders. Albumin, plasma, and solutions of colloids and crystalloids have been used.[357] Albumin has been extensively studied in experimental models of brain ischemia and does increase local CBF in ischemic zones.[358] Albumin also is a powerful antioxidant and dissolves arteriolar microthrombi, leading investigators to posit that albumin might have a neuroprotective effect in addition to expansion of blood volume and augmentation of blood flow. However, in the High-dose albumin treatment for acute ischaemic stroke (ALIAS) Part 2 trial, favorable clinical outcomes were not increased among albumin patients (44% vs. 44%), and the albumin group had more pulmonary edema complications (13% vs. 1%).[359]

Volume expansion agents seek to augment CBF by increasing blood volume. Mannitol, most often used to treat brain edema in patients with edematous brain infarcts and brain hemorrhages, may also temporarily expand intravascular volume and increase microcirculatory blood flow. Simply providing a fluid bolus or a red blood cell transfusion will increase blood volume and augment blood flow in ischemic fields after SAH.[360]

Another target for altering blood flow is blood viscosity. The two major determinants of blood viscosity within brain vessels are fibrinogen and Hct. Lowering Hct by hemodilution can reduce whole blood viscosity and increase blood flow.[361,362] The optimal Hct for blood flow and preservation of oxygen transport has been estimated to be approximately 33%.[363] Recent studies suggest that, since oxygen carrying capacity is reduced by the reduction in Hct, hemodilution may only increase CBF without increasing brain oxygen delivery.[364] Trials of hemodilution in stroke patients have all failed to show effectiveness.[365–368]

Fibrinogen contributes significantly to whole blood viscosity[369] and high fibrinogen levels have been noted to predict stroke recurrence in high-risk patients.[370–373] Reducing fibrinogen levels could also augment CBF and reduce coagulability since both white and red thrombi involve fibrinogen conversion to fibrin.[374,375] Ancrod, an agent discussed earlier in this chapter under thrombolysis, selectively acts on fibrinogen and inhibits formation of cross-linked fibrin.[255] Another method of rapidly reducing blood fibrinogen levels and whole blood viscosity is to use plasmaphoresis techniques. Investigators in Austria developed a technique that they call Heparin-induced Extracorporeal Low Density

Lipoprotein Precipitation (HELP).[375,376] In this system, blood is removed from a cubital vein and passed through a filter that separates the cellular components from the plasma. Isovolemic acetate buffer and heparin are added to the plasma. Fibrinogen, low-density lipoprotein (LDL), cholesterol, and triglycerides are removed by this process. The blood is then reinfused into the cubital vein on the opposite side. HELP treatment reduces fibrinogen levels, lowers whole blood viscosity at high and low shear rates, lowers plasma viscosity, and reduces red cell transit time.[375–377] This pharesis technique has been used for decades in the United States and Europe to treat patients with familial hypercholesterolemia.[377] It is quite effective in preventing premature atherosclerosis. Fibrinogen depletion after treatment is dramatic but temporary, lasting less than 2 weeks. Pharesis also lowers C-reactive protein quite effectively.[378] This treatment has been used acutely to augment CBF and can also be used repeatedly in patients with microvascular occlusive disease with vascular dementia who have high fibrinogen levels. The effectiveness of the fibrinogen depletion (acutely or chronically) in preventing stroke or limiting the extent of brain infarction has not been studied well in patients who have normal cholesterol levels

Omega-3 fatty acids, especially eicosopentanoic acid, can also lower blood fibrinogen levels, although the effect is quite variable.[379–381] In a preliminary study, eicosopentanoic acid also reduced blood viscosity, especially in those patients with high baseline viscosities.[379] Eicosopentanoic acid and omega-3 fatty acids, plentiful in various fish oils, have the potential to reduce platelet aggregability in addition to their effects on fibrinogen and viscosity. The low frequency of atherosclerosis in Eskimos has been posited to be related to diets rich in fish and omega-3 fatty acids. However, clinical trials of omega-3 fatty acids have not confirmed a benefit in prevention of cardiovascular disease.[382] Atromid, ticlopidine, and pentoxyphilline also have some fibrinogen-lowering effects.

Another strategy that has been used experimentally to improve microcirculatory flow and oxygen delivery is the use of perfluorochemicals. Perfluorochemicals are relatively small molecules, much smaller than erythrocytes. They can carry and release oxygen yet are not metabolized, remain chemically inert, and have low surface tension.[383] When patients or laboratory animals breathe 100% oxygen, these small molecules become saturated with oxygen. Perfluorochemicals have been used mostly as so-called white blood given to patients who are severely anemic but refuse blood transfusions for religious reasons.[384,385] Theoretically, small molecules can squeeze through vascular passages that block erythrocytes and thereby succeed in delivering needed oxygen to the ischemic stunned penumbral brain tissue. In clinical studies, however, investigators have not been able to attain concentrations of perfluorochemicals ("fluocrits") high enough to provide useful oxygen-carrying capabilities.[385] In experimental stroke models, perfusion of the ventricular and subarachnoid fluid spaces with highly oxygenated fluorocarbons decreases the extent of brain infarction.[386,387] The concept of delivering oxygen to tissues by using fluorocarbon emulsions shows promise, but the need for direct intraventricular delivery is a barrier to clinical development.[388]

Mechanical measures have also been used to augment CBF. Installation of an intra-aortic balloon has often been used in patients with acute myocardial infarction to bolster coronary artery and systemic blood flow. Partial aortic occlusion of the abdominal aorta results in a prompt increase in blood volume above the occlusion, and increases CBF.[389,390] The increase in blood flow can persist even after the balloon is removed. A special catheter was designed (Neuroflo) to partially occlude the aorta and it was preliminarily tested in small numbers of patients with vasoconstriction after SAH and in patients with acute ischemic stroke.[391,392] The Safety and Efficacy of NeuroFlo in Acute Ischemic Stroke (SENTIS) trial was designed to test the safety and effectiveness of this Neuroflo device in patients with acute brain ischemia – 230 patients treated with the device and 257 control patients.[393] The primary effectiveness end-point was global disability measured at 90 days after treatment. The trial met its primary safety end-point but not its primary effectiveness end-point. Signals of treatment effect were suggested on all-cause mortality, in patients presenting within 5 hours, in those older than age 70 years, and those with moderately severe strokes.[393]

Researchers in Hong Kong used external counterpulsation (ECP) to try to augment cerebral perfusion in patients with large artery occlusive disease.[394] The ECP technique used was delivering electrocardiogram-triggered diastolic pressures of 250 mmHg to the lower extremities through air-filled cuffs. The diastolic increase in blood flow and simultaneous decrease in systolic afterload increases blood flow to the heart, brain, and kidneys.[394,395]

Daily treatment for an hour a day was given to 50 patients either within a week after stroke or later. The treatment was safe and outcomes were better in those given ECP early after stroke.[394]

In patients with low flow, stagnation causes clot formation and embolization. Measures to prevent embolization, discussed in the following section, are also applicable to many low flow situations.

Prevention of clot formation, propagation, and embolism

The formation of a thrombus depends on a number of interrelated factors that include local vascular injury or roughening, the number of platelets and their activation, and the presence of serum coagulant and anticoagulant substances. Thrombi can be divided into red erythrocyte–fibrin clots and white platelet–fibrin clots. Red clots are treated with thrombolytic drugs and heparins, warfarin, factor Xa inhibitors, and direct thrombin inhibitors.[396] In contrast, white clot formation is prevented by so-called antiplatelet agents (aspirin, trifusal, prasugrel, clopidogrel, dipyridamole, cilostazol and others).[396–398] In general, red clots, erythrocyte–fibrin thrombi, tend to form in regions where there is low flow or stagnation, whereas smaller, so-called white platelet clots adhere to roughened places in faster-moving streams of blood.

Red thrombi are most apt to develop when flow is reduced. Dilated cardiac atria especially those with inefficient contractility as found with atrial fibrillation, regions of hypokinesia of the cardiac ventricles, and frank ventricular aneurysms often harbor red clots. Red thrombi are also often formed in heart chambers when ejection fractions are low. Red thrombi tend to form on the surface of myocardial infarcts. Thrombi formed in the leg and pelvic veins that pass through defects in the cardiac atrial and ventricular septa or pass through arteriovenous fistulas in the lungs are nearly always red thrombi. Both red and white thrombi often form along damaged heart valves especially those made of prosthetic materials.

Red thrombi are composed mostly of red blood cells and fibrin and they tend to form in areas of slowed blood flow. Their formation does not require an abnormal vessel wall or tissue thromboplastin. Red clots are formed by activation of circulating coagulation factors. The final step in the coagulation cascade is the conversion of the soluble protein fibrinogen into insoluble polymers called fibrin. Fibrin strands form a network of fibers that entangle the formed blood elements (platelets, erythrocytes, and leukocytes) into a clot. Fibrin is quite adhesive and is capable of contracting. The fibrinogen–fibrin reaction occurs when factor II, prothrombin is converted to thrombin. The amounts of circulating fibrinogen and prothrombin are important in these reactions.

Prothrombin is activated in two different ways. In the so-called extrinsic system of coagulation, a tissue or endothelial injury releases thromboplastic substances, tissue factors, which in turn cause both platelet activation and activation of blood serine protease coagulation factors, especially factors V, VII, and X. Activation of factor X catalyzes the reaction of prothrombin to thrombin. Activation of platelets causes them to agglutinate, to adhere to the injured vessel wall, and to release various intracellular substances, which in turn also activate the coagulation system.[396,399,400]

The complementary intrinsic coagulation system refers to blood-coagulation factors that circulate in inactive forms (factors V, VIII (antihemophilic globulin), IX, X, XI, XII) and are intrinsic to the blood. Activation of factor XII from an inert precursor form to an activated form triggers a series of reactions, the coagulation cascade, in which the various blood-clotting factors are sequentially converted to their active enzymatic forms. Ultimately, these reactions lead to activation of factor X, which catalyzes the prothrombin–thrombin reaction

White clots are composed of platelets and fibrin and do not contain red blood cells. White clots form almost exclusively in areas in which the endothelial surface is abnormal, characteristically in fast-moving bloodstreams. Irregular valvular and endothelial surfaces predispose to platelet–fibrin thrombi forming in areas of irregularities. In many patients thrombosis involves first the deposition of white clots on denuded or abnormal endothelium, Platelets adhere to the abnomal endothelium and aggregate forming a white clot. Platelet activation also stimulates thrombin generation which in turn can lead to the deposition of red thrombi superimposed upon the white thrombi.[401] An analysis of thrombi retrieved from cerebral arteries of patients with acute ischemic stroke most often showed a pattern of mixed white and red clots.[402] Imaging can provide clues to the composition of cerebral thrombi. The higher iron content of erythrocyte-rich red clots makes them more likely to appear hyperdense on CT imaging and hypointense on MRI.[403]

Standard "anticoagulants" including unfractionated heparin, low-molecular-weight heparins, synthetic pentasaccharides, warfarin, factor Xa inhibitors, and direct thrombin inhibitors theoretically should be more useful in preventing red clots, whereas antiplatelet agglutinating agents should be better at preventing white platelet plugs.[398] Anticoagulants should work best in occlusive disease of veins and in cardiac disorders that predispose to cardiac-origin thromboembolism, whereas agents that decrease platelet aggregation might have an advantage in arterial plaque disease. Thrombolytic agents lyse red clots but are not thought to lyse white clots. In fact they may stimulate platelet activation instead.

Polycythemia and thrombocytosis increase the probability of clot formation. Frequent blood donations, removal of causes of secondary erythremia such as cigarette smoking, and specific antineoplastic treatment of polycythemia vera are therapeutic alternatives for reduction of the Hct. In the acute situation, hemodilution decreases the Hct reducing viscosity and thrombotic tendencies. Thrombocytosis can also cause a clotting tendency and usually accompanies hematological proliferative disorders that require specific therapy. Severe anemia also may promote thrombosis.

Anticoagulants

Unfractionated and low-molecular-weight heparins

Heparin, a biological substance derived from tissues of various animals (most often bovine lungs and porcine intestines), has been used clinically since the 1940s. Heparin derives its name from the original description of it as an aqeous extract of liver (hepar) that showed anticoagulant activity in vitro.[404] Heparin decreases hyperlipemia and has a variety of different anticoagulant effects. The anticoagulant properties of heparin are due to the ability of components of the compound to bind to antithrombin III (AT III). AT III slowly binds to thrombin and the serine proteases factors VIIa, IXa, Xa, XIa, and XIIa and neutralizes these compounds. Heparin binds to AT III and dramatically accelerates the complex formation of AT III with thrombin and also with coagulation factors Xa and XIa.[405,406] Heparin also antagonizes thromboplastin and prevents thrombi from reacting with fibrinogen to form fibrin. Unfractionated heparin is a heterogeneous mixture of sulfated mucopolysaccharides containing at least 21 compounds ranging in size from 3000 to 37 500 daltons.[407]

Unfractionated heparin has been used most often during the acute phase of thrombosis or embolism. The necessity of giving the drug parenterally has limited its long-term use. Unfractionated heparin has also been used during pregnancy in patients who require anticoagulation because of the potential adverse effects of warfarin on the fetus. Unfractionated heparin can be given as an IV bolus, a continuous-drip

infusion, or, less effectively, subcutaneously. The dose is usually adjusted to keep the activated partial thromboplastin time (aPTT) at 1.5–2.5 times the mean of the normal control values.[404,408,409]

Unfractionated heparin has usually been given acutely to maintain anticoagulation until oral vitamin K antagonist anticoagulants reach therapeutic levels. There are two main reasons behind this practise. Unfractionated heparin works very quickly while oral anticoagulants, especially warfarin, take days to reach therapeutic levels. The other reason relates to prevention of hypercoagulability that occasionally develops with the initiation of warfarin without preceding heparin. Warfarin-induced skin necrosis mostly occurs in patients with hereditary protein C deficiency. It is a rare occurrence and almost invariably develops in the setting of acute thrombosis when there is inflammation and cytokine elaboration, There is no need in ambulatory patients with atrial fibrillation without thrombosis to give heparin along with warfarin or to test such individuals for protein C deficiency. The only exception would be a patient with known protein C deficiency in whom it would be wise to build up the warfarin dose slowly starting from a dose of 2 mg.

Some patients treated with unfractionated heparin develop a drop in their platelet count (thrombocytopenia) and new ischemic events.[410–414] There are two varieties of heparin-induced thrombocytopenia (HITS). The most common variety involves a slight degree of thrombocytopenia usually beginning 1–5 days after the start of heparin owing to heparin-induced platelet aggregation. Ischemia does not result and platelet counts return to normal despite continuation of heparin. In the more severe form of HITS, antibodies of the IgG and IgM groups become bound to platelets and platelet counts fall, usually during the second week of treatment. Often, thrombocytopenia is severe ($10\,000$ mm^3) and thromboembolic and hemorrhagic complications may develop owing to consumption of coagulation factors and platelets. Blockage of small arteries by white platelet–fibrin clots can cause regions of skin and visceral organ necrosis, termed the white clot syndrome. Occasionally, thrombosis seems to be precipitated by unfractionated heparin without thrombocytopenia.[415]

The anticoagulant activities of various commercial preparations of unfractionated heparin vary among sources and even within batches from the same source.[409–407] These variations lead to variability in clinical effectiveness and unexpected bleeding. Unfractionated heparin has begun to be replaced by low-molecular-weight heparins, heparinoids and synthetic heparin pentasaccharides. Crude commercial preparations of heparin can be separated into low- and high-molecular-weight fractions. Low-molecular-weight heparins are fragments of standard heparin with molecular weights of 4000–6000.[416,417] Heparinoids are heparin analogs, natural or semisynthetic sulfated glycosaminoglycans, prepared by tissue extraction or by blending various components.[417,418] They are related structurally to heparin and have similar biological functions, especially anticoagulant effects. Synthetic heparin pentasaccharides are molecules synthesized to mimic the active site of naturally occurring heparins. Unfractionated heparins, low-molecular-weight heparins, heparinoids and synthetic heparin pentasaccharides act as anticogulants by binding to plasma AT III.[419] This interaction induces a conformational change in AT III that increases its ability to inactivate coagulation enzymes, including thrombin and activated factor X (factor Xa).

Low-molecular-weight heparins are thought to have more favorable bioavailability and pharmacokinetics than standard unfractionated heparin. Their plasma half-lives are two to four times that of unfractionated heparin.[416] Low-molecular weight heparins are posited to cause fewer hemorrhagic complications than standard heparin because they have less pronounced effect on platelet function and vascular permeability.[416,417] Some evidence suggests that low-molecular-weight heparin has more anticoagulant effect than unfractionated heparin and does not activate platelets.[405,418] Unfractionated heparin's bleeding complications most likely relate to effects on platelets, especially inhibition of platelet aggregation which is mostly an action of the high-molecular-weight components in heparin.[418] Low-molecular-weight heparins also cause less heparin-related thrombocytopenia, heparin-related skin necrosis, and white clot syndromes. While heparin is monitored closely using the partial thromboplastin time (PTT), low-molecular-weight heparins, heparinoids, and synthetic heparin pentasaccharides can be monitored by measuring antifactor Xa activity. However, not all laboratories have high-quality reliably reproducible analyses of antifactor Xa. Low-molecular-weight heparins and synthetic heparin pentasaccharides are more convenient to use than standard unfractionated heparin and are often used in patients outside of acute-care hospital settings. Although high-dose low-molecular-weight heparins and synthetic heparin pentasaccharides have been well studied in patients with lower extremity phlebothrombosis and pulmonary embolism, there are few studies in stroke patients. Low-dose low-molecular-weight heparin has shown advantages as an agent to prevent deep venous thrombosis among non-ambulatory acute ischemic stroke patients. In the PREVAIL randomized trial, among 1762 randomized patients, deep venous thrombi were detected in 10% of low-molecular-weight heparin patients versus 18% of unfractionated heparin patients.[420]

The effectiveness of heparins and anticoagulants in ischemic stroke has not been well studied except in regard to atrial fibrillation. Heparin followed by warfarin has often been used in patients with cardiogenic embolism who are at high risk for early re-embolization. Recent studies also suggest that heparin is effective in patients with cerebral dural sinus thrombosis. The newer anticoagulants (direct thrombin and factor Xa inhibitors) work quickly and they do not require heparin to be used before they are prescribed.

Because the indications for anticoagulation (except for timing) relate to both parenteral and oral anticoagulants, we will review them after discussing the oral anticoagulants.

Warfarin

Warfarin is a water-soluble derivative of coumaric acid that is absorbed by the small intestine and transported in the blood loosely bound to albumin. Its therapeutic effect is to inhibit the action of vitamin K necessary for the biological synthesis of factors II (prothrombin), VII, IX, and X.[421] By depressing these procoagulant factors, warfarin affects the so-called intrinsic cascade and the extrinsic coagulation pathway.[421,422] Warfarin works quite differently from heparin. In some patients who have continued transient spells or progressive ischemic symptoms despite warfarin anticoagulation, symptoms sometimes almost miraculously stop when heparin is substituted for warfarin. The therapeutic dosing window for warfarin is the range at which it effectively prevents thromboemboli that will cause ischemic stroke without causing a high rate of bleeding. Warfarin metabolism varies widely among and within individual patients, and is modified by other drugs and dietary foods. Accordingly, regular monitoring of warfarin activity is necessary for its safe use.[421–425]

Because of the wide variation in thromboplastin reagents used, the World Health Organization designated a single batch of human brain thromboplastin as an international standard. Manufacturers calibrate their reagent against the international standard and calculate an International Sensitivity Index that relates their reagent to the international standard. Using the International Sensitivity Index and the prothrombin times, the international normalized ratio (INR) can be readily calculated. Various expert groups have published recommendations for intensity of anticoagulation based on the international system.[426,427] Two intensities of anticoagulation have often been recommended: a less intense range (INR 2.0–3.0) and a more intense range (INR 3.0–4.5).[426] The higher intensity range clearly has more risk of bleeding. The Stroke Prevention in Reversible Ischemia Trial (SPIRIT), a large Dutch trial that compared the effectiveness of aspirin versus oral anticoagulation (INR target range, 3.0–4.5) was prematurely stopped after an interim analysis showed an unacceptable rate of hemorrhage in the anticoagulant-treated group.[428] In another analysis, the frequency of bleeding increased by a factor of 1.43 for each 0.5 U increase in the INR.[424]

Genetic analysis can identify some individuals who are more sensitive to warfarin compounds. Various alleles in the genes *CYP2C9* and *VKORCI* render patients more susceptible to bleeding during warfarin administration.[429] *VKORCI* variants are especially common in patients of Asian origin. Genetic analysis can be useful in guiding the dose of warfarins.[430,431] Pharmacogenetic biomarkers may also become important in the use of direct thrombin inhibitors, other types of anticoagulants, and anticonvulsants.[432]

The Atrial Fibrillation Investigators analyzed the results of five trials of anticoagulation in patients with atrial fibrillation (INR target range, 1.4–4.2) and recommended a target range of 2.0–3.0 as having the best benefit and risk results.[433,434] Hylek and colleagues also analyzed the results of anticoagulation in atrial fibrillation trials and found that the rate of stroke increased when the INR fell below 2.0.[435] Optimal protection ocurred in patients with INRs between 2.0 and 3.0.[435] No further protection was attributable to INRs above 3.0. In most patients, we aim at an INR between 2.0 and 3.0. In patients older than 75 years, we use an INR target of 2.0–2.5. Higher doses of warfarin are needed for the prevention of cardiac emboli arising from mechanical mitral valve replacements, with a recommended INR target of 2.5–3.5.

Indications and timing of anticoagulants

Cardiac-origin embolism

The greatest body of evidence to guide antithrombotic therapy for cardiogenic embolism is for atrial fibrillation. Until the 1990s, the effectiveness of anticoagulation with heparin or warfarin had not been tested in modern randomized trials in patients with known pathologies. Early observational studies showed the effectiveness of warfarin in atrial fibrillation patients with rheumatic mitral stenosis who had brain embolism.[436–439] Trials of stroke prophylaxis in patients with atrial fibrillation who did not have valvular heart disease have now shown a dramatic benefit of anicoagulant treatment.[439–452] All trials showed a consistent and considerable risk reduction for stroke in patients treated with warfarin. Warfarin is approximately 50% more effective than aspirin in reducing the rate of stroke in patients with atrial fibrillation who do not have valvular disease.[447] Pooled analyses have identified variables that help select those patients with non-valvular atrial fibrillation. Clinical features favoring anticoagulation are older age, history of congestive heart failure, history of hypertension, diabetes, being female, and having had a prior brain or systemic embolism.[449] Echocardiographic features favoring anticoagulation are: atrial and ventricular thrombi, spontaneous echo contrast, atrial enlargement, valvular disease, ventricular regions of aneurysmal dilatation, akinesis or hypokinesis, and low cardiac ejection fraction.

The various cardiac sources besides atrial fibrillation that are potential indications for anticoagulation are listed in Box 6.9. In many the relative value of anticoagulants versus other treatments such as platelet inhibitors has not been well studied.

Controversy still exists about how soon to anticoagulate in patients with cardiac sources of embolism who have just had an ischemic stroke.[453–460] On the one hand, delaying treatment start risks the occurrence of a second episode of thromboembolism before anticoagulation is started. On the other hand, starting anticoagulation early increases the risk of bleeding into the fresh brain infarct. The risk of hemorrhagic transformation is highest in the first few days after ischemic stroke onset. The clinical trials that have investigated early anticoagulation in cardioembolic stroke have only tested crude strategies, comparing anticoagulating all patients immediately whatever their stroke size and bleeding risk versus delaying anticoagulation in all patients for a prolonged 7–14-day period. These studies found that neither of these strategies is better than the other. Often the occurrence of early bleeding with immediate anticoagulation strategy was more or less exactly counterbalanced by the occurrence of early recurrent

Box 6.9 Cardiac sources of emboli and use of antithrombotic agents

Anticoagulants indicated

Atrial fibrillation
Thrombus found in the heart on echocardiography
Ventricular aneurysm
Hypokinetic ventricle
Acute myocardial infarction
Very low ejection fraction
Mitral stenosis with large left atrium
Spontaneous echo contrast and large left atrium
Prosthetic mechanical valves

Antibiotics indicated

Bacterial endocarditis

Antiplatelets indicated

Libman–Sacks endocarditis
Fibrotic valve disease in antiphospholipid antibody syndrome
Non-thrombotic (marantic) endocarditis
Fibrous strands
Calcific aortic stenosis

Anticoagulants sometimes used

Mitral valve prolapse (with thrombi)
Mitral annulus calcification (with thrombi)
Patent foramen ovale especially with atrial septal aneurysm

embolic infarction with the delay anticoagulation strategy. For example, in the largest trial of early anticoagulation in atrial fibrillation patients, the International Stroke Trial, 3169 patients with atrial fibrillation were randomized to different doses of heparin versus no heparin and to aspirin or no aspirin.[451] The high-dose heparin group, compared with the no heparin group, had fewer ischemic strokes (2.4% vs. 4.9%) but more hemorrhagic strokes (2.8% vs. 0.4%) and no difference in the rate of being alive and independent at 6 months after stroke.[451]

We urge weighing the benefits versus the risks of any given treatment in the individual patient. Regarding the timing of anticoagulation in patients with cardiac-origin embolism, the risk of early embolic recurrence if not anticoagulated should be weighed against the risk of bleeding of early anticoagulation. The probability of early recurrence in atrial fibrillation patients depends on: the number of prior embolic events, the presence of valve abnormalities, atrial size, the presence of atrial or auricular appendage thrombi, the presence of ventricular lesions, ventricular function, ejection fraction, and blood and coagulation factors. The risk of hemorrhage with early anticoagulation relates to the patient's blood pressure, coagulation factors, use of a bolus starting dose, the route and intensity of anticoagulation, and the size of the bland or hemorrhagic infarction on CT or MRI scans. Echocardiography can help decide on the risk of early recurrence.

Anticoagulants are not routinely used as prophylaxis in patients with mitral valve prolapse (MVP), mitral annulus calcification (MAC), calcific aortic stenosis, and those with

fibrotic valve lesions (Libman–Sacks endocarditis in patients with lupus erythematosus and non-thrombotic (marantic) endocarditis), cardiac myxomas, and bacterial endocarditis. Anticoagulants are continued in patients with bacterial endocarditis if there was a pre-existing indication such as atrial fibrillation, and prosthetic heart valves. Some patients with MVP and MAC have thrombi attached to their mitral valves and so anticoagulants are then used.

The data regarding optimal prophylaxis in patients with atrial septal defects or patent foramen ovale (PFO) is to date not conclusive and also should be eclectic and depend on the individual circumstances. The data from echocardiographic studies shows that there is a strong association between atrial septal aneurysms and inter-atrial shunts, and that the presence of either atrial septal aneurysms and/or PFOs is strongly associated with the presence of cryptogenic stroke especially among young stroke patients.[461–464] The mechanism by which atrial septal aneurysms contribute to brain embolism has not been satisfactorily clarified but these lesions can harbor thrombi. Thrombus was seen within an atrial septal aneurysm in one patient,[465] and has been found within the base of atrial septal aneurysms at necropsy.[466]

The recurrence rate of stroke in patients with PFOs and the effect of various treatments on recurrence has been studied.[462,467–470] In a European multicenter study, 277 patients with PFOs and/or atrial septal aneurysms and cryptogenic stroke were followed for an average of 22.6 months while treated with only aspirin.[462,468] The recurrence rate was approximately 2.3% after 4 years for patients with PFO alone, and much higher, 15.2% at 4 years, among patients with both PFO and atrial septal aneurysm[468]

The Patent Foramen Ovale in Cryptogenic Stroke Study (PICSS)[470] was a substudy of the Warfarin Aspirin Recurrent Stroke Study (WARSS).[471] All patients in WARSS who had received a transesophageal echocardiography (TEE) were eligible. In PICSS 312 stroke patients were treated with warfarin and 318 received aspirin. Large PFOs were much more common in patients with cryptogenic strokes. Among the cryptogenic stroke patients, warfarin treatment was slightly but not significantly better than aspirin in regard to annual rate of stroke or death (4.75% vs. 8.95%; relative risk (RR) = 0.53 CI 0.18–1.58) because the numbers were small and the CIs were wide.[470]

PFO closure devices are an alternative, minimally invasive approach to stroke prevention in patients with PFO.[472–474] The devices consist of discs that are positioned by transcatheter approach on both sides of the atrial septal opening, closing the defect. Newer devices, like the Amplatzer PFO Occluder and Gore Helex, appear safer than earlier generation devices, which tended to provoke atrial fibrillation and to become surfaces for clot formation.[475] In two randomized trials, RESPECT (the Randomized Evaluation of Recurrent Stroke Comparing PFO Closure to Established Current Standard of Care Treatment) and PC (Percutaneous Closure of Patent Foramen Ovale in Cryptogenic Embolism), placement of the Amplatzer PFO Occluder was associated with numerically fewer strokes than antithrombotic therapy alone.[473–475] Strokes were few in

number in both treatment arms and these differences did not reach statistical significance.

The available data regarding optimal treatment of PFO-related strokes is inconclusive. The presence of both a PFO and an atrial septal aneurysm substantially increases the risk of stroke ocurrence. Large defect, spontaneous right-to-left shunting, and large number of bubbles shunted may indicate a higher risk of paradoxical embolism. Warfarin and surgical or transcatheter closure are posited to be more effective than drugs that affect platelet functions but studies have not definitively shown their superiority.

Dural sinus and cerebral venous thrombosis

Occlusions of the venous structures that drain the brain are due to red erythrocyte–fibrin thrombi. Since standard anticoagulants are effective in preventing peripheral phlebothrombosis and pulmonary embolism, it is logical to posit that anticoagulation would be effective in patients with venous occlusions involving nervous system structures. Case reports and reviews showed that patients do not worsen or develop new hemorrhages after heparin anticoagulation.[476–483] In one study, among 82 heparin-treated patients, there were no deaths and 77% of patients recovered completely.[477] In another study, among 79 patients given anticoagulants, 94% improved and survived while only half of 157 patients not given anticoagulants survived.[478] A meta-analysis of two trials showed an absolute risk reduction in mortality of 14% and a RR reduction of 70% in heparin-treated patients.[479,480] Among 102 patients with cerebral venous thromboses (43 of whom had intracerebral hemorrhages), those not treated with heparin fared worse and had higher mortality.[480] In a double-blind, placebo-controlled multicenter trial, central venous thrombosis patients treated with low-molecular-weight heparin had better outcomes than those given placebo.[481] No new symptomatic brain hemorrhages occurred. Prevention of pulmonary embolism is another reason to administer anticoagulants to patients with dural sinus thrombosis.[483] Most clinicians now agree that early and longer-term anticoagulants are indicated in patients with central venous thrombosis. The optimal duration of anticoagulation has not been well studied.

Large artery thrombosis and arterial dissections

The use of anticoagulants in the treatment of stroke patients with non-cardioembolic strokes continues to be controversial.[484,485] Few neurologists now use heparin routinely during the acute phase of non-cardioembolic stroke. Others use anticoagulants in selected patients with large artery disease. Because the newer anticoagulants administered orally work very quickly, they are an attractive alternative to heparin. Anticoagulants should not be indiscriminately used in all brain ischemia patients. Bleeding complications will outweigh therapeutic benefit. Acute anticoagulation should theoretically be useful in patients with fresh red erythrocyte–fibrin thrombi within large arteries to prevent the development of fresh clots and intra-arterial embolism, when the brain infarct is small, reducing the risk of hemorrhagic transformation. Acute and subacute anticoagulation is posited to be effective in preventing red clot development in the small

subgroup of patients with acute thrombosis engrafted upon stenotic lesions and those in whom vascular imaging shows reduced distal blood flow. For example, a patient with a proximal basilar occlusion and with slow to and fro flow in the mid and upper basilar may be at risk for clotting of the remainder of the basilar trunk and all its penetrators from stasis thrombosis. Also the fresh thrombus is non-adherent and so a fresh clot appended to the end of the existing thrombus may break loose and embolize into the distal basilar artery and its branches. Anticoagulants might be useful in preventing a fresh clot from forming and embolizing during the first 3–6 weeks after such an arterial occlusion. Unfortunately, randomized trials have not adequately studied anticoagulants in patients with conditions likely to respond to treatment. Reported trials lumped patients with brain ischemia together without diagnostic investigations that defined stroke etiology, stroke subtypes, or vascular lesions.

Worsening and development of new neurological deficits can occur when thrombi form, propagate, and embolize. Stroke worsening, even when thrombi are present, occurs in only about 20–33% of ischemic stroke patients.[486] Ischemic stroke progression in patients with atherothrombotic large artery occlusive disease is due to perfusion failure and propagation and embolization of occlusive thrombi. Randomized trials in patients with non-cardioembolic brain ischemia to effectively determine anticoagulant utility must be: (1) eclectic and include only patients in whom brain and cardiac and vascular imaging show high-risk artery-to-artery embolic brain infarcts in patients with documented severe extracranial or intracranial large artery occlusive disease; (2) powered to account for clinical worsening and/or new brain infarcts in less than one-third of patients; and (3) anticoagulant activity must be closely and effectively monitored to ensure an effective therapeutic dose and infrequent bleeding. No available trials even remotely meet these criteria. In the International Stroke Trial (IST) trial, the largest heparin trial, vascular and cardiac imaging were not reported, some patients had no brain imaging before treatment, heparin was given subcutaneously while elsewhere heparins are usually given IV, and levels of anticoagulation were not always closely monitored.[487] Heparin effectively prevented pulmonary embolism.[487]

The results of two trials suggest that anticoagulation might be effective in patients with acute ischemic stroke caused by large artery thromboembolism.[450,488,489] In a trial performed in Hong Kong among 312 patients with acute ischemic stroke, low-molecular-weight heparin was more effective than placebo.[488] This study found a significant dose-dependent reduction in the risk of death or dependency among patients treated with low-molecular-weight heparin. Although vascular studies were not mandated, most patients with ischemic stroke in Hong Kong have intracranial artery occlusive disease. Patients with cardiac lesions that required anticoagulation were not included in this study. However another study of low-molecular-weight heparin in Asian patients with large artery occlusive disease (mostly intracranial) did not show a benefit of nadroparin over aspirin.[490]

In the TOAST trial (Trial of ORG 10172 in Acute Stroke Treatment), the low-molecular-weight heparinoid ORG 10172

was given within 24 hours of the onset of symptoms of an acute ischemic stroke.[450,489] This heparinoid was then given by continuous IV infusion for 7 days with the dose adjusted after 24 hours to maintain the anti-Xa factor activity at 0.6–0.8 antifactor Xa units/ml. The control group received no antithrombotic therapy, including no aspirin. ORG 10172 (Danaparoid) is a mixture of glycosaminoglycans with a mean molecular weight of 5500 isolated from porcine intestinal mucosa. The antifactor Xa activity of Danaparoid is attributed to its heparin sulfate component which has a high affinity for AT III. Although Danaparoid treatment was not effective in terms of the entire group of patients with ischemic stroke, there was effectiveness in the group of patients that were diagnosed as having large artery atherosclerosis.[489] In this group, heparinoid reduced the number of recurrences of stroke during the 7 days of infusion, and the rates of favorable and very favorable outcomes were significantly higher in patients given heparinoid when compared with placebo. 68% of patients with large artery atherosclerosis treated with Danaparoid had favorable outcome versus 54.7% treated with placebo (P = 0.04); 43% of patients with large artery atherosclerosis treated with Danaparoid had very favorable outcomes versus 29.1% treated with placebo (P = 0.02). Recurrent strokes developed in 6% of Danaparoid-treated patients with large artery atherosclerosis versus 11% of those treated with placebo. In this study most of the patients with large artery disease had occlusive disease of the internal carotid arteries in the neck defined by ultrasound. Intracranial vascular imaging was not reported. Because of the small numbers the figures for recurrent strokes did not meet statistical significance.[489]

In the Warfarin–Aspirin Recurrent Stroke Study (WARSS) trial in non-cardioembolic stroke, coumadin and aspirin were equally effective in preventing new strokes.[471] The drugs were given within a month of stroke onset, not always acutely, and secondary prevention of new strokes was studied. The number of patients with documented large artery disease was small and vascular studies were not required or reported. Some patients received heparin acutely and then aspirin. Some patients did not receive heparin but were given coumadin within a month. The data does not relate well to the use of anticoagulation during the acute stroke.

In the Warfarin–Aspirin for Symptomatic Intracranial Disease (WASID) trial of patients with severe intracranial atherosclerosis, there was no significant difference in the prevention of new strokes between aspirin and warfarin.[491] Again the study drugs were initiated often weeks after the last ischemic event. Warfarin was difficult to control. In those patients who were maintained within the target therapeutic INR range, warfarin performed better than 1300 mg aspirin per day. In those who were below the target range more infarcts developed, and more hemorrhages developed in those above the target INR range.[491,492]

We administer antithrombotics to patients with acute arterial dissections. Unfortunately, there is no data from trials about the effectiveness of aspirin, unfractionated heparin or any other antiplatelet or anticoagulant treatment in patients with acute arterial dissections. Therapeutics in patients with dissection has not been studied in trials, although most stroke clinicians use either antiplatelets or anticoagulants when the diagnosis of extracranial arterial dissection is made. Although transient ocular and brain ischemia may develop when a dissection causes a complete or near complete arterial occlusion, the great majority of strokes are caused by embolization of thrombi formed in the region of the dissection. Thrombus is often present within the lumen, either as a result of communication of the intramural hematoma with the lumen or because perturbation of the endothelium leads to the release of tissue factors that promote thrombosis. The luminal clot is usually loosely adherent to the intima and can readily embolize distally. In the weeks and months after dissection, the intramural blood is absorbed and the narrowed lumen usually returns to its normal size; if the artery becomes completely occluded, it remains occluded in about 75% of patients. Anecdotally, many neurologists use anticoagulants in this situation and believe it effective, although initially there was much concern that it could enlarge the intramural clot. Available evidence suggests recurrent stroke rates are low with both antiplatelet or anticoagulant therapy.[493] Optimal anticoagulation has not been studied. During the first 4–8 weeks clots become adherent, collateral circulation solidifies, and often luminal narrowing abates, so that we usually stop anticoagulation after 9–12 weeks and prescribe an antiplatelet instead.

Clearly, more trials are needed in patients with documented cardiac and cardiovascular lesions. Until the results of such trials are available, we use and recommend the use of anticoagulants in patients who have or are at risk of developing red clots. In some patients we prescribe anticoagulants for a period of 4–8 weeks until clots become organized and adhere to the vascular wall. In other patients with chronic conditions that continue to pose a risk for red thrombus formation, mostly those with cardiac thrombi, arrhythmias, or cardiac lesions promoting thrombus formation, anticoagulants are given indefinitely until the risk of thrombosis diminishes or anticoagulants become contraindicated. Our present practice is to monitor vascular occlusive lesions by ultrasound or vascular imaging (CTA or MRA). We stop oral anticoagulants approximately a month after vessel segments with stasis flow are shown to have recanalized, increase flow speed, or remain completely occluded. Anticoagulation is also used for some patients with congenital or acquired hypercoagulable states.

Warfarin has proven to be a difficult drug to use. Studies in non-academic community settings[494] (Figure 6.5), and even in anticoagulation clinics (Figure 6.6),[495] have shown that many patients remain under or over anticoagulated even in the best of situations. Warfarin anticoagulation is difficult to control because of individual variance in dose and the effect of a variety of foods and pharmaceutical agents on vitamin K, prothrombin, and liver functions. Especially worrisome is the observation that important INR changes may develop just before major hemorrhages. One study showed that when INRs were

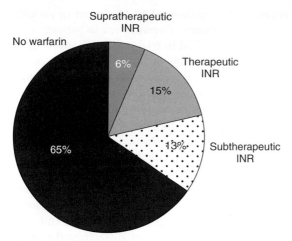

Figure 6.5 Use of warfarin in a primary care population. All patients analyzed were judged to be appropriate candidates for warfarin according to guidelines. There were no contraindications to warfarin treatment. INR, international normalized ratio. From Samsa GP, Matchar DB, Goldstein LB, et al. Quality of anticoagulation management among patients with atrial fibrillation. *Arch Intern Med* 2000;160:967–973.

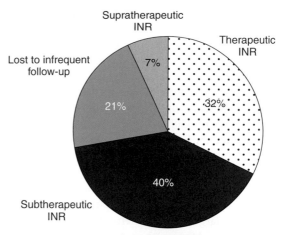

Figure 6.6 Adequacy of warfarin control achieved in an anticoagulation clinic. Distribution of international normalized ratio (INR) values based on a target range of 2–3. From Chiquette E, Amato MG, Bussey HI, et al. Comparison of an anticoagulation clinic with usual medical care: Anticoagulation control, patient outcomes and health care costs. *Arch Intern Med* 1998;15:1641–1647.

plotted in relation to the time before the onset of bleeding, a marked increase in the patients' INRs was observed only shortly before the bleeding began.[496]

The adequacy of anticoagulation is important. In the WASID study of the prevention of recurrent stroke in patients with intracranial occlusive vascular disease, although there were no differences in stroke recurrence in patients treated with warfarin versus aspirin, those in the target anticoagulation range had less strokes and less bleeding than those patients treated with aspirin and those outside of the INR range chosen.[491,492] Although warfarin anticoagulation has been definitively shown to be effective in a number of conditions including atrial fibrillation, many primary care physicians and internists are reluctant to prescribe it because of the perceived difficulty in keeping the INR in target range, the seriousness of complications, and medicolegal implications of adverse events.

Newer anticoagulants: factor Xa and thrombin inhibitors

Red thrombi are composed mostly of red blood cells and fibrin. They are formed by activation of circulating coagulation factors; their formation does not require an abnormal vessel wall or tissue thromboplastin. The final step in the coagulation cascade is the conversion of the soluble protein fibrinogen into insoluble polymers called fibrin. Fibrin strands form a network of fibers that entangle the formed blood elements (platelets, erythrocytes, and leukocytes) into a clot. Fibrin is quite adhesive and is capable of contracting. Activation of factor X to Xa catalyzes the conversion of prothrombin (factor II) to thrombin. Thrombin in turn catalyzes the fibrinogen to fibrin conversion.

Several key components in the coagulation system – prothrombin, factor Xa, and thrombin – are targets for pharmacological anticoagulation. The new anticoagulant agents mostly target inhibition of factor Xa or thrombin.

Direct inhibitors of thrombin offer many potential advantages. Argatroban is an IV agent that has been used often in Asia instead of heparin.[497] It has also been used in the United States and Europe, mostly in patients with HITS.[498] One trial showed that it could be effective in patients with acute ischemic stroke.[499] Argatroban's safety record and control are comparable or better than heparins. Ximelagatran is an oral direct thrombin inhibitor that was studied in trials and approved in Europe but not in the United States. In studies of patients with deep vein thrombosis[500] and atrial fibrillation,[501–503] ximelagatran was as effective or more effective than warfarin and caused less bleeding. Ximelagatran and other direct thrombin inhibitors act quickly so that heparins are not needed. The dose was constant and did not require monitoring by either aPTT or INR determinations. The US FDA failed to authorize release of ximelagatran in the United States because of liver enzyme abnormalities. After the failure of ximelagatran to be marketed in the United States, another oral direct thrombin inhibitor dabigatran, which had fewer side effects in early experiments, was introduced and has now been tested in trials.

The direct oral anticoagulant agents mostly target inhibition of factor Xa or thrombin. The major oral direct thrombin inhibitor now on the market is dabigatran.[504–596] The oral factor Xa inhibitors include rivaroxaban, apixaban, and edoxaban.[507–511] The direct oral anticoagulant agents offer several advantages compared with warfarin. Their metabolism is much more predictable, with fewer interactions with food and with other drugs. Accordingly, they can be taken at fixed doses without needing regular blood tests and dose adjustment. They have shorter half-lives and faster onset and offset of action, so usually do not require bridging treatment with parenteral anticoagulants until they reach therapeutic effect. The direct thrombin inhibitors and factor Xa inhibitors are mostly excreted by the kidney so dosage must be adjusted in patients with renal insufficiency. These agents cause bleeding less often then vitamin K inhibitors. Recently, antidotes have been tested and proven to be effective in controlling bleeding.

The direct oral anticoagulants have been most extensively tested for stroke prevention in atrial fibrillation. All of these agents, when compared to warfarin in patients with atrial fibrillation, were found to be equally or more effective in preventing embolic stroke and equally or more safe in avoiding intracerebral hemorrhage.[506–511] For example, in the Apixaban for Reduction in Stroke and Other Thromboembolic Events in Atrial Fibrillation (ARISTOTLE) trial, 18 201 patients with atrial fibrillation were randomized to apixaban or warfarin and followed for an average of 1.8 years.[508,509] The rate of combined ischemic and hemorrhagic stroke was lower in the apixaban group (1.27% versus 1.60% per year). The apixaban group also had lower rates of major bleeding (2.13% vs. 3.09% per year) and of death (3.52% vs. 3.94%).[508] Trials of rivaroxaban (ROCKET AF)[510] and edoxaban (ENGAGE AF)[511] also showed that these factor Xa inhibitors were more effective and safer than warfarin in patients with non-valvular atrial fibrillation. The trials of newer anticoagulants had enough differences in patient selection and methodology that they are not directly comparable. Much uncertainty remains about which newer anticoagulants to use in which patients for which indications.[512]

Fondaparinux is a pentasaccharide given subcutaneously that causes less bleeding than heparins and does not cause thrombocytopenia. It is an indirect inhibitor of factor Xa. Fondaparinux has been very effective in trials to prevent phlebothrombosis and pulmonary emboli in patients who have had recent surgery[513] and in hospitalized patients.[514] Fondaparinux has been more effective than low-molecular-weight heparin in patients with acute coronary syndromes.[515–517] Fondaparinux is excreted through the kidneys and accumulates in patients with renal impairment.

Drugs that modify platelet functions

Aspirin

The first clinical observations on aspirin as an antithrombotic agent was probably made by a practitioner named Craven.[518] Craven, observing that dental patients bled more if they had used aspirin, urged friends and his patients to take one or two aspirin tablets a day. He later published the effectiveness of this strategy in preventing coronary and cerebral thrombosis among 8000 men in articles in the *Mississippi Valley Medical Journal*, not a periodical on many neurologist's bookshelf.[519,520] Twenty years later, case reports from the United States and Britain on the effectiveness of aspirin in preventing attacks of transient monocular blindness brought more attention to the subject.[521,522] The American[523] and Canadian[524] aspirin trials soon ensued in the late 1970s.

Aspirin and other non-steroidal anti-inflammatory drugs, such as indomethacin, phenylbutazone, and ibuprofen, inhibit platelet release reactions secondary to adenosine diphosphate-induced platelet aggregation and platelet adhesion to collagen when tested in vitro.[525] Aspirin inhibits platelet aggregation and secretion by preventing the synthesis of prostaglandins and thromboxane A$_2$. This action is achieved by inhibiting the cyclo-oxygenase enzyme that converts arachidonic acid to prostaglandin G$_2$, the precursor of thromboxane A$_2$.[526] Aspirin, however, also inhibits the production of prostacyclin by endothelial cells. Prostacyclin has a potent platelet anti-aggregant and vasodilator effect.[527]

The optimal therapeutic dosage of aspirin is still controversial. The American,[523] Canadian[524] and WASID[491] trials used four 5-grain aspirin tablets (approx. 1300 mg) each day. Some investigators posit that smaller doses produce the desired inhibition of platelet functions and do not inhibit production of prostacyclin by endothelial cells.[528,529] In-vitro studies of the effects of small and larger dose aspirin on prostaglandin and prostacyclin formation have used normal, young animal vessels; however, in patients with extracranial vascular disease, the endothelium is frequently damaged and might no longer be able to synthesize prostacyclin. In the British UK-TIA Trial, one 300-mg aspirin a day was as effective as higher doses.[530] In the Swedish Aspirin Low-Dose Trial, 75 mg of aspirin a day resulted in a statistically significant 18% reduction in stroke and death,[531] while in the Dutch TIA trial, even 30 mg was as effective and better tolerated than 300 mg of aspirin a day.[532]

Patients given aspirin do not all have the same effect on platelet functions as measured in vitro.[533–538] Helgason and colleagues studied the effectiveness of aspirin on platelet function measured in vitro.[535] Among 107 patients who received 325 mg of aspirin per day, inhibition of platelet aggregation was complete in 85 (79%) and partial in 22 (20.5%). Among 9 patients who did not respond to 325 mg of aspirin, escalating the dose to 650 mg per day resulted in complete platelet inhibition in 5 (56%). An increase to 975 mg caused complete inhibition in 1 of the 4 patients who did not respond to 650 mg. The 3 patients who did not respond to 975 mg had only partial inhibition at a 1300-mg aspirin dose.[535] Others have also shown a a variability of response on platelet aggregation tested in vitro according to the dose of aspirin.[536] Genetic factors clearly play a role in aspirin effects and those of virtually all other drugs. Some patients require more aspirin than others. Platelets interact with the endothelium and arterial wall, so platelet function is only one of the factors that relates to the deposition of platelet–fibrin and erythrocyte–fibrin thrombi. The presence and importance of "aspirin resistance" continues to be debated.[536,539] Most neurologists now use aspirin doses that vary from 50 to 325 mg per day. Gastrointestinal bleeding and gastritis are important and common side effects of aspirin. The frequency of these side effects is dose-related.

Phosphodiesterase inhibitors – dipyridamole and cilostazol

Phosphodiesterase inhibitors modestly reduce platelet function[398,540] and important endothelial activity, and act as vasodilators.[398,540] In Western populations, dipyridamole, a pyramidopyrimidine compound, has been most extensively studied for stroke treatment, while cilastazol has been a focus of studies in Asian populations. Dipyridamole inhibits the attachment of platelets to the endothelium. In rabbits, a combination of aspirin and dipyridamole protected against thrombosis induced by combined chemical and electrical stimuli when neither drug did so separately.[541] In a study reported in 1971, Sullivan and colleagues showed a beneficial effect of

adding dipyridamole in a dose of 400 mg per day to warfarin anticoagulation to effectively prevent brain embolic strokes in patients who had prosthetic heart valves.[542] Two trials reported during the early 1980s showed no benefit of dipyridamole even when added to aspirin.[543,544] In the Canadian–American trial, dipyridamole in doses of 300 mg per day had no significant therapeutic effect when added to 1300 mg per day aspirin in patients with TIA or minor stroke.[543] In a French trial 225 mg dipyridamole used with 1000 mg aspirin was not better than aspirin alone.[544]

Dipyridamole in the form given in these two trials had variable gastrointestinal absorption related to gastric acidity, and required four times a day dosing because of its pharmacokinetics. The dose of dipyridamole was relatively low and likely did not produce adequate sustained blood levels. An extended release form of dipyridamole has longer activity and much improved absorption. Two trials – the European Stroke Prevention Studies (ESPS 1 and ESPS 2) – reported a beneficial effect on stroke prevention of extended-release dipyridamole when used with aspirin.[545–548] In ESPS 1, dipyridamole 75 mg 3 times a day + aspirin 330 mg 3 times a day given for 2 years showed a 38% reduction in stroke compared to placebo in patients with ischemic strokes or TIAs.[545] In the ESPS 2 trial, 6602 patients took either placebo, aspirin (25 mg twice a day), dipyridamole in a modified-release form 200 mg twice a day, or aspirin and dipyridamole 25 mg aspirin + 200 mg modified-release dipyridamole twice a day.[546] The RR reduction for the combined end-points of stroke and death were 13.2% for aspirin, 15.4% for dipyridamole, and 24.4% for the combination of aspirin and dipyridamole.[546] The combined therapy reduced the stroke risk 23.1% over aspirin alone and 24.7% over dipyridamole alone.[546–548]

A later trial, carried out in the Netherlands, also studied the effectiveness of dipyridamole in stroke prevention of patients who had recent TIAs or minor strokes.[549] Several features distinguish this trial (ESPRIT) from the ESPS trials: varied dose of aspirin (30–325 mg, median dose 75 mg), 17% of patients assigned to dipyridamole did not receive the extended-release form; and the trial was not initiated or funded by a pharmaceutical company. The primary outcome studied was the composite of death from all vascular causes, non-fatal stroke, non-fatal myocardial infarction, and major bleeding. These outcomes occurred in 13% of patients assigned to aspirin–dipyridamole versus 16% of those in the aspirin group.[549] Ischemic stroke developed in 7% of those assigned to aspirin–dipyridamole versus 8.4% of those assigned to aspirin. Cardiac events were also more common in those on aspirin.[549] A meta-analysis concluded that "the combination of aspirin and dipyridamole was more effective than aspirin alone in preventing stroke and other serious vascular events in patients with minor strokes and TIAs."[550]

Cilostazol is a phosphodiesterase inhibitor that, like dipyridamole, has both antiplatelet and vasodilator effects.[551,552] In a trial in Japan, which included greater than 1000 patients with brain infarcts acquired 1–6 months before entry, cilostazol 100 mg twice daily showed a 42.3% relative risk reduction (from 10.3% to 62.9% CI, $P = 0.013$) in reducing the frequency of recurrent brain infarction in an intention-to-treat analysis.[553] In a trial in 278 sites in Japan, 2757 patients with non-cardioembolic stroke were randomized to cilostazol 100 mg twice daily or aspirin 81 mg once daily and followed for up to 5 years, average of 29 months.[554] Combined ischemic and hemorrhagic strokes occurred less often in the cilastazol group, 2.76% versus 3.71% per year.[554] Cilostazol has been shown to increase CBF in patients with atherosclerotic risk factors.[555] Cilostazol is often used in patients with peripheral vascular occlusive disease. In a Korean trial, cilostazole and aspirin were more effective than aspirin alone in preventing progression of atherosclerotic stenosis.[556] To date the effect of cilostazole or cilostazole + aspirin on stroke prevention has been mainly studied in Asians, and the patients studied have had a high frequency of penetrating artery disease (lacunar strokes) and intracranial large artery disease. Its effect in white patients in the United States and Europe has not been studied in any depth.

Thienopyridines: clopidogrel and ticlopidine

Ticlopidine hydrochloride was the first thienopyridine derivate studied in trials and introduced into practise. The thienopyridines inhibit the adenosine diphosphate pathway of platelet aggregation; unlike aspirin they do not inhibit the cyclooxygenase pathway.[476,557] In the Ticlopidine–Aspirin Stroke Study (TASS), a large, randomized trial, ticlopidine showed a RR reduction of approximately 30% in decreasing the rate of stroke, myocardial infarction, and vascular death in men and women who had a previous minor stroke.[558] In the Canadian–American Ticlopidine Study (CATS), ticlopidine (500 mg daily) was slightly more effective than aspirin (1300 mg daily) in reducing the rate of stroke in patients with TIAs or minor strokes.[559] In these clinical trials, ticlopidine had a relatively high rate of side effects, especially diarrhea and skin rash. Neutropenia, sometimes severe, was a serious but infrequent complication of ticlopidine (approx. 1% of patients).[558,559] Patients taking ticlopidine had a slightly elevated cholesterol level.[558] Bennett et al. reported 60 patients with thrombotic thrombocytopenic purpura after using ticlopidine,[560] and thrombocytopenia has been noted by others as a ticlopidine side effect.[557] Ticlopidine was introduced into stroke prophylaxis in the early 1990s but recognition of serious side effects and the introduction of clopidogrel (a thienopyridine with a closely related chemical structure that differs from ticlopidine by the addition of a carboxymethyl side group) an agent that had similar effectiveness but fewer severe side effects led to the gradual disappearance of ticlopidine as a newly prescribed antiplatelet agent.

The Clopidogrel versus Aspirin in Patients at Risk of Ischemic Events (CAPRIE) trial was a randomized, double-blinded trial of clopidogrel (75 mg/day) versus aspirin (325 mg/day) in preventing ischemic events (ischemic stroke, myocardial infarction, and vascular death).[561] During 3 years, 19 185 patients were entered, including 6421 ischemic stroke patients, 6302 patients with myocardial infarcts, and 6452 patients who had atherosclerotic peripheral vascular occlusive disease. Clopidogrel had a relative risk reduction over aspirin

of 8.7%, considering all end-points.[561] The frequency of stroke was 405 out of 17 636 (2.30%) for clopidogrel versus 430 out of 17 519 (2.45%) for aspirin. The frequency of myocardial infarction was more effectively reduced by clopidogrel than the frequency of stroke.[561] Clopidogrel had an excellent safety record in this large trial; the frequency of neutropenia and thrombocytopenia in patients using clopidogrel were no different than for aspirin, but clopidogrel was later reported to be associated with thrombotic thrombocytopenic purpura in another report.[562]

Reasoning that decreasing platelet activities by two different mechanisms might prove superior to single agents alone, the MATCH trial tested aspirin (75 mg/day) + clopidogrel (75 mg/day) against clopidogrel (75 mg/day) alone in patients with brain ischemia.[563,564] The combination was not superior in decreasing the primary outcome measure (reduction in ischemic stroke, myocardial infarction, vascular death, and rehospitalization for acute ischemic events) and caused more life-threatening bleeding, often intracranial.[563,564] Similarly, the Clopidogrel and Aspirin versus Aspirin Alone for the Prevention of Atherothrombotic Events (CHARISMA) trial studied the effectiveness of adding clopidogrel to aspirin for stroke prevention.[565] The trial included 15 063 patients with either clinically evident cardiovascular disease (coronary, cerebrovascular, or peripheral vascular) or multiple risk factors. Overall, clopidogrel plus aspirin was not more effective than aspirin alone in reducing the rate of myocardial infarction, stroke, or death from cardiovascular causes. Moderate and severe bleeding were more common in those taking both clopidogrel and aspirin.[565]

While long-term combined clopidogrel and aspirin therapy has not shown benefit over single agent treatment, recent data suggest that short-term combined therapy in the first few weeks after a minor stroke or TIA may be beneficial. The first several weeks after a non-cardioembolic cerebral ischemic event is the period of highest risk of recurrent ischemia, as atherosclerotic plaques remain in unstable condition and collaterals have not yet fully matured. The greater bleeding risk associated with combined antiplatelet therapy may be outweighed by added benefit in averting ischemic events during these first, high risk weeks. In an Asian population, a brief course of combined clopidogrel and aspirin was shown superior to aspirin alone in the Clopidogrel in High-Risk Patients with Acute Nondisabling Cerebrovascular Events (CHANCE) trial.[566] At 114 centers in China, 5170 patients with minor ischemic stroke or TIA were randomized to combined clopidogrel and aspirin for 21 days followed by clopidogrel alone through 90 days versus aspirin alone for 90 days. Recurrent ischemic stroke occurred in 8.2% of patients in the combined clopidogrel–aspirin group compared to 11.7% in the aspirin group.[566] The rate of hemorrhagic stroke was low and equal in both groups (0.3%). In the United States and Europe, the Platelet-Oriented Inhibition in New TIA and minor ischemic stroke (POINT) trial is currently under way testing short-term combined clopidogrel and aspirin for non-cardioembolic minor stroke and TIA in a Western population.[567]

Trials in patients with coronary artery stents, especially those that are drug-eluted, have shown that double antiplatelets are important in decreasing the frequency of in-stent thrombosis, and most often aspirin and clopidogrel are given for 6–12 months.[568] Double antiplatelets are also routinely given for patients with carotid artery stents.[569] Stents cover the vascular intima so they remove the contact of platelets with the endothelium; agents that affect the attachment of platelets to the endothelium (cilostazole and dipyridamole) are likely not to be effective in patients with stents. The requirement in stented patients for relatively long-term double antiplatelets is important when considering adding an anticoagulant.

Glycoprotein IIb/IIIa antagonists

The advent of drugs that are antagonists of the glycoprotein (GP) platelet IIb/IIIa complex gives promise of even more effective inhibition of platelet functions. The platelet GP IIb/IIIa complex is the site of binding to adhesive proteins including fibrinogen. Binding to fibrinogen activates platelet aggregation and adhesion to blood vessels. Abciximab is a humanized monoclonal antibody that binds to the GP IIb/IIIa complex on platelets.[570,571] Abciximab has been used mostly IV and acutely in patients after invasive coronary and cerebral revascularization procedures.[570,572,573] This agent causes a profound impairment of the function of platelets similar to a temporary thrombasthenia so that the rate of bleeding is potentially high.[570] The use of abciximab during the first 24 hours after stroke proved safe in a preliminary study.[574] The Abciximab in Emergent Stroke Treatment Trial II (AbESTT-II), a double-blind randomized phase III trial designed to compare abciximab with placebo for the treatment of acute ischemic stroke patients, did not show efficacy and was terminated prematurely for safety reasons – excessive bleeding.[304]

Some patients develop a veritable carpet of white platelet–fibrin thrombi after vascular surgery and interventional vascular treatments. In that setting abciximab may prove very useful. Abciximab has also been used during interventional procedures to accomplish reperfusion in acute stroke patients as an adjunct to thrombolytic agents.[575–577] Cardiologists often use abciximab or other GP IIb/IIIa antagonists along with thrombolytics, other antiplatelets, and anticoagulants as a potent IV "cocktail" in patients with acute coronary-related cardiac ischemia.[578,579]

Other parenteral small molecule, non-antibody GP IIb/IIIa antagonists, tirofiban and eptifibatide have shorter duration of antiplatelet activity but have been shown to improve outcomes after coronary procedures and have less bleeding complications than abciximab.[570,580] GP IIb/IIIa inhibiting agents that can be used orally and chronically are now being tested but to-date have been associated with excess bleeding and have not been introduced into clinical practice. Lotrafiban, an orally administered GP IIb/IIIa inhibitor was studied in a trial (Blockade of the Glycoprotein IIb/IIIa Receptor to Avoid Vascular Occlusion (BRAVO)) that included 9190 patients admitted with coronary or cerebrovascular disease.[580] Lotrafiban was given 30 or 50 mg twice a

day or placebo was given with aspirin. Lotrafiban administration was associated with a significantly higher death rate due to vascular disease and more serious bleeding. Lotrafiban use was not associated with a significant decrease in the composite end-point of all-cause mortality, myocardial infarction, recurrent ischemia requiring hospitalization or urgent revascularization.[581]

Antiplatelet therapies for specific vessel sites

Most early trials of antiplatelet therapy in ischemic stroke prevention lumped all non-cardioembolic stroke patients together. A decade ago, the Antiplatelet Trialists Collaboration,[582,583] the Antithrombotic Trialists' Collaboration,[584] and the Cochrane[585] and other reviews[586,587] analyzed the results among 285 trials (>135 000 patients) that examined the effectiveness and safety of antiplatelet drugs in stroke prevention and other vascular events. None of the early published studies mandated rigorous evaluation of the heart, aorta, and craniocerebral arteries or technology-assisted diagnosis of stroke mechanisms. None of the early studies showed which drugs were effective for which vascular lesions.

Trials have recently begun to appear that are more sophisticated in their approach. Large trials have evaluated well-evaluated patients found to have ischemic stroke due to specific arterial sites, and have begun to provide a more nuanced guide to therapy.

Aortic arch atherosclerosis: The Aortic Arch Related Cerebral Hazard (AARCH) trial enrolled 349 patients with ischemic stroke, TIA, or peripheral embolism, plaque in the thoracic aorta greater than 4 mm in thickness, and no other identified embolic source.[588] Patients were randomized to receive either double antiplatelet therapy with aspirin 75–150 mg/day and clopidogrel 75 mg/day or warfarin with a target INR of 2–3. After an average of 3.4 years of follow-up, adverse vascular events tended to occur less often with double antiplatelet therapy, 7.6% (13/172), than with warfarin therapy, 11.3% (20/177).[588] Aortic arch atherosclerosis is typically characterized by rapid dyslaminar flow over an irregular atherosclerotic surface, a setting more likely to produce white than red clots and to be responsive to platelet antiaggregant therapy. Although not large enough to be definitive, the AARCH results suggest that intensive, double antiplatelet therapy is indeed better than anticoagulation for aortic arch atherosclerosis. In some patients with protruding mobile large aortic arch lesions anticoagulants might be indicated.

Intracranial large artery atherosclerosis: The Warfarin–Aspirin for Symptomatic Intracranial Disease (WASID) trial enrolled 569 patients with ischemic stroke related to 50–99% atherosclerotic stenosis of a large intracranial artery.[489] Patients were randomized to high-dose aspirin, 1300 mg/day, or warfarin with a target INR 2–3. During an average of 1.8 years, the rate of recurrent ischemic stroke was similar in the aspirin versus warfarin groups. The warfarin group had higher rates of myocardial infarction (7.3% vs. 2.9%), major hemorrhage (8.3% vs. 3.2%), and death (9.7% vs. 4.3%). Patients in the warfarin-treated group with subtherapeutic INRs had an overabundance of ischemic strokes, and those with supratherapeutic INRs had a high frequency of hemorrhages.[489,490] Intracranial large artery stenoses sometimes produce rapid dsylaminar flow over irregular surfaces, predisposing to white clots, and sometimes produce slow flow, predisposing to red clots. As a result, both antiplatelet and anticoagulant therapy prevent ischemic stroke somewhat, but antiplatelet agents better prevent coronary events and have fewer hemorrhagic complications than vitamin K antagonists. The newer anticoagulants (direct thrombin and factor Xa inhibitors) show promise of more reliable control and less bleeding. They should have a better benefit–risk ratio than vitamin K antagonists and may prove superior to antiplatelets in selected patients with severe flow-reducing stenosis and acute occlusions.

Small penetrator micro-atherosclerosis and lipohyalinosis: The Secondary Prevention of Small Subcortical Strokes (SPS 3) trial enrolled 3020 patients with recent lacunar infarcts confirmed by magnetic resonance imaging.[589] Patients were randomized to receive dual antiplatelet therapy with aspirin 325 mg daily + clopidogrel 75 mg daily, or single antiplatelet therapy with aspirin 325 mg daily. After a mean follow-up of 3.4 years, there tended to be fewer recurrent ischemic strokes with double antiplatelet therapy (2.0% vs. 2.4% per year) but also more hemorrhagic strokes (0.42% vs. 0.25% per year), so that the overall stroke rate did not differ between the groups.[589] The risk of any major hemorrhage was almost doubled with dual antiplatelet therapy (2.1% vs. 1.1% per year) and deaths were increased in the double antiplatelet arm (2.1% vs. 1.4% per year). These findings suggest that the double antiplatelet therapy with both aspirin and clopidogrel does not have sufficient advantages over aspirin alone to outweigh the increased bleeding risk. Because cilostazole and dipyridamole have different actions than aspirin and clopidogrel, and cause less bleeding, LRC posits that they may have a better benefit–risk ratio than aspirin and/or clopidogrel in patients with penetrating artery disease. Cilostazole has been given with aspirin and has been shown to have salutary effects in patients with intracranial disease.[556]

More studies are needed comparing antiplatelet drugs with other strategies in patients with well-defined vascular lesions. Some investigators and clinicians have used a combination of warfarin anticoagulants and platelet antiaggregants, usually aspirin, in patients with severe atherosclerosis who did not respond to more conventional treatments.[590] This combination was effective but resulted in a higher bleeding-complication rate.[590,591] We have also used this strategy in patients in whom warfarin was indicated but was ineffective when used alone.

A useful strategy may be to use platelet antiaggregants when there is no documented flow reduction and ischemia is most likely due to the process of platelet plugs and small white (or white and red) clots. The newer anticoagulants are reserved for situations with arterial flow stasis or clots within the heart. Results of the use of these stratagies to date are anecdotal and have not been tested scientifically. Box 6.10 reviews our present recommendations for the use of platelet antiaggregants and anticoagulants.

Box 6.10 Present recommended use of platelet aggregants and anticoagulants

Immediate anticoagulation therapy

1. Patients with ischemic stroke or TIA due to definite cardiac-origin brain embolism (severe hypertension, bacterial endocarditis, or sepsis would delay or contraindicate this use)
2. Large artery severe stenosis or occlusion, with no or only small–moderate size established infarction
3. Venous prophylaxis using low-molecular-weight heparin, low-dose unfractionated heparin or dabigatran or a factor Xa inhibitor for prevention of deep vein occlusion in patients immobilized by stroke (unless contraindicated)
4. Delayed therapy of brain infarction due to definite cardiac-origin brain embolism (for small infarcts <1.5 cm in diameter) (uncontrolled hypertension, bacterial endocarditis, or sepsis would delay or contraindicate this use)

Immediate antiplatelet therapy

1. Double antiplatelet therapy with aspirin and clopidogrel or aspirin with cilostazole, or the combination of aspirin and modified release dipyridamole (Aggrenox) for TIA and minor stroke patients with plaque disease of the extracranial and intracranial arteries. In patients with stents, aspirin and clopidogrel are preferred. Cilostazole and aspirin or aspirin and modified-release dipyridamole are preferred for penetrating artery disease related brain ischemia
2. Single antiplatelet therapy (aspirin unless allergic; if so, then clopidogrel with loading dose) for all others

Delayed anticoagulation therapy

After initial antiplatelet therapy, begin anticoagulant therapy for definite cardiac-origin brain embolism (severe hypertension, bacterial endocarditis, or sepsis would delay or contraindicate this use). Start 48 hours after onset when infarct is small, 7 days after onset when infarct is large, 14 days after onset when there has been initial hemorrhagic transformation

Long-term anticoagulation

1. Patients with cardiogenic brain embolization and rheumatic heart disease, atrial fibrillation with large atria or prior brain embolism, prosthetic valves, and some hypercoagulable states
2. Patients with stasis flow demonstrated in basilar, ICA, or MCA shown on flow-sensitive imaging (time-of-flight MRA, catheter angiography) due to large artery severe stenosis

Long-term platelet antiaggregants (aspirin, clopidogrel, combined aspirin–dipyridamole, cilostazol)

1. For patients with plaque disease of the extracranial and intracranial arteries without severe stenosis
2. For patients with lacunar ischemic strokes
3. For patients with polycythemia or thrombocytosis and related ischemic attacks

Increasing the brain's resistance to ischemia ("neuroprotection")

Theoretically, there might be substances or strategies that make the brain relatively resistant, at least for some time, to the deleterious effect of lack of oxygen and energy delivery; that is keeping brain cells alive despite poor perfusion. If these neuroprotective agents could be administered soon after the ischemic insult, it might delay neuronal death and allow a longer time window for thrombolysis or other reperfusion strategies. We have discussed some of these so-called neuroprotection strategies that have been used in combination with thrombolysis earlier in this chapter. Trials of putative neuroprotectants, when used alone without adjunctive measures to enhance reperfusion, have all resulted in failure as of this writing. Many failed because animal experiments were not rigorously blinded and controlled to prevent observer bias.[592,593] Some agents that were effective in experimental animal models of acute ischemia simply had no or little benefit in humans with brain ischemia. Many failures are likely due to suboptimal trial design and testing.[594]

Neuronal death depends on multiple factors[595] including: (1) level of activity (the more work that goes on, the more fuel is needed); (2) presence of local metabolites such as lactic acid[596,597] and oxygen-free radicals;[598–601] (3) temperature of the system (at low temperatures there is less metabolism and less need for fuel);[601–603] (4) integrity of the neuronal cell membranes; and (5) influx of calcium into cells and the extracellular-to-intracellular gradient for calcium.[604–606]

Experimental evidence from global ischemia experiments in young animals indicates that hyperglycemia makes the brain more vulnerable to ischemia.[597] Sugar increases metabolism and leads to the production of lactic acid. Acidosis can be destructive to brain tissue.[607] Hyperglycemia is known to be associated with poor outcomes in patients with brain ischemia and brain hemorrhage.[608–611] A high concentration of extracellular calcium can also contribute to final neuronal death. Lowering of blood sugars and reducing calcium influx into cells are among the many means posited to protect neurons from cell death.

Neurotransmitters, especially glutamate, released at sites of ischemia might overexcite neurons and cause toxic damage increasing the effects of the initial ischemia.[612–616] This theory, often referred to as the excitotoxin hypothesis, has stimulated much research concerning neurotransmitters and ischemia and attempts to counter the harmful effects of excess neurotransmitter release. The excitotoxin hypothesis was introduced by Olney and colleagues to describe the mechanism by which

glutamate and some other acidic amino acids caused neuronal lesions in periventricular structures when given systemically to mice.[612–615] Electrophysiological studies showed that these compounds functioned as neuronal excitants and damaged the periventricular structures studied. Hypothetically, hypoxia and ischemia caused energy depletion and release of glutamate into the tissues. Glutamate then was taken up by receptors and excited the cells already depleted of blood supply, ultimately leading to neuronal death. Putative neurotoxins include glutamate, kainic acid, N-methyl-D-aspartate (NMDA), and homocysteic acid. By far, glutamate has been the most studied. These compounds have various receptor types, usually referred to as NMDA and non-NMDA receptors, including quisqualate and kainate receptors.

Experimental evidence supports the role of excitotoxins in potentiating ischemia. When kainic acid is injected into the hippocampus of experimental animals it causes a pattern of cell death similar to hypoxic–ischemic damage.[615] The concentration of glutamate in the extracellular compartment in ischemic brain is increased. Deafferentation of specific intrahippocampal excitatory pathways seems to protect against ischemic damage. Drugs that block excitatory neurotransmission are sometimes protective when given to animals early after experimentally induced ischemia.

Glutamate opens membrane sodium conductance allowing a large influx of sodium to enter cells. Chloride ion and water follow the sodium causing cytotoxic edema. Transmembrane influx of calcium into cells leads to a toxic increase in cytosolic free calcium that can kill cells.[604,605] Experimentally, a number of compctitive and non-competitive NMDA-receptor antagonists have been used, including MK 801, dextrorphan, dextromethorphan, ketamine, magnesium, memantine, selfotel, aptiganel, felbamate, and phencyclidine.[617–619] Although the vast bulk of the work on excitatory neurotransmitters has been in laboratory animals, the studies that carried out in human stroke patients have been disappointing.[617–619] Many of the agents used have had prominent central nervous system or cardiovascular toxicity. Agitation, confusion, sedation, hallucinations, catatonia, and psychotic behavior occur during therapy with many of the NMDA-channel antagonists. Unfortunately the agents used have been associated with unacceptable frequencies of side effects especially psychosis.

Some investigators posit that free radicals found during hypoxic injury may lead to further neuronal damage.[598–600] A free radical is an atom, group of atoms, or molecule having one or more unpaired electrons in its outermost orbit. Covalent chemical bonds usually have paired electrons; free radicals are molecules with an open bond, which accounts for their extreme reactivity. The free radicals of importance in brain ischemia are superoxide and hydroxyl radicals. Hydrogen peroxide can generate hydroxyl radicals in reaction with superoxide. Xanthine oxidase is the major enzyme that generates superoxide radicals. Free radicals can react with and damage proteins, nucleic acids, lipids, and other molecules and can initiate destructive chain reactions.[598–600] Oxygen radicals can also damage blood vessels and cause vasodilation, increased vascular permeability, endothelial and smooth muscle injury, and increased platelet aggregation.[600]

Strategies to prevent and neutralize oxygen free radicals have been attempted mostly in experimental animals. The agents used are often referred to as free radical scavengers. Unfortunately none have proved effective in man in preliminary trials. The most recent free radical scavengers tested in human trials were NXY-059 and albumin. NXY-059 appeared to be safe and effective in the Stroke–Acute Ischemic NXY Treatment I (SAINT I) trial[620–622] but was not effective in the SAINT II trial,[623] and the pharmaceutical company that produced and studied the drug has said that it will not pursue its use for stroke neuroprotection. Albumin did not improve outcome and increased pulmonary edema in the High-Dose Albumin Treatment For Acute Ischaemic Stroke (ALIAS) Part 2 trial.[359]

One cytoprotective strategy is to give a substrate that might help injured neurons to recover. Citicoline (cytidine-5-diphosphocholine) is the agent in this category that has been used most often in experimental animals and humans. Citicoline is an intermediary in the biosynthesis of the membrane phospholipid phosphatidylcholine and is used to enhance the synthesis of this lipid in the brain. Citicoline has been used alone and in combination with thrombolysis.[624–628] Citicoline was studied in preliminary clinical trials in acute ischemic stroke patients that showed the substance was very safe and there were some suggestions of effectiveness.[625,626] However, in a trial enrolling 2298 patients in Europe, citicoline did not improve outcome.[627]

The most important substrates used by nerve cells are oxygen and sugar. We have already noted the problems with adminstration of sugar. Hyperglycemia increases lactate production and likely has adverse rather than protective effects.[606,608–611] Adminstration of oxygen was thought to potentially induce vasoconstriction in arteries feeding ischemic brain tissue so that only recently has its use been explored in patients with acute brain ischemia. Another theoretical concern is that extra oxygen could increase generation of damaging oxygen free radicals in ischemic fields. Because hyperbaric oxygen therapy was known to be effective in divers who developed bends – a disorder in which gas was introduced into blood vessels during pressure changes during diving – it seemed worth trying in patients with brain ischemia. Unfortunately preliminary trials of hyperbaric oxygen in acute stroke patients showed no benefit and the pressure chamber could cause harm by reducing arterial input flow.[629,630] Bedside inhaled oxygen (normobaric oxygen) also failed to demonstrate benefit.[631–634]

Another neuroprotective strategy has been to reduce the metabolic needs of brain tissue thus allowing survival despite less energy delivery. This strategy also hopes to enlarge the time window during which reperfusion would be effective. The two most common strategies in this category are to induce hypothermia[635–643] and to use barbiturates at or near anesthesia levels.[644,645] These interventions reduce cerebral energy and metabolism and thereby reduce the brain's requirements for fuel, oxygen, and blood. However, each can lead to circulatory

changes and can complicate the examination and management of stroke patients. Hypothermia has been used effectively in reducing brain injury in patients after cardiac arrest, and this has been its most commonly used clinical application.[636,637] Open series and trials have shown that hypothermia is beneficial in reducing edema in large brain infarcts, but it is not as effective an intervention as hemicraniectomy decompression.[638–640] Hypothermia also shows potential promise as a treatment to reduce initial ischemic injury and reperfusion injury after tPA in more moderate sized ischemic strokes. Cooling to effective hypothermic levels is not simple. When deep hypothermia is targeted, shivering and discomfort usually require heavy sedation, intubation, and the administration of muscle paralyzing agents, and changes in electrolytes are common, as are potential cardiac arrythmias. Newer techniques of administering hypothermia have made its use more promising for moderate ischemic strokes.[641] Antishivering drugs permit patients to undergo moderate cooling without needing to be intubated and paralyzed.[646] Hypothermia should not be used as a neuroprotective strategy except in medical centers that have considerable experience with its use. Barbiturate use also involves practical problems in managing patients with induced coma and has not been pursued clinically in acute stroke patients.

At the time of writing, no neuroprotective strategy for focal ischemic stroke has proved effective in man. Armchair ideas and theories abound and far outweigh the data, but this field of investigation still may prove fruitful in the future. More rigorous, unbiased testing in animal models is needed before treatments are brought to human testing. Trials in human stroke patients have not always been well designed to show an effect of the various therapies. They have customarily been given to all patients with acute stroke late after onset, and in the vast majority of trials and studies full brain and vascular imaging have not been mandated at entry or follow-up.

Among all patients with acute brain ischemia:

1. Many would already have large infarcts. Dead brain would likely not respond to neuroprotection. Treating hyper-early would help. Treating in the ambulance, in the first minutes after onset, would ensure that patients still have salvageable brain to save. Among patients seen later after onset, those who already have developed large infarcts could be identified by DWI MRI scans or full CT protocols.

2. In many the blood vessels supplying the ischemic brain would be occluded. The neuroprotective agents might not reach the ischemic neurons because the roads are blocked. Administering the agents to patients who have open arteries or are undergoing thrombolysis or other reperfusion techniques would be most effective.

3. White matter infarcts especially lacunes might not respond to neuroprotective agents that are cytoprotective since the white matter consists of tracts and not neurons.

Neuroprotective agents are unlikely to ever be as powerful a treatment for ischemic stroke as restoring normal blood flow to the threatened field. However, they could possibly play a useful complementary role to thrombolytic and catheter reperfusion techniques if they could be given early after onset, stabilizing the threatened field until reperfusion treatment is started, or they can help prevent reperfusion injury after blood vessels are reopened.[647–649]

Statins (HMG-CoA reductase inhibitors)

Because of their pleotrophic effects in stroke and vascular disease prevention and their potential in neuroprotection, statins are worth separate consideration in this chapter. The 3-hydroxy-3-methylglutaryl coenzyme A reductase (HMG-CoA) inhibitors (statins) were initially prescribed because of their potent effect in lowering serum cholesterol, especially the low-density lipoprotein component. Early trials showed that statin drugs not only reduced cholesterol levels but also were effective in reducing coronary artery disease-related events and mortality, even in patients with average levels of cholesterol.[650–652] Analysis of randomized trials of statins also shows a clear and rather dramatic reduction in the incidence of stroke.[653–655] Use of statin drugs slows progression of coronary artery lesions[656] and carotid artery atherosclerotic plaques.[657–659] High doses of statins (equivalent of 80 mg of atorvastatin) have been shown to be more effective than lower doses in patients with coronary artery disease[656] and in preventing strokes in those patients who had TIAs or strokes.[660,661] In a review of over 8800 patients who had a history of cerebrovascular disease and were treated with statins, there was a reduction in subsequent ischemic strokes and total strokes but an increase in hemorrhagic strokes.[662] Other studies that contained fewer patients who had cerebrovascular disease did not show an increase in hemorrhagic strokes.[662]

Preliminary studies suggest that statins may also have potent neuroprotective effects.[661,663–667] Large doses of statins increase CBF at the ischemic core and penumbra. One mechanism of this increase in blood flow is related to an increase in endothelium-derived nitric oxide synthase (eNOS).[666,668,669] The beneficial effects of the statins on nearly all aspects of atherosclerotic disease morbidity and mortality are not entirely explained by reduction in serum lipid levels. Basic research indicates some other important salutory effects of the statins including: (1) normalization of the vascular endothelium; (2) anti-inflammatory effects: Statins reduce C-reactive protein (CRP) as well as LDL cholesterol,[656] and high CRP levels are strong predictors of the occurrence of coronary and cerebrovascular events;[670–672] (3) depletion and stabilization of the lipid core content of plaques; (4) strengthening of the fibrous cap of plaques; (5) decrease in formation of platelet–fibrin thrombi and decreased deposition of white clots on endothelial surfaces; (6) reduction in the thrombogenicity of plaque elements;[673] and (7) increase in cerebrovascular reactivity which might prove effective in reducing vasospasm after SAH,[674] and could improve blood flow in patients with lacunar infarction due to penetrating artery disease.[675] Although a randomized trial did not find statins beneficial in acute SAH,[676] there are many potential indications for statin use in patients with focal ischemic stroke.[661,666,677–679]

High-dose statins have proved very safe with less than 1% serious complications.[663] Discontinuation of statin administration in patients with coronary or cerebrovascular events can promote the development of myocardial and brain damage.[680–682] In one trial that included 215 patients in whom statins were not given for the first 3 days after an acute ischemic stroke, statin withdrawal was associated with increased brain infarct volumes, higher Rankin scores, and an increased risk of death or dependency at 3 months.[682] Neuromuscular symptoms and findings include: asymptomatic creatine kinase (CK) elevations, cramps, stiffness, exercise intolerance, proximal muscle weakness, and rhabdomyolysis.[683,684] Severe myopathy is rare. Hydrophilic statins (pravastatin and atorvastatin), when used at high doses are associated with elevated transaminases but not CK, while lipophilic statins (simvastatin, lovastatin) in high doses are associated with high CK levels and not transaminase.[683]

Increased intracranial pressure and brain edema and their control

Large ischemic and hemorrhagic strokes often increase the volume and pressure inside the cranium. Herniations, shifts in intracranial contents, and generalized increase in intracranial pressure (ICP) are all common causes of death in patients with large strokes. Treatment of these patients often includes strategies to control changes in ICP. SAH is also accompanied by increased blood within the cranium, often complicated by decreased drainage of cerebrospinal fluid (CSF). Patients with subarachnoid hemorrhage almost always have increased ICP.

The cranium can be thought of as an almost completely closed structure within a rigid container. The brain and its interstitial fluid account for approximately 80% of the intracranial volume, whereas CSF and blood within vessels each account for approximately 10% of the volume.[685] When ICP rises, adaptation occurs mostly by altering the CSF and vascular compartments. Less CSF can be produced or more can be absorbed. Blood volume inside the cranium can also be reduced. Most blood is contained in the low-pressure venous system, and this volume can be reduced.[685]

ICP has a major effect on pressure and flow in brain blood vessels. To maintain viability of brain tissue, there must be adequate cerebral perfusion pressure. In supine patients, cerebral perfusion pressure is approximately equal to the mean systemic arterial blood pressure minus the mean ICP.[685] Either an increase in ICP or a decrease in systemic blood pressure can further compromise rCBF to brain regions that are already ischemic. For practical purposes, there are only a few mechanisms of ICP elevation in stroke patients. These include: (1) introduction of new contents into the cranium, such as a hematoma within the brain or SAH; (2) edema in and around infarcts and hemorrhages; (3) obstruction of the ventricular system leading to hydrocephalus; and (4) decreased absorption of CSF caused by subarachnoid bleeding or inflammation. Each of these problems dictates different treatment strategies.

Reducing or limiting the size of an intracerebral hemorrhage

Unlike brain infarction, a hemorrhage always introduces extra volume into the closed cranial cavity. The larger the hemorrhage, the more the intracranial volume is expanded. In addition, the local blood collection induces surrounding edema, which further increases the volume of extra matter within the brain. Serial brain imaging studies have confirmed that hematomas often expand during the first hours after symptom onset.[686–688] About 35–40% of hematomas expand within a 3–6 hour period after onset. Expansion of hematoma volume is an important factor that increases morbidity and mortality in patients with intracerebral hemorrhages.[689] Edema usually develops around the hematoma beginning within the first 48 hours and often increases during the first week. The CT "spot sign," a locus of extra density at a hemorrhage margin, indicates active ongoing bleeding. It is present in one out of five acute hemorrhage patients and identifies patients much more likely to have hemorrhage expansion in the next minutes and hours.[690,691] Larger hematomas have more surrounding edema than smaller ones. Hemoglobin products and thrombin may promote edema formation. The volume of perihematomal edema also correlates with outcome.[692] ICP is generally elevated, especially in the region of the hematoma; the pressure changes can lead to a shift of midline structures and herniation into other dural compartments. The aim of therapy is to limit the size of the hemorrhage. This can be accomplished by limiting the bleeding, treating the accompanying edema, or draining the hematoma. In the case of hemorrhage caused by a vascular malformation or aneurysm, removing the offending vascular lesion also prevents recurrent hemorrhage.

The most important method to stop the bleeding is to reduce arterial tension. When LRC was a stroke fellow, before the advent of CT scanning, Dr Miller Fisher would sometimes transiently occlude with his finger the ipsilateral carotid artery in a patient with a clinical hypertensive basal ganglionic hemorrhage in order to diminish blood flow and stop the bleeding. The strategy is similar to the placement of a tourniquet on a limb proximal to bleeding. Overzealous blood pressure reduction, however, can be harmful because the elevated blood pressure helps perfuse brain tissue remote from the hemorrhage. The increased ICP is transmitted passively to the cerebral veins and dural sinuses increasing the pressures in those structures. The arterial pressure must rise to produce an effective arteriovenous pressure differential to perfuse the brain. Excessive reduction in blood pressure could decrease brain perfusion. The patient's alertness and neurological findings must be carefully monitored as the blood pressure is lowered.

Preliminary trials show that early lowering of blood pressure to normal range in acute intracerebral hemorrhage may reduce hemorrhage expansion and potentially improve outcome.[693–696] In the Second Intensive Blood Pressure Reduction in Acute Cerebral Hemorrhage Trial (INTERACT2), 2839 patients with intracerebral hemorrhage and elevated systolic blood pressure within 6 hours of onset

were randomized to receive intensive treatment to lower their blood pressure to a target systolic less than 140 mmHg within 1 hour or less aggressive treatment to lower their blood pressure to a target systolic less than 180 mmHg, with the use of agents of the physician's choosing.[696] Death or major disability tended to be lower in the intensive blood-pressure lowering arm, 52.0% versus 55.6%.[696]

When hemorrhage is caused by a bleeding diathesis, correction of the coagulopathy is critical in containing the hemorrhage. Use of antihemophilic globulin in hemophiliacs and reversal of warfarin-induced hypoprothrombinemia by fresh frozen plasma, vitamin K, activated factor VII, or prothrombin-complex concentrate are examples of such therapeutic interventions. Antidotes are now available in patients with hemorrhages who were taking dabigatran, apixaban, and rivaroxaban.

Clinicians and investigators have attempted to limit hematoma expansion even in patients without coagulopathies by administering recombinant activated factor VII (rFVIIa) to patients early in the course of intracerebral hemorrhages.[697–700] Two randomized trials of rFVIIa showed some effectiveness in reducing hemorrhage size but also some risk related to the induced hypercoagulability. In the first trial, 399 patients with CT confirmed intracerebral hematomas were randomly assigned within 3 hours after onset to receive placebo (96 patients) or 40 μg of rFVIIa per kg (108 patients), 80 μg/kg (92 patients), or 160 μg/kg (103 patients) within 1 hour after the initial CT scan.[698] The primary outcome measure was the percent change in the volume of the intracerebral hemorrhage measured at 24 hours. Hematoma volume increased more in the placebo group than in the rFVIIa groups. The mean increase was 29% in the placebo group, contrasted with 16%, 14%, and 11% in those given 40 μg, 80 μg, and 160 μg of rFVIIa/kg, respectively ($P = 0.01$ for the comparison of the three rFVIIa groups with the placebo group). Growth in the volume of intracerebral hemorrhage was reduced by 3.3 ml, 4.5 ml, and 5.8 ml in the three treatment groups, compared with the placebo group ($P = 0.01$).[698] Serious thromboembolic adverse events, mainly myocardial or cerebral infarction, occurred in 7% of rFVIIa-treated patients, compared with 2% of those given placebo ($P = 0.12$).[698,701] In the larger second trial, 841 patients were randomized to placebo, 20 μg of rFVIIa/kg, or 80 μg of rFVIIa/kg within 4 hours after onset.[700] The growth in volume of the hemorrhage was reduced by 2.6 ml in the 20 μg/kg group and by 3.8 ml in the 80 μg/kg group (95% CI, 0.9–6.7, $P = 0.009$). However, arterial thromboembolic events were more frequent in the high-dose group than controls, (9% vs. 4%). Overall, there was no difference among the three groups in the rate of poor clinical outcome, 24% in placebo, 26% in the low-dose group, and 29% in the high-dose group. For patients with pre-existing severe vascular occlusive disease involving the coronary or peripheral arteries, or past venous thromboembolism, the administration of rFVIIa poses a risk of myocardial infarction or venous occlusion with pulmonary embolism. Given these risks, a promising approach under investigation is to treat with

hemostatic agents only those patients at very high risk for hemorrhage expansion, as evidenced by both early presentation and the presence of the CT spot sign.

Drainage of hematomas can provide rapid decompression. Drainage can be performed by open craniotomy or stereotactically through small burr holes. Some patients may decompress their own lesions through spontaneous dissection of the hematoma into the ventricle or the subarachnoid space. Ease of surgical drainage will depend on the location of the lesion and its proximity to the surface. Lobar, putaminal, and cerebellar hemorrhages are easiest to drain surgically; thalamic and pontine hemorrhages are difficult to drain effectively.[702,703] The purpose of drainage is to reduce critical volume expansion that threatens life. Drainage of the hematoma leaves a residual cavity that disconnects brain pathways. Although allowing survival, drainage probably does not reduce the final neurological deficit. In comparable-sized infarcts, the cortex is invariably destroyed, whereas hematomas usually spare the cortex. For this reason, recovery from hemorrhages is usually better than from infarcts of equal size but recovery takes longer.

Open surgical drainage of intracerebral hematomas remains controversial. Unfortunately clinical series and trials have not settled the issues concerning surgical drainage of intracerebral hematomas.[704] A meta-analysis[705] and a Cochrane review[706] conclude that there was insufficient evidence regarding surgical treatment. Case series lump together patients with different location hemorrhages, of different sizes, operated on by different surgeons, using different surgical techniques, at different times. No wonder conclusions are difficult. The prevailing opinion of most neurologists has been that patients with very large hematomas who have reduced consciousness are not helped by drainage since the outcome is so bleak with or without surgical decompression. Similarly there is little use in draining very small hematomas since patients recover well without drainage. Patients with moderate-sized lobar and cerebellar hemorrhages, especially when associated with hematoma enlargement, mass effect, and clinical worsening, are those most likely to respond to decompressive surgery.

The largest randomized trials to date, the STICH I and STICH II (Surgical Trials in Lobar Intracerebral Haemorrhage) trials, failed to show a definite superiority of either medical or surgical treatment.[704,707,708] In the large STICH I trial, 1033 patients from 83 centers in 27 countries were randomized to surgery within 24 hours of randomization or initial conservative treatment. Among those randomized to early surgery, 26% had a favourable outcome compared with 24% randomized to initial conservative treatment (OR 0.89 (95% CI 0.66–1.19), $P = 0.414$). In this analysis deep and lobar hemorrhages were considered together.[707] Among the 530 patients randomized to initial conservative treatment, 140 crossed over and had surgery, complicating the analysis and interpretation of the results.[709] The investigators concluded that overall "patients with spontaneous supratentorial intracerebral haemorrhage in neurosurgical units show no overall benefit from early surgery when compared with initial

conservative treatment.[707] The STICH I trial did show that the presence of intraventricular bleeding and hydrocephalus adversely affected outcomes.[710]

The timing of surgical drainage of hematomas is clearly important. Initially the intracerebral blood is liquid. Later the blood coagulates and solidifies and is more difficult to remove. Much later the intracerebral clot again becomes softer and more liquid. Unfortunately, the present CT and MRI technologies do not reliably reflect the liquidity unless there is a fluid level within the hematoma. Clinicians posited that very early surgery, within 4 hours after symptom onset, might allow drainage of liquid blood and lead to better outcomes than surgery after 12 hours.[711] A planned study to test this hypothesis was stopped prematurely after 11 patients in the 4-hour arm had surgery.[711] Median time to surgery was 180 minutes; median hematoma volume was 40 ml; median baseline NIHSS score was 19. Postoperative rebleeding occurred in four patients, three of whom died. Rebleeding occurred in 40% of the patients treated within 4 hours, compared with 12% of the patients treated within 12 hours. A relationship between postoperative rebleeding and mortality was apparent.[711] Too early surgery often led to rebleeding which adversely affected outcome. The ideal time to operate is unknown.

Stereotactic drainage with or without thrombolytic softening of intracerebral and intraventricular clots is posited to provide better outcomes than open drainage. Stereotactic surgery has been performed for ICH for nearly 2 decades.[712–715] It has been used more often in Asian countries than in the west. Drainage is performed through a small burr hole and no cortisectomy is involved. Stereotactic surgery has been performed with and without a stereotactic frame and with and without administration of a thrombolytic agent directly into the intracerebral clot. The results show promise and are likely to prove superior in the hands of experienced surgeons to direct surgical drainage. Endoscopic drainage of blood is another promising technique.[716,717]

Drainage of subacute hemorrhages, by reducing ICP can improve alertness and reduce the frequency and severity of medical complications that often develop in stuporous patients.[714] In the largest randomized trial to date of minimally invasive surgery for intracerebral hemorrhage, patients were randomized to stereotactic aspiration with tPA instilled in the hematoma to break up clot versus medical therapy.[718] After stereotactic drainage, the average hemorrhage size was 20 cc in the first 79 patients randomized to the intervention versus 41 cc in the first 39 patients randomized to medical therapy. The amount of edema around the hemorrhage was also reduced in the surgical group, 28 versus 42 cc.[718]

Since intraventricular blood, especially a large amount, adversely effects outcome, clinicians have posited that more aggressive drainage of the ventricular blood might improve outcomes in patients with brain hemorrhages that involved the cerebral ventricles.[719,720] Preliminary trials show that intraventricular thrombolysis with urokinase or tPA was able to speed the resolution of intraventricular blood clots, compared with treatment with ventricular drainage alone or with medical therapy.[719,720]

We believe that, in the foreseeable future, more aggressive drainage of hematomas using advanced stereotactic and endoscopic techniques and thrombolytic agents to liquefy clots will result in improved outcomes for patients with intracerebral hematomas. Brain edema surrounding the hematomas can be treated with agents discussed in the next section.

Treatment of brain edema and increased intracranial pressure

Brain infarcts, hemorrhages, and subarachnoid bleeding can cause secondary effects that lead to swelling of the brain. The resulting increase in ICP contributes to reduction in consciousness and increases the likelihood of a bad outcome. The three major processes that swell the brain are vascular congestion, so-called vasogenic brain edema, and cytotoxic edema. The potential volume of distended brain capillaries is great. When consciousness is reduced, patients may hypoventilate, thus raising the partial pressure of arterial CO_2. Carbon dioxide is a potent vasodilator. The potential importance of vascular congestion can be shown by the use of mechanical hyperventilation in rapidly reducing elevated ICP.[685,721] Hyperventilation causes an almost immediate decrease in ICP but the peak decrement occurs approximately 30 minutes after the carbon dioxide partial pressure (P_{CO_2}) is reduced.[685,721] The initial acute reduction in P_{CO_2} of 5–10 mmHg often reduces ICP by 25–30%.[685] The P_{CO_2} should be kept between 25 and 35 mmHg. Blood gases should be monitored using capillary oximetry in patients with reduced consciousness. The ICP-reducing effect of hyperventilation is temporary and lasts only 1–2 days.[722] In many patients, it may be necessary to use sedation and a curarelike drug to adequately control mechanical hyperventilation. Reducing the volume of blood in the head reduces ICP irrespective of the cause. Even when there is no important vascular dilation or congestion, decreasing the amount of venous blood volume in the cranium allows acute decompression of intracranial contents.

Infarcts and hematomas are often accompanied by considerable edema during the acute period. The two basic types of brain edema are customarily classified as vasogenic and cytotoxic.[723] Vasogenic edema predominates in intracerebral hemorrhage and cytotoxic edema predominates in brain infarcts. Water in the interstitial or extracellular compartment has been traditionally called vasogenic edema after Klatzo.[724] This type of edema responds to osmotic diuretics, such as mannitol and glycerol. Glycerol is an effective osmotic dehydrating agent that reduces ICP and can be given either orally or IV.[725–727] When given IV, glycerol should be infused every 2 hours but can be given every 4–6 hours orally.[685] Glycerol is a purified preparation of glycerine. Glycerine is readily obtained over-the-counter in most pharmacies and the impurities are not absorbed and are excreted in the feces. Glycerine is a very useful agent in outpatients who continue to have brain edema after hospital discharge.

A 20–25% solution of mannitol has been the most common osmotic agent used to reduce ICP. Although dosage varies, the

typical initial dose of mannitol is 0.75–1.0 g/kg followed by 0.25–0.50 g/kg every 3–5 hours depending on the ICP.[685] Small doses of 0.25g/kg may decrease ICP as well as higher doses, but the effect of small doses lasts a shorter time.[685,728] Mannitol may also improve microcirculatory perfusion in the regions directly surrounding hematomas. There is theoretical concern that large molecule hypertonic agents like mannitol could diffuse into the hematoma during continued bleeding and increase the volume of the hematoma. Recently, many neurology intensivists have begun to use hypertonic saline (about 23% solution) to reduce brain edema. This strategy has been effective in reversing brain herniation symptoms and has been well tolerated.[729–732] Elevated head position and barbiturate sedation also reduce ICP. Patients with intracerebral hematomas and increased ICP should be nursed in a sitting position.

The effect of corticosteroids in stroke patients is controversial, but most studies show no benefit of steroids in patients with brain hemorrhages and infarcts.[685] Corticosteroids stabilize the blood–brain barrier that is disrupted in vasogenic edema, and are useful for edema due to tumors and other chronic lesions. However, although hematomas are commonly surrounded by vasogenic edema, steroid therapy has not proven helpful.[733]

The second type of brain edema, so-called cytotoxic edema, is caused by swelling of the cells so that the water is intracellular.[723] Most of the edema in patients with ischemia is intracellular and does not respond to corticosteroids. Glyburide has shown some promise as an agent that can limit cytotoxic edema in infarct patients.[734] Cytotoxic edema is said to account for the positivity of brain images seen on DWI-MRI scans in patients with acute brain infarcts. Ischemia can also produce some vasogenic edema. This develops later, however, when brain cell necrosis has released substances that compromise the blood–brain barrier and lead to extracellular edema.

In some animal models, both vasogenic and cytotoxic edema can be potentiated by reperfusion of brain tissue.[723,735] When the arterial supply to a brain region is blocked, the capillaries and small blood vessels may be damaged by the resulting ischemia. When this region is reperfused, the damaged capillaries leak fluid because of injury to the endothelium and basement membranes. Increased brain edema and brain hemorrhage are potential complications of reperfusion after thrombolytic treatment. The reperfused blood may also carry or promote circulation of substances to the region, such as excitotoxins and Ca^{2+} ions that might enhance cell damage leading to more cytotoxic edema.[3]

Clinical trials have not shown a beneficial effect from corticosteroids in ischemic stroke or primary supratentorial inracerebral hemorrhage.[685,733,736–738] Most authorities do not recommend their use in patients with brain infarcts. In most infarct patients, edema is not clinically important except when there is massive infarction and the prognosis is already poor. For these patients, hypothermia can be helpful in controlling edema extent, and hemicraniectomy can be life-saving by reducing the mechanical consequences of edema. Dramatic edema does develop in certain younger patients, however,

despite seemingly limited infarction. In this circumstance, osmotic agents and steroids are probably helpful.

Physicians working in ICUs now seem to prefer hypertonic saline to mannitol infusions.[685,739] Solutions of IV fluid that contain 1.25–3.00% saline can be used to produce a slow but hopefully sustained rise in osmolality. Alternatively, bolus infusions of varying amounts of saline (e.g., 23.4% or 10.0%) saline can be used instead of mannitol.[731,732,740–743] Phlebitis is a problem with hypertonic saline infusions unless a central catheter is used. Congestive heart failure can also develop as a complication of expansion of the intravascular fluid volume.[741,743]

For selected patients, surgical decompression with removal of infarcted and edematous brain can be helpful in patients with impending herniations. When the infarction extensively involves the cerebellum, compression of the brain stem and IVth ventricle may result.[744–747] The infarcted cerebellum acts much like a hematoma causing critical mass effect in the posterior cranial fossa, a relatively small, enclosed compartment. Hemicraniectomy has been increasingly used to treat patients with large cerebral infarcts.[640,748–753] Decompressive hemicraniectomy involves removing a large bone flap of approximately 12 cm that usually includes the frontal, parietal, and temporal bones and part of the occipital squama.[750] The dura mater is opened and a dural patch is used for closure.

At first, the surgery was limited to patients with large right cerebral hemispherc infarcts because it was thought that survivors with large left hemisphere infarcts would remain hopelessly disabled by aphasia and right hemiplegia.[748] Initially, surgery was only performed after a major shift in brain contents had occurred and the patient became stuporous. Later studies showed that survival from massive cerebral infarction is better when hemicraniectomy is performed early before herniation occurs.[748,749,751–753] Some series with surprisingly good results could be obtained even in patients with large left hemisphere infarcts.[640,749,750] The prognosis of patients with large MCA territory infarcts is so poor[754] that aggressive therapy is warranted, especially in young, previously healthy individuals. In a pooled analysis of 3 trials of hemicraniectomy for very large MCA infarcts, 134 patients 60 years or younger were analyzed.[755] Surgery was life-saving, with deaths occurring in 22% of surgical patients versus 64% of medically treated patients. Most patients kept alive had moderate-to-severe final disability, but surgery did increase the frequency of patients having a non-disabled final outcome, 38% versus 25%. Occasional patients, even those with uncal herniation, do respond and survive after the use of acute hyperventilation followed by mannitol.[748,749,751–753,756] Ethical concerns do remain since individuals and families have different personal opinions and choices of whether severe disability survival is preferred over a peaceful non-suffering death.[757]

Hydrocephalus can be caused by ventricular drainage system blockage, most often at the level of the aqueduct or IVth ventricle, or by failure of CSF absorption caused by plugging of the meninges by blood and blood products. In SAH, the ventricles may enlarge early in the course, and some patients

develop persistent hydrocephalus.[758] Ventricular shunting is needed in only a minority of patients with SAH because, in many patients, the hydrocephalus is temporary. Most other patients respond to repeated lumbar punctures and the use of acetazolamide to decrease CSF production. Large cerebellar infarcts and hemorrhages distort the IVth ventricle, leading to obstructive hydrocephalus.[744,759] Insertion of a ventricular drain or shunt can be life-saving in that situation and can allow recovery in some patients, without the need for direct surgery on the posterior fossa lesion.[759] The decision whether to treat patients with large cerebellar infarcts with ventricular drainage or removal of a large portion of the infarct depends on the clinical and neuroimaging findings in the individual patient.[747,760,761]

Promoting recovery

The previous sections discussed prevention and minimization of ischemic brain damage. What if damage has already occurred and an infarct or hemorrhage is already present? The incidence of stroke is projected to increase considerably during the next few decades because of the rapidly increasing number of individuals over 70 in the population.[762–764] Stroke is predicted to account for 6.2% of the total burden of illness by the year 2020.[765] Even with optimal treatment of patients with acute brain ischemia and hemorrhages, many will have residual brain damage. Are there agents or strategies that might improve function or accelerate and promote maximum recovery? The study of recovery from brain injuries has been greatly facilitated by new technologies such as functional MRI (fMRI) and transcranial magnetic stimulation (TMS). Stem cell and brain electrical stimulation research has kindled a reawakening of research on the plasticity of the nervous system and regeneration. These advances in research and technology have stimulated research and clinical interest in neurological recovery.[766–768] We will briefly mention herein various strategies for facilitating recovery but will cover this topic in more detail in Chapter 20. We will not discuss standard physical or occupational therapy in this chapter but will limit the discussion to novel strategies now being pursued and studied.

The most dramatic new research in promoting recovery relates to transplantation of primitive stem cells into patients with stroke.[769–771] Early transplantation experiments in animals showed that grafted neurons survive and remain viable only if they are immature before they have elaborated axonal connections. Preliminary studies in man, using post-mitotic human neuron-like cells (NT2N) derived originally from a human testicular germ cell tumor, showed the feasibility of implanting these cells into humans after striato-capsular infarcts and hemorrhages.[769,770,772,773] Cyclosporine immunosuppression was given to the transplanted patients. Some patients seemed to improve.[772,773] There were no major safety issues. In subsequent years, it was determined that progenitor cells injected into systemic blood vessels would cross the blood–brain barrier and preferentially migrate to a recent infarct bed. Accordingly, less invasive routes for administering progenitor cells to patients are being explored, including IA or simple IV injection of bone marrow stromal cells.[774–776] Researchers are also exploring removing patients' own cells and reinjecting them after extracting stem cell components and having them proliferate ex-vivo. This strategy would avoid immunosuppression.

Stem cell research in stroke patients is clearly very preliminary. Full integration of injected cells into synaptic networks may not be necessary for recovery. These cells also release abundant growth factors that could stimulate endogenous proliferation of neural elements. Researchers are exploring the potential for using bone marrow stromal cells,[769,770,777–779] and blood from the human umbilical cord,[770,772,778] as potential donor sources of cells and accompanying growth factors. Many questions arise[771]:(1) When to transplant? If too early, ischemia may reduce the potential for the implants to take and cytokines and leukocytes could impair implantation. Also prognosis is often less evident during the acute period making it less likely that patients and physicians would opt for an experimental procedure soon after stroke onset. Transplantation weeks or months after the stroke may not be very effective and be too late. (2) Which cells to use as a donor source and how many? (3) Which strokes? Should only patients with infarcts limited to one area, e.g., the putamen, be chosen: Would transplants be effective if a number of divergent neuronal cells are infarcted (cortical, putaminal, hippocampal, etc). What about size? What if the infarction is predominantly white matter or involves important white matter tracts such as those that travel in the internal capsule? (4) Which route should be used for administration? IV, IA, intraventricular, or directly into the stroke bed? Inducing brain plasticity with progenitor cells and, more recently with magnetic and electrical stimulation,[780] has become a fertile area of research and advance.

Another strategy to promote recovery is a derivation of the old saying "Use it or lose it." Stimulating the brain region damaged by the stroke might promote plasticity and encourage assumption of the functions of the damaged areas by other brain regions. Researchers have explored the effectiveness of forcing use of a hemiparetic arm by constraining the good arm.[781–783] Preliminary studies investigated the effect of therapeutic interventions for the arm in the acute phase after stroke, with follow-ups at a maximum of 12 months.[781] A much larger multisite randomized clinical trial conducted at 7 US academic centers between January 2001 and January 2003, entitled the Extremity Constraint Induced Therapy Evaluation (EXCITE) trial, enrolled 222 patients with predominantly ischemic stroke.[782] Participants were assigned to receive either constraint-induced movement therapy wearing a restraining mitt on the less-affected hand while engaging in therapy on the weak arm and hand (N = 106), or usual and customary care that ranged from no treatment after formal acute stroke rehabilitation to pharmacological or physiotherapeutic interventions (N = 116). Among patients who had a stroke within the previous 3–9 months, restraint and physical therapy on the affected hand produced statistically significant and clinically relevant improvements in arm motor function that persisted for at least 1 year.[782]

Others have examined the effect of sensory and sensory motor stimulation of paretic limbs. One early study examined the effect of repetitive sensorimotor training of the arm after stroke.[784,785] One hundred consecutive stroke patients were randomly assigned either to an experimental group that received daily additional sensorimotor stimulation of the arm or to a control group. The treatment period was 6 weeks. Assessments of the patients were made before and after treatment and at 6 and 12 months after stroke, and 62 patients at 5 years after stroke. At the 5-year follow-up, there was a statistically significant difference in function tests favoring the treatment group that received early, repetitive, and targeted stimulation of the paretic arm. Extra stimulation of the arm during the acute phase after a stroke resulted in a clinically meaningful and long-lasting salutary effect on motor function.[784] Another study showed that 100-Hertz (Hz) current applied to finger surfaces in patients with chronic post-stroke deficits improved the use of utensils with the involved hand.[786,787] Many different types of sensory input – optokinetic, neck proprioceptive, vestibular, and somatosensory – show improvement in neglect in stroke patients.[786,787]

Another way to attempt to facilitate functional recovery is to directly stimulate the brain.[780,788–792] Repetitive transcranial magnetic stimulation (rTMS) and direct electrical stimulation have potential long-term effects on cerebral cortex excitability. Researchers have begun to explore the potential of this in facilitating recovery. Both inhibitory and facilitatory effects can result from rTMS depending on the frequency range of the stimulation. When applied to the primary motor cortex M1, low-frequency (1 Hz) stimulation inhibits excitability while high-frequency (5–20 Hz) stimulation increases cortical excitability. Two studies showed that low-frequency rTMS applied to the motor cortex on the side opposite a brain infarct improved function in the hand that was weakend by the stroke.[789,790] The authors posited that inhibition of activity contralateral to the infarct facilitated activity in the hemisphere harboring the brain infarct.[789,790] Other studies showed that rTMS, applied at a frequency of 3 Mz[791] and 10 Mz[792] to the motor cortex on the side of a brain infarct, improved function of the contralateral weak hand. Often rTMS was applied along with routine standard physical and occupational therapy.

Direct current stimulation can have similar effects to magnetic stimulation.[793–795] Direct current can also be applied transcranially. During transcranial direct current stimulation (tDCS) a constant low-amplitude DC current is transmitted to the cerebral cortex by way of surface mounted scalp electrodes.[793] Stimulation or inhibition depends on whether the direct current stimulation is anodal or cathodal. Anodal stimulation increases brain activity and excitability while cathodal stimulation is inhibitory. The patient cannot tell if the current is turned on or off. Preliminary studies show that direct current stimulation can facilitate movement of paretic limbs.[793–795] Direct current stimulation has been tested concurrent with other rehabilitative therapies in promoting recovery.

Pharmacological interventions to enhance stroke recovery have also been explored. Stroke-related injury to nerve cells affects their ability to secrete or respond to neurotransmitters. One popular strategy is to attempt to restore function by replacing neurotransmitters known to be active in damaged regions. Results to-date of this approach are mostly anecdotal experiences or small trials. Levodopa is given to patients with Parkinson's disease to replace depleted dopamine because of nigrostriatal degeneration. Acetylcholine-like drugs have been tried in an attempt to treat the hypothesized cholinergic deficit in Alzheimer's disease. After this lead, a few clinicians have tried neurotransmitters in stroke patients. In one patient with bilateral paramedian thalamic infarcts who was apathetic and habitually assumed sleeping postures, bromocriptine, a dopamine agonist, led to improvement in spontaneity and less time in bed.[796] In a patient who had been aphasic since a left frontal-lobe hemorrhage 3.5 years before study, bromocriptine led to an improvement in speech fluency and a reduction in hesitancy when talking.[797] Several small studies suggested that bromocriptine using an average dose of 30 mg alone or with carbidopa/levodopa preparations can improve speech fluency in some patients with Broca's and transcortical motor aphasia.[798,799] Bromocriptine was also effective in a patient with neglect of the left side of space owing to a right frontoparietal and striatal infarct.[799] Neglect and lack of attention were improved while taking bromocriptine and worsened after the drug was withdrawn. Bromocriptine and lisuride have been used effectively to treat abulia in four patients with degenerative diseases and strokes.[800] In all of these circumstances, bromocriptine presumably had no healing effect on the damaged tissues; it merely improved functional capacity.

Amphetamines have also been given to promote recovery and enhance function. After the animal experiments of Feeney and colleagues,[801,802] who found that amphetamines coupled with motor activity accelerated recovery of beam-walking ability in rats, some investigators began to try amphetamines in stroke patients.[787,803–807] In rats, neither saline (if the rats had low blood volumes, also used as a control) nor amphetamine alone facilitated recovery after sensorimotor-cortex lesions. A single 2 mg/kg injection of amphetamines and continued experience walking on the beam were needed.[804,805] In contrast, animals given haloperidol performed far worse than controls.[801,802] Amphetamines were also effective in promoting recovery of function in animals with experimental sensorimotor-cortex lesions.[806] In a preliminary human study, 10 mg of D-amphetamine sulfate and physical therapy led to accelerated recovery when compared with patients given placebo and therapy.[804] Amphetamine had to be given early to be effective. A single 10 mg dose of D-amphetamine followed by training improved hand function capabilities in some normal individuals when training alone had not done so.[808] In another study that used normal young volunteers, a single dose of a selective norepinephrine reuptake inhibitor enhanced motor skill acquisition and corticomotor excitability as studied by TMS.[809] From the available studies, it is not clear whether amphetamine has a specific effect in promoting recovery or merely a general stimulatory function when combined with physical activity.[810] Amphetamine administration might lead to long-term potentiation of cell function or merely promote non-specific stimulation of less-than-normal cells.

Some pharmacological agents have the potential of retarding recovery. Haloperidol has a definite negative effect on recovery.[802] Similarly, drugs that enhance gamma-aminobutyric acid transmission, such as diazepam, might increase inhibition of function and also delay recovery.[810] Stroke patients are often exposed to polypharmacy.[811,812] Some drugs have been prescribed before the stroke and others are given after the stroke to treat various symptoms and general medical conditions. In general, the acute and chronic effects of concurrent drugs on recovery have been poorly studied but are clearly important.[812,813] Sedatives, anticonvulsants, haloperidol, and opiates should be avoided when possible.

Brain–machine computer interfaces offer an alternative approach to improving patient function, giving patients' minds control over an artificial prosthesis or an alternative pathway to control their own limbs.[814,815]

Concluding comments and rules

Stroke is a complex disease. Care should include: (1) stroke and general atherosclerosis risk assessment and stroke prevention strategies; (2) rapid clinical evaluation and diagnosis; (3) rapid complete brain and vascular imaging studies and blood tests; (4) management of blood pressure and fluid balance; (5) medical or surgical treatment (or both) of the process causing the acute stroke; (6) early use of rehabilitation techniques; (7) surveillance and treatment to prevent common stroke complications (e.g., aspiration, phlebothrombosis, urinary and pulmonary infections, and bed sores); and (8) education for patients and their families regarding their specific problems and stroke in general.

Because patients with strokes often develop second and third strokes that are different in etiology from the initial stroke,[816] all patients should be fully investigated for conditions that may cause future strokes. Consideration should be given to prophylaxis of all of the risks found.[817]

The field of stroke treatment is changing so quickly that we have included much armchair theorizing and investigational strategies. We suggest the following rules clinicians should use when approaching treatment in their patients with strokes and cerebrovascular disease:

1. Begin preventive strategies early. Educate patients and families about stroke risk factors and their control early during hospitalization.
2. Treatment of the acute stroke, prevention of the next stroke, and rehabilitation should be concurrent themes throughout hospitalization and recovery.

3. Avoid common stroke complications, such as deep vein thrombosis, aspiration, hypovolemia, pressure sores, contractures, and urinary tract infections. These problems are easier to prevent than treat.
4. Plan treatment of the acute stroke by analyzing the mechanism and pathophysiology in the individual patient. The time course of the symptoms should never be the sole guide to treatment.
5. The clinician should determine the location and severity of the vascular lesion, the blood constituents and coagulation functions, and the state of the brain (e.g., normal, stunned, or irreversibly damaged).
6. Determine precisely what is wrong with every stroke patient. Stroke is a cerebrovascular disease and diagnosis involves finding the cardiac-cerebrovascular–hematological cause. Precise diagnosis has great intrinsic value. It allows better estimates of prognosis and guides logical treatment.
7. Unblocking occlusive arterial lesions in patients who have brain ischemia with endarterectomy or thrombolysis or clot retrieval should be considered when there is no brain damage or when ischemia is recent and possibly reversible.
8. Prevention of thrombus formation, propagation, and embolization is often possible by using drugs that modify platelet aggregation and adhesion and by using parenteral and oral anticoagulants. We suggest using antiplatelet aggregants (e.g., aspirin) to prevent white clots and anticoagulants to counteract red clots.
9. Anticoagulants may be useful after an acute large artery occlusion. Anticoagulation is prescribed.[4–8] Longer-term anticoagulants are warranted in some patients with severe arterial stenosis and in patients who have chronic cardiac lesions that produce flow stasis and in mechanical cardiac valves.
10. Try to maximize blood flow to ischemic regions during the acute stroke. Avoid excessive reduction of blood pressure and hypovolemia during the acute stage of infarction.
11. Cardiac disease and mortality are frequent in most stroke patients. Always consider the heart and its blood supply in addition to the brain.

Discussion of these general treatments and strategies is expanded in Part II (Stroke syndromes) and III (Prevention, complications, and recovery–rehabilitation) of this book.

References

1. Caplan LR. Evidence based medicine: Concerns of a clinical neurologist. *J Neurol Neurosurg Psychiatry.* 2001;**71**:569–574

2. Thibault GE. Too old for what? *N Engl J Med.* 1993;**328**:946–950

3. Caplan LR. Reperfusion of ischemic brain: Why and why not? In W Hacke GDZ, M Hirschberg, eds. *Thrombolytic therapy in acute ischemic stroke.* Berlin: Springer; 1991:36–45

4. Pan J, Konstas A-A, Bateman B, Ortolano G, Pile-Spellman J.

Reperfusion injury following cerebral ischemia: Pathophysiology, MR imaging, and potential therapies. *Neuroradiology.* 2007;**49**:93–102

5. Albers GW, Thijs VN, Wechsler L, Kemp S, Schlaug G, Skalabrin E, et al. Magnetic resonance imaging profiles

predict clinical response to early reperfusion: The diffusion and perfusion imaging evaluation for understanding stroke evolution (DEFUSE) study. *Ann Neurol.* 2006;**60**:508–517

6. Caplan LR. Are terms such as completed stroke or RIND of continued usefulness? *Stroke.* 1983;**14**:431–433

7. Caplan LR. TIAs: We need to return to the question, "What is wrong with Mr Jones?" *Neurology.* 1988;**38**:791–793

8. Cebul RD, Snow RJ, Pine R, Hertzer NR, Norris DG. Indications, outcomes, and provider volumes for carotid endarterectomy. *JAMA.* 1998;**279**:1282–1287

9. Wennberg DE, Lucas FL, Birkmeyer JD, Bredenberg CE, Fisher ES. Variation in carotid endarterectomy mortality in the medicare population: Trial hospitals, volume, and patient characteristics. *JAMA.* 1998;**279**:1278–1281

10. Robinson RG, Spalletta G. Poststroke depression: A review. *Can J Psychiatry.* 2010;**55**:341–349

11. Robinson RG, Lipsey JR, Price TR. Diagnosis and clinical management of post-stroke depression. *Psychosomatics.* 1985;**26**:769–772, 775–768

12. Alberts MJ, Hademenos G, Latchaw RE, Jagoda A, Marler JR, Mayberg MR, et al. Recommendations for the establishment of primary stroke centers. Brain attack coalition. *JAMA.* 2000;**283**:3102–3109

13. Alberts MJ, Latchaw RE, Selman WR, Shephard T, Hadley MN, Brass LM, et al. Recommendations for comprehensive stroke centers: A consensus statement from the brain attack coalition. *Stroke.* 2005;**36**:1597–1616

14. Song S, Saver J. Growth of regional acute stroke systems of care in the United States in the first decade of the 21st century. *Stroke.* 2012;**43**:1975–1978

15. Indredavik B, Slordahl SA, Bakke F, Rokseth R, Haheim LL. Stroke unit treatment. Long-term effects. *Stroke.* 1997;**28**:1861–1866

16. Diez-Tejedor E, Fuentes B. Acute care in stroke: Do stroke units make the difference? *Cerebrovasc Dis.* 2001;**11** Suppl 1:31–39

17. Birbeck GL, Zingmond DS, Cui X, Vickrey BG. Multispecialty stroke services in California hospitals are associated with reduced mortality. *Neurology.* 2006;**66**:1527–1532

18. Leys D, Ringelstein EB, Kaste M, Hacke W. The main components of stroke unit care: Results of a European expert survey. *Cerebrovasc Dis.* 2007;**23**:344–352

19. Candelise L, Gattinoni M, Bersano A, Micieli G, Sterzi R, Morabito A. Stroke-unit care for acute stroke patients: An observational follow-up study. *Lancet.* 2007;**369**:299–305

20. Stroke Unit Trialists' Collaboration. Organised inpatient (stroke unit) care for stroke. *Cochrane Database Syst Rev.* 2013;**9**: CD000197

21. Indredavik B, Bakke F, Solberg R, Rokseth R, Haaheim LL, Holme I. Benefit of a stroke unit: A randomized controlled trial. *Stroke.* 1991;**22**:1026–1031

22. Stroke Unit Trialists' Collaboration. Collaborative systematic review of the randomised trials of organised inpatient (stroke unit) care after stroke. *BMJ.* 1997;**314**:1151–1159

23. Stroke Unit Trialists' Collaboration. How do stroke units improve patient outcomes? A collaborative systematic review of the randomized trials. *Stroke.* 1997;**28**:2139–2144

24. Xian Y, Holloway RG, Chan PS, Noyes K, Shah MN, Ting HH, et al. Association between stroke center hospitalization for acute ischemic stroke and mortality. *JAMA.* 2011;**305**:373–380

25. Caplan LR, Sergay S. Positional cerebral ischaemia. *J Neurol Neurosurg Psychiatry.* 1976;**39**:385–391

26. Toole JF. Effects of change of head, limb and body position on cephalic circulation. *N Engl J Med.* 1968;**279**:307–311

27. Wojner-Alexander AW, Garami Z, Chernyshev OY, Alexandrov AV. Heads down: Flat positioning improves blood flow velocity in acute ischemic stroke. *Neurology.* 2005;**64**:1354–1357

28. Favilla CG, Mesquita RC, Mullen M, Durduran T, Lu X, Kim MN, et al. Optical bedside monitoring of cerebral blood flow in acute ischemic stroke patients during head-of-bed manipulation. *Stroke.* 2014;**45**:1269–1274

29. Rordorf G, Cramer SC, Efird JT, Schwamm LH, Buonanno F, Koroshetz WJ. Pharmacological elevation of blood pressure in acute stroke. Clinical effects and safety. *Stroke.* 1997;**28**:2133–2138

30. Hillis AE, Ulatowski JA, Barker PB, Torbey M, Ziai W, Beauchamp NJ, et al.

A pilot randomized trial of induced blood pressure elevation: Effects on function and focal perfusion in acute and subacute stroke. *Cerebrovasc Dis.* 2003;**16**:236–246

31. Chalela JA, Dunn B, Todd JW, Warach S. Induced hypertension improves cerebral blood flow in acute ischemic stroke. *Neurology.* 2005;**64**:1979

32. Hillis AE, Kane A, Tuffiash E, Ulatowski JA, Barker PB, Beauchamp NJ, et al. Reperfusion of specific brain regions by raising blood pressure restores selective language functions in subacute stroke. *Brain Lang.* 2001;**79**:495–510

33. Lehv MS, Salzman EW, Silen W. Hypertension complicating carotid endarterectomy. *Stroke.* 1970;**1**:307–313

34. Holton P, Wood JB. The effects of bilateral removal of the carotid bodies and denervation of the carotid sinuses in two human subjects. *J Physiol.* 1965;**181**:365–378

35. Breen JC, Caplan LR, DeWitt LD, Belkin M, Mackey WC, O'Donnell TP. Brain edema after carotid surgery. *Neurology.* 1996;**46**:175–181

36. Caplan LR, Skillman J, Ojemann R, Fields WS. Intracerebral hemorrhage following carotid endarterectomy: A hypertensive complication? *Stroke.* 1978;**9**:457–460

37. Ogasawara K, Sakai N, Kuroiwa T, Hosoda K, Iihara K, Toyoda K, et al. Intracranial hemorrhage associated with cerebral hyperperfusion syndrome following carotid endarterectomy and carotid artery stenting: Retrospective review of 4494 patients. *Journal of Neurosurgery.* 2007;**107**:1130–1136

38. North American Symptomatic Carotid Endarterectomy Trial Collaborators. Beneficial effect of carotid endarterectomy in symptomatic patients with high-grade carotid stenosis. *N Engl J Med.* 1991;**325**:445–453

39. European Carotid Surgery Trialists' Collaborative Group. MRC European Carotid Surgery Trial: Interim results for symptomatic patients with severe (70–99%) or with mild (0–29%) carotid stenosis. *Lancet.* 1991;**337**:1235–1243

40. Brott TG, Halperin JL, Abbara S, Bacharach JM, Barr JD, Bush RL, et al. ASA/ACCF/AHA/AANN/AANS/ACR/ASNR/CNS/SAIP/SCAI/SIR/SNIS/SVM/SVS Guideline on the management of patients with extracranial carotid and vertebral artery

disease: Executive summary. *Circulation.* 2011;**124**:489–532

41. Barnett HJ, Taylor DW, Eliasziw M, Fox AJ, Ferguson GG, Haynes RB, et al. Benefit of carotid endarterectomy in patients with symptomatic moderate or severe stenosis. North American Symptomatic Carotid Endarterectomy Trial collaborators. *N Engl J Med.* 1998;**339**:1415–1425

42. European Carotid Surgery Trialists' Collaborative Group. Randomised trial of endarterectomy for recently symptomatic carotid stenosis: Final results of the MRC European Carotid Surgery Trial (ECST). *Lancet.* 1998;**351**:1379–1387

43. Spetzler RF, Hadley MN, Martin NA, Hopkins LN, Carter LP, Budny J. Vertebrobasilar insufficiency. Part 1: Microsurgical treatment of extracranial vertebrobasilar disease. *J Neurosurg.* 1987;**66**:648–661

44. Kieffer E, Koskas F, Bahnini A, et al. Long-term results after reconstruction of the cervical vertebral artery. In LR Caplan, EG Shifrin, AN Nicolaides, WS Moore, eds. *Cerebrovascular Ischaemia – Investigation and Management.* London: Med-Orion; 1996: 617–625

45. Berguer R, Flynn LM, Kline RA, Caplan LR. Surgical reconstruction of the extracranial vertebral artery: Management and outcome. *J Vasc Surg.* 2000;**31**:9–18

46. Executive Committee for the Asymptomatic Carotid Atherosclerosis Study. Endarterectomy for asymptomatic carotid artery stenosis. *JAMA.* 1995;**273**:1421–1428

47. Halliday A, Mansfield A, Marro J, Peto C, Peto R, Potter J, et al. Prevention of disabling and fatal strokes by successful carotid endarterectomy in patients without recent neurological symptoms: Randomised controlled trial. *Lancet.* 2004;**363**:1491–1502

48. Hopkins LN, Martin NA, Hadley MN, Spetzler RF, Budny J, Carter LP. Vertebrobasilar insufficiency. Part 2. Microsurgical treatment of intracranial vertebrobasilar disease. *J Neurosurg.* 1987;**66**:662–674

49. Ausman JI, Diaz FG, Pearce JE, de los Reyes RA, Leuchter W, Mehta B, et al. Endarterectomy of the vertebral artery from C2 to posterior inferior cerebellar artery intracranially. *Surg Neurol.* 1982;**18**:400–404

50. Meyer FB, Piepgras DG, Sundt TM, Jr., Yanagihara T. Emergency embolectomy for acute occlusion of the middle cerebral artery. *J Neurosurg.* 1985;**62**:639–647

51. Kerber C W, Cromwell L D, Loehden O L. Catheter dilatation of proximal carotid stenosis during distal bifurcation endarterectomy. *AJNR Am J Neuroradiol.* 1980;**1**:348–349

52. Kachel R. Results of balloon angioplasty in the carotid arteries. *J Endovasc Surg* 1996;**3**:22–30

53. Caplan LR, Meyers PM, Schumacher HC. Angioplasty and stenting to treat occlusive vascular disease. *Rev Neurol Dis.* 2006;**3**:8–18

54. Wholey MH, Wholey M, Mathias K, Roubin GS, Diethrich EB, Henry M, et al. Global experience in cervical carotid artery stent placement. *Catheter Cardiovasc Interv.* 2000;**50**:160–167

55. Roubin GS, New G, Iyer SS, Vitek JJ, Al-Mubarak N, Liu MW, et al. Immediate and late clinical outcomes of carotid artery stenting in patients with symptomatic and asymptomatic carotid artery stenosis: A 5-year prospective analysis. *Circulation.* 2001;**103**:532–537

56. Crawley F, Clifton A, Buckenham T, Loosemore T, Taylor RS, Brown MM. Comparison of hemodynamic cerebral ischemia and microembolic signals detected during carotid endarterectomy and carotid angioplasty. *Stroke.* 1997;**28**:2460–2464

57. Eckert B, Thie A, Valdueza J, Zanella F, Zeumer H. Transcranial Doppler sonographic monitoring during percutaneous transluminal angioplasty of the internal carotid artery. *Neuroradiology.* 1997;**39**:229–234

58. Markus HS, Clifton A, Buckenham T, Brown MM. Carotid angioplasty. Detection of embolic signals during and after the procedure. *Stroke.* 1994;**25**:2403–2406

59. McCleary AJ, Nelson M, Dearden NM, Calvey TA, Gough MJ. Cerebral haemodynamics and embolization during carotid angioplasty in high-risk patients. *Br J Surg.* 1998;**85**:771–774

60. Ribo M, Molina CA, Alvarez B, Rubiera M, Alvarez-Sabin J, Matas M. Transcranial Doppler monitoring of transcervical carotid stenting with flow reversal protection: A novel carotid revascularization technique. *Stroke.* 2006;**37**:2846–2849

61. Hofmann R, Niessner A, Kypta A, Steinwender C, Kammler J, Kerschner K, et al. Risk score for peri-interventional complications of carotid artery stenting. *Stroke.* 2006;**37**:2557–2561

62. Endovascular versus surgical treatment in patients with carotid stenosis in the Carotid and Vertebral Artery Transluminal Angioplasty Study (CAVITAS): A randomised trial. *Lancet.* 2001;**357**:1729–1737

63. Brown MM. Vascular Surgical Society of Great Britain and Ireland: Results of the Carotid and Vertebral Artery Transluminal Angioplasty Study. *Br J Surg.* 1999;**86**:710–711

64. Coward LJ, McCabe DJ, Ederle J, Featherstone RL, Clifton A, Brown MM. Long-term outcome after angioplasty and stenting for symptomatic vertebral artery stenosis compared with medical treatment in the Carotid and Vertebral Artery Transluminal Angioplasty Study (CAVITAS): A randomized trial. *Stroke.* 2007;**38**:1526–1530

65. Ederle J, Bonati LH, Dobson J, Featherstone RL, Gaines PA, Beard JD, et al. Endovascular treatment with angioplasty or stenting versus endarterectomy in patients with carotid artery stenosis in the Carotid and Vertebral Artery Transluminal Angioplasty Study (CAVITAS): Long-term follow-up of a randomised trial. *Lancet Neurol.* 2009;**8**:898–907

66. Bonati LH, Ederle J, McCabe DJ, Dobson J, Featherstone RL, Gaines PA, et al. Long-term risk of carotid restenosis in patients randomly assigned to endovascular treatment or endarterectomy in the Carotid and Vertebral Artery Transluminal Angioplasty Study (CAVATAS): Long-term follow-up of a randomised trial. *Lancet Neurol.* 2009;**8**:908–917

67. Yadav JS, Wholey MH, Kuntz RE, Fayad P, Katzen BT, Mishkel GJ, et al. Protected carotid-artery stenting versus endarterectomy in high-risk patients. *N Engl J Med.* 2004;**351**:1493–1501

68. Ringleb PA, Allenberg J, Bruckmann H, Eckstein HH, Fraedrich G, Hartmann M, et al. 30 day results from the space trial of stent-protected angioplasty versus carotid endarterectomy in symptomatic patients: A randomised non-inferiority trial. *Lancet.* 2006;**368**:1239–1247

69. Mas JL, Chatellier G, Beyssen B, Branchereau A, Moulin T, Becquemin JP, et al. Endarterectomy versus stenting in patients with symptomatic severe carotid stenosis. *N Engl J Med.* 2006;**355**:1660–1671

70. Qureshi AI. Carotid angioplasty and stent placement after EVA-3S trial. *Stroke.* 2007;**38**:1993–1996

71. Brott TG, Hobson RW, 2nd, Howard G, Roubin GS, Clark WM, Brooks W, et al. Stenting versus endarterectomy for treatment of carotid-artery stenosis. *N Engl J Med.* 2010;**363**:11–23

72. Voeks JH, Howard G, Roubin GS, Malas MB, Cohen DJ, Sternbergh WC, 3rd, et al. Age and outcomes after carotid stenting and endarterectomy: The Carotid Revascularization Endarterectomy Versus Stenting Trial. *Stroke.* 2011;**42**:3484–3490

73. Choi JC, Johnston C, Kim AS. Early outcomes after carotid artery stenting compared with endarterectomy for asymptomatic carotid stenosis. *Stroke* 2015;**46**:120–125

74. Hadjipetrou P, Cox S, Piemonte T, Eisenhauer A. Percutaneous revascularization of atherosclerotic obstruction of aortic arch vessels. *J Am Coll Cardiol.* 1999;**33**:1238–1245

75. Motarjeme A. Percutaneous transluminal angioplasty of supra-aortic vessels. *J Endovasc Surg.* 1996;**3**:171–181

76. Wada T, Takayama K, Taoka T, Nakagawa H, Myouchin K, Miyasaka T, et al. Long-term treatment outcomes after intravascular ultrasound evaluation and stent placement for atherosclerotic subclavian artery obstructive lesions. *Neuroradiol J.* 2014;**27**:213–221

77. Henry M, Amor M, Henry I, Ethevenot G, Tzvetanov K, Chati Z. Percutaneous transluminal angioplasty of the subclavian arteries. *J Endovasc Surg.* 1999;**6**:33–41

78. Schillinger M, Haumer M, Schillinger S, Ahmadi R, Minar E. Risk stratification for subclavian artery angioplasty: Is there an increased rate of restenosis after stent implantation? *J Endovasc Ther.* 2001;**8**:550–557

79. Chastain HD, 2nd, Campbell MS, Iyer S, Roubin GS, Vitek J, Mathur A, et al. Extracranial vertebral artery stent placement: In-hospital and follow-up results. *J Neurosurg.* 1999;**91**:547–552

80. Piotin M, Spelle L, Martin JB, Weill A, Rancurel G, Ross IB, et al. Percutaneous transluminal angioplasty and stenting of the proximal vertebral artery for symptomatic stenosis. *AJNR Am J Neuroradiol.* 2000;**21**:727–731

81. Higashida R, Tsai F, Halbach V, Dowd C, Hieshima G. Transluminal angioplasty, thrombolysis, and stenting for extracranial and intracranial cerebral vascular disease. *Journal of Interventional Cardiology.* 1996;**9**:245–255

82. SSYLVIA Study Investigators. Stenting of symptomatic atherosclerotic lesions in the vertebral or intracranial arteries (SSYLVIA): Study results. *Stroke.* 2004;**35**:1388–1392

83. Edgell RC, Zaidat OO, Gupta R, Abou-Chebl A, Linfante I, Xavier A, et al. Multicenter study of safety in stenting for symptomatic vertebral artery origin stenosis: Results from the Society of Vascular and Interventional Neurology Research Consortium. *Journal of Neuroimaging.* 2013;**23**:170–174

84. Meyers PM, Schumacher HC, Tanji K, Higashida RT, Caplan LR. Use of stents to treat intracranial cerebrovascular disease. *Annu Rev Med.* 2007;**58**:107–122

85. Higashida R, Meyers, PM, Connors, JJ 3rd, Sacks D, Strother CM, Barr JD, et al. Intracranial angioplasty and stenting for cerebral atherosclerosis: A position statement of the American Society of Interventional and Therapeutic Neuroradiology, Society of Interventional Radiology, and the American Society of Neuroradiology. *J Vasc Interv Radiol.* 2005;**16**:1281–1285

86. Gress DR, Smith WS, Dowd CF, Van Halbach V, Finley RJ, Higashida RT. Angioplasty for intracranial symptomatic vertebrobasilar ischemia. *Neurosurgery.* 2002;**51**:23–27; discussion 27–29

87. Marks MP, Marcellus M, Norbash AM, Steinberg GK, Tong D, Albers GW. Outcome of angioplasty for atherosclerotic intracranial stenosis. *Stroke.* 1999;**30**:1065–1069

88. Connors JJ, 3rd, Wojak JC. Percutaneous transluminal angioplasty for intracranial atherosclerotic lesions: Evolution of technique and short-term results. *J Neurosurg.* 1999;**91**:415–423

89. Takis C, Kwan ES, Pessin MS, Jacobs DH, Caplan LR. Intracranial angioplasty: Experience and complications. *AJNR Am J Neuroradiol.* 1997;**18**:1661–1668

90. Gomez CR, Misra VK, Liu MW, Wadlington VR, Terry JB, Tulyapronchote R, et al. Elective stenting of symptomatic basilar artery stenosis. *Stroke.* 2000;**31**:95–99

91. Yu W, Smith WS, Singh V, Ko NU, Cullen SP, Dowd CF, et al. Long-term outcome of endovascular stenting for symptomatic basilar artery stenosis. *Neurology.* 2005;**64**:1055–1057

92. Kessler IM, Mounayer C, Piotin M, Spelle L, Vanzin JR, Moret J. The use of balloon-expandable stents in the management of intracranial arterial diseases: A 5-year single-center experience. *AJNR Am J Neuroradiol.* 2005;**26**:2342–2348

93. Marks MP, Marcellus ML, Do HM, Schraedley-Desmond PK, Steinberg GK, Tong DC, et al. Intracranial angioplasty without stenting for symptomatic atherosclerotic stenosis: Long-term follow-up. *AJNR Am J Neuroradiol.* 2005;**26**:525–530

94. Wojak JC, Dunlap DC, Hargrave KR, DeAlvare LA, Culbertson HS, Connors JJ, 3rd. Intracranial angioplasty and stenting: Long-term results from a single center. *AJNR Am J Neuroradiol.* 2006;**27**:1882–1892

95. Henkes H, Miloslavski E, Lowens S, Reinartz J, Liebig T, Kuhne D. Treatment of intracranial atherosclerotic stenoses with balloon dilatation and self-expanding stent deployment (WingSpan). *Neuroradiology.* 2005;**47**:222–228

96. Bose A, Hartmann M, Henkes H, Liu HM, Teng MM, Szikora I, et al. A novel, self-expanding, nitinol stent in medically refractory intracranial atherosclerotic stenoses: The WingSpan study. *Stroke.* 2007;**38**:1531–1537

97. Fiorella D, Levy EI, Turk AS, Albuquerque FC, Niemann DB, Aagaard-Kienitz B, et al. US multicenter experience with the WingSpan stent system for the treatment of intracranial atheromatous disease: Periprocedural results. *Stroke.* 2007;**38**:881–887

98. Chimowitz MI, Lynn MJ, Derdeyn CP, Turan TN, Fiorella D, Lane BF, et al. Stenting versus aggressive medical therapy for intracranial arterial stenosis. *N Engl J Med.* 2011;**365**:993–1003

99. Derdeyn CP, Chimowitz MI, Lynn MJ, Fiorella D, Turan TN, Janis LS, et al. Aggressive medical treatment with or without stenting in high-risk patients with intracranial artery stenosis (SAMMPRIS): The final results of a randomised trial. *Lancet.* 2014;**383**:333–341

100. Zaidat O. VISSIT trial final results. Sixth Annual Meeting of the Society of Vascular and Interventional Neurology. October 26–27, Houston, TX, 2013

101. Liebeskind DS, Cotsonis GA, Saver JL, Lynn MJ, Turan TN, Cloft HJ, et al. Collaterals dramatically alter stroke

risk in intracranial atherosclerosis. *Ann Neurol.* 2011;**69**:963–974

102. Montorsi P, Galli S, Ravagnani PM, Trabattoni D, Fabbiocchi F, Lualdi A, et al. Drug-eluting balloon for treatment of in-stent restenosis after carotid artery stenting: Preliminary report. *J Endovasc Ther.* 2012;**19**:734–742

103. Vajda Z, Aguilar M, Göhringer T, Horváth-Rizea D, Bäzner H, Henkes H. Treatment of intracranial atherosclerotic disease with a balloon-expandable paclitaxel eluting stent. *Clin Neuroradiol.* 2012;**22**:227–233

104. Gupta R, Al-Ali F, Thomas AJ, Horowitz MB, Barrow T, Vora NA, et al. Safety, feasibility, and short-term follow-up of drug-eluting stent placement in the intracranial and extracranial circulation. *Stroke.* 2006;**37**:2562–2566

105. Shuchman M. Trading restenosis for thrombosis? New questions about drug-eluting stents. *N Engl J Med.* 2006;**355**:1949–1952

106. Collen D. On the regulation and control of fibrinolysis. Edward Kowalski memorial lecture. *Thromb Haemost.* 1980;**43**:77–89

107. Sloan MA. Thrombolysis and stroke. Past and future. *Arch Neurol.* 1987;**44**:748–768

108. del Zoppo G, Hosomi, N. Mechanisms of thrombolysis. In P Lyden, ed. *Thrombolytic Therapy for Acute Stroke.* Totowa, NJ: Humana Press; 2005:3–27

109. Meyer JS, Gilroy J, Barnhart MI, Johnson JF. Anticoagulants plus streptokinase therapy in progressive stroke. *JAMA.* 1964;**189**:373

110. Meyer JS GJ, Barnhart ME, Johnson JF. Therapeutic thrombolysis in cerebral thromboembolism: Randomized evaluation of streptokinase. In C Millikan, JP Whisnant, eds. *Cerebral Vascular Disease, Fourth Princeton Conference.* New York, NY: Grune & Stratton; 1965:200–213

111. Del Zoppo GJ. Thrombolytic therapy in cerebrovascular disease. *Stroke.* 1988;**19**:1174–1179

112. Pessin MS, del Zoppo GJ, Furlan AJ. Thrombolytic treatment in acute stroke: Review and update of selected topics. In MA Moskowitz, LR Caplan, eds. *Cerebrovascular Diseases, 19th Princeton Conference, 1994.* Boston, MA: Butterworth–Heinemann; 1995:409–418

113. Caplan LR. *Caplan's Stroke: A Clinical Approach.* Boston, MA: Butterworth–Heinemann; 2000

114. Caplan LR. Thrombolysis 2004: The good, the bad, and the ugly. *Rev Neurol Dis.* 2004;**1**:16–26

115. Grond M, Rudolf J, Schmulling S, Stenzel C, Neveling M, Heiss WD. Early intravenous thrombolysis with recombinant tissue-type plasminogen activator in vertebrobasilar ischemic stroke. *Arch Neurol.* 1998;**55**:466–469

116. Wardlaw JM, Murray V, Berge E, Del Zoppo GJ. Thrombolysis for acute ischaemic stroke. *Cochrane Database Syst Rev.* 2009:CD000213

117. Sandercock P, Wardlaw JM, Lindley RI, Dennis M, Cohen G, Murray G, et al. The benefits and harms of intravenous thrombolysis with recombinant tissue plasminogen activator within 6 h of acute ischaemic stroke (The Third International Stroke Trial [IST-3]): A randomised controlled trial. *Lancet.* 2012;**379**:2352–2363

118. Hacke W, Kaste M, Fieschi C, Toni D, Lesaffre E, von Kummer R, et al. Intravenous thrombolysis with recombinant tissue plasminogen activator for acute hemispheric stroke. The European Cooperative Acute Stroke Study (ECASS). *JAMA.* 1995;**274**:1017–1025

119. Fisher M, Pessin MS, Furian AJ. ECASS: Lessons for future thrombolytic stroke trials. European Cooperative Acute Stroke Study. *JAMA.* 1995;**274**:1058–1059

120. Steiner T, Bluhmki E, Kaste M, Toni D, Trouillas P, von Kummer R, et al. The ECASS 3-hour cohort. Secondary analysis of ECASS data by time stratification. ECASS study group. European Cooperative Acute Stroke Study. *Cerebrovasc Dis.* 1998;**8**:198–203

121. The National Institute of Neurological Disorders and Stroke rt-PA Stroke Study Group. Tissue plasminogen activator for acute ischemic stroke. *N Engl J Med.* 1995;**333**:1581–1587

122. Ingall TJ, O'Fallon WM, Asplund K, Goldfrank LR, Hertzberg VS, Louis TA, et al. Findings from the reanalysis of the NINDS tissue plasminogen activator for Acute Ischemic Stroke Treatment Trial. *Stroke.* 2004;**35**:2418–2424

123. Lansberg MG, Schrooten M, Bluhmki E, Thijs VN, Saver JL. Treatment time-specific number needed to treat estimates for tissue plasminogen activator therapy in acute stroke based on shifts over the entire range of the modified Rankin Scale. *Stroke.* 2009;**40**:2079–2084

124. Lees KR, Bluhmki E, von Kummer R, Brott TG, Toni D, Grotta JC, et al. Time to treatment with intravenous alteplase and outcome in stroke: An updated pooled analysis of ECASS, ATLANTIS, NINDS, and EPITHET trials. *Lancet.* 2010;**375**:1695–1703

125. Wardlaw JM, Murray V, Berge E, del Zoppo G, Sandercock P, Lindley RL, et al. Recombinant tissue plasminogen activator for acute ischaemic stroke: An updated systematic review and meta-analysis. *Lancet.* 2012;**379**:2364–2372

126. Lansberg M, Bluhmki E, Saver J. Number needed to treat estimates for tPA per 90-minute time interval. *Stroke.* 2008;**39**:560

127. Hacke W, Kaste M, Fieschi C, von Kummer R, Davalos A, Meier D, et al. Randomised double-blind placebo-controlled trial of thrombolytic therapy with intravenous alteplase in acute ischaemic stroke (ECASS II). Second European–Australasian Acute Stroke Study Investigators. *Lancet.* 1998;**352**:1245–1251

128. Clark WM, Wissman S, Albers GW, Jhamandas JH, Madden KP, Hamilton S. Recombinant tissue-type plasminogen activator (alteplase) for ischemic stroke 3 to 5 hours after symptom onset. The ATLANTIS study: A randomized controlled trial. Alteplase thrombolysis for acute noninterventional therapy in ischemic stroke. *JAMA.* 1999;**282**:2019–2026

129. Hacke W, Donnan G, Fieschi C, Kaste M, von Kummer R, Broderick JP, et al. Association of outcome with early stroke treatment: Pooled analysis of ATLANTIS, ECASS, and NINDS rt-Pa stroke trials. *Lancet.* 2004;**363**:768–774

130. Flaherty ML JE, Kothari RU, Broderick JP. Intravenous thrombolytic therapy for acute ischemic stroke: Results of large, randomized clinical trials. In P Lyden, ed. *Thrombolytic Therapy for Acute Stroke.* Totowa, NJ: Humana Press; 2005:111–127

131. Donnan GA, Davis SM, Chambers BR, Gates PC, Hankey GJ, McNeil JJ, et al. Trials of streptokinase in severe acute ischaemic stroke. *Lancet.* 1995;**345**:578–579

132. del Zoppo GJ, Higashida RT, Furlan AJ, Pessin MS, Rowley HA, Gent M. PROACT: A phase II randomized trial of recombinant pro-urokinase by

direct arterial delivery in acute middle cerebral artery stroke. PROACT investigators. Prolyse in acute cerebral thromboembolism. *Stroke.* 1998;**29**:4–11

133. Furlan A, Higashida R, Wechsler L, Gent M, Rowley H, Kase C, et al. Intra-arterial prourokinase for acute ischemic stroke. The PROACT II study: A randomized controlled trial. Prolyse in acute cerebral thromboembolism. *JAMA.* 1999;**282**:2003–2011

134. Furlan AJ, Katzan I, Abou-Chebl A, Russman A. Intra-arterial thrombolysis in acute ischemic stroke. In P Lyden, ed. *Thrombolytic Therapy for Acute Stroke.* Totowa, NJ: Humana Press; 2005:159–184

135. Ogawa A, Mori E, Minematsu K, Taki W, Takahashi A, Nemoto S, et al. Randomized trial of intraarterial infusion of urokinase within 6 hours of middle cerebral artery stroke: The Middle Cerebral Artery Embolism Local Fibrinolytic Intervention Trial (MELT) Japan. *Stroke.* 2007;**38**:2633–2639

136. Saver JL. Intra-arterial fibrinolysis for acute ischemic stroke: The message of MELT. *Stroke.* 2007;**38**:2627–2628

137. Adams HP, Jr., Brott TG, Furlan AJ, Gomez CR, Grotta J, Helgason CM, et al. Guidelines for thrombolytic therapy for acute stroke: A supplement to the guidelines for the management of patients with acute ischemic stroke. A statement for healthcare professionals from a special writing group of the Stroke Council, American Heart Association. *Stroke.* 1996;**27**:1711–1718

138. Practice advisory: Thrombolytic therapy for acute ischemic stroke – summary statement. Report of the quality standards subcommittee of the American Academy of Neurology. *Neurology.* 1996;**47**:835–839

139. Jauch EC, Saver JL, Adams HP, Jr., Bruno A, Connors JJ, Demaerschalk BM, et al. Guidelines for the early management of patients with acute ischemic stroke: A guideline for healthcare professionals from the American Heart Association/ American Stroke Association. *Stroke.* 2013;**44**:870–947

140. Adams HP, Jr., del Zoppo G, Alberts MJ, Bhatt DL, Brass L, Furlan A, et al. Guidelines for the early management of adults with ischemic stroke: A guideline from the American Heart Association/American Stroke Association Stroke Council, Clinical Cardiology Council, Cardiovascular Radiology and Intervention Council, and the Atherosclerotic Peripheral Vascular Disease and Quality of Care Outcomes in Research Interdisciplinary Working Groups: The American Academy of Neurology affirms the value of this guideline as an educational tool for neurologists. *Stroke.* 2007;**38**:1655–1711

141. Horowitz SH. Thrombolytic therapy in acute stroke: Neurologists, get off your hands! *Arch Neurol.* 1998;**55**:155–157

142. Burton T. Doctors push for more scans in stroke cases. *Wall Street Journal.* 2009:**D1**

143. American College of Emergency Physicians. Use of intravenous tPA for the management of acute stroke in the emergency department. www.acep.org, 2002

144. Adams HP, Jr, Kenton EJ, 3rd, Scheiber SC, Juul D. Vascular neurology: A new neurologic subspecialty. *Neurology.* 2004;**63**:774–776

145. Josephson SA, Engstrom JW, Wachter RM. Neurohospitalists: An emerging model for inpatient neurological care. *Ann Neurol.* 2008;**63**:135–140

146. Scott PA, Xu Z, Meurer WJ, Frederiksen SM, Haan MN, Westfall MW, et al. Attitudes and beliefs of Michigan emergency physicians toward tissue plasminogen activator use in stroke: Baseline survey results from the increasing stroke treatment through interactive behavioral change tactic (INSTINCT) trial hospitals. *Stroke.* 2010;**41**:2026–2032

147. Schwamm LH, Pancioli A, Acker JE, 3rd, Goldstein LB, Zorowitz RD, Shephard TJ, et al. Recommendations for the establishment of stroke systems of care: Recommendations from the American Stroke Association's task force on the development of stroke systems. *Stroke.* 2005;**36**:690–703

148. Demaerschalk BM, Durocher DL. How diagnosis-related group 559 will change the US medicare cost reimbursement ratio for stroke centers. *Stroke.* 2007;**38**:1309–1312

149. Wahlgren N, Ahmed N, Davalos A, Ford GA, Grond M, Hacke W, et al. Thrombolysis with alteplase for acute ischaemic stroke in the safe implementation of thrombolysis in stroke-monitoring study (SITS-MOST): An observational study. *Lancet.* 2007;**369**:275–282

150. Fonarow GC, Smith EE, Saver JL, Reeves MJ, Bhatt DL, Grau-Sepulveda MV, et al. Timeliness of tissue-type plasminogen activator therapy in acute ischemic stroke: Patient characteristics, hospital factors, and outcomes associated with door-to-needle times within 60 minutes. *Circulation.* 2011;**123**:750–758

151. Saver JL, Fonarow GC, Smith EE, Reeves MJ, Grau-Sepulveda MV, Pan W, et al. Time to treatment with intravenous tissue plasminogen activator and outcome from acute ischemic stroke. *JAMA.* 2013;**309**:2480–2488

152. Nakagawara J, Minematsu K, Okada Y, Tanahashi N, Nagahiro S, Mori E, et al. Thrombolysis with 0.6 mg/kg intravenous alteplase for acute ischemic stroke in routine clinical practice: The Japan post-marketing alteplase registration study (J-MARS). *Stroke.* 2010;**41**:1984–1989

153. Chao AC, Hsu HY, Chung CP, Liu CH, Chen CH, Teng MM, et al. Outcomes of thrombolytic therapy for acute ischemic stroke in Chinese patients: The Taiwan Thrombolytic Therapy for Acute Ischemic Stroke (TTT-AIS) study. *Stroke.* 2010;**41**:885–890

154. Schwamm LH, Reeves MJ, Pan W, Smith EE, Frankel MR, Olson D, et al. Race/ethnicity, quality of care, and outcomes in ischemic stroke. *Circulation.* 2010;**121**:1492–1501

155. Alberts MJ, Latchaw RE, Jagoda A, Wechsler LR, Crocco T, George MG, et al. Revised and updated recommendations for the establishment of primary stroke centers: A summary statement from the brain attack coalition. *Stroke.* 2011;**42**:2651–2665

156. LaMonte MP, Bahouth MN, Hu P, Pathan MY, Yarbrough KL, Gunawardane R, et al. Telemedicine for acute stroke: Triumphs and pitfalls. *Stroke.* 2003;**34**:725–728

157. Audebert HJ, Kukla C, Clarmann von Claranau S, Kuhn J, Vatankhah B, Schenkel J, et al. Telemedicine for safe and extended use of thrombolysis in stroke: The telemedic pilot project for integrative stroke care (TEMPIS) in Bavaria. *Stroke.* 2005;**36**:287–291

158. Audebert HJ, Kukla C, Vatankhah B, Gotzler B, Schenkel J, Hofer S, et al. Comparison of tissue plasminogen

activator administration management between telestroke network hospitals and academic stroke centers: The telemedical pilot project for integrative stroke care in Bavaria/Germany. *Stroke.* 2006;**37**:1822–1827

159. Meyer BC, Raman R, Hemmen T, Obler R, Zivin JA, Rao R, et al. Efficacy of site-independent telemedicine in the stroke doc trial: A randomised, blinded, prospective study. *Lancet Neurol.* 2008;**7**:787–795

160. Silva GS, Farrell S, Shandra E, Viswanathan A, Schwamm LH. The status of telestroke in the United States: A survey of currently active stroke telemedicine programs. *Stroke.* 2012;**43**:2078–2085

161. Alberts MJ, Wechsler LR, Jensen ME, Latchaw RE, Crocco TJ, George MG, et al. Formation and function of acute stroke-ready hospitals within a stroke system of care recommendations from the brain attack coalition. *Stroke.* 2013;**44**:3382–3393

162. Hachinski V, Donnan GA, Gorelick PB, Hacke W, Cramer SC, Kaste M, et al. Stroke: Working toward a prioritized world agenda. *Int J Stroke.* 2010;**5**:238–256

163. Moynihan B, Davis D, Pereira A, Cloud G, Markus HS. Delivering regional thrombolysis via a hub-and-spoke model. *J R Soc Med.* 2010;**103**:363–369

164. Gladstone DJ, Rodan LH, Sahlas DJ, Lee L, Murray BJ, Ween JE, et al. A citywide prehospital protocol increases access to stroke thrombolysis in Toronto. *Stroke.* 2009;**40**:3841–3844

165. Song S, Saver J. Growth of regional stroke systems of care in the United States in the first decade of the 21st century. *Stroke.* 2011;**42**:e340

166. Schwamm LH, Smith E, Saver JL, Reeves M, Messe S, Bhatt D, et al. Temporal trends in the use of IV tPA among all ischemic stroke patients presenting to GWTG-stroke hospitals (abstract). *Stroke.* 2011;**42**:e104

167. Addo J, Bhalla A, Crichton S, Rudd AG, McKevitt C, Wolfe CDA. Provision of acute stroke care and associated factors in a multiethnic population: Prospective study with the South London Stroke Register. *BMJ* 2011;**342**:d744

168. Grau AJ, Eicke M, Biegler MK, Faldum A, Bamberg C, Haass A, et al. Quality monitoring of acute stroke care in Rhineland–Palatinate, Germany, 2001–2006. *Stroke.* 2010;**41**:1495–1500

169. Gumbinger C, Reuter B, Stock C, Sauer T, Wietholter H, Bruder I, et al. Time to treatment with recombinant tissue plasminogen activator and outcome of stroke in clinical practice: Retrospective analysis of hospital quality assurance data with comparison with results from randomised clinical trials. *BMJ.* 2014;**348**:g3429

170. Marler JR, Winters Jones P, EMR M. *The National Institute of Neurological Disorders and Stroke: Proceedings of National Symposium on Rapid Identification and Treatment of Acute Stroke.* Bethesda, MD: National Institute of Neurological Disorders and Stroke; 1997

171. Summers D, Leonard A, Wentworth D, Saver JL, Simpson J, Spilker JA, et al. Comprehensive overview of nursing and interdisciplinary care of the acute ischemic stroke patient: A scientific statement from the American Heart Association. *Stroke.* 2009;**40**:2911–2944

172. Xian Y, Smith EE, Zhao X, Peterson ED, Olson DM, Hernandez AF, et al. Strategies used by hospitals to improve speed of tissue-type plasminogen activator treatment in acute ischemic stroke. *Stroke.* 2014;**45**:1387–1395

173. Ford AL, Williams JA, Spencer M, McCammon C, Khoury N, Sampson TR, et al. Reducing door-to-needle times using Toyota's lean manufacturing principles and value stream analysis. *Stroke.* 2012;**43**:3395–3398

174. Fonarow GC, Zhao X, Smith EE, Saver JL, Reeves MJ, Bhatt DL, et al. Door-to-needle times for tissue plasminogen activator administration and clinical outcomes in acute ischemic stroke before and after a quality improvement initiative. *JAMA.* 2014;**311**:1632–1640

175. Qureshi AI, Suri MF, Nasar A, He W, Kirmani JF, Divani AA, et al. Thrombolysis for ischemic stroke in the United States: Data from national hospital discharge survey 1999–2001. *Neurosurgery.* 2005;**57**:647–654

176. Albers GW, Bates VE, Clark WM, Bell R, Verro P, Hamilton SA. Intravenous tissue-type plasminogen activator for treatment of acute stroke: The Standard Treatment with Alteplase to Reverse Stroke (STARS) Study. *JAMA.* 2000;**283**:1145–1150

177. Demchuk AM, Tanne D, Hill MD, Kasner SE, Hanson S, Grond M, et al. Predictors of good outcome after intravenous tPA for acute ischemic stroke. *Neurology.* 2001;**57**:474–480

178. Katzan IL, Furlan AJ, Lloyd LE, Frank JI, Harper DL, Hinchey JA, et al. Use of tissue-type plasminogen activator for acute ischemic stroke: The Cleveland area experience. *JAMA.* 2000;**283**:1151–1158

179. Katzan IL, Hammer MD, Furlan AJ, Hixson ED, Nadzam DM. Quality improvement and tissue-type plasminogen activator for acute ischemic stroke: A Cleveland update. *Stroke.* 2003;**34**:799–800

180. Weimar C, Kraywinkel K, Maschke M, Diener HC. Intravenous thrombolysis in German stroke units before and after regulatory approval of recombinant tissue plasminogen activator. *Cerebrovasc Dis.* 2006;**22**:429–431

181. Heuschmann PU, Berger K, Misselwitz B, Hermanek P, Leffmann C, Adelmann M, et al. Frequency of thrombolytic therapy in patients with acute ischemic stroke and the risk of in-hospital mortality: The German Stroke Registers Study Group. *Stroke.* 2003;**34**:1106–1113

182. Sobesky J, Frackowiak M, Zaro Weber O, Hahn M, Moller-Hartmann W, Rudolf J, et al. The Cologne stroke experience: Safety and outcome in 450 patients treated with intravenous thrombolysis. *Cerebrovasc Dis.* 2007;**24**:56–65

183. Toni D, Lorenzano S, Puca E, Prencipe M. The SITS-MOST Registry. *Neurol Sci.* 2006;**27** Suppl 3:S260–262

184. Lisboa RC, Jovanovic BD, Alberts MJ. Analysis of the safety and efficacy of intra-arterial thrombolytic therapy in ischemic stroke. *Stroke.* 2002;**33**:2866–2871

185. Qureshi AI, Ali Z, Suri MF, Kim SH, Shatla AA, Ringer AJ, et al. Intra-arterial third-generation recombinant tissue plasminogen activator (reteplase) for acute ischemic stroke. *Neurosurgery.* 2001;**49**:41–48; discussion 48–50

186. Arnold M, Schroth G, Nedeltchev K, Loher T, Remonda L, Stepper F, et al. Intra-arterial thrombolysis in 100 patients with acute stroke due to middle cerebral artery occlusion. *Stroke.* 2002;**33**:1828–1833

187. Edwards MT, Murphy MM, Geraghty JJ, Wulf JA, Konzen JP. Intra-arterial cerebral thrombolysis for acute ischemic stroke in a community hospital. *AJNR Am J Neuroradiol.* 1999;**20**:1682–1687

188. Suarez JI, Sunshine JL, Tarr R, Zaidat O, Selman WR, Kernich C, et al. Predictors of clinical improvement, angiographic recanalization, and intracranial hemorrhage after intra-arterial thrombolysis for acute ischemic stroke. *Stroke.* 1999;**30**:2094–2100

189. Molina CA, Saver JL. Extending reperfusion therapy for acute ischemic stroke: Emerging pharmacological, mechanical, and imaging strategies. *Stroke.* 2005;**36**:2311–2320

190. Rajajee V, Saver J. Prehospital care of the acute stroke patient. *Tech Vasc Interv Radiol.* 2005;**8**:74–80

191. Crocco T, Gullett T, Davis SM, Flores N, Sauerbeck L, Jauch E, et al. Feasibility of neuroprotective agent administration by prehospital personnel in an urban setting. *Stroke.* 2003;**34**:1918–1922

192. Saver JL, Starkman S, Eckstein M, Stratton SJ, Franklin D, Pratt TM, et al. for the FAST-MAG Investigators and Coordinators. Prehospital use of magnesium sulfate as neuroprotection in acute stroke. *N Engl J Med* 2015;**372**:528–536

193. Saver JL. The 2012 Feinberg lecture: Treatment swift and treatment sure. *Stroke.* 2013;**44**:270–277

194. Ankolekar S, Fuller M, Cross I, Renton C, Cox P, Sprigg N, et al. Feasibility of an ambulance-based stroke trial, and safety of glyceryl trinitrate in ultra-acute stroke: The Rapid Intervention with Glyceryl Trinitrate in Hypertensive Stroke Trial. *Stroke.* 2013;**44**:3120–3128

195. Hougaard KD, Hjort N, Zeidler D, Sorensen L, Norgaard A, Hansen TM, et al. Remote ischemic preconditioning as an adjunct therapy to thrombolysis in patients with acute ischemic stroke: A randomized trial. *Stroke.* 2014;**45**:159–167

196. Walter S, Kostopoulos P, Haass A, Keller I, Lesmeister M, Schlechtriemen T, et al. Diagnosis and treatment of patients with stroke in a mobile stroke unit versus in hospital: A randomised controlled trial. *Lancet Neurol.* 2012;**11**:397–404

197. Weber JE, Ebinger M, Rozanski M, Waldschmidt C, Wendt M, Winter B, et al. Prehospital thrombolysis in acute stroke: Results of the PHANTOM-S pilot study. *Neurology.* 2013;**80**:163–168

198. Ebinger M, Winter B, Wendt M, Weber JE, Waldschmidt C, Rozanski M, et al. Effect of the use of ambulance-based thrombolysis on time to thrombolysis in acute ischemic stroke: A randomized clinical trial. *JAMA.* 2014;**311**:1622–1631

199. Rajan S, Baraniuk S, Parker S, Wu T-C, Bowry R, Grotta JC. Implementing a mobile stroke unit program in the United States. Why, how and how much? *JAMA Neurology* 2015;**72**(2):229–234

200. del Zoppo GJ, Poeck K, Pessin MS, Wolpert SM, Furlan AJ, Ferbert A, et al. Recombinant tissue plasminogen activator in acute thrombotic and embolic stroke. *Ann Neurol.* 1992;**32**:78–86

201. Wolpert SM, Bruckmann H, Greenlee R, Wechsler L, Pessin MS, del Zoppo GJ. Neuroradiologic evaluation of patients with acute stroke treated with recombinant tissue plasminogen activator. The rt-PA Acute Stroke Study Group. *AJNR Am J Neuroradiol.* 1993;**14**:3–13

202. Montavont A, Nighoghossian N, Derex L, Hermier M, Honnorat J, Philippeau F, et al. Intravenous rt-PA in vertebrobasilar acute infarcts. *Neurology.* 2004;**62**:1854–1856

203. Lindsberg PJ, Soinne L, Tatlisumak T, Roine RO, Kallela M, Happola O, et al. Long-term outcome after intravenous thrombolysis of basilar artery occlusion. *JAMA.* 2004;**292**:1862–1866

204. Kent DM, Selker HP, Ruthazer R, Bluhmki E, Hacke W. Can multivariable risk–benefit profiling be used to select treatment-favorable patients for thrombolysis in stroke in the 3 -to 6-hour time window? *Stroke.* 2006;**37**:2963–2969

205. Davis SM, Donnan GA, Parsons MW, Levi C, Butcher KS, Peeters A, et al. Effects of alteplase beyond 3 h after stroke in the echoplanar imaging thrombolytic evaluation trial (EPITHET): A placebo-controlled randomised trial. *Lancet Neurol.* 2008;**7**:299–309

206. Fink JN, Kumar S, Horkan C, Linfante I, Selim MH, Caplan LR, et al. The stroke patient who woke up: Clinical and radiological features, including diffusion and perfusion MRI. *Stroke.* 2002;**33**:988–993

207. Manawadu D, Bodla S, Keep J, Jarosz J, Kalra L. An observational study of thrombolysis outcomes in wake-up ischemic stroke patients. *Stroke.* 2013;**44**:427–431

208. Barber PA, Zhang J, Demchuk AM, Hill MD, Buchan AM. Why are stroke patients excluded from tPA therapy? An analysis of patient eligibility. *Neurology.* 2001;**56**:1015–1020

209. Smith EE, Abdullah AR, Petkovska I, Rosenthal E, Koroshetz WJ, Schwamm LH. Poor outcomes in patients who do not receive intravenous tissue plasminogen activator because of mild or improving ischemic stroke. *Stroke.* 2005;**36**:2497–2499

210. Rajajee V, Kidwell C, Starkman S, Ovbiagele B, Alger JR, Villablanca P, et al. Early MRI and outcomes of untreated patients with mild or improving ischemic stroke. *Neurology.* 2006;**67**:980–984

211. Urra X, Ariño H, Llull L, Amaro S, Obach V, Cervera Á, et al. The outcome of patients with mild stroke improves after treatment with systemic thrombolysis. *PLoS One.* 2013;**8**:e59420

212. Selim M, Kumar S, Fink J, Schlaug G, Caplan LR, Linfante I. Seizure at stroke onset: Should it be an absolute contraindication to thrombolysis? *Cerebrovasc Dis.* 2002;**14**:54–57

213. Saqqur M, Uchino K, Demchuk AM, Molina CA, Garami Z, Calleja S, et al. Site of arterial occlusion identified by transcranial Doppler predicts the response to intravenous thrombolysis for stroke. *Stroke.* 2007;**38**:948–954

214. Schellinger PD, Fiebach JB, Jansen O, Ringleb PA, Mohr A, Steiner T, et al. Stroke magnetic resonance imaging within 6 hours after onset of hyperacute cerebral ischemia. *Ann Neurol.* 2001;**49**:460–469

215. Koroshetz WJ, Lev MH. Contrast computed tomography scan in acute stroke: "You can't always get what you want but . . . You get what you need". *Ann Neurol.* 2002;**51**:415–416

216. Wintermark M, Reichhart M, Thiran JP, Maeder P, Chalaron M, Schnyder P, et al. Prognostic accuracy of cerebral blood flow measurement by perfusion computed tomography, at the time of emergency room admission, in acute stroke patients. *Ann Neurol.* 2002;**51**:417–432

217. Kidwell CS, Alger JR, Saver JL. Beyond mismatch: Evolving paradigms in

imaging the ischemic penumbra with multimodal magnetic resonance imaging. *Stroke*. 2003;**34**:2729–2735

218. Sanak D, Nosal V, Horak D, Bartkova A, Zelenak K, Herzig R, et al. Impact of diffusion-weighted MRI-measured initial cerebral infarction volume on clinical outcome in acute stroke patients with middle cerebral artery occlusion treated by thrombolysis. *Neuroradiology*. 2006;**48**:632–639

219. Kohrmann M, Juttler E, Fiebach JB, Huttner HB, Siebert S, Schwark C, et al. MRI versus CT-based thrombolysis treatment within and beyond the 3 h time window after stroke onset: A cohort study. *Lancet Neurol*. 2006;**5**:661–667

220. Davis SM, Donnan GA, Butcher KS, Parsons M. Selection of thrombolytic therapy beyond 3 h using magnetic resonance imaging. *Curr Opin Neurol*. 2005;**18**:47–52

221. Prosser J, Butcher K, Allport L, Parsons M, MacGregor L, Desmond P, et al. Clinical–diffusion mismatch predicts the putative penumbra with high specificity. *Stroke*. 2005;**36**:1700–1704

222. Butcher KS, Parsons M, MacGregor L, Barber PA, Chalk J, Bladin C, et al. Refining the perfusion–diffusion mismatch hypothesis. *Stroke*. 2005;**36**:1153–1159

223. Hacke W, Albers G, Al-Rawi Y, Bogousslavsky J, Davalos A, Eliasziw M, et al. The Desmoteplase In Acute Ischemic Stroke Trial (DIAS): A phase II MRI-based 9-hour window acute stroke thrombolysis trial with intravenous desmoteplase. *Stroke*. 2005;**36**:66–73

224. Hjort N, Butcher K, Davis SM, Kidwell CS, Koroshetz WJ, Rother J, et al. Magnetic resonance imaging criteria for thrombolysis in acute cerebral infarct. *Stroke*. 2005;**36**:388–397

225. Schellinger PD, Thomalla G, Fiehler J, Kohrmann M, Molina CA, Neumann-Haefelin T, et al. MRI-based and CT-based thrombolytic therapy in acute stroke within and beyond established time windows: An analysis of 1210 patients. *Stroke*. 2007;**38**:2640–2645

226. Lansberg MG, Thijs VN, Bammer R, Kemp S, Wijman CA, Marks MP, et al. Risk factors of symptomatic intracerebral hemorrhage after tPA therapy for acute stroke. *Stroke*. 2007;**38**:2275–2278

227. Fiehler J, Albers GW, Boulanger JM, Derex L, Gass A, Hjort N, et al. Bleeding risk analysis in stroke imaging before thrombolysis (BRASIL): Pooled analysis of T2*-weighted magnetic resonance imaging data from 570 patients. *Stroke*. 2007;**38**:2738–2744

228. Lee SJ, Saver JL, Liebeskind DS, Ali L, Ovbiagele B, Kim D, et al. Safety of intravenous fibrinolysis in imaging-confirmed single penetrator artery infarcts. *Stroke*. 2010;**41**:2587–2591

229. Lansberg MG, Lee J, Christensen S, Straka M, De Silva DA, Mlynash M, et al. Rapid automated patient selection for reperfusion therapy: A pooled analysis of the echoplanar imaging thrombolytic evaluation trial (EPITHET) and the diffusion and perfusion imaging evaluation for understanding stroke evolution (DEFUSE) study. *Stroke*. 2011;**42**:1608–1614

230. Scalzo F, Alger JR, Hu X, Saver JL, Dani KA, Muir KW, et al. Multi-center prediction of hemorrhagic transformation in acute ischemic stroke using permeability imaging features. *Magn Reson Imaging*. 2013;**31**:961–969

231. Warach S, Al-Rawi Y, Furlan AJ, Fiebach JB, Wintermark M, Lindstén A, et al. Refinement of the magnetic resonance diffusion-perfusion mismatch concept for thrombolytic patient selection: Insights from the desmoteplase in acute stroke trials. *Stroke*. 2012;**43**:2313–2318

232. Furlan AJ, Eyding D, Albers GW, Al-Rawi Y, Lees KR, Rowley HA, et al. Dose escalation of desmoteplase for acute ischemic stroke (DEDAS): Evidence of safety and efficacy 3 to 9 hours after stroke onset. *Stroke*. 2006;**37**:1227–1231

233. Hacke W, Furlan AJ, Al-Rawi Y, Davalos A, Fiebach JB, Gruber F, et al. Intravenous desmoteplase in patients with acute ischaemic stroke selected by MRI perfusion–diffusion weighted imaging or perfusion CT (DIAS-2): A prospective, randomised, double-blind, placebo-controlled study. *Lancet Neurol*. 2009;**8**:141–150

234. Liberatore GT, Samson A, Bladin C, Schleuning WD, Medcalf RL. Vampire bat salivary plasminogen activator (desmoteplase): A unique fibrinolytic enzyme that does not promote neurodegeneration. *Stroke*. 2003;**34**:537–543

235. Wintermark M, Reichhart M, Cuisenaire O, Maeder P, Thiran JP, Schnyder P, et al. Comparison of admission perfusion computed tomography and qualitative diffusion- and perfusion-weighted magnetic resonance imaging in acute stroke patients. *Stroke*. 2002;**33**:2025–2031

236. Obach V, Oleaga L, Urra X, Macho J, Amaro S, Capurro S, et al. Multimodal CT-assisted thrombolysis in patients with acute stroke: A cohort study. *Stroke*. 2011;**42**:1129–1131

237. Parsons M, Spratt N, Bivard A, Campbell B, Chung K, Miteff F, et al. A randomized trial of tenecteplase versus alteplase for acute ischemic stroke. *N Engl J Med*. 2012;**366**:1099–1107

238. Hu HH, Teng MM, Hsu LC, Wong WJ, Wang LM, Luk YO, et al. A pilot study of a new thrombolytic agent for acute ischemic stroke in Taiwan within a five-hour window. *Stroke*. 2006;**37**:918–919

239. Alexandrov AV, Demchuk AM, Burgin WS, Robinson DJ, Grotta JC. Ultrasound-enhanced thrombolysis for acute ischemic stroke: Phase l. Findings of the CLOTBUST trial. *J Neuroimaging*. 2004;**14**:113–117

240. Barlinn K, Barreto AD, Sisson A, Liebeskind DS, Schafer ME, Alleman J, et al. Clotbust-hands free: Initial safety testing of a novel operator-independent ultrasound device in stroke-free volunteers. *Stroke*. 2013;**44**:1641–1646

241. Lewandowski CA, Frankel M, Tomsick TA, Broderick J, Frey J, Clark W, et al. Combined intravenous and intra-arterial r-tPA versus intra-arterial therapy of acute ischemic stroke: Emergency Management of Stroke (EMS) Bridging Trial. *Stroke*. 1999;**30**:2598–2605

242. Ernst R, Pancioli A, Tomsick T, Kissela B, Woo D, Kanter D, et al. Combined intravenous and intra-arterial recombinant tissue plasminogen activator in acute ischemic stroke. *Stroke*. 2000;**31**:2552–2557

243. The IMS II Trial Investigators. Combined intravenous and intra-arterial recanalization for acute ischemic stroke: The Interventional Management of Stroke Study. *Stroke*. 2004;**35**:904–911

244. The IMS Study Investigators. Hemorrhage in the Interventional Management of Stroke Study. *Stroke*. 2006;**37**:847–851

245. Sekoranja L, Loulidi J, Yilmaz H, Lovblad K, Temperli P, Comelli M, et al. Intravenous versus combined (intravenous and intra-arterial) thrombolysis in acute ischemic stroke: A transcranial color-coded duplex sonography – guided pilot study. *Stroke*. 2006;**37**:1805–1809

246. The IMS II Trial Investigators. The Interventional Management of Stroke (IMS) II Study. *Stroke*. 2007;**38**:2127–2135

247. Keris V, Rudnicka S, Vorona V, Enina G, Tilgale B, Fricbergs J. Combined intraarterial/intravenous thrombolysis for acute ischemic stroke. *AJNR Am J Neuroradiol*. 2001;**22**:352–358

248. Butcher K, Shuaib A, Saver J, Donnan G, Davis SM, Norrving B, et al. Thrombolysis in the developing world: Is there a role for streptokinase? *Int J Stroke*. 2013;**8**:560–565

249. Ducrocq X, Bracard S, Taillandier L, Anxionnat R, Lacour JC, Guillemin F, et al. Comparison of intravenous and intra-arterial urokinase thrombolysis for acute ischaemic stroke. *J Neuroradiol*. 2005;**32**:26–32

250. Sugg RM, Noser EA, Shaltoni HM, Gonzales NR, Campbell MS, Weir R, et al. Intra-arterial reteplase compared to urokinase for thrombolytic recanalization in acute ischemic stroke. *AJNR Am J Neuroradiol*. 2006;**27**:769–773

251. Macleod MR, Davis SM, Mitchell PJ, Gerraty RP, Fitt G, Hankey GJ, et al. Results of a multicentre, randomised controlled trial of intra-arterial urokinase in the treatment of acute posterior circulation ischaemic stroke. *Cerebrovasc Dis*. 2005;**20**:12–17

252. Inoue T, Kimura K, Minematsu K, Yamaguchi T. A case-control analysis of intra-arterial urokinase thrombolysis in acute cardioembolic stroke. *Cerebrovasc Dis*. 2005;**19**:225–228

253. Tirschwell DL, Coplin WM, Becker KJ, Vogelzang P, Eskridge J, Haynor D, et al. Intra-arterial urokinase for acute ischemic stroke: Factors associated with complications. *Neurology*. 2001;**57**:1100–1103

254. Fanale PL. *Thrombolytic Therapy for Acute Ischemic Stroke in Acute Stroke, Bench to Bedside*. New York, NY: Informa Healthcare; 2007

255. The Ancrod Stroke Study Investigators. Ancrod for the treatment of acute ischemic brain infarction. *Stroke*. 1994;**25**:1755–1759

256. Sherman DG, Atkinson RP, Chippendale T, Levin KA, Ng K, Futrell N, et al. Intravenous ancrod for treatment of acute ischemic stroke: The STAT study: A randomized controlled trial. Stroke Treatment with Ancrod Trial. *JAMA*. 2000;**283**:2395–2403

257. Hossmann V, Heiss WD, Bewermeyer H, Wiedemann G. Controlled trial of ancrod in ischemic stroke. *Arch Neurol*. 1983;**40**:803–808

258. Olinger CP, Brott TG, Barsan WG, Hedges JR, Glas-Greenwalt P, Pollak VE, et al. Use of ancrod in acute or progressing ischemic cerebral infarction. *Ann Emerg Med*. 1988;**17**:1208–1209

259. Hennerici MG, Kay R, Bogousslavsky J, Lenzi GL, Verstraete M, Orgogozo JM. Intravenous ancrod for acute ischaemic stroke in the European Stroke Treatment with Ancrod Trial: A randomised controlled trial. *Lancet*. 2006;**368**:1871–1878

260. Van De Werf F, Adgey J, Ardissino D, Armstrong PW, Aylward P, Barbash G, et al. Single-bolus tenecteplase compared with front-loaded alteplase in acute myocardial infarction: The ASSENT-2 double-blind randomised trial. *Lancet*. 1999;**354**:716–722

261. Haley EC, Thompson JLP, Grotta JC, Lyden PD, Hemmen TG, Brown DL, et al. Phase IIB/III trial of tenecteplase in acute ischemic stroke: Results of a prematurely terminated randomized clinical trial. *Stroke*. 2010;**41**:707–711

262. Parsons M, Spratt N, Bivard A, Campbell B, Chung K, Miteff F, et al. A randomized trial of tenecteplase versus alteplace for acute ischemic stroke. *N Engl J Med* 2012;**366**:1099–1107

263. Leary MC, Saver JL, Gobin YP, Jahan R, Duckwiler GR, Vinuela F, et al. Beyond tissue plasminogen activator: Mechanical intervention in acute stroke. *Ann Emerg Med*. 2003;**41**:838–846

264. Saver JL. Improving reperfusion therapy for acute ischaemic stroke. *J Thromb Haemost*. 2011;**9** Suppl 1:333–343

265. Baltsavias G, Yella S, Al Shameri RA, Luft A, Valvanis A. Intra-arterial administration of papaverine during mechanical thrombectomy for acute ischemic stroke. *J Stroke Cerebrovasc Dis* 2015;**24**:41–47

266. Rha JH, Saver JL. The impact of recanalization on ischemic stroke outcome: A meta-analysis. *Stroke*. 2007;**38**:967–973

267. Levy EI, Siddiqui AH, Crumlish A, Snyder KV, Hauck EF, Fiorella DJ, et al. First food and drug administration-approved prospective trial of primary intracranial stenting for acute stroke: SARIS (Stent-Assisted Recanalization in acute Ischemic Stroke). *Stroke*. 2009;**40**:3552–3556

268. Velat GJ, Hoh BL, Levy EI, Mocco J. Primary intracranial stenting in acute ischemic stroke. *Curr Cardiol Rep*. 2010;**12**:14–19

269. The Penumbra Pivotal Stroke Trial Investigators. The Penumbra Pivotal Stroke Trial: Safety and effectiveness of a new generation of mechanical devices for clot removal in intracranial large vessel occlusive disease. *Stroke*. 2009;**40**:2761–2768

270. Kulcsár Z, Bonvin C, Pereira VM, Altrichter S, Yilmaz H, Lövblad KO, et al. Penumbra system: A novel mechanical thrombectomy device for large-vessel occlusions in acute stroke. *Am J Neuroradiol*. 2010;**31**:628–633

271. Psychogios M-N, Kreusch A, Wasser K, Mohr A, Gröschel K, Knauth M. Recanalization of large intracranial vessels using the penumbra system: A single-center experience. *Am J Neuroradiol*. 2012;**33**:1488–1493

272. Jankowitz B, Grandhi R, Horev A, Aghaebrahim A, Jadhav A, Linares G, et al. Primary manual aspiration thrombectomy (MAT) for acute ischemic stroke: Safety, feasibility and outcomes in 112 consecutive patients. *J NeuroIntervent Surg*. 2014; doi:10.1136/neurintsurg-2013–011024

273. Turk AS, Frei D, Fiorella D, Mocco J, Baxter B, Siddiqui A, et al. Adapt FAST study: A direct aspiration first pass technique for acute stroke thrombectomy. *J NeuroIntervent Surg*. 2014;**6**:260–264

274. Smith WS, Sung G, Starkman S, Saver JL, Kidwell CS, Gobin YP, et al. Safety and efficacy of mechanical embolectomy in acute ischemic stroke: Results of the MERCI trial. *Stroke*. 2005;**36**:1432–1438

275. Smith WS, Sung G, Saver J, Budzik R, Duckwiler G, Liebeskind DS, et al. Mechanical thrombectomy for acute ischemic stroke: Final results of the Multi MERCI trial. *Stroke*. 2008;**39**:1205–1212

276. Smith WS. Safety of mechanical thrombectomy and intravenous tissue plasminogen activator in acute ischemic stroke. Results of the Multi Mechanical Embolus Removal In

Cerebral Ischemia (MERCI) trial, part I. *AJNR Am J Neuroradiol.* 2006;**27**:1177–1182

277. Jahan R. Solitaire flow-restoration device for treatment of acute ischemic stroke: Safety and recanalization efficacy study in a swine vessel occlusion model. *AJNR Am J Neuroradiol.* 2010;**31**:1938–1943

278. Hausegger K, Hauser M, Kau T. Mechanical thrombectomy with stent retrievers in acute ischemic stroke. *Cardiovasc Intervent Radiol.* 2014;**37**:863–874

279. Saver JL, Jahan R, Levy EI, Jovin TG, Baxter B, Nogueira RG, et al. Solitaire flow restoration device versus the MERCI retriever in patients with acute ischaemic stroke (SWIFT): A randomised, parallel-group, non-inferiority trial. *Lancet.* 2012;**380**:1241–1249

280. Nogueira RG, Lutsep HL, Gupta R, Jovin TG, Albers GW, Walker GA, et al. TREVO versus MERCI retrievers for thrombectomy revascularisation of large vessel occlusions in acute ischaemic stroke (TREVO 2): A randomised trial. *Lancet.* 2012;**380**:1231–1240

281. Ciccone A, Valvassori L. Endovascular treatment for acute ischemic stroke. *N Engl J Med.* 2013;**368**:2433–2434

282. Broderick JP, Palesch YY, Demchuk AM, Yeatts SD, Khatri P, Hill MD, et al. Endovascular therapy after intravenous t-PA versus t-PA alone for stroke. *N Engl J Med.* 2013;**368**:893–903

283. Kidwell CS, Jahan R, Gornbein J, Alger JR, Nenov V, Ajani Z, et al. A trial of imaging selection and endovascular treatment for ischemic stroke. *N Engl J Med.* 2013;**368**:914–923

284. Berkheimer OA, Fransen PSS, Beumer D, van den Berg LA, Lingsma HF, Yoo AJ, et al. for the Mr CLEAN Investigators. A randomized trial of intraarterial treatment for acute ischemic stroke. *N Engl J Med.* 2015;**372**:11–20

285. Goyal M, Demchuk AM, Menon BK, Eesa M, Rempel JL, Thronton J, et al. for the ESCAPE Trial Investigators. Randomized assessment of rapid endovascular treatment of ischemic stroke. *N Engl J Med.* 2015;**372**:1019–1030

286. Saver J, Goyal M, Bonafe A, Diener H-C, Levy EI, Pereira VM, et al. for the SWIFT PRIME Investigators.

SolitaireTM with the intention for Thrombectomy as Primary Endovascular Treatment for Acute Ischemic Stroke (SWIFT PRIME) trial: protocol for randomized, controlled, multicenter study comparing the SolitaireTM revascularization device with IV tPA with IV tPA alone in acute ischemic stroke. *Int J Stroke.* 2015;**10**:439–448

287. Campbell BC. EXTEND-IA: Endovascular therapy after intravenous t-PA versus t-PA alone for ischemic stroke using CT perfusion imaging selection. International Stroke Conference, 2015: http://my.american heart.org/idc/groups/ahamah-public/@wcm/@sop/@scon/documents/down loadable/ucm_471810.pdf

288. Delgado-Mederos R, Rovira A, Alvarez-Sabin J, Ribo M, Munuera J, Rubiera M, et al. Speed of tPA-induced clot lysis predicts DWI lesion evolution in acute stroke. *Stroke.* 2007;**38**:955–960

289. Mazighi M, Chaudhry SA, Ribo M, Khatri P, Skoloudik D, Mokin M, et al. Impact of onset-to-reperfusion time on stroke mortality: A collaborative pooled analysis. *Circulation.* 2013;**127**:1980–1985

290. Wunderlich MT, Goertler M, Postert T, Schmitt E, Seidel G, Gahn G, et al. Recanalization after intravenous thrombolysis: Does a recanalization time window exist? *Neurology.* 2007;**68**:1364–1368

291. Uchino K, Anderson DC. Better late than never?: The story of arterial recanalization in acute ischemic stroke. *Neurology.* 2007;**68**:1335–1336

292. Sacco RL, Chong JY, Prabhakaran S, Elkind MS. Experimental treatments for acute ischaemic stroke. *Lancet.* 2007;**369**:331–341

293. Hemmen TM, Raman R, Guluma KZ, Meyer BC, Gomes JA, Cruz-Flores S, et al. Intravenous thrombolysis plus hypothermia for acute treatment of ischemic stroke (ICTUS-l): Final results. *Stroke.* 2010;**41**:2265–2270

294. Lyden PD, Hemmen TM, Grotta J, Rapp K, Raman R. Endovascular therapeutic hypothermia for acute ischemic stroke: ICTUS 2/3 protocol. *Int J Stroke.* 2014;**9**:117–125

295. Steiner T, Hacke W. Combination therapy with neuroprotectants and thrombolytics in acute ischaemic stroke. *Eur Neurol.* 1998;**40**:1–8

296. Alexandrov AV, Grotta JC. Arterial reocclusion in stroke patients

treated with intravenous tissue plasminogen activator. *Neurology.* 2002;**59**:862–867

297. Qureshi AI, Saad M, Zaidat OO, Suarez JI, Alexander MJ, Fareed M, et al. Intracerebral hemorrhages associated with neurointerventional procedures using a combination of antithrombotic agents including abciximab. *Stroke.* 2002;**33**:1916–1919

298. Abciximab Emergent Stroke Treatment Trial (ABESTT) Investigators. Emergency administration of abciximab for treatment of patients with acute ischemic stroke: Results of a randomized phase 2 trial. *Stroke.* 2005;**36**:880–890

299. Mangiafico S, Cellerini M, Nencini P, Gensini G, Inzitari D. Intravenous glycoprotein IIB/IIIA inhibitor (tirofiban) followed by intra-arterial urokinase and mechanical thrombolysis in stroke. *AJNR Am J Neuroradiol.* 2005;**26**:2595–2601

300. Straub S, Junghans U, Jovanovic V, Wittsack HJ, Seitz RJ, Siebler M. Systemic thrombolysis with recombinant tissue plasminogen activator and tirofiban in acute middle cerebral artery occlusion. *Stroke.* 2004;**35**:705–709

301. Seitz RJ, Meisel S, Moll M, Wittsack HJ, Junghans U, Siebler M. The effect of combined thrombolysis with rtPA and tirofiban on ischemic brain lesions. *Neurology.* 2004;**62**:2110–2112

302. Pancioli AM, Broderick J, Brott T, Tomsick T, Khoury J, Bean J, et al. The combined approach to lysis utilizing eptifibatide and rt-PA in acute ischemic stroke: The CLEAR Stroke Trial. *Stroke.* 2008;**39**:3268–3276

303. Pancioli AM, Adeoye O, Schmit PA, Khoury J, Levine SR, Tomsick TA, et al. Combined approach to lysis utilizing eptifibatide and recombinant tissue plasminogen activator in Acute Ischemic Stroke-Enhanced Regimen Stroke Trial. *Stroke.* 2013;**44**:2381–2387

304. Adams HP, Jr., Effron MB, Torner J, Davalos A, Frayne J, Teal P, et al. Emergency administration of abciximab for treatment of patients with acute ischemic stroke: Results of an international phase III trial: Abciximab in Emergency Treatment of Stroke Trial (ABESTT-II). *Stroke.* 2008;**39**:87–99

305. Sugg RM, Pary JK, Uchino K, Baraniuk S, Shaltoni HM, Gonzales NR, et al. Argatroban tPA stroke study: Study design and results in the first treated

cohort. *Arch Neurol.* 2006;**63**:1057–1062

306. Barreto AD, Alexandrov AV, Lyden P, Lee J, Martin-Schild S, Shen L, et al. The argatroban and tissue-type plasminogen activator stroke study: Final results of a pilot safety study. *Stroke.* 2012;**43**:770–775

307. Diener HC, Foerch C, Riess H, Rother J, Schroth G, Weber R. Treatment of acute ischaemic stroke with thrombolysis or thrombectomy in patients receiving anti-thrombotic treatment. *Lancet Neurol.* 2013;**12**:677–688

308. Grond M, Rudolf J, Neveling M, Stenzel C, Heiss WD. Risk of immediate heparin after rt-PA therapy in acute ischemic stroke. *Cerebrovascular Diseases.* 1997;**7**:318–323

309. Schmulling S, Rudolf J, Strotmann-Tack T, Grond M, Schneweis S, Sobesky J, et al. Acetylsalicylic acid pretreatment, concomitant heparin therapy and the risk of early intracranial hemorrhage following systemic thrombolysis for acute ischemic stroke. *Cerebrovasc Dis.* 2003;**16**:183–190

310. Zinkstok SM, Roos YB. Early administration of aspirin in patients treated with alteplase for acute ischaemic stroke: A randomised controlled trial. *Lancet.* 2012;**380**:731–737

311. Alexandrov AV, Demchuk AM, Felberg RA, Grotta JC, Krieger DW. Intracranial clot dissolution is associated with embolic signals on transcranial Doppler. *J Neuroimaging.* 2000;**10**:27–32

312. Alexandrov AV, Demchuk AM, Felberg RA, Christou I, Barber PA, Burgin WS, et al. High rate of complete recanalization and dramatic clinical recovery during tpa infusion when continuously monitored with 2-Mhz transcranial Doppler monitoring. *Stroke.* 2000;**31**:610–614

313. Eggers J, Koch B, Meyer K, Konig I, Seidel G. Effect of ultrasound on thrombolysis of middle cerebral artery occlusion. *Ann Neurol.* 2003;**53**:797–800

314. Tsivgoulis G, Eggers J, Ribo M, Perren F, Saqqur M, Rubiera M, et al. Safety and efficacy of ultrasound-enhanced thrombolysis: A comprehensive review and meta-analysis of randomized and nonrandomized studies. *Stroke.* 2010;**41**:280–287

315. Alexandrov AV, Molina CA, Grotta JC, Garami Z, Ford SR, Alvarez-Sabin

J, et al. Ultrasound-enhanced systemic thrombolysis for acute ischemic stroke. *N Engl J Med.* 2004;**351**:2170–2178

316. Molina CA, Barreto AD, Tsivgoulis G, Sierzenski P, Malkoff MD, Rubiera M, et al. Transcranial Ultrasound in Clinical Sonothrombolysis (TUCSON) Trial. *Ann Neurol.* 2009;**66**:28–38

317. Polak JF. Ultrasound energy and the dissolution of thrombus. *N Engl J Med.* 2004;**351**:2154–2155

318. Eggers J, Seidel G, Koch B, Konig IR. Sonothrombolysis in acute ischemic stroke for patients ineligible for rt-PA. *Neurology.* 2005;**64**:1052–1054

319. Molina CA, Ribo M, Rubiera M, Montaner J, Santamarina E, Delgado-Mederos R, et al. Microbubble administration accelerates clot lysis during continuous 2-Mhz ultrasound monitoring in stroke patients treated with intravenous tissue plasminogen activator. *Stroke.* 2006;**37**:425–429

320. Furlan AJ, Little JR, Dohn DF. Arterial occlusion following anastomosis of the superficial temporal artery to middle cerebral artery. *Stroke.* 1980;**11**:91–95

321. Gumerlock MK, Ono H, Neuwelt EA. Can a patent extracranial–intracranial bypass provoke the conversion of an intracranial arterial stenosis to a symptomatic occlusion? *Neurosurgery.* 1983;**12**:391–400

322. The EC/IC bypass study group. Failure of extracranial–intracranial arterial bypass to reduce the risk of ischemic stroke. Results of an international randomized trial. *N Engl J Med.* 1985; **313**:1191–1200

323. Caplan LR, Piepgras DG, Quest DO, Toole JF, Samson D, Futrell N, et al. EC-IC bypass 10 years later: Is it valuable? *Surg Neurol.* 1996;**46**:416–423

324. Przybylski GJ, Yonas H, Smith HA. Reduced stroke risk in patients with compromised cerebral blood flow reactivity treated with superficial temporal artery to distal middle cerebral artery bypass surgery. *J Stroke Cerebrovasc Dis.* 1998;**7**:302–309

325. Diaz FG, Umansky F, Mehta B, Montoya S, Dujovny M, Ausman JI, et al. Cerebral revascularization to a main limb of the middle cerebral artery in the sylvian fissure. An alternative approach to conventional anastomosis. *J Neurosurg.* 1985;**63**:21–29

326. Diaz F. Technique for extracranial–intracranial bypass grafting. In

W Moore, ed. *Surgery for Cerebrovascular Disease.* Philadelphia, PA: W B Saunders; 1996:638–654

327. Tulleken CA, Verdaasdonk RM, Beck RJ, Mali WP. The modified Excimer laser-assisted high-flow bypass operation. *Surg Neurol.* 1996;**46**:424–429

328. Klijn CJ, Kappelle LJ, van der Zwan A, van Gijn J, Tulleken CA. Excimer laser-assisted high-flow extracranial/intracranial bypass in patients with symptomatic carotid artery occlusion at high risk of recurrent cerebral ischemia: Safety and long-term outcome. *Stroke.* 2002;**33**:2451–2458

329. Derdeyn CP, Grubb RL, Jr., Powers WJ. Cerebral hemodynamic impairment: Methods of measurement and association with stroke risk. *Neurology.* 1999;**53**:251–259

330. Grubb RL, Jr., Derdeyn CP, Fritsch SM, Carpenter DA, Yundt KD, Videen TO, et al. Importance of hemodynamic factors in the prognosis of symptomatic carotid occlusion. *JAMA.* 1998;**280**:1055–1060

331. Powers WJ. Cerebral hemodynamics in ischemic cerebrovascular disease. *Ann Neurol.* 1991;**29**:231–240

332. Yokota C, Hasegawa Y, Minematsu K, Yamaguchi T. Effect of acetazolamide reactivity on long-term outcome in patients with major cerebral artery occlusive diseases. *Stroke.* 1998;**29**:640–644

333. Vernieri F, Pasqualetti P, Passarelli F, Rossini PM, Silvestrini M. Outcome of carotid artery occlusion is predicted by cerebrovascular reactivity. *Stroke.* 1999;**30**:593–598

334. Grubb RL, Jr., Powers WJ, Derdeyn CP, Adams HP, Jr., Clarke WR. The carotid occlusion surgery study. *Neurosurg Focus.* 2003;**14**:e9

335. Grubb RL, Jr. Extracranial–intracranial arterial bypass for treatment of occlusion of the internal carotid artery. *Curr Neurol Neurosci Rep.* 2004;**4**:23–30

336. Adams HP, Jr., Powers WJ, Grubb RL, Jr., Clarke WR, Woolson RF. Preview of a new trial of extracranial-to-intracranial arterial anastomosis: The carotid occlusion surgery study. *Neurosurg Clin N Am.* 2001;**12**:613–624

337. Dusick JR, Liebeskind DS, Saver JL, Martin NA, Gonzalez NR. Indirect revascularization for nonmoyamoya intracranial arterial stenoses: Clinical

201

and angiographic outcomes. *J Neurosurg.* 2012;**117**:94–102

338. Garg BP, Biller J. Moyamoya disease and cerebral ischemia. In HH Batjer, L Friberg, RG Greenlee Jr, TA Kopitnik, WL Young, eds. *Cerebrovascular Disease.* Philadelphia, PA: Lippincott-Raven; 1997:489–499

339. Scott RM, Smith JL, Robertson RL, Madsen JR, Soriano SG, Rockoff MA. Long-term outcome in children with moyamoya syndrome after cranial revascularization by pial synangiosis. *J Neurosurg.* 2004;**100**:142–149

340. Miyamoto S, Yoshimoto T, Hashimoto N, Okada Y, Tsuji I, Tominaga T, et al. Effects of extracranial–intracranial bypass for patients with hemorrhagic moyamoya disease: Results of the Japan adult moyamoya trial. *Stroke.* 2014;**45**:1415–1421

341. Miyamoto S. Study design for a prospective randomized trial of extracranial–intracranial bypass surgery for adults with moyamoya disease and hemorrhagic onset - the Japan adult moyamoya trial group. *Neurol Med Chir (Tokyo).* 2004;**44**:218–219

342. Caplan L. Use of vasodilating drugs for cerebral symptomatology. In R Miller, D Greenblatt, eds. *Drug Therapy Reviews.* Amsterdam: Elsevier; 1979:305–317

343. Golino P, Piscione F, Willerson JT, Cappelli-Bigazzi M, Focaccio A, Villari B, et al. Divergent effects of serotonin on coronary-artery dimensions and blood flow in patients with coronary atherosclerosis and control patients. *N Engl J Med.* 1991;**324**:641–648

344. Piepgras A, Schmiedek P, Leinsinger G, Haberl RL, Kirsch CM, Einhaupl KM. A simple test to assess cerebrovascular reserve capacity using transcranial Doppler sonography and acetazolamide. *Stroke.* 1990;**21**:1306–1311

345. Mette D, Strunk R, Zuccarello M. Cerebral blood flow measurement in neurosurgery. *Transl Stroke Res.* 2011;**2**:152–158

346. Hojer-Pedersen E. Effect of acetazolamide on cerebral blood flow in subacute and chronic cerebrovascular disease. *Stroke.* 1987;**18**:887–891

347. Braunwald E. Mechanism of action of calcium-channel-blocking agents. *N Engl J Med.* 1982;**307**:1618–1627

348. Gorelick PB, Caplan LR. Calcium, hypercalcemia and stroke. Current concepts in cerebrovascular disease. *Stroke.* 1985:**20**:13–17

349. Allen GS, Ahn HS, Preziosi TJ, Battye R, Boone SC, Boone SC, et al. Cerebral arterial spasm – a controlled trial of nimodipine in patients with subarachnoid hemorrhage. *N Engl J Med.* 1983;**308**:619–624

350. Philippon J, Grob R, Dagreou F, Guggiari M, Rivierez M, Viars P. Prevention of vasospasm in subarachnoid haemorrhage. A controlled study with nimodipine. *Acta Neurochir (Wien).* 1986;**82**:110–114

351. Jan M, Buchheit F, Tremoulet M. Therapeutic trial of intravenous nimodipine in patients with established cerebral vasospasm after rupture of intracranial aneurysms. *Neurosurgery.* 1988;**23**:154–157

352. Pickard JD, Murray GD, Illingworth R, Shaw MD, Teasdale GM, Foy PM, et al. Effect of oral nimodipine on cerebral infarction and outcome after subarachnoid haemorrhage: British aneurysm nimodipine trial. *BMJ.* 1989;**298**:636–642

353. Trust Study Group. Randomised, double-blind, placebo-controlled trial of nimodipine in acute stroke. *Lancet.* 1990;**336**:1205–1209

354. The American Nimodipine Study Group. Clinical trial of nimodipine in acute ischemic stroke. *Stroke.* 1992;**23**:3–8

355. Pandey P, Steinberg GK, Dodd R, Do HM, Marks MP. A simplified method for administration of intra-arterial nicardipine for vasospasm with cervical catheter infusion. *Neurosurgery.* 2012;**71**:77–85

356. Yancy H, Lee-Iannotti JK, Schwedt TJ, Dodick DW. Reversible cerebral vasoconstriction syndrome. *Headache.* 2013;**53**:570–576

357. Heros RC, Korosue K. Hemodilution for cerebral ischemia. *Stroke.* 1989;**20**:423–427

358. Huh PW, Belayev L, Zhao W, Busto R, Saul I, Ginsberg MD. The effect of high-dose albumin therapy on local cerebral perfusion after transient focal cerebral ischemia in rats. *Brain Res.* 1998;**804**:105–113

359. Ginsberg MD, Palesch YY, Hill MD, Martin RH, Moy CS, Barsan WG, et al. High-dose albumin treatment for acute ischaemic stroke (ALIAS) part 2:

A randomised, double-blind, phase 3, placebo-controlled trial. *Lancet Neurol.* 2013;**12**:1049–1058

360. Dhar R, Scalfani MT, Zazulia AR, Videen TO, Derdeyn CP, Diringer MN. Comparison of induced hypertension, fluid bolus, and blood transfusion to augment cerebral oxygen delivery after subarachnoid hemorrhage. *J Neurosurg.* 2012;**116**:648–656

361. Thomas DJ. Hemodilution in acute stroke. *Stroke.* 1985;**16**:763–764

362. Thomas DJ, Marshall J, Russell RW, Wetherley-Mein G, du Boulay GH, Pearson TC, et al. Effect of haematocrit on cerebral blood-flow in man. *Lancet.* 1977;**2**:941–943

363. Wood JH, Kee DB, Jr. Hemorheology of the cerebral circulation in stroke. *Stroke.* 1985;**16**:765–772

364. Chittiboina P, Guthikonda B, Wollblad C, Conrad SA. A computational simulation of the effect of hemodilution on oxygen transport in middle cerebral artery vasospasm. *J Cereb Blood Flow Metab.* 2011;**31**:2209–2217

365. Strand T, Asplund K, Eriksson S, Hagg E, Lithner F, Wester PO. A randomized controlled trial of hemodilution therapy in acute ischemic stroke. *Stroke.* 1984;**15**:980–989

366. Staedt U, Schlierf G, Oster P. Hypervolemic hemodilution with 10% HES 200/0.5 and 10% dextran 40 in patients with ischemic stroke. In A Hartmann, Kuschinsky E, eds. *Cerebral Ischemia and Hemorheology.* New York, NY: Springer; 1987:429–435

367. Scandinavian Stroke Study Group. Multicenter trial of hemodilution in acute ischemic stroke. Results of subgroup analyses. *Stroke.* 1988;**19**:464–471

368. Aichner FT, Fazekas F, Brainin M, Polz W, Mamoli B, Zeiler K. Hypervolemic hemodilution in acute ischemic stroke: The Multicenter Austrian Hemodilution Stroke Trial (MAHST). *Stroke.* 1998;**29**:743–749

369. Grotta J, Ackerman R, Correia J, Fallick G, Chang J. Whole blood viscosity parameters and cerebral blood flow. *Stroke.* 1982;**13**:296–301

370. Coull BM, Beamer N, de Garmo P, Sexton G, Nordt F, Knox R, et al. Chronic blood hyperviscosity in subjects with acute stroke, transient

ischemic attack, and risk factors for stroke. *Stroke*. 1991;**22**:162–168

371. Beamer N, Coull BM, Sexton G, de Garmo P, Knox R, Seaman G. Fibrinogen and the albumin–globulin ratio in recurrent stroke. *Stroke*. 1993;**24**:1133–1139

372. Ernst E, Resch KL. Fibrinogen as a cardiovascular risk factor: A meta-analysis and review of the literature. *Ann Intern Med*. 1993;**118**:956–963

373. Rothwell PM, Howard SC, Power DA, Gutnikov SA, Algra A, van Gijn J, et al. Fibrinogen concentration and risk of ischemic stroke and acute coronary events in 5113 patients with transient ischemic attack and minor ischemic stroke. *Stroke*. 2004;**35**:2300–2305

374. Liu M, Counsell C, Wardlaw J, Sandercock P. A systematic review of randomized evidence for fibrinogen-depleting agents in acute ischemic stroke. *J Stroke Cerebrovasc Dis*. 1998;**7**:63–69

375. Schuff-Werner P, Schutz E, Seyde WC, Eisenhauer T, Janning G, Armstrong VW, et al. Improved haemorheology associated with a reduction in plasma fibrinogen and LDL in patients being treated by heparin-induced extracorporeal LDL precipitation (HELP). *Eur J Clin Invest*. 1989;**19**:30–37

376. Walzl M, Lechner H, Walzl B, Schied G. Improved neurological recovery of cerebral infarctions after plasmapheretic reduction of lipids and fibrinogen. *Stroke*. 1993;**24**:1447–1451

377. Bambauer R, Schiel R, Latza R. Low-density lipoprotein apheresis: An overview. *Ther Apher Dial*. 2003;**7**:382–390

378. Wieland E, Schettler V, Armstrong VW. Highly effective reduction of c-reactive protein in patients with coronary heart disease by extracorporeal low density lipoprotein apheresis. *Atherosclerosis*. 2002;**162**:187–191

379. Radack K, Deck C, Huster G. Dietary supplementation with low-dose fish oils lowers fibrinogen levels: A randomized, double-blind controlled study. *Ann Intern Med*. 1989;**111**:757–758

380. Kobayashi S, Hirai A, Terano T, Hamazaki T, Tamura Y, Kumagai A. Reduction in blood viscosity by eicosapentaenoic acid. *Lancet*. 1981;**2**:197

381. Vanschoonbeek K, Feijge MA, Paquay M, Rosing J, Saris W, Kluft C, et al. Variable hypocoagulant effect of fish oil intake in humans: Modulation of fibrinogen level and thrombin generation. *Arterioscler Thromb Vasc Biol*. 2004;**24**:1734–1740

382. Kwak SM, Myung SK, Lee YJ, Seo HG. Efficacy of omega-3 fatty acid supplements (eicosapentaenoic acid and docosahexaenoic acid) in the secondary prevention of cardiovascular disease: A meta-analysis of randomized, double-blind, placebo-controlled trials. *Arch Intern Med*. 2012;**172**:686–694

383. Geyer RP. Oxygen transport in vivo by means of perfluorochemical preparations. *N Engl J Med*. 1982;**307**:304–305

384. Tremper KK, Friedman AE, Levine EM, Lapin R, Camarillo D. The preoperative treatment of severely anemic patients with a perfluorochemical oxygen-transport fluid, Fluosol-DA. *N Engl J Med*. 1982;**307**:277–283

385. Gould SA, Rosen AL, Sehgal LR, Sehgal HL, Langdale LA, Krause LM, et al. Fluosol-DA as a red-cell substitute in acute anemia. *N Engl J Med*. 1986;**314**:1653–1656

386. Bose B, Osterholm JL, Triolo A. Focal cerebral ischemia: Reduction in size of infarcts by ventriculo-subarachnoid perfusion with fluorocarbon emulsion. *Brain Res*. 1985;**328**:223–231

387. Bell RD, Frazer GD, Osterholm JL, Duckett SW. A novel treatment for ischemic intracranial hypertension in cats. *Stroke*. 1991;**22**:80–83

388. Bell RD, Powers BL, Brock D, Provencio JJ, Flanders A, Benetiz R, et al. Ventriculo-lumbar perfusion in acute ischemic stroke. *Neurocrit Care*. 2006;**5**:21–29

389. Hammer M, Jovin T, Wahr J, Heiss WD. Partial occlusion of the descending aorta increases cerebral blood flow in a non-stroke porcine model. *Cerebrovasc Dis*. 2009;**28**:406–410

390. Liebeskind DS. Aortic occlusion for cerebral ischemia: From theory to practice. *Curr Cardiol Rep*. 2008;**10**:31–36

391. Lylyk P, Vila JF, Miranda C, Ferrario A, Romero R, Cohen JE. Partial aortic obstruction improves cerebral perfusion and clinical symptoms in patients with symptomatic vasospasm. *Neurol Res*. 2005;**27**(Suppl 1):S129–S135

392. Emery DJ, Schellinger PD, Selchen D, Douen A, Chan R, Shuaib A, et al. Safety and feasibility of collateral blood flow augmentation following intravenous thrombolysis. *Stroke*. 2011;**42**:1135–1137

393. Shuaib A, Bornstein NM, Diener H-C, et al. Partial aortic occlusion for cerebral perfusion augmentation: safety and efficacy of Neuroflo in acute ischemic stroke. *Stroke*. 2011;**42**:1680–1690

394. Han JH, Leung TW, Lam WL et al. Preliminary findings of external counterpulsation for ischemic stroke patients with large artery occlusions. *Stroke*. 2008;**39**:1340–1343

395. Bonetti PO, Holmes DR Jr, Lerman A, Barsness GW. Enhanced external counterpulsation for ischemic heart disease: What's behind the curtain? *J Am Coll Cardiol*. 2003;**41**;1918–1925

396. del Zoppo GJ. Vascular hemostasis and brain embolism In LR Caplan WJ Manning, eds. *Brain Embolism*. New York, NY: Informa Healthcare; 2006:243–258

397. Weksler B. Antithrombotic therapies in the management of cerebral ischemia. In F Plum, W Pulsinelli, eds. *Cerebrovascular Diseases: Proceedings of the Fourteenth Princeton Conference*. New York, NY: Raven Press, 1985:211–223

398. Caplan LR. Antiplatelet therapy in stroke prevention: Present and future. *Cerebrovasc Dis*. 2006;**21** Suppl 1:1–6

399. Bloom AL, Thomas DP. *Haemostasis and Thrombosis*. Edinburgh: Churchill-Livingstone; 1987

400. Deykin D. Thrombogenesis. *N Engl J Med*. 1967;**276**:622–628

401. Hemker HC, Lindhout T. Interaction of platelet activation and coagulation. In V Fuster, Topol EN, Nabel EG, eds. *Atherothrombosiss and Coronary Artery Disease*. Philadelphia, PA: Lippincott–Williams & Wilkins; 2005:569–581

402. Marder VJ, Chute DJ, Starkman S, Abolian AM, Kidwell C, Liebeskind D, et al. Analysis of thrombi retrieved from cerebral arteries of patients with acute ischemic stroke. *Stroke*. 2006;**37**:2086–2093

403. Liebeskind DS, Sanossian N, Yong WH, Starkman S, Tsang MP, Moya

AL, et al. CT and MRI early vessel signs reflect clot composition in acute stroke. *Stroke.* 2011;**42**:1237–1243

404. Francis CW, Kaplan KL. Principles of antithrombotic therapy. In MA Lichtman, TJ Kipps, K Kaushansky, eds. *Williams Hematology*, 7th ed. New York, NY: McGraw-Hill; 2006:283–300

405. Caplan LR. Anticoagulation for cerebral ischemia. *Clin Neuropharmacol.* 1986;**9**:399–414

406. Damus PS, Hicks M, Rosenberg RD. Anticoagulant action of heparin. *Nature.* 1973;**246**:355–357

407. Wu KK. New pharmacologic approaches to thromboembolic disorders. *Hosp Pract (Off Ed).* 1985;**20**:101–104, 107–108, 117–120

408. Hirsh J. Heparin. *N Engl J Med.* 1991;**324**:1565–1574

409. Salzman EW, Deykin D, Shapiro RM, Rosenberg R. Management of heparin therapy: Controlled prospective trial. *N Engl J Med.* 1975;**292**:1046–1050

410. Warkentin TE, Levine MN, Hirsh J, Horsewood P, Roberts RS, Gent M, et al. Heparin-induced thrombocytopenia in patients treated with low-molecular-weight heparin or unfractionated heparin. *N Engl J Med.* 1995;**332**:1330–1335

411. Becker PS, Miller VT. Heparin-induced thrombocytopenia. *Stroke.* 1989;**20**:1449–1459

412. Arepally GM, Ortel TL. Clinical practice. Heparin-induced thrombocytopenia. *N Engl J Med.* 2006;**355**:809–817

413. Das P, Ziada K, Steinhubl SR, Moliterno DJ, Hamdalla H, Jozic J, et al. Heparin-induced thrombocytopenia and cardiovascular diseases. *Am Heart J.* 2006;**152**:19–26

414. Lovecchio F. Heparin-induced thrombocytopenia. *Clinical Toxicology.* 2014;**52**:579–583

415. Phelan BK. Heparin-associated thrombosis without thrombocytopenia. *Ann Intern Med.* 1983;**99**:637–638

416. Weitz JI. Low-molecular-weight heparins. *N Engl J Med.* 1997;**337**:688–698

417. Gordon DL, Linhardt R, Adams HP, Jr. Low-molecular-weight heparins and heparinoids and their use in acute or progressing ischemic stroke. *Clin Neuropharmacol.* 1990;**13**:522–543

418. Rosenberg RD, Lam L. Correlation between structure and function of heparin. *Proc Natl Acad Sci U S A.* 1979;**76**:1218–1222

419. Bick RL, Frenkel EP, Walenga J, Fareed J, Hoppensteadt DA. Unfractionated heparin, low molecular weight heparins, and pentasaccharide: Basic mechanism of actions, pharmacology, and clinical use. *Hematol Oncol Clin North Am.* 2005; **19**:1–51, v

420. Sherman DG, Albers GW, Bladin C, Fieschi C, Gabbai AA, Kase CS, et al. The efficacy and safety of enoxaparin versus unfractionated heparin for the prevention of venous thromboembolism after acute ischaemic stroke (PREVAIL study): An open-label randomised comparison. *Lancet.* 2007;**369**:1347–1355

421. Wessler S, Gitel SN. Warfarin. From bedside to bench. *N Engl J Med.* 1984;**311**:645–652

422. Deykin D. Warfarin therapy. 1. *N Engl J Med.* 1970;**283**:691–694

423. Hull R, Hirsh J, Jay R, Carter C, England C, Gent M, et al. Different intensities of oral anticoagulant therapy in the treatment of proximal-vein thrombosis. *N Engl J Med.* 1982;**307**:1676–1681

424. Taberner DA, Poller L, Burslem RW, Jones JB. Oral anticoagulants controlled by the British comparative thromboplastin versus low-dose heparin in prophylaxis of deep vein thrombosis. *Br Med J.* 1978;**1**:272–274

425. Francis CW, Marder VJ, Evarts CM, Yaukoolbodi S. Two-step warfarin therapy. Prevention of postoperative venous thrombosis without excessive bleeding. *JAMA.* 1983;**249**:374–378

426. Hirsh J, Poller L, Deykin D, Levine M, Dalen JE. Optimal therapeutic range for oral anticoagulants. *Chest.* 1989;**95**:5s–11s

427. The Boston Area Anticoagulation Trial for Atrial Fibrillation Investigators. The effect of low-dose warfarin on the risk of stroke in patients with nonrheumatic atrial fibrillation. *N Engl J Med.* 1991;**325**:129–132

428. The Stroke Prevention In Reversible Ischemia Trial (SPIRIT) Study Group. A randomized trial of anticoagulants versus aspirin after cerebral ischemia of presumed arterial origin. *Ann Neurol.* 1997;**42**:857–865

429. Sconce EA, Khan TI, Wynne HA, Avery P, Monkhouse L, King BP, et al.

The impact of *CYP2C9* and *VKORC1* genetic polymorphism and patient characteristics upon warfarin dose requirements: Proposal for a new dosing regimen. *Blood.* 2005;**106**:2329–2333

430. Rieder MJ, Reiner AP, Gage BF, Nickerson DA, Eby CS, McLeod HL, et al. Effect of *VKORC1* haplotypes on transcriptional regulation and warfarin dose. *N Engl J Med.* 2005;**352**:2285–2293

431. Yin T, Miyata T. Warfarin dose and the pharmacogenomics of *CYP2C9* and *VKORC1* – rationale and perspectives. *Thromb Res.* 2007;**120**:1–10

432. Ingelman-Sundberg M. Pharmacogenomic biomarkers for prediction of severe adverse drug reactions. *N Engl J Med.* 2008;**358**:637–639

433. Risk factors for stroke and efficacy of antithrombotic therapy in atrial fibrillation. Analysis of pooled data from five randomized controlled trials. *Arch Intern Med.* 1994;**154**:1449–1457

434. Hart RG. Oral anticoagulants for secondary prevention of stroke. *Cerebrovascular Diseases.* 1997;7(Suppl 6):24–29

435. Hylek EM, Skates SJ, Sheehan MA, Singer DE. An analysis of the lowest effective intensity of prophylactic anticoagulation for patients with nonrheumatic atrial fibrillation. *N Engl J Med.* 1996;**335**:540–546

436. Fleming HA, Bailey SM. Mitral valve disease, systemic embolism and anticoagulants. *Postgrad Med J.* 1971;**47**:599–604

437. Adams GF, Merrett JD, Hutchinson WM, Pollock AM. Cerebral embolism and mitral stenosis: Survival with and without anticoagulants. *J Neurol Neurosurg Psychiatry.* 1974;**37**:378–383

438. Carter AB. Prognosis of cerebral embolism. *Lancet.* 1965;**2**:514–519

439. Caplan LR. Brain embolism. In LR Caplan MC, JW Hurst, MI Chimowitz, eds. *Clinical Neurocardiology.* New York, NY: Marcel Dekker; 1999:35–185

440. The Boston Area Anticoagulation Trial for Atrial Fibrillation Investigators. The effect of low-dose warfarin on the risk of stroke in patients with nonrheumatic atrial fibrillation. *N Engl J Med.* 1990;**323**:1505–1511

441. The European Atrial Fibrillation Trial (EAFT) Study Group. Silent brain infarction in nonrheumatic atrial fibrillation. *Neurology*. 1996;**46**:159–165

442. European Atrial Fibrillation Trial Study Group. Secondary prevention in non-rheumatic atrial fibrillation after transient ischaemic attack or minor stroke. *Lancet*. 1993;**342**:1255–1262

443. Petersen P, Boysen G, Godtfredsen J, Andersen ED, Andersen B. Placebo-controlled, randomised trial of warfarin and aspirin for prevention of thromboembolic complications in chronic atrial fibrillation. The Copenhagen AFASAK study. *Lancet*. 1989;**1**:175–179

444. The Stroke Prevention in Atrial Fibrillation Investigators. Stroke Prevention in Atrial Fibrillation Study. Final results. *Circulation*. 1991;**84**:527–539

445. The Stroke Prevention in Atrial Fibrillation Investigators. Warfarin versus aspirin for prevention of thromboembolism in atrial fibrillation: Stroke Prevention in Atrial Fibrillation II Study. *Lancet*. 1994;**343**:687–691

446. The Stroke Prevention in Atrial Fibrillation Investigators. Adjusted-dose warfarin versus low-intensity, fixed-dose warfarin plus aspirin for high-risk patients with atrial fibrillation: Stroke Prevention in Atrial Fibrillation III randomised clinical trial. *Lancet*. 1996;**348**:633–638

447. Albers GW. Atrial fibrillation and stroke. Three new studies, three remaining questions. *Arch Intern Med*. 1994;**154**:1443–1448

448. Manning W. *Cardiac Source of Embolism: Treatment in Brain Embolism*. New York, NY: Informa Healthcare; 2006

449. Lip GY. Can we predict stroke in atrial fibrillation? *Clin Cardiol*. 2012;**35** Suppl 1:21–27

450. The Publications Committee for the Trial of Org 10172 in Acute Stroke Treatment (TOAST) Investigators. Low molecular weight heparinoid, Org 10172 (Danaparoid), and outcome after acute ischemic stroke: A randomized controlled trial. *JAMA*. 1998;**279**:1265–1272

451. Saxena R, Lewis S, Berge E, Sandercock PA, Koudstaal PJ. Risk of early death and recurrent stroke and effect of heparin in 3169 patients with acute ischemic stroke and atrial fibrillation in the International Stroke Trial. *Stroke*. 2001;**32**:2333–2337

452. Berge E, Abdelnoor M, Nakstad PH, Sandset PM. Low molecular-weight heparin versus aspirin in patients with acute ischaemic stroke and atrial fibrillation: A double-blind randomised study. HAEST Study Group. Heparin in Acute Embolic Stroke Trial. *Lancet*. 2000;**355**:1205–1210

453. Cerebral Embolism Study Group. Immediate anticoagulation of embolic stroke: A randomized trial. *Stroke*. 1983;**14**:668–676

454. Chamorro A, Vila N, Saiz A, Alday M, Tolosa E. Early anticoagulation after large cerebral embolic infarction: A safety study. *Neurology*. 1995;**45**:861–865

455. Chamorro A, Vila N, Ascaso C, Blanc R. Heparin in acute stroke with atrial fibrillation: Clinical relevance of very early treatment. *Arch Neurol*. 1999;**56**:1098–1102

456. Cerebral Embolism Task Force. Cardiogenic brain embolism. *Arch Neurol*. 1986;**43**:71–84

457. Cerebral Embolism Task Force. Cardiogenic brain embolism. The second report of the Cerebral Embolism Task Force. *Arch Neurol*. 1989;**46**:727–743

458. Cerebral Embolism Study Group. Immediate anticoagulation of embolic stroke: Brain hemorrhage and management options. *Stroke*. 1984;**15**:779–789

459. Furlan AJ, Cavalier SJ, Hobbs RE, Weinstein MA, Modic MT. Hemorrhage and anticoagulation after nonseptic embolic brain infarction. *Neurology*. 1982;**32**:280–282

460. Pessin MS, Estol CJ, Lafranchise F, Caplan LR. Safety of anticoagulation after hemorrhagic infarction. *Neurology*. 1993;**43**:1298–1303

461. Cabanes L, Mas JL, Cohen A, Amarenco P, Cabanes PA, Oubary P, et al. Atrial septal aneurysm and patent foramen ovale as risk factors for cryptogenic stroke in patients less than 55 years of age. A study using transesophageal echocardiography. *Stroke*. 1993;**24**:1865–1873

462. Mas JL, Arquizan C, Lamy C, Zuber M, Cabanes L, Derumeaux G, et al. Recurrent cerebrovascular events associated with patent foramen ovale, atrial septal aneurysm, or both. *N Engl J Med*. 2001;**345**:1740–1746

463. Thaler DE, Saver JL. Cryptogenic stroke and patent foramen ovale. *Curr Opin Cardiol*. 2008;**23**:537–544

464. Kent DM, Ruthazer R, Weimar C, Mas JL, Serena J, Homma S, et al. An index to identify stroke-related vs. incidental patent foramen ovale in cryptogenic stroke. *Neurology*. 2013;**81**:619–625

465. Grosgogeat Y, Lhermitte F, Carpentier A, Facquet J, Alhomme P, Tran T. [Aneurysm of the interauricular septum revealed by a cerebral embolism]. *Arch Mal Coeur Vaiss*. 1973;**66**:169–177

466. Silver MD, Dorsey JS. Aneurysms of the septum primum in adults. *Arch Pathol Lab Med*. 1978;**102**:62–65

467. Bogousslavsky J, Garazi S, Jeanrenaud X, Aebischer N, Van Melle G. Stroke recurrence in patients with patent foramen ovale: The Lausanne Study. Lausanne Stroke with Paradoxal Embolism Study Group. *Neurology*. 1996;**46**:1301–1305

468. Mas JL, Zuber M. Recurrent cerebrovascular events in patients with patent foramen ovale, atrial septal aneurysm, or both and cryptogenic stroke or transient ischemic attack. French Study Group on Patent Foramen Ovale and Atrial Septal Aneurysm. *Am Heart J*. 1995;**130**:1083–1088

469. Bridges ND, Hellenbrand W, Latson L, Filiano J, Newburger JW, Lock JE. Transcatheter closure of patent foramen ovale after presumed paradoxical embolism. *Circulation*. 1992;**86**:1902–1908

470. Homma S, Sacco RL, Di Tullio MR, Sciacca RR, Mohr JP. Effect of medical treatment in stroke patients with patent foramen ovale: Patent Foramen Ovale in Cryptogenic Stroke Study. *Circulation*. 2002;**105**:2625–2631

471. Mohr JP, Thompson JL, Lazar RM, Levin B, Sacco RL, Furie KL, et al. A comparison of warfarin and aspirin for the prevention of recurrent ischemic stroke. *N Engl J Med*. 2001;**345**:1444–1451

472. Furlan AJ, Reisman M, Massaro J, Mauri L, Adams H, Albers GW, et al. Closure or medical therapy for cryptogenic stroke with patent foramen ovale. *N Engl J Med*. 2012;**366**:991–999

473. Carroll JD, Saver JL, Thaler DE, Smalling RW, Berry S, MacDonald LA, et al. Closure of patent foramen ovale versus medical therapy after cryptogenic stroke. *N Engl J Med*. 2013;**368**:1092–1100

474. Meier B, Kalesan B, Mattle HP, Khattab AA, Hildick-Smith D, Dudek D, et al. Percutaneous closure of patent foramen ovale in cryptogenic embolism. *N Engl J Med.* 2013;**368**:1083–1091

475. Li Y, Zhou K, Hua Y, Wang C, Xie L, Fang J, et al. Amplatzer occluder versus cardioSEAL/STARFlex occluder: A meta-analysis of the efficacy and safety of transcatheter occlusion for patent foramen ovale and atrial septal defect. *Cardiol Young.* 2013;**23**:582–596

476. Bousser M-G, Ross Russell, R. *Cerebral Venous Thrombosis.* Philadelphia, PA: W B Saunders; 1997

477. Ameri A, Bousser M-G. Cerebral venous thrombosis. *Neurol Clin.* 1992;**10**:87–111

478. Jacewicz M, Plum F. Aseptic cerebral venous thrombosis. In K Einhaupl, O Kempski, Baethmann A, eds. *Cerebral Sinus Thrombosis. Experimental and Clinical Aspects.* New York, NY: Plenum; 1990:157–170

479. Einhaupl KM, Villringer A, Meister W, Mehraein S, Garner C, Pellkofer M, et al. Heparin treatment in sinus venous thrombosis. *Lancet.* 1991;**338**:597–600

480. Meister W, Einhaupl K, Villringer A. Treatment of patients with cerebral sinus and vein thrombosis with heparin. In K Einhaupl, O Kempski, Baethmann A, eds. *Cerebral Sinus Thrombosis. Experimental and Clinical Aspects.* New York, NY: Plenum; 1990:225–230

481. de Bruijn SF, Stam J. Randomized, placebo-controlled trial of anticoagulant treatment with low-molecular-weight heparin for cerebral sinus thrombosis. *Stroke.* 1999;**30**:484–488

482. Caplan LR. Venous and dural sinus thrombosis. In LR Caplan, ed. *Posterior Circulation Disease. Clinical Findings, Diagnosis, and Management.* Boston, MA: Blackwell Science; 1996:569–592

483. Diaz JM, Schiffman JS, Urban ES, Maccario M. Superior sagittal sinus thrombosis and pulmonary embolism: A syndrome rediscovered. *Acta Neurol Scand.* 1992;**86**:390–396

484. Caplan LR. Resolved: Heparin may be useful in selected patients with brain ischemia. *Stroke.* 2003;**34**:230–231

485. Caplan LR. Anticoagulants to prevent stroke occurrence and worsening. *Isr Med Assoc J.* 2006;**8**:773–778

486. Caplan LR. Worsening in ischemic stroke patients: Is it time for a new strategy? *Stroke.* 2002;**33**:1443–1445

487. International Stroke Trial Collaborative Group. The International Stroke Trial (IST): A randomised trial of aspirin, subcutaneous heparin, both, or neither among 19 435 patients with acute ischaemic stroke. *Lancet.* 1997;**349**:1569–1581

488. Kay R, Wong KS, Yu YL, Chan YW, Tsoi TH, Ahuja AT, et al. Low-molecular-weight heparin for the treatment of acute ischemic stroke. *N Engl J Med.* 1995;**333**:1588–1593

489. Adams HP, Jr., Bendixen BH, Leira E, Chang KC, Davis PH, Woolson RF, et al. Antithrombotic treatment of ischemic stroke among patients with occlusion or severe stenosis of the internal carotid artery: A report of the Trial of Org 10172 in Acute Stroke Treatment (TOAST). *Neurology.* 1999;**53**:122–125

490. Wong KS, Chen C, Ng PW, Tsoi TH, Li HL, Fong WC, et al. Low-molecular-weight heparin compared with aspirin for the treatment of acute ischaemic stroke in asian patients with large artery occlusive disease: A randomised study. *Lancet Neurol.* 2007;**6**:407–413

491. Chimowitz MI, Lynn MJ, Howlett-Smith H, Stern BJ, Hertzberg VS, Frankel MR, et al. Comparison of warfarin and aspirin for symptomatic intracranial arterial stenosis. *N Engl J Med.* 2005;**352**:1305–1316

492. Koroshetz WJ. Warfarin, aspirin, and intracranial vascular disease. *N Engl J Med.* 2005;**352**:1368–1370

493. Georgiadis D, Arnold M, von Buedingen HC, Valko P, Sarikaya H, Rousson V, et al. Aspirin vs. anticoagulation in carotid artery dissection: A study of 298 patients. *Neurology.* 2009;**72**:1810–1815

494. Samsa GP, Matchar DB, Goldstein LB, Bonito AJ, Lux LJ, Witter DM, et al. Quality of anticoagulation management among patients with atrial fibrillation: Results of a review of medical records from two communities. *Arch Intern Med.* 2000;**160**:967–973

495. Chiquette E, Amato MG, Bussey HI. Comparison of an anticoagulation clinic with usual medical care: Anticoagulation control, patient outcomes, and health care costs. *Arch Intern Med.* 1998;**158**:1641–1647

496. Kucher N, Connolly S, Beckman JA, Cheng LH, Tsilimingras KV, Fanikos J, et al. International normalized ratio increase before warfarin-associated hemorrhage: Brief and subtle. *Arch Intern Med.* 2004;**164**:2176–2179

497. Kobayashi S, Tazaki Y. Effect of the thrombin inhibitor argatroban in acute cerebral thrombosis. *Semin Thromb Hemost.* 1997;**23**:531–534

498. Lewis BE, Wallis DE, Leya F, Hursting MJ, Kelton JG. Argatroban anticoagulation in patients with heparin-induced thrombocytopenia. *Arch Intern Med.* 2003;**163**:1849–1856

499. LaMonte MP, Nash ML, Wang DZ, Woolfenden AR, Schultz J, Hursting MJ, et al. Argatroban anticoagulation in patients with acute ischemic stroke (ARGIS-1): A randomized, placebo-controlled safety study. *Stroke.* 2004;**35**:1677–1682

500. Fiessinger JN, Huisman MV, Davidson BL, Bounameaux H, Francis CW, Eriksson H, et al. Ximelagatran vs. low-molecular-weight heparin and warfarin for the treatment of deep vein thrombosis: A randomized trial. *JAMA.* 2005;**293**:681–689

501. Olsson SB. Stroke prevention with the oral direct thrombin inhibitor ximelagatran compared with warfarin in patients with non-valvular atrial fibrillation (SPORTIF III): Randomised controlled trial. *Lancet.* 2003;**362**:1691–1698

502. Albers GW, Diener HC, Frison L, Grind M, Nevinson M, Partridge S, et al. Ximelagatran vs. warfarin for stroke prevention in patients with nonvalvular atrial fibrillation: A randomized trial. *JAMA.* 2005;**293**:690–698

503. Akins PT, Feldman HA, Zoble RG, Newman D, Spitzer SG, Diener HC, et al. Secondary stroke prevention with ximelagatran versus warfarin in patients with atrial fibrillation: Pooled analysis of SPORTIF III and V clinical trials. *Stroke.* 2007;**38**:874–880

504. Ahmed S, Levin V, Malacoff R, Martinez MW. Dabigatran: A new chapter in anticoagulation. *Cardiovasc Hematol Agents Med Chem.* 2012;**10**:116–123

505. Di Nisio M, Middeldorp S, Buller HR. Direct thrombin inhibitors. *N Engl J Med.* 2005;**353**:1028–1040

506. Connolly SJ, Ezekowitz MD, Yusuf S, Eikelboom J, Oldgren J, Parekh A, et al. Dabigatran versus warfarin in patients with atrial fibrillation. *N Engl J Med.* 2009;**361**:1139–1151

507. Yeh CH, Fredenburgh JC, Weitz JI. Oral direct factor Xa inhibitors. *Circ Res.* 2012;**111**:1069–1078

508. Connolly SJ, Eikelboom J, Joyner C, Diener HC, Hart R, Golitsyn S, et al.

Apixaban in patients with atrial fibrillation. *N Engl J Med.* 2011;364:806–817

509. Granger CB, Alexander JH, McMurray JJ, Lopes RD, Hylek EM, Hanna M, et al. Apixaban versus warfarin in patients with atrial fibrillation. *N Engl J Med.* 2011;365:981–992

510. Patel MR, Mahaffey KW, Garg J, Pan G, Singer DE, Hacke W, et al. Rivaroxaban versus warfarin in nonvalvular atrial fibrillation. *N Engl J Med.* 2011;365:883–891

511. Giugliano RP, Ruff CT, Braunwald E, Murphy SA, Wiviott SD, Halperin JL, et al. Edoxaban versus warfarin in patients with atrial fibrillation. *N Engl J Med.* 2013;369:2093–2104

512. Bauer KA. New anticoagulants: Anti IIa vs. anti Xa – is one better? *J Thromb Thrombolysis.* 2006;21:67–72

513. Turpie AG, Bauer KA, Eriksson BI, Lassen MR. Fondaparinux vs. enoxaparin for the prevention of venous thromboembolism in major orthopedic surgery: A meta-analysis of four randomized double-blind studies. *Arch Intern Med.* 2002;162:1833–1840

514. Cohen AT, Davidson BL, Gallus AS, Lassen MR, Prins MH, Tomkowski W, et al. Efficacy and safety of fondaparinux for the prevention of venous thromboembolism in older acute medical patients: Randomised placebo controlled trial. *BMJ.* 2006;332:325–329

515. Yusuf S, Mehta SR, Chrolavicius S, Afzal R, Pogue J, Granger CB, et al. Comparison of fondaparinux and enoxaparin in acute coronary syndromes. *N Engl J Med.* 2006;354:1464–1476

516. Yusuf S, Mehta SR, Chrolavicius S, Afzal R, Pogue J, Granger CB, et al. Effects of fondaparinux on mortality and reinfarction in patients with acute ST-segment elevation myocardial infarction: The OASIS-6 randomized trial. *JAMA.* 2006;295:1519–1530

517. Rajagopal V, Bhatt DL. Factor Xa inhibitors in acute coronary syndromes: Moving from mythology to reality. *J Thromb Haemost.* 2005;3:436–438

518. Fields WS, Lemak NA. *A History of Stroke: Its Recognition and Treatment.* New York, NY: Oxford University Press; 1989

519. Craven LL. Experiences with aspirin (acetylsalicylic acid) in the nonspecific prophylaxis of coronary thrombosis. *Miss Valley Med J.* 1953;75:38–44

520. Craven LL. Prevention of coronary and cerebral thrombosis. *Miss Valley Med J.* 1956;78:213–215

521. Mundall J, Quintero P, Von Kaulla KN, Harmon R, Austin J. Transient monocular blindness and increased platelet aggregability treated with aspirin. A case report. *Neurology.* 1972;22:280–285

522. Harrison MJ, Marshall J, Meadows JC, Russell RW. Effect of aspirin in amaurosis fugax. *Lancet.* 1971;2:743–744

523. Fields WS, Lemak NA, Frankowski RF, Hardy RJ. Controlled trial of aspirin in cerebral ischemia. *Stroke.* 1977;8:301–314

524. The Canadian Cooperative Study Group. A randomized trial of aspirin and sulfinpyrazone in threatened stroke. *N Engl J Med.* 1978; 299:53–59

525. Moncada S, Vane JR. Arachidonic acid metabolites and the interactions between platelets and blood-vessel walls. *N Engl J Med.* 1979;300:1142–1147

526. Nurden AT, Guyonnet Duperat V, Nurden P. Platelet function and pharmacology of antiplatelet drugs. *Cerebrovasc Dis.* 1997;7 Suppl 6:2–9

527. Moncada S. Biology and therapeutic potential of prostacyclin. *Stroke.* 1983;14:157–168

528. Preston FE, Whipps S, Jackson CA, French AJ, Wyld PJ, Stoddard CJ. Inhibition of prostacyclin and platelet thromboxane A$_2$ after low-dose aspirin. *N Engl J Med.* 1981;304:76–79

529. Weksler BB, Pett SB, Alonso D, Richter RC, Stelzer P, Subramanian V, et al. Differential inhibition by aspirin of vascular and platelet prostaglandin synthesis in atherosclerotic patients. *N Engl J Med.* 1983;308:800–805

530. United Kingdom Transient Ischaemic Attack (UK-TIA) aspirin trial: Interim results. UK-TIA study group. *Br Med J (Clin Res Ed).* 1988;296:316–320

531. The SALT Collaborative Group. Swedish Aspirin Low-Dose Trial (SALT) of 75 mg aspirin as secondary prophylaxis after cerebrovascular ischaemic events. *Lancet.* 1991;338:1345–1349

532. The Dutch TIA Trial Study Group. A comparison of two doses of aspirin (30 mg vs. 283 mg a day) in patients after a transient ischemic attack or minor ischemic stroke. *N Engl J Med.* 1991;325:1261–1266

533. Schwartz KA. Aspirin resistance: A review of diagnostic methodology, mechanisms, and clinical utility. *Adv Clin Chem.* 2006;42:81–110

534. Helgason CM, Hoff JA, Kondos GT, Brace LD. Platelet aggregation in patients with atrial fibrillation taking aspirin or warfarin. *Stroke.* 1993;24:1458–1461

535. Helgason CM, Tortorice KL, Winkler SR, Penney DW, Schuler JJ, McClelland TJ, et al. Aspirin response and failure in cerebral infarction. *Stroke.* 1993;24:345–350

536. Dalen JE. Aspirin resistance: Is it real? Is it clinically significant? *Am J Med.* 2007;120:1–4

537. Chen WH, Cheng X, Lee PY, Ng W, Kwok JY, Tse HF, et al. Aspirin resistance and adverse clinical events in patients with coronary artery disease. *Am J Med.* 2007;120:631–635

538. Hohlfeld T, Weber AA, Junghans U, Schumacher M, Boucher M, Schror K, et al. Variable platelet response to aspirin in patients with ischemic stroke. *Cerebrovasc Dis.* 2007;24:43–50

539. Gaglia MA, Jr., Clavijo L. Cardiovascular pharmacology core reviews: Aspirin. *J Cardiovasc Pharmacol Ther.* 2013;18:505–513

540. FitzGerald GA. Dipyridamole. *N Engl J Med.* 1987;316:1247–1257

541. Honour AJ, Hockaday TD, Mann JI. The synergistic effect of aspirin and dipyridamole upon platelet thrombi in living blood vessels. *Br J Exp Pathol.* 1977;58:268–272

542. Sullivan JM, Harken DE, Gorlin R. Pharmacologic control of thromboembolic complications of cardiac-valve replacement. *N Engl J Med.* 1971;284:1391–1394

543. The American–Canadian Co-operative Study Group. Persantine aspirin trial in cerebral ischemia. *Stroke.* 1983;14:99–103

544. Bousser M-G, Eschwege E, Haguenau M, Lefauconnier JM, Thibult N, Touboul D, et al. "AICLA" controlled trial of aspirin and dipyridamole in the secondary prevention of athero-thrombotic cerebral ischemia. *Stroke.* 1983;14:5–14

545. The ESPS Group. The European Stroke Prevention Study (ESPS). Principal end-points. *Lancet.* 1987;2:1351–1354

546. Diener HC, Cunha L, Forbes C, Sivenius J, Smets P, Lowenthal A. European Stroke Prevention Study. 2. Dipyridamole and acetylsalicylic acid in the secondary prevention of stroke. *J Neurol Sci*. 1996;**143**:1–13

547. Leonardi-Bee J, Bath PM, Bousser M-G, Davalos A, Diener HC, Guiraud-Chaumeil B, et al. Dipyridamole for preventing recurrent ischemic stroke and other vascular events: A meta-analysis of individual patient data from randomized controlled trials. *Stroke*. 2005;**36**:162–168

548. Sacco RL, Sivenius J, Diener HC. Efficacy of aspirin plus extended-release dipyridamole in preventing recurrent stroke in high-risk populations. *Arch Neurol*. 2005;**62**:403–408

549. Halkes PH, van Gijn J, Kappelle LJ, Koudstaal PJ, Algra A. Aspirin plus dipyridamole versus aspirin alone after cerebral ischaemia of arterial origin (ESPRIT): Randomised controlled trial. *Lancet*. 2006;**367**:1665–1673

550. Verro P, Gorelick PB, Nguyen D. Aspirin plus dipyridamole versus aspirin for prevention of vascular events after stroke or TIA: A meta-analysis. *Stroke*. 2008;**39**:1358–1363

551. Ikeda Y, Kikuchi M, Murakami H, Satoh K, Murata M, Watanabe K, et al. Comparison of the inhibitory effects of cilostazol, acetylsalicylic acid and ticlopidine on platelet functions ex vivo. Randomized, double-blind cross-over study. *Arzneimittelforschung*. 1987;**37**:563–566

552. Tanaka T, Ishikawa T, Hagiwara M, Onoda K, Itoh H, Hidaka H. Effects of cilostazol, a selective camp phosphodiesterase inhibitor on the contraction of vascular smooth muscle. *Pharmacology*. 1988;**36**:313–320

553. Gotoh F, Tohgi H, Hirai S, Terashi A, Fukuuchi Y, Otomo E, et al. Cilostazol stroke prevention study: A placebo-controlled double-blind trial for secondary prevention of cerebral infarction. *J Stroke Cerebrovasc Dis*. 2000;**9**:147–157

554. Shinohara Y, Katayama Y, Uchiyama S, Yamaguchi T, Handa S, Matsuoka K, et al. Cilostazol for prevention of secondary stroke (CSPS 2): An aspirin-controlled, double-blind, randomised non-inferiority trial. *Lancet Neurol*. 2010;**9**:959–968

555. Ameriso SF, Lagos R, Ferreira LM, Fernandez Cisneros L, La Mura AR. Cerebrovascular effects of cilostazol in patients with atherosclerotic disease. *J Stroke Cerebrovasc Dis*. 2006;**15**:273–276

556. Kwon SU, Cho Y-J, Koo J-S, Bae H-J, Lee Y-S, Hong K-S, et al. Cilostazol prevents the progression of the symptomatic intracranial arterial stenosis: The multicenter double-blind placebo-controlled trial of cilostazol in symptomatic intracranial arterial stenosis. *Stroke*. 2005;**36**:782–786

557. Sharis PJ, Cannon CP, Loscalzo J. The antiplatelet effects of ticlopidine and clopidogrel. *Ann Intern Med*. 1998;**129**:394–405

558. Hass WK, Easton JD, Adams HP, Jr., Pryse-Phillips W, Molony BA, Anderson S, et al. A randomized trial comparing ticlopidine hydrochloride with aspirin for the prevention of stroke in high-risk patients. Ticlopidine Aspirin Stroke Study Group. *N Engl J Med*. 1989;**321**:501–507

559. Gent M, Blakely JA, Easton JD, Ellis DJ, Hachinski VC, Harbison JW, et al. The Canadian–American Ticlopidine Study (CATS) in thromboembolic stroke. *Lancet*. 1989;**1**:1215–1220

560. Bennett CL, Weinberg PD, Rozenberg-Ben-Dror K, Yarnold PR, Kwaan HC, Green D. Thrombotic thrombocytopenic purpura associated with ticlopidine. A review of 60 cases. *Ann Intern Med*. 1998;**128**:541–544

561. CAPRIE Steering Committee. A randomised, blinded, trial of clopidogrel versus aspirin in patients at risk of ischaemic events (CAPRIE). *Lancet*. 1996;**348**:1329–1339

562. Bennett CL, Connors JM, Carwile JM, Moake JL, Bell WR, Tarantolo SR, et al. Thrombotic thrombocytopenic purpura associated with clopidogrel. *N Engl J Med*. 2000;**342**:1773–1777

563. Diener HC, Bogousslavsky J, Brass LM, Cimminiello C, Csiba L, Kaste M, et al. Aspirin and clopidogrel compared with clopidogrel alone after recent ischaemic stroke or transient ischaemic attack in high-risk patients (MATCH): Randomised, double-blind, placebo-controlled trial. *Lancet*. 2004;**364**:331–337

564. Hankey GJ, Eikelboom JW. Adding aspirin to clopidogrel after TIA and ischemic stroke: Benefits do not match risks. *Neurology*. 2005;**64**:1117–1121

565. Bhatt DL, Fox KA, Hacke W, Berger PB, Black HR, Boden WE, et al. Clopidogrel and aspirin versus aspirin alone for the prevention of atherothrombotic events. *N Engl J Med*. 2006;**354**:1706–1717

566. Wang Y, Zhao X, Liu L, Wang D, Wang C, Li H, et al. Clopidogrel with aspirin in acute minor stroke or transient ischemic attack. *N Engl J Med*. 2013;**369**:11–19

567. Johnston SC, Easton JD, Farrant M, Barsan W, Battenhouse H, Conwit R, et al. Platelet-oriented inhibition in new TIA and minor ischemic stroke (POINT) trial: Rationale and design. *Int J Stroke*. 2013;**8**:479–483

568. Steinhubl SR, Berger PB, Mann JT, 3rd, Fry ET, DeLago A, Wilmer C, et al. Early and sustained dual oral antiplatelet therapy following percutaneous coronary intervention: A randomized controlled trial. *JAMA*. 2002;**288**:2411–2420

569. Chaturvedi S, Yadav JS. The role of antiplatelet therapy in carotid stenting for ischemic stroke prevention. *Stroke*. 2006;**37**:1572–1577

570. Weksler BB. Antiplatelet agents in stroke prevention. Combination therapy: Present and future. *Cerebrovasc Dis*. 2000;**10** Suppl 5:41–48

571. Tcheng JE. Differences among the parenteral platelet glycoprotein IIB/IIIA inhibitors and implications for treatment. *Am J Cardiol*. 1999;**83**:7e–11e

572. Lefkovits J, Plow EF, Topol EJ. Platelet glycoprotein IIB/IIIA receptors in cardiovascular medicine. *N Engl J Med*. 1995;**332**:1553–1559

573. Wallace RC, Furlan AJ, Moliterno DJ, Stevens GH, Masaryk TJ, Perl J, 2nd. Basilar artery rethrombosis: Successful treatment with platelet glycoprotein IIB/IIIA receptor inhibitor. *AJNR Am J Neuroradiol*. 1997;**18**:1257–1260

574. The Abciximab in Ischemic Stroke Investigators. Abciximab in acute ischemic stroke. A randomized, double-blind, placebo-controlled, dose-escalation study. *Stroke*. 2000;**31**:601–609

575. Qureshi AI, Harris-Lane P, Kirmani JF, Janjua N, Divani AA, Mohammad YM, et al. Intra-arterial reteplase and intravenous abciximab in patients with acute ischemic stroke: An open-label, dose-ranging, phase I study. *Neurosurgery*. 2006;**59**:789–796; discussion 796–787

576. Eckert B, Koch C, Thomalla G, Kucinski T, Grzyska U, Roether J, et al. Aggressive therapy with intravenous abciximab and intra-arterial rtPA and

additional PTA/stenting improves clinical outcome in acute vertebrobasilar occlusion: Combined local fibrinolysis and intravenous abciximab in acute vertebrobasilar stroke treatment (FAST): Results of a multicenter study. *Stroke.* 2005;**36**:1160–1165

577. Velat GJ, Burry MV, Eskioglu E, Dettorre RR, Firment CS, Mericle RA. The use of abciximab in the treatment of acute cerebral thromboembolic events during neuroendovascular procedures. *Surg Neurol.* 2006;**65**:352–358, discussion 358–359

578. Heer T, Zeymer U, Juenger C, Gitt AK, Wienbergen H, Zahn R, et al. Beneficial effects of abciximab in patients with primary percutaneous intervention for acute STsegment elevation myocardial infarction in clinical practice. *Heart.* 2006;**92**:1484–1489

579. De Luca G, Suryapranata H, Stone GW, Antoniucci D, Tcheng JE, Neumann FJ, et al. Abciximab as adjunctive therapy to reperfusion in acute ST-segment elevation myocardial infarction: A meta-analysis of randomized trials. *JAMA.* 2005;**293**:1759–1765

580. Coller BS. Anti-gpIIB/IIIA drugs: Current strategies and future directions. *Thromb Haemost.* 2001;**86**:427–443

581. Topol EJ, Easton D, Harrington RA, Amarenco P, Califf RM, Graffagnino C, et al. Randomized, double-blind, placebo-controlled, international trial of the oral IIB/IIIA antagonist lotrafiban in coronary and cerebrovascular disease. *Circulation.* 2003;**108**:399–406

582. Antiplatelet Trialists' Collaboration. Secondary prevention of vascular disease by prolonged antiplatelet treatment. *Br Med J (Clin Res Ed).* 1988;**296**:320–331

583. Antiplatelet Trialists' Collaboration. Collaborative overview of randomised trials of antiplatelet therapy – I: Prevention of death, myocardial infarction, and stroke by prolonged antiplatelet therapy in various categories of patients. Antiplatelet Trialists' Collaboration. *BMJ.* 1994;**308**:81–106

584. Antiplatelet Trialists' Collaboration. Collaborative meta-analysis of randomised trials of antiplatelet therapy for prevention of death, myocardial infarction, and stroke in high risk patients. *BMJ.* 2002;**324**:71–86

585. Gubitz G, Sandercock P, Counsell C. Antiplatelet therapy for acute ischaemic stroke. *Cochrane Database Syst Rev.* 2000:Cd000029

586. Tran H, Anand SS. Oral antiplatelet therapy in cerebrovascular disease, coronary artery disease, and peripheral arterial disease. *JAMA.* 2004;**292**:1867–1874

587. Diener HC. Secondary stroke prevention with antiplatelet drugs: Have we reached the ceiling? *Int J Stroke.* 2006;**1**:4–8

588. Amarenco P, Davis S, Jones EF, Cohen AA, Heiss WD, Kaste M, et al. for The Aortic Arch Related Cerebral Hazard Trial Investigators. Clopidogrel plus aspirin versus warfarin in patients with stroke and aortic arch plaques. *Stroke.* 2014;**45**:1248–1257

589. The SPS 3 Investigators. Effects of clopidogrel added to aspirin in patients with recent lacunar stroke. *N Engl J Med.* 2012;**367**:817–825

590. Miller A, Lees RS. Simultaneous therapy with antiplatelet and anticoagulant drugs in symptomatic cardiovascular disease. *Stroke.* 1985;**16**:668–675

591. Chesebro JH, Fuster V, Elveback LR, McGoon DC, Pluth JR, Puga FJ, et al. Trial of combined warfarin plus dipyridamole or aspirin therapy in prosthetic heart valve replacement: Danger of aspirin compared with dipyridamole. *Am J Cardiol.* 1983;**51**:1537–1541

592. O'Collins VE, Macleod MR, Donnan GA, Horky LL, van der Worp BH, Howells DW. 1,026 experimental treatments in acute stroke. *Ann Neurol.* 2006;**59**:467–477

593. Macleod MR, Fisher M, O'Collins V, Sena ES, Dirnagl U, Bath PM, et al. Good laboratory practice: Preventing introduction of bias at the bench. *Stroke.* 2009;**40**:e50–52

594. Ovbiagele B, Kidwell CS, Starkman S, Saver JL. Neuroprotective agents for the treatment of acute ischemic stroke. *Curr Neurol Neurosci Rep.* 2003;**3**:9–20

595. Garcia J. Mechanisms of cell death in ischemia. In LR Caplan, ed. *Brain Ischemia, Basic Concepts and Clinical Relevance.* London: Springer; 1995:7–18

596. Plum F. What causes infarction in ischemic brain?: The Robert Wartenberg lecture. *Neurology.* 1983;**33**:222–233

597. Myers R. Lactic acid accumulation as a cause of brain edema and cerebral necrosis resulting from oxygen deprivation. In R Korobkin, C Guilleminault, eds. *Advances in Perinatal Neurology.* New York: Spectrum; 1979:88–114

598. McCord JM. Oxygen-derived free radicals in postischemic tissue injury. *N Engl J Med.* 1985;**312**:159–163

599. Floyd R. Production of free radicals. In KMA Welch LR Caplan, DJ Reis, BK Siesjo, B Weir, eds. *Primer on Cerebrovascular Diseases.* San Diego, CA: Academic Press; 1997:165–169

600. Kontos HA. Oxygen radicals in cerebral ischemia: The 2001 Thomas Willis lecture. *Stroke.* 2001;**32**:2712–2716

601. Ginsberg MD. Adventures in the pathophysiology of brain ischemia: Penumbra, gene expression, neuroprotection: The 2002 Thomas Willis lecture. *Stroke.* 2003;**34**:214–223

602. Busto R, Dietrich WD, Globus MY, Ginsberg MD. The importance of brain temperature in cerebral ischemic injury. *Stroke.* 1989;**20**:1113–1114

603. WD Dietrich RB. Hyperthermia and brain ischemia. In KMA Welch, LR Caplan, DJ Reis, BK Siesjo, B Weir, eds. *Primer on Cerebrovascular Diseases.* San Diego, CA: Academic Press; 1997:165–169

604. Siesjo BK, Bengtsson F. Calcium fluxes, calcium antagonists, and calcium-related pathology in brain ischemia, hypoglycemia, and spreading depression: A unifying hypothesis. *J Cereb Blood Flow Metab.* 1989;**9**:127–140

605. Tymianski M, Sattler RG. Is calcium involved in excitotoxic or ischemic neuronal damage? In KMA Welch, LR Caplan, DJ Reis, BK Siesjo, B Weir, eds. *Primer on Cerebrovascular Diseases.* San Diego, CA: Academic Press; 1997:190–192

606. Siesjo BK. Historical overview. Calcium, ischemia, and death of brain cells. *Ann N Y Acad Sci.* 1988;**522**:638–661

607. Siesjo B, Smith M-L. Mechanism of acidosis-related damage. In KMA Welch, LR Caplan, DJ Reis, BK Siesjo, B Weir, eds. *Primer on Cerebrovascular Diseases.* San Diego, CA: Academic Press; 1997:223–226

608. Adams HP, Jr., Olinger CP, Marler JR, Biller J, Brott TG, Barsan WG, et al. Comparison of admission serum glucose concentration with neurologic outcome in acute cerebral infarction. A study in patients given naloxone. *Stroke*. 1988;**19**:455–458

609. Woo J, Lam CW, Kay R, Wong AH, Teoh R, Nicholls MG. The influence of hyperglycemia and diabetes mellitus on immediate and 3-month morbidity and mortality after acute stroke. *Arch Neurol*. 1990;**47**:1174–1177

610. Alvarez-Sabin J, Molina CA, Montaner J, Arenillas JF, Huertas R, Ribo M, et al. Effects of admission hyperglycemia on stroke outcome in reperfused tissue plasminogen activator-treated patients. *Stroke*. 2003;**34**:1235–1241

611. Passero S, Ciacci G, Ulivelli M. The influence of diabetes and hyperglycemia on clinical course after intracerebral hemorrhage. *Neurology*. 2003;**61**:1351–1356

612. Choi D. The excitotoxic concept. In KMA Welch, LR Caplan, DJ Reis, BK Siesjo, B Weir, eds. *Primer on Cerebrovascular Diseases*. San Diego, CA: Academic Press; 1997:187–190

613. Choi D. Excitotoxicity and stroke. In LR Caplan, ed. *Brain Ischemia, Basic Concepts and Clinical Relevance*. London: Springer; 1995:29–36

614. Olney JW. Brain lesions, obesity, and other disturbances in mice treated with monosodium glutamate. *Science*. 1969;**164**:719–721

615. Meldrum B. Excitotoxicity in ischemia: An overview. In MD Ginsberg, WD Dietrich, eds. *Cerebrovascular Diseases*. New York, NY: Raven Press; 1989:47–60

616. Lai TW, Zhang S, Wang YT. Excitotoxicity and stroke: Identifying novel targets for neuroprotection. *Prog Neurobiol*. 2014;**115**:157–188

617. Small DL, Buchan AM. NMDA and AMPA receptor antagonists in global and focal ischemia. In KMA Welch, LR Caplan, DJ Reis, BK Siesjo, B Weir, eds. *Primer on Cerebrovascular Diseases*. San Diego, CA: Academic Press; 1997:244–247

618. Onai MZ, Fisher M. Thrombolytic and cytoprotective therapies for acute ischemic stoke: A clinical overview. *Drugs Today*. 1996;**32**:573–592

619. Lees KR. Cerestat and other NMDA antagonists in ischemic stroke. *Neurology*. 1997;**49**:S66–S69

620. Lees KR, Zivin JA, Ashwood T, Davalos A, Davis SM, Diener HC, et al. NXY-059 for acute ischemic stroke. *N Engl J Med*. 2006;**354**:588–600

621. Hess DC. NXY-059: A hopeful sign in the treatment of stroke. *Stroke*. 2006;**37**:2649–2650

622. Fisher M. NXY-059 for acute ischemic stroke: The promise of neuroprotection is finally realized? *Stroke*. 2006;**37**:2651–2652

623. Shuaib A, Lees KR, Lyden P, Grotta J, Davalos A, Davis SM, et al. NXY-059 for the treatment of acute ischemic stroke. *N Engl J Med*. 2007;**357**:562–571

624. Overgaard K, Meden P. Citicoline – the first effective neuroprotectant to be combined with thrombolysis in acute ischemic stroke? *J Neurol Sci*. 2006;**247**:119–120

625. Clark WM, Wechsler LR, Sabounjian LA, Schwiderski UE. A phase III randomized efficacy trial of 2000 mg citicoline in acute ischemic stroke patients. *Neurology*. 2001;**57**:1595–1602

626. Warach S, Pettigrew LC, Dashe JF, Pullicino P, Lefkowitz DM, Sabounjian L, et al. Effect of citicoline on ischemic lesions as measured by diffusion-weighted magnetic resonance imaging. Citicoline 010 investigators. *Ann Neurol*. 2000;**48**:713–722

627. Davalos A, Alvarez-Sabin J, Castillo J, Diez-Tejedor E, Ferro J, Martinez-Vila E, et al. Citicoline in the treatment of acute ischaemic stroke: An international, randomised, multicentre, placebo-controlled study (ICTUS trial). *Lancet*. 2012;**380**:349–357

628. Alonso de Lecinana M, Gutierrez M, Roda JM, Carceller F, Diez-Tejedor E. Effect of combined therapy with thrombolysis and citicoline in a rat model of embolic stroke. *J Neurol Sci*. 2006;**247**:121–129

629. Nighoghossian N, Trouillas P, Adeleine P, Salord F. Hyperbaric oxygen in the treatment of acute ischemic stroke. A double-blind pilot study. *Stroke*. 1995;**26**:1369–1372

630. Rusyniak DE, Kirk MA, May JD, Kao LW, Brizendine EJ, Welch JL, et al. Hyperbaric oxygen therapy in acute ischemic stroke: Results of the hyperbaric oxygen in acute ischemic stroke trial pilot study. *Stroke*. 2003;**34**:571–574

631. Ronning OM, Guldvog B. Should stroke victims routinely receive supplemental oxygen? A quasi-randomized controlled trial. *Stroke*. 1999;**30**:2033–2037

632. Hughes S. SO2S: No benefit of routine oxygen in acute stroke. XXIII European Stroke Conference. Presented May 7, 2014

633. Kim HY, Singhal AB, Lo EH. Normobaric hyperoxia extends the reperfusion window in focal cerebral ischemia. *Ann Neurol*. 2005;**57**:571–575

634. Singhal AB, Benner T, Roccatagliata L, Koroshetz WJ, Schaefer PW, Lo EH, et al. A pilot study of normobaric oxygen therapy in acute ischemic stroke. *Stroke*. 2005;**36**:797–802

635. Ginsberg M. Hypothermic neuroprotection in cerebral ischemia. In KMA Welch, LR Caplan, DJ Reis, BK Siesjo, B Weir, eds. *Primer on Cerebrovascular Diseases*. San Diego, CA: Academic Press; 1997:272–275

636. Bernard SA, Gray TW, Buist MD, Jones BM, Silvester W, Gutteridge G, et al. Treatment of comatose survivors of out-of-hospital cardiac arrest with induced hypothermia. *N Engl J Med*. 2002;**346**:557–563

637. Mayer SA. Hypothermia for neuroprotection after cardiac arrest. *Curr Neurol Neurosci Rep*. 2002;**2**:525–526

638. Schwab S, Schwarz S, Spranger M, Keller E, Bertram M, Hacke W. Moderate hypothermia in the treatment of patients with severe middle cerebral artery infarction. *Stroke*. 1998;**29**:2461–2466

639. Schwab S, Georgiadis D, Berrouschot J, Schellinger PD, Graffagnino C, Mayer SA. Feasibility and safety of moderate hypothermia after massive hemispheric infarction. *Stroke*. 2001;**32**:2033–2035

640. Georgiadis D, Schwarz S, Aschoff A, Schwab S. Hemicraniectomy and moderate hypothermia in patients with severe ischemic stroke. *Stroke*. 2002;**33**:1584–1588

641. Abou-Chebl A, DeGeorgia MA, Andrefsky JC, Krieger DW. Technical refinements and drawbacks of a surface cooling technique for the treatment of severe acute ischemic stroke. *Neurocrit Care*. 2004;**1**:131–143

642. Krieger DW, De Georgia MA, Abou-Chebl A, Andrefsky JC, Sila CA, Katzan IL, et al. Cooling for acute ischemic brain damage (COOL AID): An open pilot study of induced

hypothermia in acute ischemic stroke. *Stroke.* 2001;32:1847–1854

643. Lyden MP, Colbourne PF, Lyden P, Schwab S. Preclinical and clinical studies targeting therapeutic hypothermia in cerebral ischemia and stroke. *Ther Hypothermia Temp Manag.* 2013;3:3–6

644. Safar P. Amelioration of post-ischemic brain damage with barbiturates. *Stroke.* 1980;11:565–568

645. Black KL, Weidler DJ, Jallad NS, Sodeman TM, Abrams GD. Delayed pentobarbital therapy of acute focal cerebral ischemia. *Stroke.* 1978;9:245–249

646. Wu TC, Grotta JC. Hypothermia for acute ischaemic stroke. *Lancet Neurol.* 2013;12:275–284

647. Stroke Therapy Academic Industry Roundtable 11 (STAIR-11). Recommendations for clinical trial evaluation of acute stroke therapies. *Stroke.* 2001;32:1598–1606

648. Fisher M. Recommendations for advancing development of acute stroke therapies: Stroke Therapy Academic Industry Roundtable 3. *Stroke.* 2003;34:1539–1546

649. Fisher M, Albers GW, Donnan GA, Furlan AJ, Grotta JC, Kidwell CS, et al. Enhancing the development and approval of acute stroke therapies: Stroke Therapy Academic Industry Roundtable. *Stroke.* 2005;36:1808–1813

650. Shepherd J, Cobbe SM, Ford I, Isles CG, Lorimer AR, MacFarlane PW, et al. Prevention of coronary heart disease with pravastatin in men with hypercholesterolemia. West of Scotland Coronary Prevention Study Group. *N Engl J Med.* 1995;333:1301–1307

651. Randomised trial of cholesterol lowering in 4444 patients with coronary heart disease: The Scandinavian Simvastatin Survival Study (4S). *Lancet.* 1994;344:1383–1389

652. Sacks FM, Pfeffer MA, Moye LA, Rouleau JL, Rutherford JD, Cole TG, et al. The effect of pravastatin on coronary events after myocardial infarction in patients with average cholesterol levels. Cholesterol and recurrent events trial investigators. *N Engl J Med.* 1996;335:1001–1009

653. Hebert PR, Gaziano JM, Chan KS, Hennekens CH. Cholesterol lowering with statin drugs, risk of stroke, and total mortality. An overview of randomized trials. *JAMA.* 1997;278:313–321

654. Blauw GJ, Lagaay AM, Smelt AH, Westendorp RG. Stroke, statins, and cholesterol. A meta-analysis of randomized, placebo-controlled, double-blind trials with HMG-CoA reductase inhibitors. *Stroke.* 1997;28:946–950

655. Bucher HC, Griffith LE, Guyatt GH. Effect of HMG CoA reductase inhibitors on stroke. A meta-analysis of randomized, controlled trials. *Ann Intern Med.* 1998;128:89–95

656. Nissen SE, Tuzcu EM, Schoenhagen P, Crowe T, Sasiela WJ, Tsai J, et al. Statin therapy, LDL cholesterol, C-reactive protein, and coronary artery disease. *N Engl J Med.* 2005;352:29–38

657. Furberg CD, Adams HP, Jr., Applegate WB, Byington RP, Espeland MA, Hartwell T, et al. Effect of lovastatin on early carotid atherosclerosis and cardiovascular events. Asymptomatic Carotid Artery Progression Study (ACAPS) Research Group. *Circulation.* 1994;90:1679–1687

658. Crouse JR, 3rd, Byington RP, Bond MG, Espeland MA, Craven TE, Sprinkle JW, et al. Pravastatin, lipids, and atherosclerosis in the carotid arteries (PLAC-II). *Am J Cardiol.* 1995;75:455–459

659. Hodis HN, Mack WJ, LaBree L, Selzer RH, Liu C, Liu C, et al. Reduction in carotid arterial wall thickness using lovastatin and dietary therapy: A randomized controlled clinical trial. *Ann Intern Med.* 1996;124:548–556

660. Amarenco P, Bogousslavsky J, Callahan A, 3rd, Goldstein LB, Hennerici M, Rudolph AE, et al. High-dose atorvastatin after stroke or transient ischemic attack. *N Engl J Med.* 2006;355:549–559

661. Amarenco P, Goldstein LB, Szarek M, Sillesen H, Rudolph AE, Callahan A, 3rd, et al. Effects of intense low-density lipoprotein cholesterol reduction in patients with stroke or transient ischemic attack: The Stroke Prevention by Aggressive Reduction in Cholesterol Levels (SPARCL) Trial. *Stroke.* 2007;38:3198–3204

662. Vergouwen MD, de Haan RJ, Vermeulen M, Roos YB. Statin treatment and the occurrence of hemorrhagic stroke in patients with a history of cerebrovascular disease. *Stroke.* 2008;39:497–502

663. Sanossian N, Ovbiagele B. Drug insight: Translating evidence on statin

therapy into clinical benefits. *Nat Clin Pract Neurol.* 2008;4:43–49

664. Schwartz GG, Olsson AG, Ezekowitz MD, Ganz P, Oliver MF, Waters D, et al. Effects of atorvastatin on early recurrent ischemic events in acute coronary syndromes: The MIRACL study: A randomized controlled trial. *JAMA.* 2001;285:1711–1718

665. Elkind MS, Flint AC, Sciacca RR, Sacco RL. Lipid-lowering agent use at ischemic stroke onset is associated with decreased mortality. *Neurology.* 2005;65:253–258

666. Amarenco P, Moskowitz MA. The dynamics of statins: From event prevention to neuroprotection. *Stroke.* 2006;37:294–296

667. Fisher M, Moonis M. Neuroprotective effects of statins: Evidence from preclinical and clinical studies. *Curr Treat Options Cardiovasc Med.* 2012;14:252–259

668. Endres M, Laufs U, Huang Z, Nakamura T, Huang P, Moskowitz MA, et al. Stroke protection by 3-hydroxy-3-methylglutaryl (HMG)-CoA reductase inhibitors mediated by endothelial nitric oxide synthase. *Proc Natl Acad Sci U S A.* 1998;95:8880–8885

669. Endres M, Laufs U, Liao JK, Moskowitz MA. Targeting eNOS for stroke protection. *Trends Neurosci.* 2004;27:283–289

670. Ridker PM, Rifai N, Rose L, Buring JE, Cook NR. Comparison of C-reactive protein and low-density lipoprotein cholesterol levels in the prediction of first cardiovascular events. *N Engl J Med.* 2002;347:1557–1565

671. Eikelboom JW, Hankey GJ, Baker RI, McQuillan A, Thom J, Staton J, et al. C-reactive protein in ischemic stroke and its etiologic subtypes. *J Stroke Cerebrovasc Dis.* 2003;12:74–81

672. Arenillas JF, Alvarez-Sabin J, Molina CA, Chacon P, Montaner J, Rovira A, et al. C-reactive protein predicts further ischemic events in first-ever transient ischemic attack or stroke patients with intracranial large-artery occlusive disease. *Stroke.* 2003;34:2463–2468

673. Rosenson RS, Tangney CC. Antiatherothrombotic properties of statins: Implications for cardiovascular event reduction. *JAMA.* 1998;279:1643–1650

674. Carod-Artal FJ. Statins and cerebral vasomotor reactivity: Implications

for a new therapy? *Stroke.* 2006;**37**:2446–2448

675. Pretnar-Oblak J, Sabovic M, Sebestjen M, Pogacnik T, Zaletel M. Influence of atorvastatin treatment on l-arginine cerebrovascular reactivity and flow-mediated dilatation in patients with lacunar infarctions. *Stroke.* 2006;**37**:2540–2545

676. Kirkpatrick PJ, Turner CL, Smith C, Hutchinson PJ, Murray GD. Simvastatin in aneurysmal subarachnoid haemorrhage (STACH): A multicentre randomised phase 3 trial. *Lancet Neurol.* 2014;**13**:666–675

677. Ovbiagele B, Kidwell CS, Saver JL. Expanding indications for statins in cerebral ischemia: A quantitative study. *Arch Neurol.* 2005;**62**:67–72

678. Elkind MS, Sacco RL, Macarthur RB, Peerschke E, Neils G, Andrews H, et al. High-dose lovastatin for acute ischemic stroke: Results of the phase I dose escalation neuroprotection with statin therapy for acute recovery trial (NEUSTART). *Cerebrovasc Dis.* 2009;**28**:266–275

679. Biffi A, Devan WJ, Anderson CD, Cortellini L, Furie KL, Rosand J, et al. Statin treatment and functional outcome after ischemic stroke: Case-control and meta-analysis. *Stroke.* 2011;**42**:1314–1319

680. Endres M, Laufs U. Discontinuation of statin treatment in stroke patients. *Stroke.* 2006;**37**:2640–2643

681. Colivicchi F, Bassi A, Santini M, Caltagirone C. Discontinuation of statin therapy and clinical outcome after ischemic stroke. *Stroke.* 2007;**38**:2652–2657

682. Blanco M, Nombela F, Castellanos M, Rodriguez-Yanez M, Garcia-Gil M, Leira R, et al. Statin treatment withdrawal in ischemic stroke: A controlled randomized study. *Neurology.* 2007;**69**:904–910

683. Dale KM, White CM, Henyan NN, Kluger J, Coleman CI. Impact of statin dosing intensity on transaminase and creatine kinase. *Am J Med.* 2007;**120**:706–712

684. Radcliffe KA, Campbell WW. Statin myopathy. *Curr Neurol Neurosci Rep.* 2008;**8**:66–72

685. Ropper A, Gress D, Diringer M, Green D, Mayer S. *Neurological and Neurosurgical Intensive Care.* New York, NY: Raven Press; 2003

686. Kazui S, Naritomi H, Yamamoto H, Sawada T, Yamaguchi T. Enlargement of spontaneous intracerebral hemorrhage. Incidence and time course. *Stroke.* 1996;**27**:1783–1787

687. Brott T, Broderick J, Kothari R, Barsan W, Tomsick T, Sauerbeck L, et al. Early hemorrhage growth in patients with intracerebral hemorrhage. *Stroke.* 1997;**28**:1–5

688. Qureshi AI, Tuhrim S, Broderick JP, Batjer HH, Hondo H, Hanley DF. Spontaneous intracerebral hemorrhage. *N Engl J Med.* 2001;**344**:1450–1460

689. Davis SM, Broderick J, Hennerici M, Brun NC, Diringer MN, Mayer SA, et al. Hematoma growth is a determinant of mortality and poor outcome after intracerebral hemorrhage. *Neurology.* 2006;**66**:1175–1181

690. Delgado Almandoz JE, Yoo AJ, Stone MJ, Schaefer PW, Goldstein JN, Rosand J, et al. Systematic characterization of the computed tomography angiography spot sign in primary intracerebral hemorrhage identifies patients at highest risk for hematoma expansion: The spot sign score. *Stroke.* 2009;**40**:2994–3000

691. Huynh TJ, Demchuk AM, Dowlatshahi D, Gladstone DJ, Krischek O, Kiss A, et al. Spot sign number is the most important spot sign characteristic for predicting hematoma expansion using first-pass computed tomography angiography: Analysis from the predict study. *Stroke.* 2013;**44**:972–977

692. Gebel JM, Jr., Jauch EC, Brott TG, Khoury J, Sauerbeck L, Salisbury S, et al. Relative edema volume is a predictor of outcome in patients with hyperacute spontaneous intracerebral hemorrhage. *Stroke.* 2002;**33**:2636–2641

693. Anderson CS, Huang Y, Wang JG, Arima H, Neal B, Peng B, et al. Intensive blood pressure reduction in acute cerebral haemorrhage trial (INTERACT): A randomised pilot trial. *Lancet Neurol.* 2008;**7**:391–399

694. Antihypertensive Treatment of Acute Cerebral Hemorrhage (ATACH) Investigators. Antihypertensive treatment of acute cerebral hemorrhage. *Crit Care Med.* 2010;**38**:637–648

695. Arima H, Huang Y, Wang JG, Heeley E, Delcourt C, Parsons M, et al. Earlier blood pressure-lowering and greater attenuation of hematoma growth in acute intracerebral hemorrhage: Interact pilot phase. *Stroke.* 2012;**43**:2236–2238

696. Anderson CS, Heeley E, Huang Y, Wang J, Stapf C, Delcourt C, et al. Rapid blood-pressure lowering in patients with acute intracerebral hemorrhage. *N Engl J Med.* 2013;**368**:2355–2365

697. Mayer SA. Ultra-early hemostatic therapy for intracerebral hemorrhage. *Stroke.* 2003;**34**:224–229

698. Mayer SA, Brun NC, Broderick J, Davis S, Diringer MN, Skolnick BE, et al. Safety and feasibility of recombinant factor VIIa for acute intracerebral hemorrhage. *Stroke.* 2005;**36**:74–79

699. Mayer SA, Brun NC, Begtrup K, Broderick J, Davis S, Diringer MN, et al. Recombinant activated factor VII for acute intracerebral hemorrhage. *N Engl J Med.* 2005;**352**:777–785

700. Mayer SA, Brun NC, Begtrup K, Broderick J, Davis S, Diringer MN, et al. Efficacy and safety of recombinant activated factor VII for acute intracerebral hemorrhage. *N Engl J Med.* 2008;**358**:2127–2137

701. Sugg RM, Gonzales NR, Matherne DE, Ribo M, Shaltoni HM, Baraniuk S, et al. Myocardial injury in patients with intracerebral hemorrhage treated with recombinant factor VIIa. *Neurology.* 2006;**67**:1053–1055

702. Kase CS, Cromwell RM. Prognosis and treatment of patients with intracerebral hemorrhage. In CS Kase, LR Caplan, eds. *Intracerebral Hemorrhage.* Boston, MA: Butterworth–Heinemann; 1994:467–489

703. Kase CS, Caplan LR. Therapy of intracerebral hemorrhage. In T Brandt, LR Caplan, J Dichgans, HC Diener, C Kennard, eds. *Neurological Disorders, Course and Treatment.* San Diego, CA: Academic Press; 1996:277–288

704. Rabinstein AA, Wijdicks EF. Surgery for intracerebral hematoma: The search for the elusive right candidate. *Rev Neurol Dis.* 2006;**3**:163–172

705. Prasad K, Browman G, Srivastava A, Menon G. Surgery in primary supratentorial intracerebral hematoma: A meta-analysis of randomized trials. *Acta Neurol Scand.* 1997;**95**:103–110

706. Prasad K, Shrivastava A. Surgery for primary supratentorial intracerebral haemorrhage. *Cochrane Database Syst Rev.* 2000:Cd000200

707. Mendelow AD, Gregson BA, Fernandes HM, Murray GD, Teasdale GM, Hope DT, et al. Early surgery versus initial conservative treatment in patients with spontaneous supratentorial intracerebral haematomas in the international surgical trial in intracerebral haemorrhage (STICH): A randomised trial. *Lancet*. 2005;**365**:387–397

708. Mendelow AD, Gregson BA, Rowan EN, Murray GD, Gholkar A, Mitchell PM. Early surgery versus initial conservative treatment in patients with spontaneous supratentorial lobar intracerebral haematomas (STICH II): A randomised trial. *Lancet*. 2013;**382**:397–408

709. Prasad KS, Gregson BA, Bhattathiri PS, Mitchell P, Mendelow AD. The significance of crossovers after randomization in the STICH trial. *Acta Neurochir Suppl*. 2006;**96**:61–64

710. Bhattathiri PS, Gregson B, Prasad KS, Mendelow AD. Intraventricular hemorrhage and hydrocephalus after spontaneous intracerebral hemorrhage: Results from the STICH trial. *Acta Neurochir Suppl*. 2006;**96**:65–68

711. Morgenstern LB, Demchuk AM, Kim DH, Frankowski RF, Grotta JC. Rebleeding leads to poor outcome in ultra-early craniotomy for intracerebral hemorrhage. *Neurology*. 2001;**56**:1294–1299

712. Shields CB, Friedman WA. The role of stereotactic technology in the management of intracerebral hemorrhage. *Neurosurg Clin N Am*. 1992;**3**:685–702

713. Niizuma H, Shimizu Y, Yonemitsu T, Nakasato N, Suzuki J. Results of stereotactic aspiration in 175 cases of putaminal hemorrhage. *Neurosurgery*. 1989;**24**:814–819

714. Marquardt G, Wolff R, Sager A, Janzen RW, Seifert V. Subacute stereotactic aspiration of haematomas within the basal ganglia reduces occurrence of complications in the course of haemorrhagic stroke in non-comatose patients. *Cerebrovasc Dis*. 2003;**15**:252–257

715. Thiex R, Rohde V, Rohde I, Mayfrank L, Zeki Z, Thron A, et al. Frame-based and frameless stereotactic hematoma puncture and subsequent fibrinolytic therapy for the treatment of spontaneous intracerebral hemorrhage. *J Neurol*. 2004;**251**:1443–1450

716. Cho DY, Chen CC, Chang CS, Lee WY, Tso M. Endoscopic surgery for spontaneous basal ganglia hemorrhage: Comparing endoscopic surgery, stereotactic aspiration, and craniotomy in noncomatose patients. *Surg Neurol*. 2006;**65**:547–555; discussion 555–546

717. Miller CM, Vespa P, Saver JL, Kidwell CS, Carmichael ST, Alger J, et al. Image-guided endoscopic evacuation of spontaneous intracerebral hemorrhage. *Surg Neurol*. 2008;**69**:441–446;discussion 446

718. Mould WA, Carhuapoma JR, Muschelli J, Lane K, Morgan TC, McBee NA, et al. Minimally invasive surgery plus recombinant tissue-type plasminogen activator for intracerebral hemorrhage evacuation decreases perihematomal edema. *Stroke*. 2013;**44**:627–634

719. Naff NJ, Hanley DF, Keyl PM, Tuhrim S, Kraut M, Bederson J, et al. Intraventricular thrombolysis speeds blood clot resolution: Results of a pilot, prospective, randomized, double-blind, controlled trial. *Neurosurgery*. 2004;**54**:577–583; discussion 583–574

720. Webb AJ, Ullman NL, Mann S, Muschelli J, Awad IA, Hanley DF. Resolution of intraventricular hemorrhage varies by ventricular region and dose of intraventricular thrombolytic: The clot lysis: Evaluating accelerated resolution of IVH (CLEAR IVH) program. *Stroke*. 2012;**43**:1666–1668

721. Zervas NT, Hedley-Whyte J. Successful treatment of cerebral herniation in five patients. *N Engl J Med*. 1972;**286**:1075–1077

722. D Krieger, Hacke W. *The Intensive Care of the Stroke Patient. Stroke Pathophysiology, Diagnosis, and Management*. New York, NY: Churchill Livingstone; 1998:1133–1154

723. O'Brien M. Ischemic cerebral edema. In LR Caplan, ed. *Brain Ischemia, Basic Concepts and Clinical Relevance*. London: Springer; 1995:43–50

724. Klatzo I. Presidental address. Neuropathological aspects of brain edema. *J Neuropathol Exp Neurol*. 1967;**26**:1–14

725. Newkirk TA, Tourtellotte WW, Reinglass JL. Prolonged control of increased intracranial pressure with glycerin. *Arch Neurol*. 1972;**27**:95–96

726. Buckell M, Walsh L. Effect of glycerol by mouth on raised intracranial pressure in man. *Lancet*. 1964;**2**:1151–1152

727. Frank MS, Nahata MC, Hilty MD. Glycerol: A review of its pharmacology, pharmacokinetics, adverse reactions, and clinical use. *Pharmacotherapy*. 1981;**1**:147–160

728. Marshall LF, Smith, RW, Rauscher LA, Shapiro HM. Mannitol dose requirements in brain-injured patients. *J Neurosurg*. 1978;**48**:169–172

729. Qureshi AI, Suarez JI. Use of hypertonic saline solutions in treatment of cerebral edema and intracranial hypertension. *Crit Care Med*. 2000;**28**:3301–3313

730. Koenig MA, Bryan M, Lewin JL, 3rd, Mirski MA, Geocadin RG, Stevens RD. Reversal of transtentorial herniation with hypertonic saline. *Neurology*. 2008;**70**:1023–1029

731. Wagner I, Hauer EM, Staykov D, Volbers B, Dorfler A, Schwab S, et al. Effects of continuous hypertonic saline infusion on perihemorrhagic edema evolution. *Stroke*. 2011;**42**:1540–1545

732. Fink ME. Osmotherapy for intracranial hypertension: Mannitol versus hypertonic saline. *Continuum (Minneap Minn)*. 2012;**18**:640–654

733. Feigin VL, Anderson N, Rinkel GJ, Algra A, van Gijn J, Bennett DA. Corticosteroids for aneurysmal subarachnoid haemorrhage and primary intracerebral haemorrhage. *Cochrane Database Syst Rev*. 2005: CD004583

734. Sheth KN, Kimberly WT, Elm JJ, Kent TA, Mandava P, Yoo AJ, et al. Pilot study of intravenous glyburide in patients with a large ischemic stroke. *Stroke*. 2014;**45**:281–283

735. Kuroiwa T, Shibutani M, Okeda R. Blood–brain barrier disruption and exacerbation of ischemic brain edema after restoration of blood flow in experimental focal cerebral ischemia. *Acta Neuropathol*. 1988;**76**:62–70

736. Mulley G, Wilcox RG, Mitchell JR. Dexamethasone in acute stroke. *Br Med J*. 1978;**2**:994–996

737. O'Brien MD. Ischemic cerebral edema. A review. *Stroke*. 1979;**10**:623–628

738. Poungvarin N, Bhoopat W, Viriyavejakul A, Rodprasert P, Buranasiri P, Sukondhabhant S, et al. Effects of dexamethasone in primary supratentorial intracerebral

hemorrhage. *N Engl J Med.* 1987;**316**:1229–1233

739. Bardutzky J, Schwab S. Antiedema therapy in ischemic stroke. *Stroke.* 2007;**38**:3084–3094

740. Shackford SR, Bourguignon PR, Wald SL, Rogers FB, Osler TM, Clark DE. Hypertonic saline resuscitation of patients with head injury: A prospective, randomized clinical trial. *J Trauma.* 1998;**44**:50–58

741. Suarez JI, Qureshi AI, Bhardwaj A, Williams MA, Schnitzer MS, Mirski M, et al. Treatment of refractory intracranial hypertension with 23.4% saline. *Crit Care Med.* 1998;**26**:1118–1122

742. Schwarz S, Georgiadis D, Aschoff A, Schwab S. Effects of hypertonic (10%) saline in patients with raised intracranial pressure after stroke. *Stroke.* 2002;**33**:136–140

743. Suarez JI. Hypertonic saline for cerebral edema and elevated intracranial pressure. *Cleve Clin J Med.* 2004;**71** Suppl 1:S9–13

744. Caplan LR. Cerebellar infarcts. In LR Caplan, ed. *Posterior Circulation Disease: Clinical Findings, Diagnosis, and Management.* Boston, MA: Blackwell Science; 1996:492–543

745. Lehrich JR, Winkler GF, Ojemann RG. Cerebellar infarction with brain stem compression. Diagnosis and surgical treatment. *Arch Neurol.* 1970;**22**:490–498

746. Feely MP. Cerebellar infarction. *Neurosurgery.* 1979;**4**:7–11

747. Neugebauer H, Witsch J, Zweckberger K, Juttler E. Space-occupying cerebellar infarction: Complications, treatment, and outcome. *Neurosurg Focus.* 2013;**34**:E8

748. Delashaw JB, Broaddus WC, Kassell NF, Haley EC, Pendleton GA, Vollmer DG, et al. Treatment of right hemispheric cerebral infarction by hemicraniectomy. *Stroke.* 1990;**21**:874–881

749. Schwab S, Rieke K, Aschoff A, Albert F, von Kummer R, Hacke W. Hemicraniotomy in space-occupying hemispheric infarction: Useful early intervention or desperate activism? *Cerebrovasc Dis.* 1996;**6**:325–329

750. Schwab S, Steiner T, Aschoff A, Schwarz S, Steiner HH, Jansen O, et al. Early hemicraniectomy in patients with complete middle cerebral artery infarction. *Stroke.* 1998;**29**:1888–1893

751. Vahedi K, Vicaut E, Mateo J, Kurtz A, Orabi M, Guichard JP, et al. Sequential-design, multicenter, randomized, controlled trial of early decompressive craniectomy in malignant middle cerebral artery infarction (DECIMAL trial). *Stroke.* 2007;**38**:2506–2517

752. Vahedi K, Hofmeijer J, Juettler E, Vicaut E, George B, Algra A, et al. Early decompressive surgery in malignant infarction of the middle cerebral artery: A pooled analysis of three randomised controlled trials. *Lancet Neurol.* 2007;**6**:215–222

753. Mayer SA. Hemicraniectomy: A second chance on life for patients with space-occupying MCA infarction. *Stroke.* 2007;**38**:2410–2412

754. Heinsius T, Bogousslavsky J, Van Melle G. Large infarcts in the middle cerebral artery territory. Etiology and outcome patterns. *Neurology.* 1998;**50**:341–350

755. Cruz-Flores S, Berge E, Whittle IR. Surgical decompression for cerebral oedema in acute ischaemic stroke. *Cochrane Database Syst Rev.* 2012: CD003435

756. Wijdicks EFM, Schievink WI, McGough PF. Dramatic reversal of the uncal syndrome and brain edema from infarction in the middle cerebral artery territory. *Cerebrovasc Dis.* 1997;**7**:349–352

757. Lukovits TG, Bernat JL. Ethical approach to surrogate consent for hemicraniectomy in older pateints with extensive middle cerebral artery stroke. *Stroke* 2014;**45**:2833–2835

758. Graff-Radford NR, Torner J, Adams HP, Jr., Kassell NF. Factors associated with hydrocephalus after subarachnoid hemorrhage. A report of the cooperative aneurysm study. *Arch Neurol.* 1989;**46**:744–752

759. Greenberg J, Skubick D, Shenkin H. Acute hydrocephalus in cerebellar infarct and hemorrhage. *Neurology.* 1979;**29**:409–413

760. Khan M, Polyzoidis KS, Adegbite AB, McQueen JD. Massive cerebellar infarction: "Conservative" management. *Stroke.* 1983;**14**:745–751

761. Rieke K, Krieger D, Adams HP, Aschoff A, Meyding-Lamade U, Hacke W. Therapeutic strategies in space-occupying cerebellar infarction based on clinical, neuroradiological and neurophysiological data. *Cerebrovasc Dis.* 1993;**3**:45–55

762. Meairs S, Wahlgren N, Dirnagl U, Lindvall O, Rothwell P, Baron JC, et al. Stroke research priorities for the next decade – a representative view of the European scientific community. *Cerebrovasc Dis.* 2006;**22**:75–82

763. Menken M, Munsat TL, Toole JF. The global burden of disease study: Implications for neurology. *Arch Neurol.* 2000;**57**:418–420

764. Ovbiagele B, Goldstein LB, Higashida RT, Howard VJ, Johnston SC, Khavjou OA, et al. Forecasting the future of stroke in the United States: A policy statement from the American Heart Association and American Stroke Association. *Stroke.* 2013;**44**:2361–2375

765. Caplan LR. Treatment of patients with stroke. *Arch Neurol.* 2002;**59**:703–707

766. Savitz SI, Rosenbaum DM, Dinsmore JH, Wechsler LR, Caplan LR. Cell transplantation for stroke. *Ann Neurol.* 2002;**52**:266–275

767. Cramer SC. Brain repair after stroke. *N Engl J Med.* 2010;**362**:1827–1829

768. Cramer SC, Sur M, Dobkin BH, O'Brien C, Sanger TD, Trojanowski JQ, et al. Harnessing neuroplasticity for clinical applications. *Brain.* 2011;**134**:1591–1609

769. Kondziolka D, Wechsler L, Goldstein S, Meltzer C, Thulborn KR, Gebel J, et al. Transplantation of cultured human neuronal cells for patients with stroke. *Neurology.* 2000;**55**:565–569

770. Bliss T, Guzman R, Daadi M, Steinberg GK. Cell transplantation therapy for stroke. *Stroke.* 2007;**38**:817–826

771. Savitz SI, Cramer SC, Wechsler L. Stem cells as an emerging paradigm in stroke 3: Enhancing the development of clinical trials. *Stroke.* 2014;**45**:634–639

772. Kondziolka D, Steinberg GK, Wechsler L, Meltzer CC, Elder E, Gebel J, et al. Neurotransplantation for patients with subcortical motor stroke: A phase 2 randomized trial. *J Neurosurg.* 2005;**103**:38–45

773. Savitz SI, Dinsmore J, Wu J, Henderson GV, Stieg P, Caplan LR. Neurotransplantation of fetal porcine cells in patients with basal ganglia infarcts: A preliminary safety and feasibility study. *Cerebrovasc Dis.* 2005;**20**:101–107

774. Misra V, Ritchie MM, Stone LL, Low WC, Janardhan V. Stem cell therapy in ischemic stroke: Role of IV and

intra-arterial therapy. *Neurology.* 2012;**79**:S207–212

775. Yavagal DR, Lin B, Raval AP, Garza PS, Dong C, Zhao W, et al. Efficacy and dose-dependent safety of intra-arterial delivery of mesenchymal stem cells in a rodent stroke model. *PLoS One.* 2014;**9**:e93735

776. Chopp M, Li Y. Transplantation of bone marrow stromal cells for treatment of central nervous system diseases. *Adv Exp Med Biol.* 2006;**585**:49–64

777. Chen J, Chopp M. Neurorestorative treatment of stroke: Cell and pharmacological approaches. *NeuroRx.* 2006;**3**:466–473

778. Chen J, Sanberg PR, Li Y, Wang L, Lu M, Willing AE, et al. Intravenous administration of human umbilical cord blood reduces behavioral deficits after stroke in rats. *Stroke.* 2001;**32**:2682–2688

779. Shen LH, Li Y, Chen J, Cui Y, Zhang C, Kapke A, et al. One-year follow-up after bone marrow stromal cell treatment in middle-aged female rats with stroke. *Stroke.* 2007;**38**:2150–2156

780. Sandrini M, Cohen LG. Noninvasive brain stimulation in neurorehabilitation. *Handb Clin Neurol.* 2013;**116**:499–524

781. van der Lee JH, Wagenaar RC, Lankhorst GJ, Vogelaar TW, Deville WL, Bouter LM. Forced use of the upper extremity in chronic stroke patients: Results from a single-blind randomized clinical trial. *Stroke.* 1999;**30**:2369–2375

782. Wolf SL, Winstein CJ, Miller JP, Taub E, Uswatte G, Morris D, et al. Effect of constraint-induced movement therapy on upper extremity function 3 to 9 months after stroke: The EXCITE randomized clinical trial. *JAMA.* 2006;**296**:2095–2104

783. Dobkin BH. Interpreting the randomized clinical trial of constraint-induced movement therapy. *Arch Neurol.* 2007;**64**:336–338

784. Feys H, De Weerdt W, Verbeke G, Steck GC, Capiau C, Kiekens C, et al. Early and repetitive stimulation of the arm can substantially improve the long-term outcome after stroke: A 5-year follow-up study of a randomized trial. *Stroke.* 2004;**35**:924–929

785. Dannenbaum RM, Dykes RW. Sensory loss in the hand after sensory stroke: Therapeutic rationale. *Arch Phys Med Rehabil.* 1988;**69**:833–839

786. Dobkin B. Stroke. In: B Dobkin, ed. *Neurologic Rehabilitation.* Philadelphia, PA: FA Davis Co.; 1996:157–217

787. Teasell RW, Kalra L. What's new in stroke rehabilitation. *Stroke.* 2004;**35**:383–385

788. Takeuchi N, Chuma T, Matsuo Y, Watanabe I, Ikoma K. Repetitive transcranial magnetic stimulation of contralesional primary motor cortex improves hand function after stroke. *Stroke.* 2005;**36**:2681–2686

789. Kobayashi M, Hutchinson S, Theoret H, Schlaug G, Pascual-Leone A. Repetitive TMS of the motor cortex improves ipsilateral sequential simple finger movements. *Neurology.* 2004;**62**:91–98

790. Khedr EM, Ahmed MA, Fathy N, Rothwell JC. Therapeutic trial of repetitive transcranial magnetic stimulation after acute ischemic stroke. *Neurology.* 2005;**65**:466–468

791. Kim YH, You SH, Ko MH, Park JW, Lee KH, Jang SH, et al. Repetitive transcranial magnetic stimulation-induced corticomotor excitability and associated motor skill acquisition in chronic stroke. *Stroke.* 2006;**37**:1471–1476

792. Kluger BM, Triggs WJ. Use of transcranial magnetic stimulation to influence behavior. *Curr Neurol Neurosci Rep.* 2007;**7**:491–497

793. Wagner T, Valero-Cabre A, Pascual-Leone A. Noninvasive human brain stimulation. *Annual Rev Biomed Eng* 2007;**9**:527–565

794. Alonso-Alonso M, Fregni F, Pascuazl-Leone A. Brain stimulation in post-stroke rehabilitation. *Cerebrovasc Dis* 2007; **24** Suppl 1:157–166

795. Hummel F, Celnik P, Giraux et al. Effects of non-invasive cortical stimulation on skilled motor function in chronic stroke. *Brain* 2005;**128**:490–499

796. Catsman-Berrevoets CE, von Harskamp F. Compulsive pre-sleep behavior and apathy due to bilateral thalamic stroke: Response to bromocriptine. *Neurology.* 1988;**38**:647–649

797. Albert ML, Bachman DL, Morgan A, Helm-Estabrooks N. Pharmacotherapy for aphasia. *Neurology.* 1988;**38**:877–879

798. Sabe L, Leiguarda R, Starkstein SE. An open-label trial of bromocriptine in nonfluent aphasia. *Neurology.* 1992;**42**:1637–1638

799. Fleet WS, Valenstein E, Watson RT, Heilman KM. Dopamine agonist therapy for neglect in humans. *Neurology.* 1987;**37**:1765–1770

800. Barrett K. Treating organic abulia with bromocriptine and lisuride: Four case studies. *J Neurol Neurosurg Psychiatry.* 1991;**54**:718–721

801. Feeney DM, Gonzalez A, Law WA. Amphetamine, haloperidol, and experience interact to affect rate of recovery after motor cortex injury. *Science.* 1982;**217**:855–857

802. Hovda DA, Feeney DM. Haloperidol blocks amphetamine induced recovery of binocular depth perception after bilateral visual cortex ablation in cat. *Proc West Pharmacol Soc.* 1985;**28**:209–211

803. Davis JN, Crisostomo EA, Duncan P. Amphetamine and physical therapy facilitate recovery of function from stroke: Correlative animal and human studies. In ME Raichle, W Powers, eds. *Cerebrovascular Diseases.* New York, NY: Raven Press; 1987:297–304

804. Goldstein L. Amphetamine-facilitated functional recovery after stroke. In MD Ginsberg, WD Dietrich, eds. *Cerebrovascular Diseases.* New York, NY: Raven Press; 1989:303–308

805. Hurwitz BE, Dietrich WD, McCabe PM, Alonso O, Watson BD, Ginsberg MD, et al. Amphetamine promotes recovery from sensory-motor integration deficit after thrombotic infarction of the primary somatosensory rat cortex. *Stroke.* 1991;**22**:648–654

806. Reding MJ, Solomon B, Borucki S. The effect of dextroamphetamine on motor recovery after stroke. *Neurology.* 1995;**45**:A222

807. Sawaki L, Cohen LG, Classen J, Davis BC, Butefisch CM. Enhancement of use-dependent plasticity by d-amphetamine. *Neurology.* 2002;**59**:1262–1264

808. Plewnia C, Hoppe J, Cohen LG, Gerloff C. Improved motor skill acquisition after selective stimulation of central norepinephrine. *Neurology.* 2004;**62**:2124–2126

809. Walker-Batson D. Amphetamine and post-stroke rehabilitation: Indications and controversies. *Eur J Phys Rehabil Med.* 2013;**49**:251–260

810. Hernandez TC, Kiefel J, Barth TM. Disruption and facilitation of recovery of behavioral function: Implication of the gamma-aminobutyric acid/

benzodiazepine receptor complex. In MD Ginsberg, WD Dietrich, eds. *Cerebrovascular Diseases*. New York, NY: Raven Press; 1989:327–334

811. Goldstein LB, Davis JN. Physician prescribing patterns following hospital admission for ischemic cerebrovascular disease. *Neurology*. 1988;**38**:1806–1809

812. Goldstein LB. Potential effects of common drugs on stroke recovery. *Arch Neurol*. 1998;**55**:454–456

813. Goldstein LB. Common drugs may influence motor recovery after stroke. The Sygen in acute stroke study investigators. *Neurology*. 1995;**45**:865–871

814. Lee B, Liu CY, Apuzzo ML. A primer on brain–machine interfaces, concepts, and technology: A key element in the future of functional neurorestoration. *World Neurosurg*. 2013;**79**:457–471

815. Lee B, Attenello FJ, Liu CY, McLoughlin MP, Apuzzo ML. Recapitulating flesh with silicon and steel: Advancements in upper extremity robotic prosthetics. *World Neurosurg*. 2014;**81**:730–741

816. Yamamoto H, Bogousslavsky J. Mechanisms of second and further strokes. *J Neurol Neurosurg Psychiatry*. 1998;**64**:771–776

817. Caplan LR. Prevention of strokes and recurrent strokes. *J Neurol Neurosurg Psychiatry*. 1998;**64**:716

Large artery occlusive disease of the anterior circulation

Louis R Caplan and Lawrence Wechsler

Specific clinical and laboratory aspects of occlusive disease of the commonly involved arteries are analyzed in this chapter. Examples of typical patients are included to discuss management and illustrate the most common clinical and imaging findings. The general epidemiological, etiological, and pathological features that relate to large artery occlusive lesions are discussed in Part I of this book.

Disease of the internal carotid artery

Atherosclerotic internal carotid artery disease in the neck

The modern era in ischemic cerebrovascular disease began in 1951 with C Miller Fisher's key report that called attention to the clinical findings in patients with occlusion of the internal carotid artery (ICA) in the neck.[1,2] Previously, ischemic strokes in the anterior circulation were invariably attributed to middle cerebral artery (MCA) disease. Fisher called attention to warning episodes in patients with carotid artery disease that preceded strokes. He recognized that attacks of eye and hemispheral ischemic symptoms were diagnostic of carotid artery disease in the neck. He dubbed these episodes transient ischemic attacks (TIAs).[1,3] Fisher commented, "It is even conceivable that some day surgery will find a way to bypass the occluded portion of the artery during the period of ominous fleeting symptoms." At that time, angiography required a surgical cut-down and only single-frame, hand-pulled films were available. During the next decades, the advent of safer and more widespread angiography led to increased recognition of the frequency and importance of ICA disease in the neck. Newer, non-invasive techniques including computed tomography angiography (CTA), magnetic resonance angiography (MRA) and ultrasound (US) now make possible reliable detection of carotid artery lesions in outpatients.

The first carotid surgical procedures were performed during the early 1950s.[1,4] During the 1960s and 1970s, improved diagnostic capability, safer anesthesia, advanced surgical techniques, and an increase in the number of vascular surgeons caused an explosion in the amount of operative procedures performed on the carotid arteries. In 1985, more than 107 000 endarterectomies were performed in the United States, making it one of the three most common surgical procedures.[4] After 1987, the number of endarterectomies began to decrease in response to widespread concern about the indications, use, and complications of the procedure.[5,6] In 1991, North American and European randomized controlled trial results showed an important therapeutic benefit of endarterectomy in symptomatic patients with high-grade (>70%) stenosis.[7,8] These reports gave the procedure more credibility and served as an impetus for more vascular surgery. Subsequent reports from the North American[9] and European[10] carotid surgery trials showed that endarterectomy was beneficial in selected patients who had moderately severe stenosis (50–69%) when operated on by surgeons who had documented records of low surgical morbidity and mortality. Patients who have hemispheric attacks, non-diabetics and males with moderate stenosis were more likely to benefit.[9] Trials also showed that selected patients who had severe carotid artery disease without recognized symptoms also could benefit from carotid artery surgery compared to the existent standard medical therapy.[11,12] Selection of the surgeon is most important since the frequency of complications, morbidity, and mortality figures still vary widely among surgeons and medical centers, even within the same city.[13,14]

During the last decade interventional procedures to open stenosed carotid arteries – angioplasty and stenting – have increasingly been performed instead of surgery in symptomatic and asymptomatic patients considered appropriate candidates. Angioplasty and stenting are now performed by many different specialists including neuroradiologists, vascular surgeons, cardiologists, neurologists, and neurosurgeons. Trials now attempt to sort out the relative risks and benefits of angioplasty/stenting compared to open surgical repair.[15,16] Improvements in medical therapy over the past decade have stimulated re-examination of carotid revascularization particularly in asymptomatic individuals.[17,18] We return to the important question of treatment after reviewing the epidemiological, clinical, and laboratory features of ICA occlusive disease in the neck.

A 58-year-old man, HL, awakened with a numb and weak left hand. He had a myocardial infarction 6 years earlier and continued to have angina pectoris on moderate exertion. During the past year, he developed pain in the left calf that abated when he stopped to rest or walked more than two blocks.

The major cause of ICA occlusive disease in the neck is atherosclerotic narrowing of the vessel. The lesion usually begins in the distal common carotid artery (CCA) and extends to the first few proximal centimeters of the ICA and external carotid artery (ECA), almost always more severely narrowing the ICA. The usual site of the lesion is shown in Figure 4.7. This lesion is found more often in whites than in African-Americans or Asians, and in men more than women.[19,20] Occlusive disease of the large systemic arteries, especially the coronary, iliac, and femoral arteries, often accompanies carotid atherosclerosis. Coexisting angina pectoris, myocardial infarction, and limb claudication are common.[21] Risk factors for the development of proximal ICA disease are similar to those for coronary artery disease and include hypertension, smoking, diabetes, and hypercholesterolemia. Mortality in patients with ICA disease is usually cardiac. Attention is appropriately focused on the heart and brain, and the brain's circulation.

Although HL did not volunteer other symptoms, direct questioning revealed several important warning signs. In the months before presentation, he had two brief episodes of transient obscuration of vision in his right eye. A dark shade descended from above, rather quickly blocking vision completely on one occasion, and obscuring only the upper half of vision during the other episode. The attacks were brief and lasted less than a minute each. He also had three episodes of transient neurological dysfunction. These episodes consisted of stumbling after his left leg gave way during one episode, and slurred speech, and numbness of the left arm, hand, and face in the other two episodes. The initial episode was 3 months earlier, the most recent 3 days earlier. He noted unaccustomed, frequent headaches in the weeks before presentation.

Atherosclerotic plaques most often gradually narrow the ICA lumen. Ulceration, attachment of platelet nidi and clots to crevices in plaques, and hemorrhage into plaques become more common as the arterial lumen becomes increasingly narrowed. Plaques usually contain a lipid core and fibrous cap. When there is a break in the fibrous cap, contact of the lipid core with the contents of the lumen activates platelets and can activate the coagulation cascade, promoting the deposition of white and red thrombi onto the plaque surface. Plugs of platelets and thrombin may detach from the arterial wall and embolize to distal vessels, causing transient or prolonged brain and eye dysfunction. Reduction in blood flow can also lead to periodic insufficiency in distal perfusion. For these reasons, TIAs often occur as the artery narrows and so warn of an impending stroke. Many times when an artery occludes, adequate collateral circulation develops and no permanent neurological damage ensues.

The single most important clue to an ICA localization of the occlusive process is an attack of transient monocular blindness also called amaurosis fugax. Often, the vision loss is described as a dimming, darkening, or obscuration. An apparent shade or curtain usually falls from above, but may move from the side like a theater curtain. After a brief period of seconds or a few minutes, the curtain lifts or recedes. This usually leaves no permanent visual loss. These attacks of transient visual obscuration are caused by decreased blood flow through the ophthalmic artery, the first branch of the ICA. Amaurosis fugax occurs when the lesion affects the ICA proximal to the ophthalmic artery (in the neck or proximal carotid siphon) or involves the ophthalmic artery itself. Diminished flow or pressure in the ophthalmic artery is a clue to the presence of carotid artery disease.

In migraine attacks, the most common differential diagnostic consideration, patients usually describe brightness, glittering, flickering, and movement within the visual field, which lasts 15–30 minutes and is seldom monocular. Occasionally, patients with severe ICA occlusive disease report unilateral spells of reduced vision after exposure to bright light, a type of retinal claudication.[22] In some patients with bilateral ICA disease, the transient loss of vision can be bilateral. As in HL, individuals may not volunteer information about temporary visual loss because they consider it completely unrelated to the present problem. The physician must directly and repeatedly ask about specific symptoms of ocular and brain ischemia.

Episodes of hemispheral ischemia are also usually brief. Attacks may be quite varied and include various deficits in different limbs during individual attacks. Sometimes, however, the spells are stereotyped. In some patients with critical stenosis, the attacks are frequent and may be precipitated by suddenly standing or a drop in blood pressure.[23] Frequent, brief, machine-gun-like attacks usually mean low flow caused by proximal severe stenosis. Emboli generally produce longer, less frequent attacks. In disease of larger vessels, such as the ICA, TIAs may occur during a period of months, as compared with a briefer span of hours, days, or a week in patients with lacunar infarction caused by disease of smaller blood vessels. As the ICA narrows, collateral circulation develops, leading to dilation of arteries and the onset of unaccustomed headache. It is unusual, however, for headache to be the only symptom; in our experience, headache is usually accompanied by TIAs. The most common symptoms of ICA disease in the neck are listed in Table 7.1.

On examination, HL had moderate weakness of the left arm, slight weakness of the left psoas muscle, and severe weakness of the left hand. Position sense was decreased in the left hand and HL could not accurately localize left-limb touch stimuli, nor recognize objects in the left hand. He drew a clock poorly (Figure 7.1, top) and also copied inaccurately (Figure 7.1, bottom). A soft, high-pitched bruit was audible at the right carotid bifurcation in the neck. A right Horner's syndrome was noted.

Physical examination of the blood vessels and eyes often yields important clues to an ICA location of the lesion (Table 7.2). Palpation of the neck is not helpful unless the CCA

Table 7.1 Symptoms of ICA disease

Attacks of transient monocular blindness
TIAs, sometimes variegated, and occurring during a span of weeks or months
Frequent, unaccustomed headache
Commonly associated history of coronary or peripheral vascular disease

Table 7.2 Signs of ICA disease

Neck
High-pitched, focal, long bruit at bifurcation
Face
Increased angular, brow, cheek (ABC) pulses[25]
Frontal artery sign[26]
Increase in superficial temporal artery
Retina
Cholesterol crystals[27]
Platelet plugs[28]
Retinal infarcts
Reduced caliber of arteries
Less severe hypertensive changes
Venous stasis retinopathy[29,30]
Reduced retinal artery pressure

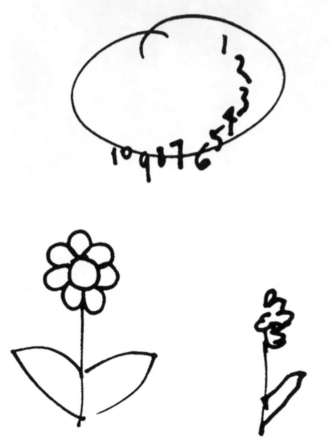

Figure 7.1 At top is a clock drawn by a patient with a right parietal lobe lesion. At the bottom is the patient's copy (right) of a daisy drawn by the examiner (left).

is occluded, in which case there is no palpable carotid pulse on that side. Even when the ICA is occluded, the CCA pulse is usually transmitted to the ICA in the neck. The presence of a typical bruit (i.e., a high-pitched, long, focal sound heard loudest over the carotid bifurcation) is virtually diagnostic of localized ICA disease. In some patients with severe ICA occlusive disease, blood flow is so severely diminished that no bruit is audible. When a bruit at the bifurcation is also audible over the ipsilateral eye, the physician can be confident that the bruit is of ICA origin and that the artery is patent. A bruit also can arise from the proximal ECA. In this case, the bruit usually radiates toward the jaw and can be diminished by pressure on ECA branches.[24] When the ICA is occluded or severely stenosed, ECA collaterals may feed into the orbit and may be palpable at the angular, brow, and cheek (ABC) regions (see

Figure 3.5).[25] Blood flow may be found to flow retrograde down the frontal artery into the orbit[26] (see Figure 3.6).

Ischemia to the iris or retina on the side of the carotid occlusive lesion is another helpful clue. Retinal arteries on the side of the carotid lesion may be reduced in caliber or show fewer hypertensive changes than their counterparts in the opposite retina. White, fluffy exudates or focal retinal atrophy can represent infarction. Small cholesterol crystal emboli are highly refractile bodies that usually lodge at bifurcations of retinal arteries.[27] White platelet plugs can also be transiently seen within retinal arteries.[28] Occasionally a fleck of calcium can be seen within retinal arteries originating from calcific valve disease or calcium within the ICA in the neck. Figures 3.8, 3.9, and 3.10 show examples of retinal vascular changes in patients with severe ICA disease in the neck.

Venous stasis retinopathy is a descriptive term for the ophthalmoscopic appearance found in patients with chronic ICA occlusion, and is characterized by microaneurysms, small-dot retinal hemorrhages, and dilated, dark retinal veins, sometimes of irregular caliber[29,30] (Figures 3.11 and 7.2). The retina in this condition resembles diabetic retinopathy but can usually be distinguished by unilaterality, location in the midportion of the retina, and its association with low retinal arterial pressure as measured by diminished ophthalmic blood-flow velocities by transcranial Doppler (TCD). The presence of venous stasis retinopathy always means that flow reduction in the ophthalmic artery is severe and longstanding.

Neurological findings are caused by infarction of brain regions within the ICA circulation. Signs in patients with ICA disease are difficult to separate clinically from those found in patients with intrinsic lesions of the MCA.[31,32] The most common loci of infarction are within the MCA territory. Weakness is common and usually affects the contralateral hand and face more than the leg. When

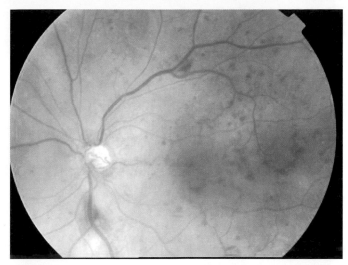

Figure 7.2 A photograph of the optic fundus in a patient with a carotid artery occlusion showing central venous retinopathy. There are dilated veins and many blot and dot hemorrhages mostly in the periphery of the retina. Courtesy of Thomas Hedges III, MD. A black and white version of this figure will appear in some formats. For the color version, please refer to the plate section.

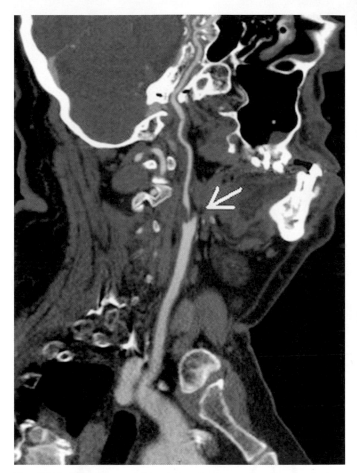

Figure 7.3 CTA of the neck, lateral view showing very severe stenosis at the origin of the ICA.

sensory loss is present, it usually is of the cortical type with loss of position sense, point localization, and stereognosis on the opposite side of the body. The hand and face often show more sensory abnormalities than the trunk and lower extremity. When bilateral simultaneous tactile stimuli are presented to the arms, the stimulus contralateral to the lesion is often not reported by the patient. Neglect of the opposite side of visual space and an attentional hemianopia are also common findings, especially when the infarct is in the right cerebral hemisphere. Poor drawing and copying, impersistence with tasks, diminished emotional responsiveness, and anosognosia (lack of awareness of the deficit) also frequently accompany right ICA-territory infarction.[33,34] Aphasia is a common sequel to left-sided infarction.

Occasionally, the infarct is located predominantly in the territory of the anterior cerebral artery (ACA); foot, leg, and shoulder weakness predominate. Rarely, when the posterior cerebral artery (PCA) is supplied directly by the ICA, an infarct caused by ICA occlusion can lie solely within the PCA territory and can manifest as a hemianopia without other signs.[35,36]

A duplex US scan was performed. B-mode showed some flat plaques within the distal right CCA and severe atherosclerotic disease at the right ICA origin with near occlusion. The Doppler frequencies also suggested high-grade stenosis of the right ICA. The left carotid artery showed only minor disease. TCD examination revealed lower flow velocities in the right ICA siphon, and the right MCA and ACA. CT showed a hypodensity in the cortical parietal lobe affecting the postcentral gyrus and superior parietal lobule. CTA showed severe, irregular narrowing of the ICA at its origin with a residual lumen of approximately 1 mm (95% luminal narrowing) (Figure 7.3). The carotid siphon and MCA were normal. Echocardiography and Holter cardiac rhythm monitoring for 48 hours were normal.

Non-invasive diagnostic tests are discussed in Chapter 4. Figures 4.6, 4.10, 4.12, and 4.13 show US studies of the ICA in the neck. In this patient, ultrasonography showed a severe flow-reducing lesion at the ICA origin and CTA confirmed the finding and showed the artery quite well. The concordance of the two vascular tests made it unnecessary to proceed to diagnostic catheter angiography. If angioplasty and/or stenting is performed, angiographic images of the artery would be performed as an adjunct to the therapeutic procedure. MRA is also a useful screening test when the arteries appear normal, but may not be reliable for determining the severity of stenosis as it typically overestimates the degree of stenosis due to the confounding effect of turbulent flow.[37] Figure 7.4A shows an ICA stenotic lesion imaged by MRA. Figure 7.4B shows the same lesion shown in Figure 7.4A studied by catheter contrast-digital angiography.

In patients with ICA atherosclerotic occlusive disease, there are several frequent patterns of disease. When the ICA is occluded, the vessel may be angiographically absent or show a pointed, tapering, or rounded stump.[38] Barnett and colleagues called attention to embolization from the stump of previously occluded carotid arteries.[39] Stenotic lesions can be ulcerated, smooth, or irregular. The lesions may be long and tapered or may slope abruptly like a shelf. B-mode scans and color-Doppler-flow ultrasound imaging (CDFI) studies of the

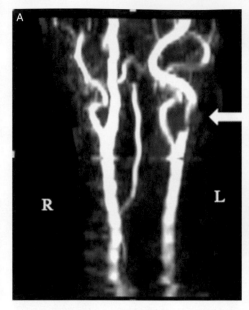

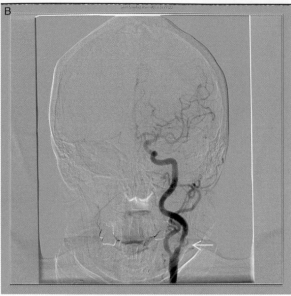

Figure 7.4 (A) MRA of the neck showing a severe stenosis at the left ICA origin (white arrow). (B) Dye-contrast cerebral angiogram in the same patient showing a localized cylindrical region of stenosis in the ICA (white arrow).

carotid origin can help define the nature of plaques, presence of ulceration, and dynamics of flow. An example of a CDFI study is shown in Figure 4.13. Calcific, smooth plaques are less often the source of intra-arterial emboli and usually do not show rapid enlargement, whereas irregular, heterogeneous, ulcerated, soft plaques often progress and are frequently the source of emboli. Cross-section images of the carotid artery using advanced magnetic resonance imaging (MRI) and computed tomography (CT) techniques can also yield useful information about the nature of plaques. When angiography is complete, it is often possible to detect embolic occlusion of the MCA or its branches, so-called occlusio supra occlusionem.[40]

Brain imaging findings in patients with internal carotid artery disease

CT scans of patients with carotid artery occlusion or severe stenosis show several common patterns of distribution of infarction (Figure 7.5). These patterns include: (1) watershed or borderzone infarction between the territories of the ACA and MCA, and between the MCA and PCA; (2) subcortical white matter infarcts often referred to as "internal borderzone" infarcts; (3) wedge-shaped, pial-artery territory infarcts; and (4) infarction of the basal ganglia and lentiform nucleus.[40]

The borderzone and subcortical white matter lesions are probably caused by a combination of reduced flow and embolism. TCD monitoring of patients with symptomatic ICA disease often shows frequent microemboli passing through the MCA.[41,42] Most such microemboli are composed of white platelet–fibrin thrombi. As the ICA narrows, blood flow velocity increases within the center of the artery and flow-separation becomes more prominent. Flow is reduced in some parts of the artery especially on the outer perimeter of the residual lumen. When subtotal or complete occlusion of the ICA develops, the bloodstream flow diminishes because of reduced volume of flow and blood

flow velocity also is decreased. Antegrade perfusion becomes less effective. This reduced perfusion and pressure decreases washout and throughput of emboli especially in arterial borderzones.[43,44] MRI using diffusion-weighted imaging (DWI) often shows tiny dot lesions often in the internal and cortical borderzone regions that result from these small emboli. Figure 7.6A and B shows such small dot infarcts. At times these small dot lesions are accompanied by larger infarcts in the center of the MCA distribution resulting from larger emboli as shown in Figure 7.7A and B, or as a vertical linear distribution within the internal borderzone on the side of the ICA occlusion (Figure 7.7C).

Larger pial and basal ganglia infarcts are caused by emboli to the mainstem MCA, its superior or inferior division trunks, or penetrating artery branches. These larger emboli most likely contain red clots, sometimes engrafted on white clots. Emboli removed from cerebral arteries by an embolus retrieving technique usually showed mixed elements of white and red clots.[45,46] In our experience, watershed infarction and large, superficial infarcts in the MCA territory are the most common lesions found on CT and MRI in patients with severe ICA obstructive disease. The mechanism of stroke in patient HL was a small superior parietal-lobe infarct caused by an embolus from the ICA stenosis in the neck. Cardiac testing did not show an alternative embologenic donor source in the heart.

HL was placed on heparin therapy for 1 week of treatment and was then switched to warfarin. The international normalized ratio (INR) was maintained between 2.0 and 2.5. At 4 weeks, an uncomplicated carotid endarterectomy was performed. Blood pressure was carefully monitored postoperatively, but did not elevate. The patient had minimal residual neurological signs of clumsiness and slight numbness of his left hand, but was able to return to his former work.

In our present practice, choice of treatment for patients with ICA disease in the neck depends on the following:

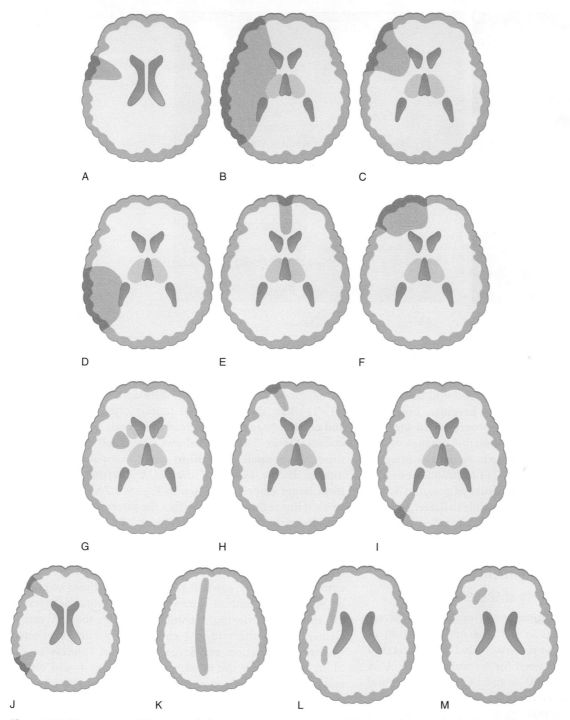

Figure 7.5 Most common CT locations of infarcts in the anterior circulation (infarcts are shown by hatched gray): (A) wedge-shaped MCA infarct, (B) entire MCA territory, (C) superior-division MCA, (D) inferior division MCA, (E) ACA, (F) ACA and MCA, (G) striatocapsular infarct, (H) wedge-shaped anterior watershed infarct, (I) wedge-shaped posterior watershed infarct, (J) anterior and posterior watershed infarcts, (K) linear watershed infarct, (L) ovular deep watershed infarct, and (M) small white matter watershed infarct.

1. Severity of the stenosis.
2. Anatomy of the carotid artery and stenosing plaque. A high carotid artery bifurcation and a long stenotic lesion increase the difficulty of surgery and are factors that favor stenting if aggressive treatment of the lesion is warranted.
3. Presence of a recent cerebral infarct as determined by a persistent clinical deficit and an appropriate CT, or MRI lesion.
4. General health of the patient, especially any contraindication to surgery, warfarin anticoagulation, or agents that decrease platelet agglutination.
5. Patient age: over age 74 favors carotid endarterectomy.
6. Morbidity and mortality record of the surgeon who would undertake surgery and of the hospital where the surgery would take place.

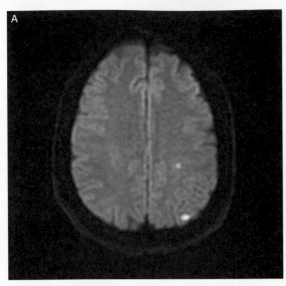
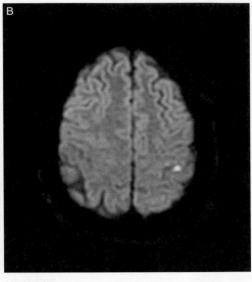

Figure 7.6 Diffusion-weighted MRI scans showing small-dot regions of hyperintensity in patients with unilateral severe carotid artery occlusive lesions. (A) Two dot lesions are seen within the posterior borderzone region. (B) There is a single dot lesion near the hand area of the cerebral cortex.

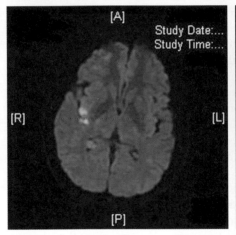
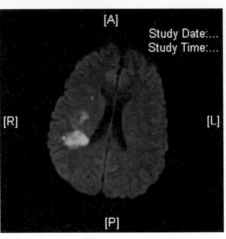
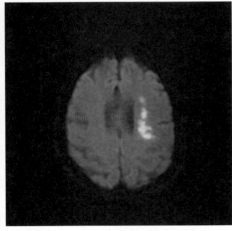

Figure 7.7 Diffusion-weighted MRI scans that show regions of infarction in patients with ICA occlusions. (A) A small-dot infarct is seen just below a slightly larger infarct in the posterior part of the insular cortex. (B) An infarct of several centimeters is seen adjacent to the most posterior portion of the lateral ventricle and smaller-dot infarcts are seen within the internal borderzone anterior to the larger infarct. (C) A line of small-dot hyperintensities is shown within the internal borderzone region.

7. Experience and record of the interventionalist who would perform angioplasty or stenting of the carotid artery lesion.
8. Attitude of the patient and family toward the situation after the alternative courses of action have been discussed.

Physicians and surgeons at the Mayo clinic carefully analyzed the neurological, medical, and angiographic risks of carotid surgery (Table 7.3). We rely heavily on their analysis in patients in whom we consider aggressive repair of the ICA (surgery or angioplasty/stenting).[47] The general topic of carotid artery surgery and stenting, including the results of observational studies and trials, has already been discussed at length in Chapter 6. Recent randomized trials, particularly the Carotid Revascularization Endarterectomy versus Stenting Trial (CREST),[48,49] provide a great deal of information regarding the relative role of stenting and surgery for symptomatic and asymptomatic carotid artery disease. Management of symptomatic patients with TIAs or small, non-disabling strokes who have various ICA lesions are considered in the following section.

Complete occlusion of the internal carotid artery in the neck

We do not recommend surgery or stenting for complete occlusion of the ICA in the neck. When the ICA occludes, clot eventually propagates high into the neck, often as far as the carotid siphon and beyond. Because there are no ICA branches in the neck, collateral flow patterns promote extension of clot toward the first branch, the ophthalmic artery. It is technically difficult to open completely occluded ICAs, and attempts to suction clots can lead to distal embolization. If it were known that an occlusion had become complete minutes or a few hours before, as might happen after angiography, or after surgery, exploration of the neck would be reasonable. In patients with acute stroke evaluated within a few hours of stroke onset, an endovascular approach often shows minimal thrombus burden above the site of occlusion and recanalization with angioplasty and stenting is usually possible. In occasional patients who have continued ischemic symptoms or

Table 7.3 Risks of carotid endarterectomies

Neurological risks
Progressive course of brain ischemia
Recent stroke
Vascular anatomy risks
High carotid bifurcation
Long lesion (3 cm distally in ICA or 5 cm into CCA)
Thrombus within the ICA
Contralateral ICA stenosis or occlusion
Intracranial stenosis or occlusion

Medical risks
Hypertension
Coronary artery disease
Diabetes
Obesity
Smoking
Chronic obstructive pulmonary disease
Congestive heart failure

Adapted from Sundt TM, Sandok BA, Whisnant JP. Carotid endarterectomy complications and preoperative assessment of risk. *Mayo Clin Proc* 1975;50:301–306.

signs, an aggressive endovascular approach can be considered. A recent study reported good results from endovascular therapy for occlusions up to 5 days from stroke onset in patients with progressive or unstable neurological symptoms.[50]

Angiography can yield clues as to the extent of the occlusive thrombosis. If opacification of the contralateral ICA shows retrograde filling of the occluded ICA down into the neck, it is more likely that the surgeon might be able to open the ICA surgically or the interventionist might successfully open the artery using thrombolysis and stenting.

When the patient arrives at the hospital soon after the onset of stroke symptoms, and CT or MRI do not show a large region of infarction, thrombolytic therapy can be considered. Intravenous recombinant tissue plasminogen activator (tPA) has often failed to recanalize occlusions of the ICA in the neck or intracranially.[51,52] In the Interventional Management of Stroke (IMS) III study, recanalization of terminal carotid occlusions occurred in only 28% of patients with intravenous tPA alone.[51] Combined therapy with intravenous tPA and endovascular treatment in this study improved recanalization rates to 83%. Similarly, good outcomes defined as a modified Rankin score (mRS) 0–2 improved from 4% with intravenous tPA alone to 27% with combined therapy.[52] The recent development of stent retrievers may achieve even better results. Most MCA occlusions recanalized by CTA at 24 hours in the

IMS III study and good outcomes were more frequent, occurring in 42% and 46% of patients treated with intravenous tPA and intravenous/intra-arterial therapy respectively.[52] When neck or intracranial thrombi are superimposed on severe atherostenotic lesions, thrombi almost always reoccur, unless the stenosis is treated by angioplasty or stenting shortly after successful thrombolysis. The use of thrombolysis in the setting of ICA thrombosis has never been compared with anticoagulant therapy.

We treat patients with acute ICA thrombosis with bed rest, keeping the head flat or slightly lower than the feet, to augment blood flow to the head. We try to avoid hypotension and have used agents that raise blood pressure in some patients. In some cases a fluid bolus is sufficient to maintain adequate blood pressure. We avoid antihypertensive drugs during the first day or two unless the blood pressure is in the malignant range (e.g., >225/125 mmHg). If the patient is normotensive and there is no contraindication to the use of anticoagulants, we use intravenous heparin, particularly if there is progression of neurological deficits or fluctuations. We now also consider using one of the newer oral anticoagulants (direct thrombin or factor Xa inhibitors) instead of heparin/warfarin but have little experience with this strategy. After the acute period, we do not use anticoagulants, but rather aspirin in doses of one 325 mg tablet per day, plavix 75 mg/day, or cilostazole 200 mg/day, or aspirin 25 mg/modified-release dipyridamole 200 mg twice a day

Caution must be exercised in the diagnosis of complete ICA occlusion because a severe reduction in flow can lead to collapse of the artery above the high-grade block. Angiography produces a picture that closely resembles occlusion (so called pseudo-occlusion[53]), but late films usually show a trickle of dye ascending anterograde toward the siphon. Color-flow Doppler US also sometimes visualizes flow through a pseudo-occlusion not seen with standard angiography.[54] Figure 4.13 shows such a circumstance. CT in cross-section of the high neck after contrast can show blood in the ICA, documenting preserved anterograde flow.[55] In pseudo-occlusion, the residual flow, albeit small, makes it possible for the surgeon to open the artery. Patients with pseudo-occlusion are considered to have very severe stenosis. Analysis of the data from the North American Symptomatic Carotid Endarterectomy Trial (NASCET) showed that patients with near occlusion do not have an increased risk of acute stroke compared with those with lesser degrees of severe stenosis (70–94%), nor do they have a higher rate of surgical complications.[56] In our experience, the course of patients with pseudo-occlusion is identical to that of occlusion and the artery has in fact collapsed. We treat them in the same way that we manage patients with complete occlusions.

In patients with ICA occlusion, the deficit usually develops at, or shortly after, the time of occlusion when embolization and low flow are maximal. A chronic low flow state, so-called misery perfusion may occur but only rarely persists.[57] Occasionally, patients with known ICA occlusion develop transient symptoms, especially if they become hypotensive from overzealous antihypertensive treatment,

or from dehydration or hypovolemia. The most common symptoms are transient obscurations of vision in the ipsilateral eye and/or weakness or numbness of the contralateral limbs. An unusual, but characteristic, sign of hypoperfusion is a so-called limb-shaking TIA.[58,59] Usually when standing or active, the patient develops a flapping flexion-extension tremor with impressive shaking and oscillation of the arm and hand contralateral to the occluded ICA. Occasionally, the lower extremity is involved. The shaking stops when the patient sits or lies down, and is caused by ischemia rather than a seizure.

We have not referred patients with ICA occlusion for extracranial-to-intracranial artery (ECA-ICA) bypass, but would consider doing so if there were persistent, recurrent ischemic attacks or if positron emission tomography (PET), single-photon emission computed tomography (SPECT), or other new technology documented persistent misery perfusion. Sequential TCD studies of blood-flow velocity in the MCA and ACA, especially after acetazolamide infusion, also yield information about distal flow and the reserve capacity of the carotid tributaries to dilate. These laboratory techniques are discussed in Chapter 4.

The Carotid Occlusion Surgery Study (COSS) randomized patients identified by PET to EC-IC bypass and best medical therapy or best medical therapy alone and failed to show any benefit to surgery even in this highly selected population.[60,61] The surgical group had more perioperative strokes than expected and the medical treatment group had a lower event rate than predicted.[60,61] Whether improved surgical results and/or other selection criteria of patients likely to benefit from bypass would achieve different results is unclear. Since acetazolamide augments blood flow in some patients with ICA occlusions, we have treated some patients with oral acetazolamide although there are no trial data on this approach.

Severe stenosis of the internal carotid artery in the neck

In our opinion, severe stenosis of the ICA in the neck, when symptomatic, requires aggressive treatment (surgery or angioplasty/stenting) unless there is a severe, disabling brain infarction in the territory of the stenotic ICA. The reported results of North American[7,9] and European trials[8,10] support carotid endarterectomy in these patients. Most clinicians apply the same inclusion criteria to interventional angioplasty/stenting treatment. What constitutes a severe stenosis? The two principal criteria are: (1) the degree of anatomical narrowing of the artery; and (2) the presence of significant reduction in flow velocity and pressure in tributary vessels shown by TCD.[62] A residual lumen of less than 1.5 mm (70–99% stenosis) invariably represents severe stenosis and nearly always impedes intracranial blood flow in the ICA branches. When the severely stenotic ICA is examined histologically, compound ulcers are often found.[63,64] Although these lesions may also be found in non-stenosed vessels, they become more frequent as the artery narrows.

When patients have TIAs, or minor stroke and severe stenosis of the ICA with a residual lumen of less than 1.5 mm (70–99% stenosis), we believe that aggressive treatment should be performed urgently. The benefit of revascularization is greatest when performed within 2 weeks but unless there is a severe neurological deficit or large infarct on CT or MRI, treatment should be initiated quickly.[65] Many instances of postendarterectomy ICH are explained by hypertension after manipulation of the carotid receptors in the neck.[65–67] Careful postoperative monitoring of blood pressure and effective treatment of hypertension (if it develops) should prevent ICH. Intracranial hemorrhage is less common after carotid stenting, perhaps because the frequency of severe hypertension after percutaneous manipulation of the ICA is less frequent than after surgery.

Endarterectomy in patients with severe stenosis can also be followed by a "hyperperfusion syndrome."[68,69] Sudden flooding of previously underperfused brain with blood can overwhelm the autoregulatory capacity of the region and lead to headache, seizures, focal neurological signs, brain edema, and brain hemorrhage.[69] Hypertension, often acute and severe, is also usually present in patients with severe effects of the hyperperfusion syndrome. Recognition of the syndrome and rapid, effective treatment of hypertension usually prevents serious brain edema and hemorrhage. Hyperperfusion may also develop after carotid stenting, but is less common than after surgery.[70]

The choice between carotid endarterectomy and angioplasty/stenting is evolving because of the many ongoing trials comparing the two treatments. The results of these trials are discussed and analyzed in Chapter 6. At present carotid endarterectomy appears to be a better choice for most patients over age 70, and carotid stenting seems a better choice in younger patients especially those with known active coronary artery disease. Improvements in the stents used, newer techniques to eliminate passage of catheters through the aorta, and the use of better distal protection devices may alter the benefit–risk ratio of interventional treatment and make it an excellent option for treatment of patients with severe carotid artery disease. Now the choice between surgery and angioplasty/stenting depends on: (1) the availability and experience, training, and past results of the individual who will perform the surgery or the percutaneous interventional treatment; (2) the nature, location, and severity of the ICA lesion and the presence of other arterial lesions; (3) the age and sex of the patient (carotid endarterectomy has poorer results in women compared to men, especially those >65); (4) vascular anatomy; (5) comorbidities that would preclude surgery or interventional treatment; and (6) the wishes of the patient after information is shared. Patients with long lesions, smooth lesions, and very high carotid bifurcations, especially those with coronary artery disease might better be treated using interventional techniques. Patients with focal irregular ulcerated lesions might better be treated surgically.

In patients with severe ICA stenosis, if surgery and angioplasty/stenting cannot be performed or if the patient refuses these procedures, we choose to anticoagulate with warfarin or

one of the newer oral anticoagulants. We also treat risk factors aggressively and prescribe a 3-hydroxy-3-methylglutaryl coenzyme A reductase inhibitor (statin) in high dose (e.g., 40–80 mg atorvastatin) and often an angiotensin-converting enzyme (ACE) inhibitor. The duration of anticoagulation is uncertain and should be individualized. We use the results of sequential duplex scans to guide the duration of anticoagulation. Arteries with tight stenosis frequently occlude on follow-up scans, often without new symptoms.[71,72] During the 4–6 weeks after occlusion, thrombi become organized and adherent, after which embolization is rare. We switch from warfarin to one aspirin per day, or two capsules of aspirin 25 mg combined with modified release dipyridamole 200 mg, 4–6 weeks after scans show complete occlusion. While the lumen remains narrowed but patent, we continue warfarin or one of the newer oral anticoagulants. In some patients, plaques regress and the lumen may become less narrowed. In these individuals, a switch to antiplatelet therapy also seems logical. No studies have been undertaken to test the strategy that we have outlined.

Plaque disease of the internal carotid artery in the neck with slight or moderate stenosis

We suggest prophylactic treatment with 3-hydroxy-3-methylglutaryl coenzyme A reductase inhibitors (statins) and an agent that decreases platelet aggregation for ICA plaque disease in the neck. Recent evidence favors rather high doses of statins.[73] Recommendations for lifestyle modification including smoking cessation, weight reduction, exercise and control of risk factors are also very important. Changes in lifestyle and success in optimizing blood pressure, blood glucose metabolism, and weight should be closely monitored. We do not recommend anticoagulation or aggressive surgical or endovascular treatment. Although it is true that ulceration can occur in non-stenotic lesions, and that ulcers can be the source of artery-to-artery embolization, this occurs less often in patients without severe stenosis. In the presence of a severe stenosing lesion, the physician can be more confident that this is the responsible lesion rather than another plaque. Furthermore, the natural history of plaques has not been well studied. They may reendothelialize and heal. Plaques are ubiquitous in individuals older than 40 years, and current angiographic and non-invasive techniques do not infallibly predict the presence of ulceration on histological examination. Agents that decrease platelet aggregation are posited to be most effective when there are non-stenosing plaques and high-velocity flow continues.

Antiplatelet agents (aspirin, aspirin combined with modified-release dipyridamole, clopidogrel, and cilostazole) have theoretical advantages over warfarin, an agent that probably works best in slow-moving vascular streams to prevent red thrombi. At present, we prefer aspirin, to other agents. The dose of aspirin is uncertain. We usually prescribe one 325 mg tablet per day, although there is no clear evidence that 325 mg of aspirin is superior to 81 mg daily.[74] Clopidogrel 75 mg/day, aspirin combined with modified-release dipyridamole or cilostazol 200 mg twice a day are alternative antiplatelet agents. An accurate, reproducible in-vitro test of the effectiveness of the platelet antiaggregants might lead clinicians to titrate the dose in individual patients, and so monitor effectiveness of the drug. However, no study to date has shown an improvement in stroke prevention by adjusting antiplatelet dosing based on platelet-function testing.

When plaques are shallow, the decision to use platelet antiaggregant agents is clear. As plaques become larger, more irregular, or clearly ulcerated, and luminal narrowing approaches 50–70%, the therapeutic decision becomes more difficult and should be individualized. The North American Symptomatic Carotid Endarterectomy Trial (NASCET) and the European Carotid Surgery Trial showed modest benefit from surgery in patients with this severity of stenosis. The benefit–risk ratio, however, is highly dependent on the individual patient and surgeon characteristics.[9,10] In a young patient with a lesion in this gray zone of near-critical stenosis, who has several TIAs and is a good candidate for aggressive vascular opening, we probably would choose surgery or angioplasty/stenting.

Carotid artery clots

Some patients with atherosclerotic plaques in the neck, with or without severe stenosis, have thrombi that are grossly visible on angiography.[75,76] Figure 7.8A and B are angiograms that show filling defects due to clot formation within the ICA; Figure 2.4 is a carotid artery specimen removed at autopsy that contains a large clot. In some of these patients, free-floating thrombi are attached to plaques and coagulation functions are normal, whereas in others, a hypercoagulable state has promoted the formation of carotid thrombi. Cancer, active inflammatory disease such as Crohn's disease, and ulcerative colitis can increase acute-phase reactants and promote thrombosis on endothelial lesions. These patients should be treated urgently. In a review of prior cases of patients with intraluminal clot, both surgery and warfarin anticoagulation were effective in preventing further stroke.[75] Clot recurred after surgery, however, in patients with coagulopathy.[76] The blood coagulation profiles of these patients should be carefully studied before treatment. Screening for common cancers especially adenocarcinomas is often indicated. In the NASCET study, the presence of ICA thrombi increased the surgical risk.[77]

Asymptomatic patients with internal carotid artery disease in the neck

The preceding discussion of treatment concerned symptomatic patients with TIA or stroke. It now has become commonplace to document ICA disease in the neck in patients who have no apparent central nervous system symptoms. The most common circumstances provoking carotid artery investigation are an audible neck bruit or imminent surgical procedures on the aorta, coronary, or peripheral-limb vessels. Some patients have cervical US examinations as part of an evaluation of systemic atherosclerosis. Some instances are discovered at angiography for indications other than vascular disease, or when an

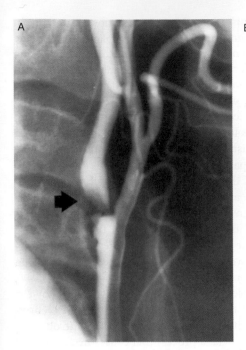
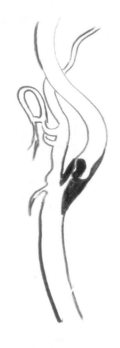
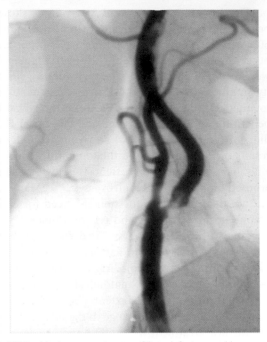

Figure 7.8 Dye-contrast digital subtraction cerebral angiograms showing thrombi within the ICA. (A) The black arrow points to a filling defect caused by a thrombus. (B) The angiogram on the right shows a filling defect at the origin of the ICA. On the left is a cartoon in which the plaque and thrombus are shown in black.

angiogram shows ICA disease on the asymptomatic side in a patient with symptoms of brain ischemia. Should these lesions be repaired before symptoms develop?

We seldom recommend carotid endarterectomy or angioplasty/stenting in asymptomatic patients. These patients do not have an unusual risk of stroke during surgery on other major vessels. Furthermore, stroke is unusual without preceding TIAs. In most medical centers, the risk of surgery and angiography (approx. 6% combined morbidity and mortality) or angioplasty/stenting is probably as great as, if not greater than, the risk of stroke without prior TIA. Analysis of a large series of patients followed for years showed that the annual stroke risk was likely less than 2%.[78] Several studies suggest that improvements in medical therapy in the past decade including statins and more aggressive blood pressure control result in even lower stroke rates in patients with asymptomatic stenosis.[17,18] A recent analysis that included 41 studies of over 16 000 patients who had moderate to severe carotid artery stenosis and were treated medically showed a rate of ipsilateral carotid territory strokes of 1.7 per 100 person-years.[79] The incidence rates of cardiovascular occurrences had improved over those cited in prior analyses.[79] A TCD detection of micro-emboli may identify patients at higher risk and those without such emboli have a very low risk of subsequent stroke.[80,81] Given these low stroke rates with aggressive medical therapy, re-evaluation of the benefits of revascularization in patients with asymptomatic stenosis is warranted.

Results of several studies of asymptomatic lesions are important to consider. In one series of 168 prospectively studied patients with known ICA stenosis, 26 patients (15%) had TIAs only; 3 patients had TIAs but refused surgery and had subsequent strokes; and just 1 patient developed sudden stroke

without warning.[82] In another series of asymptomatic patients with carotid stenosis followed for 2 years, among 318 patients, 5% developed TIAs, but only 2 patients had a stroke without a preceding TIA.[83] Sequential studies show that stenotic arteries often occlude without symptoms.[71,72] In patients undergoing endarterectomy who have bilateral carotid artery stenosis, subsequent stroke on the unoperated side is uncommon.[83] Even when a bruit is detected before elective non-cardiac vascular surgery, the incidence of postoperative stroke is not increased.[84] In patients who must have cardiac surgery, postoperative strokes are usually caused by cardiogenic emboli.

Treatment of asymptomatic patients must be individualized.[85] We do not think surgery or interventional repair of the ICA in asymptomatic patients should be seriously considered unless the stenosis is severe (>80% luminal narrowing). When made aware of a definite risk of stroke, some patients become quite anxious and psychologically tolerate knowledge of that risk poorly. They prefer the small gamble of an intraprocedural complication to the sword that they sense hangs perpetually over them. The situation must be fully discussed with the patient, and the benefits and risks of medical and surgical therapy explained. In patients who do not elect surgery, we teach them about TIAs and urge them to immediately report any attacks. We prescribe statin drugs and antiplatelet aggregants and lifestyle changes when appropriate and follow the carotid artery disease with sequential duplex US examinations. Significant increase in severity of the stenosis does increase the risk of a stroke and there is some evidence favoring aggressive treatment in those patients.[86] The occurrence of TIAs puts patients in the symptomatic category and makes them potential surgical candidates.

The Asymptomatic Carotid Artery Study showed a modest benefit for carotid endarterectomy in men who had more than 60% carotid stenosis, and did not have important cardiac or other comorbidity.[87] Surgeons who participated in this study were carefully selected, and the perioperative surgical morbidity and mortality was low (2.3%). The risk of stroke attributed to angiography was 1.2%.[87] A European study also reported a benefit for surgery, but women and those over 65 years of age did not fare as well as men and younger individuals.[88] The results of these studies and the topic of treatment of patients who have carotid artery stenosis with no symptoms has aroused considerable controversy.[89–91] Many neurologists and vascular surgeons question the need for catheter angiography in these patients and rely on duplex US and vascular imaging with MRA or CTA. The decision remains an individual one for each patient. Factors that should be considered when deciding between medical or surgical or interventional treatment include the anatomical aspects of the plaque (e.g., location in the neck, extent, degree of stenosis, heterogeneity, and echodensity), change in the plaque during conservative medical treatment with statins and platelet antiaggregants, comorbidities, especially the presence of hypertension and coronary artery disease, the experience and results of the surgeon and the interventionalist chosen, and the biases and wishes of the well-informed patient.[85]

Data are now accruing about the results of angioplasty/ stenting in patients with asymptomatic ICA atherosclerotic disease. Registry data now indicates that the morbidity and mortality from carotid artery stenting (CAS) has achieved the target of less than 3% recommended for revascularization of asymptomatic stenosis.[92] In the CREST trial, periprocedural stroke and death and postprocedural ipsilateral stroke occurred in 2.5% (+0.6%) of asymptomatic patients undergoing carotid artery stenting.[48] A detailed discussion of the relative benefits of carotid artery stenting versus carotid endarterectomy for asymptomatic stenosis is provided in Chapter 6.

Extracranial carotid artery dissections

After atherosclerosis, dissection is the next most common lesion that affects the carotid artery in the neck. Dissections are discussed in more detail in Chapter 12. Carotid artery dissections usually involve the pharyngeal portion of the artery above the origin but below entry into the skull. Dissections are tears in arteries, almost always involving the medial coat. Dissections are customarily referred to as traumatic or spontaneous in origin. The great majority of dissections probably involve some trauma or mechanical stress.[93,94] Sudden neck movements and stretching are likely to cause dissection. Some inciting events are trivial, such as lunging for a tennis shot or turning the neck while driving to see other cars to the side and rear. Many patients forget such events or believe them to be too inconsequential to mention. Congenital and acquired abnormalities of the arterial media and elastic tissue, especially fibromuscular dysplasia, make patients more vulnerable to dissection. Most patients with dissection, however, do not

have concurrent disorders. Migraine is more common in patients with dissection. The posited explanation for the relationship between migraine and dissection is that edema of the vessel wall during a migraine attack makes the involved artery more vulnerable to tearing.

Arterial dissections probably begin with a tear in the media that then leads to bleeding within the arterial wall. Intramural blood then dissects longitudinally, spreading along the vessel proximally and distally. Dissections can tear through the intima, allowing partially coagulated intramural blood to enter the lumen of the artery. The arterial wall, expanded by intramural blood, also compresses the lumen. Dissections probably begin from the luminal side at the intimal surface in some patients and dissect into the media. Intimal flaps are often present on the intimal surface. At times, the major dissection plane is between the media and the adventitia, causing an aneurysmal outpouching of the arterial wall.

Extracranial dissections cause symptoms primarily by the presence of luminal compromise and luminal clot. Dissections through the adventitia lead to rupture into the surrounding neck, muscles, and fascia, a process that causes neck pain and formation of a pseudoaneurysm, but usually does not further compromise blood flow. Thrombus is present within the lumen because of rupture of intramural clot into the lumen or thrombus formation in situ within the lumen. Narrowing of the lumen by the intramural blood, with alteration in blood flow and irritation of the endothelium causing release of endothelins and tissue factors, and activation of platelets and the coagulation cascade, all contribute to formation of intraluminal thrombus. Brain ischemia can result from hypoperfusion (usually from acute luminal compromise), embolism, or both. Hypoperfusion usually causes transient ischemia, but seldom is prolonged enough to cause infarction. Infarction is more often caused by embolization or propagation of luminal thrombus.

The major symptoms of carotid artery dissection in the neck are: (1) neck, head, and face pain; (2) Horner's syndrome; (3) pulsatile tinnitus; (4) transient ipsilateral monocular vision loss; (5) transient hemispheral attacks with contralateral limb numbness or weakness; (6) sudden onset strokes; and (7) palsy of lower cranial nerves (IX–XII).[93–97]

We separate symptoms related to the arterial wall lesion from those related to brain ischemia. The commonest symptoms not indicative of brain ischemia are pain, Horner's syndrome, pulsatile tinnitus, and loss of function of lower cranial nerves.[98] Many patients present with pain and headache as their only symptoms and do not have neurological findings. The pain is often in the neck, face, or jaw. Headaches may be generalized, but are most often on the side of the dissection. Features of Horner's syndrome are caused by involvement of the sympathetic fibers along the dilated carotid artery segments. Pulsatile tinnitus is explained by the course of the ICA near the tympanic membrane. We personally have not seen a patient present with non-ischemic findings (other then pain and headache) that were present for a week or more who later developed brain ischemia.

Neurological symptoms related to hypoperfusion are usually multiple, brief TIAs, referred to as carotid allegro by

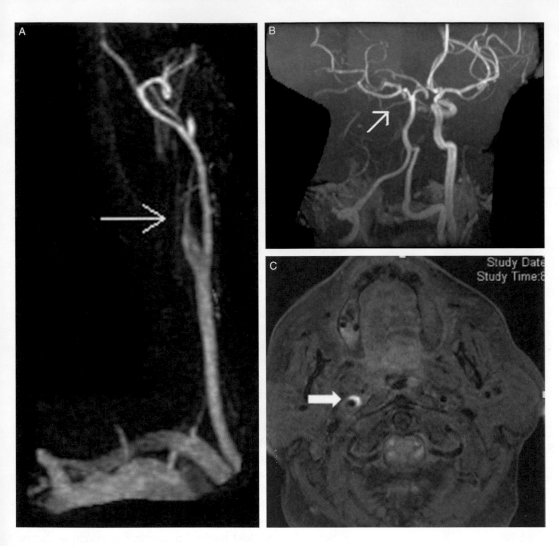

Figure 7.9 Dissection of the ICA. (A) Magnetic resonance angiogram showing narrowing with tapering of the ICA (white arrow) above its origin. (B) Magnetic resonance angiogram showing that the distal right ICA does not opacify. The white arrow indicates where the vessel should be visible. (C) Fat-saturated MRI image showing a half-moon-shaped hyperintensity (white arrow) that represents blood or edema within the dissected right ICA.

Miller Fisher because of their rapidity. Sudden-onset strokes are usually caused by embolism of clot from the region of dissection. The distended, dilated carotid artery at the skull base can compress the lower cranial nerves (IX–XII) that exit this region.[98]

The diagnosis of carotid artery dissection can be suggested by US when the ultrasonographer explores the neck with the probe from above the carotid bifurcation to the skull base.[99] MRA, CTA, and standard angiography are helpful. Figure 7.9A and B shows MRAs of a patient with a carotid dissection. A cross-section of fat-saturated MRI scans of the neck can show a characteristic change in the signal intensity in the wall of the artery (Figure 7.9C). Figure 7.10 is an angiogram that shows a characteristic aneurysm in the pharyngeal ICA from a patient with a carotid dissection. A montage of angiograms in patients with carotid artery dissections is found in Figure 12.3.

Table 7.4 lists various treatments given in large series of patients with cervical, mostly carotid artery dissections.[95,97,100,101] Fully 87% of the 572 patients were treated with anticoagulants in these series. Prevention of embolization of thrombus at or shortly after the dissection should prevent stroke. Anticoagulants have not seemed to increase the extent of the dissections, a major theoretical concern. The non-randomized

arm of the Cervical Artery Dissection in Stroke Study (CADISS-NR) included 88 patients treated either with antiplatelet therapy or anticoagulants.[102] The subsequent stroke rate was low in both groups and no differences were found. However the patients were mostly entered beyond 7 days after the diagnosis of dissection.[102] Whether one therapy is superior during the acute phase which is known to have the highest risk of stroke, has not been studied in randomized therapeutic trials. The recently completed randomized phase of Cervical Artery Dissection in Stroke Study (CADISS) included patients within 7 days of symptom onset; however, the results are not yet available.[102]

Physicians had worried that anticoagulants could increase the bleeding within the arterial wall and so promote arterial luminal occlusions. One report gives some evidence that occasionally anticoagulation can be problematic by showing delayed carotid artery occlusion after heparin use.[103] We use heparin then warfarin in those patients who have neurological ischemic symptoms, in those with severe narrowing of the arterial lumen, and those with intracranial embolic occlusions. Our reasons for choosing anticoagulants over antiplatelets follow: (1) evidence that red clot (erythrocyte–fibrin) thromboemboli enter the arterial lumen in dissection patients and

Table 7.4 Acute treatment in patients with neck arterial dissections in three series

Series	N	Antiplatelets	Anticoagulants	tPA	Surgery
Biousse et al.[95]	80	15 (19%)	58 (73%)	0	1 (1%)
Engelter et al.[100]	33	8 (24%)	25 (76%)	0	0
Touze et al.[101]	459	24 (5%)	416 (91%)*	2 (0.4%)	0
Totals	**572**	**47 (8%)**	**499 (87%)**	**2 (0.3%)**	**1 (0.2%)**

*405 heparin and 11 warfarin.
tpA, tissue plasminogen activator.

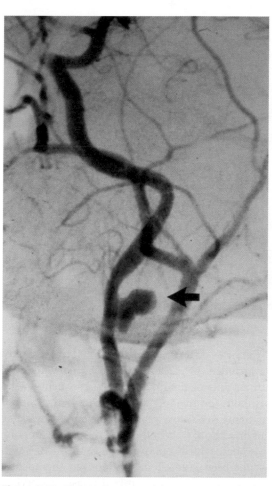

Figure 7.10 Right internal carotid dye-contrast digital subtraction cerebral angiogram showing an aneurysmal outpouching within the pharyngeal portion of the ICA in a patient with a carotid artery dissection.

anticoagulants are more effective against red clots than antiplatelets; (2) many reports of others that anticoagulants are effective and relatively safe; and (3) personal experience with more than 200 dissection patients treated with anticoagulants. We do favor a randomized trial testing this choice of anticoagulant treatment. Because the risk of embolization is only during the acute period, we use heparin, followed by warfarin or use of a newer oral anticoagulant, and try to maximize cerebral blood flow (CBF) during the acute period, to augment collateral circulation. Healing of dissections can be monitored using MRI, MRA, CTA, and US. We stop anticoagulants after 6 weeks in patients with dissected arteries that remain occluded. We continue anticoagulants in patients with patent arteries until luminal stenosis improves and blood flow is not importantly obstructed. When arterial blood flow is improved, we switch to drugs that modify platelet function such as aspirin, clopidogrel, cilostazole or aspirin with modified-release dipyridamole.

Thrombolytics have been given to a few patients with ICA neck dissections. They might be effective in patients with intracranial red clot embolization who do not have obstruction of the pharyngeal ICA, who are seen soon after neurological symptom onset and do not already have large brain infarcts. These circumstances are very unusual in our experience. Intravenous tissue plasminogen activator (tPA) is likely to be ineffective when the ICA is occluded. Stenting is rarely indicated since in patients without occlusions, the arterial lumens usually open well with time and anticoagulants are effective in preventing further thrombi from forming and embolizing. Stenting may be useful in the very rare carotid artery dissection patient who has tight luminal narrowing or recent occlusion and continues to have progressing or fluctuating neurological symptoms despite anticoagulants.[104,105]

Intracranial internal carotid artery disease

Narrowing and thrombotic occlusion of the ICA occur at the siphon far less often than at the ICA origin. The siphon includes the S-shaped portion of the carotid artery from its entry through the carotid foramen into the petrous bone to its exit from the cavernous sinus above the petrous clinoid. The ophthalmic artery originates from the ICA within the siphon. Less is known about the pathology of the artery in its entirely intraosseous course because the bone is seldom removed for study. Calcification of the ICA in the siphon is common.[106] Studies of groups of patients with ICA siphon disease report a high frequency of strokes, frequent coexistent extracranial vascular disease, and a high death rate from coronary artery disease.[107–112]

RY, a 70-year-old African-American man, had an attack of transient weakness of his right leg one week before he awakened with weakness of the right face and leg. This was accompanied by an unaccustomed reluctance to speak. He repeated spoken language normally and comprehension of written and spoken language was good. There was a past history of hypertension, angina pectoris and a high-pitched focal bruit was audible over the right neck.

The epidemiology of carotid siphon disease is probably similar to ICA-origin disease. African-Americans, however, have an unexpectedly high incidence of this lesion.[19] Accompanying disease at the ICA and vertebral artery origins is common. In one series of ICA-siphon disease patients, tandem ICA origin and siphon disease occurred in 62% of patients.[107] TIAs are less frequent and fewer in number in patients with siphon disease when compared with ICA-origin disease. The ratio of strokes to TIAs and asymptomatic patients is higher in carotid-siphon disease.

The presence of amaurosis fugax depends on the level of the lesion in the siphon. In our experience, the occlusive lesion is most often distal to the ophthalmic artery origin, so that ICA siphon disease is an uncommon cause of transient monocular visual loss.

On examination, there are usually no signs of collateral circulation through the ECA vessels of the face. The ocular and retinal pathologies discussed in ICA-origin disease are uncommon. We have seen a number of patients with angiographically verified thrombotic occlusion of the carotid siphon, who days later developed signs of decreased ophthalmic flow and reduced central retinal artery pressure. The mechanism of delayed ophthalmic ischemia is retrograde extension of the clot below the ophthalmic artery branch, a phenomenon documented at necropsy in patients with stenosis and thrombosis of the ICA siphon.[113] The thrombus can also extend retrograde into the neck and mimic occlusive disease at the ICA origin. Retrograde extension of clot is, however, rare if the siphon occlusion is caused by embolism.[113]

Too few patients have been well studied to allow a comparison of the topography and distribution of cerebral infarcts in patients with ICA-siphon disease, as compared with disease of the ICA origin or the MCA. Our impression is that separate infarcts in portions of the ACA and MCA territories are more common in carotid siphon disease. The leg is more often paretic in siphon disease, indicating ACA-territory damage. Sometimes, the lesions affect the center of the ACA and MCA territories, causing weakness of the lower extremity and face with relative sparing of the hand, whereas in ICA-origin disease, upper-extremity weakness is most common.

In RY, a carotid duplex scan showed moderate stenosis (50%) of the right ICA origin. TCD showed increased blood-flow velocities through the orbital window at the left carotid siphon, and reduced velocities in the left MCA and ACA. Velocities in the right intracranial arteries were normal. Angiography by femoral catheterization revealed severe stenosis of the left ICA just as it entered the siphon, well below the ophthalmic-artery origin (Figure 7.11). The left ICA origin had a shallow plaque without stenosis. No definite distal-branch artery occlusion was seen. MRI showed small infarcts in the paramedian frontal lobe and in the left posterior parietal lobe.

US studies confirmed severe carotid-siphon disease on the side appropriate to the symptoms and the infarcts found on MRI. TCD is effective for detecting and quantifying stenotic lesions of the intracranial ICA.[114,115] MRAs of the carotid siphon are often difficult to interpret. Tortuosity makes this a common area for artifacts. CTAs are more useful than MRAs in this region. The contralateral ICA-origin lesion was asymptomatic and not severe enough to reduce flow. The clinical signs of leg and foot weakness and transcortical motor aphasia were caused by ACA-territory ischemia. The infarct was caused by either low flow with good MCA collaterals or embolism originating from the irregular siphon stenosis.

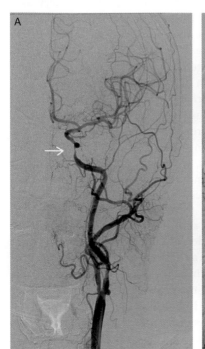
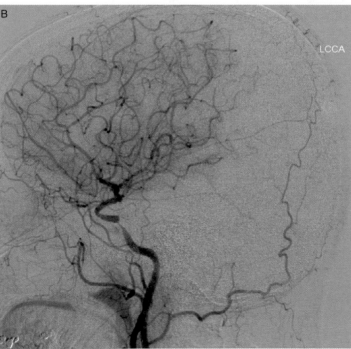

Figure 7.11 Dye contrast digital subtraction left carotid artery cerebral angiogram. (A) Anteroposterior view showing a severe area of narrowing of the ICA as it enters the carotid siphon (arrow). (B) Lateral view of the lesion. Courtesy of Dr Ajith Thomas, Neurosurgery, Beth Israel Deaconess Medical Center, Boston, MA.

RY was given intravenous heparin. After a slight increase in leg weakness during the first day, he stabilized. Warfarin was begun on day 5. On day 7, heparin was discontinued. The patient was maintained on warfarin therapy for one year, at which time he developed a fatal myocardial infarction.

Reviews in the 1980s confirm that ICA-siphon disease has a worse prognosis than ICA-origin disease.[107–112] Intracranial occlusive disease in general carries a worse prognosis than disease in the neck.[116] The closer the obstructing lesion to the brain, the more likely that infarction will occur. At the same time, when infarction is related to localized in-situ atherosclerosis, the infarcts tend to be relatively smaller than those caused by intra-arterial emboli originating in the neck, aorta, or heart.

Late strokes and cardiac death are common. Stenosis of the ICA in the siphon seems to be more stable than other intracranial lesions. Follow-up angiography shows a low rate of progression or regression of stenotic carotid siphon atherosclerotic lesions.[117] Lesions within the siphon cannot be treated surgically. Therapeutic alternatives include thrombolytics for patients who arrive soon after stroke onset, and to prevent worsening and for secondary stroke prevention antiplatelet agglutinating agents, warfarin, angioplasty, and ECA-ICA bypass to MCA branches. There have been no prospective controlled studies to fully document the effectiveness, or lack thereof, of any medical treatment in patients with disease of the carotid siphon, mostly because the number of recognized patients is relatively small. In some series, white men with TIAs relating to siphon disease had a relatively good outcome after warfarin therapy.[108,109]

The WASID trial randomized patients with intracranial stenosis to treatment with warfarin or 1300 mg of aspirin daily.[118–120] The study included 119 patients with stenosis of the intracranial ICA. Specific outcomes for this relatively small group of patients with ICA disease were not presented; however, in patients with all intracranial lesions there was no significant reduction in ischemic strokes and an increase in hemorrhages in patients treated with warfarin.[118–120] A higher mortality was observed in the warfarin group although many of the deaths in the warfarin group were not vascular deaths.

The tortuous, windy course and calcification within the siphon makes angioplasty or stenting of stenotic lesions difficult and risky. Some balloon angioplasties, however, have been performed without stents.[121–124] The Stenting and Aggressive Medical Management for Preventing Recurrent Stroke in Intracranial Stenosis (SAMMPRIS) trial randomized patients with intracranial stenosis to angioplasty and stenting (PTAS) and aggressive medical therapy or aggressive medical therapy alone.[125] Only 94 patients had 70–99% stenosis of the intracranial ICA. The study was terminated after enrollment of 451 patients due to a higher early stroke and hemorrhage rate in patients treated with percutaneous angioplasty and stenting. Outcomes were better in patients treated with aggressive medical therapy alone.[125] Although technical limitations of the stent and procedural skills may have contributed to the worse outcomes in the interventional group, at present it is difficult to justify endovascular treatment of intracranial stenosis except perhaps in the case of recurrent ischemia despite maximal medical therapy.

In patients who have occlusion of the ICA siphon and who arrive within 6–8 hours of neurological symptom onset, revascularization should be considered in those patients who have no or small brain infarcts. In many of these patients an embolus has reached the top of the carotid artery (Carotid T portion) and retrograde clot is found in the siphon. Within the first 3 hours, intravenous treatment should be used. If unsuccessful, endovascular therapy with mechanical devices such as stent retrievers can then be pursued. In published therapeutic trials, intracranial ICA occlusions are not separated into different siphon and Carotid T groups. We review the results of intracranial ICA occlusion interventions when discussing the Carotid T region. Promonitory TIAs that preceded the occlusion favor an in-situ thrombosis engrafted upon a previously very stenotic intracranial ICA. These patients are very difficult to recanalize by any method and anticoagulants and maximizing CBF are pursued.

Based on the results of the Warfarin–Aspirin Symptomatic Intracranial Disease (WASID) study, most patients with ICA siphon stenosis should be treated with antiplatelet therapy such as aspirin, clopidogrel, cilostazole, and/or combined low-dose aspirin and dipyridamole. For patients with tight ICA siphon stenosis and progressing or fluctuating symptoms despite antiplatelet therapy, anticoagulation can be considered. As with disease of the ICA origin, attention should also be directed to the heart because of the high incidence of associated cardiac morbidity (as in the case of RY).

In some patients, there is associated severe disease of the ICA origin in addition to the siphon stenosis. In these patients with tandem lesions, operation on the ICA in the neck is sometimes followed by opening of the siphon lesion on follow-up angiography.[126] This occurrence is explained by preoperative distal collapse or narrowing of the artery as a result of diminished flow. In the face of complete occlusion of the ICA siphon, there is no gain in opening an ICA-origin stenosis. If, however, the ICA stenosis at the siphon is not critical, carotid endarterectomy or stenting of the more proximal ICA-origin lesion might greatly augment flow.

In the presence of severe critical stenosis at both neck and intracranial sites, angioplasty/stenting can be performed at both sites during a single procedure. When tandem ICA occlusive lesions are present along with other occlusive extracranial and/or intracranial lesions, we usually choose anticoagulants or antiplatelet therapy and high-dose statins rather than aggressive attempts to open the tandem lesions. Aggressive surgery or interventional treatment mandates cessation of anticoagulants before and shortly after interventions and the use of anticoagulants plus double antiplatelets after stent placement. This scenario carries a relatively high risk of occlusion of other stenotic arteries during the cessation of anticoagulants and/or hemorrhage during the weeks and few months after the interventional procedures. In our estimate, the risks outweigh the benefits in most patients with widespread occlusive disease. We usually choose to prescribe warfarin or one of the newer oral anticoagulants for these patients.

Top of the carotid artery occlusions

Occlusions of the intracranial carotid artery bifurcation are predominantly embolic.[127,128] This portion of the ICA is often called the T portion because of its shape. When an embolus blocks the distal intracranial ICA, the result is usually a large infarct that includes the ACA and MCA territories. Often the thrombus propagates into the MCA. Death or severe disability often results. Occlusions of the distal intracranial carotid artery have been thought in the past to seldom recanalize with either intravenous or endovascular treatment. More recent analyses have been more optimistic about the potential for carotid T recanalization after thrombolysis.[129] In the IMS III trial, only 28% of carotid T occlusions recanalized with intravenous tPA alone, but the rate increased to 83% with the combined intravenous and intra-arterial approach.[51] Good outcome defined as mRS 0–2 was observed in only 4% of those treated with intravenous tPA and 27% of patients treated with combined therapy.[52] Two reviews analyzed the results of intra-arterial thrombolysis with or without mechanical clot extraction in large numbers of patients.[130,131] Among 201 patients with acute symptomatic ICA occlusions, 107 (53%) had ICA-T occlusions, and among these only 17 (16%) patients had favorable outcomes.[130] Mechanical extraction was more effective than thrombolytics in opening the artery.[130] In another endovascular series, among 623 patients the 75 patients with carotid T occlusions had the worst outcomes in the entire series.[131]

In the Diffusion Weighted Imaging Evaluation for Understanding Stroke Evolution Study-2 (DEFUSE-2) study, patients were eligible if they had a National Institutes of Health Stroke Scale (NIHSS) score of 5 or more, and a baseline MRI could be obtained within 90 minutes before endovascular therapy, and if the endovascular procedure could begin within 12 hours after stroke onset.[132] In this study, reperfusion rates were comparable in those with ICA (61%) and MCA (59%) occlusions. When reperfusion was obtained the percentages of favorable clinical response were similar between patients with stroke due to ICA (65%) and MCA (63%) occlusions. When reperfusion was not achieved, favorable outcomes were less frequent with obstructions of the ICA (9%) than the MCA (52%).[132,133]

Prophylactic management of patients with emboli to the carotid T depends on the nature and site of the lesion from which the thromboembolus originated. Severe stenosis and thrombotic occlusion of the supraclinoid carotid artery before its intracranial bifurcation into MCA and ACA branches (top of the carotid) rarely occurs. In our experience, an unusual number of patients with a lesion at this site have had coagulation abnormalities, such as sickle cell disease or circulating lupus anticoagulant.

Intracranial dissections involving the carotid artery

Intracranial anterior circulation dissections are much less common than those that involve the extracranial (mostly pharyngeal portion) of the ICA. When intracranial dissections do occur they often involve the ICA within or above the carotid siphon. Past reports of intracranial ICA dissections emphasize severe morbidity and mortality. LRC and colleagues recently reported 10 patients who had spontaneous intracranial ICA dissections.[134] Their ages ranged from 15 to 59 years (mean age 28 years). Severe retro-orbital or temporal headache followed by contralateral hemiparesis was the most common initial clinical presentation. No patient had vascular risk factors or a history of neck or head trauma. One patient had only a TIA, but the other nine had brain infarcts, one accompanied by some subarachnoid bleeding. The most common location of the dissection was in the supraclinoid ICA (eight patients) with extension to the MCA or anterior cerebral artery in two patients each. Aneurysm formation in the ipsilateral anterior cerebral artery was seen in one patient. Two patients had a total occlusion of the supraclinoid portion of the ICA. All patients did well, with no ($N = 3$), mild ($N = 4$), or moderate ($N = 3$) disability on the mRS during a 3-month follow-up period.[134] Others have also reported patients, often children and young adults, with intracranial ICA dissections that resulted in relatively good outcomes.[135,136] Dissections may also begin in the MCAs.

In those patients who present with ischemia and do not have any evidence of subarachnoid bleeding, we use anticoagulants acutely to prevent propagation and embolization of luminal thrombi. We have not found that subsequent aneurysmal rupture is an important risk in patients who present with ischemic symptoms.

Occlusion or severe stenosis of the middle cerebral artery stem or its major upper and lower trunks

Occlusion of the MCA was a common diagnosis in the era before cerebral angiography. After Fisher and others called attention to the high incidence of extracranial ICA disease[1-3] and angiography became prevalent, most patients formerly diagnosed with MCA occlusion were found instead to have ICA disease in the neck. The vast majority of MCA occlusions are embolic, arising from a proximal ICA plaque or from the heart or aorta. The observations on the rarity of occlusive lesions in the intracranial anterior circulation were generated at hospitals with a predominance of white patients. Studies of African-American[19,20,137,138] and Asian[139-144] patients show a higher frequency of intracranial occlusive disease of the MCA and its major trunk branches than is found in white patients. A necropsy study in Paris of the MCAs in 339 predominantly white stroke patients showed that 11% had non-stenotic atherosclerotic plaques, 13% had plaques causing 30–74% stenosis, and 6% had 75–99% stenosis or in-situ occlusion.[145] Figure 7.12 shows the most common patterns of infarction in patients with MCA occlusions.

A 48-year-old Chinese woman, AC, awakened with weakness of the right face and was unable to speak. These symptoms cleared during the day. Three days later, during the morning, she became unable to speak normally and recognized

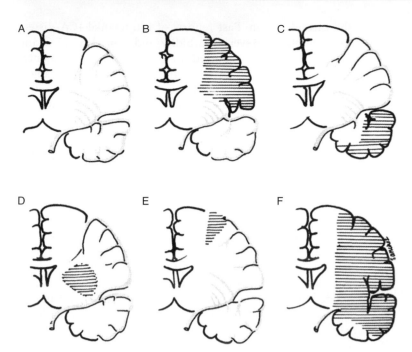

Figure 7.12 Common patterns of infarction with MCA occlusion: (A) normal cerebral hemisphere in coronal section; (B) occlusion of the upper trunk of the MCA; (C) occlusion of the lower trunk of the MCA; (D) infarct of the deep basal ganglia; (E) wedge infarct in the pial territory; and (F) whole MCA occlusion.

weakness of her right limbs. She had a past history of slight hypertension, but had no history of coronary or peripheral vascular disease. She came to the hospital 10 hours after the symptoms began.

In our experience, patients with MCA occlusive disease, when compared with patients with ICA disease, are more often African-American or Asian, young, female, hypertensive, and diabetic.[20,31,142,146] They also have had a lower incidence of hypercholesterolemia and associated coronary and peripheral vascular disease. Patients of Japanese, Chinese, Korean, and Thai descent, as well as diabetics and women taking contraceptive pills, share a propensity for MCA pathology with African-Americans. As in atherosclerotic neck disease, active lipid-laden plaques and ulcerations predispose to deposition of white and red thrombi and thrombosis of the artery.[147,148] The loosely attached thrombi can propagate and embolize distally as well as occlude the orifices of the penetrating lenticulostriate arteries.

Although TIAs do occur in patients with MCA disease, they are probably less frequent than with ICA disease and occur during a shorter time span.[31] The frequency of TIAs in patients with MCA disease also seems to vary with race. In four series of predominantly white patients with MCA occlusive disease, TIAs were a more frequent presentation than stroke.[149–152] The TIA-to-stroke ratios in these studies were 15 to 1,[149] 15 to 6,[150] 13 to 11,[151] and 9 to 4.[152] In contrast, the TIA–stroke ratio in a predominantly African-American patient series was 4 to 16.[31] It was 3 to 20 in a series of mostly Chinese-origin patients,[146] and 8 to 28 in a series of Japanese patients.[153] Smoking was an important risk factor in a large study that reported its frequency.[143] Eighty percent of patients with MCA occlusion and 72% of patients with MCA stenosis had a history of cigarette smoking.[143] Because the vascular lesion is intracranial and, of course, beyond the ophthalmic artery supply, transient monocular blindness does not occur.

During the first 3 days in the hospital, AC progressively worsened, gradually developing a complete right hemiplegia, minor tingling of the right limbs, and mutism. Examination revealed no bruits, facial, or limb-pulse abnormalities.

Patients with MCA disease often develop their deficits more gradually than comparable series of patients with ICA disease.[31,146] Patients with MCA disease often note their abnormalities on awakening in the morning or after a nap and often have subsequent fluctuations or progression during the next 1–7 days. This gradual onset and progressive course support a low flow contribution to the ischemia. Deficits begin when flow is most sluggish, and collateral circulation takes time to develop and equilibrate. Recent studies using TCD show that microemboli often originate from regions of MCA stenosis.[154–156] As in the ICA, reduced perfusion results in poor washout of emboli. Production of thromboemboli and reduced clearance both contribute to infarction.[43,44] In contrast, patients with ICA disease more often have sudden-onset deficits while awake and thereafter remain stable (a course better explained by embolism of large white, red, or mixed clots from their ICA lesion than by reduced perfusion alone). Intrinsic MCA occlusive lesions cause symptoms by: (1) being the intra-arterial source of emboli mostly to pial branches on the convexal surface; (2) decreased perfusion causing borderzone region ischemia both involving deep and superficial borderzone regions; and (3) by plaques and thrombi blocking flow through deep lenticulostriate branches causing deep gray and white matter infarcts. In many patients these mechanisms are combined.

Because the occlusive process is intracranial, there are no important associated signs of extracranial disease. Neurological findings vary, depending on the location of the vascular occlusion and the location and extent of brain

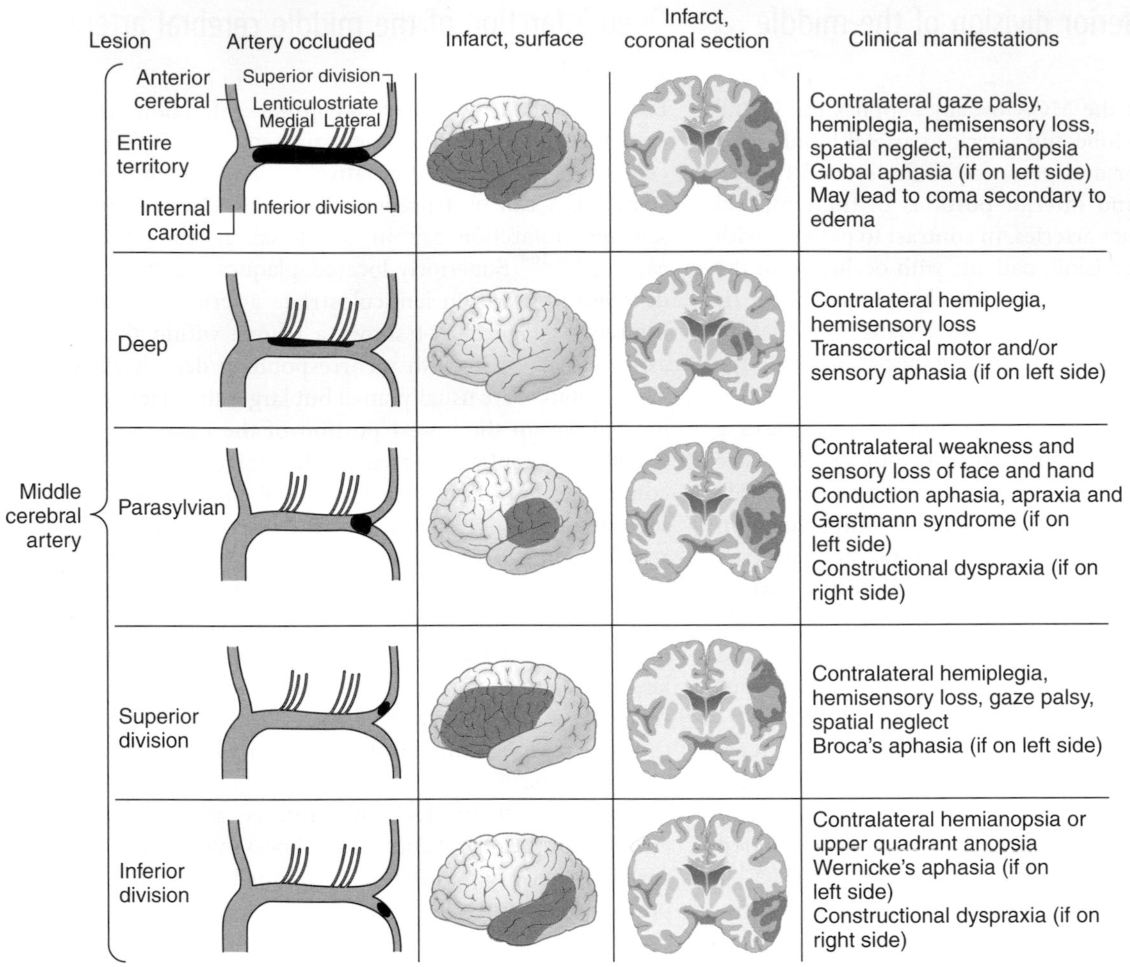

Lesion	Artery occluded	Infarct, surface	Infarct, coronal section	Clinical manifestations
Middle cerebral artery — Entire territory (Anterior cerebral, Superior division, Lenticulostriate Medial Lateral, Internal carotid, Inferior division)				Contralateral gaze palsy, hemiplegia, hemisensory loss, spatial neglect, hemianopsia Global aphasia (if on left side) May lead to coma secondary to edema
Deep				Contralateral hemiplegia, hemisensory loss Transcortical motor and/or sensory aphasia (if on left side)
Parasylvian				Contralateral weakness and sensory loss of face and hand Conduction aphasia, apraxia and Gerstmann syndrome (if on left side) Constructional dyspraxia (if on right side)
Superior division				Contralateral hemiplegia, hemisensory loss, gaze palsy, spatial neglect Broca's aphasia (if on left side)
Inferior division				Contralateral hemianopsia or upper quadrant anopsia Wernicke's aphasia (if on left side) Constructional dyspraxia (if on right side)

Figure 7.13 Patterns of occlusion of the MCA and their anatomical correlates.

ischemia.[157] The following sections discuss the most common patterns of neurological deficits seen in patients with MCA disease. Although these syndromes are discussed under the heading of intrinsic MCA-occlusive disease, the patterns are more commonly caused by embolism to the MCA territory. Figure 7.13 shows the common patterns of MCA occlusion and their anatomical and clinical correlates.

Occlusion or stenosis of upper division of the MCA

The superior division of the MCA supplies the frontal and superior parietal lobes. It can be thought of as supplying the MCA territory above the sylvian fissure. Occasionally, when the mainstem MCA is short, the lenticulostriate vessels arise from the proximal portion of the superior trunk.[31,158,159] In that case, the internal capsule and lateral basal ganglia are also nourished by the superior trunk.

The findings include: (1) hemiplegia, more severe in the face, hand, and upper extremity, with relative sparing of the lower extremity; (2) hemisensory loss, usually including decreased pinprick and position sense, sometimes sparing the leg; (3) conjugate eye deviation, with the eyes resting toward the side of the brain lesion; and (4) neglect of the contralateral side of space, especially to visual stimuli. Visual neglect is usually more severe in patients with right hemisphere lesions.

When the lesion is in the left dominant hemisphere, there invariably is an accompanying aphasia. Verbal output is sparse and patients do not do what they are asked to do with either hand. They may follow whole-body commands such as turn over, sit, and stand. They may be able to nod appropriately to yes and no questions, but comprehension of written material is poor. With time, a pattern of Broca's aphasia evolves with sparse, effortful speech, poor pronunciation of syllables, and omission of filler words. Comprehension of spoken language is usually preserved.

Patients who have superior-division MCA infarcts in the right hemisphere often seem unaware of their deficit (anosognosia) and may not admit they are hemiplegic or impaired in any way.[33,34,160] Some patients are also impersistent; they perform requested tasks quickly, but fail to persevere and terminate tasks prematurely.[33,34,161] When asked to read, patients with right superior-trunk occlusions often omit the left of the page or paragraph, and do not heed people or objects to their left.

Occlusion of the inferior division of the middle cerebral artery

The inferior division of the MCA usually supplies the lateral surface of the temporal lobe and inferior parietal lobule. The supply is mostly inferior and posterior to the sylvian fissure. The anterior, medial, and inferior portions of the temporal lobes are supplied by other arteries. In contrast to patients with lesions of the superior division, patients with occlusion of the MCA inferior division usually have no elementary motor or sensory abnormalities. They often have a visual field defect, either a hemianopia or an upper quadrantanopia, affecting the contralateral visual field.

When the left hemisphere is involved, patients have a Wernicke-type aphasia. Speech is fluent, and syllables are well pronounced. Patients use wrong or non-existent words and often what is said makes little sense. Comprehension and repetition of spoken language are poor. There may be relative sparing of written comprehension, with the patient preferring that words be written rather than spoken.[162,163] When the right hemisphere is affected, patients draw and copy poorly, and may have difficulty finding their way about or reading a map.

Behavioral abnormalities also frequently accompany temporal-lobe infarctions. Patients with Wernicke's aphasia are sometimes irascible, paranoid, and may become violent. Patients with right temporal infarcts often have an agitated hyperactive state resembling delirium tremens.[164–166] Diagnosis of right inferior-trunk occlusion is sometimes difficult unless patients are examined thoroughly. The key neurological findings are a left visual-field defect and poor drawing and copying in an agitated person.[166]

Deep infarction of the middle cerebral artery territory

Basal ganglia and internal-capsule infarction is usually explained by occlusion of the mainstem MCA before its lenticulostriate branches. Alternatively, plaques within the mainstem MCA can obstruct lenticulostriate branches leading to selective infarction within the basal ganglia and internal capsule.[167,168] Superiorly-located plaques are most likely to decrease flow within lenticulostriate arteries and cause deep infarcts.[168] Figure 7.14 shows a plaque within the superior aspect of an MCA with a corresponding deep brain infarct. These infarcts are usually small but larger than lacunes and are located within the lowest portion of the basal ganglia.[167,168] Excellent potential exists for collateral circulation over the convexities but there is poor collateral circulation potential in the deep basal gray nuclei and the internal capsule. For this reason, some patients with MCA occlusion have selective ischemia of the deep lenticulostriate territory. Collateral circulation is often adequate to prevent cortical infarction. On CT or MRI scans, the lesions can be confused with lacunes, but are larger and often extend to the inferior brain surface. Some have called these lesions giant lacunes.[31,169] The preferred term for these deep MCA lenticulostriate-territory lesions is striatocapsular infarcts.[146,170,171]

Patients with stratiocapsular infarcts are invariably hemiparetic, but the distribution of weakness in face, arm, and leg is variable. Sensory loss is usually minor because the posterior portion of the internal capsule is spared. When the lesion is in the left hemisphere, after a short period of temporary mutism, speech is sparse and dysarthric, but repetition of spoken language is preserved. Comprehension of spoken and written

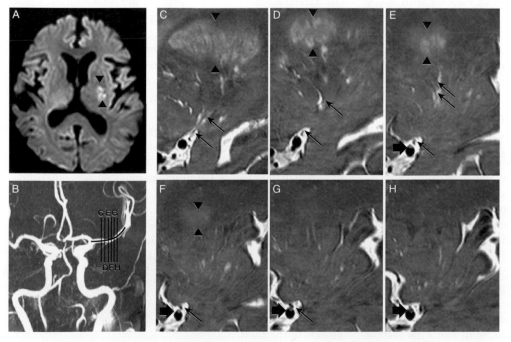

Figure 7.14 An illustrative patient showing superior plaque in the MCA causing single subcortical infarction. Diffusion-weighted MRI (A) and sagittal images of high resolution MRI (C–F) show single subcortical infarction (arrowheads). MRA (B) shows no significant stenosis in the left MCA. Lines C–H indicate the location of each panel. High resolution MRI (C–H) shows the traceable perforators (thin arrows) originating from the superiorly located plaque (thick arrows) that blocks the perforators (F–H). Kindly submitted by Professor Jong Kim.

language depends on the size and anteroposterior extent of the lesion.[172,173] When the right hemisphere is involved, there often is neglect of contralateral visual and tactile stimuli, but this is usually more transient than with parietal cortical infarction.

Mainstem occlusion with total infarction of the middle cerebral artery territory

Mainstem occlusion with total infarction of the MCA territory is most common in patients with embolism to the proximal MCA (Figure 4.19). In most patients with intrinsic occlusive disease of the MCA, there is sufficient collateral circulation to spare at least the outer borders of the territory.

These patients are usually devastated. Among 208 patients with large MCA-territory infarcts in one series, the mortality rate was 17%. Fifty percent of patients had severe disability.[174] Severe paralysis, hemisensory loss, attentional hemianopia, and conjugate eye deviation to the opposite side were found. When the left hemisphere is involved, there is a global aphasia. Right hemisphere lesions produce severe neglect, anosognosia, disinterest or poor motivation, apathy, and severe constructional apraxia. Recovery to useful function is unusual.[175]

Brain edema with swelling of the infarcted hemisphere, causing a midline shift and brain herniations, is an important complication in patients with large MCA-territory infarction.[174] This complication is especially apt to develop in young patients with large embolic MCA-territory infarcts. Coma usually heralds a fatal outcome. Many young and older patients with large MCA-territory infarcts and severe brain edema have been treated with hemicraniectomy and have survived.[176–178] Survivors often have severe neurological deficits and are dependent on others for activities of daily living.

Segmental infarction in the middle cerebral artery territory

Segmental infarctions in the MCA territory are caused by occlusion of the distal cortical branches of the upper or lower division of the MCA. They are almost invariably embolic and are seldom caused by intrinsic atheromatous occlusion of a convexity branch. The syndromes are quite variable and depend on the branch affected.[157]

Insula of reil infarction

Infarction of a portion of the insular cortex is quite common in patients with embolic occlusion of the MCA. One of the clues to MCA infarction, known for some time, is the so-called "insular ribbon" sign on CT scans of patients with acute brain ischemia. Figure 7.15 is an MRI of an infarct involving predominantly a portion of the insular cortex. Among 150 consecutive patients with acute non-lacunar brain ischemia studied at the Beth Israel Deaconess Medical Center in Boston using modern multimodal MRI, we found that 72 (48%) had insular infarcts on DWI.[179] Major insular lesions were present in 34 (23%) and 38 (25%) had minor lesions. Insula infarcts were associated with lenticulostriate territory

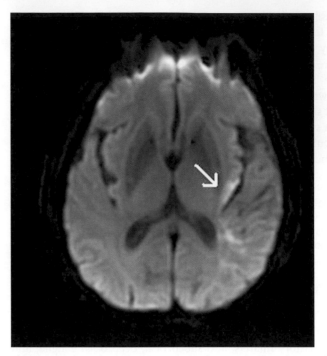

Figure 7.15 MRI–DWI image showing an infarct involving predominantly the inferior portion of the left insular cortex (white arrow).

infarction, more severe neurological deficits, and proximal MCA occlusion detected on MRA.[179]

Several patterns were apparent: (1) infarction limited to the anterior portion of the insula, often accompanied by infarcts in the suprasylvian territory of the MCA; (2) infarcts limited to the posterior insula, often accompanied by temporal and inferior parietal lobe infarction in territory supplied by the inferior division of the MCA; (3) and major infarcts involving the anterior and posterior insula, often accompanied by striato-capsular infarcts and/or involvement of cortical and subcortical territories supplied by the superior and/or inferior division of the MCA.[179] The superior division of the MCA supplies the anterior insular cortex, and the inferior division supplies the posterior insular cortex. When the entire insula (or parts of the anterior and posterior insula) are infarcted, the occlusive lesion must have at some time involved the mainstem MCA.

Animal and some human observations indicate that the insular cortex has important autonomic and cardiovascular control functions.[180–184] Oppenheimer and colleagues stimulated the insular cortex of human epileptic patients.[180,181] They found that when they electrically stimulated areas of the left human insular cortex, bradycardia, and blood pressure depression responses resulted, while stimulation of the right insular cortex elicited tachycardia and pressor effects.[180] Stimulation of the left insula decreased protective parasympathetic effects and increased cardiovascular sympathetic effects on the heart rate and blood pressure. This asymmetry of autonomic function was also shown by Yoon and colleagues who studied autonomic function in patients evaluated for epilepsy surgery.[182] They found that the right cerebral hemisphere predominantly modulated sympathetic nervous system activity. Hachinski et al. showed that rats with experimentally induced, right-MCA occlusions developed an increase in Q-T intervals and

had elevated plasma norepinephrine levels, while sham-operated and left-MCA occlusion animals had neither of these findings.[183] They concluded that right-cerebral hemisphere infarcts caused more sympathetic nervous system perturbations than comparable left hemisphere infarcts.[183] Other investigators have shown using power spectrum analysis of heart rate variability that stroke patients with MCA territory infarcts have a significant sympathetic/parasympathetic imbalance.[184] These cardiovascular changes have usually been predominantly attributed to the insula of Reil in the respective cerebral hemispheres.

> Neck US in patient AC was normal. Blood-sugar levels were high on admission and remained elevated until insulin was begun. DWI-MRI showed a deep striatocapsular infarct. Perfusion MRI showed a large perfusion defect occupying most of the deep and superficial MCA territory. TCD showed an absence of flow velocities in the left MCA with normal ACA and right-sided values. Angiography showed occlusion of the left mainstem MCA after a tapered, irregular origin.

CT patterns of MCA-territory infarction have already been described. The most common patterns are wedge-shaped, pial-territory infarcts, and subcortical, deep basal ganglia, and internal-capsule infarcts.[157] Hyperdensity of the MCA in non-contrast-enhanced CT scans is an important and relatively common finding in patients with acute-onset MCA-territory infarcts (see Figure 4.19). In one series among 55 patients, one-third had the hyperdense MCA sign.[185] TCD is a useful technique for showing MCA disease.[114,115,186,187] Stenosis often causes high velocities when insonating at the depth of the lesion. When the MCA is occluded, flow and velocities decline, and often no signal can be obtained. TCD can be used to rapidly diagnose embolic MCA occlusion and monitor recanalization during and after thrombolysis.[187] TCD monitoring sometimes shows microembolic signals in patients with MCA stenosis.[155,156,187,188] This indicates embolism from the MCA lesion, a situation also documented to occur at necropsy in patients with thrombi engrafted on MCA stenotic lesions.[189]

MRA and CTA, with concentration on intracranial views, can also usually document severe MCA occlusive lesions.[190,191] MRA tends to overestimate the degree of stenosis although complete signal dropout at the site of stenosis usually signifies a severe stenosis.[192] When MRA or CTA shows widely patent arteries it is unlikely that any significant stenosis would be found by angiography. Using standard dye-contrast angiography, MCA occlusion is best seen on the anteroposterior view of a selective ICA injection. At times, the occlusion is near the MCA trifurcation, so oblique views are needed. The area of poorest supply of MCA tributaries is best identified on lateral views. At times, poor opacification of inferior and superior trunk arteries is seen, and it is difficult to identify the precise point of narrowing or occlusion.

> AC was treated with heparin. The neurological deficit continued to progress. She remained on warfarin for 2 months. Repeat angiography showed good collateral filling of the MCA from ACA and PCA branches. The infarct on a T2-weighted MRI scan at 2 months matched the perfusion defect on the perfusion-weighted MRI performed initially.

Therapy of intrinsic MCA disease is uncertain because there have been few series of patients studied and seldom have the studies included treatment begun during the acute period of ischemia. In patients with acute thrombotic or embolic MCA occlusion, thrombolytic treatment is sometimes effective if given early enough. Thrombolytic therapy is more likely to lead to recanalization in patients with MCA emboli than in those with in-situ thrombosis engrafted on atherosclerosis. Early studies showed that intravenous[193–196] and intra-arterial[197] thrombolysis could be effective in recanalizing MCA embolic occlusions. Subsequent studies have shown that the rate of recanalization of intracranial anterior circulation occlusions is relatively low after intravenous tPA. Table 7.5 shows the rate of recanalization in patients with ICA-T, M1 MCA, and M2 MCA occlusions shown by CTA and/or TCD after intravenous tPA and after interventional treatments, data acquired at the Calgary stroke center between 2002 and 2009.[198] In patients with thrombotic disease within the MCA, thrombi often reform within the MCA after thrombolysis unless angioplasty is performed after the clot is lysed.

During the past two decades. angioplasty and stenting were increasingly often performed to dilate occlusive MCA-stenotic lesions.[121–124,199–201] Figure 6.2 contains angiograms of a patient with an irregular MCA mainstem stenosis that was treated successfully with a WingSpan stent. Angioplasty can be complicated by occlusion of lenticulostriate branches with resultant striatocapsular infarction.[200] Dissection and vasoconstriction are other complications of angioplasty on the mainstem MCA.[200] The success of angioplasty depends greatly on the location, length, angulation, and morphology of the

Table 7.5 The overall rate of partial and complete TCD and angiographic evidence of acute recanalization in patients with intracranial anterior circulation arterial occlusions

Occlusion location	Recanalization (all)	Recanalization after intravenous tPA	Recanalization after interventional Rx	No recanalization
ICA-T	43.5%	4%	39%	56.5%
M1 MCA	75%	32%	43%	25%
M2 MCA	92%	31%	61.5%	8%

Modified from Bhatia R, Hill MD, Shobha N, et al. Low rates of acute recanalization with intravenous recombinant tissue plasminogen activator in ischemic stroke: Real-world experience and a call for action. *Stroke* 2010;41:2254–2258.

MCA-occlusive lesion.[201] Despite the potential for treatment of intracranial stenosis with stenting, the Stenting and Aggressive Medical Management for Preventing Recurrent stroke in Intracranial Stenosis (SAMMPRIS) trial failed to show any significant benefit over intensive medical therapy.[125,202] Much of the reason for the superior result of medical therapy was the unexpected success of aggressive medical treatment, which included monitoring the results of treatments and used lifestyle coaches. Whether angioplasty alone would result in fewer complications and better outcomes than stenting remains to be determined.

Heparin, low-molecular-weight heparin, and heparinoids have been given to patients with acute-thrombotic and embolic-MCA occlusions. Warfarin is then used to attempt to prevent propagation and embolization from the MCA thrombus during a period of 6 weeks to 3 months. The newer anticoagulants could also theoretically be used instead of heparin and warfarin, but there is no present experience with this strategy. During anticoagulation, the clot becomes organized and adherent, and collateral circulation maximizes. Warfarin has been also used to prevent total occlusion of a stenosed MCA.

In the series of Hinton et al., white patients often stabilized while taking warfarin.[149] However, in series of black and Asian patients, anticoagulation has been reported to be less successful.[31,110,146] MCA pathology and pathophysiology may differ among whites, blacks, Asians, and others. In the WASID trial, which retrospectively compared outcome in patients with intracranial occlusive disease treated with aspirin or warfarin, warfarin was more effective.[203] In this study, MCA-stenotic lesions were the most common intracranial stenotic lesions studied and the patients were treated acutely usually with heparin followed by warfarin.[203] In the prospective randomized WASID trial, aspirin (1300 mg/day) was as effective and caused less hemorrhage than warfarin.[118,119] This trial was a secondary prevention trial and patients were enrolled after the acute ischemic period. Warfarin was a bit more effective than aspirin, and did not cause excessive bleeding in those patients in whom the INR values remained in the therapeutic range.[119]

We tend to use warfarin anticoagulation in patients with severe MCA stenosis, keeping the INR between 2.0 and 2.5, particularly if deficits are fluctuating or progressing. If ischemic symptoms are not controlled with intensive medical therapy, we consider angioplasty or stenting in selected patients with lesions amenable to this treatment.

Occlusion or severe stenosis of the anterior cerebral artery

Intrinsic occlusive disease of the ACA is unusual. Most ACA-territory infarcts are caused by embolism from the heart or the ICA. Many patients with intrinsic disease of the ACA also have extensive ICA and MCA disease, often with multiple infarcts, making clinicopathological correlation of the ACA lesions difficult.[204,205] In Asian countries, especially Japan, many ACA-territory infarcts are attributable to intracranial

dissections of the ACA or its branches.[206–213] Among 17 intracranial dissections, found among 194 patients with isolated ACA, MCA, and PCA infarcts studied by angiography in one Japanese center, two-thirds involved the ACA.[212] In another report, 43% of patients with isolated ACA territory infarcts had ACA dissections.[211] The A2 and A3 segments were predominantly involved in these reports. These locations are infrequent sites of intrinsic atherosclerosis and also infrequently involved with emboli. Other ACA-territory infarcts are caused by vasospasm-related ischemia in patients with SAH who have aneurysms of the anterior communicating artery.[214]

In one study of cerebral infarcts documented by CT, 13 of 413 (3%) were in the ACA territory.[215] Eight of the 13 patients with ACA-territory ischemia had angiography that showed five ACA occlusions. In three other patients, angiography showed ACA occlusion, but the CT showed no infarction in this territory. Nearly all patients in this series with occlusion of the ACA had severe occlusive disease at the origin of the ICA in the neck or in the carotid siphon on the side of the ACA lesion.[215] The most likely mechanism of ACA-territory infarction in this group of patients was intra-arterial embolism arising from the more proximal ICA lesions. In one patient, the authors postulated that intra-arterial embolic material traveled from an occluded ICA origin to the contralateral ACA, through a widely patent anterior communicating artery.

In the Lausanne Stroke Registry, 27 of 1490 patients (1.8%) with first-ever strokes had infarcts limited to the ACA territory.[216] Ten of the 27 patients had ICA-occlusive lesions and seven had cardiac-origin embolism. Only one patient, a Vietnamese man, had intrinsic ACA-occlusive disease. In the remainder of the patients, the cause of the ACA-territory infarcts was not discovered.[216]

Our experience and that of others[205,215–217] leads us to the following opinions about the mechanisms of ACA-territory infarction: (1) ACA-territory infarction is most often embolic; (2) embolism is most often artery to artery, arising from proximal ICA occlusive disease; (3) when intrinsic atherostenosis affects the ACA, patients usually have widespread extracranial and intracranial occlusive disease with multiple brain infarcts; (4) patients of Asian extraction often have predominantly intracranial occlusive disease, sometimes involving the ACA; and (5) stenotic lesions of the ACA are not always in the horizontal first portion of the artery, but can involve the pericallosal artery and other branches. Figure 7.16 depicts patterns of ACA occlusion and their anatomical correlates.

The ACA, after its brief horizontal A1 segment, gives off penetrating arteries that supply anteromedial portions of the caudate nucleus, anterior limb of the internal capsule, and the anterior perforated substance.[218–221] One group of these penetrators is usually termed "the artery of Heubner," but analyses of anatomical specimens shows that there are more often a group of relatively parallel Heubner and medial striate arteries rather than a single artery.[219,221] After reaching the midline, the ACA swings posteriorly and divides to form the pericallosal and callosomarginal arteries that supply the paramedian frontal lobe above the corpus callosum. Figures 2.11, 2.12, and 2.15 show the ACA and its

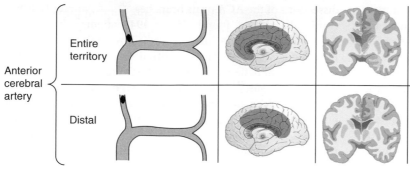

| | Incontinence
Contralateral hemiplegia
Abulia
Transcortical motor aphasia or
motor and sensory aphasia
Left limb dyspraxia |

Figure 7.16 Patterns of occlusion of the anterior cerebral artery and their anatomical correlates.

| | Contralateral weakness of leg, hip, foot and shoulder
Sensory loss in foot
Transcortical motor aphasia or motor and sensory aphasia
Left limb dyspraxia |

usual region of supply. At times, the A1 segment of the ACA on one side may be absent or hypoplastic, so that both ACAs are supplied by one ICA. The extent of infarction after ACA occlusion depends on the location of the obstruction and the pattern of the anterior circle of Willis.

> A 75-year-old man, CF, awakened from a nap with paralysis of his left leg and foot. He also had slight tingling in his left toes. Examination showed complete paralysis of the left lower extremity. When asked to salute, wave goodbye, or pretend to throw a ball, he performed these functions normally with the right arm, but used incorrect movements with the left arm. His arms, however, were not weak or clumsy. The patient was surprised to find that, on occasion, the left hand would grasp the right hand in the midst of an activity and seemed to do things without his will.

The single most important clue to an ACA-territory infarct is the distribution of motor weakness. Paralysis is usually greatest in the foot, but is also severe in the proximal thigh. Shoulder shrug is weak on the involved side, but the hand and face are usually normal if the deep ACA territory is spared. Some patients with anterior or large ACA-territory infarcts have a hemiplegia.[205] Some patients with medial frontal infarcts in the ACA territory have prominent motor neglect.[222] These individuals have little voluntary movement on the hemiparetic side. Despite the lack of spontaneous movement, strong prodding induces slow, clumsy arm movements. In these patients, the lower-extremity paralysis is explained by involvement of the precentral gyrus motor cortex. The upper limb motor dysfunction, however, is related to infarction of the premotor cortex anterior to the precentral gyrus.[222] Cortical sensory loss is also present in the weak limbs but is usually slight. The patient may have difficulty touching the spot on his or her lower extremity touched by the examiner, be unable to identify numbers written on his or her foot with a blunt pencil, or extinguish bilateral tactile stimuli on the paralyzed foot and leg. A grasp reflex is often present in the hand contralateral to the infarct.

Another helpful sign is apraxia of the left arm. Normally, speech is received in the posterior portions of the left cerebral hemisphere. To communicate language to regions of the right hemisphere that control the left limbs, the information goes forward toward the left frontal region and then across the corpus callosum to the right frontal region. In ACA-territory infarcts, the corpus callosum or its adjacent white matter is often infarcted. This interrupts the pathway, regardless of whether the right or left ACA territory is infarcted.[223–225] This anterior disconnection can be detected by the following simple bedside tests:

1. Ask the patient to perform spoken commands with the right and left arms. Patients with ACA infarction may be unable to perform the commands correctly using the left hand. The fact that they follow the commands normally with the right hand proves they understand the commands.
2. Ask the patient to write or print first with the right hand, then with the left hand. Some patients with ACA infarction make aphasic errors when they write using the left hand.
3. Ask the patient to name objects placed first in the left hand, then in the right hand. Patients with an ACA infarct may be unable to name objects in their left hand, but can select the same objects by vision or touch and can name them correctly when placed in the right hand. The topic of left limb apraxia was reviewed by Geschwind and Kaplan,[223,224] and has often been referred to as an anterior disconnection syndrome.

When the infarct involves the left ACA territory and supplementary motor cortex, a transcortical motor and sensory aphasia often results.[205,226–228] Despite reduced spontaneous speech, the patient can repeat spoken language well. Incontinence that is characterized by inability to control micturition, although the urge to urinate is preserved, may occur especially in patients with bilateral lesions. Patients with unilateral ACA infarcts or bilateral frontal infarcts are often abulic. They are apathetic with decreased spontaneity, show slowness in responding to queries or commands, and use terse speech that is limited in amount.[229–231] These patients have difficulty counting quickly from 20 to 1, or in persevering with any protracted task such as crossing off all the letter A's in a paragraph or telling the examiner without prodding each time their finger is moved or touched. In some patients, the decreased activity is intermittent. At one moment patients speak. The next moment they stare blankly and pay no heed to queries or conversation, as if their brain were temporarily shut off.[229–232]

Another phenomenon found in some patients with frontal-lobe infarction related to ACA disease has been called the alien hand sign.[205,233–235] CF had noticed that his left hand had a mind of its own, often doing things that he did not will it to do. This sign is most common in the right hand that interferes with

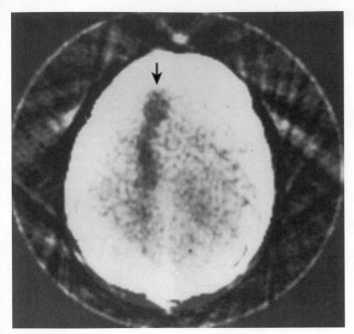

Figure 7.17 CT scan showing linear infarct in the right anterior cerebral artery territory (black arrow).

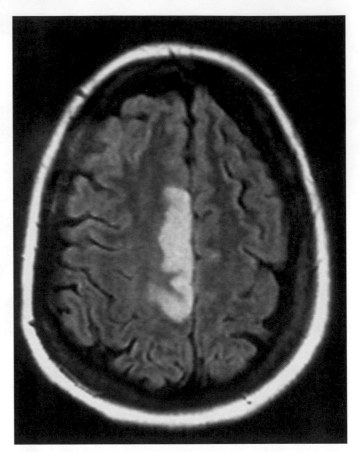

Figure 7.18 MRI FLAIR image showing a typical anterior cerebral artery cortical infarct located along the paramedian cerebral cortex.

willed movements of the left hand. One hand acts against the other or acts involuntarily. Similar findings occur in patients with epilepsy after surgical cutting of the corpus callosum, making it likely that the phenomenon is caused by defective interhemispheric connections. Forced grasping and a heightened grasp reflex found often contralateral to frontal-lobe lesions may also play a role in causing this sign.

> The CT scan in patient CF showed a moderate-sized, right medial frontal infarct in CF (Figure 7.17), and angiography documented severe stenosis of the right ACA before it formed the callosomarginal artery. After physical therapy, he was able to walk with a brace.

MRI is able to show the topography of ACA-territory infarction quite well. Figure 7.17 is a CT scan and Figure 7.18 is an MRI showing typical paramedian ACA-territory infarcts in patients who had paralysis of the contralateral foot, leg, and thigh. Little is known about treatment for intrinsic ACA disease. LRC elected not to expose this older gentleman with an already sizable infarct to the risk of anticoagulation because little additional damage would ensue, even if the remainder of the right ACA territory were infarcted.

Occasionally, patients have the sudden development of bilateral ACA-territory infarction.[236–238] Figure 7.19 is a CT scan that shows a large, bilateral ACA-territory infarct. Figure 7.20 is a necropsy specimen of a patient with asymmetric large right and left ACA-territory infarcts. Bilateral ACA-territory infarction is most often explained by hypoplasia or absence of the A1 segment of the ACA on one side. In that circumstance, the territories of the ACA on both sides are supplied by one ACA. On angiography, dye instillation into one ICA produces bilateral ACA opacification. Occlusion of the ICA or ACA supplying both sides leads to bilateral

frontal-lobe infarction. The resulting clinical picture is sudden apathy, abulia, and incontinence.[236–238] When the paracentral lobule is involved, weakness on one or both sides occurs. This predominantly affects the lower extremities. The sudden onset of a frontal lobe type of dementia presents a striking clinical picture, especially to those unfamiliar with this rare syndrome.

Caudate infarcts

One of the major branch territories of the ACA is that of the recurrent arteries of Heubner, which supply the head of the caudate nucleus and the anterior limb of the internal capsule.[220,239,240] Much of the lateral portion of the caudate nucleus is supplied by the lateral lenticulostriate branches of the MCA. Although older descriptions spoke of a single Heubner's artery, newer dissections show there usually are multiple, parallel penetrating arteries arising from the ACA near the anterior communicating artery junction. In approximately 25% of individuals, there is a single Heubner's artery; often, there are two, three, or even four recurrent arteries.[218,219] Occlusion of one of these penetrating arteries, or of the parent ACA before the origin of the perforators, leads to infarcts in the head of the caudate nucleus. The infarction also often involves the anterior limb of the internal capsule and the most anterior part of the putamen. Medial and lateral lenticulostriate artery branches of the MCA supply the caudate

241

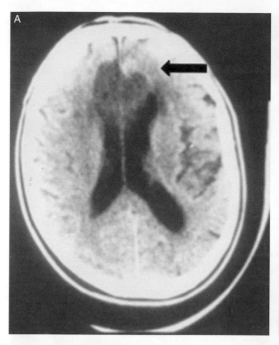

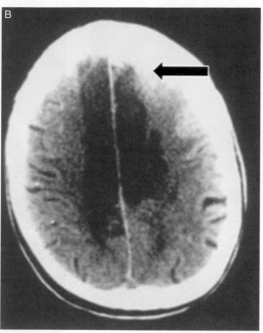

Figure 7.19 CT scan showing large bilateral paramedian anterior cerebral artery territory infarcts in a patient who suddenly developed bilateral lower-limb paralysis and mutism. (A) CT scan showing bilateral infarction involving the corpus callosum and cingulate gyri just anterior to the lateral ventricles. (black arrow) (B) Higher CT scan section showing extensive bilateral paramedian anterior cerebral artery territory infarction (black arrow). Courtesy of Noble, David MD.

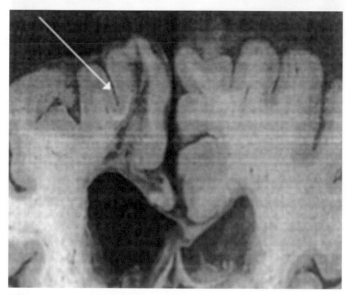

Figure 7.20 Post-mortem necropsy coronal slice of brain showing a large anterior cerebral artery-territory infarct above the very enlarged left lateral ventricle (white arrow). The corpus callosum is necrotic, and the infarct extends toward the right cingulate gyrus.

nucleus, anterior limb of the internal capsule, and the putamen. Figure 7.21 shows a montage of the findings from CT scans from a series of patients with caudate infarcts.[220]

The clinical signs of caudate infarction are quite variable. Motor weakness is not prominent, although many patients have slight, but usually transient, hemiparesis. Among 18 patients in one series, 13 patients (72%) had some weakness in the limbs contralateral to the infarct. In most patients, however, the motor dysfunction was minor and recovered quickly.[221] Dysarthria is a more common finding and was present in 11 of 18 patients (61%) with caudate infarcts in one series,[220] and in 18 of 21 patients (86%) in another series.[239] Occasionally,

patients with caudate infarcts have a movement disorder, usually choreoathetosis in the contralateral limbs, as the major clinical manifestation of caudate nucleus infarction.[241]

Most important are changes in behavior.[220,231,239,240,242] The most common behavioral change, in our experience, has been abulia.[220,231,239,240] Families describe the patients as more apathetic, uninterested, inert, laconic, and inactive than they were before the stroke. Slowness is a frequent theme; each activity takes longer and requires more concentration and effort. Another frequent abnormality, especially in patients with right caudate infarcts, is restlessness and hyperactivity. Some patients speak incessantly, call out, and appear agitated, confused, and delirious, closely resembling patients with right temporal-lobe infarcts.[165,166,220,242] In some patients with caudate infarction, restlessness and agitation alternate with apathy and inertia. Slight aphasia can be found in left caudate infarcts. Some patients with right caudate lesions have left visual neglect.[220,242]

The cognitive and behavioral abnormalities found in patients with caudate infarcts closely resemble the clinical signs found in patients with lesions in the medial thalamus and the frontal and temporal lobes. Anatomical and physiological studies have shown strong interconnections between the caudate nucleus and various cortical regions, and between the caudate nucleus and the thalamus, globus pallidus, and substantia nigra.[212,243,244] Caudato-nigro-thalamo-cortical circuits are intimately related to planning, thinking, acting, and other higher cortical functions.[220,243]

The causes of caudate infarction are diverse. The most lateral portion is supplied by the medial and lateral striate penetrators of the MCA. Occlusion of these branches, or of the parent proximal MCA, can lead to striatocapsular infarction, including the caudate nucleus. Occlusion of the ACA, by intrinsic atherosclerosis or more often by

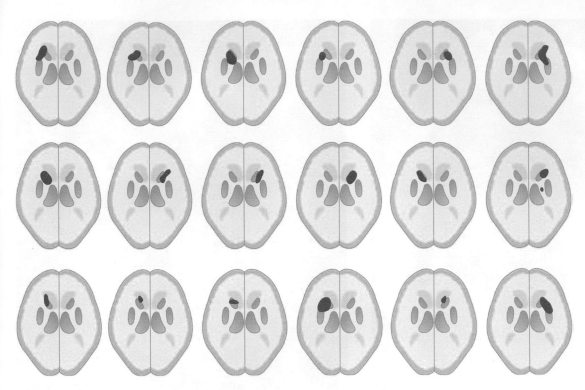

Figure 7.21 Montage of drawings of CT scans showing caudate-nucleus infarcts.

embolism, is another important mechanism of caudate infarction. In most patients, the lesions are probably caused by atheromatous branch disease at the origins of these penetrating arteries.[220,245] In a 1990 series of patients with caudate infarcts, risk factors for small artery disease were prevalent.[220] Among the 18 patients, hypertension (77%) and diabetes (33%) were common, 5 patients had both diabetes and hypertension, and only 3 of 18 patients had neither hypertension nor diabetes. Only one of the 18 patients had confirmed large-artery disease (ICA siphon stenosis). One patient had a cardiac source of embolism (mitral stenosis).[220] These data suggest that most caudate infarcts are caused by atheromatous branch disease. This conclusion, however, must be tentative without more clinical and necropsy data. At present, we suggest screening patients with caudate infarcts with cardiac testing, US, or CTA or MRA before diagnosing a small artery etiology.

Occlusion of the anterior choroidal artery

Neuroimaging (CT and MRI) often shows infarction limited to the territory of the anterior choroidal artery (AChA). Often AChA territory infarction is accompanied by infarcts in the MCA territory as part of an occlusion of the intracranial ICA. The AChA originates from the ICA after its ophthalmic and posterior communicating branches, and courses posteriorly and laterally to supply the globus pallidus, lateral geniculate body, posterior limb of the internal capsule, and medial temporal lobe.[246,247] There is a small supply to the thalamus. Figure 2.17 shows the AChA and its supply regions. Occasionally, there are anomalies of the AChA.[248] The artery can occasionally arise from the MCA or from the posterior

communicating artery. Sometimes, the AChA is a larger-than-normal vessel that supplies the temporo-occipital lobes, the usual territory of the posterior cerebral artery.[248]

Before CT, occlusion of the anterior choroidal artery had seldom been diagnosed during life. Cooper, at first inadvertently and later purposefully, tied this vessel in Parkinsonian patients to stop tremor. The results were variable.[249] Analyses of various series of patients[250–255] shows that the syndrome of the AChA includes the following:

- hemiparesis affecting the face, arm, and leg
- prominent hemisensory loss that is often temporary
- homonymous hemianopia
- when the lateral geniculate body is infarcted, an unusual hemianopia, with sparing of a beak-shaped tongue of vision, within the center of the hemianopic visual field[256]
- absence of persistent neglect, aphasia, or other higher cortical-function abnormalities.

Hemiparesis is the most consistent finding. Dysarthria and hemisensory abnormalities are present less often and usually do not persist. Hemianopia is the least common sign. Some patients with bilateral AChA-territory capsular infarcts have severe dysarthria and may even become mute.[257]

The diagnosis of AChA territory infarction is verified by CT (Figure 7.22) or MRI (Figure 7.23), which shows infarction in the pallidum and lateral geniculate body adjacent to the temporal horn,[250,255,258] and by occlusion of the AChA demonstrated angiographically. Many of the reported patients with AChA-territory infarcts have been diabetic or hypertensive.[250,255,259] Most often, infarction in AChA territory is caused by occlusion of the AChA. The pathology is

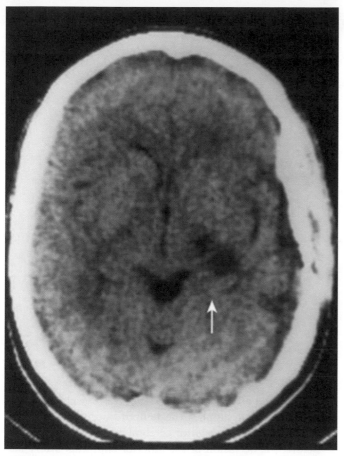

Figure 7.22 CT scan showing an anterior choroidal artery territory infarct (white arrow).

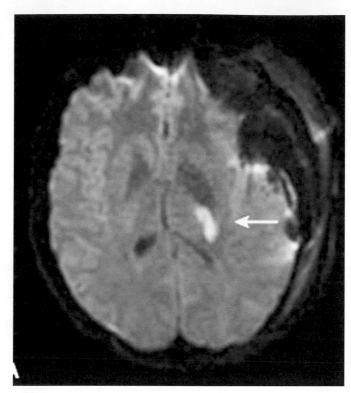

Figure 7.23 Diffusion-weighted MRI scan showing an infarct in the territory of the anterior choroidal artery (white arrow). The patient had had epilepsy surgery removing a portion of the frontal lobe.

probably that of intracranial branch atheromatous disease.[245] Carotid artery occlusion, vasospasm in patients with carotid artery aneurysms, and cardiac-origin embolism are occasionally responsible for AChA-territory infarction, often coupled with MCA-territory infarcts.[260,261]

The PCA is occasionally supplied directly through the posterior communicating branch of the ICA. This vessel is considered in Chapter 8 because it usually arises from the basilar artery.

References

1. Estol CJ: Dr C Miller Fisher and the history of carotid artery disease. *Stroke* 1996;**27**:559–566.

2. Fisher CM: Occlusion of the internal carotid artery. *Arch Neurol Psychiatry* 1951;**65**:346–377.

3. Fisher CM: Occlusion of the carotid arteries. *Arch Neurol Psychiatry* 1954;**72**:187–204.

4. Thompson JE: The evolution of surgery for the treatment and prevention of stroke: The Willis lecture. *Stroke* 1996;**27**:1427–1434.

5. Dyken M: Carotid endarterectomy studies: A glimmering of science. *Stroke* 1986;**17**:355–358.

6. Barnett HJ, Plum F, Walton J: Carotid endarterectomy – an expression of concern. *Stroke* 1984;**15**:941–943.

7. NASCET Collaborators: Beneficial effect of carotid endarterectomy in symptomatic patients with high-grade carotid stenosis. *N Engl J Med* 1991;**325**:445–453.

8. European Carotid Surgery Trialists Collaborative Group: Interim results for symptomatic patients with severe (70–99%) or with mild (0–19%) carotid stenosis. *Lancet* 1991;**337**:1235–1243.

9. Barnett HJM, Taylor DW, Eliasziw M, et al: Benefit of carotid endarterectomy in patients with symptomatic moderate or severe stenosis. North American Symptomatic Carotid Endarterectomy Trial Collaborators. *N Engl J Med* 1998;**339**:1415–1425.

10. European Carotid Surgery Trialists' Collaborative Group: Randomised trial of endarterectomy for recently symptomatic carotid stenosis: Final results of the MRC European Carotid Surgery Trial (ECST). *Lancet* 1998;**351**:1379–1387.

11. Executive Committee for the Asymptomatic Carotid Atherosclerosis Study: Endarterectomy for symptomatic carotid artery stenosis. *JAMA* 1995;**273**:1421–1428.

12. Halliday A, Mansfield A, Marro J, et al: Prevention of disabling and fatal strokes by successful carotid endarterectomy in patients without

recent neurological symptoms: Randomised controlled trial. *Lancet* 2004;**363**:1491–1502.

13. Wennberg DE, Lucas FL, Birkmeyer JD, et al: Variation in carotid endarterectomy mortality in the Medicare population. *JAMA* 1998;**279**:1278–1281.

14. Kempczinski RF, Brott TG, Labutta RJ: The influence of surgical specialist and caseload on the results of carotid endarterectomy. *J Vasc Surg* 1986;**3**:911–916.

15. Meyers PM, Schumacher C, Higashida RT, et al: Use of stents to treat extracranial cerebrovascular disease. *Ann Rev Med* 2006;**57**:437–454.

16. Caplan LR, Meyers PM, Schumacher HC: Angioplasty and stenting to treat occlusive vascular disease. *Rev Neurol Dis* 2006;**3**:8–18.

17. Abbott AL: Medical (nonsurgical) intervention alone is now best for prevention of stroke associated with asymptomatic severe carotid stenosis: Results of a systematic review and analysis. *Stroke* 2009;**40**:e573–e583.

18. Marquardt L, Geraghty OC, Mehta Z, Rothwell PM: Low risk of ipsilateral stroke in patients with asymptomatic carotid stenosis on best medical treatment: A prospective, population-based study. *Stroke* 2010;**41**:e11–e17.

19. Gorelick PB, Caplan LR, Hier DB, et al: Racial differences in the distribution of anterior circulation occlusive disease. *Neurology* 1984;**34**:54–59.

20. Caplan LR, Gorelick PB, Hier DB: Race, sex, and occlusive cerebrovascular disease: A review. *Stroke* 1986;**17**:648–655.

21. Mohr JP, Caplan LR, Melski J, et al: The Harvard Cooperative Stroke Registry: A prospective registry. *Neurology* 1978;**28**:752–754.

22. Furlan A, Whisnant J, Kearns T: Unilateral visual loss in bright light. *Arch Neurol* 1979;**36**:675–676.

23. Caplan LR, Sergay S: Positional cerebral ischemia. *J Neurol Neurosurg Psychiatry* 1976;**39**:385–391.

24. Reed C, Toole J: Clinical technique for identification of external carotid bruits. *Neurology* 1981;**31**:744–746.

25. Fisher CM: Facial pulses in internal carotid artery occlusion. *Neurology* 1970;**20**:476–478.

26. Caplan LR: The frontal artery sign. *N Engl J Med* 1973;**288**:1008–1009.

27. Hollenhorst R: Ocular manifestations of insufficiency or thrombosis of the internal carotid artery. *Am J Ophthalmol* 1959;**47**:753–767.

28. Fisher CM: Observations of the fundus oculi in transient monocular blindness. *Neurology* 1959;**9**:333–347.

29. Kearns T, Hollenhorst R: Venous stasis retinopathy of occlusive disease of the carotid artery. *Mayo Clin Proc* 1963;**38**:304–312.

30. Carter JE: Chronic ocular ischemia and carotid vascular disease. In Bernstein EF (ed): *Amaurosis Fugax*. New York: Springer, 1988, pp 118–134.

31. Caplan LR, Babikian V, Helgason C, et al: Occlusive disease of the middle cerebral artery. *Neurology* 1985;**35**:975–982.

32. Neau J-P, Bogousslavsky J: Superficial middle cerebral artery syndromes. In Bogousslavsky J, Caplan LR (eds): *Stroke Syndromes*, 2nd ed. Cambridge: Cambridge University Press, 2001, pp 405–427.

33. Caplan LR, Bogousslavsky J: Abnormalities of the right cerebral hemisphere. In Bogousslavsky J, Caplan LR (eds): *Stroke Syndromes*. Cambridge: Cambridge University Press, 1995, pp 162–168.

34. Hier DB, Mondlock J, Caplan LR: Behavioral abnormalities after right hemisphere stroke. *Neurology* 1983;**33**:337–344.

35. Pessin MS, Kwan E, Scott RM, Hedges TR: Occipital infarction with hemianopsia from carotid occlusive disease. *Stroke* 1989;**20**:409–411.

36. Linn FH, Chang H-M, Caplan LR: Carotid artery disease: A rare cause of posterior cerebral artery territory infarction. *J Neurovasc Dis* 1997;**2**:31–34.

37. Townsend TC, Saloner D, Pan XM, Rapp JH: Contrast material-enhanced MRA overestimates severity of carotid stenosis, compared with 3D time-of-flight MRA. *J Vasc Surg* 2003;**38**:36–40.

38. Pessin M, Duncan G, Davis K, et al: Angiographic appearance of carotid occlusion in acute stroke. *Stroke* 1980;**11**:485–487.

39. Barnett HJM, Peerless S, Kaufmann J: "Stump" of internal carotid artery: A source for further cerebral embolic ischemia. *Stroke* 1978;**9**:448–452.

40. Ringelstein E, Zeumer H, Angelou D: The pathogenesis of strokes from internal carotid artery occlusion: Diagnostic and therapeutic implications. *Stroke* 1983;**14**:867–875.

41. Orlandi G, Parenti G, Bertolucci A, Murri L: Silent cerebral microembolism in asymptomatic and symptomatic carotid artery stenoses of low and high degree. *Eur Neurol* 1997;**38**:39–43.

42. Droste DW, Dittrich R, Kerveny V, et al: Prevalence and frequency of microembolic signals in 105 patients with extracranial carotid artery occlusive disease. *J Neurol Neurosurg Psychiatry* 1999;**67**:525–528.

43. Caplan LR, Hennerici M: Impaired clearance of emboli (washout) is an important link between hypoperfusion, embolism, and ischemic stroke. *Arch Neurol* 1998;**55**:1475–1482.

44. Caplan LR, Wong K-S, Gao S, et al: Is hypoperfusion an important cause of strokes? If so, how? *Cerebrovasc Dis* 2006;**21**:145–153.

45. Marder VJ, Chute DJ, Starkman S, et al: Analysis of thrombi retrieved from cerebral arteries of patients with acute ischemic stroke. *Stroke* 2006;**37**:2086–2093.

46. Liebeskind D, Sanossian N, Young WH et al. CT and MRI early vessel signs reflect clot composition in acute stroke. *Stroke* 2011;**42**:1237–1243.

47. Sundt T, Sandok BA, Whisnant JP: Carotid endarterectomy: Complications and preoperative assessment. *Mayo Clin Proc* 1975;**50**:301–306.

48. Brott TG, Hobson RW, 2nd, Howard G, et al. and the CREST Investigators: Stenting versus endarterectomy for treatment of carotid-artery stenosis. *N Engl J Med* 2010;**63**:11–23.

49. Caplan LR, Brott TG: Of horse races, trials, meta-analyses, and carotid artery stenosis. (Editorial). *Arch Neurol* 2011;**68**:157–159.

50. Aghaebrahim A, Jovin T, Jadhav AP, Noorian A, Gupta R, Nogueira RG: Endovascular recanalization of complete subacute to chronic atherosclerotic occlusions of intracranial arteries. *J Neurointerv Surg* 2014;**6**:645–648.

51. Broderick JP, Palesch YY, Demchuk AM, et al. for the Interventional Management of Stroke (IMS) III Investigators: Endovascular therapy after intravenous t-PA versus t-PA alone for stroke. *N Engl J Med* 2013;**368**:893–903.

52. Demchuk AM, Goyal M, Yeatts SD, et al. for the interventional

Management of Stroke (IMS) III Investigators: Recanalization and clinical outcome of occlusion sites at baseline CT angiography in the Interventional Management of Stroke III trial. *Radiology* 2014;**273**:202–210.

53. Sekhar L, Heros R: Atheromatous pseudo-occlusion of the internal carotid artery. *J Neurosurg* 1980;**52**:782–789.

54. Steinke W, Kloetzsch C, Hennerici M: Symptomatic and asymptomatic high-grade carotid stenosis in Doppler color-flow imaging. *Neurology* 1992;**42**:131–138.

55. Riles T, Posner M, Cohen W, et al: Rapid sequential CT scanning of the occluded internal carotid artery. *Stroke* 1982;**13**:124.

56. Morganstern LB, Fox AJ, Sharpe BL, et al: The risks and benefits of carotid endarterectomy in patients with near occlusion of the carotid artery. *Neurology* 1997;**48**:911–915.

57. Baron JC: Stroke research in the modern era: Images versus dogma. *Cerebrovasc Dis* 2005;**20**:154–163.

58. Baquis GD, Pessin MS, Scott RM: Limb shaking – a carotid TIA. *Stroke* 1985;**16**:444–448.

59. Yanigahara T, Piepgras DG, Klass DW: Repetitive involuntary movement associated with episodic cerebral ischemia. *Ann Neurol* 1985;**18**:244–250.

60. Powers WJ, Clarke WR, Grubb RL, Jr, Videen TO, Adams HP, Jr, Derdeyn CP, and the COSS. Investigators: Extracranial–intracranial bypass surgery for stroke prevention in hemodynamic cerebral ischemia: The Carotid Occlusion Surgery Study randomized trial. *JAMA* 2011;**306**:1983–1992.

61. Caplan LR: Bypassing trouble. *Arch Neurol* 2012;**69**:518–520.

62. Can U, Furie K, Suwanwela N, et al: Transcranial Doppler ultrasound criteria for hemodynamically significant internal carotid artery stenosis based on residual lumen diameter calculated from en bloc endarterectomy specimens. *Stroke* 1997;**28**:1966–1971.

63. Fisher CM, Ojemann RG: A clinico-pathological study of carotid endarterectomy plaques. *Rev Neurol (Paris)* 1986;**39**:273–299.

64. Fisher M, Paganini-Hill A, Martin A, et al: Carotid plaque pathology: Thrombosis, ulceration, and stroke pathogenesis. *Stroke* 2005;**36**:253–257.

65. Caplan LR, Skillman J, Ojemann R, et al: Intracerebral hemorrhage following carotid endarterectomy: A hypertensive complication. *Stroke* 1978;**9**:457–460.

66. Piepgras DG, Morgan MK, Sundt TM, et al: Intracerebral hemorrhage after carotid endarterectomy. *J Neurosurg* 1988;**68**:532–536.

67. Wade J, Larson C, Hickey R, et al: Effect of carotid endarterectomy on carotid chemoreceptor and baroreceptor function in man. *N Engl J Med* 1970;**282**:823–829.

68. Reigel MM, Hollier LH, Sundt TM, et al: Cerebral hyperperfusion syndrome: A cause of neurologic dysfunction after carotid endarterectomy. *J Vasc Surg* 1987;**5**:628–634.

69. Breen JC, Caplan LR, DeWitt LD, et al: Brain edema after carotid surgery. *Neurology* 1996;**46**:175–181.

70. Abou-Chebl A, Yadav JS, Reginelli JP, et al: Intracranial hemorrhage and hyperperfusion syndrome following carotid artery stenting: Risk factors, prevention, and treatment. *J Am Coll Cardiol* 2004;**43**:1596–1561.

71. Hennerici M, Rautenberg W, Struck R: Spontaneous clinical course of asymptomatic vascular processes of the extracranial cerebral arteries. *Klin Wochenschr* 1984;**62**:570–576.

72. Hennerici M, Hulsbower HB, Hefter K, et al: Natural history of asymptomatic extracranial disease: Results of a long-term prospective study. *Brain* 1987;**110**:777–791.

73. Stroke Prevention by Aggressive Reduction in Cholesterol Levels (SPARCL) Investigators: High-dose atorvastatin after stroke or transient ischemic attack. *N Engl J Med* 2006;**355**:549–559.

74. Johnson ES, Lanes SF, Wentworth CE, 3rd, Satterfield MH, Abebe BL, Dicker W: A metaregression analysis of the dose-response effect of aspirin on stroke. *Arch Intern Med* 1999;**159**:1248–1253.

75. Caplan LR, Stein R, Patel D, et al: Intraluminal clot of the carotid artery detected angiographically. *Neurology* 1984;**34**:1175–1181.

76. Pessin MS, Abbott BF, Prager R, et al: Clinical and angiographic features of carotid circulation thrombus. *Neurology* 1986;**36**:518–523.

77. Buchan A, Gates P, Pelz D, Barnett HJM: Intraluminal thrombus in the cerebral circulation. Implications for surgical management. *Stroke* 1988;**19**:681–687.

78. Nadareishvili ZG, Rothwell PM, Beletsky V, et al: Long-term risk of stroke and other vascular events in patients with asymptomatic carotid artery stenosis. *Arch Neurol* 2002;**59**:1162–1166.

79. Hadar N, Raman G, Moorthy D et al: Asymptomatic carotid artery stenosis treated with medical therapy alone: Temporal trends and implications for risk assessment and the design of future studies. *Cerebrovasc Dis* 2014;**38**:163–173.

80. Markus HS, King A, Shipley M et al: Asymptomatic embolisation for prediction of stroke in the Asymptomatic Carotid Emboli Study (ACES): A prospective observational study. *Lancet Neurol* 2010;**9**:663–671.

81. Spence JD, Coates V, Li, H, et al: Effects of intensive medical therapy on microemboli and cardiovascular risk in asymptomatic carotid stenosis. *Arch Neurol* 2010;**67**:180–186.

82. Humphries A, Young J, Santilli P, et al: Unoperated asymptomatic significant carotid artery stenosis: A review of 182 instances. *Surgery* 1976;**80**:694–698.

83. Durward Q, Ferguson G, Barr H: The natural history of asymptomatic carotid bifurcation plaques. *Stroke* 1982;**13**:459–464.

84. Ropper A, Wechsler L, Wilson L: Carotid bruits and the risk of stroke in elective surgery. *N Engl J Med* 1982;**307**:1387–1390.

85. Caplan LR: A 79-year-old musician with asymptomatic carotid artery disease. *JAMA* 1995;**274**:1383–1389.

86. Chambers BR, Norris JW: Outcome in patients with asymptomatic neck bruits. *N Engl J Med* 1986;**315**:860–865.

87. Executive Committee for the Asymptomatic Carotid Atherosclerosis Study (ACAS): Endarterectomy for asymptomatic carotid artery stenosis. *JAMA* 1995;**273**:1421–1428.

88. Halliday A, Mansfield A, Marro J, et al: Prevention of disabling and fatal strokes by successful carotid endarterectomy in patients without recent neurological symptoms: Randomised controlled trial. *Lancet* 2004;**363**:1491–1502.

89. Brott T, Toole J: Medical compared with surgical treatment of asymptomatic carotid artery stenosis. *Ann Intern Med* 1995;**123**:720–722.

90. Warlow C: Surgical treatment of asymptomatic carotid stenosis. *Cerebrovasc Dis* 1996;**6**(Suppl 1):7–14.

91. Perry JR, Szalai JP, Norris JW: Consensus against both endarterectomy and routine screening for asymptomatic carotid artery stenosis. *Canadian Stroke Consortium. Arch Neurol* 1997;**54**:25–28.

92. Gray WA, Verta P: The impact of regulatory approval and Medicare coverage on outcomes of carotid stenting. *Catheter Cardiovasc Interv* 2014;**83**:1158–1166.

93. Caplan LR: Dissections of brain-supplying arteries. *Nat Clin Pract Neurol* 2008;**4**:34–42.

94. Debette S, Leys D: Cervical-artery dissections: Predisposing factors, diagnosis, and outcome. *Lancet Neurol.* 2009;**8**:668–678.

95. Biousse V, D'Anglejan-Chatillon, Toboul P-J, et al: Time course of symptoms in extracranial carotid artery dissections. A series of 80 patients. *Stroke* 1995;**26**:235–239.

96. Bogousslavsky J, Despland PA, Regli F: Spontaneous carotid dissection with acute stroke. *Arch Neurol* 1987;**44**:137–140.

97. Baumagartner RW, Bogousslavsky J: Clinical manifestations of carotid dissection. In Baumgartner RW, Bogousslavsky J, Caso V, Paciaroni M (eds): *Handbook on Cerebral Artery Dissection.* Basel: Karger, 2005, pp 70–76.

98. Caplan LR, Gonzalez RG, Buonanno FS: Case 18–2012: A 35-year-old man with neck pain, hoarseness, and dysphagia. *N Engl J Med* 2012;**366**:2306–2313.

99. Sturznegger M: Ultrasound findings in spontaneous carotid artery dissection: The value of Duplex sonography. *Arch Neurol* 1991;**48**:1057–1063.

100. Engelter ST, Lyrer PA, Kirsch EC, Steck AJ: Long-term follow-up after extracranial internal carotid artery dissection. *Eur Neurol* 2000;**44**:199–204.

101. Touze E, Gauvrit J-Y, Moulin T, et al: Risk of stroke and recurrent dissection after a cervical artery dissection. A multicenter study. *Neurology* 2003;**61**:1347–1351.

102. Kennedy F, Lanfranconi S, Hicks C, and the Cervical Artery Dissection in Stroke Study (CADISS-NR) Investigators: Antiplatelets vs. anticoagulation for dissection: CADISS

nonrandomized arm and meta-analysis *Neurology* 2012;**79**:686–689.

103. Dreier JP, Lurtzing F, Kappmeier M, et al: Delayed occlusion after internal carotid artery dissection under heparin. *Cerebrovasc Dis* 2004;**18**:296–303.

104. Kadkhodayan Y, Jeck DT, Moran CJ, et al: Angioplasty and stenting in carotid dissection with and without pseudoaneurysm. *AJNR Am J Neuroradiol* 2005;**26**:2328–2335.

105. Lavallée PC, Mazighi M, Saint-Maurice J-P, et al. Stent-assisted endovascular thrombolysis versus intravenous thrombolysis in internal carotid artery dissections with tandem internal carotid and middle cerebral artery occlusion. *Stroke* 2007;**38**:2270–2274.

106. Fisher CM, Gore I, Okabe N, et al: Calcification of the carotid siphon. *Circulation* 1965;**32**:538–548.

107. Marzewski D, Furlan A, St Louis P, et al: Intracranial internal carotid artery stenosis: Long-term prognosis. *Stroke* 1982;**13**:821–824.

108. Craig D, Meguro K, Watridge G, et al: Intracranial internal carotid artery stenosis. *Stroke* 1982;**13**:825–828.

109. Wechsler LR, Kistler JP, Davis KR, et al: The prognosis of carotid siphon stenosis. *Stroke* 1986;**17**:714–718.

110. Caplan LR: Cerebrovascular disease: Larger artery occlusive disease. In Appel S (ed): *Current Neurology*, vol **8**. Chicago: Yearbook Medical, 1988, pp 179–226.

111. Borozan PG, Schuler JJ, LaRosa MP, et al: The natural history of isolated carotid siphon stenosis. *TJ Vasc Surg* 1984;**1**:744–749.

112. Bogousslavsky J: Prognosis of carotid siphon stenosis. *Stroke* 1987;**18**:537.

113. Castaigne P, Lhermitte F, Gautier JC, et al: Internal carotid artery occlusion: A study of 61 instances in 50 patients with postmortem data. *Brain* 1970;**93**:231–258.

114. Ley-Pozo J, Ringelstein EB: Noninvasive detection of occlusive disease of the carotid siphon and middle cerebral artery. *Ann Neurol* 1990;**28**:640–647.

115. Sloan MA, Alexandrov AV, Tegeler CH, et al: Assessment: Transcranial Doppler ultrasonography: Report of the Therapeutics and Technology Assessment Subcommittee of the American Academy of Neurology. *Neurology* 2004;**62**:1468–1481.

116. Thijs VN, Albers GW: Symptomatic intracranial atherosclerosis: outcome of patients who fail antithrombotic therapy. *Neurology* 2000;**55**:490–497.

117. Akins PT, Pilgram TK, Cross DT, Moran CJ: Natural history of stenosis from intracranial atherosclerosis by serial angiography. *Stroke* 1998;**29**:433–438.

118. Chimowitz MI, Lynn MJ, Howlett-Smith H, et al: Comparison of warfarin and aspirin for symptomatic intracranial arterial stenosis. *N Engl J Med* 2005;**352**:1305–1316.

119. Kasner SE, Chimowitz MI, Lynn MJ, et al: Predictors of ischemic stroke in the territory of a symptomatic intracranial arterial stenosis. Warfarin Aspirin Symptomatic Intracranial Disease Trial Investigators. *Circulation* 2006;**113**:555–563.

120. Kasner SE, Lynn MJ, Chimowitz MI, et al: Warfarin vs. aspirin for symptomatic intracranial stenosis: Subgroup analyses from WASID. *Neurology* 2006;**67**:1275–1278.

121. Callahan III AS, Berger BL: Balloon angioplasty of intracranial arteries for stroke prevention. *J Neuroimaging* 1997;**7**:232–235.

122. Marks MP, Marcellus M, Norbash AM, et al: Outcome of angioplasty for atherosclerotic intracranial stenosis. *Stroke* 1999;**30**:1065–1069.

123. Connors 3rd JJ, Wojak JC: Percutaneous transluminal angioplasty for intracranial atherosclerotic lesions: Evolution of technique and short-term results. *J Neurosurg* 1999;**91**:415–423.

124. Marks MP, Marcellus ML, Do HM, et al: Intracranial angioplasty without stenting for symptomatic atherosclerotic stenosis: Long-term follow-up. *AJNR Am J Neuroradiol* 2005;**26**:525–530.

125. Chimowitz MI, Lynn MJ, Derdeyn CP, et al. for the SAMMPRIS Investigators: Stenting versus aggressive medical therapy for intracranial arterial stenosis. *N Engl J Med* 2011;**365**:993–1003.

126. Day A, Rhoton A, Quisling R: Resolving siphon stenosis following endarterectomy. *Stroke* 1980;**11**:278–281.

127. Bladin PF, Berkovic SF: Striatocapsular infarction. *Neurology* 1984;**34**:1423–1430.

128. Jansen O, von Kummer R, Forsting M, et al: Thrombolytic therapy in acute occlusion of the intracranial internal carotid artery bifurcation. *AJNR Am J Neuroradiol* 1995;**16**:1977–1986.

129. Zaidat OO, Suarez JI, Santillan C, et al: Response to intra-arterial and combined intravenous and intra-arterial thrombolytic therapy in patients with distal internal carotid artery occlusion. *Stroke* 2002;**33**:1821–1827.

130. Fisher U, Mono ML, Schroth G, et al: Endovascular therapy in 201 patients with acute symptomatic occlusion of the internal carotid artery. *Eur J Neurol* 2013;**20**:1017–1024.

131. Galimanis A, Jung S, Mono M-L, et al: Endovascular therapy of 623 patients with anterior circulation stroke. *Stroke* 2012;**43**:1052–1057.

132. Lansberg MG, Straka M, Kemp S, et al: MRI profile and response to endovascular reperfusion after stroke (DEFUSE 2): a prospective cohort study. *Lancet Neurol* 2012;**11**:860–867.

133. Lemmens R, Mlvnash M, Straka M, et al: Comparison of the response to endovascular reperfusion in relation to site of arterial occlusion. *Neurology.* 2013;**81**:614–618.

134. Chaves C, Estol C, Esnaola MM, et al: Spontaneous intracranial internal carotid artery dissection: Report of 10 patients. *Arch Neurol* 2002;**59**:977–981.

135. Pelkonen O, Tikkakoski T, Leinonen S, et al: Intracranial arterial dissection. *Neuroradiology* 1998;**40**:442–447.

136. Estol C, Caplan LR: Intracranial arterial dissections. In Caplan LR, van Gijn J (eds): *Stroke Syndromes*, 3rd ed. Cambridge, UK: Cambridge University Press, 2012, pp 566–573.

137. Russo L: Carotid system transient ischemic attacks: Clinical, racial, and angiographic correlations. *Stroke* 1981;**12**:470–473.

138. Bauer R, Sheehan S, Wechsler N, et al: Arteriographic study of sites, incidence, and treatment of arteriosclerotic cerebrovascular lesions. *Neurology* 1962;**12**:698–711.

139. Kieffer S, Takeya Y, Resch J, et al: Racial differences in cerebrovascular disease: Angiographic evaluation of Japanese and American populations. *AJR Am J Roentgenol* 1967;**101**:94–99.

140. Brust R: Patterns of cerebrovascular disease in Japanese and other population groups in Hawaii: An angiographic study. *Stroke* 1975;**6**:539–542.

141. Kubo H: Transient cerebral ischemic attacks: An arteriographic study. *Naika* 1968;**22**:969–978.

142. Feldmann E, Daneault N, Kwan E, et al: Chinese–white differences in the distribution of occlusive cerebrovascular disease. *Neurology* 1990;**40**:1541–1545.

143. Bogousslavsky J, Barnett JHM, Fox AJ, et al: Atherosclerotic disease of the middle cerebral artery. EC-IC Bypass Study Group. *Stroke* 1986;**17**:1112–1120.

144. Gorelick P, Han J, Huang Y, Wong K-SL: Epidemiology. In Kim J, Caplan LR, Wong K-SL (eds): *Intracranial Atherosclerosis*. Oxford: Wiley-Blackwell, 2008, pp 33–44.

145. Mazighi M, Labreuche J, Gongora-Rivera F, et al: Autopsy prevalence of intracranial atherosclerosis in patients with fatal stroke. *Stroke* 2008;**39**:1142–1147.

146. Yoo K-M, Shin H-K, Chang H-M, Caplan LR: Middle cerebral artery occlusive disease: The New England Medical Center Stroke Registry. *J Stroke Cerebrovasc Dis* 1998;**7**:344–351.

147. Chen XY, Wong KS, Lam WWM, et al: Middle cerebral artery atherosclerosis: histological comparison between plaques associated with and not associated with infarct in a postmortem study. *Cerebrovasc Dis* 2008;**25**:74–80.

148. Ogata J, Yutani C, Otsubo R, et al: Heart and vessel pathology underlying brain infarction in 142 stroke patients. *Ann Neurol* 2008;**63**:770–781.

149. Hinton R, Mohr JP, Ackerman R, et al: Symptomatic middle cerebral artery stenosis. *Ann Neurol* 1979;**5**:152–157.

150. Corston RN, Kendall BE, Marshall J: Prognosis in middle cerebral artery stenosis. *Stroke* 1984;**15**:237–241.

151. Moulin DE, Lo R, Chiang J, et al: Prognosis in middle cerebral artery occlusion. *Stroke* 1985;**16**:282–284.

152. Feldmeyer JJ, Merendaz C, Regli F: Stenosis symptomatiques de l'artère cerebrale moyenne. *Rev Neurol (Paris)* 1983;**139**:725–736.

153. Naritomi H, Sawada T, Kuriyama Y, et al: Effect of chronic middle cerebral artery stenosis on the local cerebral hemodynamics. *Stroke* 1985;**16**:214–219.

154. Segura T, Serena J, Molins A, Davalos A: Clusters of microembolic signals: A new form of cerebral microembolism in a patient with middle cerebral artery stenosis. *Stroke* 1998;**29**:722–724.

155. Wong KS, Gao S, Chan YL, et al: Mechanisms of acute cerebral infarctions in patients with middle cerebral artery stenosis: A diffusion-weighted imaging and microemboli monitoring study. *Ann Neurol* 2002;**52**:74–81.

156. Gao S, Wong KS, Hansberg T, et al: Microembolic signal predicts recurrent cerebral ischemic events in acute stroke patients with middle cerebral artery stenosis. *Stroke* 2004;**35**:2832–2836.

157. Mohr JP, Kedja-Scharlein J: Middle cerebral artery syndromes. In Caplan LR, van Gijn (eds): *Stroke Syndromes*, 3rd ed. Cambridge, UK: Cambridge University Press, 2012, pp 344–363.

158. Jain K: Some observations on the anatomy of the middle cerebral artery. *Can J Surg* 1964;**7**:134–139.

159. Kaplan H: Anatomy and embryology of the arterial system of the forebrain. In Vinken P, Bruyn G (eds): *Handbook of Clinical Neurology*, vol **11**. Amsterdam: North Holland, 1972, pp 1–23.

160. Hier DB, Gorelick PB, Shindler AG: *Topics in Behavioral Neurology and Neuropsychology*. Boston: Butterworth, 1987.

161. Fisher CM: Left hemiplegia and motor impersistence. *J Nerv Ment Dis* 1956;**123**:201–218.

162. Hier DB, Mohr JP: Incongruous oral and written naming: Evidence for a subdivision of the syndromes of Wernicke's aphasia. *Brain Lang* 1977;**4**:115–126.

163. Sevush S, Roeltgen D, Campanella D, et al: Preserved oral reading in Wernicke's aphasia. *Neurology* 1983;**33**:916–920.

164. Awada A, Poncet M, Signoret J: Confrontation de la Salpêtrière 4 Mai 1983: Troubles des compartement soudains avec agitation chez un homme de 68 ans. *Rev Neurol (Paris)* 1984;**140**:446–451.

165. Schmidley J, Messing R: Agitated confusional states in patients with right hemisphere infarctions. *Stroke* 1984:**15**;883–885.

166. Caplan LR, Kelly M, Kase CS, et al: Infarcts of the inferior division of the

right middle cerebral artery. *Neurology* 1986;**36**:1015–1020.

167. Kim JS, Yoon Y: Single subcortical infarction associated with parental arterial disease: important yet neglected sub-type of atherothrombotic stroke. *Int J Stroke* 2013;**8**:197–203.

168. Yoon Y, Lee DH, Kang DW, Kwon SU, Kim JS: Single subcortical infarction and atherosclerotic plaques in the middle cerebral artery: High-resolution magnetic resonance imaging findings. *Stroke* 2013;**44**:2462–2467.

169. Adams H, Damasio H, Putnam S, et al: Middle cerebral artery occlusion as a cause of isolated subcortical infarction. *Stroke* 1983;**14**:948–952.

170. Weiller C, Ringelstein EB, Reiche W, et al: The large striatocapsular infarct: A clinical and pathological entity. *Arch Neurol* 1990;**47**:1085–1091.

171. Caplan LR: The large striato-capsular infarct: A clinical and pathophysiologic entity: Critique. *Neurol Chronicle* 1991;**1**:12–13.

172. Damasio A, Damasio H, Rizzo M, et al: Aphasia with nonhemorrhagic lesions in the basal ganglia and internal capsule. *Arch Neurol* 1982;**89**:15–20.

173. Naesser M, Alexander M, Estabrooks N, et al: Aphasia with predominantly subcortical lesion sites. *Arch Neurol* 1982;**39**:2–14.

174. Heinsius T, Bogousslavsky J, van Melle G: Large infarcts in the middle cerebral artery territory. Etiology and outcome patterns. *Neurology* 1998;**50**:341–350.

175. Hier DB, Mondlock J, Caplan LR: Recovery of behavioral abnormalities after right hemisphere stroke. *Neurology* 1983;**33**:345–350.

176. Staykov D, Gupta R: Hemicraniectomy in malignant middle cerebral artery infarction. *Stroke* 2011; **42**:513–516.

177. Kolias A, Kirkpatrick PJ, Hutchinson PJ: Decompressive craniectomy: Past, present and future. *Nature Rev Neurol* 2013;**9**:405–415.

178. Jüttler E, Unterberg A, Woitzik J, et al. for the Destiny II Investigators. Hemicraniectomy in older patients with extensive middle-cerebral-artery stroke. *N Engl J Med* 2014;**370**:1091–1100.

179. Fink JN, Selim MH, Kumar S, et al: Insular cortex infarction in acute middle cerebral artery territory stroke: Predictor of stroke severity and vascular lesion. *Arch Neurol* 2005;**62**:1081–1085.

180. Oppenheimer SM, Cechetto DF, Hachinski VC: Cerebrogenic cardiac arrythmias: Cerebral ECG influences and their role in sudden death. *Arch Neurol* 1990;**47**:513–519.

181. Oppenheimer SM, Wilson JX, Guiraudon C, Cechetto DF: Insular cortex stimulation produces lethal cardiac arrhythmias: A mechanism of sudden death. *Brain Res* 1991;**550**:115–121.

182. Yoon R-W, Morillo CA, Cechetto DF, Hachinski V: Cerebral hemispheric lateralization in cardiac autonomic control. *Arch Neurol* 1997;**54**:741–744.

183. Hachinski VC, Oppenheimer SM, Wilson JX, et al: Assymetry of sympathetic consequences of experimental stroke. *Arch Neurol* 1992;**49**:697–702.

184. Giubilei F, Strano S, Lino S, et al: Autonomic nervous system activity during sleep in middle cerebral artery infarction. *Cerebrovasc Dis* 1998;**8**:118–123.

185. Tomsick T, Brott T, Barsan W, et al: Prognostic value of the hyperdense middle cerebral artery sign and stroke scale score before ultra-early thrombolytic therapy. *AJNR Am J Neuroradiol* 1996;**17**:79–85.

186. Alexandros AV, Bladin CF, Norris JW: Intracranial blood flow velocities in acute ischemic stroke. *Stroke* 1994;**25**:1378–1383.

187. Molina CA, Alexandrov AV: Transcranial Doppler ultrasound. In Caplan LR, Manning WJ (eds): *Brain Embolism*. New York: Informa Healthcare, 2006, pp 113–128.

188. Segura T, Serena J, Molins A, Davalos A: Clusters of microembolic signals: A new form of cerebral microembolism presentation in a patient with middle cerebral artery stenosis. *Stroke* 1998;**29**:722–724.

189. Masuda J, Yutani C, Miyashita T, Yamaguchi T: Artery-to-artery embolism from a thrombus formed in a stenotic middle cerebral artery. Report of an autopsy case. *Stroke* 1987;**18**:680–684.

190. Wong KS, Lam WWM, Liang E, et al: Variability of magnetic resonance angiography and computed tomography angiography in grading middle cerebral artery stenosis. *Stroke* 1996;**27**:1084–1087.

191. Bash S, Villablanca JP, Duckwiler G, et al: Intracranial vascular stenosis and occlusive disease. Evaluation with CT angiography, MR angiography, and digital subtraction angiography. *AJNR Am J Neuroradiol* 2005;**26**:1012–1021.

192. Nederkoorn PJ, van der Graaf Y, Eikelboom BC, van der Lugt A, Bartels LW, Mali WP: Time-of-flight MR angiography of carotid artery stenosis: does a flow void represent severe stenosis? *AJNR Am J Neuroradiol* 2002;**23**:1779–1784.

193. Mori E, Yoneda Y, Tabuchi M, et al: Intravenous recombinant tissue plasminogen activator in acute carotid artery territory stroke. *Neurology* 1992;**42**:976–982.

194. Trouillas P, Nighogossian N, Getenet J, et al: Open trial of intravenous tissue plasminogen activator in acute carotid territory stroke. *Stroke* 1996;**27**:882–890.

195. Wolpert SM, Bruckman H, Greenlee R, et al: Neuroradiologic evaluation of patients with acute stroke treated with recombinant tissue plasminogen activator. *AJNR Am J Neuroradiol* 1993;**14**:3–13.

196. Albers GW, Thijs VN, Wechsler L, et al: MRI profiles predict clinical response to early reperfusion: The Diffusion and Perfusion Imaging Evaluation for Understanding Stroke Evolution (DEFUSE) Study. *Ann Neurol* 2006;**60**:508–517.

197. del Zoppo GJ, Higashida R, Furlan AJ, et al: PROACT: A phase II randomized trial of recombinant pro-urokinase by direct arterial delivery in acute middle cerebral artery stroke. *Stroke* 1998;**29**:4–11.

198. Bhatia R, Hill MD, Shobha N et al: Low rates of acute recanalization with intravenous recombinant tissue plasminogen activator in ischemic stroke: real-world experience and a call for action. *Stroke* 2010;**41**:2254–2258.

199. Meyers PM, Schumacher HC, Tanji K, et al: Use of stents to treat intracranial cerebrovascular disease. *Ann Rev Med* 2007;**58**:107–122.

200. Chaturvedi S, Caplan LR: Angioplasty for intracranial atherosclerosis: Is the treatment worse than the disease? *Neurology* 2003;**61**:1647–1648.

201. Mori T, Fukuoka M, Kazita K, Mori K: Follow-up study after intracranial percutaneous transluminal cerebral balloon angioplasty. *AJNR Am J Neuroradiol* 1998;**19**:1525–1533.

202. Derdeyn CP, Chimowitz MI, Lynn MJ, for the Stenting and Aggressive Medical Management for Preventing Recurrent Stroke in Intracranial Stenosis Trial Investigators. Aggressive medical treatment with or without stenting in high-risk patients with intracranial artery stenosis (SAMMPRIS): the final results of a randomised trial. *Lancet* 2014;**383**:333–341.

203. Chimowitz MI, Kokkinos J, Strong J, et al: The Warfarin–Aspirin Symptomatic Intracranial Disease Study. *Neurology* 1995;**45**:1488–1493.

204. Critchley M: The anterior cerebral artery, and its syndromes. *Brain* 1930;**53**:120–165.

205. Brust JCM. Anterior cerebral artery. In Caplan LR, van Gijn J (eds): *Stroke Syndromes*, 3rd ed. Cambridge UK, Cambridge University Press, 2012, pp 364–374.

206. Ohkuma H, Suzuki S, Kikkawa T, et al: Neuroradiologic and clinical features of arterial dissection of the anterior cerebral artery. *Am J Neuroradiol* 2003;**24**:691–699.

207. Sasaki O, Koike T, Takeuchi S, Tanaka R: Serial angiography in a spontaneous dissecting anterior cerebral artery aneurysm. *Surg Neurol* 1991;**36**:49–53.

208. Guridi J, Gallego J, Monzon F, Aguilera F: Intracerebral hemorrhage caused by intramural dissection of the anterior cerebral artery. *Stroke* 1993;**24**:1400–1402.

209. Koyama S, Kotani A, Sasaki J: Spontaneous dissecting aneurysm of the anterior cerebral artery: report of two cases. *Surg Neurol* 1996;**46**:55–61.

210. Matsumoto S, Takada T, Kazui S, et al: Rotational angiographic demonstration of dissection of the anterior cerebral artery. *Cerebrovasc Dis* 2005;**20**:55–58.

211. Sato S, Toyoda K, Matsuoka H, et al: Isolated anterior cerebral artery territory infarction: dissection as an etiological mechanism. *Cerebrovasc Dis* 2010;**29**:170–177.

212. Shimoyama T, Kimura K, Iguchi Y, et al: Spontaneous intra-cranial arterial dissection frequently causes anterior cerebral artery dissection. *J Neurol Sci* 2011;**304**:40–43.

213. Nagamine Y, Fukuoka T, Hayashi T et al: Research article: Clinical characteristics of isolated anterior cerebral artery territory infarction due to arterial dissection. *J Stroke Cerebrovasc Dis* 2014;**23**:2907–2913.

214. Uihlein A, Thomas R, Cleary J: Aneurysms of the anterior communicating artery complex. *Mayo Clin Proc* 1967;**42**:73–87.

215. Gacs G, Fox A, Barnett HJM, et al: Occurrence and mechanisms of occlusion of the anterior cerebral artery. *Stroke* 1983;**14**:952–959.

216. Bogousslavsky J, Regli F: Anterior cerebral artery territory infarction in the Lausanne Stroke Registry. Clinical and etiologic patterns. *Arch Neurol* 1990;**47**:144–150.

217. Nagaratnam N, Davies D, Chen E: Clinical effects of anterior cerebral artery infarction. *J Stroke Cerebrovasc Dis* 1998;**7**:391–397.

218. Rhoton AL, Sacki N, Pearlmutter D, Zeal A: Microsurgical anatomy of common aneurysm sites. *Clin Neurosurg* 1978;**26**:248–306.

219. Gorczyca W, Mohr G: Microvascular anatomy of Heubner's recurrent artery. *J Neurosurg* 1976;**44**:359–367.

220. Caplan LR, Schmahmann JD, Kase CS, et al: Caudate infarcts. *Arch Neurol* 1990;**47**:133–143.

221. Dunker R, Harris A: Surgical anatomy of the proximal anterior cerebral artery. *J Neurosurg* 1976;**44**:359–367.

222. Chamarro A, Marshall RS, Valls-Sole J, et al: Motor behavior in stroke patients with isolated medial frontal ischemic infarction. *Stroke* 1997;**28**:1755–1760.

223. Geschwind N, Kaplan E: A human cerebral deconnection syndrome. *Neurology* 1962;**12**:675–695.

224. Geschwind N: Disconnection syndromes in animals and man. *Brain* 1965;**88**:237–294, 585–644.

225. Pereira A, Schomer A, Feng W, et al: Anterior disconnection syndrome revisited using modern technologies. *Neurology* 2012;**79**:290–291.

226. Rubens A: Aphasia with infarction in the territory of the anterior cerebral artery. *Cortex* 1975;**11**:239–250.

227. Alexander M, Schmitt M: The aphasia syndrome of stroke in the left anterior cerebral artery territory. *Arch Neurol* 1980;**37**:97–100.

228. Ross E: Left medial parietal lobe and receptive language functions: Mixed transcortical aphasia after left anterior cerebral artery infarction. *Neurology* 1980;**30**:144–151.

229. Fisher CM: Abulia minor versus agitated behavior. *Clin Neurosurg* 1983;**31**:9–31.

230. Fesenmeier JT, Kuzniecky R, Garcia J: Akinetic mutism caused by bilateral anterior cerebral tuberculous arteritis. *Neurology* 1990;**40**:1005–1006.

231. Ghoshal S, Gokhale S, Rebovich G, Caplan LR: The neurology of decreased activity: abulia. *Rev Neurol Dis* 2011;**8**:55–67.

232. Fisher CM: Intermittent interruption of behavior. *Trans Am Neurol Assoc* 1968;**93**:209–210.

233. Brion S, Jedynak C-P: Trouble du tranfer inter-hemispherique a propos de trois observations de tumeurs du corps calleux. Le signe de al main etrangere. *Rev Neurol (Paris)* 1972;**126**:257–266.

234. Goldberg G, Mayer NH, Toglia JU: Medial frontal cortex infarction and the alien hand sign. *Arch Neurol* 1981;**38**:683–686.

235. Geschwind DH, Iacoboni M, Mega MS, et al: Alien hand syndrome: Interhemispheric motor disconnection due to a lesion in the midbody of the corpus callosum. *Neurology* 1995;**45**:802–808.

236. Freeman FR: Akinetic mutism and bilateral anterior cerebral artery occlusion. *J Neurol Neurosurg Psychiatry* 1971;**34**:693–694.

237. Borggreve F, De Deyn PP, Marien P, et al: Bilateral infarction in the anterior cerebral artery vascular territory due to an unusual anomaly of the circle of Willis. *Stroke* 1994;**25**:1279–1281.

238. Ferbert A, Thorn A: Bilateral anterior cerebral territory infarction in the differential diagnosis of basilar artery occlusion. *J Neurology* 1992;**239**:162–164.

239. Caplan LR: Caudate infarcts. In Donnan G, Norrving B, Bamford J, Bogousslavsky J (eds): *Subcortical Stroke*, 2nd ed. Oxford: Oxford University Press, 2002, pp 209–223.

240. Chung C-S, Caplan LR: Caudate nucleus infarcts and hemorrhages. In Caplan LR, van Gijn J (eds): *Stroke Syndromes*, 3rd ed. Cambridge, UK: Cambridge University Press, 2012, pp 397–404.

241. Saris S: Chorea caused by caudate infarction. *Arch Neurol* 1983;**40**:590–591.

242. Mendez M, Adams N, Lewandowski K: Neurobehavioral changes

associated with caudate lesions. *Neurology* 1989;**39**:349–354.

243. Alexander GE, DeLong MR, Strick PL: Parallel organization of functionally segregated circuits linking basal ganglia and cortex. *Ann Rev Neurosci* 1986;**9**:357–381.

244. Alexander GE, Delong MR: Microstimulation of the primate neostriatum: I: Physiological properties of striatal microexcitable zones. *J Neurophysiol* 1985;**53**:1417–1432.

245. Caplan LR: Intracranial branch atheromatous disease. *Neurology* 1989;**39**:1246–1250.

246. Rhoton A, Fuji K, Fradd B: Microsurgical anatomy of the anterior choroidal artery. *Surg Neurol* 1979;**12**:171–187.

247. Mohr JP, Steinke W, Timsit SG, et al: The anterior choroidal artery does not supply the corona radiata and lateral ventricular wall. *Stroke* 1991;**22**:1502–1507.

248. Takahashi S, Suga T, Kawata Y, Sakamoto K: Anterior choroidal artery: Angiographic analysis of variations and anomalies. *AJNR Am J Neuroradiol* 1990;**11**:719–729.

249. Cooper I: Surgical occlusions of the anterior choroidal artery in Parkinsonism. *Surg Gynecol Obstet* 1954;**99**:207–219.

250. Helgason C, Caplan LR, Goodwin V, et al: Anterior choroidal territory infarction: Case reports and review. *Arch Neurol* 1986;**43**:681–686.

251. Helgason C, Caplan LR: Anterior choroidal artery territory strokes. In Caplan LR, van Gijn J (eds): *Stroke Syndromes*, 3rd ed. Cambridge, UK: Cambridge University Press, 2012, pp 375–386.

252. Ward T, Bernat J, Goldstein A: Occlusion of the anterior choroidal artery. *J Neurol Neurosurg Psychiatry* 1984;**47**:1046–1049.

253. Masson M, DeCroix JP, Henin D, et al: Syndrome de l'artère choroidienne anterieure: Etude clinique et tomodensitometrique de 4 cas. *Rev Neurol (Paris)* 1983;**139**:553–559.

254. Decroix JP, Graveleau PH, Masson M, Cambier J: Infarction in the territory of the anterior choroidal artery: A clinical and computerized tomographic study of 16 cases. *Brain* 1986;**109**:1071–1085.

255. Helgason CM: Anterior choroidal artery territory infarction. In Donnan G, Norrving B, Bamford J, Bogousslavsky J (eds): *Lacunar and Other Subcortical Infarctions.* Oxford: Oxford University Press, 1995, pp 131–138.

256. Frisen L: Quadruple sector anopia and sectorial optic atrophy: A syndrome of the distal anterior choroidal artery. *J Neurol Neurosurg Psychiatry* 1979;**42**:590–594.

257. Helgason C, Wilbur A, Weiss A, et al: Acute pseudobulbar mutism due to discrete bilateral capsular infarction in the territory of the anterior choroidal artery. *Brain* 1988;**111**:507–524.

258. Damasio H: A computed tomographic guide to the identification of cerebral vascular territories. *Arch Neurol* 1983;**40**:138–142.

259. Bruno A, Graff-Radford NR, Biller J, Adams HP: Anterior choroidal artery territory infarction: A small vessel disease. *Stroke* 1989;**20**:616–619.

260. Mayer JM, Lanoe Y, Pedetti L, Fabry B: Anterior choroidal-artery territory infarction and carotid occlusion. *Cerebrovasc Dis* 1992;**2**:315–316.

261. Leys D, Mounier-Vehier F, Lavenu I, et al: Anterior choroidal artery territory infarcts. Study of presumed mechanisms. *Stroke* 1994;**25**:837–842.

Chapter 8

Large vessel occlusive disease of the posterior circulation

Louis R Caplan and Jong S Kim

Following the suggestions of American[1–5] and British[1,6] authors during the late 1950s and early 1960s, physicians lumped posterior circulation ischemia under the catch-all terms *vertebrobasilar insufficiency* (VBI) or *vertebrobasilar territory infarction*. Various treatments were tried in groups of patients with VBI.[1,7] As was found in the case of large, heterogeneous groups of patients with anterior and posterior circulation disease lumped under the categories of transient ischemic attack (TIA), progressing, or so-called completed stroke, no single treatment strategy proved helpful for the group as a whole. With the advent of better brain imaging, more angiography, better surgery, and safe, non-invasive diagnostic techniques, physicians and surgeons began to consider treatment of individual patients with anterior circulation disease, depending on the: (1) nature, severity, and location of their vascular lesions; (2) degree of infarction; (3) hematologic-coagulation findings; and (4) general health of the patient.

The same strategy should be applied to patients with vertebrobasilar disease because this category is even more heterogeneous than anterior-circulation ischemic disease.[1,2,8,9] This chapter follows this idea and categorizes posterior circulation occlusive disease, depending on the causative vascular lesions. Remember that in the posterior circulation, considerably more tissue is fed by small, penetrating arteries, so the proportion of small-artery to large-artery disease is higher than in the anterior circulation. Lacunes and penetrating branch territory infarcts within the vertebrobasilar system are considered in Chapter 9. A monograph devoted entirely to posterior circulation disease discusses this topic in much more detail than is possible in this chapter.[1]

Occlusion or severe stenosis of the subclavian and innominate arteries

The extracranial vertebral arteries (ECVAs) arise from the proximal subclavian arteries. The subclavian artery arises in the great majority of patients as the last brachiocephalic branch of the aortic arch, while the right subclavian artery originates from the innominate artery. Thus, disease of the subclavian or innominate arteries before the ECVA origins can lead to changes in vertebral artery blood flow. Reivich et al.[10] and others[11–13]

brought this practical fact to the attention of physicians when they recognized the subclavian steal syndrome. In this syndrome, obstruction to the proximal subclavian artery led to a low-pressure system within the ipsilateral vertebral artery and in blood vessels of the ipsilateral upper extremity. Blood from a higher-pressure system, the contralateral vertebral artery and basilar artery, was diverted and flowed retrograde down the ipsilateral vertebral artery into the arm (Figure 8.1). Figure 8.2 shows an arteriogram from a patient with subclavian steal.

Most patients with subclavian artery disease are asymptomatic. In those with symptoms, most complaints relate to arm ischemia. Fatigue, aching after exercise, and coolness are described by some patients, especially those that use their arms vigorously during athletics or work. Among a large series of patients with subclavian steal, studied in 1988 by Hennerici and colleagues using ultrasound documentation of vertebral artery reversed flow, one-third of patients reported pain,

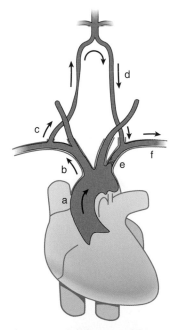

Figure 8.1 Subclavian steal: (a) aortic arch, (b) innominate artery, (c) right vetebral artery, (d) left vertebral artery, (e) occlusion of subclavian artery proximal to the left vertebral artery, (f) subclavian artery. Arrows represent direction of flow.

Caplan's Stroke: A Clinical Approach, 5th Edition, ed. Louis R Caplan. Published by Cambridge University Press. © Cambridge University Press, 2016.

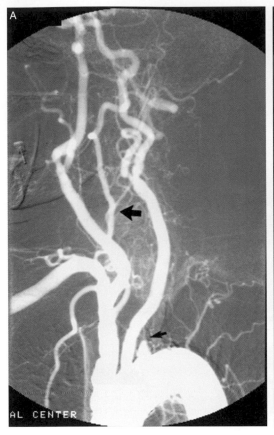
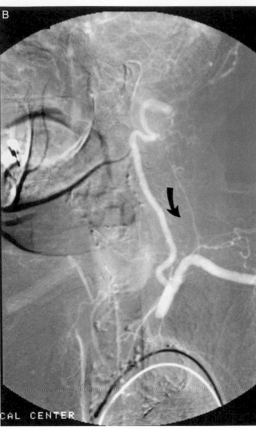

Figure 8.2 Subtraction arch angiograms from a patient with subclavian steal syndrome. (A) Arch angiogram early phase. The right subclavian artery and right vertebral artery (large black arrow) fill normally. The left subclavian artery is occluded just above its origin (lower, small black arrow). (B) Arch angiogram, later films. The left vertebral artery is now opacified after filling from the right ICVA, and blood is flowing retrograde down the left vertebral artery into the left subclavian artery beyond the occlusion (large curved arrow). From Caplan LR. *Posterior Circulation Disease: Clinical Findings, Diagnosis, and Management.* New York: Blackwell Science, 1996 with permission of Blackwell Publishing Ltd.

numbness, or fatigue in the arm.[14] Only 15 of the 324 patients (4.6%) studied, however, had objective physical signs of brachial ischemia or embolism.[14] Neurological symptoms are not common unless there is accompanying carotid artery disease. Among 155 patients, 116 patients (74%) with a unilateral subclavian steal shown by ultrasonography had no neurological symptoms.[14]

> JK, a 53-year-old laborer, noted occasional dizziness, sometimes with diplopia and fuzzy vision, when he worked. The attacks were brief, and always went away within seconds when he stopped working. For 6 months, his left hand felt cool and occasionally ached after he exercised.

The most frequent symptoms of subclavian artery disease relate to the ipsilateral arm and hand. Coolness, weakness, and pain on use of the arm are common, but may not be severe enough for the patient to consult a doctor. When there is impairment of vertebral artery flow (decreased antegrade flow or retrograde flow), patients may report spells of dizziness. Dizziness is by far the most common neurological symptom of subclavian steal syndrome, and usually has a spinning or vertiginous character. Diplopia, decreased vision, oscillopsia, and staggering occur but less frequently, often accompanying the dizziness. The attacks are brief and are occasionally brought on by exercising the ischemic arm, a diagnostic point that is sometimes useful during examination. In patients who underwent coronary artery bypass surgery using the internal mammary artery, blood flow to the heart may be diverted during ipsilateral

upper extremity exercise, thereby leading to symptoms of angina (coronary-subclavian steal phenomenon).[15] In most patients, however, exercise of the ischemic limb does not provoke neurological symptoms or signs.

> On examination of JK, the left radial pulse was smaller in volume and delayed relative to the carotid and right radial pulses. Blood pressure was 160/90 mmHg in the right arm, and 120/50 mmHg in the left. The left hand felt cool. There was a loud bruit in the left supraclavicular region that decreased slightly as the blood pressure cuff on the left arm was inflated to a pressure exceeding 120 mmHg. There also was a loud, high-pitched focal bruit at the right carotid bifurcation. Neurological examination was normal.

The diagnosis of subclavian artery occlusive disease can usually be made by physical examination. Invariably, there is a difference in the wrist and the antecubital pulses in the two arms. The pulse in the affected limb is of smaller volume and is delayed relative to the contralateral arm. The blood pressure is also reduced asymmetrically. In our experience, the pulse asymmetry has usually been more obvious than the blood pressure difference. We believe that it is more important to carefully feel both wrist pulses simultaneously than it is to routinely measure blood pressure in both arms. A supraclavicular bruit may be present. When the bruit originates from an ECVA stenosis without subclavian artery narrowing, inflating a blood pressure cuff above systolic pressure may augment the bruit by directing more blood into the ECVA. When the bruit

253

is caused by subclavian or innominate artery stenosis, similarly inflating the cuff reduces flow into the arm, so the bruit becomes softer.

Atherosclerotic subclavian artery stenosis occurs in 0.5–2.0% of patients. The left side is more often affected than the right, and the segment proximal to the vertebral artery is more often involved than the segment distal to the vertebral artery origin. Atherosclerosis of the proximal subclavian artery is usually associated with occlusive disease in other large arteries, typically the coronary, lower extremity, and other extracranial arteries. In JK, the loud, focal, right carotid bruit indicated important concomitant right internal carotid artery (ICA) disease.

Other diseases, especially temporal arteritis[16] and Takayasu's disease,[17,18] can cause subclavian artery stenosis. Temporal arteritis with involvement of aortic arch branches is rare and is limited to geriatric patients. Takayasu's arteritis is most common in young Asian girls and women, and middle-aged men in India. Takayasu's is also known as pulseless disease because of the almost invariable loss of arterial pulses at the wrist. In these patients, arterial blood pressure measurements taken in the usual way are not a reliable reflection of systemic blood pressure.

Baseball pitchers and cricket bowlers are also at risk for developing innominate and subclavian artery disease because of their arm mechanics during throwing. A cervical rib or chronic use of an arm crutch can also lead to stenosis or aneurysmal dilation of the subclavian artery. Clots can form in the diseased vessel and periodically embolize to individual finger arteries, causing a syndrome that can be confused with unilateral Raynaud's syndrome. When the lesion affects the innominate artery, signs and symptoms of decreased carotid artery flow can also occur. Innominate artery disease is much less common than subclavian artery disease.[19,20] Figure 8.3 is a magnetic resonance angiogram (MRA) of a patient with severe innominate artery stenosis.

A large proportion of patients with innominate artery disease are cigarette smokers. In series of patients with innominate artery disease, women are more often affected than men, in contrast to patients with carotid, subclavian, and peripheral vascular occlusive disease, in which there is a male preponderance.[19] Although right subclavian steal is much less frequent than left, it is more serious and more important to treat. Two early patients, reported by Symonds, had right subclavian-artery occlusion with spread of clot into the innominate and carotid arterial systems.[21] Since then, occasional patients who had recurrent arm and brain ischemia, caused by embolization of floating thrombi within the innominate artery, have been reported.[1,22,23]

An illustrative case report described the events in a well-known professional baseball pitcher.[24] Symptoms began when the pitcher noted his throwing arm suddenly went "dead" and his first three digits felt numb. Angiography showed complete occlusion of the right subclavian artery just proximal to the medial edge of the first rib. Five days later while exercising, he suddenly developed a left hemiplegia and confusion.[24] A new angiogram showed that the clot had propagated proximally to

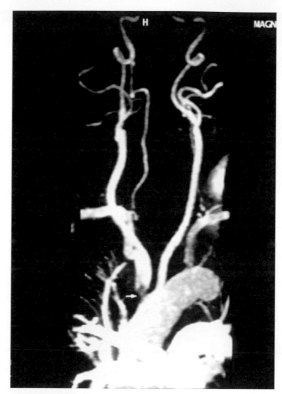

Figure 8.3 Gadolinium-enhanced MRA of the aortic arch region showing a severe stenosis of the proximal innominate artery (white arrow).

block the innominate artery, and had embolized into ICA branches intracranially.[24]

LRC had a patient whose clinical symptoms and signs allowed him to posit an innominate artery occlusion. She presented with a remarkable constellation of symptoms and signs including transient right monocular visual loss, coldness of the right arm, left upper-extremity weakness, double vision, dizziness, ataxia, and a left homonymous hemianopia. Evaluation, including magnetic resonance imaging (MRI) and angiography, showed a stenosis of the right innominate artery with a superimposed thrombus. Infarcts were present within the right MCA territory, right posterior cerebral artery (PCA) territory, and the cerebellar territory supplied by the superior cerebellar artery (SCA). The patient had embolization through the right carotid artery branch of the innominate artery, to the ipsilateral eye and the MCA, and through the ipsilateral subclavian-ECVA to the distal basilar artery and its PCA and SCA branches. The array of ipsilateral arm and eye ischemia, accompanied by anterior and posterior circulation ischemia (or both), is diagnostic of innominate artery disease.

Although frequent attacks of posterior circulation ischemia may occur in patients with subclavian steal, development of a posterior circulation stroke is rare.[1,14,25] There is usually much smoke but little fire. I could find only two documented, reported examples of serious brainstem or cerebellar infarction in patients with subclavian steal, and each followed severe hypotension. Among 407 patients with posterior circulation TIAs and ischemic strokes in the New England Medical Center Posterior Circulation Registry, only two had symptoms (TIAs)

attributable to significant subclavian or innominate artery disease.[1,2,26,27]

Non-invasive testing of JK's arms showed reduced left forearm blood flow measured by oscillography. Duplex ultrasonography showed severe stenosis 2 cm beyond the origin of the left subclavian artery. Continuous wave (CW) Doppler examination at C2 revealed a reversal of flow in the left ECVA. Transcranial Doppler (TCD) blood-flow velocities were normal. MRI was normal. Angiography confirmed a high-grade stenosis of the left subclavian artery, with retrograde flow down the left vertebral artery on delayed films. A moderately severe stenosis (2.5-mm residual lumen) of the right ICA and slight stenosis of the left ICA at their origins were also evident. The intracranial arteries were normal. He was treated with a combination of 25 mg of aspirin and 200 mg of modified-release dipyridamole twice a day and was urged to limit vigorous exercising of the left arm. The episodes of dizziness persisted for 2 months and then stopped. He has been followed for symptoms of anterior circulation ischemia.

Non-invasive testing of flow in the arm should allow the diagnosis of subclavian artery stenosis. Helpful are oscillographic measurements of forearm blood flow, venous occlusive plethysmography of the arm,[28] and analysis of the relative velocities of pulse-wave propagation in the two arms.[29] Doppler sonography gives an accurate indication of flow in the proximal ECVA system. Hennerici et al. studied the accuracy of CW Doppler in detecting innominate and subclavian artery lesions.[20] All 21 patients with Doppler-detected innominate artery stenosis and all 66 patients with subclavian steal had angiography that confirmed the ultrasound findings.[20] In patients with slight or moderate subclavian artery stenosis, reduction of flow is found in the ECVA during systole. The flow, however, is usually antegrade. With increasingly severe subclavian artery stenosis, blood flow reverses during systole, but remains cephalad in diastole, or blood flow is persistently decreased.[14,30–33] The subclavian and proximal portion of the vertebral arteries are often well shown by duplex sonography and CW Doppler[34] (see Figures 4.9, 4.10, and 4.11). The left subclavian artery B-mode images are usually obtained 1–4 cm above the subclavian artery origin. Duplex scanning of the right subclavian artery is more problematic because the proximal right subclavian artery makes a posterolateral curve.[34]

TCD recordings give information about the intracranial effects of the proximal arterial diease.[14,32,33] Hennerici et al. reported the TCD findings in 50 patients with subclavian steal: 47 unilateral and 3 bilateral.[14] Most patients had normal brachial artery blood flow velocities and retrograde flow, irrespective of the flow pattern in the proximal ECVA. CTA and MRA can also show the innominate and subclavian arteries as well as the ECVAs, especially when arch films are taken after gadolinium infusions. Figure 4.23 is a gadolinium-enhanced MRA that shows normal subclavian, innominate, and vertebral arteries. Figure 8.3 is a gadolinium-enhanced study that shows severe innominate artery disease. Figure 4.26 is a CTA showing the left subclavian artery and the origin of the vertebral artery.

When angiography is performed, it is especially important to obtain delayed films of ECVA flow; otherwise, the retrograde phase of flow might be missed. It is also important to assess the carotid arteries carefully because often there is associated occlusive disease in other arteries.

Subclavian artery disease is usually relatively benign. The spells of posterior circulation ischemia and the arm symptoms often improve with time, as collateral circulation to the arm develops. Operations on the proximal subclavian or innominate artery, when performed by thoracotomy, are more serious operative procedures than vascular surgery involving only a neck incision. Angioplasty and stenting have recently almost entirely replaced surgery on the innominate and subclavian arteries.

Surgery on the subclavian and innominate arteries is much more difficult than carotid artery surgery and has more frequent complications. In a systematic review of 2496 patients, the average complication rate associated with surgery was 16%, with a stroke rate of 3%, and mortality rate of 2%.[35] Studies of balloon angioplasty and/or stenting for treatment of subclavian artery stenosis report more favorable results than surgery with improvement or cessation of presenting symptoms in 72–100%, technical success in 90–100%, periprocedural complications in 0–10%, and stroke and death in 0–4%.[36–42] Stenting has been performed in patients with subclavian artery stenosis with very good technical success and patency rates. In one series, Henry et al. reported the results among 113 patients treated for subclavian stenosis or occlusion with either angioplasty alone ($N = 57$) or stenting ($N = 46$) with 91% technical success and 2.6% complication rate.[38] Procedural failures were mostly in patients with occluded vessels. Over 4.3 years of average follow-up, restenosis occurred in 16%, the majority of whom had been treated with angioplasty only.[38] In contrast, Schillinger et al. found a higher rate of initial technical success in 115 patients in whom stents were applied for subclavian stenosis: 95% of stented vessels remained patent at 1 year versus 76% treated with angioplasty; however, by 4 years, only 59% of stented vessels remained patent compared with 68% for angioplasty alone.[43] Currently, there is insufficient evidence to determine whether stenting is more effective than angioplasty alone for stenosis of the subclavian artery.[44]

Sometimes, the intriguing radiological demonstration of reversal of VA flow seduces surgeons into operating on the subclavian artery (by repair of the subclavian artery or ligation of the proximal ECVA) or interventionalists into angioplasty or stenting of the narrowed artery. When the patient is incapacitated by arm ischemia (e.g., if the syndrome occurs in a golfer or a pitcher), repair is indicated. When the disease affects the right innominate or subclavian artery, serious carotid-territory infarction can ensue, so aggressive treatment is often indicated. In most other patients, we suggest watchful waiting. Subclavian artery stenosis, even when symptomatic, is a marker for atherosclerosis burden. The presence of subclavian artery stenosis is associated with increased total mortality (hazard ratio 1.40) and cardiovascular disease mortality (hazard ratio 1.57).[45]

When patients with subclavian or innominate artery stenosis are encountered, we try to reduce risk factors, such as smoking, hypertension, and hyperlipidemia, and observe the patient for attacks related to the anterior circulation. LRC usually prescribes a statin in high doses (equivalent of 80 mg of atorvastatin), an antiplatelet agent, and often an angiotensin-converting enzyme (ACE) inhibitor or ACE receptor blocker.

Occlusion or severe stenosis of the vertebral artery in the neck

Proximal atherosclerotic extracranial vertebral artery disease

The most frequent location for atherosclerotic disease of the ECVAs is at their origin from the subclavian arteries. Atherosclerosis at this site shares epidemiological features with its close cousin, atherosclerosis of the ICA origin. In fact, the two sites are frequently affected in the same individuals.[46–48] LRC and his colleagues found that stenosis at the ECVA origins is found less often in African-Americans and Asians than in whites.[1,49] JSK and colleagues found that ECVA disease (4%) was a less common cause of ischemic stroke than distal vertebral artery (6 %) or posterior cerebral artery (6 %) or basilar artery disease (8%) in Korean patients.[50] Proximal ECVA stenosis is often accompanied by hypertension, smoking, coronary artery disease, and peripheral vascular occlusive disease. ECVA was the most common site of atherosclerotic narrowing in the New England Medical Center Posterior Circulation Registry series among 407 patients with vertebrobasilar TIAs and strokes.[1,26,27] A total of 131 patients (32%) had significant (>50%) narrowing of the ECVA, 29 bilaterally. Many patients with severe ECVA disease also had severe occlusive disease within the intracranial vertebrobasilar arterial system, sometimes at multiple sites.[26,27] Among patients who had occlusive lesions at only one site, 52 had only proximal ECVA disease (15 bilaterally).[26,27]

> LM, a 63-year-old white man, had repeated attacks of spinning dizziness during the past 2 weeks. In some spells, the only symptom was dizziness. In others, diplopia and staggering occurred. In one attack, his right limbs felt transiently weak. The attacks were brief, lasting 30 seconds to 4 minutes. They tended to occur while he was quietly resting, and never occurred during exertion. He also had occasional left occipital headaches.

The most frequently reported symptom during TIAs caused by ECVA-origin disease is dizziness. The attacks are indistinguishable from those described by patients with subclavian steal, except that ECVA-origin TIAs are not precipitated by effort or by arm exertion. Although dizziness is the most common symptom, it is seldom the only neurological symptom. Usually, in at least some attacks, dizziness is accompanied by other definite signs of hindbrain ischemia. Diplopia, oscillopsia, hemiparesis, or numbness are often mentioned if the patient is closely questioned. Repeated spells of dizziness or vertigo unaccompanied by other neurological symptoms are rarely associated with occlusive posterior circulation lesions.[51–53] Because dizziness is a common neurological symptom and is in most cases not caused by cerebrovascular disease, we seldom diagnose ECVA disease in patients with repeated, unaccompanied dizziness. True benign positional vertigo, present only on rising and retiring, are almost never caused by ECVA-origin disease. In patients with risk factors for stroke, however, ultrasound or CTA or MRA may be needed to detect lesions of the vertebral arteries in the neck or intracranially.

Vertebral artery atheromas often originate in the subclavian artery and spread to the proximal few centimeters of the ECVA. They may also arise at the origin of the ECVA. Little has been written about the morphology of VA-origin lesions. Although ulceration and plaque hemorrhage are commonly recognized when carotid endarterectomy specimens are examined, ECVA lesions are said to be fibrous and smooth and seldom ulcerate.[54,55] Scant pathological data about ECVA-origin lesions exist because endarterectomy is not often performed in patients with ECVA disease, so the vessel is not available for pathological examination. Careful necropsy examinations of the ECVAs have not been reported subsequent to recognition of the importance of plaque ulceration and hemorrhage. ICA- and ECVA-origin lesions may not be morphologically identical. The geometry of the two origins is quite different. The ECVA arises at nearly 90 degrees from the subclavian artery, whereas the ICA is almost a direct 180-degree extension of the common carotid artery (CCA). Caliber and flow disparities between the ICA and ECVA origins also exist. Only a small fraction of subclavian artery flow goes into each ECVA, a much smaller artery, whereas a high proportion of CCA blood goes into the ICA, a vessel of nearly the same size.

In 1989, Pelouze reported a man who had multiple attacks of vertigo and brainstem ischemia that continued despite prescription of aspirin.[56] Angiography showed irregular stenosis near the ECVA origin and a B-mode ultrasound scan suggested an ulcerated plaque. An ECVA endarterectomy was performed, and the surgical specimen showed an ulcerated, irregular plaque that represented the source of multiple intracranial posterior circulation emboli.[56] The question of the frequency of ECVA-origin plaque ulceration is of great importance, but remains unsolved until more necropsy or surgical specimens are carefully examined. Do small platelet–fibrin and erythrocyte–fibrin emboli arise frequently from the proximal ECVA and embolize to distal arteries in the posterior circulation? Would agents that reduce platelet aggregability or anticoagulants (or both) be effective for patients with ECVA-origin TIAs?

Two important anatomical facts explain why ECVA-origin lesions seldom cause chronic, hemodynamically significant low flow to the vertebrobasilar system:

1. The vertebral arteries are paired vessels that unite to form a single basilar artery; only rarely is there complete atresia of one vertebral artery, although asymmetries are frequent.

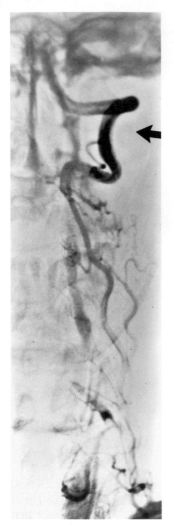

Figure 8.4 Subclavian artery angiogram showing filling of the distal extracranial VA (black arrow) from collaterals. From Caplan LR. *Posterior Circulation Disease: Clinical Findings, Diagnosis, and Management.* New York: Blackwell Science, 1996 with permission of Blackwell Publishing Ltd.

2. The ECVA gives off numerous muscular and other branches as it ascends in the neck. In contrast, there are no nuchal branches of the ICA.

In the vertebral artery system, there is much more potential for development of adequate collateral circulation than when a carotid artery occludes. Figure 8.4 shows collaterals filling the distal ECVA in a patient with ECVA-origin occlusion. Even when there is bilateral occlusion of the ECVAs, some patients do not develop posterior circulation infarcts.[1,26,27,57–62] ECVA-origin disease is more benign than ICA-origin disease from a hemodynamic aspect. Only 13 patients who had ECVA disease among the 407 patients in the New England Medical Center Posterior Circulation Registry had a chronic, recurrent low flow mechanism of brain ischemia.[27] In 12 of these 13, there was severe bilateral, vertebral artery occlusive disease. Six had severe bilateral ECVA disease and six had severe intracranial vertebral artery (ICVA) disease contralateral to severe disease of one ECVA. The only patient who did not have bilateral vertebral artery disease, had a unilateral ECVA occlusion and

Table 8.1 Groups of patients with severe ECVA disease in the New England Medical Center Posterior Circulation Registry

ECVA group characteristics	No. of patients (%)
Coexistent severe intracranial (ICVA and/or basilar artery) occlusive disease	22 (27.5%)
Artery-to-artery embolism from the ECVA	19 (24%)
Probable artery-to-artery embolism from the ECVA*	20 (25%)
Hemodynamic TIAs	13 (16%)
Dissection	6 (7.5%)

* These patients all had other potential embolic sources but the ECVA was judged the most likely source.

bilateral ICA occlusions. All 13 patients had TIAs. Only two had brain infarcts, one affecting the occipital lobe and the other the temporal lobe and cerebellum. TIAs were multiple and recurred during one week to several months. Dizziness, often accompanied by veering to one side and gait ataxia, visual blurring, perioral paresthesias, and diplopia were the commonest TIA symptoms.[27]

Embolization of white platelet–fibrin and red erythrocyte–fibrin thrombi from atherostenotic occlusive lesions is the most important presentation of ECVA-origin disease.[1,2,27,58–62] During one 2-week period, LRC cared for 3 patients with intra-arterial posterior circulation embolism arising from an occlusive lesion at the ECVA origin. A similar situation is well known in the anterior circulation. A patient is admitted with a small MCA-territory infarct, and ultrasound or angiography shows an occlusion at the ICA origin. The recently formed occlusive thrombus has fragmented and embolized distally. Among 407 patients in the New England Medical Center Posterior Circulation Registry, 80 patients had very severe pre-occlusive stenosis or occlusion of the proximal ECVA. In 45 (56%) of these 80 patients (39 who had atherosclerotic lesions and 6 with dissections), embolization from the VA lesion was the most likely cause of brain ischemia.[58] Table 8.1 describes the posited mechanisms of brain infarction among these 80 patients. Twenty-two had coexistent severe intracranial disease that was more likely to explain the stroke than the ECVA lesion. Figure 8.5 is a CTA that shows a thrombus at the origin of the vertebral artery in the neck. Intra-arterial embolism to the intracranial posterior circulation arteries occurs much more often than is presently recognized.

Neurological examination of LM was normal. A high-pitched focal bruit was audible in the left supraclavicular fossa, and a soft bruit was heard over the right posterior mastoid region. The MRI was normal. Non-invasive testing confirmed a reduction of flow in the left ECVA. A catheter digital-subtraction angiogram showed severe stenosis of the left ECVA origin (Figure 8.6). Intracranial films showed good basilar artery filling. The right VA was normal. He was treated with warfarin

257

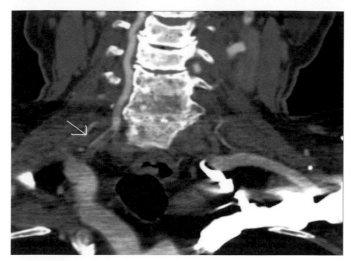

Figure 8.5 CTA showing a filling defect (white arrow) representing a thrombus that formed at the origin of the right VA.

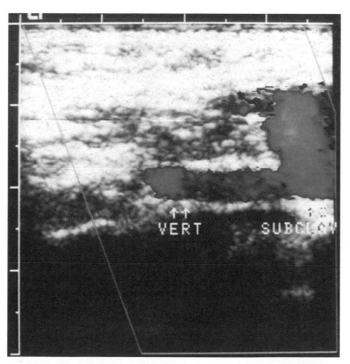

Figure 8.7 An image is shown from a color-flow Doppler study of the vertebral artery of the proximal ECVA. Blood flows from the subclavian artery (right) into the VA.

and had no further attacks. Six months later, B-mode, CW Doppler, and Color flow Doppler imaging (CFDI) suggested complete occlusion of the proximal ECVA with no antegrade flow. Warfarin was stopped a month later without subsequent ischemic spells.

In patients with proximal ECVA disease, a bruit can often be heard over the supraclavicular region. Physicians should auscultate by moving the stethoscope bell to listen over the posterior cervical muscles and mastoid. Sometimes, as in the patient LM, a bruit is heard over the contralateral side because of increased collateral blood flow. B-mode scans can image the proximal VA in the segment between the origin of the artery

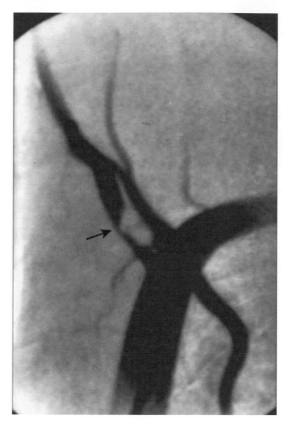

Figure 8.6 Subclavian angiogram showing severe stenosis of the left ECVA origin (arrow).

until its entrance into the foramen transversaria of the cervical vertebrae.[1,32–34] CFDI is also helpful in showing the origin of the ECVA and distal flow patterns. Figure 8.7 shows a CFDI image of the origin of the ECVA from the subclavian artery. CW Doppler insonation in the low neck and at the C2 region is the most effective means of monitoring ECVA blood flow. In the presence of a severe occlusive lesion at the ECVA origin, blood flow is usually retrograde or to-and-fro above the occlusive lesion. CTA has been able to show the vertebral artery origin from the subclavian artery, at times better than using MRA. MRA, especially with gadolinium enhancement and attention to the aortic arch branches, can also most often provide diagnostic quality images of the proximal ECVA.

Data about the natural history of disease of the ECVA origin and the response of patients with this lesion to various treatments are insufficient to warrant firm conclusions as to the best therapy. Moufarrij and colleagues reviewed the Cleveland Clinic experience with VA lesions.[63] Long-term follow-up of their series of more than 80 patients with greater than 75% stenosis of the ECVA origin showed that only two patients had brainstem strokes. These two patients also had basilar artery stenosis.[63]

Vascular surgeons with considerable experience in operating on the ECVA have shown that they can bypass ECVA-origin lesions with low morbidity and mortality.[1,55,56,64–68] Angioplasty and stenting have been performed much less often on the ECVA than on the ICA. Some reports cite a restenosis rates of 9–10% within one year.[69–73] In the

Stenting of Symptomatic Atherosclerotic Lesions in the Vertebral or Intracranial Arteries (SSYLVIA) trial, 6 of 14 (43%) ECVAs treated with stenting developed restenosis more than 50% at 6 months follow-up.[73] This preliminary experience with ECVA angioplasty/stenting has raised concerns that the restenosis rate of interventional treatment of the ECVA may be relatively high.

No data exist about the effectiveness or lack thereof of antiplatelet aggregating agents or warfarin in patients with proximal ECVA disease. In the case of LM, LRC chose warfarin to prevent thrombosis and subsequent embolization in a vessel with low-antegrade blood flow. If the lesion had been less stenotic, LRC would have chosen aspirin or aspirin combined with modified-release dipyridamole or with cilostazole to prevent fibrin–platelet emboli. JSK prefers to use aspirin plus clopidogrel for the initial few months and change to monotherapy after the patient is stabilized.

In selected patients, LRC has chosen surgical reconstruction while JSK and his colleagues prefer angioplasty/stenting. Clearly, more data are needed regarding the natural history of ECVA-origin disease and its response to medical, surgical, and interventional treatments. The advent of CTA and MRA and wider application of non-invasive techniques to the posterior circulation may provide groups of patients with ECVA-origin disease who can be followed prospectively and studied to determine the relative effectiveness and risks of various potential therapies.

Dissections of the extracranial vertebral artery

Dissections usually involve portions of arteries that are mobile and rarely occur at the origins of arteries.[74] VA dissections are also discussed in detail in Chapter 12. The carotid and vertebral arteries are relatively fixed at their origins from the common carotid and subclavian arteries. The ECVAs are anchored at their origin from the subclavian artery and during their course through bone within the intervertebral foramina (V_2 portion), and also by the dura at the point of intracranial penetration. The short movable segments between these anchored regions are most vulnerable to tearing and stretching. Dissections can involve the proximal (V_1) portion of the ECVA, usually beginning well above the vessel origin from the subclavian artery, affecting the artery before it enters the intervertebral foramina at C5 or C6. V_1 dissections are almost always unilateral. The distal extracranial portion (V_3) is the most common location for dissection. This segment is relatively mobile and so vulnerable to tearing by sudden motion and stretching as might occur during chiropractic manipulation. Distal ECVA dissections may extend into the ICVA and proximally into the V_2 segment. Distal ECVA dissections are usually bilateral, even though pain and other symptoms are often unilateral.

ECVA dissections were first recognized in patients who had either neck trauma or chiropractic manipulation, but ECVA injuries also have been reported in patients who manipulate their own necks or who have maintained their necks in a fixed position for some time. ECVA dissections also occur after surgery and resuscitation, presumably because of sustained neck positions in patients who are anesthetized or

unresponsive.[75] Cervical vertebral artery dissections most often involve the distal ECVA (V_3). Spontaneous ECVA dissections closely mimic those related to trauma. Pain in the posterior neck or occiput is common, as is generalized headache.

Pain often precedes neurological symptoms by hours, days, and, rarely, weeks.[74,76–82] Some patients with ECVA dissections have only neck pain and do not develop neurological symptoms or signs. TIAs most often include dizziness, diplopia, veering, staggering, and dysarthria. TIAs are less common in ECVA dissections than in ICA dissections. Infarcts usually cause signs that begin suddenly. The commonest patterns of ischemic brain damage are cerebellar infarction in posterior inferior cerebellar artery (PICA) territory distribution and lateral medullary infarction. As in extracranial ICA dissections, infarcts are invariably explained by embolization of fresh thrombus to the ICVA. Occasionally, dissections extend or begin intracranially. Sometimes, emboli reach the superior cerebellar arteries (SCAs), the main basilar artery, or the posterior cerebral arteries (PCAs). Young age and presentation with pain and no or minor neurological signs are features predictive of a good prognosis.[82]

ECVA dissections also can cause cervical root pain.[83,84] Aneurysmal dilatation of the ECVA adjacent to nerve roots causes the radicular pain and can lead to radicular distribution motor, sensory, and reflex abnormalities. Occasionally spinal cord infarction results because of hypoperfusion in the supply zones of arteries from the ECVA that supply the cervical spinal cord.[84,85] Many patients with ECVA dissections have headache, pain, and TIAs without lasting neurological deficits.

Duplex scans of the ECVAs can suggest dissection. Typical findings are increased arterial diameter, decreased pulsatility, intravascular abnormal echoes, and hemodynamic evidence of decreased flow.[86] CFDI can also show the regions of dissection within the neck. Diminished flow in the high neck at the level of the atlas detected by CW Doppler and decreased flow in the ICVA shown by transcranial Doppler (TCD) suggest the presence of distal ECVA dissections. Dye-contrast catheter cerebral angiography is still the optimal method of imaging the extracranial vertebral arteries in patients suspected of having vertebral artery dissections. Figure 12.5 is a montage of angiograms that show VA dissections.

Intracranial vertebral artery disease

Severe atherosclerotic narrowing is rare in the cervical portions of the vertebral arteries, except at their origins. Plaques are relatively routinely observed opposite osteophytes but rarely narrow the vessel.[1,54] The distal ECVA is vulnerable to trauma,[1] dissections, and fibromuscular dysplasia. The distal cervical ECVA is occasionally severely narrowed in patients with temporal arteritis[87] and in women taking high estrogen-content contraceptive pills.[88]

Atherosclerosis of the ICVAs is most severe in the distal segment of the arteries, often at the vertebral–basilar junction.[1,89,90] Narrowing often extends into the proximal portion of the basilar artery. Less often, stenosis involves the

ICVA just after it penetrates the dura to enter the cranium. In contrast to patients with proximal ECVA disease, there is no single typical patient with ICVA occlusive disease.

Recent reports from Asia show that ICVA dissection is more common than previously thought, and most often involves the vertebral artery near the origin of PICA.[91] The dissections often extend into the basilar artery. Less commonly, the dissection may act as a mass lesion ("dissecting aneurysm") compressing the brainstem and/or cranial nerves.[92] In one study, among 31 patients with intracranial vertebrobasilar artery dissections, 55% had headache, 48% had infarction involving the brainstem or cerebellum, and 10% presented with subarachnoid hemorrhage.[93] ICVA dissection is an important cause of lateral medullary infarction.[94]

The clinical findings in patients with ICVA atherosclerosis and dissection depend heavily on the location and extent of the occlusive process and the areas of brain rendered ischemic. We present four different patients with clinical findings that illustrate the various typical patterns often presented to clinicians.

Patient 1

A 57-year-old white man, WA, had a transient attack of dizziness and diplopia when he arose from a nap. Awakening the next day, he felt dizzy, as if the room were rocking or wavering like a ship. He felt a series of sharp, painful jabs in his left eye. His left face seemed strangely numb. He veered to the left when he tried to sit or stand. His left arm was clumsy. His voice was hoarse, and he gagged as he tried to swallow water. Vomiting and hiccups developed as the morning progressed, so he went to the hospital. Examination showed: diminished pain and temperature sensation on the left face and right body, including the limbs; nystagmus with greater amplitude on looking leftward; diminished left corneal reflex; left ptosis, and a smaller left pupil; clumsiness of the left hand and foot; and decreased palatal motion on the left.

One common pattern found in patients with ICVA occlusion is explained by ischemia of the lateral medulla, the lesion illustrated by this patient.[1,94] In patients with lateral medullary infarction, the most common vascular lesion is occlusion of the proximal or middle portion of the ICVA.[1,94,95] Penetrating branches to the lateral medulla arise from the middle and distal two-thirds of the ICVAs and penetrate through the lateral medullary fossa to reach and supply the lateral medullary tegmentum.[1,96,97] The medial branches of the PICAs supply only a small portion of the dorsal medullary tegmentum.[97] The ICVA occlusive lesions decrease flow in these penetrators. Less often, lateral medullary infarction is caused by occlusion of one of the small medullary branches.

The important symptoms and signs of lateral medullary infarction can be understood best by recalling the anatomical nuclei and tracts in the lateral medulla (Figure 8.8).

1. Nucleus and descending spinal tract of V. Symptoms include sharp jabs or stabs of pain in the ipsilateral eye and face and a feeling of numbness of the face; examination usually confirms decreased pinprick and temperature sensations on the ipsilateral face, and a reduced corneal reflex.

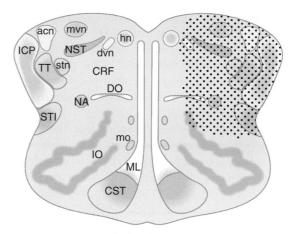

Figure 8.8 Cartoon of a dorsal lateral medullary infarct (Wallenberg's syndrome). acn, accessory cuneate nucleus; CRF, central reticular formation; CST, corticospinal tract; DO, dorsal accessory olivary nucleus; dvn, dorsal vagal nucleus; hn, hypoglossal nucleus; ICP, inferior cerebellar peduncle; IO, inferior olivary nucleus; ML, medial lemniscus; mo, medial accessory olivary nucleus; mvn, medial vestibular nucleus; NA, nucleus ambiguus; NST, nucleus of the solitary tract; STT, spinothalamic tract; stn, spinal trigeminal nucleus; TT, trigeminal tract.

2. Vestibular nuclei and their connections. Feelings of dizziness or instability of the environment result from dysfunction of the vestibular system and may invoke vomiting; careful examination usually shows nystagmus with coarse rotatory eye movements when looking to the ipsilateral side and small-amplitude, faster nystagmus when looking contralaterally;[1] sometimes, the eyes forcibly deviate to the side of the lesion, known as *ocular lateral pulsion*.[1,98,99]

3. Sensory tracts:

   Spinothalamic tract. Lesions of this structure usually produce diminished pinprick and temperature sensation in the contralateral limbs and body; this loss of function is seldom spontaneously recognized or reported by patients. Some patients note that they cannot feel hot or cold in the involved limbs. Most individuals only recognize the sensory abnormality during sensory testing when examined neurologically. Occasionally a sensory level is present on the contralateral trunk with pain and temperature loss on the trunk below that level and in the lower extremity.[1,100–102] More commonly, there is a sensory gradient, usually worse in the leg than in the arm. This is explained by a partial involvement of the spinothalamic tract of the lower brainstem, where the fibers carrying sensations from the sacral area, leg, trunk, and arm are arranged in an orderly fashion from the superficial to the medial direction.[101] At times, the pinprick and temperature loss extends to the contralateral face because of involvement of the crossed quintothalamic tract, which appends itself medially to the spinothalamic tract.[1,102] The loss of pain and temperature sensation may be totally contralateral and involves the face, arm, trunk, and leg.[1,102]

   Medial lemniscus. About 7 % of patients with lateral medullary infarction describe numbness, tightness or the sense of weakness in the ipsilateral limb especially distal

upper limb. Vibration and proprioceptive sensation are occasionally impaired. This ipsilateral sensory disturbance is almost always associated with caudal lesions extending dorsomedially that probably involve the ipsilateral dorsal column or decussating lemniscal fibers.[103]

4. Restiform body (inferior cerebellar peduncle). Symptoms include veering or leaning toward the side of the lesion and clumsiness of the ipsilateral limbs. On examination, hypotonia and exaggerated rebound of the ipsilateral arm are common, but frank intention tremor is not. On standing or sitting, patients often lean or tilt to the side of the lesion.

5. Autonomic nervous system nuclei and tracts. The descending sympathetic system traverses the lateral medulla in the lateral reticular formation; dysfunction causes an ipsilateral Horner's syndrome; and the dorsal motor nucleus of the vagus is sometimes affected, leading to tachycardia and a labile increased blood pressure. Hiccups are common.

6. Nucleus ambiguus. When the infarct extends medially, it often affects this nucleus, causing hoarseness and dysphagia. The pharynx and palate are weak on the side of the lesion, sometimes causing patients to retain food within the piriform recess of the pharynx. A crow-like cough represents an attempt to extricate food from this area.

7. Facial nuclei or tract. At times, there is ipsilateral facial weakness, perhaps related to ischemia of the caudal part of the VII-nerve nucleus or fascicles, just rostral to the nucleus ambiguus, or involvement of corticobulbar fibers going toward the VII-nerve nucleus.[1]

8. Respiratory control structures. Initiation and control of respiration are known to involve the lateral pontine and medullary tegmentum. Poliomyelitis and bilateral medullary infarcts are well known to cause decreased respiratory drive.[104] Levin and Margolis described a single patient with failure of automatic respirations ("Ondine's curse," or sleep-related apnea) caused by a one-sided lateral medullary infarct.[105] Bogousslavsky et al. described the clinical and autopsy findings in two patients with one-sided lateral medullopontine infarction who had respiratory failure.[106] Hypoventilation is probably related to involvement of the nucleus of the solitary tract, nucleus ambiguus, nucleus retroambiguus, and nuclei parvocellularis and gigantocellularis.[1,106]

MRI studies have shown that infarct patterns and clinical findings differ according to the rostal-caudal location of infarcts.[94] Rostral lesions are associated with distal vertebral artery (or vertebro-basilar junction) atherosclerotic disease and tend to involve ventral paramedian area that include the nucleus ambiguus and the crossed secondary quintothalamic sensory tract. These patients tend to have severe dysphagia, dysarthria, contralateral trigeminal sensory loss and facial palsy. On the other hand, caudally located infarcts are usually superficial and laterally located, and produce more severe gait ataxia and sensory gradient worse in the lower extremities due to involvement of the laterally located spinocerebellar tract and partial involvement of the spinothalamic tract, respectively. The intermediate lesions usually present with signs similar to WA.

When infarction is limited to the lateral medulla, prognosis for recovery is good,[1,107] although there are three exceptions to this rule:[1,108]

1. Some patients also have infarction in the ipsilateral inferior cerebellum, a region fed by the PICA. When the ICVA occlusion is long and extends to block the orifices of both PICA and the lateral medullary penetrators, both lateral medullary and cerebellar infarction develop. This occurs in about one in six patients with lateral medullary infarction.[1,109] When the infarct is large, headache, head tilt, and stupor can result. A posterior fossa pressure cone can develop and cause death from medullary compression.[1]

2. Some patients with lateral medullary infarcts die suddenly; although the etiology of sudden death is uncertain, it is most likely caused by an increase in vagal tone (secondary to involvement of the dorsal motor nucleus of the vagus), or to involvement of automatic respiratory centers.

3. Some patients with one-sided lateral medullary infarcts have occlusive lesions in both ICVAs. Development of symptomatic ischemia, in the lateral medulla contralateral to the infarct, has a serious prognosis because of the frequency of autonomic dysfunction and loss of automatic control of respiration. Some patients with bilateral ICVA disease have a poor outcome once symptoms develop.[1,89,90,110]

Because of these important problems, it has been our practice to evaluate patients with lateral medullary infarcts for cerebellar infarction and cerebellar mass effect using MRI, to study the ICVAs non-invasively using MRA, CTA, or TCD, and to monitor respiration early in the course of the illness. Figure 8.9 shows MRIs that clearly show lateral medullary infarcts.

In some patients with ICVA steno-occlusion, ischemia of the medial medulla accompanies the lateral medullary infarct. This phenomenon is explained by an ICVA occlusion that concomitantly blocks the orifice of the lateral medullary penetrators and the anterior spinal artery that supplies the medial portion of the medulla.[111] In addition to the signs already mentioned, a hemiparesis affects the contralateral arm and leg because of ischemia to the medullary pyramid. Ipsilateral weakness of the tongue and contralateral loss of position sense are less frequent findings and are explained by involvement of the hypoglossal nerve and the medial lemniscus.[112–114] The combination of medial and lateral medullary infarcts is often referred to as *hemimedullary infarction* and is caused by a long occlusion of the distal ICVA (that spares the PICA branch).

Occlusion of the distal portion of the ICVA that blocks only the orifice of the anterior spinal artery branch can cause infarction, limited to the medial medulla, without associated lateral medullary infarction.[114] In approximately 10% of the patients, medial medullary infarction is bilateral and may extend caudally into the rostral spinal cord, causing a syndrome of

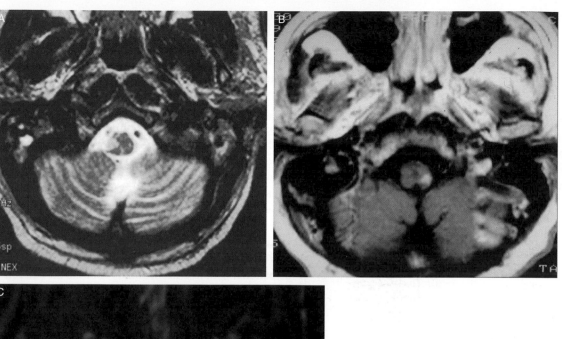

Figure 8.9 MRIs showing lateral medullary infarcts. (A) T2-weighted MRI scan. A small area of hyperintensity is shown in the left lateral medulla. The flow void in the adjacent left intracranial vertebral artery has been obliterated because of occlusion of that vessel. The right vertebral artery flow void is clearly visible and is normal. (B) T2-weighted MRI scan. A small infarct is seen in the right dorsal lateral medulla. (C) FLAIR MRI showing a triangular area of infarction in a young patient with lateral medullary infarction who died suddenly. Kindly submitted by Dr Agnieszka Ardelt, University Of Chicago, IL.

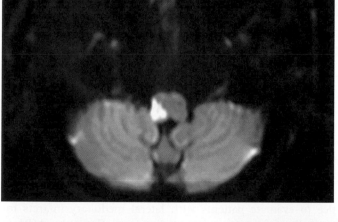

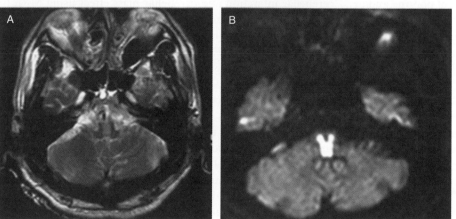

Figure 8.10 MRI scans of a patient with a bilateral medial medullary infarct. (A) A T2-weighted scan. The hyperintensity in the medial medullary base and tegmentum is visible but is slight. (B) This diffusion-weighted scan shows the abnormality much more obviously. Courtesy of Yasumasa Yamamoto, MD, Kyoto, Japan.

quadriparesis difficult to separate from basilar artery occlusion with pontine infarction.[115,116] Although contributors to the anterior spinal artery usually originate from each side, in some patients a branch from one side becomes the anterior spinal artery supply to the bilateral caudal medial medulla and rostral spinal cord. The MRI in Figure 8.10 shows a bilateral medial medullary infarct.

The ICVAs are located lateral to the brainstem when they first penetrate the dura mater to enter the cranium. They angle medially to merge together to form the basilar artery at the medullo-pontine junction. The proximal portion of the ICVAs lies adjacent to the medullary tegmentum while the distal more medially located distal portion of the ICVA lies more in relation to the ventral portion of the rostral medulla. The

medullary pyramids lie closest to the distal ICVAs. This relationship is shown in Figure 8.11. The changing relationship of the ICVAs to the portions of the caudal, middle, and rostral portions of the medulla explain why lesions of the ICVAs at different levels have a predilection for causing different clinical syndromes.

In many patients with ICVA disease, the region of stenosis is distal within the artery, often near the ICVA/basilar artery junction. Patients in whom there is only distal ICVA stenosis do not have ischemic symptoms or infarction in the medulla and posterior inferior cerebellum caused by the ICVA lesions. Table 8.2 shows the location of ICVA stenosis in the New England Medical Center Posterior Circulation Registry.

In WA, B-mode and CW Doppler of the ECVA were normal. TCD showed an increase in blood-flow velocities in the left ICVA. Right ICVA pressures were normal. MRA showed severe stenosis of the left ICVA, just after the artery entered the cranium.

TCD can give accurate indications of occlusive lesions, involving the ICVAs, using insonation through a suboccipital foramen magnum window.[32,33] After the TCD and MRA results, the patient was treated with warfarin. The arterial stenosis is being followed by serial TCD examinations.

Table 8.2 Location within the ICVA of steno-occlusive lesions in the New England Medical Center Posterior Circulation Registry

Location	Number
Proximal-third of the ICVA	14 (24%)
Middle-third of the ICVA	2 (3%)
Distal-third of the ICVA and ICVA–basilar artery junction	40 (66%)
Proximal- and middle-thirds of the ICVA	2 (3%)
Proximal-, middle-, and distal-thirds of the ICVA	17 (28%)

Patient 2

A 48-year-old woman, AD, suddenly felt dizzy and unsteady on her feet. She vomited and became unable to walk. When examined, the only abnormal findings were gait ataxia and slight conjugate gaze paresis to the left. CT was normal. The next morning, she was sleepy and reported severe headache. Her neck was stiff and she preferred to stay stationary in bed. A complete left conjugate gaze paresis to oculocephalic maneuvers was evident, and the left corneal reflex was reduced. Both plantar responses were extensor. CT showed a large area of hypodensity in the left cerebellum. The IVth ventricle was not visible, and the lateral ventricles were enlarged. MRI confirmed a large PICA-territory cerebellar infarct (Figure 8.12). She became stuporous and difficult to arouse. She was treated with intravenous steroids and mannitol, but did not awaken. Soft, necrotic, cerebellar tissue was removed through a left posterior fossa craniotomy, after which she made an excellent recovery.

The most common vascular lesion found in patients with cerebellar infarction is occlusion or severe stenosis of the ICVA.[1,117–120] Often, the ICVA occlusion is caused by embolism, the thrombus arising from a source in the heart, or proximal vascular system.[1,120–122] The syndrome of cerebellar infarction is often difficult to diagnose. Symptoms can resemble labyrinthitis and often appear deceptively slight. Gait ataxia and vomiting are often accompanied by dizziness, closely mimicking the findings in patients with cerebellar hemorrhage.[1,122,123] Most often, no signs of lateral medullary ischemia are evident. Initial CT scans may be normal. It is important to make certain that the IVth ventricle is of normal size and is in normal position. In retrospect, this was not done in this patient. Review of the initial films revealed slight rightward deviation and tilting of the IVth ventricle.

MRI is more accurate in detecting early cerebellar ischemia. Especially important for localization are T2-weighted sagittal sections. On sagittal films, localization of the vascular territory involved is relatively easy. Lesions above the horizontal fissure are in the SCA territory. Lesions below the fissure are localized to anterior inferior cerebellar artery (AICA) or

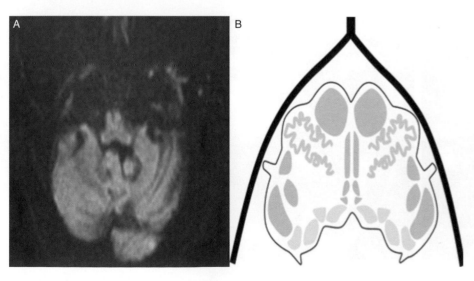

Figure 8.11 (A) This figure is a T2-weighted MRI of the medulla. Note that the pyramids are more dorsally located and the medullary tegmentum is more ventrally placed within the posterior cranial fossa. (B) The drawing shows diagrammatically the medullary components in relation to the intracranial vertebral arteries which course from lateral to medial where they join together at the top of the figure.

PICA territories, depending on anterior or posterior localization on the inferior surface of the cerebellum. Figure 8.13 shows a PICA-territory infarct on a T2-weighted sagittal MRI section. Compare this image with Figure 8.14A and B that show SCA territory cerebellar infarcts. Figure 8.15 is a sagittal MRI that shows PICA and SCA territory infarcts on the same side.

Swollen cerebellar lesions may compress the cerebellopontine angle, leading to involvement of the ipsilateral fifth, sixth, seventh, and eighth cranial nerves. Compression of the medulla and pons is the probable cause of conjugate-gaze paresis to the ipsilateral side. This finding is especially important because the presence of a conjugate-gaze palsy, without contralateral hemiplegia, is virtually diagnostic of a cerebellar space-taking lesion. With more severe compression, the plantar responses become extensor, systolic pressure rises, diastolic pressure falls, the pulse may slow, and respiration may cease.

As the cerebellum swells, hypodensity usually appears on repeat CT scans. Posterior fossa cisterns are compressed, and the ventricles become enlarged because of compression of the IVth ventricle. On MRI, compression of the contralateral vermis and brainstem are usually evident. Without treatment, death often ensues.[1,120,124-126] The preferred therapy is decompression of the swollen cerebellum. In some patients, medical decompression using steroids and osmotic agents has been helpful. Success has also been achieved in some patients by placing a ventricular drain in the lateral ventricles.[127,128] It is often difficult to separate brainstem pressure caused by cerebellar infarction, from brainstem ischemia caused by the propagation of clot into the basilar artery. MRI scans are helpful in making this distinction, but MRA or catheter angiography (or both) are often necessary to visualize the vascular lesions.

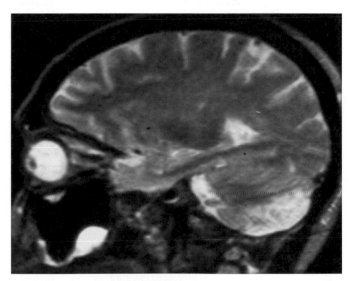

Figure 8.12 MRI T2-weighted axial image showing large PICA-territory infarct.

Figure 8.13 MRI T2-weighted sagittal view showing an infarct in the posterior inferior portion of the cerebellum.

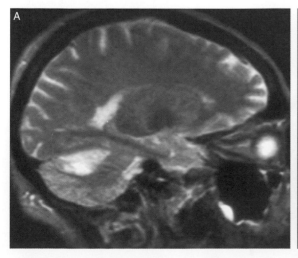

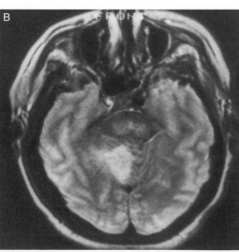

Figure 8.14 T2-weighted MRI scans. (A) An infarct is seen in the superior portion of the cerebellum in the territory of the SCA. (B) Axial scan showing an infarct in the superior portion of the cerebellar vermis in the territory of the medial branch of the SCA.

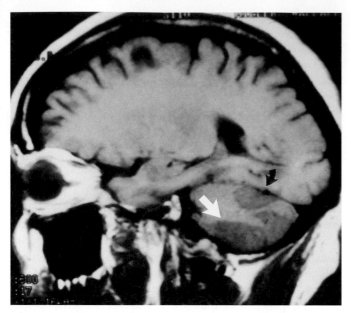

Figure 8.15 T1-weighted MRI scan sagittal projection showing infarcts in the posterior inferior cerebellar artery territory (white arrow) and also in the SCA territory (curved black arrow) on the same side. From Caplan LR. *Posterior Circulation Disease: Clinical Findings, Diagnosis, and Management.* New York: Blackwell Science, 1996 with permission of Blackwell Publishing Ltd.

Patient 2, AD, is an example of a large cerebellar infarct. In other patients, cerebellar infarcts are quite small and cause little or no abnormal neurological signs. Infarcts limited to the medial vermis in territory supplied by the medial branch of PICA often present as isolated vertigo.[53] Examination may be normal except for nystagmus and gait ataxia. The most important signs of infarction of the posterior inferior cerebellum are alteration of posture, gait ataxia, and limb hypotonia. Patients topple, lean, or veer to the ipsilateral side when they sit or stand. In many patients, standing or walking is impossible during the acute period and helpers may be needed to support them in maintaining an erect posture. When they become able to walk, patients often feel as if they are being pulled to the side of the lesion. They veer, lean, or weave to the side, especially on turns. The ipsilateral limbs usually do not show a cerebellar type of rhythmic intention tremor. Hypotonia of the ipsilateral arm can best be shown by having the patient quickly lower or raise the outstretched hands together, braking the ascent or descent suddenly. The arm on the ipsilateral side often overshoots and is not as quickly braked. In some patients, the ipsilateral arm also makes a slower ascent or descent to facilitate braking. Some patients have great difficulty in feeding themselves with the ataxic limbs. They overshoot targets and have difficulty pointing accurately to moving targets.

Embolism from the heart or ECVA can cause cerebellar infarction by blocking the ICVA, PICA, or SCA. Cardiac evaluation and MRA or standard angiography can usually delineate the nature of the causative vascular disease.

Patient 3

A 65-year-old man, BE, had transient headache and dizziness on two occasions, 7 and 10 days before admission. On the day of admission, he suddenly became blind and agitated. When examined 5 hours later, he could not recall events of the past 3 weeks. He could form no new memories and had a complete right hemianopia. No other abnormalities of brainstem or central nervous system function were evident. CT revealed infarcts in the left occipital and temporal lobes in the distribution of the left PCA. MRI also showed a small infarct in the left cerebellum, in PICA territory. Angiography revealed occlusion of the left ICVA and embolic amputation of the left PCA. All other vessels were normal or showed only minor atheroma. Cardiac evaluation was normal.

This patient had an ICVA occlusion, followed by an embolus to the distal basilar artery system. In retrospect, the two episodes of dizziness probably represented transient cerebellar or medullary ischemia. When the vertebrobasilar system has been studied at necropsy, embolic occlusions are common in the PCAs.[1,128] These emboli may arise from recent occlusion within the ECVAs or the ICVAs.[1,60,61,129,130] Koroshetz and Ropper studied 12 patients with PCA infarcts and brainstem symptoms.[130] They found that three patients had intra-arterial embolism arising from a donor site in the ICVA. The three other patients had lesions of the ICVAs and the ECVAs. All of the patients had intra-arterial embolism as the cause of PCA infarction.[130] Documentation of artery-to-artery emboli, from freshly occluded vertebral arteries, has led us to prescribe heparin or warfarin for such patients during the time it takes for the clot to solidify and attach to the artery (3–4 weeks). Insufficient data exist to determine the risk–benefit ratio of anticoagulants for preventing embolization and progressing infarction in patients with recent ICVA occlusions. Thrombolysis is another potential therapeutic strategy to treat recent ICVA occlusion, although there is no published data.

Patient 4

A 60-year-old hypertensive, diabetic African-American man, EO, noted diplopia and dizziness after arising from a nap. The symptoms were transient. Two days later, he staggered and had double vision. On examination, he had gait ataxia, nystagmus, and slight left facial weakness. When he stood, he became dizzy, felt weak, and his vision dimmed. He was treated with heparin and bed rest. Six days later, he gradually became stuporous and quadriplegic. He died soon after of pneumonia. Necropsy revealed bilateral occlusion of the ICVAs and extensive necrosis of the cerebellar hemispheres, medulla, and pons.

Bilateral ICVA disease is relatively common. Among 430 patients in the New England Medical Center Posterior Circulation Registry, 21% had severe ICVA occlusive disease[89] and 42 patients (10%) had bilateral severe ICVA occlusive disease or severe unilateral ICVA occlusive disease associated with other extracranial and/or intracranial lesions that compromised posterior circulation perfusion.[90] Table 8.3 shows the patterns of ICVA occlusive disease and the frequency of other major occlusive lesions. The diagnosis of bilateral ICVA occlusion is often difficult.[1,110] Early symptoms may be deceptively mild and are usually referable to the cerebellum and

Table 8.3 ICVA steno-occlusive disease in the New England Medical Center Posterior Circulation Registry

Location	Number
Unilateral ICVA only	18 (30%)
Bilateral ICVA	21 (35%)
Unilateral ICVA +*	21 (35%)
Accompanying basilar artery stenosis	10 (17%)
Accompanying basilar artery occlusion	6 (10%)

* ECVA stenosis-occlusion, or hypoplastic contralateral VA, or basilar artery disease.

lateral medulla, like those seen in patients 1 (WA) and 2 (AD). Because of a low flow system, the symptoms are often positionally sensitive, worsening when the patient sits or stands or when blood pressure falls spontaneously or after treatment. Usually, TIAs continue and are multiple and stereotyped.[90] Symptoms and signs may also gradually progress.[110] Heparin is most often ineffective because the progressive ischemia is caused by reduced brainstem perfusion rather than thrombus propagation or embolization. Figure 4.30A is a multimodal MRI in a patient with bilateral ICVA occlusions showing severe perfusion abnormalities in the medulla, pons, and cerebellum. Ataxia and pyramidal signs and symptoms predominate. At times, ischemia of the PCA territories also leads to abnormalities of vision, memory, and behavior. Bilateral ICVA occlusive lesions are most common in hypertensive and diabetic patients.[1,90,110] Death caused by extensive hindbrain ischemia can result.[110]

In the 1970s and 1980s, a preferred treatment for patients with persistent brainstem ischemia related to bilateral ICVA disease was surgical creation of shunts from a variety of different donor arteries – mostly the occipital and superficial temporal arterial branches of the external carotid arteries to various posterior circulation arteries distal to the ICVA obstruction.[131–133] Endarterectomy of a stenotic ICVA was also occasionally performed when the stenotic lesion was proximal in the ICVA.[134] More recently, the preferred treatment has become angioplasty with or without stenting of one of the stenotic ICVAs.[135–137]

Patients 1 through 4 illustrate serious posterior circulation infarction caused by ICVA disease. In some patients, this vascular lesion is tolerated without symptoms or with only minor TIAs. As a general rule, however, the more distally located a vascular lesion is along the path from the proximal subclavian-vertebral junction to the distal basilar artery, the more likely it is to cause infarction. The more proximal the lesion, the more likely it is to be more benign.

Little is known about optimal treatment of lesions of the ICVA.[137] Interventional radiologists are able to perform angioplasties on the ICVA. LRC has been involved in the treatment of three patients with bilateral ICVA occlusive disease in whom unilateral ICVA angioplasty effectively stopped TIAs.[135] A randomized trial of angioplasty and stenting compared with best medical treatment (SAMMPRIS) showed an advantage of medical treatment using monitored pharmacological treatment and a coach for life-style changes.[138] In SAMMPRIS, there were 36 patients who had ICVA stenting. Three of these patients had ischemic complications and 3 hemorrhagic complications during the 30 days after the procedure.[139,140] Patients who had ICVA stenting had more ischemic complications than those who had carotid and MCA stenting but less than those in whom the basilar artery was stented.[138,139] The rate of hemorrhage was highest in SAMMPRIS in the ICVA stented group.[139,140]

Thrombolytic treatment could also lyse ICVA thrombi if given early enough after occlusion. At the time of this writing there have been no trials or published series of the results of intravenous thrombolysis in patients with acute ICVA occlusions. A few series report the results of intra-arterial thrombolysis with clot retrieval mostly in patients with bilateral ICVA lesions.[137,141,142]

In the patient examples and discussion, we have emphasized the need for vigilance to detect large cerebellar infarcts and decompress these lesions. LRC often uses short-term heparin or warfarin or newer anticoagulants in patients with ICVA occlusions in an attempt to prevent clot propagation and embolization. In some patients with severe ICVA stenosis, he has prescribed longer-term anticoagulation (6 months to 1 year), keeping the international normalized ratio (INR) between 2.0 and 2.5 when warfarin is used. He follows patients with ICVA stenosis with serial TCD, and MRA examinations for progression of the vascular lesion to complete occlusion or for recanalization with disappearance of critical stenosis. LRC then stops anticoagulants approximately a month after documented occlusion or re-establishment of wide patency. Although there have are no data that support this plan of treatment, they make good sense to LRC at the present time.[136] JSK and his colleagues prefer to use dual antiplatelets, aspirin plus clopidogrel, for a few months. After stabilization of the patient, they switch treatment to either aspirin alone or aspirin plus cilostazol, depending on the severity of the ICVA disease. This treatment is chosen based partly on the higher incidence of bleeding complication in patients who received warfarin than in those having aspirin in the Warfarin–Aspirin Symptomatic Intracranial Disease (WASID) study[143] and partly on their result that aspirin plus cilostazol more effectively prevented progression of intracranial atherosclerosis than aspirin alone.[144] We await careful prospective studies of treatment of patients with ICVA disease.

Occlusion or severe stenosis of the basilar artery

Bilateral brainstem infarction

In a landmark report, Kubik and Adams called attention to the clinical and pathological features of occlusion of the basilar artery.[145] Characterized by quadriparesis and cranial nerve abnormalities, which allowed for accurate diagnosis during life, the disorder was then considered invariably fatal. We

now know that the outcome of patients with basilar-artery occlusive disease is quite variable. Some patients die or are left severely disabled, whereas others survive with little or no deficit.[1,26,62,146–149] Prognosis depends on the rapidity of the occlusion, location, and extent of the thrombosis, presence of occlusive disease in other posterior circulation arteries, and development of adequate collateral circulation.

> A 63-year-old man, OL, was unable to rise from bed because of weakness in both his legs. He had a myocardial infarction 5 years earlier. During the past 2 weeks, he had two transient episodes of diplopia, one accompanied by momentary buckling of the legs. During the past month, he had occasional, severe occipital headaches. For the past 3 days, he had noted weakness of his left leg and diplopia but refused to seek medical care.

Atherosclerosis commonly affects the first few centimeters of the basilar artery. Stenosis can also occur in the middle and distal segments.[1,147,148,150,151] Patients with basilar-artery atherosclerosis have a high frequency of atherosclerosis elsewhere, especially in the coronary, carotid, and iliofemoral arteries. In Kubik and Adams' original report,[145] most patients developed signs abruptly without previous warnings. Their paper preceded recognition of the frequency and importance of TIAs. Kubik and Adams examined the patients' organs only after death; historical data about symptoms that preceded the fatal strokes was scanty. Careful questioning of most patients with basilar-artery occlusive disease elicits descriptions of attacks of temporary brainstem dysfunction before their strokes, as in patient OL. The most common symptoms during these TIAs are: (1) diplopia; (2) dizziness, most often without true spinning; (3) weakness of both legs; and (4) weakness alternating between different limbs in different attacks. As in occlusive disease of other large extracranial and cranial arteries, some patients develop prominent headache during the weeks before and during development of a critical decrease in blood flow. With basilar-artery occlusive disease, the headache is usually occipital, often spreading to the vertex of the head.

> On examination, OL's limbs were weak, more so on his right side. He could not move his right arm and leg, but could lift the left heel off the bed to a height of 15 cm for 5 seconds before it would fall. He could adduct the left shoulder toward himself by sliding it along the bed, but could not lift the arm or move his fingers. Both plantar responses were extensor. Pinprick and touch perception were normal. He could not look to the right. On gazing to the left, only the left eye moved but with abducting nystagmus. No adduction of the right eye on attempted left gaze occurred. His voice was dysarthric, and secretions pooled in the back of his throat.

The basilar artery forms from the merging of the two ICVAs at the medullopontine junction. The basilar artery ends at the junction of the pons and midbrain. The major territory of supply of the basilar artery is the pons, especially the basis pontis. The tegmentum of the pons has a rich, collateral supply of vessels but depends primarily on the SCAs, vessels that originate from the rostral basilar artery just before it bifurcates. Occlusion of the basilar artery often causes ischemia in the pontine base

bilaterally, sometimes extending into the medial tegmentum on one or both sides. Figure 8.16 shows an example of the distribution of ischemia in basilar-artery occlusion, patterned after Kubik and Adams.[145] Note that the medulla and the cerebellar hemispheres are usually spared, in contrast to the situation when one or both ICVAs are blocked. Blockage of the midbasilar artery at the orifice of the AICAs often is accompanied by infarction in the anterior inferior cerebellum on one or both sides.[1,122,152,153] Figure 8.17 is a necropsy specimen of the pons in a patient with basilar artery occlusion that shows a pattern similar to that drawn in Figure 8.16B.

Visualizing the anatomical regions of damage helps in predicting and understanding the usual neurological signs and symptoms that accompany basilar-artery occlusion:

1. Paralysis of the limbs. Weakness is usually bilateral but may be asymmetric, as in patient OL's presentation; stiffness, hyperreflexia, and extensor plantar reflexes are found on examination of the weak limbs. Some patients present with a hemiparesis, but also usually have weakness and reflex changes in the limbs contralateral to the hemiparesis on examination.[1] Hemiparesis was more common than quadriparesis in patients with basilar artery occlusion studied in the New England Medical Center Posterior Circulation Registry.[1,147]

2. Bulbar or pseudobulbar paralysis of the cranial musculature. The infarct can directly involve cranial motor nuclei, causing paralysis of the face, palate, pharynx, neck, or tongue on one or both sides. The IX–XII nerve nuclei are located within the medullary tegmentum, which is usually below the level of the infarct. Weakness of the cranial musculature innervated by these nuclei causes dysarthria, dysphonia, hoarseness, dysphagia, and tongue weakness. These are common findings in patients with basilar artery occlusion and pontine infarction. The pontine lesion interrupts corticofugal descending fibers destined for these cranial-nerve nuclei. The resulting weakness is referred to as pseudobulbar because it involves the descending pathways controlling the bulbar nuclei rather than the nuclei themselves. Exaggerated jaw and facial reflexes, increased gag reflex, and easily induced emotional incontinence with excessive laughing and/or crying accompany the weakness. In some patients, the limb and bulbar paralysis is so severe that the patient cannot communicate verbally or by gesture. Such patients have been referred to as locked-in because of their loss of motor function.[1,154–156] Eye movement or eye-blinking signals can sometimes be arranged, which clearly prove the patient is alert and intellectually preserved despite the paralysis.

3. Absence of sensory or cerebellar abnormalities. The infarct usually affects the midline and paramedian structures in the basis pontis. Collateral circulation is generally through the circumferential vessels, which course around the lateral portions of the brainstem, and supply the lateral base, tegmentum, and cerebellum. Figure 8.18A is a cartoon that shows the potential paths of collateral supply when the basilar artery is occluded. Figure 8.18B is a digital cerebral angiogram that shows cerebellar artery collaterals filling

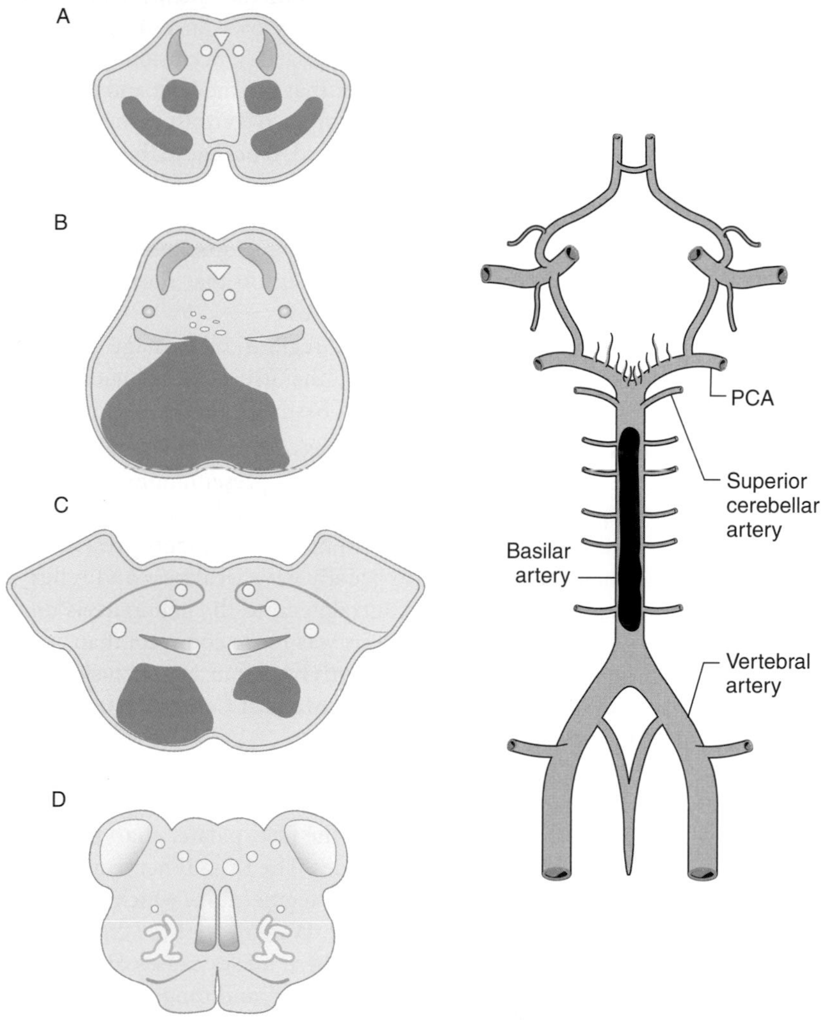

A

B

C

D

Figure 8.16 Cartoon showing the pons with an infarct caused by occlusion of the basilar artery: (A) midbrain, (B) upper pons, (C) lower pons, and (D) medulla. PCA, posterior cerebral artery.

PCA

Superior cerebellar artery

Basilar artery

Vertebral artery

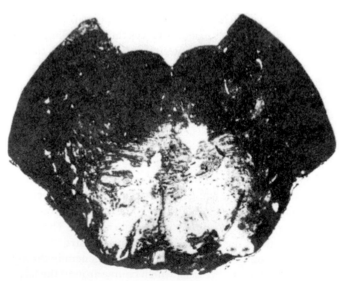

Figure 8.17 Myelin-stained section of the pons showing a large infarct limited to the paramedian portion of the base in a patient with basilar artery occlusion. From Caplan LR. *Posterior Circulation Disease: Clinical Findings, Diagnosis, and Management*. New York: Blackwell Science, 1996 with permission of Blackwell Publishing Ltd.

the upper basilar artery in a patient with proximal basilar artery occlusion. The cerebellar hemispheres are mostly nourished by the PICA, which originates before the basilar artery, and the SCA, which is preserved when the basilar-artery clot does not extend to the distal basilar artery. Infarcts involving the AICA portion of the cerebellum and the basis pontis do occur but the usual clinical cerebellar signs are overshadowed by the accompanying paralysis and pyramidal tract abnormalities. The spinothalamic tracts and the cerebellum are often spared from the ischemia.

4. Abnormalities of eye movement.[1,157–159] The VIth-nerve nuclei, medial longitudinal fasciculi (MLF), and pontine lateral gaze centers are located in the paramedian pontine tegmentum, and therefore are vulnerable to ischemia in this region. Lesions of the VIth nerve or nucleus cause paralysis of abduction of the eye. An MLF lesion produces a defect in adduction of the ipsilateral eye on gaze directed to the opposite side and nystagmus of the contralateral abducting eye. This syndrome, called an internuclear ophthalmoplegia, can be bilateral. Lesions of the paramedian pontine tegmentum may also affect the paramedian pontine reticular formation (PPRF), the

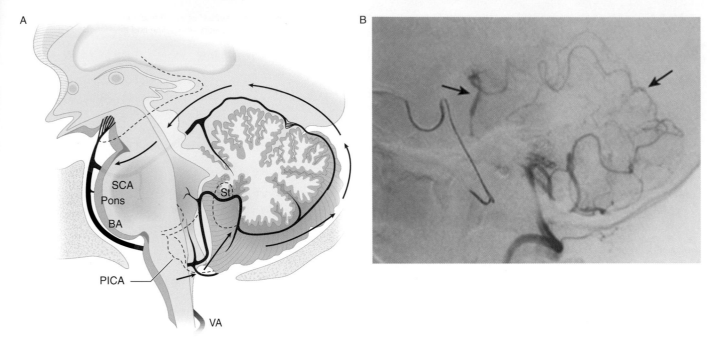

Figure 8.18 (A) Drawing of the brainstem and cerebellum in sagittal section. The cerebellar arteries are well shown. When the basilar artery occludes blood can flow from the intracranial vertebral artery (VA) to the posterior inferior cerebellar artery (PICA) over the cerebellum to the superior cerebellar artery (SCA), and from there into the distal basilar artery (BA). St represents the straight portion of PICA. (B) Vertebral angiogram, lateral view: Basilar artery is occluded; rostral basilar artery is filled (arrow, upper left) from collaterals going around the cerebellum (arrow, upper right) from PICA to SCA branches.

so-called pontine lateral gaze center that mediates gaze to the same side. A lesion of this region causes an ipsilateral conjugate-gaze paresis. A unilateral lesion can affect both the PPRF and the MLF on the same side. The resulting syndrome was present in patient OL, and has been called the one- and one-half syndrome by Fisher[1,159] because only one-half of gaze (scoring 1 for gaze to each side) is preserved. OL had paralysis of right gaze caused by a lesion of the right PPRF and paralysis of the adducting right eye on gaze to the left caused by involvement of the right MLF.

5. Nystagmus. The vestibular nuclei and their connections are also commonly affected, causing vertical and horizontal nystagmus.
6. Other eye signs. Ptosis, small pupils, and ocular skewing are also often found in patients with basilar-artery occlusion.
7. Coma. If the lesion interrupts function of the medial pontine tegmentum bilaterally, coma may develop.[1,160,161] Reduced consciousness is a poor prognostic sign, but care must be taken in differentiating reduced alertness from the locked-in state.

CT of OL was normal. MRI on the 1st day showed ischemia in the mid and lower pons bilaterally in the basis pontis. The basilar-artery flow void was absent in the lower pons. Heparin was given intravenously in a continuous-drip infusion. During the first 24 hours, the patient developed increased weakness of the right leg. He remained stable thereafter, and by day 10 he could lift both arms and speak more clearly. MRA on day 2 was technically poor but suggested a basilar artery occlusion. Catheter angiography on day 3 showed slight irregularity without stenosis of the ECVAs at their origins. The basilar artery was occluded just after its origin. An ICA injection opacified the rostral basilar artery through the posterior communicating artery. By day 14, he could sit with help and had no blood pressure drop or increased weakness when he did so. Heparin was stopped after coumadin had achieved an INR of 2.5. He recovered partially during rehabilitation and had no further worsening of signs or symptoms.

CT is not sensitive in imaging brainstem infarcts, although this capability has improved with newer-generation scanners. CT is, however, reliable in excluding primary brainstem hemorrhage, one of the differential diagnostic considerations. MRI provides better imaging of brainstem and cerebellar infarcts.[147–149,162] In the patient OL, and in others with bilateral abnormalities of brainstem function, the principal differential diagnosis is between pontine hemorrhage, basilar-artery obstruction and obliteration of basilar branch arteries bilaterally despite a patent basilar artery.[163] This distinction can usually be made by vascular imaging tests, CTA, MRA, and catheter angiography.[1,147–149,162,164]

When OL presented, the lack of a history of prior stroke and the extensive nature of the bilateral signs made it highly probable that the lesion involved the main basilar artery. He had persistent neurological signs for more than 72 hours, so he was not a candidate for thrombolysis. If he had presented within 24 hours, LRC would have considered catheter angiography followed by intra-arterial thrombolysis if his basilar artery were occluded. LRC would have performed MRA as a screening test as soon as he presented before performing angiography. Both intravenous and intra-arterial thrombolysis

Table 8.4. The BASICS Registry with 592 treated patients. Outcomes according to severity at baseline and method of treatment. The numbers in the top table indicate the time to treatment and the bottom results indicate the outcome frequencies according to severity at baseline and treatments

Time to treat	AT (*N* = 183)	IVT (*N* = 121)	IAT (*N* = 288)	Total (*N* = 592)
0–3 h	45 (25%)	67 (55%)	67 (23%)	179 (30%)
3–6 h	39 (21%)	32 (26%)	119 (41%)	190 (32%)
79 h	28 (15%)	7 (6%)	49 (17%)	84 (14%)
>9 h	71 (39%)	15 (12%)	53 (18%)	139 (23%)

	Mild to moderate at baseline			Severe at baseline			Totals
mRS	AT (*N* = 104)	IVT (*N* = 49)	IAT (*N* = 92)	AT (*N* = 79)	IVT (*N* = 72)	IAT (*N* = 196)	(*N* = 592)
0–2	38 (37%)	26 (53%)	28 (30%)	21 (27%)	15 (21%)	22 (11%)	150 (25%)
3–5	53 (51%)	15 (31%)	43 (47%)	15 (19%)	24 (33%)	78 (40%)	228 (39%)
Dead	13 (12%)	8 (16%)	21 (23%)	43 (54%)	33 (46%)	96 (49%)	214 (36%)

AT, antithrombotic; IAT, intra-arterial tPA; IVT, intravenous tPA; mRS, modified Rankin Scale.
Derived from data in Schonewille W, Wijman CAC, Michel P, et al. on behalf of the BASICS Study Group. Treatment and outcomes of acute basilar artery occlusion in the Basilar Artery International Cooperation Study (BASICS): a prospective registry study. *Lancet Neurol* 2009;8:724–730, with permission.

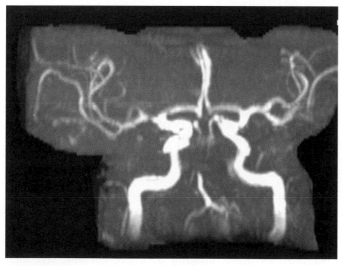

Figure 8.19 Intracranial MRA. The basilar artery stops abruptly.

have occasionally proved successful in patients with basilar artery occlusion even when treatment has been delayed for up to 24 hours.[1,165–168]

Intra-arterial therapy was once considered necessary to recanalize an occluded basilar artery, but the results of intravenous and intra-arterial thrombolytic therapy in series of patients with basilar artery occlusion are very similar.[164–168] The Basilar Artery International Cooperation Study (BASICS) registry is by far the largest of all databases that reported the results of treatment of patients with acute strokes caused by basilar artery occlusions.[168] Nearly half the patients (288/592 (49%)) were treated intra-arterially. Among those treated intra-arterially, 179 were treated only with locally administered thrombolytics, 79 were given thrombolytics and mechanical clot extraction devices were used, and 30 only had mechanical thrombectomy.[168] Table 8.4 shows the time to treat after the onset of neurological symptoms by treatment categories – antithrombotic (antiplatelet or anticoagulant), intravenous tPA or intra-arterial treatment (locally introduced thrombolytic and/ or mechanical thrombectomy). Almost two-thirds of the patients were treated within 6 hours – 369 of 592 (62%). Table 8.4 also includes outcomes according to the mRS at baseline, whether the patient had a mild or moderate deficit (mRS 0–2) or a severe deficit (mRS 3–5 – coma and/or tetraplegia or locked-in state).[168] Despite early and aggressive treatment, only one-fourth of the patients had good outcomes (mRS 0–2) and 36% of patients died. Those patients who had a mild to moderate deficit at baseline had a higher risk of poor outcome when treated intra-arterially (relative risk 1.49 95% CI 1–2.23); patients with severe deficits at treatment onset had similar outcomes whether treated intravenously or intra-arterially. Clot retrievers are often used along with intra-arterial thrombolytic agents but there are now no data concerning their effectiveness.

LRC gave OL heparin intravenously after the CT scan excluded hemorrhage. JSK prefers to use aspirin plus clopidogrel in this circumstance. CT, CTA, MR and MRA are usually sufficient to make the diagnosis of basilar artery disease and to define the extent of infarction.[169–171] Figure 8.19 shows an MRA of a patient with basilar artery stenosis and occlusion.

We prefer not to do digital catheter angiography early in the course of fluctuating brainstem ischemia, performing angiography only when the diagnosis remains uncertain, or when intra-arterial treatment (thrombolysis, stenting, or both) is considered. Reduced perfusion of the brainstem is a major problem. Attention must be given to maximizing blood flow. We keep patients at bed rest with their heads flat. Blood pressure should not be lowered unless it is in the malignant range, and cardiac failure should be treated. Dehydration and hypovolemia should be avoided. During the initial course of

the ischemia (up to 2 weeks), patients may develop additional symptoms when they sit, stand, or are merely propped up in bed.[172] We observe patients carefully when they sit or stand, checking their pulse and blood pressure and noting any change in neurological symptoms and signs. Ambulation should be gradual and carefully supervised. TCD is sometimes not accurate in showing basilar-artery disease because the lesion is often beyond the range of the suboccipital probe.

If CTA, MRA, or angiography shows a complete basilar-artery occlusion, LRC continues heparin, followed by warfarin, for a total of 6–8 weeks, and uses aspirin or combined aspirin and modified-release dipyridamole thereafter. If there is a severe stenosis of the basilar artery without occlusion, LRC usually uses long-term warfarin treatment in an attempt to prevent occlusion. If there is only minor plaque disease in the major basilar artery, LRC selects agents, such as aspirin or aspirin with dipyridamole, or clopidogrel that decrease platelet aggregation and agglutination. JSK prefers to use aspirin plus clopidogrel or aspirin plus cilostazol in patients with severe basilar artery occlusive disease. In patients with mild stenosis that produced unilateral brainstem infarction associated with branch occlusion, aspirin or aspirin plus cilostazol is usually used. LRC and JSK both prescribe a high dose of statin in these patients.

In patients with no obvious intrinsic basilar artery lesions, it is important to think of the possibility of embolism and be certain that studies are adequate to exclude a cardiogenic embolus or embolism from the aorta or the proximal innominate, subclavian or vertebral arteries. Angioplasty and stenting has been performed to open basilar-artery stenotic lesions, but this procedure can result in obliteration of paramedian and other arteries that penetrate from the basilar artery.[141,142] LRC is very wary of basilar artery stenting but does favor interventional thrombus extraction using interventional techniques when IV-tPA is unsuccessful and there is no major brainstem infarct. The vertebral arteries are smaller in diameter and more tortuous than the internal carotid artery, so their manipulation is technically more demanding. Nevertheless, JSK and his colleagues believe that angioplasty and stenting with or without thrombectomy is very efficacious if the candidate patients are well selected based on clinical and imaging data – patients with: (1) sudden devastating neurological symptoms (e.g., unconsciousness with quadriparesis) or progressively/stutteringly worsening neurological symptoms; (2) severe basilar artery stenoocclusive disease or severe vertebral artery stenoocclusive disease with non-functional contralateral vertebral artery (atresia, PICA ending or bilateral atherosclerosis); (3) diffusion-weighted MRI findings that do not show extensive brainstem lesions (clinical–diffusion mismatch). They have treated patients who show dramatic clinical improvement after successful recanalization. The earlier the recanalization is achieved the better is the result, but the therapeutic time window appears to be longer and bleeding complication rates are lower than in anterior circulation counterparts. These interventional procedures can be feasible even in the subacute stage of stroke if there is major salvageable tissue.[173]

The procedures should be done only in a well organized stroke center where there are sufficient facilities and experienced neurologists and interventionalists. A recent, non-randomized study that compared endovascular therapy with medical therapy in 99 patients with basilar artery occlusion showed that, at 90 days follow-up, good functional outcome (mRS ≤2) was reached in 45% of the endovascular treatment group and none in the conservative treatment group ($P = 0.012$).[174] Although large, controlled trials are still needed to prove the efficacy of interventional therapy, they are unlikely to be performed in patients with basilar artery occlusion because the outcome of the patients in the placebo arm is too dismal.

> A 38-year-old man, PG, was discovered comatose by his son. That morning he had been normal, according to his wife, who recalled no recent signs of ill health in her husband. He had no history of heart or vascular disease. On examination, his pupils were dilated and fixed at 8 mm each. His eyes were deviated downward and outward. Lateral motion in each eye was obtained by oculocephalic maneuvers. No abnormal motor signs were evident.

The bilateral III nerve dysfunction and coma indicate a midbrain lesion. This could be caused by a large supratentorial space-taking lesion with midbrain compression or by an intrinsic lesion within the midbrain. Because of the lack of history, absence of stroke risk factors, and limitation of the neurological examination by coma, LRC believed it mandatory to order urgent neuroimaging tests.

> The CT in patient PG was normal with and without contrast. MRI could not be performed urgently. The next day diffusion-weighted and T2-weighted images showed infarction in the paramedian thalamus and midbrain tegmentum. MRA was normal. An echocardiogram showed a left atrial myxoma.

In most patients with basilar artery occlusive thrombi engrafted upon atherosclerotic stenosis, the thrombus is limited to the proximal basilar artery. In some patients, the occlusion extends to the distal basilar-artery segment; in other patients, more often in African-Americans, occlusion or severe stenosis can predominantly affect the distal basilar artery.[1,50,150] Figure 8.20 shows a patient with a bilateral SCA territory infarct caused by a localized stenosis that was located at the orifices of the SCAs. SCA territory infarction is accompanied most often by dysarthria and limb dysmetria and intention tremor. Dizziness and gait ataxia are less prominent signs compared to patients with PICA territory cerebellar infarction.

Occlusion of the distal basilar artery is most often caused by embolism from the heart or the proximal vertebral artery system. Emboli small enough to pass through the intracranial vertebral arteries do not usually lodge in the proximal basilar artery, a vessel larger than each ICVA, but travel to the distal basilar artery or its terminal branches. The distal basilar artery supplies the midbrain and diencephalon through small vessels that pierce the posterior perforated substance. Signs of dysfunction in this territory include the following:[1,175–177]

271

1. Pupillary abnormalities. The lesion often interrupts the afferent reflex arc by interfering with fibers going toward the Edinger–Westphal nucleus. The III-nerve nucleus can also be involved, as well as the rostral descending sympathetic system. The pupils are usually abnormal and can be small, midposition, or dilated, depending on the level and extent of the lesion. Decreased pupillary reactivity and eccentricity of the pupil are also found. Sometimes a pupil attains an oval shape.[178]

2. Eye movement abnormalities. Vertical gaze abnormalities are common in patients with rostral brainstem lesions.[157,158,179–181] Paralysis of upward or downward gaze is common. The eyes may also be skewed and may be deviated at rest, most often downward and inward. Hyperconvergence, retractory nystagmus, and pseudo VI-nerve paresis are other oculomotor

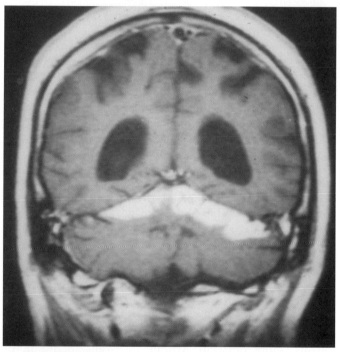

Figure 8.20 T2-weighted MRI scan, coronal view. There is bilateral infarction in the superior portion of the cerebellum in the territory of the bilateral SCAs in a patient with a basilar artery occlusion that blocks the orifices of the SCAs. This appearance resembles icing on a cake.

abnormalities.[1,157–159,175,177] The failure of ocular abduction in patients with pseudo-VI paresis is explained by hyperadduction of the eye. The adduction vector neutralizes the abduction motion and so abduction is incomplete. The lesion is of course far rostral to the VI-nerve nucleus or fibers.[1,162,180,182]

3. Altered level of alertness. Hypersomnolence or frank coma can result from bilateral paramedian rostral brainstem dysfunction. After the acute phase, the patient may remain relatively inert and apathetic. Some patients sleep many hours a day unless stimulated or coaxed into activities.

4. Eyelid abnormalities – ptosis or lid retraction. III-nerve palsies result from involvement of the nucleus or the fibers of the oculomotor nerve. When the oculomotor nucleus is involved, patients usually have bilateral ptosis.[182] The subnucleus of the levator palpebra superioris component is located medially and has crossed projections to the subnucleus controlling the levator muscle of the contralateral eye.[182] In some patients with lesions at the midbrain–thalamic junction the eyelid is retracted – Collier's sign.[182,183]

5. Amnesia. Memory loss can accompany thalamic infarction. Patients are unable to form new memories and may not be able to recall events just preceding their stroke. There may be an array of other behavioral abnormalities, including agitation, hallucinations, and abnormalities that mimic lesions of the frontal lobe. Cognitive deficits often persist in patients with left and bilateral paramedian thalamic infarcts.[184]

In PG, the bilateral III-nerve palsies identified a midbrain lesion that was confirmed by MRI. Because the most frequent cause is embolic, the cardiac and vascular investigations are important. Identification of the left atrial myxoma led to successful removal of the cardiac tumor. The patient awakened on day 4 after his stroke and was left with a unilateral III-nerve palsy and a contralateral ptosis as his only important, persistent, neurological signs. In other patients with top-of-the-basilar emboli, the distribution of infarction varies and may include the midbrain and thalami and the territories of the SCAs and PCAs. Infarction can be limited to one SCA or PCA. Figure 8.21 shows MRI and CTA scans in a patient with a top-of-the-basilar embolus. Infarcts are shown in the midbrain, superior

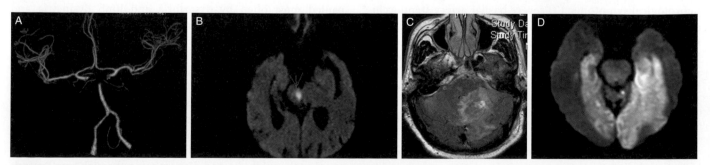

Figure 8.21 Images from a patient with an embolic occlusion of the top of the basilar artery. (A) CTA reconstructed. The very distal portion of the basilar artery and the left posterior cerebral artery do not opacify. (B) diffusion-weighted MRI image showing an infarct (arrow) in the medial midbrain. (C) DW MRI scan showing an infarct involving the left superior cerebellar artery territory of the cerebellum and the left dorsal pontine tegmentum. (D) diffusion-weighted MRI scan showing extensive occipital lobe infarction bilaterally in the territory of the posterior cerebral arteries.

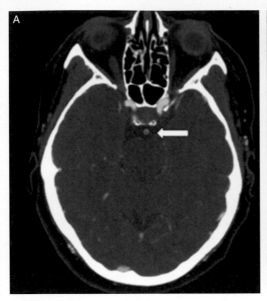 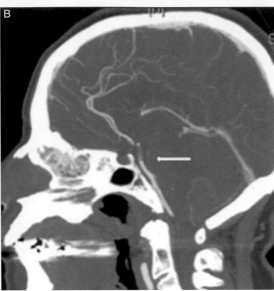

Figure 8.22 CTA of a patient with a top-of-the-basilar embolus. (A) Axial section showing a hypointense region within the basilar artery (white arrow). The outline of the peripheral circumference of the artery is visible. (B) Sagittal view showing the filling defect in the rostral basilar artery (small white arrow). Figure kindly submitted by Dr Mark McAllister, Beth Israel Deaconess Medical Center, Boson, MA.

cerebellum, and bilateral posterior cerebral artery territories. Figure 8.22 contains CTA scans that show a filling defect that represents thrombus in the distal basilar artery.

Unilateral brainstem infarction

Basilar artery atherothrombotic lesions may occlude the orifice of a perforator, thereby causing unilateral pontine or midbrain infarction (branch occlusion or branch atheromatous disease).[185–189] The lesion within the basilar artery can be shown using cross-section high resolution MRI views of the basilar artery.[188] The resultant infarcts usually abut on the ventral surface of the brainstem and primarily involve the paramedian pontine base. The most common symptoms include contralateral hemiparesis, dysarthria, and occasionally ataxia. If the lesions extend to the tegmentum, hemisensory deficits and/or ocular motor abnormalities (most often internuclear ophthlamoplegia) are added. Emotional incontinence is occasionally present, but less marked than in patients with bilateral lesions. Recent studies have shown that branch occlusions associated with basilar artery atherosclerotic disease are an important stroke mechanism for unilateral pontine infarction occurring in 23% of patients with pontine infarctions[184] and in 39–50% of patients that have lesions extending to the basal surface.[190–192] This topic is discussed in more detail in Chapter 9 on penetrating artery disease.

Basilar artery dissection

Basilar artery dissections are rare. In the past they had been thought to carry a more grave prognosis than vertebral artery dissections. A 1979 review cited the most common presentation as extensive, bilateral pontine infarction clinically manifested as sudden reduction in consciousness and quadriparesis.[193] As in other intracranial arterial dissections, patients present usually with either brainstem

ischemia or subarachnoid hemorrhage related to rupture of a dissecting aneurysm. In a review of 38 patients with basilar artery dissections published in 1993, 27 had brainstem ischemia, 5 had subarachnoid hemorrhages, and 6 patients had hemorrhages and ischemia. Thirty patients (79%) died.[194] A study published in 2010 showed that unilateral pontine infarction with a favorable outcome is actually more common.[195] In early years, basilar artery dissection was only diagnosable by catheter angiography, an invasive procedure often only performed in very ill stroke patients. With the advent of non-invasive vascular testing, many more intracranial dissections are diagnosed in patients whose presentations vary widely from minor brainstem ischemia to subarachnoid hemorrhages, to coma and quadriplegia. Our experience is that many of the intracranial posterior circulation dissections begin in the ICVA and spread into the basilar artery and that many patients have minor clinical findings.

Occlusion or severe stenosis of the posterior cerebral arteries

The posterior cerebral arteries (PCAs) are the major terminal branches of the basilar artery. In approximately 30% of patients, one basilar communicating segment is hypoplastic, and the PCA is derived primarily from the ipsilateral ICA through its posterior communicating artery branch. Intrinsic atheromatous disease of the PCA most often affects the origin of the vessel. Its epidemiology is similar to disease of the proximal MCA. Infarcts in the PCA territory are often caused by emboli to the posterior circulation.[1,62,63,131,132,196–198] Castaigne and colleagues in a necropsy study identified 30 infarcts within PCA territory.[129] The most common mechanism of infarction was embolism from a proximal occlusive lesion within the vertebrobasilar system (15/30, 50%). In eight patients, clot

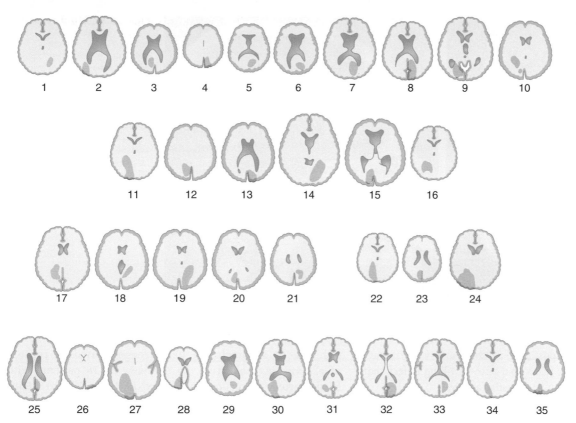

Figure 8.23 Montage of PCA occipital lobe infarcts on CT.

propagated from the basilar artery into the PCA. Only three patients had thrombosis of the PCA engrafted on previous atherosclerotic narrowing.[131]

Pessin, LRC, and colleagues studied the mechanism of infarction in 35 patients with hemianopia and a unilateral infarct on CT limited to the PCA territory on one side.[196] Figure 8.23 is a montage of the CT scans with their lesions from this study. The most frequent mechanism of infarction was embolism. A cardiac source of embolism was present in 10 patients (28.5%), and intra-arterial embolism arising from proximal posterior circulation lesions was found in six patients (17%). In 11 other patients, the clinical and angiographic findings suggested embolism, but no definite donor site was established. Among the 35 patients, 27 (77%) had embolic occlusion of PCA branches.[196] Among 79 patients with PCA-territory infarction in the New England Medical Center Posterior Circulation Registry, embolism was the most likely stroke mechanism in 65 patients (82%).[198] Series of patients with PCA-territory infarcts reported by other centers have shown that embolism is the predominant cause of these infarcts.[1,197,198]

Recent studies from Turkey[199] and Korea,[200] where MRA was performed in all stroke patients, identified PCA atherosclerosis as a cause of PCA territory infarct in 1 in 4 and 1 in 5 patients who had PCA territory infarction, respectively. These results suggest that PCA atherosclerosis may be a more important cause of PCA territory infarction than was previously recognized. Ethnic differences, inclusion of isolated deep infarcts in the series,[200] and the thoroughness of

the vascular evaluation may explain the different prevalence of PCA atherosclerosis among studies. Important stroke mechanisms of PCA atherosclerosis include generation of emboli leading to cortical infarction and occlusion of deep perforators, leading to deep (midbrain or thalamic) infarction.

Although atherosclerosis is the most important pathology affecting the PCA, dissection,[201] moyamoya disease,[202] fibromuscular dysplasia,[203] and vasospasm (reversible cerebral vasoconstriction syndrome)[204] can involve the PCA, resulting in PCA territory infarction.

An analogy can be drawn between the two brain circulations. In the anterior circulation, emboli usually lodge in MCA branches, leading to cortical infarcts; in the posterior circulation, emboli traverse the vertebral and basilar arteries and ultimately lodge in PCA branches, producing cortical infarcts. Intrinsic disease of the MCA and PCA does occur, but is far less common than cardiogenic or artery-to-artery embolization. When intrinsic atherosclerosis of the PCA is present, the clinical presentation usually consists of transient hemianopic visual symptoms, sometimes accompanied by transient hemisensory symptoms on the same side.[205]

A 64-year-old African-American woman, MA, awakened and realized she could not see to her left. She was able to read and could clearly identify objects in the room, but found it necessary to turn to the left to "see better." She also noted a dull pain behind her right eye. She was not aware of any difficulty with her limbs, walking, or thinking.

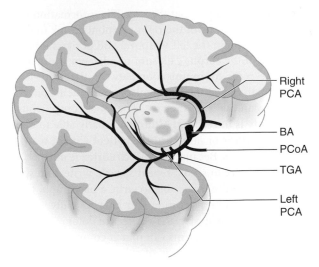

Figure 8.24 Cartoon of the posterior cerebral arteries and their branches. BA, basilar artery; PCA, posterior cerebral artery; PCoA, posterior communicating artery; TGA, thalamogeniculate artery pedicle. Drawn by Laurel Cook-Lhowe.

During the past few weeks, she had several attacks of diminished vision to her left, each lasting a few minutes. On examination, there was a left homonymous hemianopia with slight sparing of the most central portion of the left visual field. She could read, note the color and nature of objects and pictures, draw common objects, copy drawings, and accurately bisect lines scattered on a page. Motor, sensory, and reflex functions and gait were normal.

After giving off penetrating branches to the midbrain and thalamus, the PCA supplies branches to the occipital lobes and supplies the medial and inferior portions of the temporal lobes (Figure 8.24). Headache in patients with PCA disease is often retro-orbital or above the eye, probably reflecting the fact that the upper surface of the tentorium is innervated by the first division of the Vth nerve. Infarction in the cerebral territories of the PCA most often affects vision and somatic sensation, but seldom causes paralysis.[1,196–198,205,206]

Visual-field abnormalities

The single most common finding in patients with PCA-territory infarction is a hemianopia.[1,196–198,205,206] Hemianopia is caused by infarction of the striate visual cortex on the banks of the calcarine fissure, a region supplied by the calcarine branch of the PCA, or is attributable to interruption of the geniculo-calcarine tract as it nears the visual cortex.[207] If just the lower bank of the calcarine fissure is involved, the lingual gyrus, a superior quadrant-field defect results. An inferior quadrantanopia results if the lesion affects the cuneus on the upper bank of the calcarine fissure.

When infarction is restricted to the striate cortex and does not extend into the adjacent parietal cortex, the patient is fully aware of the visual field loss. Usually described as a void, blackness, or limitation of vision to one side, patients usually recognize that they must focus extra attention to the hemianopic field. When given written material or pictures, patients with hemianopia caused by occipital lobe infarction are, like patient MA described above, able to see and interpret the stimuli normally, although it may take them a bit longer to explore the hemianopic visual field. They will often cant the picture obliquely and hold it in the preserved visual field.

Hemianopia and visual neglect are not synonymous, nor is visual neglect merely a more or less severe form of hemianopia. In patients with occipital lobe infarcts, physicians can reliably map out the visual fields by confrontation. At times, the central or medial part of the field is spared, known as *macular sparing*. Optokinetic nystagmus is normal. Some patients, although they accurately report motion or the presence of objects in their hemianopic field, cannot identify the nature, location, or color of that object.[1,207]

In contrast, patients with infarction in the parietal lobe, most often in MCA territory, who have preservation of geniculo-calcarine fibers and the striate cortex, have visual neglect. Their findings are quite different from those in patients with medial occipital infarction. Patients with visual neglect are usually unaware of their visual-field defect. They often: (1) ignore objects in the abnormal visual field; (2) do not notice words in their impaired field, often reading only half of a headline or paragraph; (3) miss objects in pictures in the neglected field; and (4) have reduced optokinetic nystagmus to the side of the visual defect.[207] Poor drawing and copying are also often associated with visual neglect. When the parieto-occipital and temporal branches of the PCA are involved, leading to large infarcts in the entire PCA territory, both a hemianopia and visual neglect can be present. More often, in isolated infarcts of the striate cortex, patients have a hemianopia without neglect. In our experience, visual neglect without a hemianopia is always caused by infarction within the MCA territory.

Somatosensory abnormalities

The lateral thalamus is the site of the major somatosensory relay nuclei, the ventro-posteromedial and lateral nuclei. Ischemia to these nuclei or white matter tracts carrying fibers from the thalamus to somatosensory cortex (postcentral gyrus and the sensory 2 region in the parietal operculum) produces sensory symptoms and signs, usually without paralysis.[197,198,208] Patients describe paresthesias or numbness in the face, limbs, and trunk. On examination, their touch, pinprick, and position senses are sometimes reduced. In many patients, the sensory symptoms far outweigh abnormalities that can be shown on examination.[209] The combination of hemisensory loss, with hemianopia and without paralysis, is virtually diagnostic of infarction in the PCA territory. The occlusive lesion is within the PCA, before the thalamogeniculate branches to the lateral thalamus.[208,209]

Motor abnormalities

Rarely, occlusion of the proximal portion of the PCA can cause a hemiplegia.[1,181,197,198,210–212] Penetrating branches from the most proximal portion of the PCA penetrate into the midbrain to supply the cerebral peduncle. PCA-origin occlusions cause hemiplegia related to midbrain peduncular infarction accompanied by a hemisensory loss caused by lateral thalamic

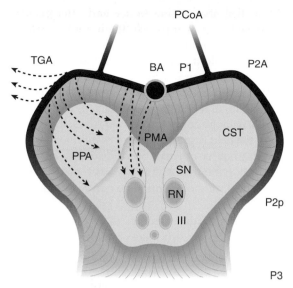

Figure 8.25 Axial diagram of the midbrain arteries. BA, basilar artery; PCoA, posterior communicating artery; P1, proximal segment of the PCA; P2A, anterior segment of the P2 part of the PCA; P2p, posterior segment of the P2 part of the PCA; P3, P3 part of the PCA; TGA, thalamogeniculate arteries; PPA, peduncular perforating arteries; PMA, paramedian arteries; CST, corticospinal tract in cerebral peduncle; SN, substantia nigra; RN, red nucleus; III, oculomotor nucleus.

infarction and hemianopia caused by occipital lobe infarction. The resultant neurological deficit is not easily distinguished clinically from MCA or anterior choroidal artery territory infarcts, but separation is made readily by CT and MRI results. Figure 8.25 from Hommel et al.[212] shows the proximal branches of the PCA.

When the lateral thalamus is infarcted and the midbrain is spared, patients often show a hemiataxia and choreic and dystonic movements on the same side as the hemisensory symptoms. The limb ataxia is likely related to interruption of cerebellofugal fibers from the superior cerebellar peduncle and red nucleus that synapse in the ventrolateral nucleus of the thalamus. The motor abnormalities of choreoathetosis and dystonia probably relate to interruption of extrapyramidal fibers from the ansa lenticularis that are destined for the ventral lateral and ventral anterior thalamic nuclei. In some patients with lateral thalamic infarcts, transient involuntary choreiform and athetotic movements are present during the first days after the stroke.[1,209]

Cognitive and behavioral abnormalities

Left PCA territory infarction

When the left PCA territory is infarcted, several additional findings may occur:

1. Alexia without agraphia. Infarction of the left occipital lobe and splenium of the corpus callosum is associated with a remarkable clinical syndrome – an inability to read despite retained ability to write correctly, first described by Dejerine,[213] and later amplified by Geschwind and Fusillo.[214] Because the left visual cortex is infarcted, patients see with their right occipital lobe and their left

visual field. To name what they see, the information must be communicated from the right occipital cortex to the language region in the left temporal and parietal lobes. Infarction of the corpus callosum or adjacent white matter paths interrupts communication between the right occipital cortex and the left hemisphere. Patients have difficulty naming what they see. The most conspicuous abnormality is in reading. Although usually able to name individual letters or numbers, the patient cannot read words or phrases. Because the speech cortex is normal, they retain the ability to speak, repeat speech, write, and spell aloud. Although they are able to write a paragraph, they often cannot read it back moments later. Usually accompanying the dyslexia is a defect in color naming.[1,207,214,215] Patients can match colors and shades, proving that their perception of colors is normal. They can also describe the usual color of familiar objects and can even color correctly when given an array of crayons. Nonetheless, they are unable to give a color its correct name.

2. Anomic or transcortical sensory aphasia.[216] Some patients with left PCA-territory infarction have difficulty naming objects. Others can repeat, but not understand, spoken language.

3. Gerstmann's syndrome. PCA-territory infarction can undercut the angular gyrus, leading to a host of findings, usually lumped together as Gerstmann's syndrome.[1] These findings include: (1) difficulty telling right from left, (2) difficulty in naming digits on their own or on others' hands, (3) constructional dyspraxia, (4) agraphia, and (5) difficulty in calculating. In any single patient, all features may appear together or one or more may occur in isolation. Gerstmann's syndrome also occurs when the angular gyrus region is infarcted during left MCA-territory infarction.

4. Altered memory. A defect in acquisition of new memories is common when both medial temporal lobes are damaged,[1,217–219] but also occurs in lesions limited to the left medial temporal lobe.[1,215,217–221] The memory deficit in unilateral lesions is usually not permanent, but has lasted up to 6 months. Patients cannot recall recent events and when given new information, they cannot recall it moments later. They often repeat statements and questions spoken only minutes before.

Memory loss is usually attributable to infarction of the hippocampus – a region supplied by temporal artery branches. Szabo and colleagues recently reported the findings among 57 consecutive patients who had hippocampal infarcts on diffusion-weighted images.[222] They characterized four different patterns of acute ischemic hippocampal lesions: complete hippocampal infarcts, lateral and dorsal infarcts that involved the hippocampal body and tail, and tiny infarcts in the lateral hippocampus. No patient had PCA territory infarction isolated only to the hippocampus. Three of the infarcts were bilateral and 54 were unilateral; 22 were right and 32 left-sided. The hippocampal infarcts were nearly complete in 25%; 32% involved the lateral length of the

hippocampal body and tail; 37% were partial lesions in the dorsal portion of the body and 7% were small dot lesions.[222] When the entire hippocampus was infarcted the occlusive lesion involved the proximal PCA and the infarcts were large and affected the temporal and occipital lobes. Smaller lesions likely represented PCA branch infarcts or small emboli. Only 11 (19%) (including 2 of the 3 patients with bilateral infarcts) showed memory loss on standard neurological bedside examination using a 3-item memory test. The left hippocampal lesion group had decreased verbal long-term memory, decreased immediate and delayed story recall, and poor scores on learning, and recognition memory.[217] The right hippocampal lesion group had reduced non-verbal memory.[222]

5. Associative visual agnosia.[1,207,215,223,224] Some patients with left PCA territory infarction have difficulty understanding the nature and use of objects presented visually. They can trace with their fingers and copy objects, demonstrating that visual perception is preserved. They can often name objects if the objects are presented in their hand and explored by touch or when the objects are described verbally. One patient, when shown a pair of scissors, had no idea what it was. When the instrument was placed in her hand, she was able to name it. When asked to list five objects that might be used for cutting, she included scissors, indicating that the name of the object was available to the patient.[215]

Right posterior cerebral artery territory infarction

Infarcts of the right PCA territory are often accompanied by prosopagnosia, difficulty in recognizing familiar faces.[1,207,224–226] At times, patients cannot recognize their spouses, children, or even their own images in a mirror. Despite the seeming inability to recognize, match, or identify faces, physiological tests of autonomic function are consistent with familiarity on a subconscious level.[226] Disorientation to place and an inability to recall routes and read or revisualize the location of places on maps are also common findings in patients with right PCA-territory infarcts.[207,227] Patients with right occipitotemporal infarcts also may have difficulty revisualizing what a given object or person should look like. Dreams may also be devoid of visual imagery. Visual neglect is much more common after lesions of the right PCA territory.

Bilateral posterior cerebral artery territory infarcts

When the PCA territory is infarcted bilaterally, the most common findings are cortical blindness, amnesia, and agitated delirium.[1,175,197,206,207,228–230] Most often, bilateral PCA-territory infarction is caused by embolism with blockage of the distal basilar artery bifurcation. Figure 8.21D is an MRI that shows bilateral PCA infarcts in a patient rendered blind by an embolus. Cortically blind patients cannot see or identify objects in either visual field, but have preserved pupillary light reflexes.[1,207,228] Although uncommon, patients may not recognize their visual deficit, and do not admit that they cannot see (visual anosognosia or Anton's syndrome).[231] It has been

hypothesized that the visual association area in the parietal lobe is posited to be concomitantly affected in these patients, which causes the lack of awareness of deficits and an inability to process information from the occipital lobes.[232] Patients with Anton's syndrome may also show confabulation or agitation and increased verbal output probably related to associated temporal lobe lesions.[233] Amnesia caused by bilateral medial temporal-lobe infarction may be permanent and closely resembles Korsakoff's syndrome.[217] Infarcting the hippocampus, fusiform, and lingual gyri, usually bilaterally, leads to an agitated hyperactive state that could be confused with delirium tremens.[1,229,230]

Upper and lower calcarine bank lesions

Physiological studies in animals and humans[1,207,234–236] and analysis of symptoms and signs in patients with lesions[237] has shown that different anatomical regions are involved in object recognition, *what* is the stimulus, than are involved in identification of the spatial features of vision, *where* is the stimulus. The visual association cortex located inferior to the calcarine fissure, the "lower bank", including parastriate and peristriate cortex in Brodmann areas 18, 19, and 37 within the lingual and fusiform gyri contain neurons activated mostly by the color, shape, and form of visual objects.[207,234–236] The occipitofugal ventral pathway for object recognition travels from the inferior occipital lobe mostly into the mid and inferior portions of the temporal lobes. The upper bank parastriate and peristriate cortex has an occipitofugal dorsal pathway directed to the parietal lobe and towards the frontal eye fields conveying information about the spatial attributes of visual percepts. Figure 8.26 shows diagrammatically these so-called "what" and "where" pathways.

The dorsal, "where" pathway carries visual information to parietal and frontal regions and is involved mostly with

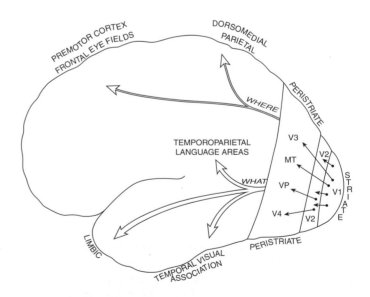

Figure 8.26 Drawing of the dorsal where and the ventral what visual pathways and their relationships. From Mesulam M-M. Higher visual functions of the cerebral cortex and their disruption in clinical practice. In Albert DM, Jakobiec FA (eds), *Principles and Practice of Ophthalmology*, Vol 4. Philadelphia: W B Saunders,1994, pp 2640–2653 with permission.

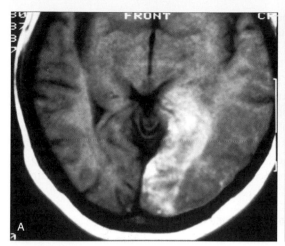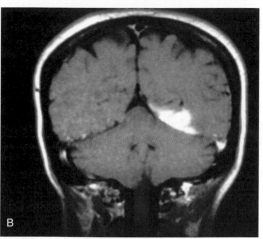

Figure 8.27 T2-weighted MRI scans showing infarction in PCA territory. (A) Axial view showing large occipital lobe infarct. (B) Coronal view showing smaller occipital lobe infarct.

processing the spatial characteristics of visual data. The ventral "what" pathway conveys visual data to the middle and inferior temporal gyri and to medial temporal limbic structures, predominantly the amygdaloid nucleus and the hippocampus, and to ventrolateral frontal lobe cortex.[207] This ventral pathway concerns mostly the nature, color, category, and functions of objects. The medial temporal lobe structures interplay with lateral temporal lobe structures in discerning the familiarity of objects and other memory-related relationships. The medial and inferior temporal occipital pathways connect closely with language cortex to categorize and name visual percepts.

When infarction is limited to the lower banks of the calcarine fissures (ventral pathway) bilaterally, the major findings are prosopagnosia and defective color vision.[1,207,224,238,239] In contrast to patients with alexia without agraphia who cannot name colors, these patients cannot recognize, match, or name colors correctly.[234,235] These patients also have difficulty revisualizing objects and people and places from memory.[237]

Bilateral infarcts primarily involving the dorsal pathway (upper bank of the calcarine cortex-cuneus) produce a variety of syndromes.[207,231] Some patients will have features of Balint's syndrome.[207,240,241] Simultanagnosia is an inability to form a panoramic view although patients can perceive individual items in the scene.[207,242] Optic ataxia is an inability to direct hand movements under visual guidance – a lack of coordination between visual input and hand motions.[207,243] Apraxia of gaze (psychic paralysis of gaze) is an inability to look directly at what the patient is instructed to focus on. Patients have difficulty in initiating saccades to visual targets on command, although they can make spontaneous scanning saccades.[207,244,245] Due to the difficulty in seeing the visual environment in panorama, and in coordinating "looking" and "seeing," patients have difficulty in reading, which should be differentiated from alexia with and without agraphia. Patients also have great difficulty in finding their way, in describing directions, and in visualizing the location of buildings, and cities on a map.[237]

CT showed an infarct in patient MA in the medial occipital lobe on the right. Angiography was not performed.

Extracranial Doppler examination at C2 did not show reversed VA flow on either side. TCD showed a focal region of increased blood-flow velocity in the right PCA. MRI showed that the occipital infarct involved striate cortex above and below the calcarine fissure. MRA showed a focal narrowing of the right PCA. Cardiac echo and rhythm monitoring were normal. She was discharged on aspirin therapy. The findings did not change during the ensuing years of follow-up.

CT can accurately reflect the vascular territory involved. In this patient, it confirmed that the lesion was in the territory of the calcarine branch of the right PCA.[1,197,206,246,247] CT scan also showed that the lesion was ischemic and not caused by intracerebral hemorrhage. MRI is better able to image small associated lesions in the thalamus, midbrain, and more proximal brainstem and cerebellum, thus helping to localize the offending vascular lesion. Sagittal T2-weighted MRI sections through the medial occipital lobes can also identify the location of the lesions in relation to the calcarine fissure and the optic radiations, and thereby help prognosticate recovery of visual field defects. Figure 8.27 contains axial and coronal MRI views of occipital lobe infarcts caused by embolism to the PCA.

The occipital lobe is a site of predilection for amyloid angiopathy. Hemorrhage from amyloid angiopathy often occurs in the absence of hypertension and can mimic an ischemic stroke. Little is known at present about optimum therapy for patients with intrinsic disease of the PCA. When infarction is limited to branches of the PCA, cardiogenic embolism should be considered and appropriate investigations performed to exclude it.

In patient MA, there was no clinical or laboratory evidence to suggest cardiac-origin embolism. Non-invasive studies gave no evidence for an ECVA occlusion in the neck, a potential source of intra-arterial embolism to the PCA. If ECVA occlusion had been suggested by non-invasive tests, or if epidemiological and ecological factors had favored an ECVA-origin lesion, a gadolinium-enhanced MRA examination of the subclavian ECVA-origin region, or CTA, or catheter angiography would have been ordered. She was African-American and had no history of coronary or peripheral vascular disease, and did

not have hypercholesterolemia. These factors weighed against the likelihood of a proximal ECVA lesion.[49] The absence of brainstem symptoms and normal ICVA blood-flow velocities on TCD examination argued against an ICVA occlusion. The TCD findings of a focal increase in blood-flow velocity in the right PCA strongly suggested a focal lesion involving the PCA. Intracranial MRA excluded an ICVA lesion and showed the intrinsic lesion within the right PCA. The preceding spells of left visual field loss also favored an intrinsic right PCA occlusive lesion.[205] Even if more extensive infarction were to occur in the right PCA territory, the likelihood of serious disability was small. The risk to the patient of further, serious, neurological disability did not, in our opinion, warrant invasive diagnostic procedures or hazardous therapy. LRC elected to prescribe aspirin.

Differential diagnosis in patients with posterior circulation ischemia

Advances in technology, especially the introduction of MRI, echocardiography, ultrasound, TCD, and CTA and MRA, have now made it possible to investigate patients with posterior circulation ischemia safely and quickly and identify the causative vascular mechanism. Diffusion and perfusion-weighted MRI can also be helpful within the posterior circulation by showing regions that are hypoperfused and identifying infarcts earlier than T2-weighted standard MRI scans.

We have found it useful to divide the posterior circulation into smaller territories that reflect the vascular distribution of the main arteries.[1,2,26,62,109] The ICVAs join at the medullopontine junction to form the basilar arteries. The territory usually perfused by the ICVAs includes the medulla and the cerebellum supplied by the PICA branch of the ICVAs. This region is designated as proximal intracranial posterior circulation territory. The basilar artery bifurcates at the pontomesencephalic junction. The territory supplied by the basilar artery, including the pons and the portion of the cerebellum supplied by the AICA branch, is designated as middle-intracranial posterior circulation territory. The portion of the posterior circulation supplied by the distal basilar artery and its SCA, PCA, and penetrating artery branches is referred to as distal intracranial posterior circulation territory. The distal territory includes the midbrain, thalamus, SCA-supplied cerebellum, and the occipital and temporal lobe regions supplied by the PCAs. Figure 8.28 shows these posterior circulation territories.

In each patient, the designation of which posterior circulation brain territory(ies) are involved is made by using both clinical and imaging data. For example, suppose a patient has clinical findings of a left lateral medullary syndrome and a right hemianopia. MRI shows only a left occipital-lobe infarct. This patient must have proximal and distal intracranial posterior circulation territory ischemia. Moreover, the left proximal-territory lesion means that the left ICVA must have been involved at some point. The combination of proximal and distal-territory infarction is most often explained by an embolus that first landed at the ICVA and then traveled to the basilar

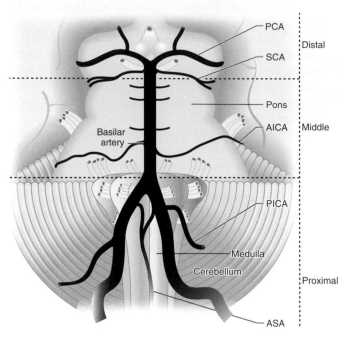

Figure 8.28 Sketch of base of the brain showing the intracranial vertebral and basilar arteries and their respective branches. The brain regions are divided into proximal, middle, and distal intracranial territories. AICA, anterior inferior cerebellar artery; ASA, anterior spinal artery; PCA, posterior cerebral artery; PICA, posterior inferior cerebellar artery; SCA, superior cerebellar artery.

artery bifurcation region, or an occlusive lesion of the ICVA causing local ischemia with distal embolism. Designation of the involved posterior circulation territory tells the clinician the rostro-caudal localization of the vascular lesion. Vascular diagnostic technology, including extracranial and transcranial ultrasound, CTA, MRA, standard angiography, and echocardiography can then be used to define the causative vascular lesions.

In the New England Medical Center Posterior Circulation Registry, distal territory lesions were the most common, either ischemia limited to the distal territory or ischemia that included the distal territory.[1,2,26,109] In other registries, the distal territory was also often involved. In the Lausanne Stroke Registry, 164 of 401 (41%) posterior circulation patients had infarcts that involved the thalamus or PCA territory.[248–250] Among 70 patients in the Lausanne Stroke registry in whom MRA was reported, 37% had distal territory infarcts while 27% had proximal territory infarcts and 23% had middle territory infarcts.[249] In the Besancon[251,252] and Athens[253] stroke registries, posterior circulation lesion localization was characterized as brainstem, cerebellum, and PCA territories. In the Besancon Stroke Registry, among 251 patients with posterior circulation ischemia, 34% were PCA, 39% brainstem, and 27% cerebellar.[251,252] In the Athens Registry, among 259 patients with posterior circulation ischemia, 27% included PCA territory, and 28% were brainstem and 24% cerebellar.[253]

In the New England Medical Center Posterior Circulation Registry, the PCA territories were the most commonly affected regions within the posterior circulation either when affected alone or when associated with other intracranial territory

lesions. A significant number of patients with distal territory ischemia also had rostral brainstem and SCA territory infarcts.[109] If rostral brainstem and SCA cerebellar infarcts are added to the PCA infarcts tabulated in the Lausanne, Besancon, and Athens Registries, it is very highly probable that the frequency of distal territory infarction would parallel that found in the New England Medical Center Posterior Circulation Registry.

In the New England Medical Center Posterior Circulation Registry, the proximal intracranial territory that included lesions involving the medulla and/or the PICA-supplied cerebellum was the next most commonly affected intracranial territory. This territory was involved mostly in patients with ECVA and ICVA occlusive disease and cardiac embolism to PICA-cerebellar territory. The middle intracranial territory which comprised the pons and AICA-supplied cerebellum

was least often involved. Middle territory lesions were caused mostly by basilar artery or basilar artery branch disease. Multiple territories were involved in a large number of patients in the Lausanne, Besancon, and Athens Stroke Registries, just as they were in the New England Medical Center Posterior Circulation Registry.[109]

Treatment has lagged far behind advances in diagnostic technology. Antiplatelet drugs, anticoagulants, surgery, angioplasty and stenting, thrombolysis, and mechanical clot extraction have all been applied but, to date, no randomized therapeutic trials have clarified optimal treatment in patients with fully characterized vascular and brain lesions. These treatments have been described in Chapter 6 and in various parts of this chapter. I hope that in the near future trials of various therapies in patients with documented vascular lesions will shed more light on treatment.

References

1. Caplan LR: *Vertebrobasilar Ischemia and Hemorrhage: Clinical Findings, Diagnosis, and Management of Posterior Circulation Disease*, 2nd ed. Cambridge: Cambridge University Press, 2015.

2. Caplan LR: Posterior circulation ischemia: Then, now, and tomorrow (Thomas Willis Lecture – 2000). *Stroke* 2000;**31**:2011–2013.

3. Millikan C, Siekert R: Studies in cerebrovascular disease. The syndrome of intermittent insufficiency of the basilar arterial system. *Mayo Clin Proc* 1955;**30**:61–68.

4. Denny-Brown D: Basilar artery syndromes. *Bull N Engl Med Center* 1953;**15**:53–60.

5. Fang H, Palmer J: Vascular phenomena involving brainstem structures. *Neurology* 1956;**6**:402–419.

6. Williams D, Wilson T: The diagnosis of the major and minor syndromes of basilar insufficiency. *Brain* 1962;**85**:741–774.

7. Millikan C, Siekert R, Shick R: Studies in cerebrovascular disease: The use of anticoagulant drugs in the treatment of insufficiency or thrombosis within the basilar arterial system. *Mayo Clin Proc* 1955;**30**:116–126.

8. Caplan LR: Vertebrobasilar disease: Time for a new strategy. *Stroke* 1981;**12**:111–114.

9. Caplan LR: Vertebrobasilar disease: Should we continue the double standard of managing patients with brain ischemia? *Heart Stroke* 1993;**2**:377–381.

10. Reivich M, Holling E, Roberts B, et al: Reversal of blood flow through the vertebral artery and its effects on cerebral circulation. *N Engl J Med* 1961;**265**:878–885.

11. Heyman A, Young W, Dillon M, et al: Cerebral ischemia caused by occlusive disease of the subclavian or innominate arteries. *Arch Neurol* 1964;**10**:581–589.

12. North R, Fisher W, DeBakey M, et al: Brachial-basilar insufficiency syndrome. *Neurology* 1962;**12**:810–820.

13. Patel A, Toole J: Subclavian steal syndrome: Reversal of cephalic blood flow. *Medicine* 1965;**44**:289–303.

14. Hennerici M, Klemm C, Rautenberg W: The subclavian steal phenomenon: A common vascular disorder with rare neurologic deficits. *Neurology* 1988;**38**:669–673.

15. Potter BJ, Pinto DS: Subclavian steal syndrome. *Circulation* 2014;**129**:2320–2323.

16. Pollock M, Blennerhassett J, Clark A: Giant cell arteritis and the subclavian steal syndrome. *Neurology* 1973;**23**:653–657.

17. Hall S, Barr W, Lie JT, et al: Takayasu arteritis. *Medicine* 1985;**64**:89–99.

18. Shinohara Y: Takayasu disease. In Caplan LR (ed): *Uncommon Causes of Stroke*, 2nd ed. Cambridge: Cambridge University Press, 2008, pp 27–31.

19. Brewster DC, Moncure AC, Darling C, et al: Innominate artery lesions: Problems encountered and lessons learned. *J Vasc Surg* 1985;**2**:99–112.

20. Hennerici M, Aulich A, Sandemann W, Freund H-J: Incidence of asymptomatic

extracranial occlusive disease. *Stroke* 1981;**12**:750–758.

21. Symonds C: Two cases of thrombosis of subclavian artery with contralateral hemiplegia of sudden onset, probably embolic. *Brain* 1927;**50**:259–260.

22. Martin R, Bogousslavsky J, Miklossy J, et al: Floating thrombus in the innominate artery as a cause of cerebral infarction in young adults. *Cerebrovasc Dis* 1992;**2**:177–181.

23. Ferriere M, Negre G, Bellecoste JF, et al: Thrombus flottant sous-clavier responsible d'un syndrome encephalo-digital, deux observations. *La Presse Med* 1984;**13**:27–29.

24. Fields WS, LeMak NA, Ben-Menachem Y: Thoracic outlet syndrome: Review and reference to a stroke in a major league pitcher. *AJNR Am J Neuroradiol* 1986;**7**:73–78.

25. Baker R, Rosenbaum A, Caplan L: Subclavian steal syndrome. *Contemp Surg* 1974;**4**:96–104.

26. Caplan LR, Wityk RJ, Glass TA, et al: New England Medical Center Posterior Circulation Registry. *Ann Neurol* 2004;**56**:389–398.

27. Caplan LR, Wityk RJ, Pazdera L, et al: New England Medical Center Posterior Circulation Stroke Registry: II. Vascular lesions. *J Clin Neurol* 2005;**1**:31–49.

28. Ekestrom S, Eklund B, Liljequist L, et al: Noninvasive methods in the evaluation of obliterative disease of the subclavian or innominate artery. *Acta Med Scand* 1979;**206**:467–471.

29. Berguer R, Higgins R, Nelson R: Noninvasive diagnosis of reversal of

vertebral artery blood flow. *N Engl J Med* 1980;**302**:1349–1351.

30. von Reutern GM, Pourcelot L: Cardiac cycle-dependent alternating flow in vertebral arteries with subclavian artery stenosis. *Stroke* 1978;**9**:229–236.

31. Liljequist L, Ekestrom S, Nordhus O: Monitoring direction of vertebral artery blood flow by Doppler shift ultrasound in patients with suspected subclavian steal. *Acta Chir Scand* 1981;**147**:421–424.

32. von Reutern G-M, von Budingen H-J: Ultrasound diagnosis of cerebrovascular disease. In von Reutern G-M, von Budingen H-J (eds): *Ultrasound Diagnosis of Cerebrovascular Disease: Doppler Sonography of the Extracranial and Intracranial Arteries: Duplex Scanning.* Stuttgart: Georg Thieme, 1993, pp 129–175.

33. von Budingen H-J, Staudacher T: Evaluation of vertebrobasilar disease. In Newell DW, Aaslid R (eds): *Transcranial Doppler.* New York: Raven Press, 1992, pp 167–195.

34. Ackerstaff RGA: Duplex scanning of the aortic arch and vertebral arteries. In Bernstein EF (ed): *Vascular Diagnosis*, 4th ed. St Louis: Mosby, 1993, pp 315–321.

35. Hadjipetrou P, Cox S, Piemonte T, Eisenhauer A: Percutaneous revascularization of atherosclerotic obstruction of aortic arch vessels. *J Am Coll Cardiol* 1999;**33**:1238–1245.

36. Dorros G, Lewin RF, Jamnadas P, Mathiak LM: Peripheral transluminal angioplasty of the subclavian and innominate arteries utilizing the brachial approach: Acute outcome and follow-up. *Catheter Cardiovasc Diagn* 1990;**19**:71–76.

37. Hebrang A, Maskovic J, Tomac B: Percutaneous transluminal angioplasty of the subclavian arteries: Long-term results in 52 patients. *AJR Am J Roentgenol* 1991;**156**:1091–1094.

38. Henry M, Amor M, Henry I, et al: Percutaneous transluminal angioplasty of the subclavian arteries. *J Endovasc Surg* 1999;**6**:33–41.

39. Millaire A, Trinca M, Marache P, et al: Subclavian angioplasty: Immediate and late results in 50 patients. *Catheter Cardiovasc Diagn* 1993;**29**:8–17.

40. Motarjeme A: Percutaneous transluminal angioplasty of supra-aortic vessels. *J Endovasc Surg* 1996;**3**:171–181.

41. Motarjeme A, Keifer JW, Zuska AJ, Nabawi P: Percutaneous transluminal angioplasty for treatment of subclavian steal. *Radiology* 1985;**155**:611–613.

42. Vitek JJ: Subclavian artery angioplasty and the origin of the vertebral artery. *Radiology* 1989;**170**:407–409.

43. Schillinger M, Haumer M, Schillinger S, et al: Risk stratification for subclavian artery angioplasty: Is there an increased rate of restenosis after stent implantation? *J Endovasc Ther* 2001;**8**:550–557.

44. Iared W, Mourao JE, Puchnick A, Soma F, Shigueoka DC: Angioplasty versus stenting for subclavian artery stenosis. *Cochrane Database Syst Rev* 2014;**5**: CD008461.

45. Aboyans V, Kamineni A, Allison MA, et al: The epidemiology of subclavian stenosis and its association with markers of subclinical atherosclerosis: the Multi-Ethnic Study of Atherosclerosis (MESA). *Atherosclerosis* 2010;**211**:266–270.

46. Fisher CM, Gore I, Okabe N, et al: Atherosclerosis of the carotid and vertebral arteries: Extracranial and intracranial. *J Neuropathol Exp Neurol* 1965;**24**:455–476.

47. Hutchinson EC, Yates PO: The cervical portion of the vertebral artery, a clinicopathological study. *Brain* 1956;**79**:319–331.

48. Hutchinson E, Yates P: Carotico-vertebral stenosis. *Lancet* 1957;**1**:2–8.

49. Gorelick PB, Caplan LR, Hier DB, et al: Racial differences in the distribution of posterior circulation occlusive disease. *Stroke* 1985;**16**:785–790.

50. Kim JS, Nah HW, Park SM, et al: Risk factors and stroke mechanisms in atherosclerotic stroke: intracranial compared with extracranial and anterior compared with posterior circulation disease. *Stroke* 2012;**43**:3313–3318.

51. Fisher CM: Vertigo in cerebrovascular disease. *Arch Otolaryngol* 1967;**85**:529–534.

52. Kerber KA, Brown D, Lisabeth LD, et al: Stroke among patients with dizziness, vertigo, and imbalance in the emergency department. A population-based study. *Stroke* 2006;**37**:2484–2487.

53. Lee H, Sohn S-I, Cho Y-W, et al: Cerebellar infarction presenting isolated vertigo. Frequency and vascular topographical patterns. *Neurology* 2006;**67**:1178–1183.

54. Moosy J: Morphology, sites, and epidemiology of cerebral atherosclerosis. *Res Publ Assoc Res Nerv Ment Dis* 1966;**51**:1–22.

55. Imparato A, Riles T, Kim G: Cervical vertebral angioplasty for brainstem ischemia. *Surgery* 1981;**90**:842–852.

56. Pelouze GA: Plaque ulcerie de l'ostium de l'artère vertebrale. *Rev Neurol* 1989;**145**:478–481.

57. Fisher CM: Occlusion of the vertebral arteries. *Arch Neurol* 1970;**22**:13–19.

58. Wityk RJ, Chang H-M, Rosengart A, et al: Proximal extracranial vertebral artery disease in the New England Medical Center posterior circulation registry. *Arch Neurol* 1998;**55**:470–478.

59. George B, Laurian C: Vertebrobasilar ischemia with thrombosis of the vertebral artery: Report of two cases with embolism. *J Neurol Neurosurg Psychiatry* 1982;**45**:91–93.

60. Caplan LR, Tettenborn B: Embolism in the posterior circulation. In Bergner R, Caplan LR (eds): *Vertebrobasilar Arterial Disease.* St Louis: Quality Medical Publishers, 1991, pp 50–63.

61. Caplan LR, Amarenco P, Rosengart A, et al: Embolism from vertebral artery origin occlusive disease. *Neurology* 1992;**42**:1505–1512.

62. Glass TA, Hennessey PM, Pazdera L, et al: Outcome at 30 days in the New England Medical Center Posterior Circulation Registry. *Arch Neurol* 2002;**59**:369–376.

63. Moufarrij N, Little JR, Furlan AJ, et al: Vertebral artery stenosis: Long-term follow-up. *Stroke* 1984;**15**:260–263.

64. Callow A: Surgical management of varying patterns of vertebral artery and subclavian artery insufficiency. *N Engl J Med* 1964;**270**:546–552.

65. Roon A, Ehrenfeld W, Cooke P, et al: Vertebral artery reconstruction. *Am J Surg* 1979;**138**:29–36.

66. Berguer R, Flynn LM, Kline RA, Caplan LR: Surgical reconstruction of the extracranial vertebral artery: Management and outcome. *J Vasc Surg* 2000;**31**:9–18.

67. Berguer R, Flynn LM, Kline RA, et al: Surgical reconstruction of the extracranial vertebral artery: Management and outcome. *J Vasc Surg* 2000;**31**:9–18.

68. Kieffer E, Koskas F, Bahnini A, et al: Long-term results after reconstruction of

the cervical vertebral artery. In Caplan LR, Shifrin EG, Nicolaides AN, Moore WS (eds): *Cerebrovascular Ischaemia: Investigations and Management*. London: Med-Orion, 1996, pp 617–625.

69. Myers PM, Schumacher HC, Higashida RT, et al: Use of stents to treat extracranial cerebrovascular disease. *Ann Rev Med* 2006;**57**:437–454.

70. Higashida R, Tsai F, Halbach V, et al: Transluminal angioplasty, thrombolysis, and stenting for extracranial and intracranial cerebral vascular disease. *J Interv Cardiol* 1996;**9**:245–255.

71. Chastain 2nd HD, Campbell MS, Iyer S, et al: Extracranial vertebral artery stent placement: In-hospital and follow-up results. *J Neurosurg* 1999;**91**:547–552.

72. Piotin M, Spelle L, Martin JB, et al: Percutaneous transluminal angioplasty and stenting of the proximal vertebral artery for symptomatic stenosis. *AJNR Am J Neuroradiol* 2000;**21**:727–731.

73. The SSLVIA Study Investigators. Stenting of Symptomatic Atherosclerotic Lesions in the Vertebral or Intracranial Arteries (SSYLVIA): Study results. *Stroke* 2004;**35**:1388–1392.

74. Caplan LR: Dissections of brain-supplying arteries. *Nat Clin Pract Neurol* 2008;**4**:34–42.

75. Tettenborn B, Caplan LR, Sloan MA, et al: Postoperative brainstem and cerebellar infarcts. *Neurology* 1993;**43**:471–477.

76. Debette S, Leys D. Cervical-artery dissections: predisposing factors, diagnosis, and outcome. *Lancet Neurol.* 2009;**8**:668–678.

77. Caplan LR, Zarins C, Hemmatti M: Spontaneous dissection of the extracranial vertebral arteries. *Stroke* 1985;**16**:1030–1038.

78. Mokri B, Houser OW, Sandok BA, Piepgras DG: Spontaneous dissections of the vertebral arteries. *Neurology* 1988;**38**:880–885.

79. Silbert PL, Mokri B, Schievink WI: Headache and neck pain in spontaneous internal carotid and vertebral artery dissection. *Neurology* 1995;**45**:1517–1522.

80. Saeed AB, Shuaib A, Al-Sulaiti G, Emery D: Vertebral artery dissection: Warning symptoms, clinical features, and prognosis in 26 patients. *Can J Neurol Sci* 2000;**27**:292–296.

81. Arnold M, Bousser M-G: Clinical manifestations of vertebral artery dissection. In Baumgartner RW,

82. Arnold M, Bousser M-G, Fahrni G, et al: Vertebral artery dissection. Presenting findings and predictors of outcome. *Stroke* 2006;**37**:2499–2503.

83. Giroud M, Gras P, Dumas R, Becker F: Spontaneous vertebral artery dissection initially revealed by a pain in one upper arm. *Stroke* 1993;**24**:480–481.

84. Dubard T, Pouchot J, Lamy C, et al: Upper limb peripheral motor deficits due to extracranial vertebral artery dissection. *Cerebrovasc Dis* 1994;**4**:88–91.

85. Goldsmith P, Rowe D, Jager R, Kapoor R: Focal vertebral artery dissection causing Brown–Séquard syndrome. *J Neurol Neurosurg Psychiatry* 1998;**64**:416–417.

86. Touboul PJ, Mas JL, Bousser M-G, Laplane D: Duplex scanning in extracranial vertebral artery dissection. *Stroke* 1987;**18**:116–121.

87. Wilkinson I, Russel R: Arteries of the head and neck in giant cell arteritis. *Arch Neurol* 1972;**27**:378–391.

88. Bickerstaff E: *Neurological Complications of Oral Contraceptives*. Oxford: Clarendon Press, 1975.

89. Muller-Kuppers M, Graf KJ, Pessin MS, et al: Intracranial vertebral artery disease in the New England Medical Center Posterior Circulation Registry. *Eur Neurol* 1997;**37**:146–156.

90. Shin H-K, Yoo K-M, Chang HM, Caplan LR: Bilateral intracranial vertebral artery disease in the New England Medical Center Posterior Circulation Registry. *Arch Neurol* 1999;**56**:1353–1358.

91. Huang YC, Chen YF, Wang YH, Tu YK, Jeng JS, Liu HM: Cervicocranial arterial dissection: Experience of 73 patients in a single center. *Surg Neurol* 2009;**72** Suppl 2:S20–77; discussion S7.

92. Caplan LR, Baquis GD, Pessin MS, et al: Dissection of the intracranial vertebral artery. *Neurology* 1988;**38**:868–877.

93. Hosoya T, Adachi M, Yamaguchi K, Haku T, Kayama T, Kato T: Clinical and neuroradiological features of intracranial vertebrobasilar artery dissection. *Stroke* 1999;**30**:1083–1090.

94. Kim JS: Pure lateral medullary infarction: clinical–radiological correlation of 130 acute, consecutive patients. *Brain* 2003;**126**:1864–1872.

95. Fisher CM, Karnes W, Kubik C: Lateral medullary infarction: The pattern of vascular occlusion. *J Neuropathol Exp Neurol* 1961;**20**:323–379.

96. Stephens RB, Stilwell DL: *Arteries and Veins of the Human Brain*. Springfield, IL: Charles C Thomas, 1969.

97. Duvernoy HM: *Human Brainstem Vessels*. Berlin: Springer, 1978.

98. Kommerall G, Hoyt W: Lateropulsion of saccadic eye movements. *Arch Neurol* 1973;**28**:313–318.

99. Meyer K, Baloh R, Krohel G, et al: Ocular lateropulsion: A sign of lateral medullary disease. *Arch Ophthalmol* 1980;**98**:1614–1616.

100. Matsumoto S, Okuda B, Imai T, Kameyama M: A sensory level on the trunk in lower lateral brainstem lesions. *Neurology* 1988;**38**:1515–1519.

101. Song I-U, Kim J-S, Lee D-G, et al: Pure sensory deficit at the T4 sensory level as an isolated manifestation of lateral medullary infarction. *J Clin Neurol* 2007;**3**:112–115.

102. Kim JS, Lee JH, Lee MC: Patterns of sensory dysfunction in lateral medullary infarction: Clinical-MRI correlation. *Neurology* 1997;**49**:1557–1563.

103. Kim JS: Sensory symptoms in ipsilateral limbs/body due to lateral medullary infarction. *Neurology* 2001;**57**:1230–1234.

104. Devereaux M, Keane J, Davis R: Automatic respiratory failure associated with infarction of the medulla: Report of two cases with pathologic study of one. *Arch Neurol* 1973;**29**:46–52.

105. Levin B, Margolis G: Acute failure of automatic respirations secondary to a unilateral brainstem infarct. *Ann Neurol* 1977;**1**:583–586.

106. Bogousslavsky J, Khurana R, Deruaz JP, et al: Respiratory failure and unilateral caudal brainstem infarction. *Ann Neurol* 1990;**28**:668–673.

107. Currier R, Giles C, Westerberg M: The prognosis of some brainstem vascular syndromes. *Neurology* 1958;**8**:664–668.

108. Caplan LR, Pessin M, Scott RM, et al: Poor outcome after lateral medullary infarcts. *Neurology* 1986;**36**:1510–1513.

109. Caplan LR, Chung CS, Wityk RJ, et al: New England Medical Center Posterior Circulation Stroke Registry: I. Methods, database, distribution of

brain lesions, stroke mechanisms, and outcomes. *J Clin Neurol* 2005;**1**:14–30.

110. Caplan LR: Bilateral distal vertebral artery occlusion. *Neurology* 1983;**33**:552–558.

111. Hauw J, Der Agopian P, Trelles L, et al: Les infarctes bulbaires. *J Neurol Sci* 1976;**28**:83–102.

112. Sawada H, Seriu N, Udaka F, Kameyama M: Magnetic resonance imaging of medial medullary infarction. *Stroke* 1990;**21**:963–966.

113. Tyler KL, Sandberg E, Baum KF: Medial medullary syndrome and meningovascular syphilis: A case report in an HIV-infected man and a review of the literature. *Neurology* 1994;**44**:2231–2235.

114. Kim JS, Kim HG, Chung CS: Medial medullary syndrome: Report of 18 new patients and a review of the literature. *Stroke* 1995;**26**:1548–1552.

115. Hagiwara N, Toyoda K, Torisu R, et al: Progressive stroke involving bilateral medial medulla expanding to spinal cord due to vertebral artery dissection. *Cerebrovasc Dis* 2007;**24**:540–542.

116. Kumral E, Afsar N, Kirbas D, et al: Spectrum of medial medullary infarction: Clinical and magnetic resonance imaging findings. *J Neurol* 2002;**249**:85–93.

117. Sypert G, Alvord E: Cerebellar infarction: A clinicopathological study. *Arch Neurol* 1975;**32**:351–363.

118. Amarenco P, Hauw JJ, Henin D, et al: Les infarctus du territoire de l'artère cerebelleuse postero-inferieure: Etude clinico-pathologique de 28 cas. *Rev Neurol* 1989;**145**:277–286.

119. Amarenco P, Hauw JJ, Gautier JC: Arterial pathology in cerebellar infarction. *Stroke* 1990;**21**:1299–1305.

120. Mazighi M, Amarenco P: Cerebellar infarcts. In Caplan LR, van Gijn J (eds): *Stroke Syndromes*, 3rd ed. Cambridge: Cambridge University Press, 2012, pp 469–479.

121. Amarenco P, Caplan LR: Vertebrobasilar occlusive disease, review of selected aspects: 3. Mechanisms of cerebellar infarctions. *Cerebrovasc Dis* 1993;**3**:66–73.

122. Caplan LR: Cerebellar infarcts: Key features. *Rev Neurol Dis* 2005;**2**:51–60.

123. Fisher CM, Picard E, Polak A, et al: Acute hypertensive cerebellar hemorrhage: Diagnosis and surgical treatment. *J Nerv Ment Dis* 1965;**140**:38–57.

124. Lehrich J, Winkler G, Ojemann R: Cerebellar infarction with brainstem compression: Diagnosis and surgical treatment. *Arch Neurol* 1970;**22**:490–498.

125. Fairburn B, Oliver L: Cerebellar softening: A surgical emergency. *BMJ* 1956;**1**:1335–1336.

126. Hornig CR, Rust DS, Busse O, et al: Space-occupying cerebellar infarction. Clinical course and prognosis. *Stroke* 1994;**25**:372–374.

127. Seelig J, Selhorst J, Young H, et al: Ventriculostomy for hydrocephalus in cerebellar hemorrhage. *Neurology* 1981;**31**:1537–1540.

128. Rieke K, Krieger D, Adams H-P, et al: Therapeutic strategies in space-occupying cerebellar infarction based on clinical, neuroradiological and neurophysiological data. *Cerebrovasc Dis* 1993;**3**:45–55.

129. Castaigne P, Lhermitte F, Gautier J, et al: Arterial occlusions in the vertebral-basilar system. *Brain* 1973;**96**:133–154.

130. Koroshetz WJ, Ropper AH: Artery-to-artery embolism causing stroke in the posterior circulation. *Neurology* 1987;**37**:292–296.

131. Sundt T, Whisnant J, Piepgras D, et al: Intracranial bypass grafts for vertebral-basilar ischemia. *Mayo Clin Proc* 1978;**53**:12–18.

132. Ausman J, Diaz F, de los Reyes R, et al: Anastomosis of occipital artery to AICA for vertebrobasilar junction stenosis. *Surg Neurol* 1981;**16**:99–102.

133. Roski R, Spetzler R, Hopkins L: Occipital artery to posterior–inferior cerebellar artery bypass for vertebrobasilar ischemia. *Neurosurgery* 1982;**10**:44–49.

134. Allen G, Cohen R, Preziosi T: Microsurgical endarterectomy of the intracranial vertebral artery for vertebrobasilar transient ischemic attacks. *Neurosurgery* 1981;**81**:56–59.

135. Takis C, Kwan ES, Pessin MS, et al: Intracranial angioplasty: Experience and complications. *AJNR Am J Neuroradiol* 1997;**18**:1661–1668.

136. Myers PM, Schumacher HC, Tanji K, et al: Use of stents to treat intracranial cerebrovascular disease. *Ann Rev Med* 2007;**58**:207–122.

137. Caplan LR: The intracranial vertebral artery: A neglected species. The Johann Jacob Wepfer Award 2012. *Cerebrovasc Dis* 2012;**34**:20–30.

138. Chimowitz MI, Lynn MJ, Derdeyn CP, et al, for the SAMPRIS Investigators: Stenting versus aggressive medical therapy for intracranial arterial stenosis. *N Engl J Med* 2011;**365**:993–1003.

139. Derdeyn CP, Fiorella D, Lynn MJ, et al: Stenting and Aggressive Medical Management for Preventing Recurrent Stroke in Intracranial Stenosis Trial Investigators. Mechanisms of stroke after intracranial angioplasty and stenting in the SAMMPRIS trial. *Neurosurg* 2013;**72**:777–795.

140. Fiorella D, Derdeyn CP, Lynn MJ, et al: SAMMPRIS Trial Investigators. Detailed analysis of periprocedural strokes in patients undergoing intracranial stenting in Stenting and Aggressive Medical Management for Preventing Recurrent Stroke in Intracranial Stenosis (SAMMPRIS). *Stroke* 2012;**43**:2682–2688.

141. Nakayama T, Tanaka K, Kaneko M, Yokoya-ma T, Uemura K: Thrombolysis and angioplasty for acute occlusion of intracranial vertebrobasilar arteries. *J Neurosurg* 1998;**88**:919–922.

142. Wang Bin, Wang Yabing, Li Shenmao, et al: Intra-arterial thrombolysis combined with angioplasty for treatment of acute ischemic cerebral infarction. *Chin J Cerebrovasc Dis* 2011;**8**:65–69.

143. Chimowitz MI, Lynn MJ, Howlett-Smith H, et al: Comparison of warfarin and aspirin for symptomatic intracranial arterial stenosis. *N Engl J Med* 2005;**352**:1305–1316.

144. Kwon SU, Cho YJ, Koo JS, et al: Cilostazol prevents the progression of the symptomatic intracranial arterial stenosis: The multicenter double-blind placebo-controlled trial of cilostazol in symptomatic intracranial arterial stenosis. *Stroke* 2005;**36**:782–786.

145. Kubik C, Adams R: Occlusion of the basilar artery: A clinical and pathologic study. *Brain* 1946;**69**:73–121.

146. Caplan LR: Occlusion of the vertebral or basilar artery. *Stroke* 1979;**10**:272–282.

147. Voetsch B, DeWitt LD, Pessin MS, et al: Basilar artery occlusive disease in the New England Medical Center Posterior Circulation Registry. *Arch Neurol* 2004;**61**:496–504.

148. Schonewille W, Wijman C, Michel P: BASICS Investigators. Treatment and clinical outcome in patients with basilar artery occlusion. *Stroke* 2006;**37**:922–928.

149. Baird TA, Muir KW, Bone I: Basilar artery occlusion. *Neurocritical care* 2004;**1**:319–329.

150. Pessin MS, Gorelick PB, Kwan ES, et al: Basilar artery stenosis: middle and distal segments. *Neurology* 1987;**37**:1742–1746.

151. LaBauge R, Pages C, Marty-Double JM, et al: Occlusion du tronc basilaire. *Rev Neurol* 1981;**137**:545–571.

152. Amarenco P, Hauw JJ: Cerebellar infarction in the territory of the anterior inferior cerebellar artery: A clinicopathological study of 20 cases. *Brain* 1990;**118**:139–155.

153. Amarenco P, Rosengart A, DeWitt LD, et al: Anterior inferior cerebellar artery territory infarcts. Mechanisms and clinical features. *Arch Neurol* 1993;**50**:154–161.

154. Nordgren RE, Markesbery WR, Fukuda K, Reeves AG: Seven cases of cerebromedullospinal disconnection: The "locked-in syndrome". *Neurology* 1971;**21**:1140–1148.

155. Nikić PM, Jovanović D, Paspalj D, Georgievski-Brkić B, Savić M: Clinical characteristics and outcome in the acute phase of ischemic locked-in syndrome: case series of twenty patients with ischemic LIS. *Eur Neurol* 2013;**69**:207–212.

156. Posner JB, Saper CB, Schiff ND, Plum F: *Plum and Posner's Diagnosis of Stupor and Coma*, 4th ed. Oxford, Oxford University Press, 2007.

157. Pierrot-Deseilligny C, Caplan LR: Eye movement abnormalities. In Caplan LR, van Gijn J (eds) *Stroke Syndromes*, 3rd ed. Cambridge: Cambridge University Press, 2012, pp 64–74.

158. Thömke F: Disorders of ocular motility. In Urban PP, Caplan LR (eds): *Brainstem Disorders*. Berlin: Springer-Verlag, 2011, pp 104–130.

159. Fisher CM: Some neuro-ophthalmological observations. *J Neurol Neurosurg Psychiatry* 1967;**30**:383–392.

160. Chase T, Moretti L, Prensky A: Clinical and electroencephalographic manifestations of a vascular lesion of the pons. *Neurology* 1968;**18**:357–368.

161. Parvizi J, Damasio AR: Neuroanatomical correlates of brainstem coma. *Brain* 2003;**126**:1524–1536.

162. Biller J, Yuh W, Mitchell GW: Early diagnosis of basilar artery occlusion using magnetic resonance imaging. *Stroke* 1988;**19**:297–306.

163. Fisher CM: Bilateral occlusion of basilar artery branches. *J Neurol Neurosurg Psychiatry* 1977;**40**:1182–1189.

164. Klein IF, Lavallee PC, Schouman-Claeys E, Amarenco P: High-resolution MRI identifies basilar artery plaques in paramedian pontine infarct. *Neurology* 2005;**64**:551–552.

165. Caplan LR: Thrombolysis in vertebrobasilar occlusive disease. In Lyden PD (ed): *Thrombolytic Therapy for Acute Stroke*, 2nd ed. Totawa, NJ: Humana Press, 2005, pp 203–209.

166. Lindsberg P, Soinne L, Tatlisumak T et al. Long-term outcome after intravenous thrombolysis of basilar artery occlusion. *JAMA* 2004;**292**:1862–1866.

167. Lindsberg PJ, Mattle HP: Therapy of basilar artery occlusion: A systematic analysis comparing intra-arterial and intravenous thrombolysis. *Stroke* 2006;**37**:922–928.

168. Schonewille WJ, Wijman CAC, Michel P et al. on behalf of the BASICS study group: Treatment and outcomes of acute basilar artery occlusion in the Basilar Artery International Cooperation Study (BASICS): A prospective registry study. *Lancet Neurol* 2009;**8**:724–730.

169. Bogousslavsky J, Regli F, Maeder P, et al: The etiology of posterior circulation infarcts: A prospective study using magnetic resonance imaging and magnetic resonance angiography. *Neurology* 1993;**43**:1528–1533.

170. Roether J, Wentz K-U, Rautenberg W, et al: Magnetic resonance angiography in vertebrobasilar ischemia. *Stroke* 1993;**24**:1310–1315.

171. Bash S, Villablanca JP, Duckwiler G, et al: Intracranial vascular stenosis and occlusive disease. Evaluation with CT angiography, MR angiography, and digital subtraction angiography. *AJNR Am J Neuroradiol* 2005;**26**:1012–1021.

172. Caplan LR, Sergay S: Positional cerebral ischemia. *J Neurol Neurosurg Psychiatry* 1976;**39**:385–391.

173. Lu PH, Park JW, Park S, et al: Intracranial stenting of subacute symptomatic atherosclerotic occlusion versus stenosis. *Stroke* 2011;**42**:3470–3476.

174. Broussalis E, Hitzl W, McCoy M, Trinka E, Killer M: Comparison of endovascular treatment versus conservative medical treatment in patients with acute basilar artery occlusion. *Vasc Endovascular Surg* 2013;**47**:429–437.

175. Caplan LR: Top of the basilar syndrome: Selected clinical aspects. *Neurology* 1980;**30**:72–79.

176. Mehler MF: The rostral basilar artery syndrome: Diagnosis, etiology, prognosis. *Neurology* 1989;**39**:9–16.

177. Mehler MF: The neuro-ophthalmologic spectrum of the rostral basilar artery syndrome. *Arch Neurol* 1988;**45**:966–971.

178. Fisher CM: Oval pupils. *Arch Neurol* 1980:**37**:502–503.

179. Hommel M, Bogousslavsky J: The spectrum of vertical gaze palsy following unilateral brainstem stroke. *Neurology* 1991;**41**:1229–1234.

180. Alemdar M, Kamaci S, Budak F: Unilateral midbrain infarction causing upward and downward gaze palsy. *J Neuro-Ophthalmol* 2006;**26**:173–176.

181. Hommel M, Besson G: Midbrain infarcts. In Bogousslavsky J, Caplan LR (eds): *Stroke Syndromes*, 2nd ed. Cambridge: Cambridge University Press, 2001, pp 512–519.

182. Caplan LR: Ptosis. *J Neurol Neurosurg Psychiatry* 1974;**37**:1–7.

183. Collier J: Nuclear ophthalmoplegia with especial reference to retraction of the lids and ptosis and to lesions of the posterior commissure. *Brain* 1927;**50**:488–498.

184. Hermann DM, Siccoli M, Brugger P, et al: Evolution of neurological, neuropsychological and sleep-wake disturbances after paramedian thalamic stroke. *Stroke* 2008;**39**:62–68.

185. Fisher CM, Caplan LR: Basilar artery branch occlusion: A cause of pontine infarction. *Neurology* 1971;**21**:900–905.

186. Fisher CM: Bilateral occlusion of basilar artery branches. *J Neurol Neurosurg Psychiatry* 1977;**40**:1182–1189.

187. Caplan LR: Intracranial branch atheromatous disease: A neglected, understudied and underused concept. *Neurology* 1989;**39**:1246–1250.

188. Klein IF, Lavallee PC, Schouman-Claeys E, Amaraenco P: High-resolution MRI identifies basilar artery plaques in paramedian pontine infarct. *Neurology* 2005;**64**:551–552.

189. Bassetti C, Bogousslavsky J, Barth A, Regli F: Isolated infarcts of the pons. *Neurology* 1996;**46**:165–175.

190. Kataoka S, Hori A, Shirakawa T, Hirose G: Paramedian pontine infarction. Neurological/topographical correlation. *Stroke* 1997;**28**:809–815.

191. Kumral E, Bayulkem G, Evyapan D: Clinical spectrum of pontine infarction. Clinical-MRI correlations. *J Neurol* 2002;**249**:1659–1670.

192. Kim JS, Cho KH, Kang DW, Kwon SU, Suh DC: Basilar artery atherosclerotic disease is related to subacute lesion volume increase in pontine base infarction. *Acta Neurol Scand* 2009;**120**:88–93.

193. Alexander CB, Burger PC, Goree JA: Dissecting aneurysms of the basilar artery in two patients. *Stroke* 1979;**10**:294–299.

194. Masson C, Krespy Y, Masson M, Colombani JM: Magnetic resonance imaging in basilar artery dissection. *Stroke* 1993;**24**:1264–1266.

195. Ruecker M, Furtner M, Knoflach M, et al: Basilar artery dissection: Series of 12 consecutive cases and review of the literature. *Cerebrovasc Dis* 2010;**30**:267–276.

196. Pessin MS, Lathi E, Cohen M, et al: Clinical features and mechanism of occipital infarction. *Ann Neurol* 1987;**21**:290–299.

197. Chaves CJ, Caplan LR: Posterior cerebral artery. In Caplan LR, van Gijn J (eds): *Stroke Syndromes*, 3rd ed. Cambridge: Cambridge University Press, 2012, pp 405–418.

198. Yamamoto Y, Georgiadis AL, Chang HM, Caplan LR: Posterior cerebral artery territory infarcts in the New England Medical Center (NEMC) Posterior Circulation Registry. *Arch Neurol* 1999;**56**:824–832.

199. Kumral E, Bayulkem G, Atac C, Alper Y: Spectrum of superficial posterior cerebral artery territory infarcts. *Eur J Neurol* 2004;**11**:237–246.

200. Lee E, Kang DW, Kwon SU, Kim JS: Posterior cerebral artery infarction: Diffusion-weighted MRI analysis of 205 patients. *Cerebrovasc Dis* 2009;**28**:298–305.

201. Caplan LR, Estol CJ, Massaro AR: Dissection of the posterior cerebral arteries. *Arch Neurol* 2005;**62**:1138–1143.

202. Hishikawa T, Tokunaga K, Sugiu K, Date I: Assessment of the difference in posterior circulation involvement between pediatric and adult patients with moyamoya disease. *J Neurosurg* 2013;**119**:961–965.

203. Frens DB, Petajan JH, Anderson R, Deblanc JH, Jr: Fibromuscular dysplasia of the posterior cerebral artery: Report of a case and review of the literature. *Stroke* 1974;**5**:161–166.

204. Calabrese LH, Dodick DW, Schwedt TJ, Singhal AB. Narrative review: Reversible cerebral vasoconstriction syndromes. *Ann Intern Med* 2007;**146**:34–44.

205. Pessin MS, Kwan E, DeWitt LD, et al: Posterior cerebral artery stenosis. *Ann Neurol* 1987;**21**:85–89.

206. Mohr JP, Pessin MS: Posterior cerebral artery disease. In Barnett HJM, Mohr JP, Stein BM, Yatsu F (eds): *Stroke Pathophysiology, Diagnosis, and Management*, 3rd ed. New York: Churchill Livingstone, 1998, pp 481–502.

207. Barton JS, Caplan LR: Cerebral visual dysfunction. In Caplan LR, van Gijn J (eds): *Stroke Syndromes*, 3rd ed. Cambridge: Cambridge University Press, 2012, pp 75–97.

208. Georgiadis AL, Yamamoto Y, Kwan ES, et al: Anatomy of sensory findings in patients with posterior cerebral artery (PCA) territory infarction. *Arch Neurol* 1999;**56**:835–838.

209. Caplan LR, DeWitt LD, Pessin MS, et al: Lateral thalamic infarcts. *Arch Neurol* 1988;**45**:959–964.

210. Benson DF, Tomlinson EB: Hemiplegic syndrome of the posterior cerebral artery. *Stroke* 1971;**2**:559–564.

211. Hommel M, Besson G, Pollak P, et al: Hemiplegia in posterior cerebral artery occlusion. *Neurology* 1990;**40**:1496–1499.

212. Hommel M, Moreaud O, Besson G, Perret J: Site of arterial occlusions in the hemiplegic posterior cerebral artery syndrome. *Neurology* 1991;**41**:604–605.

213. Dejerine J: Contribution à l'étude anatomo-pathologique et clinique des différentes variétés de cécité verbale. *Memoires de la Societe Biologique* 1892;**4**:61–90.

214. Geschwind N, Fusillo M: Color naming defect in association with alexia. *Arch Neurol* 1966;**15**:137–146.

215. Caplan LR, Hedley-White T: Cueing and memory dysfunction in alexia without agraphia. *Brain* 1974;**97**:25–262.

216. Kertesz A, Sleppard A, MacKenzie R: Localization in transcortical sensory aphasia. *Arch Neurol* 1982;**39**:475–479.

217. Victor M, Angevine J, Mancall E, et al: Memory loss with lesions of hippocampal formation. *Arch Neurol* 1961;**5**:244–263.

218. Ferro JM, Martins IP: Memory loss. In Caplan LR, van Gijn J (eds): *Stroke Syndromes*, 3rd ed. Cambridge: Cambridge University Press, 2012, pp 212–220.

219. Benson F, Marsden C, Meadows J: The amnestic syndrome of posterior cerebral artery occlusion. *Acta Neurol Scand* 1974;**50**:133–145.

220. Mohr JP, Leicester J, Stoddard L, et al: Right hemianopia with memory and color deficits in circumscribed left posterior cerebral artery territory infarction. *Neurology* 1971;**21**:1104–1113.

221. Ott B, Saver JL: Unilateral amnestic stroke. Six new cases and a review of the literature. *Stroke* 1993;**24**:1033–1042.

222. Szabo K, Forster A, Jager T et al: Hippocampal lesion patterns in acute posterior cerebral artery stroke: Clinical and imaging findings. *Stroke* 2009;**40**:2042–2045.

223. Rubens A, Benson F: Associative visual agnosia. *Arch Neurol* 1971;**24**:305–316.

224. Grusser OJ, Landis T: *Visual Agnosias and Other Disturbances of Visual Perception and Cognition*. Boston: CRC Press, 1991.

225. Damasio A, Damasio H, Van Hoesen G: Prosopagnosia: Anatomic basis and behavioral mechanisms. *Neurology* 1982;**32**:331–341.

226. Tranel D, Damasio AR: Intact recognition of facial expression, gender, and age in patients with impaired recognition of face identity. *Neurology* 1988;**38**:690–696.

227. Fisher CM: Disorientation to place. *Arch Neurol* 1982;**39**:33–36.

228. Symonds C, McKenzie I: Bilateral loss of vision from cerebral infarction. *Brain* 1957;**80**:415–455.

229. Medina J, Rubino F, Ross E: Agitated delirium caused by infarctions of the hippocampal formation and fusiform and lingual gyri: A case report. *Neurology* 1974;**24**:1181–1183.

230. Horenstein S, Chamberlain W, Conomy J: Infarction of the fusiform and calcarine regions: Agitated delirium and hemianopsia. *Trans Am Neurol Assoc* 1962;**92**:357–367.

231. Kumral E, Bayulkem G, Atac C, Alper Y: Spectrum of superficial posterior cerebral artery territory infarcts. *Eur J Neurol* 2004;**11**:237–246.

232. Kondziella D, Frahm-Falkenberg S: Anton's syndrome and eugenics. *J Clin Neurol* 2011;**7**:96–98.

233. Eby SA, Buchner EJ, Bryant MG, Mak HK: The rehabilitation of Anton syndrome. *PM R* 2012;**4**:385–387.

234. Mesulam M-M: Higher visual functions of the cerebral cortex and their disruption in clinical practice. In Albert DM, Jakobiec FA (eds): *Principles and Practice of Ophthalmology*, vol **4**. Philadelphia, WB Saunders Co., 1994, pp 2640–2653.

235. Mishkin M, Ungerleider LG, Macko KA: Object vision and spatial vision: Two cortical pathways. *Trends Neurosci* 1983;**6**:414–417.

236. Ungerleider LG, Haxby JV: "What" and "where" in the human brain. *Curr Opin Neurobiol* 1994;**4**:157–165.

237. Levine DN, Warach J, Farah M: Two visual systems in mental imagery: Dissociation of "what" and "where" in imagery disorders due to bilateral posterior cerebral lesions. *Neurology* 1985;**35**:1010–1018.

238. Meadows J: Disturbed perception of colors associated with localized cerebral lesions. *Brain* 1974;**97**:615–632.

239. Damasio A, Yamada T, Damasio H, et al: Central achromatopsia: behavioral, anatomic, and physiologic aspects. *Neurology* 1980;**30**:1064–1071.

240. Hecaen H, De Ajuriaguerra J: Balint's syndrome (psychic paralysis of visual fixation) and its minor forms. *Brain* 1954;**77**:373–400.

241. Bálint R: Seelenlahmung des `Schauens' optische ataxie, räumliche storung der aufmerksamkeit. *Monatschr Psychiatr Monatschr Psychiatr Neurol* 1909;**25**:51–191.

242. Luria AR: Disorders of "simultaneous perception" in a case of bilateral occipito-parietal brain injury. *Brain* 1959;**82**:437–449.

243. Holmes G: Disturbances of visual orientation. *Br J Ophthalmol* 1918;**2**:506–516.

244. Cogan DG: Ophthalmic manifestations of bilateral non-occipital cerebral lesions. *Br J Ophthalmol* 1965;**49**:281–297.

245. Johnston JL, Sharpe JA, Morrow MJ: Spasm of fixation: A quantitative study. *J Neurol Sci* 1992;**107**:166–171.

246. Kinkle W, Newman R, Jacobs L: Posterior cerebral artery branch occlusions: CT and anatomical considerations. In Berguer R, Bauer R (eds): *Vertebrobasilar Arterial Occlusive Disease*. New York: Raven Press, 1984, pp 117–133.

247. Goto K, Tagawa K, Uemma K, et al: Posterior cerebral artery occlusion. *Radiology* 1979;**132**:357–368.

248. Bogousslavsky J, Cachin C, Regli F, et al: Cardiac sources of embolism and cerebral infarction – clinical consequences and vascular concomitants: The Lausanne Stroke Registry. *Neurology* 1991;**41**:855–859.

249. Bogousslavsky J, Regli F, Maeder P, Meuli R, Nader J: The etiology of posterior circulation infarcts: A prospective study using magnetic resonance angiography. *Neurology* 1993;**43**:1528–1533.

250. Bogousslavsky J, Van Melle G, Regli F: The Lausanne Stroke Registry: Analysis of 1000 consecutive patients with first stroke. *Stroke* 1988;**19**:1083–1092.

251. Moulin T, Tatu L, Crepin-Leblond T, et al: The Besancon Stroke Registry: An acute stroke registry of 2500 consecutive patients. *Eur Neurol* 1997;**38**:10–20.

252. Moulin T, Tatu L, Vuillier F, et al: Role of a stroke data bank in evaluating cerebral infarction subtypes: Patterns and outcome of 1776 consecutive patients from the Besancon Stroke Registry. *Cerebrovasc Dis* 2000;**10**:261–271.

253. Vemmos K, Takis C, Georgilis K, et al: The Athens Stroke Registry: Results of a five-year hospital-based study. *Cerebrovasc Dis* 2000;**10**:133–141.

Penetrating and branch artery disease

Louis R Caplan, Geoffrey Donnan, and Marie Dagonnier

Occlusions or stenoses of large extracranial and intracranial arteries are traditional lesions usually recognized by physicians and surgeons caring for stroke patients. Abnormalities in larger arteries are easily confirmed by angiography and non-invasive tests and are readily verified by inspection of arteries removed at surgery or necropsy. In contrast, lesions in microscopic intracranial arteries, although acknowledged as genuine pathological findings, are a more controversial cause of stroke. C Miller Fisher (see Figures 1.6–1.8) reviewed the history of lacunar infarctions,[1] defined the nature and etiology of the vascular pathology causing lacunes,[2] and described many clinical syndromes that can be readily and reliably diagnosed as lacunar. Fisher almost single-handedly brought this disorder to the attention of the neurological community. Yet, some clinicians failed or refused to integrate the concept of lacunar infarction into their differential diagnosis of stroke, and others were skeptical that lacunar infarction could be reliably diagnosed clinically. Hence, the so called "lacunar hypothesis" has long been controversial.[3]

Durand-Fardel first introduced the term *lacunes* in 1843 to describe small holes, usually found in the striatum, which contain fine meshwork of tissues and vessels.[3–5] The clinical findings in patients with lacunar infarction were first described by Ferrand,[6] working in the laboratory of Pierre Marie, and by Marie himself.[7] These French authors noted that lacunes were most often located in the lentiform nuclei, thalamus, pons, internal capsule, and cerebral white matter. Hemiplegia was the major finding in acute lacunar infarction. The clinical condition of multiple lacunes was termed *état lacunaire* (lacunar state) by Marie and was characterized by pseudobulbar palsy and an abnormal small-stepped gait. Foix and colleagues added clinical details about the findings in capsular and pontine lacunar infarcts.[8–10] Little was added after Foix until Fisher's work on the pathology and clinical findings in patients with lacunar infarction.[3,4]

The importance of lacunar strokes is emphasized by their frequency and the sizable proportion of strokes that are lacunar. They account for 20–25% of all ischemic strokes, with an annual incidence of approximately 15 per 100 000 people.[11,12]

Pathology

Lacunar infarcts are small, discrete, often irregular lesions, ranging from 1 to 15 mm in size. Only 17% of lacunes are smaller than 1 cm.[1] Inspection of the tiny cavities usually reveals fine strands of connective tissue resembling cobwebs. Marie recognized that true lacunar infarcts had to

be differentiated from dilated perivascular spaces, so-called *état criblé*, and from post-mortem holes produced by gas-forming bacilli (*état vermoulu*).[7] At necropsy, gas cavities are usually numerous, perfectly round, with no cobwebs, and often retain a characteristic bad smell. Magnetic resonance imaging (MRI) often reveals dilated perivascular état criblé lesions as discrete loci of increased signal.[13] The most common locations of lacunar infarcts are the putamen and the pallidum, followed by the pons, thalamus, caudate nucleus, internal capsule, and corona radiata. Rarer are lacunes in the cerebral peduncles, pyramids, and subcortical white matter. These lesions are not found in the cerebral or cerebellar cortices.

Serial sections of the penetrating arteries that supply the territory of lacunar infarcts show a characteristic vascular pathology.[2] These tiny vessels often have focal enlargements and small hemorrhagic extravasation through the walls of the arteries. Subintimal foam cells sometimes obliterate the lumens, and pink-staining fibrinoid material lies within the vessel walls (Figure 9.1). The arteries in spots are often replaced by whorls, tangles, and wisps of connective tissue that obliterate the usual

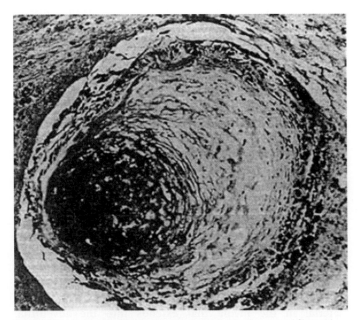

Figure 9.1 Small penetrating artery showing lipohyalinosis and fibrinoid necrosis; lumen is considerably compromised. Courtesy of C Miller Fisher, MD.

Caplan's Stroke: A Clinical Approach, 5th Edition, ed. Louis R Caplan. Published by Cambridge University Press. © Cambridge University Press, 2016.

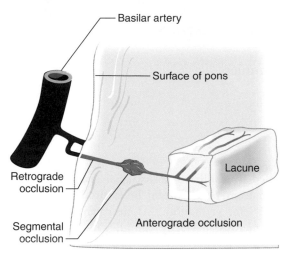

Figure 9.2 Diagram showing the relationship of a lacune in the pons to the causative penetrating artery vascular lesion. The artery beyond the region of arterial disorganization is thrombosed and thrombus has also formed in a retrograde manner extending toward the parent basilar artery. Adapted from Fisher CM. The arterial lesion underlying lacunes. *Acta Neuropathol* 1969;12:1–15.

vascular layers. Fisher called these processes *segmental arterial disorganization, fibrinoid degeneration,* and *lipohyalinosis.* Fisher also recognized that sometimes larger deep infarcts, which he dubbed *giant lacunes,* could be caused by occlusion of parent vessels, such as the middle cerebral artery (MCA) stem, causing obstruction of the orifices of lateral lenticulostriate arteries.[14] Figure 9.2 shows a cartoon modeled after Fisher of a lipohyalinatic lesion that disrupts arterial flow causing a pontine infarct.[2]

Fisher,[15,16] Cole and Yates,[17] and Rosenblum[18] recognized that small aneurysmal dilatations of these lipohyalinotic penetrating arteries could potentially rupture, causing intracerebral hemorrhage. These lesions were probably similar to those recognized by Charcot and Bouchard[19] as the cause of parenchymatous bleeding. The distribution of deep hypertensive hemorrhages was the same as the locations of lacunes (putamen, capsule, thalamus, and pons). Lipohyalinotic arteries could occlude, leading to lacunar infarction, or rupture, causing intracerebral hemorrhage.[15] Fisher reviewed the charts of 114 patients who had lacunes at necropsy. All but 3 patients had hypertension defined by a prior history of this disease, elevated blood pressure recorded on examination, or heart weight exceeding 400 g without another explanation.[1] Fisher attributed segmental arterial disorganization and lipohyalinosis to hypertension. Hypertension was very difficult to control during the 1960s at the time of Fisher's necropsy studies.

A hereditary disorder, cerebral autosomal dominant arteriopathy with subcortical infarcts and leukoencephalopathy (CADASIL), has now been convincingly shown to be a disorder of the small penetrating arteries within the brain.[20–22] The penetrating arteries in this condition contain a granular material in the media that extends into the adventitia. Periodic acid–Schiff (PAS) staining suggests the presence of glycoproteins, but staining for elastin and amyloid are invariably negative. Smooth muscle cells in the media are swollen and often degenerated.[22] The endothelium may be absent and

replaced by collagen fibers. Capillaries as well as small arterioles are involved. At times abnormalities seen in hypertensive patients are also found, including duplication and splitting of the internal elastic lamina, adventitial fibrosis and hyaline change, and fibrosis and hypertrophy of the arterial media. This hereditary condition causes lacunar infarcts in the basal ganglia and cerebral white matter similar to those found in hypertensive patients.

Cerebral autosomal recessive arteriopathy with subcortical infarcts and leukoencephalopathy (CARASIL) is a condition now known to be caused by a single-gene disorder that involves mutations in the *HTRA1* gene encoding HtrA serine peptidase/ protease 1 (HTRA1).[23] The clinical–neurological findings are similar to CADASIL except that premature baldness and back pain and severe spondylitis are additional major features. In contrast to CADASIL, the arteries in CARASIL do not contain osmiophilic materials. In CARASIL, penetrating arteries are enlarged and at times collapsed.[24] The arterial medial smooth muscle cells are diminished and there is a reduction in extracellular matrix.[24]

Another hereditary angiopathic condition, now known to be associated with mutations in a gene that encodes procollagen type IV alpha 1 (*COL4A1*), has recently been identified. This genetic mutation affects small brain arteries as well as larger retinal and cerebral arteries.[25–29] The clinical findings are heterogeneous and include: perinatal hemorrhages and porencephaly, tendency to brain hemorrhage after trauma, retinal artery tortuosity, cerebral aneurysms, penetrating artery-related infarcts, white matter gliosis, microbleeds, and kidney disease.[25–29] Unlike CADASIL, the temporal lobes are usually spared of the chronic white matter abnormalities.

There are likely other hereditary causes of vascular-related chronic white matter pathology that are as yet not well characterized. One condition was described in children who develop progressive cognitive and motor signs and brain imaging shows extensive white matter gliosis and cyst formation and calcifications in the basal ganglia, cerebellar nuclei and deep white matter.[30] On microscopy angiomatous-like changes in small penetrating arteries was found.[30] Similar findings have now been described in a 44-year-old woman.[31]

Detailed anatomical dissections during the late nineteenth century[32,33] and early twentieth century[9,10,34–38] defined the locations, anatomy, and territories of arteries that branched from the parent cerebral and basilar arteries. Pullicino reviewed and illustrated in detail the anatomy of these arteries and their usual territories of supply.[39,40] Some of these penetrating arteries are shown in Figures 2.14, 2.18, and 2.22.

Foix recognized that infarcts were often limited to the territories of one of these branches. The orifices of these branches were often obstructed by a pathology that differed from lipohyalinosis. Fisher and Caplan,[41] Fisher,[42] and Caplan[43] described the vascular pathology in these branches. Fisher and Caplan[41] reported vascular lesions causing ischemia limited to the territory of basilar artery branches, separating this vasculopathy from lipohyalinosis. This pathology is referred to as *intracranial branch atheromatous disease.* Figures 2.33, 9.3, and 9.4 contain cartoons that illustrate

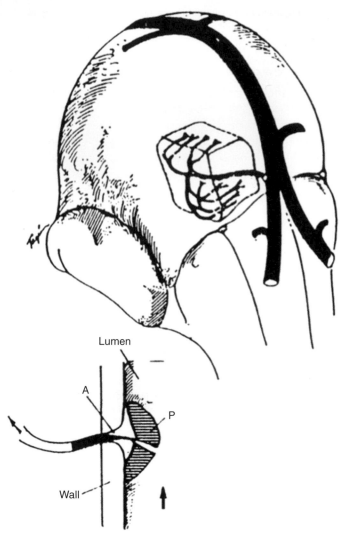

Figure 9.3 Basilar-branch occlusion. The diagram at the bottom shows a close-up of the artery shown within the cube above; a plaque is seen extending into the branch. A, atheroma; P, plaque. From Fisher CM, Caplan LR. Basilar artery branch occlusion: A cause of pontine infarction. *Neurology* 1971;21:900–905.

the location and mechanism of the pathology in the parent artery.[43] The orifices of the penetrating branches could be blocked by atheroma in the parent artery, atheroma could originate in the parent artery and extend into the branch (so-called junctional atheromatous plaques), or microatheroma could arise at the origin of the branch itself. Thrombus was sometimes superimposed on the atheromas. This vasculopathy is sometimes referred to as microatheroma and is clearly distinct on pathological grounds from the lipohyalinotic arteriopathy that also causes small deep infarcts.[44]

It is now possible to image intracerebral branch atheromatous disease using high resolution MRI. Plaques in the middle cerebral artery[45,46] and basilar artery[47] (Figure 9.5) can be shown to impinge upon or occlude penetrating branches by MRI techniques that show axial sections of the origins of branches from the parent arteries.

The ability to image during life the intracranial arteries has led to different categorizations. Kim and Yoon and their Korean colleagues[48,49] and the Chinese Intracranial

Atherosclerosis Study group[50] introduced different terms to separate different mechanisms that cause single subcortical infarcts (SSIs), which were referred to as lacunes by most prior authors. Distal single subcortical infarcts (dSSI) infers pathology within the penetrating artery itself (e.g., lipohyalinosis in Fisher's terminology). Proximal single subcortical infarcts (pSSI) infers pathology at the orifice of the penetrating artery. Patients with pSSI are then subdivided into two categories: pSSI with parent artery lesions and pSSI without parent artery lesions. The parent artery lesions are diagnosed using high-resolution intracranial vascular imaging. An example of this imaging and characterization has been shown in Figure 7.14. The category of pSSI without parent artery lesions corresponds to that of intracranial atheromatous branch disease in the Fisher and Caplan terminology discussed above.[41–43] The posited pathology is a microatheroma that forms at the orifice of a branch as illustrated in Figure 2.33C. The category pSSI with parent artery disease corresponds to the illustrations shown in Figure 2.33A and B. The parent artery disease can be minor and not encroach on the lumen of the parent artery or can be more extensive. Parent artery plaques are an important mechanism of blockage of the orifices of penetrating arteries in the pons (Chapter 8) and the lenticulostriate arteries causing deep MCA territory striato-capsular infarcts (Chapter 7).

Hypertension and diabetes are prevalent risk factors in patients with lacunar infarcts. Patients with these risk factors also often have associated occlusive lesions involving the large cervico-cranial arteries that supply the brain and the coronary arteries. Among a cohort of 108 patients with lacunar infarction, Horowitz et al. reported that, hypertension was present in 68%, diabetes in 37%; both occurred in 28% and neither occurred in 23%.[51] They also noticed that of those without these 2 cardiovascular risk factors, 32% had a possible carotid or cardiac etiology. Microemboli can also originate from the heart and aorta and cause lacunar infarcts but usually there are coexistent cortical and subcortical infarctions.

Pontine infarcts are the most frequent pathological lesion found in necropsies of diabetics and are, in most cases, caused by atheromatous branch disease.[52] Infarcts limited to the territories of the anterior choroidal arteries (AChA) and the thalamogeniculate arteries are also most often explained by atheromatous branch disease. Microatheromas, parent-artery plaques, and occlusion of parent arteries by in-situ thrombosis or embolism probably explain deep infarcts in normotensive patients.

The major important condition to separate from these "micropathologies" is occlusion of the parent artery blocking flow in penetrating artery branches. In patients of Asian origin, especially Japan, Korea, and China, small deep infarcts are often caused by occlusive disease of the large intracranial parent arteries, the occlusive lesions blocking the orifices of penetrating arteries.[53,54] In patients whose small deep infarcts are caused by severe occlusive disease of the intracranial large parent arteries, the infarcts are slightly larger, the neurological signs are slightly worse, and recurrence is more common than in infarcts caused by intrinsic disease of the penetrating

Middle cerebral

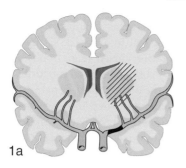

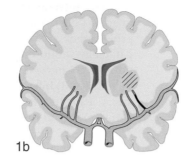

1a

1b

Posterior cerebral

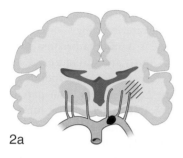

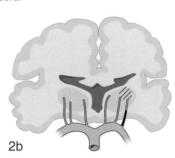

2a

2b

Figure 9.4 Mechanisms of deep infarction. 1a, Basal ganglionic capsular infarct due to MCA occlusion. 1b, Smaller deep capsular infarct due to lenticulostriate artery occlusion. 2a, Lateral thalamic infarct due to PCA occlusion. 2b, Lateral thalamic infarct due to thalamogeniculate artery occlusion. MCA, middle cerebral artery; PCA, posterior cerebral artery. From Caplan LR, DeWitt LD, Pessin MS, et al. Lateral thalamic infarcts. *Arch Neurol* 1988;45:959–964.

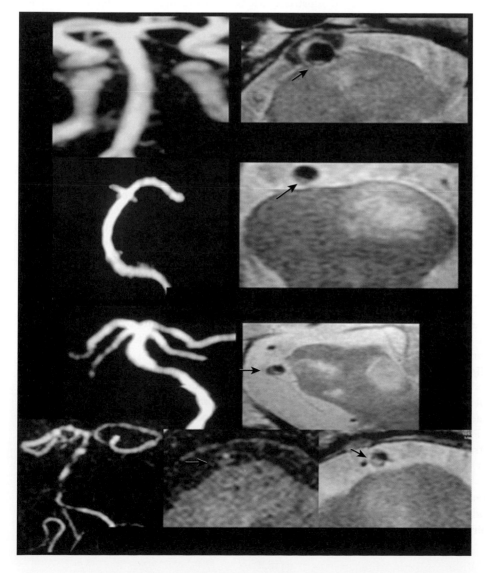

Figure 9.5 High-resolution magnetic resonance angiographies (MRAs) that show a plaque in the parent basilar artery (arrows) obstructing a penetrating branch causing an infarct in the basis pontis. From Klein IF, Lavallee PC, Schouman-Claeys E, Amaraenco P. High-resolution MRI identifies basilar artery plaques in paramedian pontine infarct. *Neurology* 2005;64:551–552.

arteries.[55,56] Vascular imaging (computed tomography angiography (CTA), magnetic resonance angiography (MRA), transcranial Doppler (TCD), and catheter contrast angiography) can now readily show occlusion of the major intracranial large arteries.

Although lipohyalinosis and microatheroma are readily separated by meticulous pathological examination, the distinction is difficult clinically. Boiten separated 100 patients with lacunes into 2 distinct groups.[57] One group had atherosclerotic risk factors and single symptomatic lacunes; the other group had hypertension, multiple lacunes (some of which were asymptomatic) and white matter abnormalities on neuroimaging scans. He posited that the former group had atheromatous branch disease and the latter group had lipohyalinosis.[57] Experience since this report confirms these observations. Clinical separation of branch occlusions at the orifice of penetrating branches and intrinsic disease of the penetrating branches themselves (lipohyalinosis) is difficult. Disease at the orifice of a branch tends to cause larger infarcts and more clinical worsening than intrinsic disease along the branches.[58]

General clinical findings

A 56-year-old, African-American man, RB, awakened with weakness of his right arm. As he stood to go to the bathroom, he became aware that his right leg was also weak. He called his wife, who noted that his voice was slightly thick. He did not have a headache, nor did he feel dizzy or otherwise unwell. As the day progressed, the weakness in his arm and leg seemed to fluctuate. By nightfall, however, he could not move his right arm or right leg. He had no prior history of stroke, heart disease, or claudication, and did not recognize any warnings during the days before the episode. Two months earlier, a physician told him that his blood pressure was high and "bore watching," but did not prescribe medication.

Fisher repeatedly emphasized in his writings that hypertension was the major cause of fibrinoid degeneration and lipohyalinosis, the arteriopathy that he considered was the cause of lacunar infarcts. Fisher noted that the same arteriopathy that caused lacunar infarcts also caused deep intracerebral hemorrhages and that these hemorrhages and lacunes involved the very same brain regions. He observed that often hypertension was of recent onset or had become recently more severe or poorly controlled. Although Fisher attributed the arteriopathy to hypertension, others have noted a lower frequency of hypertension in patients, in whom computed tomography (CT) verified the diagnosis of lacunar infarcts (52.5%,[59] 57%,[60] 65%,[61] 72%[62]). Seventy-five percent of patients clinically diagnosed as having lacunar infarcts in the Harvard Stroke Registry had hypertension.[63] In a necropsy study, 64% of patients with lacunes at post-mortem had a history of hypertension.[64] These frequencies are not importantly different from the incidence of hypertension in large registries of patients with ischemic strokes. In the Northern Manhattan Study that included a multiethnic cohort of individuals, lacunar infarct patients tended to be older, and were

more likely to have diabetes and elevated cholesterol levels than those with deep intracerebral hemorrhages.[65]

For a more thorough evaluation, Fisher used pathological criteria to diagnose lacunes and hypertension (heart weight 400 g with no other cause), and carefully searched hospital and doctors' notes for past blood-pressure recordings. Although clearly not all patients with deep infarcts are hypertensive, a diagnosing physician should be wary of attributing a lesion to intrinsic penetrating artery occlusive disease if there is no past or current evidence of hypertension or diabetes. Systolic hypertension, a finding very common in elderly individuals, may be particularly important in causing penetrating artery damage related to increased vascular pulsatility. LRC has also seen normotensive patients with elevated hematocrit (Hct) who have a clinical picture of lacunar infarction, possibly caused by clotting within small arteries. Chronic kidney disease[66] and dilatative arteriopathy[67] (large intracranial dolichoectasia) (see Chapter 12) have also been found to be associated with small-vessel brain arterial disease.

Fisher found severe large-vessel atherosclerosis in 64% of the 114 patients with lacunes, a frequency far exceeding the usual 9% found in a population without lacunes.[1] Hypertension is known to predispose patients to premature atherosclerosis of larger extracranial and intracranial arteries. Large- and small-vessel diseases frequently coexist, so the mere presence of clinical, non-invasive, or angiographic evidence of atherosclerotic stenosis does not exclude a lacunar etiology of stroke.

Lacunes are small and deep. Because there is no accompanying overdistension of superficial arteries and deep arteries have no pain fibers, headache caused by vascular distension does not occur in patients with lacunes. These small lesions produce no mass effect that might cause headache or decreased alertness. Lacunes are far from the cortex and do not produce seizures[63] or affect the surface-recorded electroencephalogram (EEG).[68] The presence of decreased alertness, unaccustomed headache, or seizures argues against a lacunar etiology of a stroke.

The course of illness in patients with lacunar infarction is also different from patients with large-artery occlusive disease and brain embolism.[63,69] Prior transient ischemic attacks (TIAs) occur in approximately 20% of patients with lacunes,[69–71] a frequency far below that for large vessel disease but more often than in patients with brain embolism. When TIAs do occur in patients with lacunar infarcts, they span a shorter time interval and are more stereotyped than in other ischemic etiologies. Brief, stereotyped TIAs may occur many times during a day. The occurrence of repeated episodes of hemiplegia preceding a pure-motor stroke was labeled the "capsular warning syndrome" by Donnan and colleagues.[72] However, these repeated TIAs can occur in subcortical lesions in other areas and in the brainstem and are not limited to the internal capsule.

The neurological deficit often evolves gradually in patients with lacunar infarcts, with frequent fluctuations and progression during the initial 72 hours of the stroke. Sudden deficits, maximal at onset, are less frequent than in patients with other

causes of ischemic stroke. Gradual worsening of paralysis over a few days is a characteristic course in some patients with pure-motor hemiparesis caused by lacunar infarction. Lacunar infarction is the most common cause of worsening of clinical neurological signs during the first week after stroke onset.[73,74]

> On examination of patient RB, the blood pressure was 165/95 mmHg. He was alert and understood, repeated, and used language normally. The patient read, wrote, and spelled words correctly. His voice was slightly slurred. His right face, shoulder, arm, hand, thigh, and foot were moderately weak. Deep tendon reflexes were exaggerated on the right, and the right plantar response was extensor. He felt touch normally in his right limbs and could identify accurately the nature of objects in his right hand. He could also localize spots touched on his right limbs. Visual fields were normal.

Lacunes have a predilection for particular anatomical sites – those nourished by penetrating arteries. Some of these deep lesions produce characteristic clinical syndromes also named lacunar syndromes,[75] whereas others are clinically silent or produce findings difficult to distinguish from superficial infarction. The clinical syndrome may not be entirely predictive of the lesion or location. Arboix et al. showed that although lacunar syndromes are highly suggestive of small deep cerebral infarction, they were not due to lacunar infarcts in 16% of the cases they investigated.[76]

In a necropsy series of 167 patients with lacunes, 93 patients (56%) had no reported related symptoms.[67] Infarcts that do not result in stroke symptoms have been dubbed silent strokes. Most silent strokes are lacunes of which hypertensive small-vessel disease is thought to be the main cause.[77] Vermeer et al. showed that silent infarcts are a major determinant of dementia. They demonstrated that the risk of developing dementia over 3.6 years of follow-up was doubled in patients with silent infarcts on MRI at baseline[78] In a systematic review, Vermeer and colleagues also reported that MRI silent brain infarcts are detected in 20% of healthy elderly people and up to 50% in some cohorts.[77]

Anatomical localization is probably most helpful in the diagnosis of lacunes. RB had paralysis of face, arm, and leg with exaggerated reflexes and an extensor toe sign. A lesion of the motor cortex causing these findings would have to extend from the face area near the sylvian fissure, a region fed by the MCA, to the paramedian frontal lobe foot area, which is fed by the anterior cerebral artery. Such a lesion would invariably affect language, sensation, or vision. A sizable superficial or deep frontal-lobe lesion would not only produce motor dysfunction, but would also likely cause conjugate eye deviation to the side of the lesion and abulia. Marie emphasized hemiplegia as the sign of lacunar infarction.[7] Fisher termed the syndrome of isolated weakness of the face, arm, and leg, *pure-motor hemiplegia*,[14] and taught that these findings were diagnostic of lacunar infarction in the pons or internal capsule.

Some authors, using radioisotope studies or CT, found lesions other than lacunes in patients with pure-motor hemiplegia.[61,79,80] MRI is more sensitive and shows cortical lesions in some patients clinically thought to have a lacunar syndrome. Remember that Fisher examined the patients thoroughly. When he called the patient's syndrome *pure motor*, he had compulsively tested sensation, visual fields, and cortical function and found them normal. Fisher also demanded that weakness include the face, arm, and leg, and that hypertension be present to make the diagnosis of a pure-motor stroke. Patient RB fulfills Fisher's criteria for pure-motor hemiplegia. Were patients with CT lesions, other than lacunes, examined in the same compulsive and thorough manner as an important requisite for the clinical diagnosis of lacunes in these other radiographic studies?

We advise a strategy similar to that taught in high school geometry: Try to prove your original diagnostic impression wrong. Seek out features (i.e., sensory, visual, or intellectual abnormalities) that would disprove your diagnosis. Mental status testing is key because most pure-motor hemiplegia patients with lesions other than lacunes have some alteration in alertness, behavior, or intellect that suggests frontal lobe disease.

Even when the lacunar syndromes are apparently pure, some patients have a small hematoma as the cause of the syndrome. Small putaminal, capsular, and pontine hematomas are known to cause pure-motor hemiparesis and other syndromes most often caused by lacunar infarction.[69,71,81–83] Before clinicians can be secure in their diagnosis of lacunar infarction, we believe neuroimaging tests (CT or MRI), that show a lacune or exclude parenchymatous hemorrhage and surface infarction, are mandatory. Diffusion-weighted MRI has the capacity for separating recent lacunar infarcts from old lesions. Vascular imaging is also important in excluding parent artery occlusive disease.

Location of lesions and clinical syndromes

Hemispheral lesions within the anterior circulation

Probably the most commonly recognized clinical syndrome in patients with lacunes in the cerebral hemispheres is pure-motor hemiparesis. Patient RB had this syndrome. The causative lesion is usually found in the internal capsule. Figure 9.6 is a necropsy specimen that shows a lacunar infarct that involves the basal ganglia and cuts through the internal capsule. The three types of capsular lesions causing pure-motor hemiparesis distinguished by Rascol and colleagues are: (1) large lesions spanning the anterior and posterior limbs of the internal capsule, caused by occlusion of large lateral lenticulostriate arteries; (2) capsulopallidal infarcts located predominantly in the posterior limb of the capsule in the territory of medial lenticulostriate arteries; and (3) lesions in the anterior limb of the internal capsule and the caudate nucleus in the supply region of the lateral lenticulostriate arteries or the recurrent arteries of Heubner.[69,71] MRI studies show that patients with pure-motor hemiparesis can also have lesions in the midbrain, pons, and medulla, affecting descending corticospinal fibers in the cerebral peduncle, basis pontis, and the medullary pyramid.[84,85]

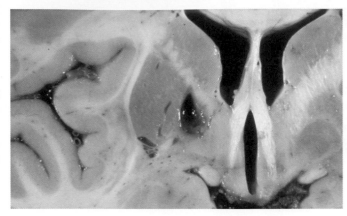

Figure 9.6 A necropsy specimen showing a cavity due to an old lacunar infarct located in the medial basal ganglia (mostly the globus pallidus) and extending through the internal capsule in a patient with a pure-motor hemiplegia during life. A black and white version of this figure will appear in some formats. For the color version, please refer to the plate section.

Motor weakness does not always equally affect the face, arm, and leg. Often, the face is at least partially spared.[69] At times, almost a pure monoparesis of the arm or leg is present with only minimal weakness or hyperreflexia of the other limb. In the Stroke Data Bank, the clinical findings related to the degree of involvement of face, arm, and leg did not correlate with the location of the lesion in the internal capsule.[69,86] Mohr summarized as follows: "There no longer seems much reason to adhere to the older dogma[71] that the motor fibers occupy the anterior half of the posterior limb of the internal capsule ... Further, the available case material does not document a series of cases with an homunculus whose face is anterior and whose leg is posterior in the plane of the internal capsule."[69]

In some patients with lacunar infarction, the clinical picture includes a combination of weakness, pyramidal signs, cerebellar-type ataxia, and incoordination of the limbs on one side of the body. This syndrome was first called *homolateral ataxia and crural paresis* in patients in whom the predominant involvement was in the lower limbs.[87] Later, Fisher dubbed the syndrome *ataxic hemiparesis*, indicating that the arm and leg could be variously involved, but the major signature of the syndrome was the combination of cerebellar and motor signs in the limbs on the same side of the body.[88] In some patients, there are also sensory symptoms ipsilateral to the motor abnormalities.[89] The relative severity of ataxia compared to weakness varies considerably, as does the relative involvement of the arm compared to the leg. Localization of lesions causing ataxic hemiparesis varies widely. Many lesions are in the posterior limb of the internal capsule. Lacunes in the midbrain and pons, however, can also cause this clinical syndrome.

At times, the clinical findings show abnormalities of motor function on one side of the body, but there is no true paralysis, reflexes are not exaggerated, and the plantar response is flexor. We refer to these findings as a *non-pyramidal hemimotor syndrome*. Some lesions that cause these clinical findings involve the striatum and the globus pallidus. Decreased spontaneous and associated movements, clumsiness, slight increased resistance to passive movement, and slowness of

the affected limbs are often found. Some patients have a minor degree of hemiparkinsonism. Others have a movement disorder with choreic features. Some patients with hemichorea have had striatal infarcts.[90,91]

Sometimes, the predominant dysfunction in patients with hemispheral lacunes is bulbar. Dysarthria, dysphagia, and even mutism may occur, caused by interruption of corticobulbar fibers in the white matter underlying the motor cortex, capsule, striatum, or pons. Limb symptoms may be minor or absent. Tapping the corner of the mouth may show heightened contraction of the orbicularis oris and the orbicularis oculi on the side of the bulbar dysfunction, or on both sides of the face. Often, the tongue and face are weak on one side. In patients with predominantly bulbar signs, the lesions are often bilateral and the syndrome is pseudobulbar.[92] The initial lesion sometimes produces no symptoms or only minor hemimotor signs. When the contralateral side of the brain becomes involved, the bilateral lesions involving corticobulbar fibers causes predominantly bulbar abnormalities, especially dysarthria and dysphagia, sometimes with exaggerated laughing and crying.

In Chapter 7, caudate[93,94] and AChA-territory infarcts are discussed.[95–98] Infarcts in these regions can be quite small, readily qualifying as lacunes, or they can be more extensive deep infarcts. Caudate lesions can be limited to the caudate nucleus or extend into the anterior limb of the internal capsule and anterior putamen.[93,94] AChA-territory infarcts can involve the globus pallidus or the posterior limb of the internal capsule.[95–98] Infarcts in these areas are probably caused by intracranial-branch atheromatous disease, affecting one or more medial lenticulostriate arteries and the AChA.[43]

Involvement of small penetrating branches of these arteries is probably most often caused by microatheromas or lipohyalinosis. Neuropathological studies of patients with lesions in the distribution of lenticulostriate arteries and the AChA are too scanty to document or refute this hypothesis.[43] Some patients with caudate infarcts have prominent dysarthria and cognitive and behavioral abnormalities, especially abulia and restlessness.[93,94,99,100] Some patients with left caudate infarcts have aphasia, usually slight and transient. In a necropsy series of patients with lacunes found at post-mortem, aphasia with right hemiparesis was one of the most frequent clinical syndromes correlating with lacunar infarction.[64] The responsible lesions were in the striatum and anterior limb of the internal capsule or thalamus.

Posterior circulation, brainstem, thalamic lacunes, and branch occlusions

Pons and medulla

Lacunes and branch-territory infarcts are often found in the pons.[84,85,101,102] In a prospective study of MRI scans in 100 patients hospitalized with lacunar infarcts in Grenoble, France, 38 of the lesions (25%) were in the pons.[84] Among 12 patients in another series studied acutely with MRI, 6 of 11 lesions were located in the pons and patients had symptoms appropriate to that localization.[103] The most common site of the pontine

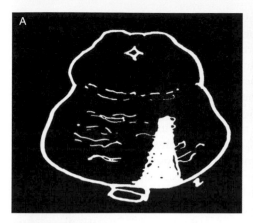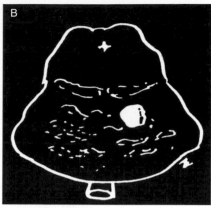

Figure 9.7 Cartoon showing pontine infarcts. A, Basilar artery branch infarct extending to the pial surface at the base of the pons. B, Infarct within the pontine parenchyma due to a lipohyalinotic lesion within the penetrating artery supplying this region. From Caplan LR. Intracranial branch atheromatous disease: A neglected understudied, and underused concept. *Neurology* 1989;39:1246–1250.

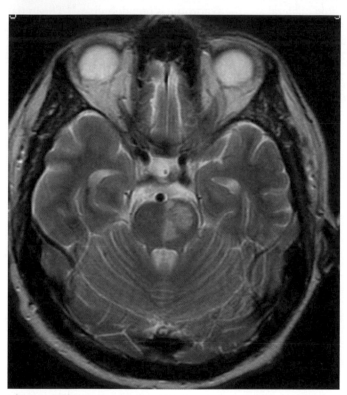

Figure 9.8 MRI T2-weighted image showing an infarct in the paramedian pons. The basilar artery flow void looks normal. Courtesy of Ladislav Pazdera, MD.

lesions is in the basis pontis on one side, most often medially in the distribution of one of the paramedian branches of the basilar artery.[101,102] The penetrating branches of the basilar artery are shown in Figure 2.22. Occlusive changes in these vessels cause pontine infarcts in the supply zone of each of these branches. Few necropsy specimens of patients with infarcts in this location have been studied. The pathology in some has been lipohyalinosis and segmental arterial disorganization of penetrating arteries within the basis pontis.[2,14]

In three patients, arterial lesions involving basilar-artery branches were studied in more detail by serially sectioning the pons, with the basilar artery and its branches still attached to the pons.[41,42] In one patient, an atheromatous plaque within the basilar artery obstructed the intramural part of the 0.5-mm-diameter basilar-artery branch.[41] Distally, in the blocked branch, there was a mass of agglutinated platelets, which arose

as a tiny intra-arterial embolus from the lesion in the parent artery or formed in situ because of reduced flow. In another patient, a plaque arising in the lumen of the basilar artery extended the mouth of a 0.5-mm-diameter branch, forming a junctional plaque.[41] In a third patient, basilar-artery branches were blocked bilaterally.[42] At the orifice of a basilar branch in this patient, a microdissection made a crevice in a plaque, and a superimposed thrombus obstructed the branch. The mechanisms of blockage of branches are depicted in Figures 2.33, 9.3, and 9.4. Flat or elevated plaques in the parent basilar artery can block the orifices of branches or provide a nidus for small embolic fragments that extend into the branches. A dilatated dolichoectatic basilar artery can also distort branch orifices.

Infarction of the medullary pyramid can give rise to a pure-motor hemiparesis, often sparing the face.[14,101,104–107] At times the medial lemniscus is also involved causing tingling of contralateral limbs. Nerve XII may be ischemic as it passes through the medullary base.

Infarcts in the pontine base caused by lipohyalinotic lesions within the course of a penetrating artery are often located within the pontine parenchyma sparing the basal pial border of the pons while occlusion of the mouth of a penetrating artery most often causes an infarct that begins at the basal pial surface. Figure 9.7 is a cartoon that illustrates the various locations of these two pathologies. Figure 9.8 is an MRI that shows an infarct in the paramedian basis pontis on one side caused by a basilar artery branch occlusion. Note that the infarct extends to the basal pial surface. Figure 9.9 is a necropsy specimen of a lacune in the dorsal portion of the basis pontis near the tegmental border.

The three major syndromes in the pons related to infarcts in the basis pontis are pure-motor hemiparesis, ataxic hemiparesis, and dysarthria clumsy-hand syndrome.[101,102,108–111] Pure-motor hemiplegia is probably the most common of the syndromes and occurs most often when the pontine infarcts are in the paramedian basis pontis. In some patients, additional findings help identify the infarct as pontine. An ipsilateral VI-nerve palsy or intranuclear ophthalmoplegia occasionally accompany the contralateral hemiparesis.[41,101,108] Involvement of the tegmentum and base can include the paramedian pontine reticular formation, causing a conjugate-gaze palsy toward the side of the lesion, accompanied by contralateral limb weakness

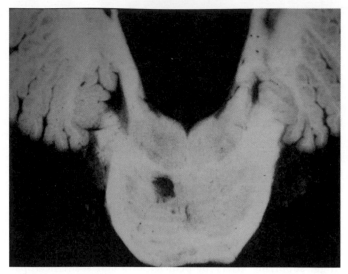

Figure 9.9 A necropsy specimen showing a lacunar infarct in the dorsal portion of the basis pontis on one side.

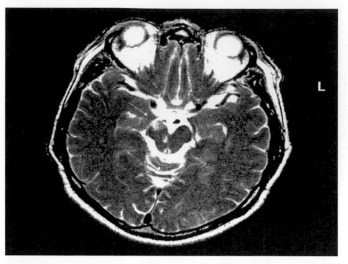

Figure 9.10 A T2-weighted MRI showing an infarct in the cerebral peduncle of the midbrain on one side.

and pyramidal signs. At times, although there is no gaze palsy, conjugate-gaze movements are asymmetric with slight abnormalities of ipsilateral conjugate gaze. Involvement of the medial lemniscus, as well as pyramidal tract fibers, leads to some sensory symptoms and signs on the side of the hemiparesis.[108,109,111] Usually, patients report minor paresthesias and sensory examination shows only slight loss of vibration sense, with preserved pinprick and temperature sensation.

The basis pontis carries fibers crossing into the brachium pontis, traveling toward the cerebellum. Interruption of pontocerebellar fibers can cause cerebellar-type incoordination and ataxia. Ataxic hemiparesis is often caused by a pontine lesion.[87,88,101,102,108,109,111] The infarcts that cause ataxic hemiparesis are usually smaller and more rostral, dorsal, and lateral than the lesions associated with pure-motor hemiparesis.[101,102,109] Subtle, minor incoordination of the ipsilateral limbs can provide a clue to this localization because pontocerebellar-crossing fibers are involved bilaterally to some extent. The dysarthria clumsy-hand syndrome is usually caused by a small lacune in the more dorsal portion of the basis pontis, affecting corticobulbar fibers near the medial lemniscus.[101,102,109–111] Often, associated facial and tongue weakness is severe, but examination of the hand and arm is nearly normal, despite the patient's report of awkwardness.

Occasionally, lacunes are located in the medial or lateral pontine tegmentum in the distribution of branches that penetrate horizontally from long, circumferential arteries or penetrate from the base of the pons.[101,102,111,112] These lacunes are the ischemic counterpart of lateral tegmental brainstem hematomas.[111,113] These lesions usually involve the sensory lemniscus that has formed from the joining of the medial lemniscus and lateral spinothalamic tracts in the rostral pons. These lesions may involve the medial lemniscus or the spinothalamic tract before formation of the sensory lemniscus. A pure, sensory, stroke-like syndrome occurs with subjective paresthesias or numbness (or both) in the contralateral face, arm, and leg. Dizziness, gait ataxia, dysarthria, and nystagmus are variable accompaniments.[111,111,114,115]

Midbrain

In the midbrain, penetrating-artery lesions involve primarily the cerebral peduncle and the paramedian zones. Figure 9.10 is an MRI that shows a cerebral peduncle infarct. Few examples have been reported in detail.[101,116–119] Some infarcts in this distribution are caused by occlusion of the parent posterior cerebral artery (PCA).[119,120] The distribution of the penetrating branches of the PCA is diagrammed in Figure 8.25. One clinical syndrome includes a third nerve palsy ipsilaterally, caused by involvement of the fascicles of the third nerve within the midbrain, accompanied by a contralateral hemiparesis (Weber's syndrome). In some patients, involvement of the red nucleus, as well as the cerebral peduncle on the same side, gives rise to a combination of motor weakness and tremor. The tremor usually develops as the hemiparesis improves and is present at rest and on intention. The affected arm is usually also quite incoordinated and ataxic. Some patients with focal lesions involving the decussation of the brachium conjunctivum in the midbrain present with bilateral limb ataxia and tremor. This syndrome is often referred to as the Wernekinck commissure syndrome and is quite rare.[121,122] Few cases of midbrain branch lesions with neuropathological confirmation have been reported.[119,120,123]

Thalamus

Thalamic lacunes are quite common. In the MRI study by Hommel and colleagues, thalamic lesions accounted for 14% of the lacunes.[84] Penetrating-artery territory infarcts are located paramedially in the distribution of the various thalamoperforating arteries and laterally in the distribution of the thalamogeniculate artery or the posterior choroidal arteries. The two most important and consistent paramedian thalamoperforating arteries are the polar (tuberothalamic) artery and the thalamic-subthalamic arteries.[101,123–132]

The polar artery arises on each side from the middle-third of the posterior communicating artery and supplies the anteromedial and anterolateral thalamic nuclei. Figure 9.11 is an

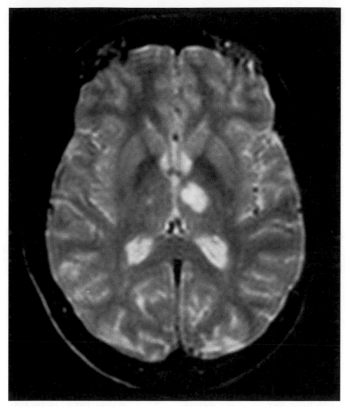

Figure 9.11 MRI T2-weighted image showing a left anterolateral polar artery territory infarct. From Bogousslavsky J, Caplan LR. Vertebrobasilar occlusive disease: Review of selected aspects. III. Thalamic infarcts. *Cerebrovasc Dis* 1993;3:193–205.

MRI that shows a polar artery territory thalamic infarct. At times, this vessel is absent, in which case its territory is supplied by the thalamic–subthalamic arteries. The predominant findings in infarcts fed by the thalamoperforating arteries are cognitive and behavioral, but the syndromes do differ, depending on the arterial territory involved.[85,101,125,127–129,131,132] Unilateral anterolateral–thalamic infarction in the distribution of the polar artery on the left or right side usually causes abulia, facial asymmetry, transient minor contralateral motor abnormalities and, at times, aphasia (left lesions) or visual neglect (right lesions). Abulia – with slowness, decreased amount of activity and speech, and long delays in responding to queries or conversation – is the predominant abnormality. Some patients are disorganized and dress in a slovenly manner. Usually, in patients with unilateral lesions, abulia and cognitive and behavioral abnormalities improve after 3–6 months. Occasionally, bilateral infarcts are found in the territory of the polar artery of each side.[133] This means that bilateral arteries probably occasionally arise from a single or loop artery, or a common rete. When the polar artery is affected bilaterally, the behavioral abnormality is more severe and persistent. Memory may also be affected.[133] The behavioral effects are probably explained by the synaptic corticothalamic relationship with the frontal lobe and other cortical regions.

The thalamic–subthalamic arteries originate from the proximal PCAs and supply the most posteromedial portion of the thalamus near the posterior commissure. The right and left-sided arteries may arise separately, but can originate from a single unilateral artery or a common pedicle.[101,123,124,130] Unilateral lesions are usually characterized by paresis of vertical gaze (upward or both upward and downward) and by amnesia. Motor and sensory signs and symptoms are absent. The pathway for vertical gaze includes the rostral interstitial nucleus of the medial longitudinal fasciculi and connections between the two eyes for vertical eye movements that travel through the commissure at the diencephalic-mesencephalic junction. A unilateral lesion interrupts these commissural fibers, thus causing conjugate vertical-gaze palsy.[134,135] Memory loss may be severe, with profound difficulty in forming new memories and encoding recent events. The amnesia often improves within 6 months in unilateral-infarct patients. Bilateral butterfly-shaped paramedian posterior thalamic infarction can result from a branch occlusion of a single supplying artery or pedicle, although scant necropsy data are available from well-studied cases.[101,123,124,130,136] Hypersomnolence and bilateral IIIrd-nerve palsies can occur in patients with bilateral infarcts.[136] The same syndrome can result from occlusion of the rostral basilar artery most often caused by brain embolism, a topic discussed in Chapters 8 and 10.

Lacunes and branch-territory infarcts are especially common in the lateral thalamus. This region which includes the somatosensory nuclei (ventral posterior lateral and ventral posterior medial) and the ventral lateral and ventral anterior nuclei, is supplied by the thalamogeniculate group of arteries. These vessels arise from the PCA and are the posterior circulation counterpart of the lenticulostriate branches of the MCA. Occlusion of these arteries or their branches leads to a variety of different clinical syndromes.[101,137]

Larger lateral thalamic infarcts were first described by Dejerine and Roussy, and the clinical findings have long been referred to as *le syndrome thalamique*.[138] The essential features of this syndrome, almost always caused by atheromatous-branch disease in our experience, are contralateral hemisensory symptoms accompanied by contralateral limb ataxia. At times, there are jumpy adventitious hemichoreic movements of the contralateral arm, and the hand may tend to assume a fisted posture. Some patients have a transient hemiparesis at onset that improves quickly.[137]

Usually, the sensory phenomena are mostly paresthesias, which involve the face, neck, trunk, and limbs. Sensory loss is usually slight. The sensory signs relate to ischemia of the somatosensory nuclei. The ataxia is caused by interruption of cerebellofugal fibers going to the ventral anterior and ventral lateral nuclei. Also interrupted are fibers from the striatum (the ansa lenticularis) that project toward these motor nuclei. Dystonia, chorea, and hemiparkinsonian-like features are probably caused by interruption of these extrapyramidal-system projections. Pain in the affected limbs and trunk may develop months after the original stroke and was one of the cardinal features mentioned by Dejerine and Roussy.[138] Many patients never have pain. Pain is almost never noted at or shortly after onset. Figure 9.12 contains MRIs that show lateral thalamic infarcts.

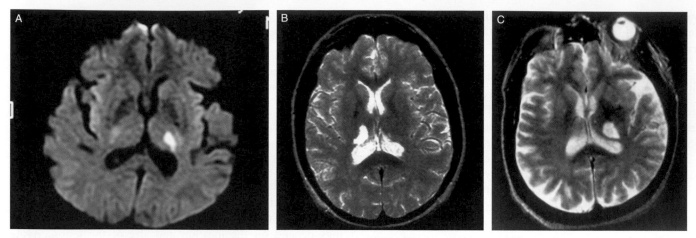

Figure 9.12 A montage of lateral thalamic infarcts. (A) MRI diffusion-weighted image (DWI) showing an acute left lateral thalamic infarct. (B) and (C) T2-weighted MRIs that show lateral thalamic infarcts.

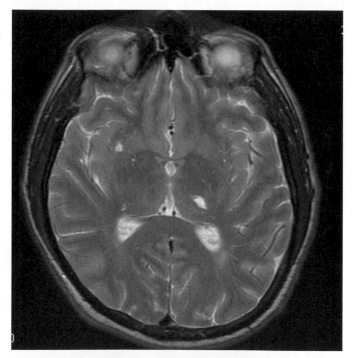

Figure 9.13 T2-weighted MRI showing a small lateral thalamic infarct in a patient with pure sensory stroke.

Occlusion of branches of the thalamogeniculate arteries supplying the somatosensory nuclei is responsible for the vast majority of patients with so-called pure sensory stroke.[139–142] The infarcts are usually smaller than those found in patients with the broader lateral thalamic syndrome. Figure 9.13 is an MRI that shows a small lateral thalamic infarct in a patient with pure sensory stroke. In this condition, the patient has somatosensory complaints without other signs or symptoms. Most often, the patient describes numbness, tingling, or pins-and-needles sensations in the face, limbs, and trunk. All hemicorporeal sensations are represented in the thalamic somatosensory-relay nuclei. In the somatosensory cortex, the hand and face have large representations, whereas little space is accorded to the trunk, scalp, and other regions not capable of fine sensory distinctions. Numbness of the inner mouth, eye,

ear, scalp, chest, back, abdomen, and genitalia is much more common in thalamic lacunes than in superficial lesions of the parietal cortex.[140,141]

After a few days, the somatic sensations may take on an unpleasant quality and may be characterized as burning, tightness, or soreness.[139,140] Sensory symptoms may be persistent or transient, even when lacunar infarction is present on MRI. Usually, subjective sensory complaints are more prominent than objective loss of sensation. Many patients with pure sensory stroke have no detectable loss of threshold to any sensory modality, whereas others show only a minimal qualitative or quantitative difference between the two sides of the body. Motor, visual, and intellectual functions are normal. Occasionally, pure sensory stroke can be caused by lateral or medial tegmental pontine or midbrain infarcts.[101,102,114,117,118,143]

Occlusion of thalamogeniculate branches, on occasion, can cause a syndrome referred to as sensory motor stroke.[144] This condition is characterized by the sensory symptoms and signs described in relation to pure sensory stroke, accompanied by paresis and pyramidal signs in the same limbs as the sensory symptoms. Few such cases have been studied at necropsy. In one well-studied case, the responsible infarct involved the somatosensory nuclei. Pallor of the adjacent posterior limb of the internal capsule was evident.[144] Review of the drawings from the original Dejerine-Roussy article clearly shows that lateral thalamic infarcts often affect the adjacent internal capsule.[101,137,138] The thalamogeniculate arteries must sometimes supply this zone, contrary to the teachings in some neuroanatomy texts. Ischemia of the internal capsule is probably responsible for the transient paresis found in some patients with lateral thalamic infarcts and for the motor abnormalities in patients with sensory motor stroke.

Infarcts in the territory of the medial and lateral posterior choroidal arteries are the least well known and most rarely reported of all thalamic infarcts. The lateral posterior choroidal arteries supply mostly the pulvinar, a portion of the lateral geniculate body, and then loop around the superior portion of the thalamus to supply the anterior nucleus. The medial arteries supply the habenula, anterior pulvinar part of the center median nucleus, and the paramedial

nuclei.[101] There have been few clinicopathological and neuroimaging reports of patients with posterior choroidal territory infarcts.[101,125,132,145–148]

Hemianopia, hemisensory symptoms, and behavioral abnormalities may occur in patients with posterior choroidal artery territory infarcts. The most specific and well-defined abnormality relates to the visual fields. The posterior choroidal arteries and their lateral choroidal artery branches supply a portion of the lateral geniculate body reciprocal to that supplied by the AChAs. The characteristic visual field defect in patients with posterior choroidal artery territory infarcts is a sectoranopia, involving a wedge-shaped defect on each side of the horizontal meridian.[146–148] In contrast, the visual field defect in patients with AChA-territory infarcts can include loss of the upper and lower quadrants, with sparing of vision in a line along the median horizontal meridian. Patients with posterior choroidal territory infarcts can also have an upper or lower quadrantanopia.[132,148] Hemisensory symptoms, usually in the form of hemianesthesia and slight hemiparesis also occur due to lesions involving or adjacent to the ventral posterior nuclei. Amnesia and transient aphasia have also been described in patients with infarcts that involve the posterior choroidal artery territory.[132,148]

Cognitive impairment

Lacunar infarcts have an overall better prognosis compared to other types of stroke, essentially because of the smaller size of the lesion and the lower severity of the symptoms. Lacunar strokes were initially described as having no acute mortality, an excellent functional outcome and a good overall long-term prognosis. It was thought that lacunar strokes might be less likely to affect cognition and behavior than more severe, larger cortical strokes. Reaffirming this view, the classic lacunar syndromes' descriptions did not include cognitive impairment as a feature. Studies now show that the development of cognitive impairment and dementia is a matter of concern in patients with cerebral small vessel infarcts. By 1992, Loeb et al. had reported that patients with lacunar infarcts developed dementia 4–12 times more frequently than the normal population.[149] The Secondary Prevention of Small Subcortical Strokes (SPS 3) trial showed that nearly half of the stroke patients recruited presented with mild cognitive impairment between 2 weeks and 6 months after the qualifying lacunar stroke.[150] In a meta-analysis that included more than 2800 patients, the prevalence of dementia after lacunar stroke was 20% and the incidence of mild cognitive impairment or dementia was 37%.[151] There is an overall estimated 11%–23% risk of developing dementia following a lacunar stroke, and this risk increases with recurrent lacunar events and the presence of concurrent white matter disease.[151–154]

Imaging and other investigations in patients suspected of having lacunar strokes

Having described the known lacunar syndromes and their usual responsible lesions, we return to patient RB, who had hypertension and the clinical findings of pure-motor hemiparesis.

> In RB, a complete blood cell count was normal. EEG showed minor symmetric slowing. CT showed a small infarct in the posterior limb of the internal capsule on the left and a tiny lesion in the right putamen. MRI also showed these lesions and another tiny lacune in the right thalamus. Magnetic resonance diffusion-weighted images (DWI) showed a bright lesion in the posterior limb of the internal capsule. MRA and ultrasound of the carotid and vertebral arteries were normal.

Because lacunes are small and deep in the hemisphere or are located in the brainstem, they usually do not have a major influence on the EEG recorded from the convexity.[68] CT findings depend on the location and size of the lesion. Acute pontine lacunes are seldom imaged well by CT, but can nearly always be seen on MRI scans. Pure-motor hemiplegia probably has the highest frequency of CT positivity among the lacunar syndromes. Rascol et al. found hypodense lesions on CT in 29 of 30 patients with pure-motor stroke.[71] They divided the lesions into large capsulo-putamino-caudate infarcts, and smaller capsulo-pallido or capsulo-caudate infarcts.[71] Some patients with larger infarcts had angiographic abnormalities in the lenticulostriate arteries. Others have reported MCA occlusive disease in patients with large basal ganglionic and capsular infarctions.[155–158] In contrast, patients with pure sensory stroke seldom have lesions visible on CT.[141]

MRI is undoubtedly superior to CT in imaging small brainstem and thalamic infarcts.[84,85,101,103,159] Rothrock and colleagues evaluated 31 patients with the clinical diagnosis of lacunar infarction. Twenty-three patients (74%) had appropriate lesions on MRI.[103] When CT and MRI were performed, MRI was superior in imaging lesions appropriate to the symptoms. In another study among 110 patients, MRI was effective in imaging one or more possibly responsible lacunar infarcts in 89 patients.[84] When gadolinium-diethylene-triamine penta-acetic acid enhancement is given, acute lacunar infarcts are usually enhanced.[159] Use of enhancement may be helpful when the clinicians find more than one lesion and are uncertain of the age of the lesions. Usually, only acute lesions are enhanced. Increasingly, the use of gadolinium enhancement is being replaced by the routine use of MRI-DWI sequences.

The overall superiority of MRI over CT for the detection of deep brain infarcts is particularly true for acute lesions. MRI DWI is especially useful in showing lacunar infarcts soon after symptoms begin, and in separating recent infarcts from old infarcts. Lacunar lesions appear hyperintense on DWI within hours of stroke onset. T2-weighted imaging or fluid-attenuated inversion recovery (FLAIR) sequences may then occur within hours or even days. The appearance of chronic deep brain infarcts is that of hypo-intensity on T1 and FLAIR sequences, often with a hyper-intense rim around them on the latter sequence.[160] Förster et al. also showed that multimodal MRI including DWI and perfusion-weighted imaging (PWI) was useful in demonstrating a mismatch associated with acute lacunar infarction and, therefore, may be useful to support acute treatment decisions for this type of stroke.[161]

Table 9.1 Findings in patient with suspected lacunar infarction (right limbs involved)

	Diagnosis highly probable	Diagnosis likely but uncertain	Lacune unlikely or excluded
Risk factors	Hypertension	Diabetic, slight hypertension	No hypertension
Neurological signs	Paralysis of right face, arm, leg	Sparing or unequal involvement of face, arm, leg	Paralysis of right hand
Other symptoms	None	Slight unaccustomed headache	Severe headache, seizure at onset
Laboratory	Compatible small deep infarct on CT or MRI	Normal CT or MRI	Hypodensity left frontal on CT or MRI; hemorrhage on CT or MRI

Although an upper limit of size of lacunes has traditionally been considered to be 15 mm, a study of 890 Korean stroke patients found that the size of the lesions alone on MRI was not indicative of a lacunar or non-lacunar etiology.[162] There is no complete consensus on the size of lacunar infarcts. A lower limit of 0.3 or 0.5 cm is widely used to differentiate lacunar infarcts from smaller perivascular spaces. An upper limit of 1.5 or 2.0 cm is used to differentiate them from other pathologies, particularly striatocapsular and embolic subcortical infarcts.[160]

CT or MRI is essential for excluding small hemorrhages from the differential diagnosis; such hemorrhages can cause findings identical to lacunar syndromes. Rajajee and colleagues compared acute CT scans and a modern multimodal MRI protocol in the diagnosis of lacunar infarction in patients presenting within 6 hours of symptom onset.[163] Among 15 patients in this series who were diagnosed as acute lacunar infarct disease using clinical and CT criteria, MRI detected a different diagnosis in 5.[163] However, large-artery occlusions were not found by MRA in any of the 15 patients implying that CT and clinical criteria are not specific for penetrating artery disease but may effectively in most instances exclude large-artery occlusion. By imaging hemosiderin, MRI is more effective than CT in determining whether old lesions were small hematomas or lacunar infarcts.

Angiographic abnormalities have been shown in some patients with lacunar infarcts, and include carotid artery and MCA disease.[158] Some large-artery lesions are incidental and unrelated to the cause of the stroke. Necropsy studies have shown that most patients with hypertension and lacunes have a high incidence of coexisting atherosclerosis. Angiography in apparently healthy prisoners also shows a high frequency of atherosclerosis.[164] Atherosclerotic plaques and stenosis in both extracranial and intracranial arteries are also found in patients with lacunar infarcts.[165] The finding of atherosclerotic occlusive disease in large extracranial and intracranial arteries does not prove an etiological relationship to the lacunar infarct. In some cases, blockage of parent arteries can produce infarction in territories of lenticulostriate, thalamogeniculate, and pontine penetrating arteries. Figure 9.4 diagrammatically depicts the vascular lesions in occlusion of penetrating and parent arteries. The lesion in the parent artery can be a plaque, in-situ thrombosis, or an embolus.[43] Parent-artery lesions are especially important to consider in

patients with lacunes exceeding 20 mm that involve the basal ganglia and capsule. In LRC's experience, the clinical syndrome usually includes more features than the usual lacunar syndrome.[43,157] Echocardiography and cardiac rhythm monitoring are also important to exclude cardiac-origin embolism to parent arteries in some patients. Larger deep infarcts are less often caused by lipohyalinosis.

Neuroimaging, preferably with MRI, is important in every patient. The need for thorough laboratory testing depends on the: (1) presence of appropriate risk factors, such as hypertension, polycythemia, or diabetes; (2) typicality of the neurological findings; (3) thoroughness of the neurological examination and the experience of the examining physician[166]; and (4) neuroimaging results. If the patient has no evidence of past or present hypertension, physicians should be skeptical of lipohyalinosis as the cause of infarction. Atypical neurological findings or the presence of unaccustomed headache, reduced alertness, or seizures argue for more complete laboratory investigations. At times, unexpected superficial infarcts, small hemorrhages, and even non-vascular conditions, such as tumors, are discovered by CT or MRI.

When the clinical diagnosis is uncertain, extracranial and transcranial ultrasound, computed tomography angiography, magnetic resonance angiography, or standard angiography may be indicated. Usually, after preliminary evaluation, which should include a detailed history and examination, blood studies, EEG, and either CT or MRI, physicians are able to place the patient with brain ischemia into one of three categories: (1) high certainty of lacune; (2) lesion consistent with a lacune but not diagnostic (atypical lacune); or (3) findings not compatible with a lacunar etiology. Examples of possible findings in these three groups are listed in Table 9.1. Patients in categories two and three require more evaluation than those in category one.

Treatment

RB was kept on bed rest. Weakness began to improve during the second week, when he was transferred to a rehabilitation hospital. He was discharged on atorvastatin 40 mg/day and a combination of 25 mg of aspirin and 200 mg of modified-release dipyridamole, taken twice a day. While he was in rehabilitation hospitalization, he was referred to an internist who carefully followed him and instituted antihypertensive treatment.

No treatment has been definitively shown to modify the acute course of lacunar infarction. The morphological nature of lipohyalinosis and fibrinoid degeneration, both of which involve lesions of the vessel wall and not the arterial intima, make it theoretically unlikely that thrombolytic agents or anticoagulants, would be effective treatments. Intracerebral hemorrhage (ICH) remains the most devastating and unpredictable complication related to thrombolysis, and it was suggested that the presence of a lacunar infarct might represent an increased risk of secondary ICH after thrombolysis. While there are no trials of thrombolysis in patients with lacunar stroke alone, there is a mounting body of evidence from large studies in which lacunar strokes have formed a significant proportion. The early report of the National Institute of Neurological Disorders and Stroke rt-PA Study (NINDS) thrombolytic trial claimed that all stroke subgroups including lacunar infarcts responded favorably to tPA,[167] but their data in relation to lacunar infarction are clearly not credible. In that trial, history and examinations were hurried and not thorough, there was no vascular imaging, only CT was used and it did not show acute infarcts well, and no follow-up imaging was mandated or reported. Furthermore, the numbers of patients in the placebo and treatment groups were very dissimilar. A committee appointed to review the data and conclusions of the NINDS study affirmed that the conclusions about stroke subgroups were not supported by the data.[168]

Some investigators have shown a non-significant trend for worse outcome at 3 months for lacunar stroke treated with thrombolysis compared to placebo within large clinical trials including other forms of ischemic stroke.[169,170] Others have shown a better outcome at 3 months for thrombolysed lacunar stroke patients.[171-173] Griebe et al. specifically compared acute lacunar stroke patients treated with recombinant tissue plasminogen activator (rt-PA) with patients who obtained standard medical care. They showed that the clinical course was more favorable in patients treated with rt-PA while functional deficit after 3 months was similar in both groups. The overall complication rates did not differ significantly between the two groups, but while they did not detect symptomatic intracranial hemorrhage, hemorrhagic transformation was more frequent in thrombolysed lacunar stroke patients.[174] Fluri et al. previously showed similar results in terms of outcome without an excess in ICH rate.[175] Although the issue is not settled, there is some evidence that intravenous thrombolysis may be beneficial in patients with lacunar infarcts and there seems to be no excess harm from its use.

Anecdotal reports indicate that heparin anticoagulation is not effective during acute lacunar stroke.[176] LRC's experience confirms that patients continue to progress while receiving heparin. The disease is far beyond the reach of the surgeon's knife.

Infarction is most likely related to impaired blood flow beyond the region of penetrating artery obstruction. Logical treatment is maximization of blood pressure, blood volume, and blood flow. Because the lesion is caused by hypertension, the most logical therapy to prevent new lipohyalinotic disease is to carefully control the blood pressure. Overzealous reduction of blood pressure during the acute ischemia, however, can decrease flow in collateral arteries and expand the region of infarction.[41,42] We prefer to wait until after the first several weeks after the stroke to institute major reductions in blood pressure.

Blood pressure management is extremely important in preventing recurrent lacunar infarcts. The investigators of the SPS 3 trial studied 3020 patients who had had a lacunar stroke within the previous 180 days and randomly assigned them to 2 different systolic blood pressure targets: 130–149 mmHg (higher group) or below 130 mmHg (lower group). The antihypertensive medication was chosen by the individual local study physicians.[177] Although the rate reductions for all stroke, and the composite outcome of myocardial infarction or vascular death was not significant with the lower systolic blood target, the rate of intracerebral hemorrhage was significantly reduced and the treatment-related serious adverse events were infrequent.[177]

Twenty-four-hour blood pressure monitoring shows that excessively high blood pressures at night with failure to show the normal nocturnal blood pressure dipping is predictive of further development of lacunes and white matter abnormalities.[178] Excessive drops in nocturnal blood pressure are also problematic. Preliminary studies suggests that perindopril and other angiotensin-converting enzyme (ACE) inhibitors may have salutary effects on vasomotor function and be preferred over other classes of antihypertensives.[179] We try to maximize blood flow during the first days and keep the patient at rest with the head flat to augment cranial flow. If the vascular etiology of the lesion is parent-vessel disease and not lipohyalinosis, then treatment of that condition is appropriate.

Some findings support the use of antiplatelet agents, especially dipyridamole and cilostazole, and statins as prophylactic agents aimed at preventing further lacunar infarction and white matter disease. In many trials, patients with lacunar infarction are overrepresented. Other causes of ischemic strokes such as cardiac embolism and carotid artery disease are usually excluded, and many patients with severe intracranial disease, such as basilar artery occlusion, are treated with anticoagulants. In the WARRS trial, lacunes made up about 40% of the patients.[180] In the European Stroke Prevention Studies 2 (ESPS 2) trial, a combination of aspirin and modified-release dipyridamole was more effective than aspirin or dipyridamole alone.[181] Lacunes were considered the most prevalent stroke type in that trial. In a Japanese trial of patients with predominantly lacunar ischemic stroke, cilostazol, a putative antiplatelet aggregant, proved quite effective.[182] Cilostazole and dipyridamole have potent vasodilator effects, and this capability might make them especially useful in patients with penetrating artery disease. A Japanese study confirmed the utility of cilostazole in patients with lacunar infarcts.[182] Aspirin has been accepted as standard antiplatelet therapy in patients with lacunar infarcts.[183] In the Prevention Regimen For Effectively avoiding Second Strokes (PRoFESS), in which more than 50% of the patients had had a small vessel infarction as the index event, there was no difference between

clopidogrel and aspirin plus extended-release dipyridamole with regard to effectiveness in prevention of recurrent strokes.[184] In SPS 3, patients with lacunar strokes were randomized in a double-blind fashion to receive either aspirin 325 mg/day or a combination of aspirin 325 mg/day and clopidogrel 75 mg/day.[185] In this study the addition of clopidogrel to aspirin did not significantly reduce the risk of recurrent stroke but significantly increased the risk of bleeding and death.[185]

In addition to their lipid-lowering capability, statins also have vasodilator effects and can augment blood flow in patients with penetrating artery disease.[186,187] The Stroke Prevention Aggressive Reduction of Cholesterol Levels (SPARCL) study showed in a subset analysis that patients with small vessel disease and increased low-density lipoprotein cholesterol have a similar risk of stroke recurrence as do patients with large vessel strokes, and that treatment with atorvastatin 80 mg daily is equally effective in reducing this risk, implying that patients with small vessel disease also benefit from statin therapy.[188] The initial SPARCL results suggested that there was an increased risk of hemorrhagic stroke in patients with lacunar stroke treated with statins.[189] The validity of this result is questionable because of the high risk of false positive findings in isolated subgroups such as these. We believe that the benefits of statins far outweigh any potential risks in the lacunar stroke subgroup.

Other than tissue plasminogen activator (tPA), there are scant data about other treatments soon after lacunar stroke onset. A trial of intravenous magnesium in patients with acute ischemic strokes (Intravenous Magnesium Efficacy in Stroke (IMAGES)) suggested that magnesium seemed to be of benefit in patients with a lacunar stroke etiology.[190] Magnesium is known to have vasoactive as well as neuroprotective properties and these may relate to the salutary effect in this population.[191]

Chronic penetrating artery disease

Historical background

The disorders that lead to single lacunar infarcts often involve multiple penetrating arteries. As a result, multiple lacunar infarcts are often found in the brain at necropsy or are visible on MRI scans. In the necropsy study of Tuszynski and colleagues, 169 patients had 327 lacunes, an average of 1.9 lacunes per patient.[64] Less than half of the patients (46%) had only one lacune, 16% had two, and 38% had three or more lacunes. Early investigators found an even higher frequency of multiple lesions,[1–7] but more widespread control of hypertension has likely altered this tendency. Most often, lacunes involve the striatum, capsule, thalamus, cerebral white matter, and pons. When extensive, they give the deeper portions of the brain a Swiss cheese-like appearance. This condition was often referred to as *état lacunaire* after Pierre Marie.[7] Traditionally, the clinical findings have been described as including: (1) pseudobulbar abnormalities of speech, swallowing, and emotional control; (2) small-stepped gait; (3) parkinsonian-like rigidity; (4) hyperreflexia; (5) extensor plantar reflexes; (6) dementia with slow thinking and responses; and (7) variable

weakness and sensory signs and symptoms. More recent experience, especially from CT and MRI, raises questions about this traditional view. First, many patients with multiple lacunes seem quite well preserved and function normally. Secondly, patients with the syndrome described almost always have associated, rather severe changes in the cerebral white matter and ventricular enlargement. Most clinicians and investigators are inclined to ascribe the dementia and clinical signs more to the white matter disease (dubbed leuko-araiosis by Hachinski[192]) than to the lacunes. The combination of lacunes, white matter gliosis, and atrophy almost invariably occur together and are associated with widespread abnormalities of penetrating small arteries.[193,194] The combination should be considered a chronic brain microvasculopathy also known in the literature as cerebral small vessel disease.

Pathology

The chronic white matter abnormalities were initially described by Binswanger.[194–196] Olszewski, in a review of the history and pathology of the condition, used the term *subcortical arteriosclerotic encephalopathy*.[194,197,198] Babikian and Ropper reviewed the pathological features in more than 40 cases described in the literature,[199] and other reviews discuss the usual pathological findings.[194,198,200,201] Grossly visible in the cerebral white matter are confluent areas of soft, puckered, and granular tissue. These areas are patchy and emphasize the occipital lobes and periventricular white matter, especially anteriorly and close to the surface of the ventricles.[194,197–201] The cerebellar white matter is also often involved. The ventricles are enlarged, and, at times, the corpus callosum is small. The volume of white matter is reduced, but the cortex is generally spared. The ventricles are enlarged as a result of atrophy of the white matter. The white matter abnormalities surrounding the ventricles may reduce the strength of the supporting tissue and allow mechanically more ventricular distension.

The white matter abnormalities are nearly always accompanied by some lacunes. These were present in one series in 39 of 42 necropsy cases of Binswanger's disease.[199] Microscopic study shows myelin pallor. Usually, the myelin pallor is not homogeneous, but islands of decreased myelination are surrounded by normal tissue. At times, the white matter abnormalities are so severe that necrosis and cavitation occur. Gliosis is prominent in zones of myelin pallor.

The walls of penetrating arteries are thickened and hyalinized. Occlusion of the small arteries is rare.[156] Some patients have a pathologically different disorder characterized by dilated perivascular spaces, the condition called *état criblé* by Pierre Marie.[7] Multiple dilated perivascular spaces can be accompanied by white matter changes and be accompanied by cognitive and behavioral abnormalities and basal ganglionic clinical dysfunction resembling Parkinson's disease.[202,203]

Occasional patients with Binswanger white matter changes have had amyloid angiopathy as the underlying vascular pathology.[204–207] In these patients, arteries within the cerebral cortex and leptomeninges are thickened and contain a congophilic substance that stains for amyloid. Arteries within the

white matter and basal ganglia are also concentrically thickened but characteristically do not contain amyloid. In a few reported patients, a granulomatous arteritis complicates amyloid angiopathy.[208–210]

Similar microangiopathic abnormalities in the cerebral white matter and lacunar infarcts can also be found in CADASIL.[21,22,211–213] The white matter abnormalities are often evident early. Relatives of patients with clinical CADASIL can show white matter abnormalities before symptoms develop. Usually localized, often nodular focal white matter lesions are found early in the course of illness. Later the white matter abnormalities become more diffuse, especially in the occipital and frontal periventricular white matter. White matter lesions in the external capsule and anterior temporal lobes are particularly characteristic of CADASIL.[214]

Clinical findings

The clinical picture in patients with microangiopathies is quite variable. Most often, patients become slow and abulic. Memory loss, aphasic abnormalities, and visuospatial dysfunction are also found. Executive functions such as planning and performing sequential tasks are affected. Pseudobulbar palsy, pyramidal signs, extensor plantar reflexes, and gait abnormalities are also common. The clinical findings often progress gradually or stepwise, with worsening during periods of days to weeks. Often, there are long plateau periods of stability of the findings.[194,198,199] Most patients also have acute lacunar strokes.

Small vessel disease is a major contributor to the growing burden of cognitive impairment, and gait abnormalities in older individuals; lacunar infarcts and white matter lesions form an important substrate for this. In a review of 16 studies, Pantoni et al. confirmed the positive association between cognitive decline and white matters lesions.[215] Neuroimaging analyses estimated that the presence of small vessel disease conveyed a more than two-times increased risk of dementia at the age of 75 years.[216] In a meta-analysis, Debette and Markus pooled the results from 22 longitudinal studies and reported an increased risk of stroke, dementia, and death associated with white matter abnormalities.[217] The Leuko-Araiosis and Disability Study (LADIS) followed a cohort of 695 patients for 3 years and showed that white matter abnormalities and lacunar infarcts were independently associated with general cognitive function. Increasing severity of white matter abnormalities and the number of lacunes were each related to poorer cognitive performance.[218] When considered together, white matter abnormalities remained significantly associated with cognitive function, whereas the association with lacunes was less prominent.[218] There is a strong association between the severity of age-related white matter changes and the severity of gait and motor compromise.[219] The LADIS investigators showed that severe white matter abnormalities more than doubled the risk of patients transitioning from an independent to a dependent status after 3 years of follow-up.[220]

Patients with cerebral amyloid angiopathy most often present with recurrent brain hemorrhages, predominantly in the cerebral white matter. Some patients present with TIAs and others show a progressive stepwise syndrome indistinguishable from the clinical picture in Binswanger disease related to hypertension.[221] Some patients with cerebral amyloid angiopathy have an accompanying granulomatous angiitis and present with progressive neurological signs.[209,210,222,223] The diagnosis is difficult to make without a brain biopsy. LRC wonders if the breakdown of blood vessels containing amyloid results in amyloid being introduced into the cerebrospinal fluid and this induces an inflammatory response. Arteries containing amyloid often show cracks and disruptions in their walls. Occasional patients with cerebral amyloid associated angiitis have responded to corticosteroid treatment.[224,225]

CADASIL has a rather early age of onset – the average is approximately 40 years of age.[211] Acute strokes and progressive cognitive, behavioral, and motor signs predominate. Depression and headache, often meeting criteria for migraine, are also frequently present in patients with CADASIL and their relatives.[211,212] Tournier-Lasserve and colleagues have shown linkage of the CADASIL disease gene to the D19S226 locus on chromosome 19q12.[213] The clinical findings vary considerably in severity. Some patients are devastated rather early in their middle years, while others have relatively slight neurological findings.

Imaging

CT often shows periventricular hypodensity. On MRI, the findings are more obvious and dramatic, with zones of periventricular increased density on T2-weighted images and patchy white matter abnormalities.[194,199,214] Figure 9.14 is an MRI of a patient with Binswanger white matter abnormalities. LRC prefers not to use the term leuko-araiosis for these white matter changes. Leuko-araiosis is a general term and many patients with white matter abnormalities do not have vascular disease. Several different patterns of white matter abnormalities include: (1) caps that occur around the ventricular system, especially in the region of the anterior horns and the occipital region; (2) a rim of abnormal white matter signal often surrounds the ventricle diffusely or more focally; and (3) discrete, small foci or patchy or confluent regions of abnormal signal are also noted and vary from single to many lesions. Awad and colleagues attempted to correlate these various lesions with the neuropathology.[13] In general, diffuse periventricular rims represent gliosis that is probably caused by transependymal flow of cerebrospinal fluid.[13] Tiny foci often are caused by *état criblé*. Lesions in the centrum semiovale and corona radiata are generally regions of chronic partial ischemia.[13]

Lacunar infarcts and white matter disease are not the only neuroimaging manifestations of cerebral small vessel disease. In addition to these ischemic consequences, macro and microscopic hemorrhagic lesions (known as microbleeds) can also be identified. Although major hemorrhages are easily recognised by conventional neuroimaging, including CT, the detection of microbleeds requires the use of appropriate magnetic resonance sequences such as T2* gradient-echo sequences.[226] Cerebral microbleeds are defined as small deep or superficial

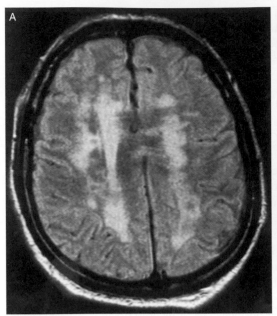
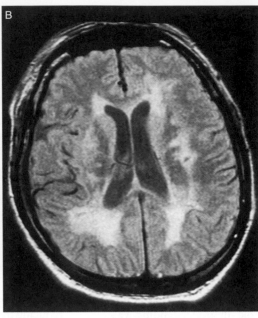

Figure 9.14 MRI T2-weighted images. Axial sections (A and B) show increased signal around the ventricles and large areas of abnormal signal in the white matter of the centrum semiovale in a patient with Binswanger's disease.

hemorrhages 2–10 mm in diameter; they represent small foci of chronic blood products such as a collection of hemosiderin around small perforating vessels in normal (or near normal) brain tissue.[227,228] Koennecke showed that these microbleeds are present in approximately 70% of patients with spontaneous ICH and 40% of those with ischemic cerebrovascular disease. Cerebral microangiopathy is associated with the highest prevalence (57%) of cerebral microbleeds among patients with ischemic stroke.[229] Microbleeds in hypertensive individuals tend to involve deep structures (the same areas involved in hypertensive hemorrhages and lacunes) while individuals with cerebral amyoid angiopathy tend to have more lobar microbleeds. Infective endocarditis patients also often have microbleeds on MRI.[230]

Pathogenesis of lacunar infarcts and chronic white matter abnormalities

The mechanism of discrete infarcts in the territory of a single penetrating artery is quite straightforward. The compromised penetrator has a reduced luminal size and further obstruction of the lumen by plaque, microdissection, or thrombus diminishes blood flow in the brain region supplied by that penetrator. Hemorheological factors could also reduce flow in that penetrator sufficiently to cause an infarct.

The mechanism of white matter abnormalities larger than the territory of a single penetrator is more difficult to explain, and may have a number of different mechanisms. The two major types of posited mechanisms involve either ischemia or vascular permeability:

1. Ischemia related to tandem penetrating arterial lesions. This explanation posits severe flow-limiting luminal compromise involving a number of parallel penetrating arteries. Then, hemorheological changes that reduce cerebral blood flow could produce ischemia and white matter damage in an area supplied by the group of

compromised arteries. Cerebral blood flow reduction could be caused by: decreased blood pressure, diminished cardiac output, decreased blood volume, or increased whole-blood viscosity. Similarly, consider the circumstance of several penetrators that were previously occluded or nearly occluded, and a single penetrator had provided collateral circulation to the region supplied by the previously compromised penetrators. Then the penetrator that supplied collateral flow becomes occluded. The resulting infarct would be larger than the supply of any of the individual penetrators.

2. Increased vascular permeability. Leakage of fluid, transudation, could occur when the blood pressure within the penetrating arteries is very high. This condition when acute is called *hypertensive encephalopathy*. This condition is characterized by transudation of fluid from small arteries and arterioles causing brain edema as well as petechial and sometimes larger intracerebral hemorrhages. When chronic, the transudated fluid could cause gliosis and damage to the cerebral white matter and basal ganglia. Some have posited that white matter damage is due to a chronic or recurrent hypertensive encephalopathy. Some patients with chronic white matter abnormalities do not have important hypertension. The media and adventitia may, in these patients, become so abnormal that fluid leaks from the damaged arteries even when the blood pressure in the arteries is normal.

Some studies support each of these two posited mechanisms. Yamamoto and colleagues analyzed the results of 24-hour blood-pressure monitoring among Japanese patients with lacunar infarcts and subcortical white matter abnormalities.[231–233] Poor control of blood pressure with high-average ambulatory blood pressures and reduced nighttime dips in blood pressure indicating excessive night time blood pressure predicted progression of both lacunar infarcts and white matter lesions. Others have also shown the importance of too-high and

too-low blood pressures on progression of white matter lesions and lacunar infarcts.[234,235] Suboptimal treatment of hypertension can clearly contribute to worsening of white matter abnormalities.

Increased whole-blood viscosity and fibrinogen levels are present in many patients with chronic severe white matter abnormalities and Binswanger disease.[194,236,237] Increased blood viscosity and slow flow through the microvasculature could compound the vascular lesions, leading to hypoperfusion in the territories of deep penetrating arteries.

Increase in vascular permeability is another potential mechanism of white matter abnormalities. Hypertension, CADASIL, CARASIL, and cerebral amyloid angiopathy all cause pathology within the vascular media and adventitia often with deposition of fibrinoid, or amyloid or other substances within the arterial walls. The components of the vascular wall especially matrix metalloproteinases are important in determining the continence of the vessels to components of the blood that is traveling through the vessels. Matrix metalloproteins have an important role in understanding vascular permeability.[238–240] Matrix metalloproteinase-9 levels are significantly elevated in the white matter and cerebrospinal fluid of patients with Binswanger-type pathology.[238,239] Matrix metalloproteinases disrupt the blood–brain barrier by degrading tight junction proteins found within blood vessels.[240] These increased levels of metalloproteinases in thickened penetrating arteries could promote leakage of fluid from these blood vessels. Another potential mechanism of brain edema in patients with white matter lesions is degenerative changes in veins within the white matter. Brown and colleagues found arteriolar tortuosity and described gradual thickening of the walls of periventricular veins and venules with collagen among 186 brains studied at necropsy.[241] Some veins and venules were occluded and others had very narrow lumens. This chronic venous collagenosis was very extensive in some patients who had leuko-araiosis.[241] Decreased venous drainage can promote brain edema. Chronic edema in

perivascular areas could stimulate gliosis and inflammation, which in turn can increase white matter damage.[242] Support for this theory of pathogenesis is that in CADACIL, white matter abnormalities precede brain infarcts.

Treatment

The optimal treatment of the chronic microangiopathies is unknown. Clearly blood pressure control is very important. Twenty-four-hour ambulatory blood pressure monitoring is a very useful way to study blood pressure levels and variations. Nocturnal blood pressure may be very important. Diabetes mellitus and high levels of Hct have also been shown to be important risk factors in patients with more than one lacunar infarct.[243] Impressed by the preliminary data about hyperviscosity, LRC has begun to treat patients with lacunar infarcts and chronic microvascular white matter disease by attempting to reduce their Hcts (by increased fluid intake, blood donation and stopping smoking) and by reducing their fibrinogen levels by prescribing eicosapentaenoic-rich fish oil preparations and other strategies. LRC encourages liberal fluid intake.

This microvasculopathy must be differentiated from multiple infarcts caused by large-artery occlusive disease and from multiple cerebral emboli as causes of vascular dementia. In these two other conditions, most of the infarcts are cortical or cortical and subcortical, and the history usually includes acute strokes. In these latter causes of vascular dementia, extracranial and transcranial ultrasound, echocardiography, cardiac rhythm monitoring, hematological screening for coagulopathies, and vascular imaging studies usually show a cardiac-origin embolic source or multiple large-artery occlusive disease. Recently, a number of genetic studies have identified that there may be specific target genes implicated in the cerebral small disease pathway such as *NOTCH3*, *HTRA1* and *APOE ε4*, and exploration of the functions of these and other genes may provide some guidance in the future for treatment.[244]

References

1. Fisher CM: Lacunes, small deep cerebral infarcts. *Neurology* 1965;**15**:774–784.

2. Fisher CM: The arterial lesions underlying lacunes. *Acta Neuropathol* 1969;**12**:1–15.

3. Besson G, Hommel M: Historical aspects of lacunes and the "lacunar controversy". In Pullicino PM, Caplan LR, Hommel M (eds): *Cerebral Small Artery Disease*. New York: Raven Press, 1993, pp 1–10.

4. Hauw J-J: The history of lacunes. In Donnan G, Norrving B, Bamford J, Bogousslavsky J (eds): *Lacunar and Other Subcortical Infarcts*. Oxford: Oxford University Press, 1995, pp 3–15.

5. Durand-Fardel M: *Traite des ramollissements du cerveau*. Paris: Bailliere, 1843.

6. Ferrand J: *Essai Sur l'Hemiplegie des Vieillards: Les Lacunes de Desintegration Cerebrale [thesis]*. Paris: University of Paris, 1902.

7. Marie P: Des foyers lacunaires de desintegration et des differents autres etats cavitaires du cerveau. *Rev Med (Paris)* 1901;**21**:281.

8. Foix C, Levy M: Les ramollissements sylviens. *Rev Neurol* 1927;**43**:1–51.

9. Foix C, Hillemand P: Contribution a l'etude des ramollissements protuberantiels. *Rev Med* 1926;**43**:287–305.

10. Caplan LR: Charles Foix – the first modern stroke neurologist. *Stroke* 1990;**21**:348–356.

11. Kolominsky-Rabas PL, Weber M, Gefeller O, Neundoerfer B, Heuschmann PU: Epidemiology of ischemic stroke subtypes according to TOAST criteria: Incidence, recurrence, and long-term survival in ischemic stroke subtypes: a population-based study. *Stroke* 2001;**32**:2735–2740.

12. Sacco S, Marini C, Totaro R, Russo T, Cerone D, Carolei A: A population-based study of the incidence and prognosis of lacunar stroke. *Neurology* 2006;**66**:1335–1338.

13. Awad I, Johnson PC, Spetzler RF, Hodak JA: Incidental subcortical lesions identified on magnetic

resonance imaging in the elderly: II. Postmortem pathological correlations. *Stroke* 1986;**17**:1090–1097.

14. Fisher CM: Pure motor hemiplegia of vascular origin. *Arch Neurol* 1965;**13**:30–44.

15. Fisher CM: Pathological observations in hypertensive cerebral hemorrhage. *J Neuropathol Exp Neurol* 1971;**30**:536–550.

16. Fisher CM: Cerebral miliary aneurysms in hypertension. *Am J Pathol* 1972;**66**:313–324.

17. Cole F, Yates P: Intracerebral microaneurysms and small cerebrovascular lesions. *Brain* 1966;**90**:759–767.

18. Rosenblum WJ: Miliary aneurysms and "fibrinoid" degeneration of cerebral blood vessels. *Hum Pathol* 1977;**8**:133–139.

19. Charcot J, Bouchard C: Nouvelles recherches sur la pathogenie de l'hemorrhagie cérébrale. *Arch Phys Norm Pathol* 1868;**1**:110–127, 643–665.

20. Baudrimont M, Dubas F, Joutel A: Autosomal dominant leukoencephalopathy and subcortical ischemic strokes: A clinicopathological study. *Stroke* 1993;**24**:122–125.

21. Lammie GA, Rakshi J, Rossor MN, et al: Cerebral autosomal dominant arteriopathy with subcortical infarcts and leukoencephalopathy – confirmation by cerebral biopsy in two cases. *Clin Neuropathol* 1995;**14**:201–206.

22. Chabriat H, Bousser M-G: Cerebral autosomal dominant arteriopathy with subcortical infarcts and leukoencephalopathy. In Donnan G, Norrving B, Bamford J, Bogousslavsky J (eds): *Subcortical Stroke*, 2nd ed. Oxford: Oxford University Press, 2002, pp 111–120.

23. Fukutake T: Cerebral autosomal recessive arteriopathy with subcortical infarcts and leukoencephalopathy (CARASIL): From discovery to gene identification. *J Stroke Cerebrovasc Dis* 2011;**20**:85–93.

24. Oide T, Nakayma H, Yanagama S, Ito N, Arima K: Extensive loss of arterial medial smooth muscle cells and mural extracellular matrix in cerebral autosomal recessive arteriopathy with subcortical infarcts and leukoencephalopathy (CARASIL). *Neuropathology* 2008;**28**:132–142.

25. Gould DB, Phalan FC, Breedveld GI, et al: Mutations in *COL4A1* cause perinatal cerebral hemorrhage and porencephaly. *Science* 2005;**308**:1167–1171.

26. van der Knaap MS, Smit LM, Barkhof F, et al: Neonatal porencephaly and adult stroke related to mutations in collagen IVA1. *Ann Neurol* 2006;**59**:504–511.

27. Gould DB, Phalan FC, van Mil SE, et al: Role of *COL4A1* in small-vessel disease and hemorrhagic stroke. *N Engl J Med* 2006;**354**:1489–1496.

28. Plaisir E, Gribouval O, Alamowitch S, et al: *COL4A1* mutations and hereditary angiopathy, nephropathy, aneurysms, and muscle cramps. *N Engl J Med* 2007;**357**:2687–2695.

29. Lanfranconi S, Markus HS: *COL4A1* mutations as a monogenic cause of cerebral small vessel disease a systematic review. *Stroke* 2010;**41**:e513–e518.

30. Labrune P, Lacroix C, Goutieres F, et al: Extensive brain calcifications, leukodystrophy, and formation of parenchymal cysts: A new progressive disorder due to diffuse cerebral microangiopathy. *Neurology* 1996;**46**:1297–1301.

31. Corboy JR, Gault J, Kleinschmidt-Demasters BK: An adult case of leukoencephalopathy with intracranial calcifications and cysts. *Neurology* 2006;**67**:1890–1892.

32. Duret H: Conclusion d'un memorie sur la circulation bulbaire. *Arch Phys Norm Pathol* 1873;**50**:88–89.

33. Duret H: Recherches anatomiques sur la circulation de l'encephale. *Arch Phys Norm Pathol* 1874;**1**:60–91, 316–353.

34. Foix C, Hillemand P: Irrigation de la protuberance. *Compt Rendu Soc Biol (Paris)* 1925;**42**:35–37.

35. Foix C, Hillemand P: Les artères de l'axe encephalique jusqu'a diencephale inclusivement. *Rev Neurol* 1925;**41**:705–739.

36. Foix C, Hillemand P: Irrigation du bulbe. *Compt Rendu Soc Biol (Paris)* 1924;**42**:33–35.

37. Stopford J: The arteries of the pons and medulla oblongata: I. *J Anat Physiol* 1915;**50**:131–164.

38. Stopford J: The arteries of the pons and medulla oblongata: II. *J Anat Physiol* 1916;**50**:255–280.

39. Pullicino PM: The course and territories of cerebral small arteries. In Pullicino PM, Caplan LR, Hommel M (eds): *Cerebral Small Artery Disease.* New York: Raven Press, 1993, pp 11–39.

40. Pullicino PM: Diagrams of perforating artery territories in axial, coronal, and sagittal planes. In Pullicino PM, Caplan LR, Hommel M (eds): *Cerebral Small Artery Disease.* New York: Raven Press, 1993, pp 41–72.

41. Fisher CM, Caplan LR: Basilar artery branch occlusion: A cause of pontine infarction. *Neurology* 1971;**21**:900–905.

42. Fisher CM: Bilateral occlusion of basilar artery branches. *J Neurol Neurosurg Psychiatry* 1977;**40**:1182–1189.

43. Caplan LR: Intracranial branch atheromatous disease: A neglected, understudied and underused concept. *Neurology* 1989;**39**:1246–1250.

44. Ostrow PT, Miller LL: Pathology of small artery disease. In Pullicino PM, Caplan LR, Hommel M (eds): *Cerebral Small Artery Disease.* New York: Raven Press, 1993, pp 93–123.

45. Klein IF, Lavallee PC, Touboul P-J, et al: In vivo middle cerebral artery plaque imaging by high-resolution MRI. *Neurology* 2006;**67**:327–329.

46. Lam WW, Wong KS, So NM, et al: Plaque volume measurement by magnetic resonance imaging as an index of remodeling of middle cerebral artery: Correlation with transcranial color Doppler and magnetic resonance angiography. *Cerebrovasc Dis* 2004;**17**:166–169.

47. Klein IF, Lavallee PC, Schouman-Claeys E, Amaraenco P: High-resolution MRI identifies basilar artery plaques in paramedian pontine infarct. *Neurology* 2005;**64**:551–552.

48. Kim JS, Yoon Y: Single subcortical infarction associated with parental arterial disease: important yet neglected sub-type of atherothrombotic stroke. *Int J Stroke* 2013;**8**:197–203.

49. Yoon Y, Lee DH, Kang DW, Kwon SU, Kim JS: Single subcortical infarction and atherosclerotic plaques in the middle cerebral artery: High-resolution magnetic resonance imaging findings. *Stroke* 2013;**44**:2462–2467.

50. Zhang C, Wang Y, Zhao X, on behalf of the Chinese Intracranial Atherosclerosis Study Group: Distal single subcortical infarction had a better clinical outcome compared with proximal single subcortical infarction. *Stroke* 2014;**45**:2613–2619.

51. Horowitz DR, Tuhrim S, Weinberger JM, Rudolph SH: Mechanisms in lacunar infarction. *Stroke* 1992;**23**:325–327.

52. Peress N, Kane W, Aronson S: Central nervous system findings in a tenth-decade autopsy population. *Prog Brain Res* 1973;**40**:473–484.

53. Bang OY, Heo JH, Kim JY, et al: Middle cerebral artery stenosis is a major clinical determinant in striatocapsular deep infarction. *Arch Neurol* 2002;**59**:259–263.

54. Wong KS, Gao S, Chan YL, et al: Mechanisms of acute cerebral infarctions in patients with middle cerebral artery stenosis: A diffusion-weighted imaging and microemboli monitoring study. *Ann Neurol* 2002;**52**:74–81.

55. Bang OY, Joo SY, Lee PH, et al: The course of patients with lacunar infarcts and a parent arterial lesion: Similarities to large artery vs. small artery disease. *Arch Neurol* 2004;**61**:514–519.

56. Baumgartner RW, Sidler C, Mosso M, Georgiadis D: Ischemic lacunar stroke in patients with and without potential mechanism other than small-artery disease. *Stroke* 2003;**34**:653–659.

57. Boiten J: *Lacunar Stroke: A Prospective Clinical and Radiologic Study [thesis].* Maastricht, 1991.

58. Yamamoto Y, Ohara T, Hamanaka M, Hosomi A, Tamura A, Akiguchi I: Characteristics of intracranial branch atheromatous disease and its association with progressive motor deficits. *J Neurol Sci* 2011;**304**:78–82.

59. Norrving B, Cronqvist S: Clinical and radiologic features of lacunar versus nonlacunar minor stroke. *Stroke* 1989;**20**:59–64.

60. Pullicino P, Nelson R, Kendall B, et al: Small deep infarcts diagnosed on computed tomography. *Neurology* 1980;**30**:1090–1096.

61. Weisberg L: Computed tomography and pure motor hemiparesis. *Neurology* 1979;**29**:490–495.

62. Donnan G, Tress B, Bladin P: A prospective study of lacunar infarction using computed tomography. *Neurology* 1982;**32**:47–56.

63. Mohr JP, Caplan LR, Melski J: The Harvard Cooperative Stroke Registry: A prospective registry. *Neurology* 1978;**28**:754–762.

64. Tuszynski MH, Petito CK, Levy DB: Risk factors and clinical manifestations of pathologically verified lacunar infarctions. *Stroke* 1989;**20**:990–999.

65. Labovitz DL, Boden-Albala B, Hauser WA, Sacco RL: Lacunar infarct or deep intracerebral hemorrhage. Who gets which? The Northern Manhattan Study. *Neurology* 2007;**68**:606–608.

66. Ikram MA, Vernooji MW, Hofman A, et al: Kidney function is related to cerebral small vessel disease. *Stroke* 2008;**39**:55–61.

67. Pico F, Labreuche J, Seilhean D, et al: Association of small-vessel disease with dilatative arteriopathy of the brain. Neuropathologic evidence. *Stroke* 2007;**38**:1197–1202.

68. Caplan LR, Young R: EEG findings in certain lacunar stroke syndromes. *Neurology* 1972;**22**:403.

69. Mohr JP: Lacunes. *Stroke* 1982;**13**:3–11.

70. Miller V: Lacunar stroke, a reassessment. *Arch Neurol* 1983;**40**:129–134.

71. Rascol A, Clanet M, Manelfe C, et al: Pure motor hemiplegia: CT study of 30 cases. *Stroke* 1982;**13**:11–17.

72. Donnan GA, O'Malley HM, Quang L, et al: The capsular warning syndrome and lacunar TIAs. In Donnan G, Norrving B, Bamford J, Bogousslavsky J (eds): *Subcortical Stroke*, 2nd ed. Oxford: Oxford University Press, 2002, pp 175–184.

73. Steinke W, Ley S: Lacunar stroke is the major cause of progressive motor deficits. *Stroke* 2002;**33**:1510–1516.

74. Caplan LR: Worsening in ischemic stroke patients: Is it time for a new strategy? *Stroke* 2002; **33**:1443–1445.

75. Donnan GA, Norrving B: Lacunes and lacunar syndromes. *Handb Clin Neurol* 2009;**93**:559–575.

76. Arboix A, Massons J, Garcia-Eroles L, Targa C, Comes E, Parra O: Clinical predictors of lacunar syndrome not due to lacunar infarction. *BMC Neurol* 2010;**10**:31.

77. Vermeer SE, Longstreth WT Jr, Koudstaal PJ: Silent brain infarcts: A systematic review. *Lancet Neurol* 2007;**6**:611–619.

78. Vermeer SE, Prins ND, denHeijer T, Hofman A, Koudstaal PJ, Breteler M: Silent brain infarcts and the risk of dementia and cognitive decline. *N Engl J Med* 2003;**348**:1215–1222.

79. Nelson R, Pullicino P, Kendall B, et al: Computed tomography in patients presenting with lacunar syndromes. *Stroke* 1980;**11**:256–261.

80. Richter R, Bruse J, Bruun B, et al: Frequency and course of pure motor hemiparesis: A clinical study. *Stroke* 1977;**8**:58–60.

81. Gobernado JM, de Molina AR, Gimeno A: Pure motor hemiplegia due to hemorrhage in the lower pons. *Arch Neurol* 1980;**37**:393.

82. Mori E, Tabuchi M, Yamadori A: Lacunar syndrome due to intracerebral hemorrhage. *Stroke* 1985;**16**:454–459.

83. Kase CS: Subcortical haemorrhages. In Donnan G, Norrving B, Bamford J, Bogousslavsky J (eds): *Subcortical Stroke*, 2nd ed. Oxford: Oxford University Press, 2002, pp 347–377.

84. Hommel M, Besson G, LeBas JF, et al: Prospective study of lacunar infarction using magnetic resonance imaging. *Stroke* 1990;**21**:546–554.

85. Besson G: *Les Infarctus Lacunaires: Evaluation Clinique et par l'Imagerie par Resonance Magnetique [thesis].* France: University of Grenoble, 1989.

86. Kase CS, Wolf PA, Hier DB, et al: Lacunar infarcts: Clinical and CT aspects. The Stroke Data Bank experience. *Neurology* 1986;**36**:178–179.

87. Fisher CM, Cole M: Homolateral ataxia and crural paresis, a vascular syndrome. *J Neurol Neurosurg Psychiatry* 1965;**28**:48–55.

88. Fisher CM: Ataxic hemiparesis. *Arch Neurol* 1978;**35**:126–128.

89. Helgason CM, Wilbur AC: Capsular hypesthetic ataxic hemiparesis. *Stroke* 1990;**21**:24–33.

90. Goldblatt D, Markesbury W, Reeves AG: Recurrent hemichorea following striatal lesions. *Arch Neurol* 1974;**32**:51–54.

91. Kase C, Maulsby G, DeJaun E: Hemichorea-hemiballism and lacunar infarction in the basal ganglia. *Neurology* 1981;**31**:452–455.

92. Helgason C, Wilbur A, Weiss A, et al: Acute pseudobulbar mutism due to discrete bilateral capsular infarction in the territory of the anterior choroidal artery. *Brain* 1988;**111**:507–524.

93. Caplan LR, Schmahmann JD, Kase CS, et al: Caudate infarcts. *Arch Neurol* 1990;**47**:133–143.

94. Caplan LR: Caudate infarcts. In Donnan G, Norrving B, Bamford J, Bogousslavsky J (eds): *Subcortical Stroke*, 2nd ed. Oxford: Oxford University Press, 2002, pp 209–223.

95. Fisher CM: Capsular infarcts. *Arch Neurol* 1979;**36**:65–73.

96. Helgason C, Caplan LR, Goodwin J, Hedges T: Anterior choroidal artery

territory infarction: Case reports and review. *Arch Neurol* 1986;**43**:681–686.

97. Mohr JP, Steinke W, Timsit SG, et al: The anterior choroidal artery does not supply the corona radiata and lateral ventricular wall. *Stroke* 1991;**22**:1502–1507.

98. Caplan LR: Anterior choroidal artery territory infarcts. In Donnan G, Norrving B, Bamford J, Bogousslavsky J (eds): *Subcortical Stroke*, 2nd ed. Oxford: Oxford University Press, 2002, pp 225–240.

99. Kumral E, Evyapan D, Balkir K: Acute caudate vascular lesions. *Stroke* 1999;**30**:100–108.

100. Mendez M, Adams N, Lewandowski K: Neurobehavioral changes associated with caudate lesions. *Neurology* 1989;**39**:349–354.

101. Caplan LR: *Vertebrobasilar Ischemia and Hemorrhage: Clinical Findings, Diagnosis and Management of Posterior Circulation Disease*. Cambridge, Cambridge University Press, 2015.

102. Bassetti C, Bogousslavsky J, Barth A, Regli F: Isolated infarcts of the pons. *Neurology* 1996;**46**:165–175.

103. Rothrock JF, Lyden PD, Hesselink JF, et al: Brain magnetic resonance imaging in the evaluation of lacunar stroke. *Stroke* 1987;**18**:781–786.

104. Leestra JE, Noronha A: Pure motor hemiplegia, medullary pyramid lesion, and olivary hypertrophy. *J Neurol Neurosurg Psychiatry* 1976;**39**:877–884.

105. Ropper AH, Fisher CM, Kleinman GM: Pyramidal infarction in the medulla: A cause of pure motor hemiplegia sparing the face. *Neurology* 1979;**29**:91–95.

106. Milandre L, Arnaud O, Khalil R: Infarction of the medullary pyramid identified on MRI. *Cerebrovasc Dis* 1992;**2**:183–184.

107. Ho KL, Meyer KR: The medial medullary syndrome. *Arch Neurol* 1981;**38**:385–387.

108. Kataoka S, Hori A, Shirakawa T, Hirose G: Paramedian pontine infarction, neurological/topographical correlation. *Stroke* 1997;**28**:809–815.

109. Kim JS, Lee JH, Im JH, Lee MC: Syndromes of pontine base infarction, a clinical–radiological correlation study. *Stroke* 1995;**26**:950–955.

110. Fisher CM: A lacunar stroke, the dysarthria-clumsy hand syndrome. *Neurology* 1967;**17**:614–617.

111. Chung C-S, Caplan LR: Pontine infarcts and hemorrhages. In Bogousslavsky J, Caplan LR (eds): *Stroke Syndromes*, 2nd ed. Cambridge: Cambridge University Press, 2001, pp 520–533.

112. Helgason CM, Wilbur AC: Basilar branch pontine infarctions with prominent sensory signs. *Stroke* 1991;**22**:1129–1136.

113. Caplan LR, Goodwin J: Lateral tegmental brainstem hemorrhages. *Neurology* 1982;**32**:252–260.

114. Shintani S, Tsuroka S, Shiigai T: Pure sensory stroke caused by a pontine infarct. Clinical, radiological, and physiological features in four patients. *Stroke* 1994;**25**:1512–1515.

115. Kim JS, Bae YH: Pure or predominant sensory stroke due to brainstem lesion. *Stroke* 1997;**28**:1761–1764.

116. Ho K-L: Pure motor hemiplegia due to infarction of the cerebral peduncle. *Arch Neurol* 1982;**39**:524–526.

117. Bogousslavsky J, Maeder P, Regli F, et al: Pure midbrain infarction: Clinical syndromes, MRI, and etiologic patterns. *Neurology* 1994;**44**:2032–2040.

118. Martin PJ, Chang H-M, Wityk R, Caplan LR: Midbrain infarction: Associations and aetiologies in the New England Medical Center Posterior Circulation Registry. *J Neurol Neurosurg Psychiatry* 1998;**64**:392–395.

119. Hommel M, Besson G: Midbrain infarcts. In Bogousslavsky J, Caplan LR (eds): *Stroke Syndromes*, 2nd ed. Cambridge: Cambridge University Press, 2001, pp 512–519.

120. Hommel B, Besson G, Pollak P, et al: Hemiplegia in posterior cerebral artery occlusion. *Neurology* 1990;**40**:1496–1499.

121. Mossuto-Agatiello L: Caudal paramedian midbrain syndrome. *Neurology* 2006;**66**:1668–1671.

122. Sato S, Toyoda K, Kawase K, et al: A caudal mesencephalic infarct presenting only tetra-ataxia and tremor. *Cerebrovasc Dis* 2008;**25**:187–189.

123. Castaigne P, Lhermitte F, Buge A, et al: Paramedian thalamic and midbrain infarcts: Clinical and

neuropathological study. *Ann Neurol* 1981;**10**:127–148.

124. Percheron G: Les arteres du thalamus humain: II. Arteres et territoires thalamique paramedians de l'arterie basilarie communicante. *Rev Neurol (Paris)* 1976;**132**:309–324.

125. Barth A, Bogousslavsky J, Caplan LR: Thalamic infarcts and hemorrhages. In Bogousslavsky J, Caplan LR (eds): *Stroke Syndromes*, 2nd ed. Cambridge: Cambridge University Press, 2001, pp 461–468.

126. Bogousslavsky J, Miklossy J, Deruaz J, et al: Unilateral left paramedian infarction of thalamus and midbrain: A clinicopathological study. *J Neurol Neurosurg Psychiatry* 1986;**49**:686–694.

127. Graff-Radford NR, Damasio H, Yamada T, et al: Nonhaemorrhagic thalamic infarction. *Brain* 1985;**108**:495–516.

128. Bogousslavsky J, Regli F, Assal G: The syndrome of tuberothalamic artery territory infarction. *Stroke* 1986;**17**:434–441.

129. Bogousslavsky J, Regli F, Uske A: Thalamic infarcts: Clinical syndromes, etiology, and prognosis. *Neurology* 1988;**38**:837–848.

130. Tatemichi T, Steinke W, Duncan C, et al: Paramedian thalamo-peduncular infarction: Clinical syndromes and magnetic resonance imaging. *Ann Neurol* 1992;**32**:162–171.

131. Bogousslavsky J, Caplan LR: Vertebrobasilar occlusive disease, review of selected aspects. III: Thalamic infarcts. *Cerebrovasc Dis* 1993;**3**:193–205.

132. de Freitas GR, Bogousslavsky J: Thalamic infarcts. In Donnan G, Norrving B, Bamford J, Bogousslavsky J (eds): *Subcortical Stroke*, 2nd ed. Oxford: Oxford University Press, 2002, pp 255–285.

133. Kaplan RF, Estol CJ, Damasio H, et al: Bilateral polar artery thalamic infarcts. *Neurology* 1991;**41**(Suppl 1):329.

134. Wall M, Slamovits TL, Weisberg LA, Trufant SA: Vertical gaze ophthalmoplegia from infarction in the area of the posterior thalamo-subthalamic paramedian artery. *Stroke* 1986;**17**:546–555.

135. Pierrot-Deseiligny C, Caplan LR: Eye movement abnormalities. In Caplan LR, van Gijn J (eds): *Stroke Syndromes*

3rd ed. Cambridge: Cambridge University Press, 2012, pp 64–74.

136. Meissner I, Sapir S, Kokmen E, Stein SD: The paramedian diencephalic syndrome: A dynamic phenomenon. *Stroke* 1987;**18**:380–385.

137. Caplan LR, DeWitt LD, Pessin MS, et al: Lateral thalamic infarcts. *Arch Neurol* 1988;**45**:959–964.

138. Dejerine J, Roussy G: Le syndrome thalamique. *Rev Neurol* 1906;**14**:521–532.

139. Fisher CM: Pure sensory stroke involving face, arm, and leg. *Neurology* 1965;**15**:76–80.

140. Fisher CM: Thalamic pure sensory stroke: A pathologic study. *Neurology* 1978;**28**:1141–1144.

141. Fisher CM: Pure sensory stroke and allied conditions. *Stroke* 1982;**13**:434–447.

142. Fisher CM: Lacunar strokes and infarcts: A review. *Neurology* 1982;**32**:871–876.

143. Hommel M, Besson G, Pollak P, et al: Pure sensory stroke due to a pontine lacune. *Stroke* 1989;**20**:406–408.

144. Mohr JP, Kase C, Meckler R, et al: Sensorimotor stroke. *Arch Neurol* 1977;**34**:734–741.

145. Mohr JP, Timsit S: Choroidal artery disease. In Barnett HJM, Mohr JP, Stein BM, Yatsu F (eds): *Stroke, Pathophysiology, Diagnosis, and Management*, 3rd ed. New York: Churchill Livingstone, 1998, pp 503–512.

146. Besson G, Bogousslavsky J, Regli F: Posterior choroidal-artery infarct with homonymous horizontal sectoranopia. *Cerebrovasc Dis* 1991;**1**:117–120.

147. Frisen I, Holmegaard L, Rosencrantz M: Sectorial optic atrophy and homonymous, horizontal sectoranopia: A lateral posterior choroidal artery syndrome. *J Neurol Neurosurg Psychiatry* 1978;**41**:374–380.

148. Neau JP, Bogousslavsky J: The syndrome of posterior choroidal artery territory infarction. *Ann Neurol* 1996;**39**:779–788.

149. Loeb C, Gandolfo C, Croce R, Conti M: Dementia associated with lacunar infarction. *Stroke.* 1992;**23**:1225–1229.

150. Jacova C, Pearce LA, Costello R, et al: Cognitive impairment in lacunar strokes: The SPS3 trial. *Ann Neurol* 2012;**72**:351–362.

151. Makin SD, Turpin S, Dennis MS, Wardlaw JM: Cognitive impairment after lacunar stroke: Systematic review and meta-analysis of incidence, prevalence and comparison with other stroke subtypes. *J Neurol Neurosurg Psychiatry* 2013;**84**:893–900.

152. Longstreth WT Jr, Arnold AM, Beauchamp NJ Jr, et al: Incidence, manifestations, and predictors of worsening white matter on serial cranial magnetic resonance imaging in the elderly: The Cardiovascular Health Study. *Stroke* 2005;**36**:56–61.

153. Schmidt R, Ropele S, Enzinger C, et al: White matter lesion progression, brain atrophy, and cognitive decline: The Austrian Stroke Prevention Study. *Ann Neurol* 2005;**58**:610–616.

154. Vermeer SE, Hollander M, van Dijk EJ, Hofman A, Koudstaal PJ, Breteler MM. Silent brain infarcts and white matter lesions increase stroke risk in the general population: The Rotterdam Scan Study. *Stroke* 2003;**34**:1126–1129.

155. Adams H, Damasio H, Putnam S, et al: Middle cerebral artery occlusion as a cause of isolated subcortical infarction. *Stroke* 1983;**14**:948–952.

156. Maki G, Mihara H, Shizuka M, et al: CT and arteriographic comparison of patients with transient ischemic attacks: Correlation with small infarcts of basal ganglia. *Stroke* 1983;**14**:276–280.

157. Caplan LR, Babikian V, Helgason C, et al: Occlusive disease of the middle cerebral artery. *Neurology* 1985;**35**:975–982.

158. Bogousavsky J, Regli F, Maeder P: Intracranial large-artery disease and "lacunar" infarction. *Cerebrovasc Dis* 1991;**1**:154–159.

159. Miyashita K, Naritomi H, Sawada T, et al: Identification of recent lacunar lesions in cases of multiple small infarction by magnetic resonance imaging. *Stroke* 1988;**29**:834–839.

160. Patel B, Markus HS: Magnetic resonance imaging in cerebral small vessel disease and its use as a surrogate disease marker. *Int J Stroke* 2011;**6**:47–59.

161. Förster A, Kerl HU, Wenz H, Brockmann MA, Nölte I, Groden, C: Diffusion- and perfusion-weighted imaging in acute lacunar infarction: Is there a mismatch? *PLoS One* 2013;**8**: e77428.

162. Bang OY, Yeo SH, Yoon JH, et al: Clinical MRI cutoff points for predicting lacunar stroke may not exist: Need for a grading rather than a dichotomized system. *Cerebrovasc Dis* 2007;**24**:520–529.

163. Rajajee V, Kidwell C, Starkman S, et al: Diagnosis of lacunar infarcts within 6 hours of onset by clinical and CT criteria versus MRI. UCLA MRI Acute Stroke Investigators. *J Neuroimag* 2008;**18**:66–72.

164. Faris A, Poser C, Wilmore D, et al: Radiologic visualization of neck vessels in healthy men. *Neurology* 1963;**13**:386–396.

165. Takahashi W, Fujii H, Ide M, et al: Atherosclerotic changes in intracranial and extracranial large arteries in apparently healthy persons with asymptomatic lacunar infarction. *J Stroke Cerebrovasc Dis* 2005;**14**:17–22.

166. Lodder J, Bamford J, Kappelle J, Boiten J: What causes false clinical prediction of small deep infarcts. *Stroke* 1994;**25**:86–91.

167. National Institute of Neurological Disorders and Stroke rt-PA Study Group: Tissue plasminogen activator for acute ischemic stroke. *N Engl J Med* 1995;**333**:1581–1587.

168. Ingall TJ, O'Fallon WM, Asplund K, et al: Findings from the reanalysis of the NINDS tissue plasminogen activator for acute ischemic stroke treatment trial. *Stroke* 2004;**35**:2418–2424.

169. Fuentes B, Martínez-Sánchez P, Alonso de Leciñana M, et al. for the Madrid Stroke Network: Efficacy of intravenous thrombolysis according to stroke subtypes: the Madrid Stroke Network data. *Eur J Neurol* 2012;**19**:1568–1574.

170. IST-3 Collaborative Group, Sandercock P, Wardlaw JM, Lindley RI, et al: The benefits and harms of intravenous thrombolysis with recombinant tissue plasminogen activator within 6 h of acute ischaemic stroke (the Third International Stroke Trial (IST-3)): A randomised controlled trial. *Lancet* 2012;**379**:2352–2363.

171. Mustanoja S, Meretoja A, Putaala J, et al. for the Helsinki Stroke Thrombolysis Registry Group: Outcome by stroke etiology in patients receiving thrombolytic treatment: descriptive subtype analysis. *Stroke* 2011;**42**:102–106.

172. Shobha N, Fang J, Hill MD: Do lacunar strokes benefit from thrombolysis? Evidence from the Registry of the Canadian Stroke Network. *Int J Stroke* 2013;**8**(Suppl A100):45–49.

173. Lahoti S, Gokhale S, Caplan LR, et al: Thrombolysis in ischemic stroke without arterial occlusions. *Stroke* 2014;**45**:2722–2727.

174. Griebe M, Fischer E, Kablau M, et al: Thrombolysis in patients with lacunar stroke is safe: an observational study. *J Neurol* 2014;**261**:405–411.

175. Fluri F, Hatz F, Rutgers MP, et al: Intravenous thrombolysis in patients with stroke attributable to small artery occlusion. *Eur J Neurol* 2010;**17**:1054–1060.

176. Dobkin B: Heparin for lacunar stroke in progression. *Stroke* 1983;**14**:421–423.

177. SPS3 Study Group: Blood-pressure targets in patients with recent lacunar stroke: The SPS3 randomised trial *Lancet* 2013;**382**:507–515.

178. Yamamoto Y, Akiguchi I, Oiwa K, et al: Twenty-four-hour blood pressure and MRI as predictive factors for different outcomes in patients with lacunar infarct. *Stroke* 2002;**33**:297–305.

179. Walters M, Muir S, Shah I, Lees K: Effect of perindopril on cerebral vasomotor reactivity in patients with lacunar infarction. *Stroke* 2004;**35**:1899–1902.

180. Mohr JP, Thompson JLP, Lazar RM, et al: A comparison of warfarin and aspirin for the prevention of recurrent ischemic stroke. Warfarin–Aspirin Recurrent Stroke Study Group. *N Engl J Med* 2001;**345**:1444–1451.

181. Diener HC, Cunha L, Forbes C, et al: European Stroke Prevention Study 2. Dipyridamole and acetylsalicylic acid in the secondary prevention of stroke. *J Neurol Sci* 1996;**143**:1–13.

182. Gotoh F, Tohgi H, Hirai S, et al: Cilostazole Stroke Prevention Study: A placebo-controlled double-blind trial for secondary prevention of cerebral infarction. *J Stroke Cerebrovasc Dis* 2000;**9**:147–157.

183. Furie KL, Kasner SE, Adams RJ, et al: Guidelines for the prevention of stroke in patients with stroke or transient ischemic attack: A guideline for healthcare professionals from the American Heart Association/American Stroke Association. *Stroke* 2011;**42**:227–276.

184. Sacco RL, Diener HC, Yusuf S, et al. for the PRoFESS Study Group: Aspirin and extended-release dipyridamole versus clopidogrel for recurrent stroke. *N Engl J Med* 2008;**359**:1238–1251.

185. SPS3 Investigators: Effects of clopidogrel added to aspirin in patients with recent lacunar stroke. *N Engl J Med* 2012;**367**:817–825.

186. Carod-Artal FJ: Statins and cerebral vasomotor reactivity. Implications for a new therapy. *Stroke* 2006;**37**:2446–2448.

187. Pretnar-Oblak J, Sabovic M, Sebestjen M, et al: The influence of atorvastatin treatment on L-arginine cerebrovascular reactivity and flow-mediated dilatation in patients with lacunar infarction. *Stroke* 2006;**37**:2540–2545.

188. Amarenco P, Benavente O, Goldstein LB, for the Stroke Prevention by Aggressive Reduction in Cholesterol Levels Investigators: Results of the Stroke Prevention by Aggressive Reduction in Cholesterol Levels (SPARCL) Trial by stroke subtypes. *Stroke* 2009;**40**:1405–1409.

189. Stroke Prevention by Aggressive Reduction in Cholesterol Levels (SPARCL) Investigators: High-dose atorvastatin after stroke or transient ischemic attack. *N Engl J Med* 2006;**355**:549–559.

190. Intravenous Magnesium Efficacy in Stroke (IMAGES) Study Investigators: Magnesium for acute stroke (Intravenous Magnesium Efficacy in Stroke Trial): Randomized controlled trial. *Lancet* 2004;**363**:439–445.

191. Aslanyan S, Weir CJ, Muir KW, Lees KR: Magnesium for treatment of acute lacunar stroke syndromes. Further analysis of the IMAGES trial. *Stroke* 2007;**38**:1269–1273.

192. Hachinski V, Potter P, Merskey H: Leuko-araiosis. *Arch Neurol* 1987;**44**:21–23.

193. Okeda R: Morphometrische Vergleichsuntersuchungen an Hirnarterien bei Binswangerscher Encephalopathie und Hochdruckencephalopathie. *Acta Neuropathol (Berlin)* 1973;**26**:23–43.

194. Caplan LR: Binswanger's disease – revisited. *Neurology* 1995;**45**:626–633.

195. Binswanger O: Die abgrenzung der allgemeinen progressiven paralyse. *Klin Wochenschr* 1894;**49**:1103–1105; 1895;50:1137–1139; 1895;52:1180–1186.

196. Blass JP, Hoyer S, Nitsch R: A translation of Otto Binswanger's article: The delineation of the generalized progressive paralysis. *Arch Neurol* 1991;**48**:961–972.

197. Olszewski J: Subcortical arteriosclerotic encephalopathy. *World Neurol* 1965;**3**:359–374.

198. Caplan LR, Schoene WC: Clinical features of subcortical arteriosclerotic encephalopathy (Binswanger's disease). *Neurology* 1978;**28**:1206–1215.

199. Babikian V, Ropper AH: Binswanger disease: A review. *Stroke* 1987;**18**:1–12.

200. Fisher CM: Binswanger's encephalopathy: A review. *J Neurol* 1989;**236**:65–79.

201. Ward NS, Brown MM: Leukoaraiosis. In Donnan G, Norrving B, Bamford J, Bogousslavsky J (eds): *Subcortical Stroke*, 2nd ed. Oxford: Oxford University Press, 2002, pp 47–66.

202. Maclullich AM, Wardlaw JM, Ferguson KJ, et al: Enlarged perivascular spaces are associated with cognitive function in healthy elderly men. *J Neurol Neurosurg Psychiatry* 2004;**75**:1519–1523.

203. Kim D-G, Oh S-H, Kim J: A case of disseminated polycystic dilated perivascular spaces presenting with dementia and parkinsonism. *J Clin Neurol* 2007;**32**:96–100.

204. Gray F, Dubas F, Roullet E, Escourolle R: Leukoencephalopathy in diffuse hemorrhagic cerebral amyloid angiopathy. *Ann Neurol* 1985;**18**:54–59.

205. Dubas F, Gray F, Roullet E, Escourolle R: Leukoencephalopathies arteriopathiques. *Rev Neurol* 1985;**141**:93–108.

206. Loes D, Biller J, Yuh WT, et al: Leukoencephalopathy in cerebral amyloid angiopathy: MR imaging in four cases. *AJNR Am J Neuroradiol* 1990;**11**:485–488.

207. DeWitt LD, Louis DN: Case records of the Massachusetts General Hospital: Case 27-1991. *N Engl J Med* 1991;**325**:42–54.

208. Fountain NB, Eberhard DA: Primary angiitis of the central nervous system associated with cerebral amyloid angiopathy: Report of two cases and review of the literature. *Neurology* 1996;**46**:190–197.

209. Caplan LR: Case records of the Massachusetts General Hospital. Case 10–2000. *N Engl J Med* 2000;**342**:957–964.

210. Marotti JD, Savitz SI, Kim W-K, Williams K, Caplan LR, Joseph JT: Cerebral amyloid angiitis progressing to generalized angiitis and leucoencephalitis. *Neuropathol Appl Neurobiol* 2007;**33**:1–5.

211. Davous P: CADASIL: A review with proposed diagnostic criteria. *Eur J Neurology* 1998;**5**:219–233.

212. Dichgans M, Mayer M, Uttner I, et al: The phenotypic spectrum of CADASIL: Clinical findings in 102 cases. *Ann Neurol* 1998;**44**:731–739.

213. Tournier-Lasserve E, Joutel A, Melki J, et al: Cerebral autosomal dominant arteriopathy with subcortical infarcts and leukoencephalopathy maps on chromosome 19q12. *Nat Gen* 1993;**3**:256–259.

214. Chabriat H, Levy C, Taillia H, et al: Patterns of MRI lesions in CADACIL. *Neurology* 1998;**51**:452–457.

215. Pantoni L, Poggesi A, Inzitari D: The relation between white matter lesions and cognition. *Curr Opin Neurol* 2007;**20**:390–397.

216. Savva GM, Wharton SB, Ince PG, Forster G, Matthews FE, Brayne C: Medical Research Council Cognitive Function and Ageing Study. Age, neuropathology, and dementia. *N Engl J Med* 2009;**360**:2302–2309.

217. Debette S, Markus HS: The clinical importance of white matter hyperintensities on brain magnetic resonance imaging: Systematic review and meta-analysis. *BMJ* 2010;**341**: c3666.

218. van der Flier WM, van Straaten EC, Barkhof F, et al: Small vessel disease and general cognitive function in nondisabled elderly: The LADIS Study. *Stroke* 2005;**36**:2116–2120.

219. Baezner H, Blahak C, Poggesi A, et al: Association of gait and balance disorders with age-related white matter changes: The LADIS Study. *Neurology* 2008;**70**:935–942.

220. The LADIS Study Group 2001–2011: A decade of the LADIS (Leukoaraiosis And DISability) Study: What have we learned about white matter changes and small-vessel disease? *Cerebrovasc Dis* 2011;**32**:577–588.

221. Greenberg SM, Vonsattel JPG, Stakes JW, et al: The clinical spectrum of cerebral amyloid angiopathy: Presentations without lobar hemorrhage. *Neurology* 1993;**43**:2073–2079.

222. Scolding NJ, Joseph J, Kirby PA, et al: Alpha-beta related angiitis: Primary angiitis of the central nervous system associated with cerebral amyloid angiopathy. *Brain* 2005;**128**:500–515.

223. Eng JA, Frosch MP, Choi K, et al: Clinical manifestations of cerebral amyloid-related inflammation. *Ann Neurol* 2004;**55**:250–256.

224. Ginsberg L, Geddes J, Valentine A: Amyloid angiopathy and granulomatous angiitis of the central nervous system: A case responding to corticosteroid treatment. *J Neurol* 1998;**235**:438–440.

225. McHugh JC, Ryan AM, Lynch T, et al: Steroid-responsive recurrent encephalopathy in a patient with cerebral amyloid angiopathy. *Cerebrovasc Dis* 2007;**23**:66–69.

226. Pantoni L: Cerebral small vessel disease: From pathogenesis and clinical characteristics to therapeutic challenges. *Lancet Neurol* 2010;**9**:689–701.

227. Greenberg SM, Vernooij MW, Cordonnier C, et al. for the Microbleed Study Group: Cerebral microbleeds: A guide to detection and interpretation. *Lancet Neurol* 2009;**8**:165–174.

228. Wardlaw JM, Smith EE, Biessels GJ, et al. for the STandards for ReportIng Vascular changes on nEuroimaging (STRIVE v1): Neuroimaging standards for research into small vessel disease and its contribution to ageing and neurodegeneration. *Lancet Neurol* 2013;**12**:822–838.

229. Koennecke HC: Cerebral microbleeds on MRI: Prevalence, associations, and potential clinical implications. *Neurology* 2006;**66**:165–171.

230. Klein I, Lung B, Labreuche J et al. for the IMAGE Study Group: Cerebral microbleeds are frequent in infective endocarditis. *Stroke* 2009;**40**:3461–3465.

231. Yamamoto Y, Akiguchi I, Oiwa K, et al: Adverse effect of nighttime blood pressure on the outcome of lacunar infarct patients. *Stroke* 1998;**29**:570–576.

232. Yamamoto Y, Akiguchi I, Oiwa K, et al: Twenty-four-hour blood pressure and MRI as predictive factors for different outcomes in patients with lacunar infarct. *Stroke* 2002;**33**:297–305.

233. Yamamoto Y, Akiguchi I, Oiwa K, et al: The relationship between 24-hour blood pressure readings, subcortical ischemic lesions and vascular dementia. *Cerebrovasc Dis* 2005;**19**:302–308.

234. Hoshide Y, Kario K, Schwartz JE, et al: Incomplete benefit of antihypertensive therapy on stroke reduction in older hypertensives with abnormal nocturnal blood pressure dipping (extreme-dippers and reverse-dippers). *Am J Hypertens* 2002;**15**:844–850.

235. Chamorro A, Pujol J, Saiz A, et al: Periventricular white matter lucencies in patients with lacunar stroke. A marker of too high or too low blood pressure. *Arch Neurol* 1997;**54**:1284–1288.

236. Schneider R, Ringelstein EB, Zeumer H, et al: The role of plasma hyperviscosity in subcortical arteriosclerotic encephalopathy (Binswanger's disease). *J Neurol* 1987;**234**:67–73.

237. Chung C-S, Caplan LR, van Swieten J, et al: White matter changes in stroke and fibrinogen levels. *Ann Neurol* 1993;**34**:260.

238. Rosenberg GA, Sullivan N, Esiri MM: White matter damage is associated with matrix metalloproteinases in vascular dementia. *Stroke* 2001;**32**:1162–1168.

239. Adair JC, Charlie J, Dencoff JE, et al: Measurement of gelatinase B (MMP-9) in the cerebrospinal fluid of patients with vascular dementia and Alzheimer disease. *Stroke* 2004;**35**: e159–e162.

240. Yang Y, Estrada EY, Thompson JF, et al: Matrix metalloproteinase-mediated disruption of tight junction proteins in cerebral vessels is reversed by synthetic matrix metalloproteinase inhibitor in focal ischemia in rat. *J Cereb Blood Flow Metab* 2007;**27**:697–709.

241. Brown WR, Moody DM, Challa VR, Thore CR, Anstrom JA: Venous collagenosis and arterial tortuosity in leukoaraiosis. *J Neurol Sci* 2002;**15**:203–204.

242. Rosenberg GA, Bjerke M, Wallin A: Multimodal markers of inflammation in the subcortical ischemic vascular disease type of vascular cognitive impairment. *Stroke* 2014;**45**:1531–1538.

243. Arauz A, Murillo L, Cantú C, Barinagarrementeria F, Higuera J: Prospective study of single and multiple lacunar infarcts using magnetic resonance imaging: Risk factors, recurrence, and outcome in 175 consecutive cases. *Stroke* 2003;**34**:2453–2458.

244. Dichgans M, Zietemann V: Prevention of vascular cognitive impairment. *Stroke* 2012;**43**:3137–3146.

Embolism is the most common cause of brain ischemia. A variety of embolic particles arise from the heart, aorta, and cervico-cranial arteries to reach the intracranial arteries, and other substances such as air, fat, tumor cells, and foreign objects are also occasionally introduced into the vascular system and reach the brain and other organs.[1] Doctors in the past thought that release of embolic materials into the circulation was unusual and had a high hit rate, that is, that emboli reaching intracranial arteries had a strong likelihood of causing stroke and brain infarction. Emboli monitoring using transcranial Doppler (TCD) ultrasound, has shown high rates of brain embolism.[2–9] Embolic particles are often found in the circulation, but the hit rate is low.[9]

Clinical findings and the recipient artery

Embolism requires a donor source and a recipient artery (Figure 2.5). The clinical presentation of a patient with brain embolism relates to the recipient site; symptoms and signs depend on the nature and size of the embolus, location of the recipient artery, and how long the embolus continues to block blood flow at the recipient site.[10] The recipient artery cannot distinguish the source and composition of the embolic material, nor do the clinical neurological findings differ among emboli of cardiac, intra-arterial, or venous origin.

> A 31-year-old carpenter, TL, was evaluated after the sudden onset of confusion and right-hand weakness. The symptoms began suddenly at work. Three years earlier, he had what had been called a minor stroke, characterized by numbness and weakness of the left arm and leg. Cerebral angiography was normal, but he was given warfarin during the 2 years after this event. Approximately 3 months after stopping coumadin, he had a brief attack of dizziness and veered to the left when he walked for approximately one week. He gave no history of cardiac or vascular disease, and examination of the heart and neck arteries was normal, except for a slight tachycardia. Blood pressure was 130/60 mmHg. On neurological examination, his speech was fluent but contained many paraphasic errors. He had difficulty repeating spoken language and he read, wrote, and spelled poorly. His right arm was weak, and he could not recognize objects placed in his right hand. His left plantar response was extensor.

TL's recent event involved the left cerebral hemisphere and most likely included the precentral and postcentral gyri and the inferior parietal lobe. The event that occurred 3 years before was also of sudden onset and involved the right cerebral hemisphere.

The dizziness and veering to one side probably represented ischemia in the left cerebellum. The three events in three different locations and vascular territories makes embolism by far the most likely diagnosis, but the source is not obvious from the clinical data.

Embolic strokes most often begin suddenly. The clinical signs evolve during seconds or a few minutes. The deficit may begin during physical activity but more often occurs during rest or activities of daily life.[10–12] Traditionally, the neurological deficit in patients with embolic stroke is described as maximal at onset. As soon as an embolus blocks a recipient brain artery, collateral circulation begins to develop and some improvement may occur. Unlike thrombi formed locally at sites of prior atherosclerotic narrowing, emboli only loosely adhere to blood vessel walls. They readily fragment, dislodge, and move to more distal arteries. The breakup and distal movement of emboli strongly affects the subsequent clinical course. Movement of emboli most often occurs during the first 24–48 hours after symptom onset.

Fragmentation and distal movement of emboli before the development of irreversible brain damage allows reperfusion ("recanalization") of ischemic brain tissue and is usually accompanied by clinical improvement. In some patients, however, the embolus or its fragments block an important distal branch, leading to further ischemia and worsening of symptoms. For example, a patient with an embolus to the left mainstem middle cerebral artery (MCA) might have the sudden onset of aphasia and right hemiplegia and hemisensory loss. When the embolus passes and the lenticulostriate arteries supplying the internal capsule and basal ganglia regions are reperfused, the hemiparesis might improve. Increased cortical blood flow could lead to better language function. If the embolus passed into the inferior division of the MCA supplying the temporal lobe and occluded a temporal artery branch, the patient might then develop a fluent Wernicke-type aphasia. When there is further worsening after initial improvement in patients with embolism, the worsening usually occurs in a single step and nearly always occurs during the first 48 hours. Multiple, stepwise worsening; gradual, smooth worsening; and delayed worsening are unusual. Late worsening after 48 hours is explained by the development of brain edema or hemorrhage into the area of infarction because hemorrhagic transformation often occurs between days 2 and 7 after stroke onset.

Another pattern quite characteristic of brain embolism has been called spectacular shrinking deficit by Mohr.[13,14] This

Caplan's Stroke: A Clinical Approach, 5th Edition, ed. Louis R Caplan. Published by Cambridge University Press. © Cambridge University Press, 2016.

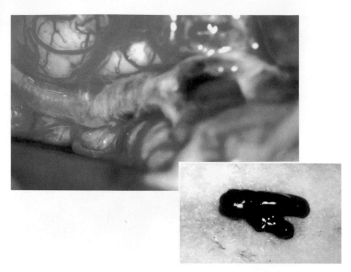

Figure 10.1 An embolus within the MCA at necropsy. The inset shows the red thrombus removed from the artery. From Caplan LR, Manning WJ. *Brain Embolism*, New York: Informa Healthcare, 2006 with permission. A black and white version of this figure will appear in some formats. For the color version, please refer to the plate section.

term describes sudden, complete, or nearly complete clearing of sudden-onset severe neurological signs. Most often, the patient has had rapid recanalization of a mainstem MCA or basilar artery embolus.[14]

Approximately four out of every five emboli that arise from the heart go into the anterior circulation equally divided between the two sides. The remaining one-fifth of emboli go into the posterior circulation,[10–12,15–17] a rate about equal to the proportion of the blood supply that goes into the vertebro-basilar arteries. The recipient artery destination depends on the size and nature of the particles. Calcific particles from heart valves and mitral annular calcifications are less mobile and adapt less well to the shape of their recipient artery than red (erythrocyte–fibrin) and white (platelet–fibrin) thrombi. Figure 10.1 shows a red thrombus that was removed from the middle cerebral artery at necropsy. The circulating bloodstream seems able to somehow bypass obstructing cholesterol crystal emboli, especially in the retinal arteries.

Within the anterior and posterior circulations, there are predilection sites for the destination of embolic particles.[10,16–18] Large emboli entering a common carotid artery (CCA) could become lodged in the CCA or internal carotid artery (ICA), especially if atheromatous plaques had already narrowed the lumens of these arteries. If the emboli successfully traversed the ICAs in the neck, the next common lodging place is the intracranial bifurcation of the ICAs (also called the carotid T and the top-of-the-carotid) into the anterior cerebral arteries (ACAs) and MCAs. Arterial bifurcations are common resting places for emboli. Emboli that pass through the carotid intracranial bifurcations most often go into the MCAs and their branches. Gacs et al. showed that balloon emboli placed in the circulation nearly always followed the same pathway and ended up in the MCAs and their branches.[16] Embolism in experimental animals caused by the introduction of silicone cylinders or spheres, elastic cylinders, and autologous blood clots also

showed a high incidence of MCA-territory localization.[17] Emboli often pass into the superior and inferior divisions of the MCA and their cortical branches. The superior division supplies the cortex and white matter above the sylvian fissure, including the frontal and superior parietal lobes. The inferior division supplies the area below the sylvian fissure, including the temporal and inferior parietal lobes. TL's recent event most likely involved the inferior division of the left MCA. His first attack probably involved the right MCA. Emboli seldom go into the MCA penetrating artery (lenticulostriate arteries) branches because these arteries originate at a nearly 90-degree angle from the parent arteries.

Embolism into the MCAs can cause a variety of patterns of infarction[10] (Figure 2.37). Cortical and cortical–subcortical infarcts are most common. In young patients whose mainstem MCA is acutely occluded, the rapid development of collateral circulation over the convexity of the brain often leads to sparing of the superficial territory of the MCA. The lenticulostriate branches are blocked by the embolus in the mainstem MCA, and collateral circulation to the deep MCA territory is poor. The resultant infarct is limited to the basal ganglia and surrounding white matter and is usually called a striatocapsular infarct. Occasionally, emboli block an ACA or its distal branches, causing an infarct in the paramedian area of one frontal lobe.

Emboli that enter the posterior circulation can block the vertebral arteries in the neck or intracranially. Emboli that are able to pass through the intracranial vertebral arteries (ICVAs) usually pass through the proximal and middle portions of the basilar artery, which are wider than the ICVAs. The basilar artery becomes narrower as it courses craniad. Emboli often block the distal basilar artery bifurcation (top-of-the-basilar) or one of its branches – the penetrating arteries to the medial portions of the thalami and midbrain, the superior cerebellar artery (SCA), which supplies the upper surface of the cerebellum, and the posterior cerebral arteries (PCAs), which supply the lateral portions of the thalami and the temporal and occipital lobe territories of the PCAs.[18–20] Figure 10.2 is a cartoon that shows the major sites of embolic occlusion within the vertebro-basilar arterial system. Figure 10.3 shows a basilar artery embolus found at necropsy. The most frequent posterior circulation brain areas infarcted are: (1) the posterior inferior portion of the cerebellum in the territory of the posterior inferior cerebellar artery branch of the ICVA; (2) the superior surface of the cerebellum in the territory of the SCA; and (3) the thalamic and hemispheral territories of the PCAs.[18] TL's second attack probably represented cerebellar ischemia.[18,21]

The clinical neurological signs depend on the location of the occluded artery and are the same as the signs described in Chapters 7 and 8. An occluded ACA causes leg weakness, abulia, and left-arm apraxia. When the occluded vessel is the upper trunk of the left MCA, Broca's aphasia and weakness of the right side of the face, and the right hand and arm result. An occluded left MCA inferior trunk causes Wernicke's aphasia and a right homonymous hemianopia. An occluded PCA causes a homonymous hemianopia, whereas an embolus at the top of the basilar artery can cause cortical blindness,

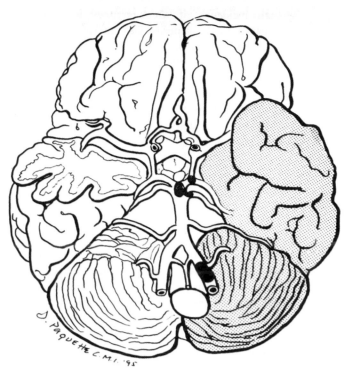

Figure 10.2 Drawing of the base of the brain showing the most frequent sites of embolism within the posterior circulation. The black clots are located within the left ICVA and in the distal basilar artery and its left superior cerebellar and PCA branches. The left temporal lobe and left cerebellum are shaded gray to show infarction. Drawn by Dari Paquette. From Caplan LR. *Posterior Circulation Disease: Clinical Findings, Diagnosis, and Management.* New York: Blackwell Science, 1996 with permission of Blackwell Publishing Ltd.

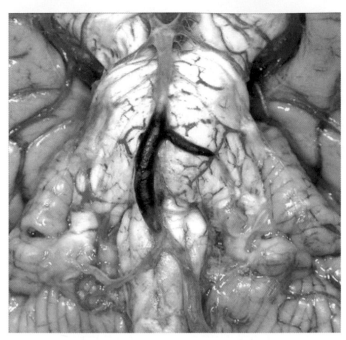

Figure 10.3 The base of the brain at necropsy showing a red embolus distending the basilar artery. A black and white version of this figure will appear in some formats. For the color version, please refer to the plate section.

lethargy or agitation, and abnormal eye movements. At times, emboli may be large enough to occlude a normal or an already stenotic ICA, MCA stem, ICVA, or basilar artery, causing more severe neurological deficits.

Emboli of cardiac origin are often larger than those arising in the cervico-cranial arteries, so the infarcts are, on average, larger than artery-to-artery infarcts.[10,22–26] In the Stroke Data Bank, the average volume of infarction on computed tomography (CT) in patients with cardiac-origin embolism was 2.4 times greater than in patients with intra-arterial embolism, a highly significant difference (*P* < 0.01).[24,26] In a study of more than 2000 stroke patients, the average size of brain infarcts caused by cardiac-source embolism was 73.7 cm^3 versus 48.9 cm^3 for non-embolic infarcts.[25] Decreased level of consciousness early during the course of the stroke, a finding probably related to the size of infarction among other factors, was also significantly more common in Stroke Data Bank patients who had cardiogenic embolism, as compared with those with intra-arterial embolism (29.8% vs. 6.1%, *P* < 0.01).[26]

TL had no history of systemic embolism. Embolism to systemic arteries has traditionally been considered an important criterion for the clinical diagnosis of brain embolism. Necropsy studies of patients with brain embolism of cardiac origin and those with fatal strokes nearly always show embolic infarcts in other organs, especially the spleen and kidneys.[27,28] In contrast, the frequency of clinical recognition of systemic embolism is quite low. The frequency of diagnosis

of systemic embolism in various stroke registries was 2% in the Harvard Stroke Registry, 2.3% in the Michael Reese Stroke Registry, 3.6% in the Stroke Data Bank, and 3% in the Lausanne Stroke Registry.[4,10–12,15,26] Eight percent, the highest frequency of systemic embolism, was found in a study of 60 patients with cardiogenic brain embolism in whom two patients had kidney embolism and three patients had peripheral limb embolism.[29]

Embolism to the brain that causes ischemia usually produces transient or persistent neurological symptoms. The brain is like litmus paper and is sensitive to perturbations. Systemic embolism also causes ischemia, but the symptoms are much less specific. Embolism to a limb might cause arm pain, leg cramps, or other transient discomfort. These symptoms are common and usually result from activity, positioning of the limb, or some other banal, everyday occurrence. Similarly, embolism to the intestinal tract might cause stomach cramps, bowel irregularity, or a stomach ache. These are rather common and non-specific symptoms. Embolism to the kidneys or spleen causes flank or abdominal discomfort and is rarely diagnosed as related to systemic embolism. Hematuria and sudden-onset severe limb ischemia are probably the only two situations that usually lead to recognition of systemic embolism, especially in patients with known heart disease. An analyis of the findings on urinalysis and renal function among 324 acute ischemic stroke patients found that patients with high urine white counts and red blood cell counts and serum creatinine determinations had a high frequency of cardiac-origin embolism.[30] Imaging using CT or magnetic resonance imaging (MRI) of the abdomen may help in differentiating embolism from a central source (heart or aorta) from intravascular lesions by showing embolic infarcts in the spleen and kidneys and other abdominal viscera.[31]

Imaging and laboratory findings related to the recipient artery and its supply

Brain imaging using CT, MRI, or both, and vascular imaging using CT angiography (CTA), MR angiography (MRA), standard catheter angiography, and TCD can yield information in relation to the recipient artery and the presence, location, and size of embolic brain infarcts.

> CT scans in TL showed a region of lucency involving the left angular and postcentral gyri. Within the lucent areas were small regions of stippling caused by hemorrhagic transformation. There were also small, old infarcts in the right frontal lobe and left cerebellum. Hematologic, serologic, and coagulation studies were normal. MRI confirmed the same regions of infarction. The hemorrhagic changes in the recent inferior parietal lobe infarct were more evident on MRI than CT. Angiography on the third hospital day revealed a sharp cutoff of the left angular artery. The proximal arteries were normal.

Brain imaging with CT and MRI can suggest brain embolism. Because emboli most often lodge in distal arteries that supply cortical zones, embolic infarcts are often V-shaped and abut on the superficial cortical surface. Multiple cortical infarcts in various vascular supply regions suggest cardiac-origin embolism. Ringelstein and colleagues analyzed the CT pattern of infarction among 60 patients with cardiogenic embolism[32] (Figure 2.37). Most infarcts were large and cortically based (41 lesions). Some patients had small cortical, subcortical, and insular infarcts. A few patients had deep infarcts in the striatocapsular region.[32] Multiple cortical and cortical–subcortical infarcts in different vascular territories are especially suggestive of brain embolism from a cardiac or aortic source. At times, acute emboli are imaged as hyperdense arteries on non-contrast CT (Figure 4.19). Most often, the hyperdensity takes the course and shape of the MCA. Occasionally, calcific fragments can also be seen within arteries on non-contrast CT scans (Figure 4.20). Emboli monitoring using TCD, (Figures 4.17 and 4.18) has shown high rates of brain embolism.[2,5–10]

Embolic infarcts may be pale, spotted with small petechial hemorrhages, or frankly hemorrhagic. Figure 10.4 is a necropsy specimen that shows a typical hemorrhagic infarct. Fisher and Adams extensively studied their necropsy material to define the mechanism of hemorrhagic infarction in the brain.[33,34] Obstruction of a nutrient artery causes brain ischemia to neurons and ischemic damage to the blood vessels within the area of ischemia. When the obstructing embolus moves distally, the previously ischemic region is reperfused with blood. The damaged capillaries and arterioles within that region are no longer competent, and blood leaks into the surrounding infarcted tissue. An example of this is shown in Figure 10.5A and B from the Fisher and Adams study. This patient had an embolus that initially blocked the mainstem MCA before its lenticulostrate branches, causing ischemia to the basal ganglia, internal capsule, and the superficial cortical territories supplied by the MCA. The embolus then moved and had passed beyond the lenticulostrate branches at necropsy

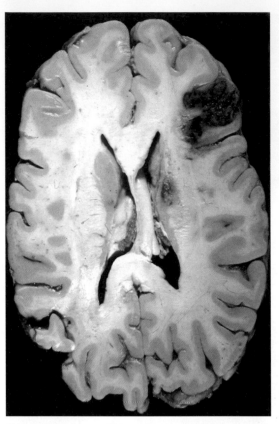

Figure 10.4 A hemorrhagic infarct involves the territory of an anterior branch of the superior division of the MCA at necropsy. There is also a small region of hemorrhagic infarction in the basal ganglia on the same side. From Caplan LR, Manning WJ. *Brain Embolism*. New York: Informa Healthcare, 2006 with permission.

but continued to obstruct the MCA more distally. The reperfused deep basal ganglionic region was hemorrhagic at necropsy, whereas the superficial territory of the MCA that was never reperfused, showed a bland infarct. In Figure 10.6, Fisher and Adams show a similar instance of hemorrhagic infarction in a reperfused region.

The essential cause of hemorrhagic infarction is reperfusion of previously ischemic tissue. The other stroke mechanism that causes hemorrhagic infarction is systemic hypoperfusion. After cardiac arrest or shock, the reinstitution of effective circulation after a prolonged period of brain hypoperfusion can cause hemorrhage within borderzone infarcts. Hemorrhagic changes are very common in patients with brain embolism. In two series, investigators prospectively studied the frequency of hemorrhagic infarction on sequential brain-imaging scans.[35,36] Yamaguchi et al. compared the findings on CT scans performed 3–10 days after stroke in 120 patients who had embolic brain infarcts with 109 patients whose infarcts were believed to be caused by local thrombotic occlusive disease.[35] Hemorrhagic infarcts were found in 45 patients (40%) with embolic infarcts, as compared with 2 patients (1.8%) with local thrombosis-related infarcts. Okada and colleagues performed CT scans every 10 days in 160 patients who had presumed embolic brain infarcts.[36] Hemorrhagic infarction was found on CT at some time during the course in 65 patients (40.6%). Hemorrhagic changes were

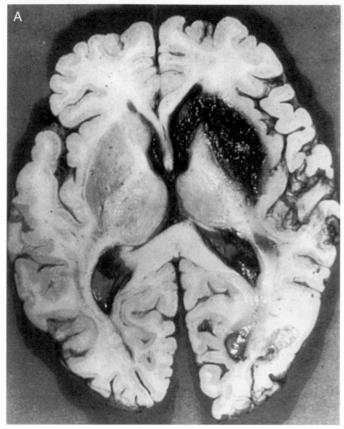

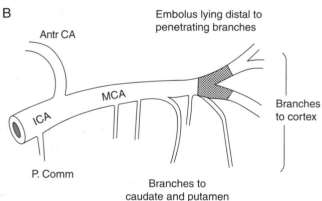

Figure 10.5 (A) Coronal section of the brain at necropsy showing a hemorrhagic infarction on the right involving the caudate nucleus and putamen, regions supplied by the lenticulostriate branches of the right MCA. (B) Cartoon of the ICA and its branches at necropsy. An embolus (hatched region) was found in the distal portion of the mainstem MCA beyond the lenticulostriate branches that supply the caudate nucleus and putamen. This embolus, at one time, must have blocked these penetrating branches and then moved more distally in the artery. Antr CA, anterior cerebral artery; ICA, internal carotid artery; MCA, middle cerebral artery; P. Comm, posterior communicating artery. From Fisher CM, Adams RD. Observations on brain embolism with special reference to hemorrhagic infarction. In Furlan AJ (ed), *The Heart and Stroke*. London: Springer, 1987, pp 17–36 with permission.

found on the initial CT scan performed during the first 4 days in only 10 patients (6%), whereas the remainder of the hemorrhagic infarcts were found on follow-up CT scans.[36] Studies at the New England Medical Center in Boston showed that all patients with cerebral and cerebellar hemorrhagic infarcts reported had embolic causes.[37,38] MRI is more sensitive than

CT in showing hemorrhagic changes, therefore sequential MRI probably would show a frequency greater than 50% for hemorrhagic changes in patients with embolic brain infarcts.

In most patients, hemorrhagic infarction consists of diapedesis of red blood cells into infarcted tissue. The appearance is that of scattered petechial hemorrhages or a confluent purpuric pattern scattered throughout the infarct. In some brain infarcts, especially large ones involving more than one lobe, localized homogeneous collections of blood (hematomas) can develop within the region of hemorrhagic infarction.[39] In most patients with hemorrhagic infarcts, the hemorrhagic transformation does not cause worsening of the clinical symptoms and signs. The hemorrhagic changes are usually found on routine follow-up scans. Bleeding into dead tissue does not alter clinical findings unless a large space-occupying hematoma develops.

Experience with acute angiography since the late 1980s has shown a high rate of demonstration of intracranial emboli in patients with cardiac-origin sources and extracranial occlusive disease.[40–42] CTA, MRA, and standard catheter angiography, especially if performed within 48 hours of stroke onset, often shows findings characteristic of embolism. A sudden sharp, abrupt termination of a distal or medium-sized vessel without visible atherosclerosis or a filling defect in the lumen of a symptomatic recipient artery are diagnostic of embolization. Figures 4.31, 4.32 and 4.33 show acute multimodal MRI and CT studies. In each patient, the vascular occlusive embolus was shown on vascular imaging (MRA and CTA), and the perfusion abnormality exceeded the diffusion abnormality, indicating the presence of brain tissue that was ischemic but not yet infarcted. Disappearance of the obstruction in subsequent films or on later angiograms substantiates the diagnosis. Dalal et al. reported nine patients that had emboli seen on initial angiography but later disappeared.[43] Others have also shown disappearance or movement of emboli.[44,45] The finding of a normal artery that supplies a region of cortical and subcortical infarction is also highly suggestive of embolism.

TCD ultrasound insonation of patients with sudden-onset hemispheric strokes has shown frequent MCA occlusion. Sequential TCD examinations that show clearing of an obstruction suggest embolism.[2,46–49] A very important but underutilized capability has entered the diagnostic arsenal of clinicians during the last decade – emboli monitoring using TCD.[2,46] Ultrasound probes are positioned over brain arteries, most often the MCA and PCA on each side. When particles pass through the arteries being monitored, they produce an audible chirping noise and high-intensity transient signals (HITS) are visible on an oscilloscope. The signal character depends on the nature of the particles (gas, thrombus, calcium, cholesterol crystal, and so forth), particle size, and particle transit time. Figures 4.17 and 4.18 show microembolic signals captured by TCD monitoring. Figure 10.7 shows a flurry of microembolic signals in an MCA in a patient during carotid artery angioplasty. Monitoring probes can be placed on the neck and brain arteries. Emboli that arise from the heart or aorta should go equally to each side, proportionately to the anterior and

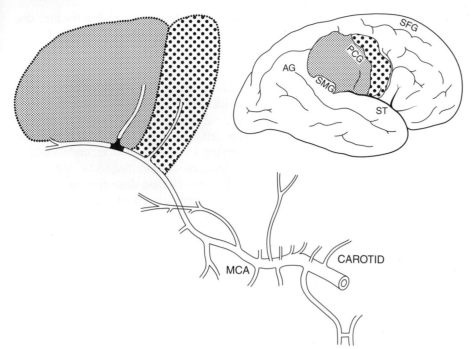

Figure 10.6 On the right is a lateral view of the right side of the brain. The stippled dotted area represents hemorrhagic transformation while the more solid gray area represents bland non-hemorrhagic infarction at necropsy. The figure on the left shows an embolus found within a branch of the MCA. The region beyond the embolus shows a bland infarct while the area reperfused is hemorrhagic. AG, angular gyrus; PCG, postcentral gyrus; SFG, superior frontal gyrus; SMG, supramarginal gyrus; ST, superior temporal gyrus. From Fisher CM, Adams RD. Observations on brain embolism with special reference to hemorrhagic infarction. In Furlan AJ (ed), *The Heart and Stroke*. London: Springer, 1987, pp 17–36 with permission.

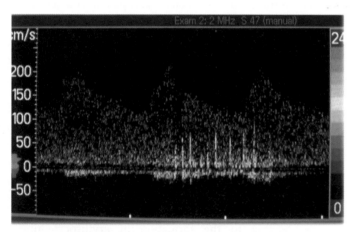

Figure 10.7 TCD monitoring during carotid angioplasty shows a flurry of microembolic signals in the MCA.

posterior circulation arteries. About 40% should go to each MCA and 20% to the posterior circulation. The signals should appear in the neck before appearing intracranially. In contrast, emboli that originate from a carotid artery should go only to the intracranial anterior circulation arterial branches on the same side. Embolic signals do not appear in the neck over that ICA. For example, emboli from the left ICA generate embolic signals detectable in the left MCA and not in the neck, PCAs, or right-sided arteries. Emboli that originate in a vertebral artery could go to either PCA. This ultrasound monitoring technique allows better identification of the nature of embolic materials and their sources. This technique also allows some quantification of the emboli load and a means of monitoring the effect of various therapies on lessening that load.

In one study, Daffertshofer and colleagues monitored 280 patients who had acute MCA-territory ischemic events, as well as 118 asymptomatic controls, for periods of 30–60 minutes.[7] Only 2 control patients (1.7%) had microembolic signals. No microembolic signals were detected among 78 patients who had no identified sources of embolism, whereas 12.9% of patients with sources of emboli had microembolic signals.[7] Microemboli were found more often in patients with vascular sources of embolism, such as ICA stenosis (17.1%), as compared with 6.2% in patients with cardiac sources of embolism. One-fifth of patients with ICA stenosis greater than 70% had microembolic signals, as compared with 13% in patients with less than 70% ICA stenosis.[7]

Sliwka et al., during a 6-month period, monitored 109 consecutive patients with atrial fibrillation or other potential cardiac sources of embolism.[8] Microembolic signals were detected in 36 of the 100 patients successfully monitored. The average number of microembolic signals was 2.69 ± 2.7 per 30 minutes (range, 1–12). Patients with atrial fibrillation who had coronary atherosclerotic heart disease with ejection fractions of less than 30%, dilatated cardiomyopathy, or mitral stenosis had the highest percentage of microemboli detection.[8]

Georgiadis and colleagues monitored 300 patients with potential cardiac sources of emboli and 100 patients with severe ICA disease using TCD.[50] They found the following frequencies of microembolic signals among their monitored patients: 43% infective endocarditis; 34% left ventricular aneurysm; 26% intracardiac thrombus; 26% dilated cardiomyopathy; 21% non-valvular atrial fibrillation; 15% native valvular disease; 55% prosthetic valves; 28% ICA disease (52% symptomatic ICA disease, 7% asymptomatic disease); and 5% among controls.[50]

CT and MR angiography can often show occlusion of major intracranial arteries. MRI, especially using T2*-weighted gradient echo images, can show clots as hypointense signals.[51,52] Using the extent of the thrombus an estmate of the "clot burden" can be made that correlates with the likelihood of clot lysis after intravenous thrombolysis.[52] The findings on MRI are

helpful in predicting whether a clot extracted from an intracraial artery using a mechanical clot retriever will be a red blood cell dominant thrombus, a fibrin–platelet rich thrombus, or a mixed clot containing both elements.[53] Some thrombi visualized using T2*-weighted images on a 3-Tesla MRI scanner have 2 layers; these thrombi are almost always red blood cell clots that have embolized from a cardiac source.[54]

> In TL, echocardiography showed an enlarged heart with a reduced ejection fraction suggestive of a cardiomyopathy. Myocardial biopsy later revealed cardiac sarcoidosis. During the next year, TL had no further brain emboli while taking warfarin.

In this patient, the multiple acute onset brain infarcts in different vascular territories, the negative hematological studies, absence of risk factors for atherosclerosis, and normal proximal extracranial and intracranial arteries suggested the likelihood of cardiac-origin brain embolism despite the absence of known cardiac disease. Cardiac evaluation finally clarified the diagnosis.

Sources of emboli

The great majority of emboli to the brain arise from the heart, aorta, and cervico-cranial arteries. Figure 2.5 illustrates these major sources. A variety of particles with different physical properties can arise from the heart, arteries, or circulation.[1,55] Table 10.1 lists the various particles that arise from cardiac and intra-arterial sources. Occasionally, foreign materials, such as air, fat, and cancer cells, enter the circulation and embolize to various systemic organs. Importantly, pharmacological prophylaxis to prevent recurrent embolization depends mostly on the nature of the substance that makes up the embolism

Table 10.1 Types of embolic materials from various sources

Cardiac origin	Arterial origin	Systemic
Red fibrin-dependent thrombi	Red fibrin-dependent thrombi	Air
White platelet–fibrin thrombi	White platelet–fibrin thrombi	Fat
Fibrin strands and bland valve vegetations (NBTE)	Combined white and red thrombi	Mucin from tumors
Bacteria from infective endocarditis	Cholesterol crystals	Talc and microcrystalline cellulose (drug injections)
Calcium from valve and mitral annulus calcifications	Atheromatous plaque debris	Foreign bodies
Tumor (myxoma and other cardiac neoplasms)	Calcium from areas of arterial calcification	

rather than its source. It's not the nest alone, but the bird that flew from the nest that deserves attention.

Cardiac sources

During the 1950s, the only two cardiac conditions accepted as having an important risk of causing embolism were rheumatic mitral stenosis with atrial fibrillation and recent myocardial infarction. Now many different cardiac lesions and disorders are recognized as carrying a risk of cardiac thrombus formation and embolism. Modern cardiac diagnostic testing has made it possible to diagnose cardiac disorders more definitively and to attempt to quantify the risk of embolism. Cardiac disorders that carry a risk of brain embolism can be divided into six groups.[4,55–57] These six groups are: (1) arrhythmias, especially atrial fibrillation and sick sinus syndrome; (2) valvular heart diseases, especially mitral stenosis, prosthetic heart valves, infective endocarditis, and marantic endocarditis; (3) ventricular myocardial abnormalities, especially related to coronary artery disease, myocarditis, and other dilatated cardiomyopathies; (4) lesions within the cavity of the ventricles, especially tumors, such as myxomas and thrombi; (5) shunts, especially intra-atrial septal defects and patent foramen ovale (PFO) that allow passage of emboli forming in the peripheral veins to enter the systemic circulation, causing so-called paradoxical embolism; and (6) atrial lesions, such as dilated atria, atrial infarcts and thrombi, and atrial septal aneurysms. Table 10.2 lists the major cardiac donor sources of embolism and Table 10.3 compares the clinical findings in patients with large artery thrombosis and embolism.

Virchow, in 1856, described three antecedent conditions for the development of thrombi within blood vessels and the chambers of the heart.[58] These three conditions are: (1) a region of circulatory stasis; (2) injury to an endothelial surface; and (3) increased blood coagulability. In areas of stasis, a low shear rate and other factors activate the classical coagulation cascade, leading to the formation of erythrocyte–fibrin thrombi. Stasis occurs most often in the atria and atrial appendages in patients with atrial fibrillation. Stasis also occurs in the ventricular chambers in patients with global and focal regions of decreased myocardial contractility. Altered myocardial endothelium occurs in patients with myocardial infarcts, ventricular aneurysms, inflammatory and other myocardiopathies, and endocardial disorders. Valvular endothelium can be damaged by many different conditions. Loss of a protective endothelial surface exposes circulating blood to the underlying tissues and causes platelet activation, adhesion, and secretion, as well as activating the coagulation cascade. Studies show increased platelet activation and blood coagulability in patients with cardiac-source embolism.[59–63]

Arrhythmias

Atrial fibrillation

Atrial fibrillation is characterized by loss of organized atrial electrical and mechanical activity resulting in stasis of blood within the body of the atria and especially within the left atrial appendage.[56,57] The ejection velocity in the left atrial

Table 10.2 Cardiac sources of emboli

Coronary artery disease
  Mural thrombi
  Ventricular aneurysms
  Hypokinetic zones

Arrhythmias
  Atrial fibrillation
  Sick sinus syndrome

Valvular disease
  Mitral stenosis, rheumatic
  Aortic stenosis, rheumatic
  Bicuspid aortic valve
  Mitral annulus calcification
  Calcific aortic stenosis
  Mitral valve prolapse
  Bacterial endocarditis
  Non-bacterial thrombotic endocarditis

Cardiomyopathies or endocardiopathies
  Endocardial fibroelastosis
  Alcoholic cardiomyopathy
  Cocaine cardiomyopathy
  Myocarditis
  Sarcoidosis
  Fabry's disease
  Amyloidosis

Intracardiac lesions
  Myxomas
  Fibroelastomas
  Malignant cardiac tumors
  Metastatic tumors
  Thrombi

Septal abnormalities (paradoxic embolism)
  Atrial septal defects
  Patent foramen ovale
  Atrial septal aneurysms

Table 10.3 Differentiating signs of thrombosis and embolism

Thrombosis	Embolism
1. Preceding brief, frequent, shotgun-like TIAs	1. Single or infrequent but longer-lasting TIAs or strokes
2. TIAs all in same vascular territory	2. Deficits maximal at onset
3. Onset of stroke after sleep	3. Onset during activity or sudden strain, cough, or sneeze
4. Postural sensitivity of the symptoms	4. Infarcts in multiple vascular territories
5. Occlusion or severe stenosis of a large artery	5. Presence of distal intra-arterial emboli
6. Absence of distal embolus by angiography	6. Hemorrhagic brain infarct
7. Infarct near borderzone of affected artery	7. Infarct in the heart of vascular territory, wedge-shaped, and abutting on cortical surface
8. Presence of risk factors for atherosclerosis: hypertension, hypercholesterolemia, angina, etc.	8. Presence of known cardiac, arterial, or venous source of embolus

appendage is markedly depressed (<20 cm/s) in patients with atrial fibrillation, and the risk of thrombus formation is inversely related to the left atrial appendage ejection velocity.[56,64] In addition to stasis, hematological studies suggest that atrial fibrillation is associated with an increased blood coagulability state.[61,62]

Atrial fibrillation is one of the most common heart conditions. Over two-and-a-half million people in the United States have atrial fibrillation, a population that greatly exceeds those with rheumatic mitral stenosis. Approximately 0.4% of the population has atrial fibrillation and the disorder becomes much more common as patients age. Perhaps as many as 5% of individuals older than 60 years have atrial fibrillation. Epidemiological studies performed since the 1970s have firmly established that atrial fibrillation is an important risk factor for stroke, that stroke in patients with atrial fibrillation is most often caused by cardiogenic embolism, and that standard antithrombotic treatment substantially reduces the frequency of brain embolism in patients with atrial fibrillation. The etiology of atrial fibrillation and associated cardiac and other

medical factors affect the risk of stroke in patients with atrial fibrillation. In the Framingham Study, the presence of rheumatic heart disease and atrial fibrillation conveyed 17.6 times the risk of stroke compared with the lone atrial fibrillation rate of 5.6 times.[65,66] Advanced age, congestive heart failure, history of hypertension, previous myocardial infarction, and prior thromboembolism increase the risk of stroke in patients with atrial fibrillation.[67–70] These features should be known from the medical history. A collaborative analysis of five atrial fibrillation stroke prevention studies analyzed the contribution of various historical risk factors on the development of stroke during follow-up.[70] The relative risks (RRs), determined by multivariate analysis of all the data, were: history of previous stroke or transient ischemic attack (TIA) (RR 2.5), diabetes mellitus (RR 1.7), history of hypertension (RR 1.6), and increasing age (RR 1.4 for each decade).[70] These calculated RRs were for the occurrence of any stroke and were not limited to those attributable to cardiogenic embolism.

Echocardiography findings are very important in assessing the risk of brain embolism in individual patients with atrial fibrillation.[56,57,71–80] Transesophageal echocardiography (TEE) can detect left atrial and left atrial appendage thrombi. Figure 4.36 is a TEE that shows a left atrial thrombus in an atrial fibrillation patient. In patients with atrial fibrillation who do not have valvular disease, thrombi often form in, and dislodge from, the left atrial appendage, whereas patients with atrial fibrillation and valvular disease have more left atrial thrombi. In patients with valvular disease and atrial fibrillation, thrombi have been detected in 9–29% of patients,

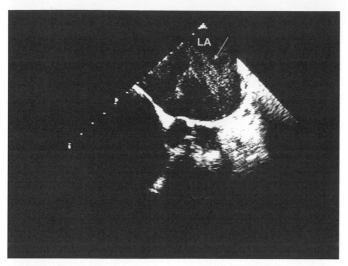

Figure 10.8 TEE in a patient with a swirling pattern of spontaneous echo contrast (white arrow) in the body of the left atrium (LA) indicating slow/stagnant flow. From Caplan LR, Manning WJ. *Brain Embolism*. New York: Informa Healthcare, 2006 with permission.

compared with 10% prevalence in patients without valvular disease.[55] Small thrombi (<2 mm) and those that have already dislodged are not readily detected. Left atrial enlargement and abnormal left atrial appendage function, as determined by Doppler TEE, also convey an increased risk for cardioembolic stroke.[71,74,75,80] The presence of mitral annulus calcification (MAC) and left ventricular dysfunction also increase the risk of stroke in patients with atrial fibrillation.

Spontaneous echo contrast (also called smoke) is an important factor that predicts the likelihood of cardiogenic embolism in patients with atrial fibrillation.[76-79] Figure 10.8 is a TEE that shows this abnormality. First described in patients with mitral valve disease, spontaneous echo contrast refers to swirling hazes of echogenicity within the cardiac chambers. The echogenic swirls can move repeatedly within the cavity and may disappear when blood flow increases or when local stasis resolves. The intensity can vary from a faint cloud-like appearance to bright echo contrast. Spontaneous echo contrast is probably caused by the interaction between plasma proteins and erythrocytes at low shear rates. It is a marker of stasis within the left atrium. The major determinants of spontaneous echogenicity are the hematocrit (Hct), fibrinogen levels, and slow intracardiac flow. Chimowitz and colleagues showed that the presence of spontaneous echo contrast was highly associated with prior strokes in patients who had either atrial fibrillation or mitral valve stenosis.[79] Spontaneous echo contrast may be seen in 60% of patients with atrial fibrillation and greater than 85% of those with atrial fibrillation and left atrial thrombi.[79-82] Prospective TEE studies show left atrial thrombi in 14% of patients with new-onset atrial fibrillation,[83-86] increasing to 27% of those with chronic atrial fibrillation,[85] and 45% in those presenting with atrial fibrillation and recent clinical thromboembolism.[86]

Cardiac rhythm monitoring is often used in patients with strokes of uncertain cause to recognize atrial fibrillation. Monitoring may be preformed only during hopsitalization, during a 24–48-hour period using a standard Holter monitor, or over a more prolonged period while the patient is ambulatory.[87-90] Still controversal is the importance of varying durations of intermittent atrial fibrillation. Very short (6–10 s) of intermittent atrial fibrillation may be insufficient to promote thrombus formation, but that might also be effected by the size and function of the left atrium and the left atrial appendage. More studies need to be performed to estimate the utility of prolonged cardiac monitoring in which patients. Two trials studied the utility of various durations of rhythm monitoring in detecting greater than 30-second instances of atrial fibrillation.[88-90] In the EMBRACE (eribulin monotherapy versus treatment of physician's choice in patients with metastatic breast cancer) trial, 16.1% of 551 patients had 30 seconds or longer instances of atrial fibrillation detected using a 30-day event-triggered belt monitor worn externally, compared to 3.2% detection using standard 24-hour monitoring.[90] In the CRYSTAL AF (cryptogenic stroke and underlying atrial fibrillation) trial, which used a device that was inserted under the skin, by 6 months of monitoring 8.9% of 441 patients had instances greater than 30 seconds of atrial fibrillation, and by a year, 12.4% of cases of intermittent atrial fibrillation were detected.[89]

Clinicians have also explored the utility of biomarkers in predicting which patients have or will develop atrial fibrillation or congestive heart failure. An analysis of the QT interval on standard electrocardiograms corrected for heart rate (QTc interval) is one strategy used to detect the likelihood of intermittent atrial fibrillation. Among 972 acute ischemic stroke patients, 69 (7.1%) of whom developed atrial fibrillation, the QTc interval was significantly longer (436 vs. 417 ms $P < 0.001$) in those that developed arial fibrillation than those that did not.[91] Measurement of the levels of brain naturetic peptide (BNP) and N-terminal-pro brain naturetic peptide (NT-proBNP) also show utility. The atria contain the highest level of BNP in healthy individuals but this is shifted to the cardiac ventricles in patients with congestive heart failure. Levels of BNP and NT-proBNP have been shown to be elevated, often considerably in patients with atrial fibrillation, congestive heart failure, and renal failure.[92-94]

The third and fourth editions of this book tabulated the results of the major trials that compared the effectiveness and frequency of hemorrhagic complications among patients with atrial fibrillation who did not have valvular disease treated with vitamin K antagonists (chiefly warfarin) and antiplatelet aggregants (mostly aspirin).[95-102] In these trials, warfarin was approximately 50% more effective than aspirin in reducing the rate of stroke in these patients. There was an overwhelming consensus among neurologists that warfarin was the drug of choice in most patients with atrial fibrillation unless there were compelling contraindications to anticoagulation. However, warfarin was a difficult drug to use. Studies in non-academic community settings[103] (Figure 6.5), and even in anticoagulation clinics (Figure 6.6),[104] showed that many patients remained under- or over-anticoagulated. Warfarin anticoagulation was difficult to control because of individual variations in dose and the effect of a variety of foods and pharmaceutical

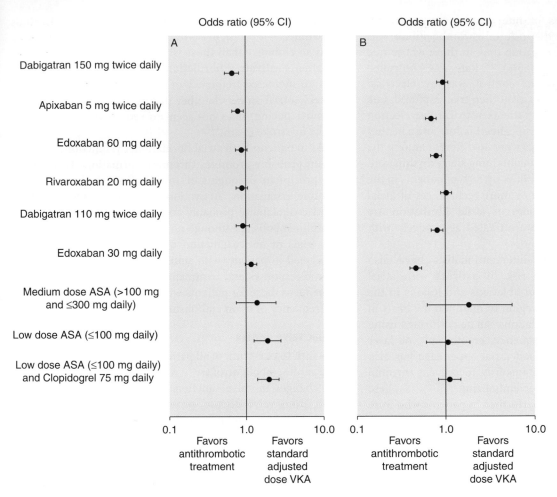

Figure 10.9 Forest plots comparing the results of trials that compared vitamin K antagonists with newer anticoagulants and aspirin. (A) In relation to prevention of all cause stroke and systemic embolism. (B) In relation to major bleeding complications. ASA, aspirin; VKA, vitamin K antagonists (warfarin). From Cameron C, Coyle D, Richter D, et al. Systematic review and network meta-analysis comparing antithrombotic agents for the prevention of stroke and major bleeding in patients with atrial fibrillation. *BMJ Open* 2014;4: e004301 with permission.

agents on vitamin K, prothrombin, and liver functions. Especially worrisome was the observation that important international normalized ratio (INR) changes may develop just before major hemorrhages. One study showed that when INRs were plotted in relation to the time before the onset of bleeding, a marked increase in the patients' INRs was observed only shortly before the bleeding began.[105]

General physicians and internists were often reluctant to anticoagulate elderly patients but studies showed that warfarin was effective and relatively safe in older individuals.[106,107] During the early years of the twenty-first century, pharmaceutical companies began to develop newer anticoagulants that did not work through vitamin K antagonism. The direct oral anticoagulant agents mostly inhibited factor Xa or thrombin. The major oral direct thrombin inhibitor used in practice is dabigatran.[108] The oral factor Xa inhibitors approved by the US Food and Drug Administration (FDA) include rivaroxaban, apixaban, and edoxaban.[109] The direct oral anticoagulant agents offer many advantages compared with warfarin. Their metabolism is much more predictable, with fewer interactions with food and with other drugs. They can be taken at fixed doses without needing regular blood tests and dose adjustments. They have shorter half-lives and faster onset and offset of action, so usually do not require bridging treatment with parenteral anticoagulants until they reach

therapeutic effect. The direct thrombin inhibitors and factor Xa inhibitors are mostly excreted by the kidney so that dosage must be adjusted in patients with renal insufficiency. These agents cause bleeding less often then vitamin K inhibitors. Recently, antidotes have been tested and approved that reverse the activity of direct oral anticoagulants if bleeding develops.

The direct oral anticoagulants have been tested for stroke prevention in atrial fibrillation. All of these agents, when compared to warfarin in patients with atrial fibrillation, were found to be equally or more effective in preventing embolic stroke and equally or more safe in avoiding intracerebral hemorrhage.[110–114] For example, in the ARISTOTLE (apixaban versus warfarin in patients with atrial fibrillation) trial, 18 201 patients with atrial fibrillation were randomized to apixaban or warfarin and followed for an average of 1.8 years.[112] The rate of combined ischemic and hemorrhagic stroke was lower in the apixaban group, 1.27% versus 1.60% per year. The apixaban group also had lower rates of major bleeding (2.13% vs. 3.09% per year) and of death (3.52% vs. 3.94%).[112] Figure 10.9 is a forest plot of studies that compared the newer anticoagulants and aspirin versus vitamin K antagonists.[115] We strongly prefer the newer anticoagulants to warfarin and predict that in the foreseeable future vitamin K antagonists will be only of historical interest.

Other treatment strategies have also been explored in patients with atrial fibrillation. Five randomized clinical trials

compared the effectiveness of rate control versus rhythm control.[116] Unexpectedly, the risk of thromboemboli was greater in the rhythm control group than in those whose rate was controlled (2.9–7.9% vs. 0.5%).[116] Rate was controlled pharmacologically and rhythm control was by electrical conversion and/or medications. Another trial explored rate versus rhythm control among patients with cardiac ejection fractions of less than 35%, congestive heart failure and a history of atrial fibrillation.[117] Outcomes were no different among the patients in the rhythm control (maintaining sinus rhythm) and rate control groups.[117] During follow-up 58% of patients in the rhythm control group had one or more recurrences of atrial fibrillation.[117] Recurrent episodes of atrial fibrillation are common even in patients who are treated aggressively with rhythm control measures.

Surgeons and cardiology interventionalists have also attempted to decrease stroke risk in patients with atrial fibrillation by producing various ablations and lesions in the pulmonary vein and left atrial region to maintain the heart in normal sinus rhythm.[118,119] Ablations can be performed using catheters that deliver radiofrequency, cryothermy, or laser energy to targeted areas. The left atrial appendage has also been removed or closed percutaneously to prevent thrombi from developing there and later embolizing.[118,120–123] These ablation procedures were first performed in patients who were having open heart surgeries for valvular heart disease at the time of the heart surgery. Now a variety of different percutaneous interventional techniques have been explored to control the atrial arrythmia and to exclude the left atrial appendage. Left atrial appendage closure using a device installed percutaneously can be complicated by pericardial effusion, atrial-esophageal fistulas, embolization of the device, and post-implant sepsis.[124] Anticoagulants and double antiplatelets are used after implantation to prevent thrombi forming on the device. The role of ablations and atrial appendage closure in the management of atrial fibrillation patients is not certain at the time of this writing.

Sick sinus syndrome

Although sinus node dysfunction has been recognized clinically since the beginning of the twentieth century, identification of the malfunctioning atrium as a source of embolism was first recognized during the 1970s.[125,126] A variety of names are used for this condition, including sick sinus syndrome, sinoatrial disorder, and bradycardia-tachycardia syndrome. Essential for the diagnosis is demonstration of sinus node dysfunctioning. Patients often present with slow or fast cardiac rhythms, or both. Lown characterized the disorder as consisting of chaotic atrial activity, changing p-wave contour, and bradycardia, admixed with multiple and recurrent ectopic beats and runs of atrial and nodal tachycardia.[127] Many patients also have atrial fibrillation or flutter with a relatively slow ventricular response (<70 beats/min).[128] An analysis of cardiovascular disease in Rochester, Minnesota showed that 2.9% of men and 1.5% of women aged 75 years or older had sick sinus syndrome.[129]

In 2 clinics that specialized in the study of cardiac dysrhythmias, systemic emboli mostly to the brain occurred in approximately 14 (18%) of patients with sick sinus syndrome.[130,131] Patients with tachyarrhythmias are more likely to embolize than those with just bradyarrhythmias. As in patients with atrial fibrillation, increasing age is associated with an increased frequency of embolism. The use of pacemakers (atrial single-chamber pacing or ventricular single-chamber pacing) does not seem to reduce the frequency of stroke or stroke death.[132]

As in patients with atrial fibrillation, dysfunction of the left atrium probably promotes thrombus formation. Tachycardia may precipitate dislodging of thrombi from the heart into the systemic circulation. Activation of platelets and increased blood coagulability probably contribute to the likelihood of thromboembolism. Although no formal, prospective, randomized trials of anticoagulation or aspirin therapy have been performed in patients with sinus node dysfunction, the therapeutic responses and treatment considerations are probably the same as those for patients with atrial fibrillation, although the frequency of brain embolism is less.

Cardiac valve disease

One-fifth to one-tenth of all patients with cardiac valve disease have cardioembolic strokes.[133] Abnormalities of valve surfaces and changes in valve function and cardiac physiology that result from valve disease, promote the formation of white platelet–fibrin thrombi and red clots on valve surfaces and in the adjacent heart chambers. Stenotic valves have decreased pliability and irregular surfaces; progressive commisural adhesions and valve leaflet dystrophic calcification develops leading to progressive narrowing of the cross-sectional area of valve orifices. Valvular outlet obstruction causes increased turbulence of blood flow. The intensity of turbulence is markedly increased in the jet stream of blood distal to a stenotic valve.[134] Platelets are activated in regions of increased turbulence; the amount of thrombus formed is directly related to valve orifice turbulence.

Distal to stenotic valves, blood flow consists of a central jet stream surrounded by annular eddies that course between the outflow tract walls and the mainstream. These eddies permit blood to remain closer to the irregular valve surfaces than occurs in regions of normal laminar flow. Platelets activated by the turbulent jet stream have prolonged contact with dystrophic irregular valve surfaces, causing adhesion of platelet–fibrin thrombi to valve surfaces, further platelet activation, and formation of thrombi. Valve incompetence also prolongs the time that blood is in contact with abnormal valve surfaces and also promotes thrombus formation. Valve disease often leads to atrial and ventricular enlargement. Left atrial enlargement is especially common in patients with mitral stenosis and mitral insufficiency and can be severe. Enlargement of the left atrium is accompanied by stasis and thrombus formation, especially in the left atrial appendage and in patients who develop atrial fibrillation.

Rheumatic mitral valve disease

Although the incidence of rheumatic fever and rheumatic heart disease has dramatically declined, rheumatic heart

disease is still an important cause of brain embolism. The mitral valve is most often involved. Second in frequency is involvement of the mitral and aortic valves. Isolated rheumatic aortic valve disease is unusual, and the pulmonic and tricuspid valves are seldom the site of important clinical rheumatic valvulitis. The strong association of rheumatic mitral stenosis and stroke has long been recognized.

The normal adult mitral valve cross-sectional area is 4–6 cm.[2,56] Clinical symptoms most often develop when the mitral valve area declines to less than 2 cm.[2,56] The predominant cause of mitral stenosis is rheumatic fever leading to predominant mitral stenosis (especially common among women), mixed mitral stenosis and mitral regurgitation, or predominant mitral regurgitation (more common among men). With rheumatic valvular disease, the mitral leaflets fuse at their edges with thickening of the chordae tendinae. The stenotic mitral valve is typically funnel shaped. Progressive mitral valve obstruction leads to increased intra-atrial pressure and progressive dilation of the left atrium. Fibrosis may also develop in the endothelium of the left atrium. Progressive left atrial dilation, blood stasis, and endocardial surface abnormalities promote thrombus formation, yet the incidence of thromboembolism does not appear to be related to the severity of mitral stenosis.[56,135] Large thrombi within the body of the left atrium, especially "ball" thrombi are almost exclusively seen among patient with rheumatic mitral stenosis (and those with prosthetic mitral valve thrombosis). Although unusual, these ball thrombi are often readily appreciated by transthoracic echocardiography.

Before the availability of anticoagulation, autopsy and surgical series showed an increased risk of clinical thromboembolism in the mitral stenosis population.[136–138] Embolization, especially to the brain, may be the earliest clinical indication of rheumatic mitral stenosis. The frequency of embolism in patients with mitral stenosis ranges in series from 10% to 20%.[139–141] Approximately 50–75% of emboli detected clinically involve the brain. Embolism is more common in patients with mitral stenosis than in those with mitral insufficiency. Although embolism does occur in patients with mitral stenosis who have normal sinus rhythm, the development of atrial fibrillation greatly increases the risk of embolism. In 194 patients with rheumatic heart disease and systemic embolism, Daley et al. found a mitral valve lesion in 97%, atrial fibrillation in 90%, and either a mitral valve lesion or atrial fibrillation in 100%.[142] In a study of 754 patients with chronic rheumatic heart disease followed for more than 5000 patient-years, the incidence of embolism was 1.5% per patient-year.[139] Embolism was seven times more frequent in patients with atrial fibrillation than in those with sinus rhythm. A third of recurrences of embolism occurred during the first month, and two-thirds of recurrences were during the first year after the onset of atrial fibrillation.[139]

Anticoagulants clearly reduce the frequency of recurrent embolism.[143] Mitral valvuloplasty, the predominant treatment of mitral stenosis during the 1960s and 1970s, did not greatly influence the frequency of embolism. The atrial appendage was sometimes removed to prevent lodging of thrombi in this region. Modern diagnostic technology, especially echocardiography, has revolutionized the diagnosis of patients with mitral stenosis and other rheumatic valve lesions. Echocardiography allows quantification of the valve orifice, as well as the effects of the mitral valve disease on the left atrium and left ventricle. These measurements can be performed sequentially to study disease progression and response to treatment. Left atrial and left atrial appendage thrombi are also reliably detected. Superimposed bacterial endocarditis can precipitate brain embolism, although the occurrence of endocarditis in patients with isolated mitral stenosis is unusual.

Rheumatic mitral regurgitation is a less frequent cause of brain embolism than mitral stenosis. Among individuals with embolism in one series, mitral insufficiency is often accompanied by progressive left ventricular hypertrophy. Mitral valve repair and mitral valve replacement are probably important considerations in the prevention of embolism in patients with rheumatic mitral insufficiency.

Aortic valve disease

Most often, the cause of acquired aortic valve disease is not determined. Progressive calcific aortic stenosis commonly develops in patients with congenital bicuspid aortic valves and can also follow rheumatic valvulitis. Calcific degenerative changes are usually well developed during the fourth and fifth decades of life in patients with bicuspid valves, whereas idiopathic calcific aortic stenosis is more prevalent during the sixth to eighth decades.[144] Idiopathic calcific aortic valve disease of the elderly may be caused by an atherosclerotic degenerative process, although definite proof of this hypothesis is not yet available. Microthrombi with evidence of organization have been found at necropsy in about half of stenotic aortic valves. Changes in the aortic valve are progressive. Thickening of previously diseased valves is thought to result from the deposition of fibrin. Fibrin deposits become organized and calcified with resultant distortion of the normal valve architecture. Bicuspid and calcific aortic valves are not able to open freely. Narrowing and irregularity of the valve orifice contributes to turbulent blood flow. Abnormal flow and valve surfaces activate platelets and induce fibrin deposition, accounting for the prevalence of microthrombi along valve surfaces.

Embolism is a much less common occurrence in patients with aortic valve disease when compared with mitral valve disease. Some clinical and necropsy studies show that embolism from calcific aortic valves is probably not rare. Soulie et al. found emboli in 33% of 81 patients with calcific aortic stenosis.[145] In another autopsy study, calcific emboli were found in 37 of 165 patients (22%) with calcific aortic stenosis.[146] Thirty-two emboli were found in the coronary arteries, 11 in the renal vessels, one in the central retinal artery, and one in the MCA. Although the MCA was occluded by a calcific embolus in one patient, no neurological signs were recorded and no infarct was found.[146] During life, calcific emboli have often been identified in the eye because of their typical morphology on fundoscopic examination of the retina. Calcific retinal emboli appear as

white, irregular, immovable densities and are usually distinguishable from bright cholesterol crystals and fibrin–platelet plugs.

In all clinical studies, symptoms that reflect embolization occur more often after cardiac procedures (catheterization and surgery) than occur spontaneously. Aortic valve surgery is especially associated with a high frequency of embolism. Embolism is also more common in patients with bacterial endocarditis superimposed on bicuspid or calcific aortic valves than it is in non-infected valves. The discrepancy between the relatively high frequency of calcific emboli found at necropsy and in the eye and the low frequency of clinically symptomatic brain and visceral organ ischemic events is probably explained by the small size of the embolic particles and the fact that visceral emboli are much harder to diagnose than brain emboli.

Hypertrophic cardiomyopathy, also called idiopathic hypertrophic subaortic stenosis, has become more frequently recognized since the advent of echocardiography. This disorder is characterized by disproportionate and asymmetric hypertrophy of the left ventricular myocardium in the region of the ventricular septum, as compared with the left ventricular free wall. Septal hypertrophy is associated with systolic anterior motion of the mitral valve and variable left ventricular outflow obstruction, depending on myocardial contractility. Structural abnormalities of the mitral valve often accompany hypertrophic cardiomyopathy.[147] The rate of stroke in patients with hypertrophic cardiomyopathy is low. Stroke rarely occurs early in the course of the disease. When stroke occurs, it is usually a result of embolism in relation to atrial fibrillation, bacterial endocarditis, mitral valve dysfunction, or mitral annular calcification. Atrial fibrillation tends to develop late in patients with hypertrophic cardiomyopathy and is often accompanied by left atrial enlargement.[147–149] Mitral annulus calcification is also associated with idiopathic hypertrophic subaortic stenosis.[150]

Little has been written about embolism in patients with aortic insufficiency. Aortic regurgitation is caused by dysfunction of the aortic valve leaflets or aortic root. Rheumatic valvulitis and infective endocarditis are probably the most common causes of aortic leaflet disease causing aortic insufficiency, whereas Marfan's syndrome, aortic dissection, and annulo-aortic ectasia caused by aging and hypertension are the usual causes of aortic root disease. Syphilis was formerly a common cause of aortic valve insufficiency but is now rare. Rheumatic aortic valvulitis and vegetations on the aortic valve are potential sources of brain and systemic embolism in patients with aortic regurgitation.

Mitral valve prolapse

Barlow and Bosman, in an early report of the midsystolic click (mitral valve prolapse (MVP)) syndrome, reported a 23-year-old woman who had transient left arm weakness. Evaluation showed MVP.[151,152] No details of the neurological symptoms or signs were included and the relationship of the neurological event to her heart condition was not considered.[151,152] Since then, a number of case-control and necropsy studies have shown that patients with MVP may have cardiogenic

embolism, but rarely. Cerebrovascular events in patients with MVP have a relatively low recurrence rate, even without treatment.

MVP is the single most frequently diagnosed cardiac valvular abnormality. Estimates of prevalence range from 5% to 21%, with the rate being slightly higher in girls and women.[153] The basic pathological process is disruption of collagen and infiltration of the valve by a myxomatous substance rich in mucopolysaccharide. The mitral valve is often thickened and the chordae tendineae and mitral annulus may also contain myxomatous deposits that can cause elongation of the chordae, sometimes with rupture and dilatation of the mitral valve annulus. Abnormal mitral valve leaflet motion can cause fibrosis and thickening of the endocardial surface of the valve leaflets.[154] The tricuspid and aortic valves sometimes also show myxomatous degeneration. When there is enough slippage, so that a portion of the mitral valve fails to coapt against the rest of the leaflet, then mitral regurgitation develops.

Patients with MVP sometimes have abnormal left ventricular contractions. At necropsy, thrombi have been found, especially in the angle between the posterior leaflet of the mitral valve and the left atrial wall.[152,155,156] Transformation of the normally rigid valve into loose myxomatous tissue results in stretching of the valve leaflets, loss of endothelial continuity, and rupture of subendothelial connective tissue fibers. These changes could promote the formation of platelet–fibrin thrombi on the valve surface.

MVP is diagnosed by echocardiography when there is abnormal posterior movement of the coapted anterior or posterior leaflets (or both) of 2 mm or more, and one or both of the mitral valve leaflets are displaced during systole into the left atrium above the plane of the mitral annulus.[152] Midsystolic "buckling" or pansystolic "hammocking" of the valve leaflets is also sometimes found.[153] Mitral valve thickening and redundancy and the presence of mitral regurgitation are important additional criteria for the presence of important myxomatous mitral valve changes.[157,158] Approximately 8% of patients with MVP develop severe mitral regurgitation, which leads to congestive heart failure and necessitates mitral valve replacement. Atrial fibrillation can occur at any time but is more common in older patients, especially those with mitral regurgitation and large left atria. Myxomatous valves can become infected during bacteremia but the frequency of infective endocarditis is low. MVP occurs in patients with inherited connective tissue disorders, such as Marfan's syndrome, Ehlers–Danlos syndrome, and osteogenesis imperfecta.[152]

The first report of a possible relation between MVP and brain ischemia was by Barnett in 1974.[159] The initial report outlined four patients, but Barnett and his colleagues later expanded the number of cases to 14 patients.[156,160] All patients were relatively young (10–48 years old), and none had cardiovascular risk factors or occlusive vascular lesions. Barnett and colleagues later published a case-control series that provided further evidence of a relationship between MVP and brain ischemia in young patients.[161] Among 6 series of patients with MVP and brain ischemic events reviewed by Lauzier and Barnett,[152] there were 114 patients, including 46 men

and 68 women. Two-thirds of the events were strokes. The remainder were TIAs. Single attacks were more common than multiple ischemic events. Sixteen of the patients had an arrhythmia detected by rhythm monitoring, including eight with atrial fibrillation.[152]

Abnormalities of platelet function have been shown in patients with MVP and thromboembolism. Shortened platelet survival time, an increase in circulating platelet aggregates, and increased levels of beta-thromboglobulin and platelet factor IV were found in patients with MVP.[152] Interaction of circulating platelets with abnormal endocardial and valve structures in patients with myxomatous valve degeneration causes increased platelet aggregation, adhesion, and secretion. Platelet fibrin aggregates adhere to abnormal valve surfaces and later embolize or promote formation of erythrocyte–fibrin clots.

The recurrence rate of stroke in patients with MVP is low. In patients with mitral regurgitation and large left atria, and in those with atrial fibrillation and atrial or valvular thrombi shown by echocardiography, warfarin anticoagulation is probably indicated. In patients who do not have atrial fibrillation, endocarditis, or severe mitral insufficiency, the treatment of choice is probably an antiplatelet aggregant, such as aspirin, aspirin combined with modified-release dipyridamole, or clopidogrel.

Mitral annulus calcification

Mitral annulus calcification (MAC) is a degenerative disorder of the fibrous support structure of the mitral valve that occurs rather commonly in the elderly, especially in women. The most common TTE finding among elderly patients referred for a cardiac source of embolism is a high reflective area in the posterior portion of the mitral annulus representing mitral annular calcification.[56,162,163] MAC is very common in the elderly. A study of over 2000 patients (mean age 81 years) found that 48% had MAC with an increased prevalence of atrial fibrillation (22% vs. 8% without MAC).[162] In addition to age, MAC is associated with hypertension and aortic atherosclerosis.

In the original description of MAC, 4 of the 14 patients described by Korn and colleagues had brain infarcts, and 3 of those 4 had multiple infarcts.[164] The first important description of MAC as a potential cause of stroke was by DeBono and Warlow who studied 151 patients with retinal or brain ischemia and found MAC in 8 patients, as compared with no instances of MAC in age and sex-matched controls who did not have brain or eye ischemia.[165] During the years 1979–1981, 426 men and 733 women in the Framingham Study Cohort (average age 70 years) who did not have strokes had M-mode echocardiograms.[166] Among these 1159 patients, 44 men (10.3%) and 116 women (15.8%) had MAC. During 8 years of follow-up, 51 patients without MAC (5.1%) had strokes, as compared with 22 patients with MAC (13.8%); MAC was associated with a 2.1 RR of stroke (95% confidence interval (CI) 1.24–3.57, $P = 0.006$).[166] A continuous relation was found in this study between frequency of stroke and severity of MAC; each millimeter of thickening on the echocardiogram

represented a RR of stroke of 1.24. Even when patients with atherosclerotic heart disease and congestive heart failure were excluded, patients with MAC still had stroke risk that was two times as high as those without MAC.[166] A recent study explored the role of MAC among 2723 Native Americans who did not have known cardiovascular disease.[167] The presence of MAC but not aortic valve sclerosis proved to be a strong risk factor for incident stroke even after adjusting for multiple other risk factors.[167]

Calcification has a predilection for the posterior portion of the mitral annulus ring. Calcific masses often extend as far as 3.5 cm into the adjacent myocardium and often project superiorly toward the atrium and centrally into the cavity of the left ventricle.[164] Ulceration and extrusion of the calcium through the overlying cusp into the ventricular cavity is found in some patients with MAC studied at necropsy, and thrombi are sometimes attached to the ulcerated regions.[168] Thrombi attached to calcified mitral annuli have also been shown by echocardiography.[167,169,170] Embolic material in patients with MAC can be calcium (as shown in calcific aortic stenosis) or thrombus. MAC is common and is often accompanied by mitral regurgitation, atrial fibrillation, and aortic atheromas. Bacterial endocarditis can be superimposed. Hypertension, coronary atherosclerotic heart disease, and occlusive cerebrovascular disease are also often present in the population of patients with MAC. There are no data on the use of any prophylactic treatment on the prevention of brain or arterial embolism in patients with MAC. The association of MAC and aortic atheroma (84% vs. 33% without MAC) may partially explain the association of MAC with stroke.[171]

Prosthetic cardiac valves

Advances in cardiac diagnosis and surgery have led to increasingly frequent replacement of heart valves. There are more than 80 different models of prosthetic valves, and more than 60 000 valve replacements are performed annually in the United States alone.[142] Some prosthetic valves are now placed percutaneously, introduced through the vascular system. Mechanical valves are made primarily with metal and carbon alloys and are quite thrombogenic. Bioprosthetic valves are most often heterografts derived from pig or cow pericardial or valve tissues mounted on metal supports. Homografts, in the form of preserved human valves, are occasionally used for valve replacements. Bioprosthetic valves have low thrombogenic tendencies (but still higher than native valves), so long-term anticoagulation is ordinarily not prescribed. Bioprosthetic valves are less durable than mechanical valves.[172]

Valve thrombosis is an important complication in patients with both mechanical and bioprosthetic valves. Important valve thrombosis causes pulmonary congestion, reduced cardiac output, and brain and systemic embolism. The frequency of prosthetic-valve thrombosis is estimated to be between 0.1% and 5.7% per year.[173,174] Alteration of blood flow related to mechanical valves, as well as the inherent thrombogenicity of the materials used, promotes thrombosis and thromboembolism. Hematological studies in patients with mechanical valves show elevation of platelet-specific proteins, which indicate

platelet activation and decreased platelet survival in patients with artificial heart valves.[175]

Thrombus formation and subsequent embolization are found most often in mechanical valve prostheses in the mitral or tricuspid position in the setting of suboptimal anticoagulation.[176,177] Evaluation of prosthetic valves, especially prostheses in the mitral position, is best performed by TEE. It is often assumed clinically that patients with mechanical prostheses who present with systemic embolization have prosthetic valve thrombi, especially if there is no other obvious cause and/or the INR is suboptimal. In patients who have thromboembolism and a therapeutic INR, TEE is often helpful in distinguishing valve dysfunction related to pannus ingrowth from thrombus.[56]

The pathophysiological events that promote thromboembolism begin during heart surgery. Prosthetic materials and injured perivalvular tissues cause platelet activation as soon as circulation is restored. Dacron sewing rings, common to all prosthetic valves, form a fertile nidus for platelet activation and adhesion. Prosthetic material also activates the intrinsic pathway of the coagulation cascade. These events promote the formation of red erythrocyte–fibrin thrombi. Degenerative changes in bioprosthetic valves can also stimulate deposition of white platelet–fibrin thrombi. Late thrombosis is also found in the cusp sinuses of bioprosthetic mitral valves that have undergone fibrosis and calcification.

Embolism is an important complication in patients with mechanical and bioprosthetic valves. The frequency of major embolism in patients with mechanical valves is estimated to be 4% per year if no antithrombotic therapy is used.[178] This frequency is reduced to approximately 2% per year by medications that decrease platelet aggregation, and to 1% per year with warfarin anticoagulation.[178] Most symptomatic emboli go to the brain. Patients with mitral mechanical valves have a slightly higher frequency of embolization than those with aortic valves, probably related to the higher frequency of associated atrial fibrillation and large left atria in patients with mitral valve prostheses. Patients with bioprosthetic valves also have a risk of embolism. In one series of 128 patients with porcine bioprosthetic valves inserted during 5–8 years of follow-up, 2 of 43 patients with aortic valve replacement, 9 of 62 with porcine mitral valves, and 4 of 18 with both mitral and aortic prosthetic valves had clinical thromboemboli.[179] Most patients with thromboemboli in this series had atrial fibrillation or heart block.[179] Large left atria, atrial fibrillation, left ventricular dysfunction, and infective endocarditis are important associated conditions in patients with prosthetic valves that cause thromboembolism.

Anticoagulation is recommended for all patients with prosthetic heart valves. Patients with bioprosthetic valves are often treated for the first 3 months after surgery using a target INR of 2.0–3.0. Oral anticoagulant therapy reduces the frequency of embolism in patients with mechanical valve prostheses and the intensity of anticoagulation has been recommended to be higher than that used with bioprosthetic valves. Patients with caged-ball prostheses may require a higher intensity of anticoagulation than those with bileaflet disk valves and those with single-tilting disk valves. Adding antiplatelet medications, such as dipyridamole, aspirin, or clopidogrel, can further reduce the frequency of embolism. Aspirin and lower-intensity anticoagulation (INR of 2.0–3.0) are probably as effective as high-intensity anticoagulation and have less risk of serious bleeding. Because prosthetic valves induce formation of white platelet–fibrin and red erythrocyte–fibrin clots, the use of combined antiplatelet aggregant and anticoagulant therapy makes sense. Pregnant women with prosthetic valves should be treated with heparin or low-molecular-weight heparin because the incidence of thromboemboli is increased while pregnant and also in the puerperium.

Infective endocarditis

Although neurological complications of infective endocarditis have been well recognized since the time of Osler,[180] the clinical spectrum of endocarditis has changed dramatically during the past decades. Compared with series of endocarditis patients performed in the 1960s, series of patients with infective endocarditis reported more recently contain older patients, more drug addicts, more examples of tricuspid valve involvement (usually in intravenous drug addicts), and more patients with infection of prosthetic valves. Diagnostic capabilities have also changed. Echocardiography and newer brain and cerebrovascular imaging techniques allow better clarification of the cardiac and brain pathology and pathophysiology. Brain ischemia, intracerebral hemorrhage, subarachnoid hemorrhage, encephalopathy, and meningitis are the major neurological complications found in series of patients with native valve and prosthetic valve endocarditis.[181–187]

Brain ischemia is invariably caused by embolism. Approximately one-fifth of patients with endocarditis develop brain infarcts. At necropsy, small, usually multiple, cortical or subcortical bland infarcts are found. Larger infarcts are usually attributable to *Staphylococcus aureus* endocarditis. Ischemia can take the form of TIAs that involve the brain or retina. Brain ischemia may be the presenting sign of endocarditis and is most common early in the course of the disease. Ischemic strokes can also occur days after antibiotic treatment has begun. Monitoring of patients with endocarditis using TCD shows that microemboli continue to occur even after antibiotic treatment, although more emboli are detected before and shortly after antibiotics are given. Brain ischemia was described in 17%,[182] 19%,[183] and 15%[186] of patients in various infective endocarditis series.

After congestive heart failure, arterial embolism is the most common life-threatening complication in patients with infective endocarditis. Embolization during the first week of antibiotic treatment is most common,[187] and becomes less frequent thereafter.[188] Late thromboembolism after completion of antibiotic treatment is rare unless recurrent infection develops. Staphylococci and streptococcus species account for greater than 80% of native valve endocarditis.[189] Staphyloccal endocarditis poses a higher risk of clinical thromboembolism compared with other bacterial causes.[182,187,188,190] Fungal endocarditis is also associated with frequent embolism. Mitral valve vegetations have a higher frequency of clinical thromboemboli than aortic valve lesions.[187,191,192]

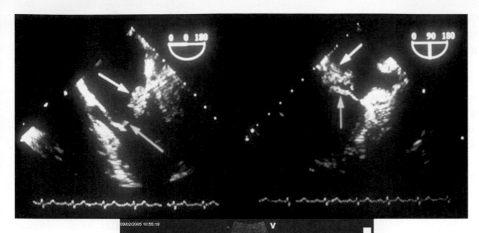

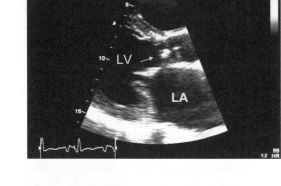

Figure 10.10 Echocardiography showing bacterial vegetations in a patient with infective endocarditis. Top row figures: TEE showing a large vegetation protruding from the posterior mitral leaflet (white arrows) and a much smaller vegetation at the tip of the anterior mitral leaflet (gray arrows). Bottom row figure: Transthoracic echocardiogram in the parasternal long axis view. Note the vegetation (arrow) on the left ventricular outflow tract side of the aortic valve. The left ventricle (LV) and left atrium (LA) are identified. From Caplan LR, Manning WJ. *Brain Embolism.* New York, Informa Healthcare, 2006 with permission.

Infective vegetations appear on echocardiograms as bright, usually mobile echo-dense lesions attached to valve leaflets. Figure 4.35 shows a large vegetation on the mitral valve in a patient with infective endocarditis. Figure 10.10 shows bacterial vegetations in a number of valve regions. The frequency of detection of vegetations on echocardiography depends on the technique used and the frequency of examinations. Lesions smaller than 2 mm are not reliably identified by echocardiography. In the series of Hart et al. (using M-mode and two-dimensional transthoracic echocardiography (TTE)), vegetations were found on 41% of initial echocardiograms in patients with *Staphylococcus aureus* endocarditis, compared with 57% of initial studies in patients with streptococcal species endocarditis.[183] An echocardiogram that fails to show a vegetation does not exclude the diagnosis of endocarditis. A negative TTE should be followed by TEE (with superior spatial resolution) if the clinical suspicion is high or moderate.[193,194] TEE evidence of large (>10 mm) vegetations and increased mobility of the lesions identify patients at high risk for clinical thromboembolism.[194]

Brain hemorrhage is much less frequent than ischemia, but the effects of hemorrhage can be devastating and fatal. Intracerebral hemorrhage was found in 6%,[182] 7%,[183] 2.8%,[185] and 5.6%[186] of patients in various endocarditis series. Series that included modern brain imaging and necropsy studies clarified the mechanisms of intracerebral hemorrhage in endocarditis.[184,195,196] Some patients bleed into bland infarcts. This usually takes the form of hemorrhagic infarction characterized by petechial and larger regions of hemorrhagic mottling within infarcts, without formation of frank, discrete hematomas. In some patients, large hematomas develop. Hematomas are often found in patients treated with anticoagulants. In other patients, intracerebral hemorrhage results from rupture of a septic arteritis caused by embolization of infected material to the artery with necrosis of the arterial wall.[195,196] In a minority of patients, intracerebral hemorrhage is caused by rupture of a mycotic aneurysm into the brain substance. Brain hemorrhage, similar to the situation in patients with brain ischemia, is most common at or near presentation and is less common after effective antibiotic treatment. Many patients who develop brain hemorrhages have had an attack of transient or persistent brain ischemia in the hours or days before the hemorrhage. This prodromal ischemia is explained by an arterial embolus causing brain infarction. Hemorrhage into an infarct or rupture of the artery that received the infected embolus causes the hemorrhage, which often proves fatal.[195,196]

The need for angiography to detect mycotic aneurysms and the indications for surgical treatment of aneurysms found by angiography remain controversial. In a review by Hart et al., among 2119 patients with endocarditis, only 5% of patients with brain hemorrhages had identified mycotic aneurysms.[195] Mycotic aneurysms are caused by embolization of infected material into the wall and adventitia of brain arteries. The aneurysms usually occur distally along arteries and tend to be multiple. The location of aneurysms in patients with infective endocarditis is similar to those found in patients with atrial myxomas, probably because of similar embolic etiologies. In contrast, ordinary saccular "berry" aneurysms occur proximally along the basal arteries of the circle of Willis. More

recently, the advent of gradient echo recall images (T2*-weighted images) shows that some patients with infective endocarditis have tiny round dark regions of susceptibility usually referred to as "microbleeds."[197,198] These are often located within sulci and probably represent small mycotic aneurysms. Angiography of patients without clinical or imaging evidence of intracranial hemorrhage seldom shows mycotic aneurysms. Mycotic aneurysms have been shown to disappear in some patients on sequential angiography performed after bacteriological cure.[199–201] Mycotic aneurysms can rupture, however, sometimes after bacteriological cure, and re-rupture can prove fatal. The decision as to whether to perform angiography and surgical treatment if an aneurysm is found must rest on the clinical findings in individual patients.

Diffuse brain-related symptoms, usually referred to as encephalopathy, are common in patients with endocarditis. Symptoms include lethargy and decreased level of consciousness, confusion, agitation, poor concentration, and reduced memory. Encephalopathy has different explanations. Often, the cause is toxi-metabolic and explained by systemic factors, such as azotemia, pulmonary dysfunction, hyponatremia, and so forth. In many patients, encephalopathy is a toxic effect related to fever and the acute infection. Patients with *S. aureus* acute endocarditis are more often encephalopathic than in endocarditis caused by other organisms. Necropsy, CT, and MRI studies of patients with encephalopathy often show multiple, small, scattered brain infarcts, microabscesses, or both.[184,202] Encephalopathy usually develops during uncontrolled infection with virulent organisms, supporting the role of microscopic septic emboli as the cause.[184]

Meningitis also occurs in patients with endocarditis. Meningeal infection is caused by embolization of infected vegetations to meningeal arteries. The presentation is often headache with fever. Because the usual infecting organism is not virulent, the patient is not as ill as in other acute forms of bacterial meningitis. Meningitis occurred in 6.4%[181] and 1.1%[182] in 2 series of patients with endocarditis.

Valvular vegetations in patients with infective endocarditis are composed of platelets, fibrin, erythrocytes, and inflammatory cells attached to damaged endothelium of native and prosthetic valves. Organisms are enmeshed within the fibrinous material, often deep within the vegetations, explaining why antibiotics have difficulty sterilizing the lesions. Vegetations range in size from several millimeters to several centimeters, and their potential for embolization relate to their size and friability. The mitral valve is most often involved. Mitral valve disease, however, is also more frequent than other valve disease. In the past, the predominant underlying valve disease was rheumatic; calcified valves, MVP, and prosthetic valves now make up a higher proportion of cases than in the past. The neurological complications of native valve and prosthetic valve endocarditis are the same.[182,184,185]

Laboratory studies are helpful in diagnosis, but the clinical findings remain protean, and most important for recognition of infective endocarditis is a strong clinical suspicion. The disease should be suspected in any patient with unexplained fever and a heart murmur. Multiple blood cultures are important in all patients suspected of having infective endocarditis. The spinal fluid may be normal or contain slightly increased protein levels and increased numbers of erythrocytes and leukocytes. Usually, the pleocytosis is moderate (<300 cells/cc) and may be predominantly lymphocytic or polymorphonuclear unless a clinical picture of meningitis is present, in which case there may be more white blood cells. Echocardiography is an important diagnostic test, but, as indicated above, a negative echocardiographic examination does not exclude the diagnosis of infective endocarditis.

The most important treatment is the rapid introduction of specific antimicrobial drugs. Most neurological complications occur before or near the time of diagnosis and initial antibiotic treatment. Recurrent strokes do occur after bacteriological cure, but rarely. In one series among 147 patients discharged from the hospital after treatment of infective endocarditis, 15 developed strokes after discharge; all except one of the stroke patients had prosthetic valve endocarditis.[182] Strokes in this series occurred long after discharge (median, 22 months) and were better explained by recurrence of endocarditis, complications of anticoagulants, and non-infective disease of the prosthetic valves than by cerebrovascular complications of the original endocarditic episode.[182]

Native valve endocarditis is not an indication for anticoagulation, even when brain or systemic embolism has occurred. Controversy surrounds the issue of maintenance of anticoagulation in patients who have mechanical valve endocarditis, but most clinicians favor cautious continuation of anticoagulants unless a brain hemorrhage develops. When a hemorrhagic infarct or brain hemorrhage develops, anticoagulation with warfarin is usually stopped for 1–2 weeks. In patients with a major risk of recurrent embolization, it may be safe to use heparin beginning soon after the hemorrhage is discovered and later switch back to warfarin. Cardiac surgery to debride or replace infected valves is performed for cardiac indications. These include mostly heart failure related to valve dysfunction, lack of control of infection, valve infection with fungal or other virulent organism not controllable by antimicrobial drugs, and valve or chordae tendineae rupture.

Non-infective fibrous and fibrinous endocardial lesions (including valve strands)

In a variety of other circumstances, fibrous valve thickening, often with grossly visible vegetations that contain mixtures of platelets and fibrin, are found on the heart valves and adjacent endocardium in patients who have no evidence of rheumatic fever or bacterial endocarditis. The first detailed description of such lesions was by Libman and Sacks, who reported four patients studied clinically and pathologically with an "atypical verrucous endocarditis."[203] Necropsy showed fibrous thickening of valves with vegetations, especially along the closure lines of the valves and on the valve leaflets. The vegetations spread to the papillary muscles and ventricular endocardium. Only one patient had prominent clinical neurological abnormalities, a unilateral paralysis and seizures that developed just before death. The authors speculated that these findings might be

caused by emboli from the valvular vegetations. Libman and Sacks were uncertain of the diagnosis but noted that the clinical findings resembled some of the erythematous diseases.[203] The next year, Klemperer et al. published the pathological findings in disseminated lupus erythematosus.[204] In 1935, Baehr and colleagues reported a series of 23 patients who had acute disseminated lupus erythematosus, among whom 13 patients had a non-rheumatic verrucous endocarditis similar to that described by Libman and Sacks.[205] These clinical and pathological reports brought the disease systemic lupus erythematosus (SLE), known previously as predominantly a skin disorder, to the attention of the medical community as an acute disseminated systemic disease.

Gross, a younger colleague of Libman and Sacks at Mount Sinai Hospital in New York in 1940, reported a detailed study of 27 hearts, 23 of which were fatal cases of SLE.[206] Gross pointed out that the patients in the original report of Libman and Sacks from the Mount Sinai Hospital[203] had the typical clinical findings of lupus erythematosus and suggested that the verrucous endocardial lesions were diagnostic of that disease.[206] Libman and Sacks[203] and Gross[206] were aware that similar endocarditic lesions also occurred in terminal or cachectic diseases, such as carcinoma, tuberculosis, and leukemia, and were called non-bacterial thrombotic endocarditis. Since these early reports, similar lesions of the cardiac valves and endocardium are known to occur in patients with SLE, antiphospholipid antibody (APLA) syndrome, and marantic non-bacterial thrombotic endocarditis (NBTE). All likely have a similar pathogenesis.

Valvular lesions are common in patients with SLE. Roldan et al. performed TEE on 69 SLE patients on 2 occasions, averaging 29 months between echocardiograms.[207] Valvular abnormalities were found in 61% of patients on the initial TEE, and in 53% on the second echocardiographic study. Valve thickening (61%), vegetations (43%), valve regurgitation (25%), and stenosis (4%) were found on the initial echocardiograms. The mitral valve was most often involved, followed closely by involvement of the aortic valve; tricuspid valve disease occurred occasionally, but pulmonic valve involvement was rare. The combined incidence of stroke, peripheral embolism, heart failure, and superimposed infective endocarditis was 22% in those with valvular disease found on TEE.[207] In a 2007 review of 38 SLE patients who had Libman–Sacks endocarditis, valvular involvement correlated with the duration of SLE and the presence of APLA and clinical thromboses.[208]

The APLA syndrome was first recognized during the 1970s as a prothrombic syndrome separate from SLE. The APLA syndrome is characterized by frequent fetal loss, strokes, myocardial infarcts, phlebothrombosis, pulmonary emboli, and thrombocytopenia. Serological testing reveals positive assays for the lupus anticoagulant, anticardiolipin antibodies, or both. Echocardiographic studies have shown that there is a relatively high frequency of cardiac valvular lesions in patients with the APLA syndrome, and that the valve lesions are indistinguishable from those found in patients with SLE. Figure 10.11 is a TEE and surgical specimen of a valve with a fibrinous vegetation in a young man with APLA syndrome. Barbut et al.

studied the prevalence of antiphospholipid antibodies among 87 patients in whom echocardiography showed mitral or aortic regurgitation, or both;[209] 26 patients (30%) had immunoglobulin G or M anticardiolipin antibodies. Focal brain ischemic events occurred in eight of these patients (seven judged embolic), including seven of the immunoglobulin G anticardiolipin-positive patients.[209] In another report, Barbut and colleagues studied 21 patients with APLA antibodies who had focal brain ischemic events.[210] Twelve of 14 stroke patients (86%), and 3 of 7 non-stroke patients (42%) had echocardiographic evidence of mitral or aortic valve abnormalities. Eight of the 21 patients with APLA had SLE in this study.[210]

In a large cooperative study performed by the Antiphospholid Antibodies in Stroke Study Group, among 128 patients who had brain or ocular ischemia and were APLA positive, 16 patients (12.5%) had mitral valve abnormalities on echocardiograms, and two patients had aortic valve lesions.[211] Phospholipids are important constituents of cardiac valve endothelium, blood platelets, vascular endothelium, and coagulation proteins. At present, most assays for antiphospholipid antibodies only include testing for lupus anticoagulant and anticardiolipin antibodies. Some patients with the clinical features of APLA syndrome have valve vegetations and cardiogenic brain embolism, but antibody assays are negative.

Hypercoagulability and NBTE have long been known to occur in patients with cancer and other debilitating chronic diseases. Most often, the cancers are mucinous adenocarcinomas.[212] In one study of 20 cancer patients who had thromboembolic disease of the brain and other organs, 16 patients (80%) had NBTE at necropsy.[213] Edoute et al. performed prospective echocardiograms on 200 cancer patients and found a 19% frequency of NBTE.[214] The valve lesions equally involved the mitral and aortic valves. Elevated plasma D-dimer levels, a marker for hypercoagulability, was also often found in cancer patients with clinical thromboembolism.[214] NBTE is characterized by friable white or tan vegetations, usually along lines of valve closure. The vegetations can be large. Microscopy usually shows degenerating platelets interwoven with strands of fibrin and some leukocytes, forming eosinophilic masses of tissue. All three conditions – SLE, APLA syndrome, and NBTE-are associated with hypercoagulability, strokes, and thrombocytopenia. The cardiac valve and endothelial lesions in these three conditions are similar and probably indistinguishable grossly and microscopically. Platelet deposition, incorporation of fibrin, and the formation of platelet thrombi on valve and endocardial surfaces are common to all three conditions. Treatment of these conditions has not been formally studied. In theory, drugs that alter platelet aggregation, secretion, and adhesion might be effective. In patients with SLE and APLA syndrome who have hypercoagulability, heparin and warfarin compounds are usually prescribed to treat the hypercoagulablity and prevent venous and arterial occlusions.

Non-infective valve lesions are also found in patients with carcinoid tumors (probably causally related to elevated serotonin levels in the blood) and after the use of some

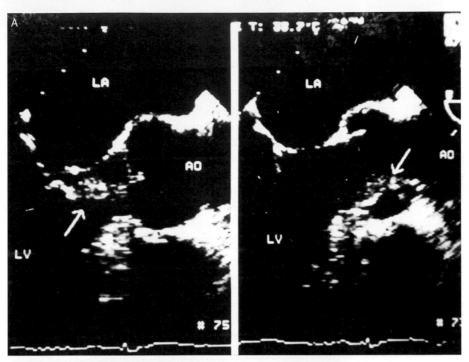

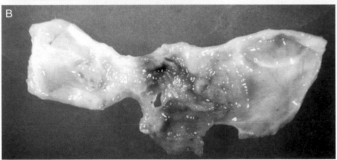

Figure 10.11 Mitral valve vegetations in a patient with APLA syndrome and multiple brain emboli. (A) Echocardiography showing a pedunculated, mobile lesion on the mitral valve (white arrows). AO, aorta; LA, left atrium; LV, left ventricle. (B) Mitral valve removed surgically showing vegetations. A black and white version of this figure will appear in some formats. From Caplan LR, Manning WJ. *Brain Embolism*. New York: Informa Healthcare, 2006 with permission. For the color version, please refer to the plate section.

drugs (ergotamine, methysergide, dexfenfluramine, and fen-fluramine and phentermine, cabergoline, and pergolide).[215,216] The valve and endocardial lesions that result are similar to each other morphologically and consist of fibrotic thickening of the valves with reduced pliability.

Echocardiographic examinations often show strands of mobile tissue attached to valve surfaces. The cause and significance of these strands remains uncertain. In 1856, Lambl had originally described such filamentous outgrowths from the ventricular surfaces of the aortic valves sometimes found at necropsy,[217] so these fibrous strand-like lesions have often been called Lambl excrescences. Later, Magarey found similar filiform strands on the atrial surface of mitral valves.[218] The strands, which were composed of a cellular connective tissue core covered by endothelium, were usually less than 1 mm thick and ranged in length from 1 to 10 mm.[218] Magarey related the strands to mitral valve thickening and posited that they originated from fibrinous deposits on valve surfaces.[218] Echocardiographic examinations show these valve excrescences as thin, elongated, mobile echoreflective structures with independent undulating hypermobility seen near the leaflet's line of closure. They are found on the atrial side of the mitral valve,

and the ventricular side of the aortic valve and are increasingly recognized in elderly patients undergoing echocardiography.[219]

Freedberg et al. reviewed retrospectively a series of 1559 patients with TEEs during a 2-year period and found mitral valve strands in 63 patients (4%) and aortic valve strands in 26 patients (1.7%).[220] Strands were found in 10.6% of patients referred because of suspected recent embolic events, compared with 2.3% of those referred for other indications.[220] Roberts and colleagues compared the frequency of strands among patients referred for TEE because of brain ischemia and those referred for other indications and also found an association between brain ischemia and strands.[221] The association was strongest for younger patients and those with mitral and aortic valve strands.[221] Cohen et al. found strands in 22.5% of 338 brain ischemia patients versus 12.1% of 276 patients who had no history of brain ischemia (OR 2, 95% CI 1.3–3.4, $P < 0.005$).[222] The risk of recurrent stroke in patients with strands was low.[222] Strands are often found in patients with mitral valve thickening.[222,223] Strands probably form because of a degenerative process that causes fibrinous deposits on valve surfaces. Emboli can arise from the abnormal valves, strands, or thrombi formed on the surface of the valve or on

the strands. In some patients, strands may share a pathogenesis with valve lesions found in patients with SLE, APLAs, and cancer.

Nighoghossian et al. reported three patients who had brain ischemic events presumably related to mitral valve strands who had cardiac surgery.[224] Extensive evaluation including cerebral angiography and serological testing showed no cause for stroke other than the valve lesions. The valve lesions were described as: a floating mass 6 mm thick on the ventricular surface of the mitral valve; a 6 mm lesion on the anterior mitral valve leaflet; and a sessile 5 mm lesion on the anterior mitral valve leaflet.[225] One patient had urgent cardiac surgery when the valve lesion was found; the other two patients had surgery when they had recurrent strokes despite anticoagulant therapy. Histopathological examinations showed that the lesions were composed of an acellular fibrous core with rings of granular material and endothelial cells. In two patients, thrombi were attached to the lesions.[224]

Treatment of patients with strands has not been formally studied but anticoagulants were unsuccessful in preventing brain emboli in two of the patients of Nighoghossian et al.[224] and may not be effective in patients with NBTE. Antiplatelet aggregants, or a combination of antiplatelet aggregants and anticoagulants, might be more effective in preventing thrombus formation and embolism than either agent alone.

Myocardial and cardiac chamber lesions

Myocardial infarction and coronary artery disease

Systemic embolism is apparent clinically in approximately 3% (range 0.6–6.4%) of patients with acute myocardial infarction.[2,56,225,226] Most clinically detected emboli involve the brain. Most strokes that occur in patients with acute myocardial infarcts are caused by embolization of thrombi formed in the left ventricle, but some strokes are caused by left atrial thrombi, hypotension, and extracranial occlusive vascular disease. Coronary artery thrombosis can cause an increase in acute phase reactants, including serine protease coagulation proteins. Venous thromboses and occlusion of atherostenotic craniocervical arteries develop in the days and weeks after myocardial infarction because of this hypercoagulability.

The risk of stroke and thrombus formation is related to infarct location (anterior at higher risk) and infarct size. In the Italian GISSI-3 trial, the incidence of left ventricle thrombus among those with an anterior infarction increased to almost 18% for patients with a left ventricle ejection fraction of less than 40% as compared with less than 10% of those with a higher ejection fraction.[227] The corresponding frequency for infarctions at non-anterior sites ranges between 1.8% and 5.4%.[55,227–230] Most thrombi form on the apical wall of the left ventricle in regions of reduced ventricular contractility. Mural thrombi are more likely to form in patients with transmural and large anterior myocardial infarcts than in those with small infarcts. Areas of decreased ventricular contractility, low ejection fraction, and development of a left ventricular aneurysm predispose to thrombus formation. Figure 10.12 shows a

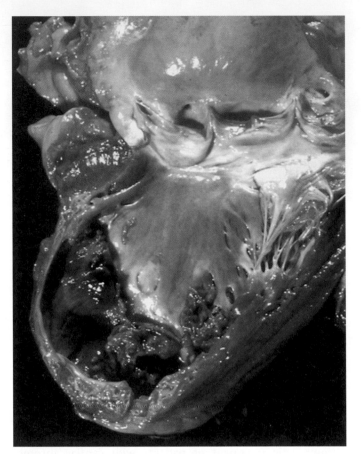

Figure 10.12 Heart at necropsy in a patient with a massive brain embolus. There is a large clot overlying a recent myocardial infarct.

large thrombus in the left ventricle of a patient with a fatal recent myocardial infarct.

Cardiac thrombi often develop within the first 3 days after myocardial infarction, especially in those patients with large infarcts, but can develop later. Using serial TTE, most thrombi are found to develop within the first 2 weeks after infarction (median 5–6 days).[231–233] While some patients develop a new left ventricle thrombus, most often it is in association with worsening left ventricle systolic function.[233,234] Thrombus mobility and protrusion are associated with increased risk of stroke.[235]

Systemic embolization occurs, on average, 14 days after myocardial infarction and is unusual after 4–6 weeks.[236] Anticoagulants reduce the frequency of stroke in patients with acute myocardial infarcts. Among 999 patients with acute myocardial infarction, short-term warfarin treatment for 28 days reduced the rate of stroke (0.8% vs. 3.8% in non-anticoagulated controls, P < 0.001).[237]

Regions of decreased ventricular contraction and frank ventricular aneurysms often persist after acute myocardial infarction. In the Coronary Artery Surgery Study (CASS), 7.6% of patients had angiographically defined left ventricular aneurysms.[238] Although aneurysms are relatively common and mural thrombi often form within aneurysms, the risk of stroke is relatively low, at approximately 5%.[239] The risk of stroke in patients with impaired left ventricular function after

myocardial infarction is substantial. In one study of 2231 patients with left ventricular dysfunction after acute myocardial infarction who were followed for an average of 42 months, 103 patients (4.6%) developed strokes.[240] Patients with ejection fractions of less than 28% were at highest risk, and for every absolute decrease of 5% in the left ventricular ejection fraction, the risk of stroke increased by 18%.[240]

Some patients with brain embolism are unexpectedly found to have thrombi within their left ventricles. These thrombi are most often detected with TTE, which has a reported sensitivity and specificity greater than 90%.[55,241–243] The use of intravenous echo contrast agents can assist with the discrimination between apical trabeculations and thrombus.[55] While detection of apical left ventricle thrombi have been reported,[228] the frequent inability of TEE to visualize the true left ventricle apex makes TEE a less appropriate imaging test for suspected left ventricle apical thrombi. Delayed enhancement cardiac magnetic resonance may be superior to both TTE and TEE for identifying left ventricular thrombi.

Some patients with left ventricular thrombi do not have a history of acute myocardial infarction, and the cardiac cavity lesions may be mistaken for myxomas or other cardiac tumors. Sequential echocardiography shows that these thrombi can gradually regress or suddenly disappear,[4] often without development of neurological or other symptoms of embolism. Thrombus formation, spontaneous endogenous fibrinolysis, and fragmentation of thrombi are dynamic processes. Thrombolytic treatment of patients with cardiac thrombi poses the theoretical risk of fragmentation of large thrombi into portions that could embolize and cause stroke, myocardial infarction, and systemic embolism. Thrombi may disappear during anticoagulation without symptoms or signs of embolism.

Myocardiopathies

Conditions that affect the endocardium and myocardium promote the formation of cardiac mural thrombi and systemic and brain embolism. The three most important factors that determine thrombus formation are: (1) involvement of the endocardial surface; (2) ventricular contractility and blood flow and ejection patterns within the ventricles; and (3) activation of platelets and the coagulation system. Among the three categories of cardiomyopathies – dilated, restrictive, and hypertrophic – mural thrombus formation and embolism are most common among the dilated cardiomyopathies. Intraventricular thrombus formation is enhanced by stasis of blood and the loss of normal subendocardial trabeculation. The network of subendocardial trabeculae functions as many small compartments that produce high levels of force within the ventricle, propelling blood away from the endocardial surface.[244]

Conditions as diverse as muscular dystrophies, cardiac amyloidosis, peripartum cardiomyopathy, Fabry's disease, cocaine-related cardiomyopathy, non-compaction of the myocardium, and cardiac sarcoidosis are sources of cardiac-origin embolism. Morbid obesity is also associated with a myocardiopathy.[245] The Japanese and others described a myocardiopathy associated with emotional distress referred to as takotsubo cardiomyopathy.[246,247] Takotsubo is the Japanese name of an octopus trap shaped like an ampulla. This name has been applied to the cardiomyopathy because of a characteristic apical ballooning of the heart recognizable on echocardiography that resembles the Japanese octopus trap. Takotsubo changes are known to occur after severe emotional duress and after subarachnoid hemorrhage. Like other disorders of the heart muscle, takotsubo cardiomyopathy is occasionally a source of brain embolism.

In patients with cardiomyopathies, mural thrombi form mostly within the trabeculae carneae near the cardiac apex. Atrial fibrillation develops in some patients with cardiomyopathies and further increases the frequency of embolism. Embolism is unusual in patients with hypertrophic cardiomyopathies unless they develop atrial fibrillation.

Cardiac myxomas and other tumors

Primary cardiac tumors are rare, occurring in less than 0.03% of autopsy studies, with myxomas constituting almost 60% of these lesions.[248] Although cardiac tumors are rare, they are an important cause of brain embolism. Myxomas are the most common heart tumor. Myxomas are histologically benign tumors that most often are found within the body of the left atrium. They are usually attached to the mid-portion of the interatrial septum at the edge of the fossa ovalis, but some originate from the posterior or anterior atrial walls or the auricular appendage.[249] Figure 10.13 is a TEE that shows a typical left atrial myxoma attached to the interatrial septum. Approximately 75% are located in the left atrium and 15–20% in the right atrium.[249] Approximately 6–8% of myxomas are found in the ventricles equally divided between the left and right ventricles.[249] Myxomas rarely arise from the heart valves. Bi-atrial myxomas have been described, in which case the tumor usually projects into the contralateral atrium through

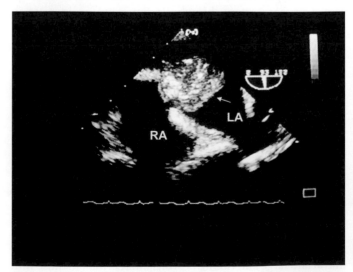

Figure 10.13 TEE in a patient with a large left atrial myxoma (white arrow) within the left atrium (LA) attached to the interatrial septum in the area of the foramen ovale. RA, right atrium. From Caplan LR, Manning WJ. *Brain Embolism*. New York: Informa Healthcare, 2006 with permission.

a PFO. Myxomas project from their endocardial attachments into cardiac chambers. Myxomas are most often found in patients between the ages of 30 and 60 years; women are affected slightly more than men, and there are instances of familial occurrence of myxomas.

Embolism occurs in 30–50% of patients with cardiac myxomas.[249,250] Most emboli arise from the left atrium and travel to the brain or systemic organs. The mobility of the myxomas is related more to the likelihood of embolism than the size of the tumors.[251] Occasionally, right atrial myxomas cause systemic embolism in the presence of a PFO. Both white and red thrombi tend to form on the surface of the myxomas. Emboli consist of tumor fragments, particles of thrombi, or both.

Occasionally, patients with brain emboli from myxomas have subarachnoid or intracerebral hemorrhage. Bleeding is related to the development of hemorrhagic infarction or rupture of aneurysms. Embolism from myxoma tissue to the wall of brain arteries causes aneurysms that are identical to mycotic aneurysms found in patients with bacterial endocarditis. Usually, the aneurysms are relatively small, multiple, and located on peripheral branches of brain arteries. Some aneurysms are quite large. The peripheral location of aneurysms in patients with myxomas and endocarditis differs from that usually found in patients with saccular ("berry") aneurysms. Delayed progressive brain ischemia and enlargement of aneurysms can develop after the initial embolic event. Although delayed growth and rupture of aneurysms and metastatic tumor growth do occur, their frequency is low. In a review of 35 patients followed at the Mayo Clinic after surgical removal of atrial myxomas, none had subsequent delayed neurological events attributable to their myxomas.[252] Recurrent cardiac tumors after surgery can, however, give rise to recurrent embolization.

Papillary fibroelastomas are another type of cardiac tumor that often give rise to brain embolism.[250,253–257] The lesions consist of multiple papillary fronds that radiate from an avascular fibrocollagenous core attached by a short pedicle to the endothelium. These tumors are usually highly spherical, highly mobile pedunculated tumors most commonly located on the aortic or mitral valves. Less often, they are found on endocardial surfaces. On echocardiograms, papillary fibroelastomas appear speckled with echolucencies near the edges.[256] These tumors classically are not associated with valvular dysfunction, but they may be a source of systemic embolization due to migration of thrombus from the tumor surface[256] or tumor embolization.[253] Angina and coronary ischemia are caused by embolism to the coronary arteries. Multiple brain infarcts usually occur before the diagnosis is made by echocardiography.

Both TTE and TEE are highly sensitive in detecting myxomas and papillary fibroelastomas, though TEE may provide more accurate anatomical details, such as the site of attachment, and, in selected patients, may help to differentiate these tumors from thrombi.[55] Rhabdomyomas are often multiple, arise from the ventricular myocardium, and project into the ventricular cavity. Tuberous sclerosis and neurofibromatosis predispose to the development of cardiac rhabdomyomas.

Emboli are often composed of tumor fragments. Theoretically, white platelet–fibrin nidi might develop on the surface and crevices of cardiac tumors, as might red erythrocyte–fibrin thrombi. For this reason, agents that affect platelet aggregation and function and standard anticoagulants might have some therapeutic effect, but no studies of their use in patients with myxomas or other cardiac neoplasms have been performed. The only definitive treatment is surgery.

Paradoxical embolism and cardiac septal lesions

The topic of paradoxical embolism and PFO has received much greater attention recently than in the past, largely because of the improved cardiac technology that can recognize the presence of a PFO. Paradoxical emboli are those that enter the systemic circulation through right-to-left shunting of blood. By far, the most common potential intracardiac shunt is a residual PFO. The high frequency of PFOs in the normal population makes it difficult to be certain in an individual stroke patient with a PFO whether paradoxic embolism through the PFO was the cause of their stroke or whether the PFO was merely an incidental finding.

Because the nomenclature is confusing it is worthwhile to review the embryology of the division of the common atrium into left and right atria. The interatrial septum begins to form during the fifth week of uterine life.[258] The septum primum grows caudally from the superior portion of the single atrium and fuses with the endocardial cushion closing the defect called the ostium primum. Another potential defect forms from partial resorption of the septum primum and is called the ostium secundum. A second septum, the septum secundum, arises from the superior portion of the atrium and descends on the right side of the septum primum to cover the ostium secundum. The ostium secundum is not covered completely because of the presence of the foramen ovale. The foramen ovale consists of the septum primum and septum secundum which are joined parallel to a slitlike valve. This valve allows oxygenated blood to bypass the pulmonary circulation of the fetus during intrauterine life.[258] A PFO is necessary during fetal life to facilitate shunting of blood from the right atrium to the left atrium, thereby bypassing the high resistance pulmonary circuit. The lungs are not aerated during intrauterine existence. At birth or shortly thereafter, the septum primum and the septum secundum usually fuse, closing the interatrial septum to the flow of blood. Ostium secundum atrial septal defects occur when there is excess resorption of the septum primum or inadequate formation of the septum secundum. A PFO occurs when fusion of the septum primum with the septum secundum is inadequate.

In a significant number of individuals the foramen ovale remains somewhat patent during adult life. The prevalence of a patent foramen ovale (PFO) varies depending on its definition. Autopsy series have shown that approximately 30% of adults have a probe PFO at necropsy.[259] Hagen et al. studied 956 patients with clinically and pathologically normal hearts and found a PFO in 27.3%.[259] The frequency of PFOs declined with age – 34.3% during the first 3 decades of life, 25.4% during the 4th–8th decades, and 20.2% during the 9th and 10th decades. The average diameter of PFOs was 4.9 mm, and the size tended to increase with age.[259] Echocardiographic studies have shown that PFOs are found more often in patients with stroke than in

Table 10.4 Conditions predisposing to venous thrombosis and pulmonary and paradoxical embolism

Blood coagulation disorders
  Deficiencies of antithrombin III, protein C, protein S, plasminogen
  Activated protein C resistance with or without factor V Leiden
  Prothrombin gene mutation
  Dysfibrinogenemia
  Elevated levels of factors VIII, IX, XI
  Very high blood fibrinogen levels
  Very high homocysteine levels

Lower limb paralysis

Prolonged sitting, e.g., airplane or car trip

Cancer

Acute inflammatory conditions (e.g., Crohn's disease, ulcerative colitis)

Surgery

Limb trauma

Pregnancy

Antiphospholipid antibody syndrome

Female hormone use

Immobilization often with a cast

Obesity

Central venous catheters

controls, and PFOs are more common in patients with an undetermined cause of stroke ("cryptogenic stroke") than in those in whom another etiology has been defined.[260–262]

Table 10.4 lists the major risk factors for venous thrombosis. We use the following five criteria for paradoxic embolism: (1) situations that promote thrombosis of leg or pelvic veins (e.g., sitting in one position for a long period, recent surgery, and so forth); (2) increased coagulability (e.g., the use of oral contraceptives, presence of Leiden factor with resistance to activated protein C, dehydration); (3) sudden onset of stroke during sexual intercourse, straining at stool, or other activity that includes a Valsalva's maneuver or promotes right-to-left shunting of blood; (4) pulmonary embolism within a short time before or after the neurological ischemic event; and (5) the absence of other putative causes of stroke after thorough evaluation. When at least four of these criteria are met, the diagnosis of paradoxical embolism is highly probable.

One typical patient was a 29-year-old woman who returned home from a trip with her husband and 4 children. The day was hot and she had nothing to drink during the 8-hour car ride. Much of the ride was spent disciplining the children while she kneeled on her seat facing the children, who cavorted in the back of the station wagon. When she and her husband got home, they fed the children and put them to bed. She showered and, immediately thereafter, had sex with her husband. At the point of climax, she became unable to speak and her right arm was weak and numb. Examination

showed a right hemiparesis and aphasia. CT showed a left-upper division MCA-territory infarct. Echocardiography showed a large PFO with increased flow during a Valsalva's maneuver. The heart and aorta were otherwise normal, and an MRA examination of the cervico-cranial arteries was normal. She made a good recovery but had residual right hand numbness and dysnomia.

Gautier and colleagues reported on 29 patients who had paradoxical embolism and reviewed 31 patients reported by others.[263] Situations that promoted venous occlusions among these 60 patients included surgery, postpartum, lower extremity injury, and jugular vein catheterization. Strokes occurred after sex, straining at stool, weight lifting, vigorous nose blowing, asthmatic attacks, gymnastics, decompressing the ears, and martial arts. Venous thrombosis was detected in few patients, and few had clinical pulmonary emboli. Pulmonary radionuclide scans, angiography, and necropsy showed pulmonary emboli in many patients.[263] The most common territory of stroke was the MCA, which was involved in 25 patients. Fifteen patients (37.5%) had vertebrobasilar-territory embolic infarcts, a proportion more than expected by chance, because only 20% of blood flow to the brain goes through the posterior circulation. A study of the distribution of microemboli in patients with PFOs also showed that there is an unexplained predilection for embolic material to go to posterior circulation arteries.[264] Another study showed that patients in whom shunting through a PFO was provoked by a valsalva maneuver (as compared to those who had constant shunting at rest) had a predisposition to posterior circulation embolism (73% vs. 28%).[265]

Paradoxic embolism also occurs through ventricular septal defects, atrial septal defects, and pulmonary arteriovenous fistulas. Venous thrombosis can be detected if studies are performed early in the course. Some venous thrombi involve the pelvic veins and might be detected by abdominal and pelvic imaging techniques.

A PFO can be identified non-invasively using TTE and/or TEE with intravenous agitated saline contrast. Microbubbles appear in the left atrium within 3–5 beats of full opacification of the right atrium. Imaging is usually performed at rest and with maneuvers that transiently increase right atrial pressure so as to promote right-to-left shunting – including Valsalva maneuver release and cough. Imaging with cough provides the highest sensitivity. The size of the shunt is graded semi-qualitatively with less than 10 bubbles considered "trivial," 10–30 bubbles considered a "small shunt" and greater than 30 bubbles suggesting a large shunt.[260] TEE is more sensitive than TTE.[55,266] Administration of saline contrast from the groin is probably superior to introduction from the antecubital fossa.[267] The relative quantity of contrast (or severity of right-to-left shunting) appearing in the left atrium after venous injection appears to be associated with increased risk.[268,269] Occasionally an echocardiogram can capture the presence of a thrombus traversing a PFO as is shown in Figure 10.14.

TCD has also been used effectively to diagnose the presence of right-to-left cardiac or pulmonary shunting.[270–272] The technique involves injection of a small amount of saline that has been agitated vigorously with a small amount of air, or

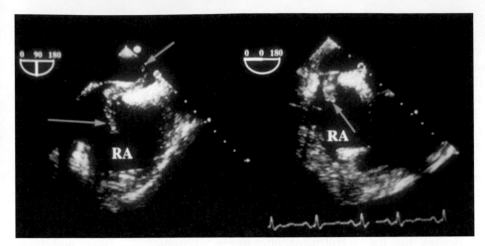

Figure 10.14 TEE in a patient who presented with an ischemic stroke. A thrombus (white arrows) is imaged in transit through the intra-atrial septum. RA, right atrium. From Caplan LR, Manning WJ. *Brain Embolism.* New York: Informa Healthcare, 2006 with permission.

mixed with a polygeline contrast agent, and injected into a cubital vein.[271] During and after the injection, the MCA is insonated using TCD. Appearance of microbubbles in the MCA within the first 3–5 cardiac cycles (<10 s) indicates the presence of right-to-left shunting of blood. Figure 4.18 shows the appearance of microembolic signals produced by air bubbles during a test for the presence of right-to-left blood shunting. The test is usually done with and without a Valsalva's maneuver. The technique has the advantage of being able to be used at the bedside because TCD is portable. Real-time MRI during injection of a gadolinium-based contrast agent is another method of showing a right-to-left shunt.[273]

Atrial septal aneurysms (ASAs) have recently received increased attention in relation to their possible role in contributing to brain embolism. Fusion of the septum primum closes the foramen ovale and leads to a depression on the right side of the interatrial septal wall. Bulging of the septum primum tissue of the atrial septum through the fossa ovalis into either the right or left atria is an ASA. A strong association exists between ASAs and interatrial shunts. ASAs are less common than a PFO and are usually defined by echocardiography as bulging/septal mobility in the region of the fossa ovalis due to redundant atrial septal tissue.[274] The amount of septal excursion for an ASA is usually defined as the sum of the greatest leftward and rightward deflections of at least 10 or 15 mm. Prevalence in the normal population is estimated to be 0.5% by TTE[275] and up to 5% by TEE.[276,277] An ASA is often associated with a PFO, with over 50% of patients with an ASA having a coexistent PFO.[278,279] The mechanism for stroke in ASA has been ascribed to coexistent PFO, tendency for atrial arrhythmias,[280] and formation of a thrombus in the neck of the aneurysm due to an irregular surface.[281] The risk of ASA in the absence of PFO is uncertain.

Cabanes et al. studied the frequency of ASAs, PFO, and MVP among 100 fully evaluated stroke patients younger than 55 years and 50 controls.[282] ASAs were found in 28% of stroke patients and 8% of controls. A PFO was found in 72% of patients with ASAs and 25% of patients without ASAs. The presence of an ASA (OR 4–3, 95% CI 1.3–14.6, $P = 0.01$) or a PFO (OR 3–9, 95% CI 1.5–10.0, $P = 0.003$) was strongly associated with cryptogenic stroke. The stroke OR of a patient with both an ASA and a PFO were 33.3 times (95% CI 4.1–270.0) the stroke OR of a patient who had neither. ASAs with more than 10 mm excursion

were 8 times more likely to be associated with stroke than those with smaller excursions.[282] The presence of MVP in this study did not increase the odds of cryptogenic stroke. One prospective intraoperative study found that the incidence of embolic strokes associated with an atrial septal defect was quite low.[277]

Predictors for the likelihood of paradoxic embolism through PFOs have been sought using TEE.[269,283] In one study, the presence of an ASA accompanying the PFO was an important finding, favoring the presence of paradoxic embolism.[283] In another study, PFOs were significantly larger, and more microbubbles were present in patients with cryptogenic stroke than in those with identified causes of stroke.[269] Electrocardiographic findings can also suggest the presence of PFOs and ostium secundum atrial septal defects. An M-shaped notch on the ascending branch or on the peak of the R-wave in inferior electrocardiographic leads (II, III, aVF) is often found in patients with PFOs or atrial septal defects.[284] This notched pattern has been called *crochetage* because of its resemblance morphologically to a crochet needle.

Some studies analyzed the recurrence rate of stroke in patients with PFOs and the effect of various treatments on recurrence.[4,285,286] Bogousslavsky and his Swiss colleagues studied stroke recurrence among 140 consecutive patients who had PFOs and brain ischemic events.[285] One-fourth of the patients also had ASAs. During a mean follow-up period of 3 years, the stroke or death rate was 2.4% per year. Among these patients, only 8 had a recurrent brain infarct (1.9% per year).[285] Ninety-two patients (66%) took aspirin (250 mg/day), 37 patients (26%) were given anticoagulants, and 11 patients (8%) had surgical closure of the PFO within 12 weeks of the stroke after being treated with anticoagulants. No significant difference was found in the effect of any of the treatments on recurrence. The relatively low rate of recurrence contrasted with the severity of the initial stroke, which left disabling effects in one-half of the patients.[285]

In a French multicenter study, 132 cryptogenic stroke patients with PFOs, ASAs, or both, were followed for an average of 22.6 months.[286] The recurrence rate was approximately 2–3% at 2 years and was higher in patients with both PFOs and ASAs. Recurrences occurred in four patients who were taking antiplatelet agents, and in one patient treated with anticoagulants.[286] Lausanne investigators found no recurrence of stroke during an average follow-up of 2 years among

30 patients who had suture closure of PFOs during cardiopulmonary bypass surgery.[287] None of the patients were given antiaggregants or anticoagulants after surgery. No serious surgical complications occurred. After surgery, two patients had interatrial shunting determined by TCD and TEE, but the shunts were much smaller than before surgery.[287] Presently some cardiothoracic surgeons are closing PFOs through small incisions – so-called minimally invasive surgery – but the success and complication rates are unknown as yet.

PFOs have been increasingly closed percutaneously using a variety of different devices.[288,289] PFO closure devices are an alternative, minimally invasive approach to stroke prevention in patients with PFO. The devices consist of discs that are positioned by transcatheter approach on both sides of the atrial septal opening, closing the defect. Newer devices, like the Amplatzer PFO Occluder and Gore Helex, appear safer than earlier generation devices, which tended to provoke atrial fibrillation and to become surfaces for clot formation.[290] In two randomized trials, RESPECT[291] and PC,[292] placement of the Amplatzer PFO Occluder was associated with numerically fewer strokes than antithrombotic therapy alone. Strokes were few in number in both treatment arms and these differences did not reach statistical significance. In the CLOSURE I trial, 909 patients with cryptogenic strokes or TIAs were randomized to medical treatment or percutaneous closure with the STARFlex device.[293] The stroke rates were 2.9% in the closure group and 3.1% in the medical therapy group ($P = 0.79$) and 3.1% and 4.1% respectively for TIA ($P = 0.44$). A cause other than paradoxical embolism was often found in patients with recurrent neurological events.[293]

The available data regarding treatment are inconclusive, but all studies have shown a low recurrence rate (approximately 2% per year) among stroke patients with PFOs. The presence of both a PFO and an ASA substantially increases the risk of stroke recurrence. Warfarin and surgical or transcatheter closure are posited to be more effective than drugs that affect platelet functions, but retrospective studies have not shown their superiority. Debate and controversy surround decisions on whether or not to close PFOs and by what method. Experience with percutaneous closure devices has improved the technique of management and their placement in the hands of experienced cardiologists who perform many procedures is now safer than when these devices were first introduced. Key is selection of patients. Kent, Thaler, and colleagues generated a Risk of Paradoxical Embolism (RoPE) score to allow an estimate of the likelihood that an observed PFO is related to an index stroke in patients characterized as having cryptogenic strokes.[294,295] In the beginning of this section on PFOs, LRC shared his rules for determining whether paradoxical embolism was the cause of a given stroke. Much more work needs to be done regarding choice of medical treatment and mechanical closure.

Frequency of sources

Atrial arrhythmias, congestive heart failure, and akinetic regions were the most common cardiac sources of brain embolism in the Stroke Data Bank.[24] Atrial arrhythmias and left ventricular akinetic regions were the most frequent potential cardiac sources of brain emboli in the Lausanne Stroke Registry.[15,296] Atrial arrhythmias, myocardial abnormalities related to coronary artery disease, and congestive heart failure with low cardiac ejection fractions are probably the most important cardiac abnormalities that predispose to embolism.

Aorta

Studies of patients with stroke and TIAs have firmly established that the thoracic aorta is an important source of brain embolism. Although it was well known that the aorta was an important site of atheromatous disease, almost no mention was made of aortic atherosclerotic disease as an important cause of stroke until the 1990s. Tunick and colleagues reported four patients with unexplained brain ischemic events in whom TEE showed large, protruding, often mobile atheromas.[297,298] Tunick and colleagues then reported the TEE results among 122 patients who had stroke, TIAs, or peripheral emboli, and 122 age- and sex-matched controls.[299] Protruding atheromas were strongly related to the occurrence of embolic events (OR 3–2, 95% CI 1.6–6.5, $P < 0.001$), and atheromas with mobile components were only found in patients with embolic events.[299]

Observational studies and case reports alerted the medical community to the possible importance of aortic atheromas as a cause of stroke and peripheral embolism. In 1992, Pierre Amarenco and his Paris colleagues published two reports that showed definitively that aortic atheromatous disease was an important cause of stroke and could be identified clinically.[300,301] Amarenco et al. first published a necropsy study of 500 patients who had stroke or other neurological diseases. Ulcerated aortic plaques were found in 26% of 239 patients with cerebrovascular disease, compared with only 5% of 261 patients with other neurological diseases ($P < 0.001$).[300] The prevalence of aortic atheromas was 61% among patients with brain infarcts and no demonstrated cause and 22% among those with other defined causes ($P < 0.001$).[300] The presence of ulcerated plaques in the aortic arch did not correlate with the presence of carotid artery stenosis, suggesting that aortic and carotid artery disease were independent stroke risk factors. Amarenco and colleagues also reported a study of 12 consecutive patients with cryptogenic stroke studied by TEE.[301] Six patients (50%) had intraluminal echogenic masses in the aortic arch, most often at the junction of the ascending aorta and the arch. In one patient, the mass was pedunculated, but, in the other five patients, the attachment was broad-based with an irregular surface. The masses extended from 3 mm to 15 mm into the aortic lumens. Cholesterol emboli were found in quadriceps muscle biopsies in two patients with aortic masses.[301]

Tobler et al. studied at necropsy the presence and distribution of atherosclerotic plaques in the ascending aorta.[302] Among 97 ascending aortas, 38% had atherosclerotic plaques larger than 8 mm in diameter; the average diameter of plaques was 19 mm. Most of the 66 plaques were distributed anteriorly or posteriorly on the right side of the ascending aorta, and the upper and lower halves of the ascending aorta were equally involved.[302] Plaques were also often found in the aortic arch, especially at the orifice of the innominate artery (21% of 48 arch specimens).[302]

Two studies investigated the frequency of occurrence of vascular events in patients who had TEE-documented aortic

arch atherosclerosis.[303,304] The French Study Group followed 331 patients who presented with brain infarcts for 2–4 years.[304] The frequency of subsequent brain infarction and other vascular events was closely correlated with the thickness of the aortic wall. After controlling for other confounding factors, the RR of brain infarction was 3.8 (95% CI 1.8–7.8, $P = 0.0012$) and of all vascular events 3.5 (95% CI 2.1–5.9, $P = <0.001$) in patients with aortic wall plaques larger than 4 mm.[304] In a prospective study conducted in 2 German university hospitals, physicians followed 136 patients with flat plaques less than 5 mm in thickness and 47 patients with thick plaques more than 5 mm thick, or complex plaques with mobile components for an average of 16 months.[305] Embolic events occurred in 15 patients; the incidence was 4.1 out of 100 patient-years in patients with flat plaques versus 13.7 out of 100 patient-years in those with complex, thick, or mobile plaques.[305]

TEE has become the usual standard way to image the aorta. Figure 4.38 shows a number of different aortic plaques imaged by TEE. There is very good concordance between TEE images and pathology of the aorta.[305,306] The limitations of TEE are that it is invasive and there is an area of the aorta that is obscured because of the bronchus and is not readily imaged. TEE can show large plaques and floating mobile thrombi within the lumen of the aorta. A study by Vaduganathan et al. showed a 73% agreement between intraoperative TEE imaging of the thoracic aorta and histology.[307] TEE does not always detect ulceration but is able to show complex atheroma and mobile debris. Epiaortic ultrasound applied at the beginning of surgery is also a useful method for detecting severe atheromas and intima-medial thickness of the aorta at various locations.[306]

The ascending aorta can also be insonated using a Duplex ultrasound probe placed in the right supraclavicular fossa; the arch and proximal descending thoracic aorta can be imaged using a left supraclavicular ultrasound probe.[308] The results are preliminary but promising. The technique requires training to master and is not used in most centers. Most plaques are located in the curvature of the arch from the distal ascending aorta to the proximal descending aorta, regions well shown using B-mode ultrasound.[308] The aorta has also been imaged by a suprasternal approach during transthoracic echocardiography using harmonic imaging. In one study large protruding plaques were found with a 91% positive predictive value and negative findings had a 98% predictive value, but unfortunately adequate image quality for interpretation could only be obtained in 89% of patients studied.[309]

MRA and MRI have also been used to image the proximal aorta. Kutz et al. compared the sensitivity of detection of large plaques (>5 mm) using gadolinium-enhanced MRA during breath-holding versus TEE.[310] The sensitivity was 54% with MRA versus 92% with TEE. Techniques that show the lumen of the aorta such as MRA and standard angiography usually do not show the wall of the aorta and so underestimate atherosclerotic plaques. Some researchers have experimented with techniques that enhance atherosclerotic plaques and the vascular endothelium. In a rabbit model gadofluorine enhances plaques and allows for detection of early atherosclerotic lesions.[311] In a 2007 study, 3 Tesla MRI was superior to TEE in recognizing important aortic abnormalities.[312] MRI showed high-risk aortic lesions greater than 4 mm in 37 of 74 patients compared to 23 by TEE ($P = 0.029$).[312] High-resolution MRI using plaque and endothelial-enhancing agents has promise for becoming the preferred imaging technique for detecting and quantifying aortic atherosclerosis in the near future.

Advances in CT angiography has made this technique an alternate attractive method of detecting aortic plaques. CT angiograms have the capability of showing plaques in the aortic arch, a blind area on TEE because of the trachea. A study that included 64 patients with cryptogenic strokes who were studied by both CTA and TEE, showed that CTA showed more aortic abnormalities than TEE.[313] Figure 4.38A is a figure from this study of a CTA showing aortic plaques and Figure 4.38B compares the number and location of aortic plaques shown by the two techniques in the ascending aorta, arch, and proximal descending aorta.[313] Flow MRI studies show that plaque material from the proximal portion of the descending aorta often flows retrograde and can be a potential source of brain and peripheral embolism.[314] TEE and contrast-enhanced CT scans of the aorta can show protruding mass lesions that are usually thrombi, but on rare occasions represent neoplastic lesions such as a sarcoma arising from the wall of the aorta that can be the donor source for brain emboli.[315]

Treatment of aortic atheromatous disease is unsettled. Although anticoagulants have been posited to aggravate cholesterol crystal embolism in several patients, aortic thrombotic masses have disappeared after anticoagulant therapy.[316,317] By preventing the formation of thrombi over ulcerated areas of aortic atheromas, heparin, coumadin, or direct thrombin inhibitors could theoretically facilitate contact of the atheromatous material with the lumen and promote cholesterol embolism. Cholesterol embolism has also been described after thrombolytic treatment of patients with acute myocardial infarction.[318] Similar to anticoagulants, thrombolytic agents could expose ulcerated areas to the circulation if thrombi were lysed. Intravenous thrombolytic treatment[319] and surgical removal of protruding atheromas[320] have also been reported to be successful in treating patients with aortic atheromas.

Agents that affect platelet aggregation and function and combinations of antiplatelet drugs and anticoagulants might be effective in preventing embolism from aortic plaques, but they have not been systematically studied. Antiplatelet agents might be successful in preventing white platelet–fibrin thrombi which, in turn, stimulate the development of superimposed red thrombi. The Aortic Arch Related Cerebral Hazard (ARCH) Trial was a prospective randomized controlled, open-labeled trial, with blinded end-point evaluation that tested the superiority of aspirin 75–150 mg/day plus clopidogrel 75 mg/day over warfarin therapy (INR 2–3) in patients with ischemic stroke, transient ischemic attack, or peripheral embolism who had plaques in the thoracic aorta greater than 4 mm and no other identified embolic source.[321] The trial was stopped prematurely. Hemorrhages were common in both groups and there was no clear superiority of either antiplatelets or anticoagulant therapy.[320] We suggest treating most patients with large protruding (>4 mm), and mobile atheromata with anticoagulants and patients with flat and smaller plaques with antiplatelet agents.

Cardiac surgery

We place the section on complications of cardiac surgery at this point in this brain embolism chapter because most complications are due to brain embolism, and because the aorta and the heart are the major donor sources of that embolism. The reported incidence of neurological abnormalities during the postoperative period varies from 7% to 61% for transient, and from 1.6% to 23% for permanent complications.[322–324] The complication rate is much higher in prospective series, in which patients are routinely examined postoperatively, rather than in retrospective reviews of charts. In one study among 312 patients, transient complications were noted in fully 61% of patients.[324] At the Cleveland Clinic among a series of 421 coronary artery bypass grafting (CABG) patients, 16.8% had prolonged encephalopathy or stroke.[325] Complications can be readily divided into four groups: (1) encephalopathy; (2) stroke; (3) cognitive dysfunction; and (4) peripheral nervous system complications.

Encephalopathy and stroke

A wide spectrum of neuropsychiatric findings, including delirium, confusion, disorientation, drowsiness, and altered behavior without focal neurological abnormalities, are often bundled together under the broad term encephalopathy. Imaging tests in these patients usually do not show new large focal brain infarcts. In the Cleveland Clinic series of CABG operations, 11.6% of patients were considered encephalopathic on the fourth postoperative day.[324] In another large series, 57 of 1669 CABG patients (3.4%) had severe postoperative mental changes, including delirium and encephalopathy.[326] The causes are multiple. Microembolism is a major cause. Encephalopathy is especially common among older patients and those with a history of alcohol abuse and renal disease. Some patients have a hypoxic-ischemic encephalopathy caused by prolonged time on the pump, during which their brain was poorly perfused. An important number of cases are explained by medications. Sedatives, analgesics, especially narcotics, and, most importantly, haloperidol and other antipsychotics are common offenders. Haloperidol often produces depressed alertness, stiffness, inertia, and drowsiness, and the drug stays in the body a long time. Haloperidol has been shown to retard recovery in animals with brain lesions.[327,328] In our opinion, this drug should not be used in older surgical and medical patients, especially those with abnormal brains.

The initial recognition that the neurobehavioral changes were not psychiatric in origin was made by Gilman when he prospectively followed a series of open heart surgery patients.[323] Early research led to the conclusion that embolization of particulate matter related to the pump and its filters was the cause of the encephalopathy.[329] The introduction of membrane, rather than bubble, oxygenators and in-line filtration led to a decrease in the risk of large macroembolic particles reaching the systemic circulation.[329]

A 1990 report of the necropsy findings in five patients and six dogs who had cardiac surgery aroused new interest in this subject.[330] Focal small capillary and arteriolar dilatations were widely scattered in 10 of these 11 brains. Approximately one-half of the focal small capillary and arteriolar dilatations contained birefringent crystalline material within the dilatated capillary regions.[330] The vascular lesions affected medium-sized arterioles, terminal arterioles, and capillaries; they were often distributed in multiples in the same vessels or in clusters near each other. Two other patients had a small number of focal small capillary and arteriolar dilatations. The authors thought that the findings were most consistent with iatrogenically induced release into the system of small particles of air or fat.[330] Microemboli are likely to be an important cause of encephalopathy and persistent cognitive abnormalities after cardiopulmonary bypass surgery.

During and shortly after cardiac surgery, many microemboli are detectable and correlate with the occurrence of strokes, encephalopathy, and cognitive abnormalities.[331–334] When patients are monitored using echocardiography and transcranial Doppler ultrasound, a myriad of microemboli are detected in the MCAs and in the aortic lumen. Most of the microembolic particles are recorded during clamping and unclamping of the aorta but flurries of emboli are also detected during cannulation of the aorta and at the beginning and end of cardiac bypass.[332,333] The particles are of diverse composition and probably consist of air, atheromatous debris, lipid, and platelet–fibrin thrombi. Cardiac and aortic origin embolism undoubtedly contribute to the brain damage often noted after cardiac surgery.

Brain perfusion during cardiac surgery is also an important factor in predicting the presence and severity of ischemic brain damage after surgery.[332] Hypoperfusion augments brain ischemia by lessening the throughput and washout of these microemboli. Among 100 cardiopulmonary bypass surgery patients, Tufo et al. found neurological signs in 78% of patients maintained at a mean arterial pressure of 40 mmHg, but in only 27% of those whose mean pressure was 60 mmHg.[335] The duration of hypotension below 60 mmHg averaged 46 minutes in patients with neurological signs compared to 21 minutes in those without signs.[335] In another study, the importance of both the severity and duration of hypotension below a mean arterial pressure of 50 mmHg were important factors in the development of neurological abnormalities after cardiac surgery.[336] In a randomized study, patients whose mean arterial pressure was maintained in the 50–60 mmHg range had a stroke frequency of 7.2% compared to 2.4% in patients whose mean arterial pressures were maintained in the 80–100 mmHg range.[337] In a review of 15 patients who were considered at high risk for postoperative stroke who had on-pump coronary artery bypass surgery, a drop in mean arterial pressure from a preoperative baseline predicted cognitive dysfunction found early after surgery.[338]

Monitoring of basal cerebral artery blood flow velocities by TCD provides a better measure of brain perfusion than mean arterial blood pressure. Among 100 patients continuously monitored using TCD during heart surgery, the reduction in baseline blood flow velocities was 17% for patients who had no neurological deficits, 34% for those who had diffuse encephalopathy, and 43% for patients who had strokes.[332] The duration

in minutes of perfusion less than 50% of baseline was 36 minutes for those without neurological signs compared to 71 minutes for those with encephalopathy, and 105 minutes for those with strokes.[332]

Pugsley and colleagues studied 100 patients who had cardiopulmonary bypass, 50 with an arterial line filter and 50 without a filter.[331] TCD was used to monitor microemboli. All patients were given neuropsychological tests before and after surgery. Neuropsychological deficits at 8 days and 8 weeks postoperatively were more common in patients who had cardiopulmonary bypass without the arterial filter, and neuropsychological abnormalities correlated with the number of microemboli.[331]

The frequency of clinical focal deficits that qualify as strokes ranges from 4.7% to 5.2% in various series.[323–325,332] Intracardiac operations, such as valve replacements, carry a higher risk of postoperative strokes, ranging from 4.2% to 13%.[332] Among 2264 patients having CABG with and without intracardiac procedures, the frequency of neurological deficits was approximately doubled in those who had intracardiac procedures in addition to CABG.[332] Among the Cleveland Clinic series were 22 of 421 patients (5.2%) who had postoperative strokes, but the deficits were severe in only 2% of the total series.[325] Twelve infarcts involved a cerebral hemisphere (seven right, five left), five involved the brainstem, five involved the retina, and two involved an optic nerve.[325] Using neuroimaging data, infarcts are multiple in 65% of patients. Infarcts are typically small and numerous and involve preferentially the cerebellum, occipital lobes, borderzone territories between the MCAs and PCAs, and territories supplied by MCA branches.[332] Many strokes are first noted after the patient awakens from anesthesia, but strokes also often develop during the first few postoperative days.

The vast majority of brain infarcts after cardiac surgery are caused by embolism from the heart and aorta. A major worry of cardiac surgeons, cardiologists, and neurologists has been that hemodynamic circulatory stress during heart surgery might lead to underperfusion of tenuous zones of pre-existing extracranial vascular stenosis. This concern was the driving force behind early use of preoperative auscultation for bruits and later use of non-invasive and angiographic demonstration of the extracranial vascular system before cardiac surgery. If carotid artery disease was found, carotid artery surgery was performed before or during the same anesthetic as cardiac surgery. The morbidity and mortality of this approach proved high.[339]

Studies of patients with carotid stenosis documented by ultrasound confirmed that there was a low frequency of ipsilateral ischemic infarcts in the perioperative periods.[340–342] In a retrospective study of CABG patients with known carotid artery disease, 144 patients had severe atherostenosis (>50% luminal narrowing) affecting 155 arteries, as shown by preoperative angiography.[343] Strokes ipsilateral to the stenosis occurred in only 1.1% of arteries with 50–90% stenosis, in 6.2% of arteries with greater than 90% stenosis, and in only 2% of arteries with carotid occlusion.[343] Von Reutern and colleagues monitored the MCA of patients using TCD during

cardiac surgery. Even patients with severe carotid stenosis usually showed no important changes during surgery.[344]

Brain infarcts often develop in the period after cardiac surgery. Because hemodynamic stress is maximal intraoperatively, underperfusion should cause damage noted on awakening after surgery. In one study, 5 of 30 postoperative strokes (17%) were noted immediately after cardiac surgery; 14 others developed deficits within 24 hours, and 7 did so during the subsequent 24- to 48-hour period.[345] In 2 patients, strokes occurred 5 and 11 days, respectively, after surgery. The distribution and multiplicity of the postoperative infarcts on CT scans were most consistent with embolism.[345]

Some emboli originate from cardiac lesions known to exist before heart surgery, such as valve lesions, ventricular aneurysms, and myocardial akinetic zones. Atrial fibrillation and other arrhythmias may have been present before surgery or may first appear during the postoperative period. Atrial fibrillation often develops after surgery and may be transient. Some patients had taken warfarin or aspirin before surgery, but this was discontinued before and during the operation and was not restarted until after the embolic stroke had occurred.

Mounting evidence links postoperative embolism to ulcerative atherosclerotic lesions of the ascending aorta.[332,346–353] Aortotomy or cross-clamping of the aorta to anastomose the vein graft may liberate cholesterol crystals and calcific plaque debris. Yellow aortic plaques are often visible and can be palpated by the surgeon. When the aorta is clamped, an audible crunch is often heard. Figure 10.15 is a photograph of the descending aorta at necropsy that contains many ulcerative lesions in a patient who did not awaken after CABG surgery. The TEE of this patient showed severe aortic disease with multiple mobile plaques. Atheromatous material from the proximal portion of the descending aorta can be carried retrograde into the aortic arch and embolize to the brain.

The most important risk factor for stroke after cardiopulmonary bypass surgery is aortic atheromatosis. The frequency of aortic atheromas increases dramatically with age, from 20%

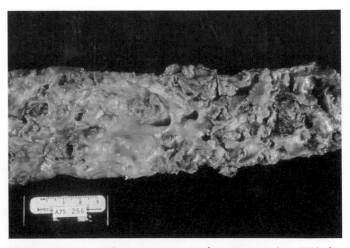

Figure 10.15 Descending aorta at necropsy from a patient whose TEE before surgery showed severe disease of the ascending aorta and aortic arch with mobile protruding plaques. This patient died after CABG surgery having never awakened after the procedure. Courtesy of Dr Denise Barbut.

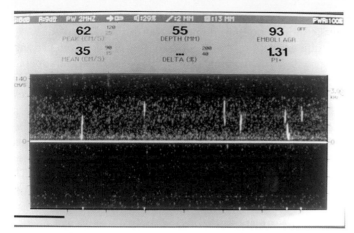

Figure 10.16 TCD recording from the MCA during steady state cardiac bypass surgery at a time when the aorta was being manipulated. The white streaks represent microemboli. Courtesy of Dr Denise Barbut.

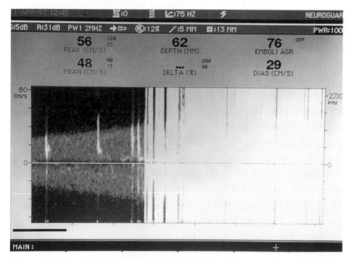

Figure 10.18 TCD recording from the MCA during cardiac bypass surgery. A few distinct emboli (white streaks in the left of the figure) are followed by a massive shower of emboli ("white-out") at the time of the release of aortic clamps. Courtesy of Dr Denise Barbut.

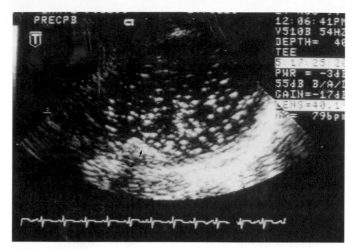

Figure 10.17 TEE recording during cardiac surgery from the aorta at the level of the origin of the left subclavian artery. A mobile plaque is seen protruding into the aortic lumen (small black arrow). This recording was taken after the release of aortic clamps and shows a "shower" of emboli within the aortic lumen beyond where the aorta was previously clamped. Courtesy of Dr Denise Barbut.

in the 5th decade at necropsy, to 80% in patients older than 75 years.[332,354] The stroke rate after CABG also increases sharply with age, from 1% in patients aged 51–60 years, to 9% in patients older than 80 years.[333] The correlation between aortic atheromas and stroke after CABG was first shown at necropsy in a study that involved 221 patients.[354] Atheroemboli were found in 37% of patients who had severe atherosclerosis of the ascending aorta, but in only 2% of patients who did not have significant ascending aortic atheromas.[354] In another study, cardiac surgeons retrospectively reviewed the records of 3279 consecutive patients with CABG at Johns Hopkins, seeking risk factors for postoperative stroke.[351] Severe atherosclerosis of the ascending aorta was one of the most definitive risk factors found.[352]

Embolization can be detected and quantified before, during, and after surgery using ultrasound. TCD recording over the MCAs can detect the arrival of microemboli in the cranial arteries. Figure 10.16 is a TCD recording taken during cardiac

surgery that shows high-intensity transient signals (HITS) that represent microemboli passing under the transducer. Intraoperative transesophageal echocardiography can be used to detect the passage of emboli into and through the aorta. Figure 10.17 is transesophageal echocardiography recorded during cardiac surgery that shows a shower of emboli entering the aortic lumen. More emboli are detected during intracardiac surgery because these patients often have valve calcifications, valve vegetations, and intracardiac thrombi. By using TCD monitoring during closed cardiac operations, the number of microemboli vary from 0 to 1200 within one MCA (average, 130).[332] The numbers of emboli detected in the aorta by TTE is in the thousands, reflecting the fact that only a fraction of the microembolic particles reach the brain.[332,355]

Embolization is not evenly distributed during the various stages of surgery. Maneuvers that involve manipulation of the aorta, such as clamping and unclamping, account for more than 60% of the total number of emboli.[333,355] Flurries of emboli are detected during aortic cannulation and at the start and termination of cardiopulmonary bypass. During open cardiac procedures, the number of emboli detected by TCD is especially high during cardiac ejection, after the release of aortic crossclamps, and immediately after bypass.[332] Figure 10.18 is a TCD recording during cardiac surgery that shows a "white-out" created by a massive shower of emboli that occurred immediately after release of aortic clamps. Many of the microemboli are gaseous particles. Aortic clamping and clamp release are followed by a snowstorm-like appearance of intensely echogenic, well-defined particles within the aorta and a corresponding flurry of particles within the brain arteries.[332] The mean diameter of these particles is 0.85 mm. These microembolic particles are most likely atheromatous debris from the aorta. They are small enough to enter the brain circulation, although only a small fraction do so. Off-pump coronary artery bypass surgery in which the aorta is not clamped is associated with a much smaller quantity of microembolic signals.[356]

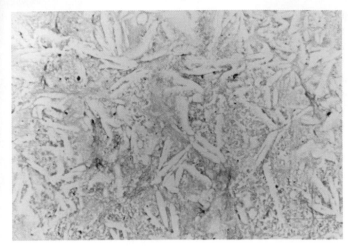

Figure 10.19 Cholesterol crystals and other particulate debris are caught in a filter placed in the aorta at the time that aortic clamps are removed. Courtesy of Dr Denise Barbut.

Transesophageal echocardiography and CTA can detect and quantitate ulcerative aortic plaques before surgery. Some cardiac surgeons use transesophageal echocardiography during surgery (before clamping) to detect aortic atheromas and so indicate the regions of the aorta to avoid during clamping. Marshall and colleagues used an intraoperative B-mode ultrasound probe placed on the aorta to search for protruding plaques.[357] Ultrasonic imaging was more effective in showing plaques than visual inspection and palpation. Furthermore, the amount and location of plaque often altered the procedure performed.[357] Cardiac surgeons have begun to introduce filter devices into the aorta when the aortic clamps are removed to catch debris and cholesterol crystals. Figure 10.19 shows cholesterol crystals and other particulate debris caught in one of these filters.

Cognitive dysfunction without accompanying focal motor, sensory, or visual dysfunction is the most common complication of CABG surgery. Some patients have obvious loss of intellect, whereas others have subtle problems detectable only by formal neuropsychological evaluation. Advanced age and length of bypass are important risk factors for cognitive dysfunction after cardiopulmonary bypass.[358] Prospective studies provide evidence that microembolism is the most important cause of cognitive deficits after cardiac surgery using cardiopulmonary bypass.[331,332,359,360] Patients with cognitive deficits have more microemboli during surgery, compared with patients who have no cognitive decline. Pugsley and colleagues found that 43% of patients with intraoperative embolic counts greater than 1000 had cognitive abnormalities at 8 weeks after cardiac surgery, compared with only 8% of patients with less than 200 emboli.[331] Barbut et al. found that the average number of microemboli at the time of removal of aortic clamps was 166 in 6 patients with cognitive abnormalities, compared with 73 microemboli in 11 patients who showed no loss of cognitive function.[359]

Another syndrome that has been found occasionally after cardiac surgery is a selective paralysis of saccadic eye movements.[361–364] Shortly after awakening from surgery the patients cannot voluntarily initiate conjugate horizontal eye movements. Vertical eye movements are also sometimes involved. Smooth pursuit and reflex eye movements are preserved. The patients often initiate eye movements by moving their heads inducing a passive reflex eye movement. At times other deficits coexist. Some patients have had small localized infarcts in the paramedian pontine tegmentum.[361–364]

In our opinion, all patients who are going to have cardiac surgery should have preoperative transesophageal echocardiography.[353] This should allow detection of potential cardiac and aortic sources of embolization. At the same time left ventricular function, atrial size, and ejection fraction can be measured. When the chest is opened, epiaortic ultrasound is also helpful. The presence of potential cardiac sources helps guide the use of heparin during and after surgery. Knowledge of aortic disease guides clamping sites and technique. Some patients can be operated on without aortic clamping – so-called off-pump surgery. A study that compared on- and off-pump surgery showed no difference in late cognitive effects, but no data about the aorta and left ventricular function were included.[365] Off-pump surgery takes a bit longer than on-pump operations but does not involve aortic clamping. On pump surgery is quicker but does involve clamping of the aorta. It seems likely that patients with severe aortic disease and good ventricular function would do best with off-pump surgery. Those with normal aortas and impaired ventricular function might do better with on-pump bypass surgery. Knowledge of left ventricular function and ejection fraction and of the aorta should be very useful information in addition to the location of the occlusive coronary artery disease in planning and carrying out surgery.[353] Placement of a filtering device in the aorta during and after release of aortic clamps is another useful maneuver to prevent microemboli from reaching the brain and other organs.

Arterial sources of embolism

Extracranial and intracranial large arteries often serve as the donor source for embolism to the brain. Arterial-source embolism is referred to as artery-to-artery, intra-arterial, or local embolism. The location and frequency of atherosclerotic lesions within the large arteries of the anterior and posterior circulations are discussed in Chapters 7 and 8. Ulcerated and stenotic lesions, and recent occlusions within the proximal extracranial and intracranial arteries are most often incriminated as embolic sources.

Although atherosclerosis is by far the most common condition that leads to intra-arterial embolism, other vascular diseases can also serve as donor sources. Trauma and dissections of arteries leads to local thrombus formation and embolism. Dissections are probably the second most frequent source of intra-arterial embolism. Occasionally, inflammatory diseases of the brachiocephalic branches of the aortic arch, such as temporal arteritis and Takayasu's disease, can lead to intra-arterial embolism. Thrombi sometimes form within arterial aneurysms, saccular,[366,367] dissecting, and fusiform dolichocephalic aneurysms,[368] and can then break off and embolize to distal-branch arteries.

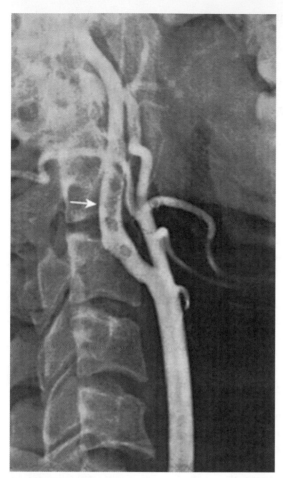

Figure 10.20 Carotid arteriogram, lateral view: dark filling defects within the artery (white arrow) represent luminal embolic clots.

Fibromuscular dysplasia is an important but relatively uncommon vascular disease that affects the pharyngeal and occasionally the intracranial portions of the carotid and vertebral arteries, which also can serve as a source of distal intra-arterial embolism. Thrombi can, on occasion, form within large arteries in the absence of important arterial disease in patients with cancer and other causes of hypercoagulability.[369] These luminal thrombi then embolize to intracranial arteries, causing strokes. Figure 10.20 shows a large thrombus within the ICA.

Imaging and laboratory evaluation of potential donor sources

When the clinical findings, brain imaging, and vascular tests suggest brain embolism, a thorough evaluation of all potential sources – cardiac, aortic, and cerebrovascular – is usually indicated. Clinical distinction between brain embolism and in-situ thrombosis are discussed in Chapter 3. Table 10.3 listed the common differential diagnostic features of these two stroke mechanisms. Some patients have more than one potential embolic donor source. Atherosclerotic plaques and occlusive lesions often coexist in the heart, aorta, and brachiocephalic arteries. Patients with cerebrovascular occlusive lesions have a high frequency of coronary atherosclerotic heart disease, and

their coronary disease is often a more serious threat for mortality and disability than their cerebrovascular disease. Also, patients with coronary atherosclerotic heart disease have a high frequency of occlusive lesions within their extracranial and intracranial vascular beds. Prophylactic treatment to prevent subsequent thromboembolism should include measures to prevent embolism from all potential donor sources, not only the one that caused the present embolism.

Many patients with severe heart disease have abnormalities uncovered by history, physical examination, electrocardiograms, and chest x-ray. TTE, including Doppler insonation and the injection of microbubbles searching for intracardiac shunts, is ordinarily indicated. Some patients, especially young adults who have a well-defined vascular donor source of embolism, such as a cervical dissection, do not need echocardiography.

In order to decide on the utility of echocardiography and to choose between a transthoracic and transesophageal approach, it is useful to review cardiac anatomy.[56] The left atrium is a thin-walled, ovoid chamber that lies immediately behind the ascending aorta. The endocardial surface of the left atrium is usually smooth and continuous as it developed from the fetal common pulmonary vein.[56,370] Body-size normograms for transthoracic left atrial measurements in men and women have been published, but absolute dimension and length value are reported by most clinical echocardiographic laboratories. With normal aging, the left atrial cavity dimensions increase. The body of the left atrium is well visualized from multiple perspectives on TTE.[56] The left atrial appendage is a highly trabeculated and often multilobulated cul-de-sac that arises from the midportion of the lateral wall of the left atrium near the entrance of the left upper pulmonary vein. The LAA is often not visualized on TTE, but the close proximity of the esophagus to the posterior portion of the left atrium and the absence of intervening bone or lung makes TEE the ideal imaging tool for visualization of both the left atrium and the left atrial appendage. Several studies have documented the very high accuracy of TEE in showing left atrial and left atrial-appendage thrombi when echocardiography has been compared with intraoperative visualization of these structures.[56,371,372]

TTE performed with saline contrast is a minimally invasive procedure, while TEE is a moderately invasive procedure during which a modified gastroscope (containing an ultrasound crystal at its tip) is positioned within the esophagus. Imaging is performed within the esophagus and the gastric fundus. Sedation is often required. The close proximity of the esophagus to the posterior portion of the heart, the lack of intervening lung and bone, and the use of higher-frequency imaging transducers results in enhanced spatial resolution.[56] TEE is preferred for identification or exclusion of pathology that is particularly relevant for detecting cardiac and aortic sources of thromboembolism, including identification of intra-atrial thrombi and tumors, PFOs, valvular vegetations, atheromatous plaques within the aorta, and spontaneous echo contrast.[56] TTE remains preferred for identification of left ventricular regional systolic function and apical left ventricular thrombi. For many

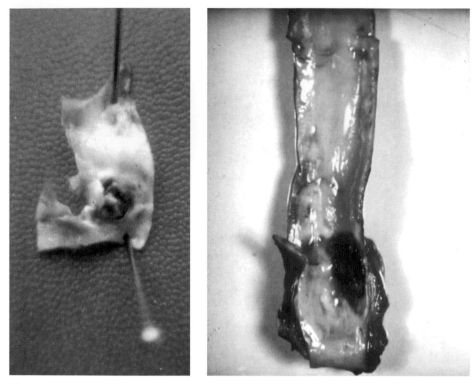

Figure 2.41 Ulcerated internal carotid artery (ICA) plaques in specimens of arteries removed at surgery.

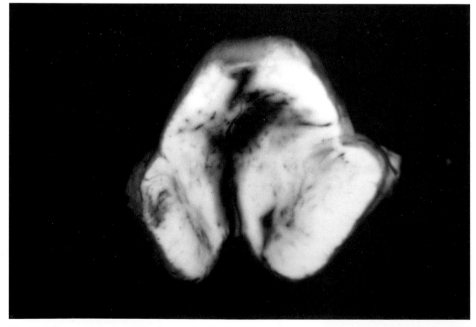

Figure 2.47 A necropsy specimen of a Düret midbrain hemorrhage. A left subdural hematoma was present on the lateral surface of the cerebral hemisphere.

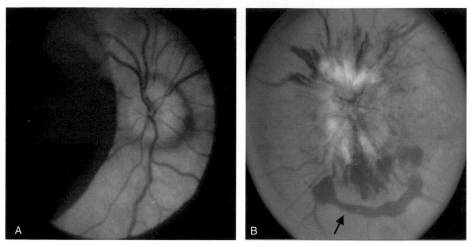

Figure 3.7 (A) This retinal photograph of the right eye shows a large subhyaloid hemorrhage. (B) Papilledema and multiple retinal flame-shaped hemorrhages are present (black arrow) in the retina of the left eye. Photographs kindly submitted by Kathleen Digre, MD, University of Utah.

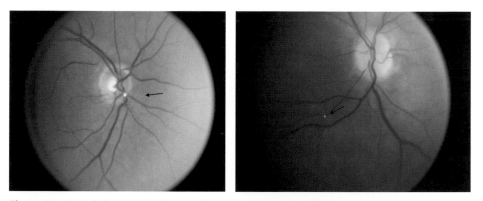

Figure 3.8 Retinal photographs showing cholesterol crystal emboli (black arrows point to the emboli).

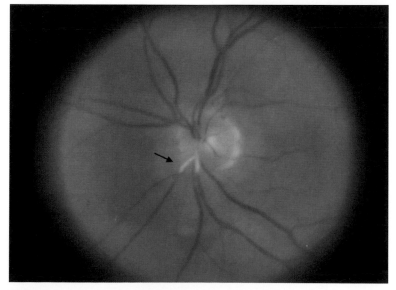

Figure 3.9 Retinal photograph showing a long white platelet–fibin plug (black arrow) impacted in two arterial branches.

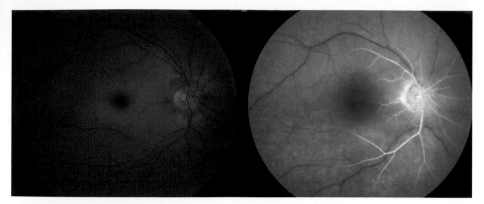

Figure 3.10 Retinal photographs showing acute central retinal artery occlusion in the right eye. (left) The arteries are very attenuated and the ischemic retina appears pale and edematous. The fovea remains red because it receives its blood supply from the choroid (so-called cherry red spot). (right) Retinal fluorescein angiogram 30 seconds after injection of fluorescein showing delayed filling of all retinal vessels which appear dark. Photograph kindly submitted by Dr Valerie Biousse, Emory University.

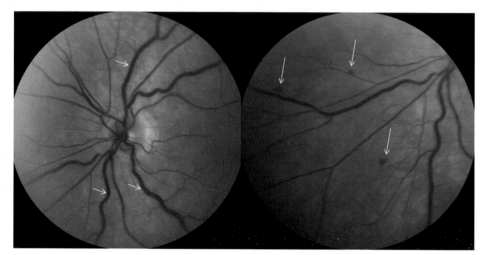

Figure 3.11 Venous stasis retinopathy in the left eye in a patient with a left internal carotid artery occlusion. (left) The posterior pole of the eye appears normal, but the veins are dilated and tortuous (arrows). (right) There are numerous dot-blot hemorrhages (arrows) in the mid-periphery of the retina, beyond the vascular arcades. The right eye is normal. Photograph kindly submitted by Dr Valerie Biousse, Emory University.

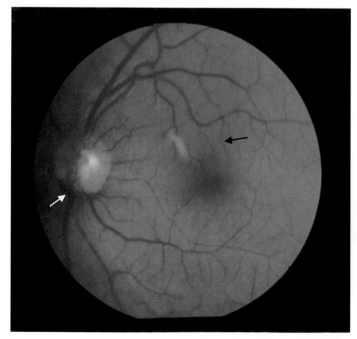

Figure 3.12 Retinal photograph showing neovascularization of the optic disc (white arrow) and retina and a cotton-wool spot retinal infarct (black arrow). Photograph kindly submitted by Kathleen Digre, MD, University of Utah.

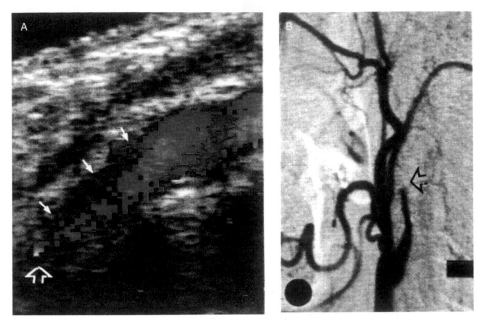

Figure 4.13 An image is shown from a color-flow Dopplar study of an ICA. (A) Blood flows from right-to-left. Blood flow in the image is red. The lumen is severely narrowed and flow is diminished (white open arrows) by an extensive atherosclerotic plaque (dark zone above the region of diminished flow to which small white arrows point). The image in (B) is a cerebral angiogram in the same patient that seems to show a complete occlusion of the artery (open arrow).

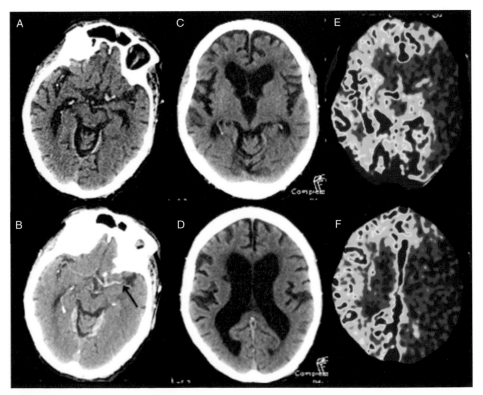

Figure 4.31 Multimodal CT protocol in a patient taken 90 minutes after the onset of dysphasia and right hemiparesis. (A) Thin slice non-contrast CT showing hyperdense thrombus in the intracranial left ICA. (B) Maximum intensity projection image showing full extent of the hyperdense thrombus in the carotid T and the MCA (black arrow). (C&D) Non-contrast CT showing minimal evidence of ischemia at this early stage. (E&F) CT perfusion showing severely reduced cerebral blood volume due to very poor collateral flow indicating a large irreversibly injured ischemic core.

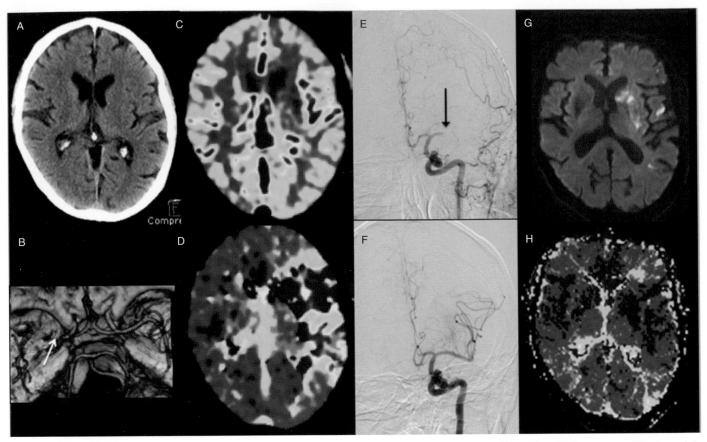

Figure 4.32 Multimodal CT protocol in a patient with the acute onset of a MCA occlusion who had good collateral blood flow. (A). Non-contrast CT brain – subtle loss of gray–white differentiation in the left caudate and putamen. (B) CT angiogram showing proximal left MCA occlusion (white arrow). (C) CT perfusion scan showing reduced cerebral blood volume in the left caudate and putamen confirming the suspicion on non-contrast CT of an ischemic core. (D) CT perfusion showing delayed flow (increased time to peak) in the MCA territory indicating the region supplied by collateral flow which is contributing to the severe clinical deficit but is potentially salvageable with rapid reperfusion. (E) Digital subtraction angiogram with left carotid injection showing persistent MCA occlusion (black arrow) 1 hour after a tPA infusion was begun. (F) Repeat angiogram after mechanical thrombectomy showing recanalization of the MCA. (G) MRI diffusion imaging 24 hours later showing the expected left striatal infarct but salvage of most of the MCA territory. (H) MRI perfusion 24 hours after treatment showing normalization of flow in the left MCA (time to peak map).

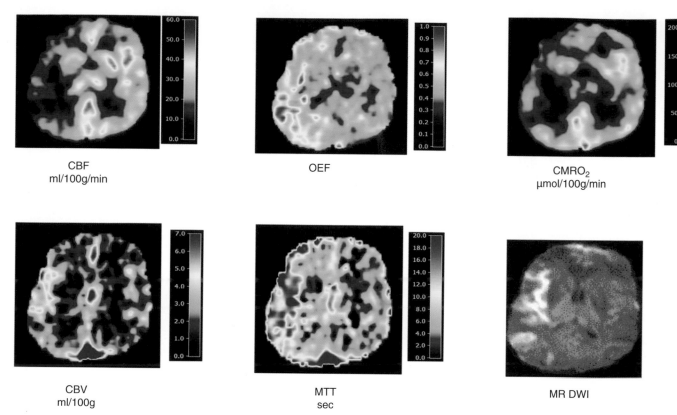

CBF
ml/100g/min

OEF

CMRO₂
μmol/100g/min

CBV
ml/100g

MTT
sec

MR DWI

Figure 4.34 PET parametric maps of cerebral blood flow (CBF), oxygen extraction fraction (OEF), oxygen consumption (CMRO$_2$), cerebral blood volume (CBV) and mean transit time (MTT), as well as the diffusion-weighted (DWI) scan, obtained in a 51-year-old man, 7–9 hours after acute-onset right-sided hemiparesis, homonymous hemianopia and neglect, and global dysphasia. One axial plane is shown for illustration. Images are shown in neurological orientation (i.e., right is shown on the right side). Quantitative gray–white intensity scales are shown to the right of each PET image for interpretation. There is extensive hypoperfusion over the entire left MCA territory, with CBF below the penumbra threshold of 20 ml/100 g/min in large parts of the affected cortex. The CMRO$_2$ is also reduced in the entire MCA territory, but less so than predicted by the CBF with massively increased OEF ("misery perfusion"). The CMRO$_2$ lies above the threshold for irreversible damage (around 39 μmol/100 g/min) throughout except around the posterior insula and surrounding white matter. The CBV and the MTT are also increased throughout, indicating overridden autoregulation from low perfusion pressure. The DWI lesion is heterogeneous and extensive but smaller than the area of hypoperfusion ("mismatch"); although it is partly congruent with the areas of very low CMRO$_2$ indicating irreversible damage, it also straddles areas of penumbra, characterized by CBF <20 ml/100 g/min, high OEF, and CMRO$_2$ above the irreversibility threshold. Courtesy of J-C Baron, J V Guadagno, M Takasawa, E A Warburton, et al., University of Cambridge, UK.

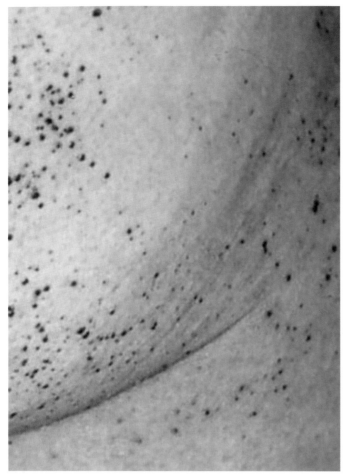

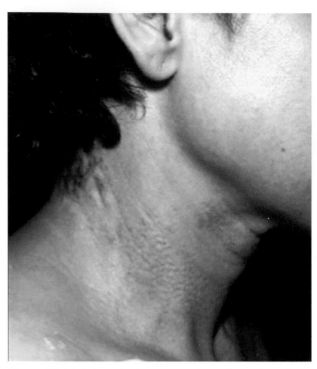

Figure 5.3 Neck skin redundancy in a patient with pseudoxanthoma elasticum. Kindly submitted by Dr Graeme Hankey, Perth, Australia.

Figure 5.2 Angiokeratomas on the buttocks region in a patient with Fabry's disease.

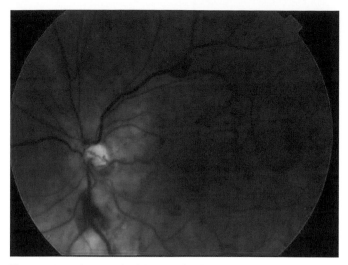

Figure 7.2 A photograph of the optic fundus in a patient with a carotid artery occlusion showing central venous retinopathy. There are dilated veins and many blot and dot hemorrhages mostly in the periphery of the retina. Courtesy of Thomas Hedges III, MD.

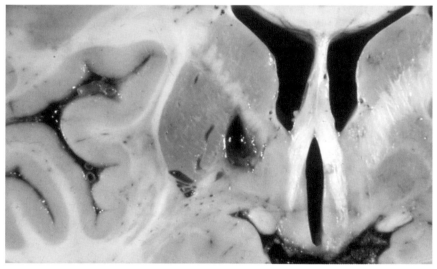

Figure 9.6 A necropsy specimen showing a cavity due to an old lacunar infarct located in the medial basal ganglia (mostly the globus pallidus) and extending through the internal capsule in a patient with a pure-motor hemiplegia during life.

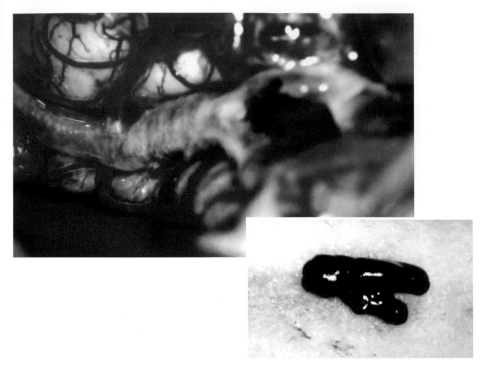

Figure 10.1 An embolus within the MCA at necropsy. The inset shows the red thrombus removed from the artery. From Caplan LR, Manning WJ. *Brain Embolism*, New York: Informa Healthcare, 2006 with permission.

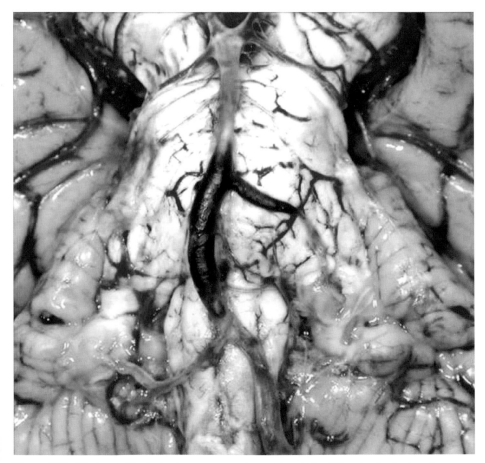

Figure 10.3 The base of the brain at necropsy showing a red embolus distending the basilar artery.

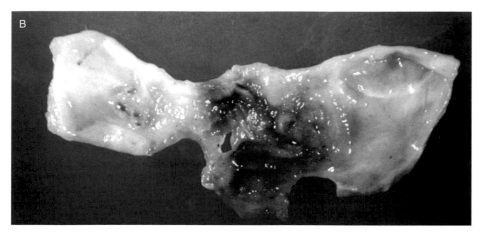

Figure 10.11b Mitral valve vegetations in a patient with APLA syndrome and multiple brain emboli. (A) Echocardiography showing a pedunculated, mobile lesion on the mitral valve (white arrows). AO, aorta; LA, left atrium; LV, left ventricle. (B) Mitral valve removed surgically showing vegetations. From Caplan LR, Manning WJ. *Brain Embolism*. New York: Informa Healthcare, 2006 with permission.

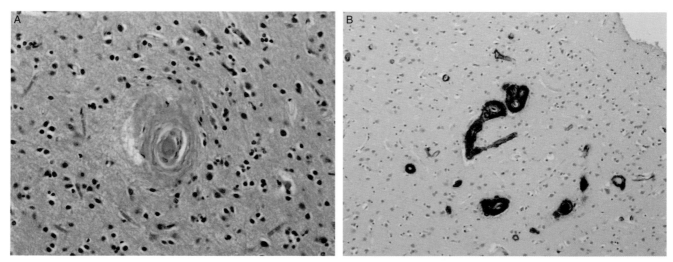

Figure 12.10 (A) Photomicrograph of the cerebral cortex, hematoxylin-eosin stain showing splitting of the amyloid-laden wall of a small artery. (B) Photomicrograph of the cerebral cortex immunostained for beta-amyloid with a hematoxylin counterstain. Amyloid is seen in many small vessels. Courtesy of Dr Steven Greenberg.

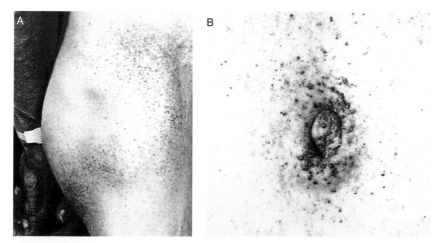

Figure 12.21 Angiokeratomas in Fabry's disease. (A) Photograph of the buttocks showing typical small lesions. (B) Periumbilical angiokeratomas. Courtesy of Dr Edward Kaye.

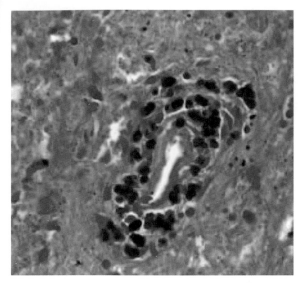

Figure 14.3 Remnant of an old pontine microhemorrhage, incidental autopsy finding in a 70-year-old woman. An elongated deep intracerbral artery with surrounding hemosiderin-laden macrophages. (hematoxylin/eosin stain). From Fiehler J. Cerebral microbleeds: Old leaks and new haemorrhages. *Int J Stroke* 2006;1:122–130 with permission.

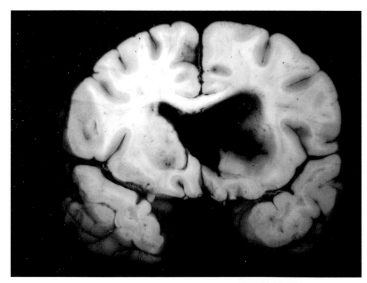

Figure 14.10 Necropsy brain specimen showing a caudate hemorrhage that extended into the adjacent lateral ventricle. From Caplan LR. Caudate hemorrhage. In Kase CS, Caplan LR (eds), *Intracerebral Hemorrhage*. Boston: Butterworth–Heinemann, 1994, pp 329–340 with permission.

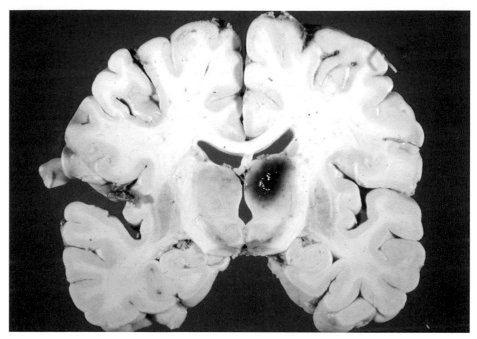

Figure 14.12 Necropsy specimen showing a small anterior thalamic hemorrhage. From Caplan LR. Thalamic hemorrhage. In Kase CS, Caplan LR (eds), *Intracerebral Hemorrhage*. Boston: Butterworth–Heinemann, 1994, pp 341–362 with permission.

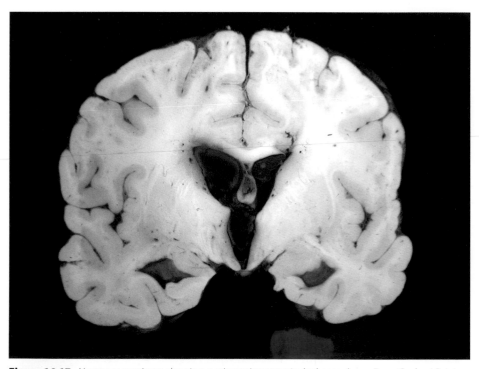

Figure 14.17 Necropsy specimen showing a primary intraventricular hemorrhage. From Caplan LR. Intraventricular hemorrhage. In Kase CS, Caplan LR (eds), *Intracerebral Hemorrhage*. Boston: Butterworth–Heinemann, 1994, pp 383–401 with permission.

patients, direct TEE (with omission of the TTE) may be the most expeditious route to identify a cardiac source of embolism.[56,373-376]

TEE sometimes fails to identify cardiac sources of emboli. Some thromboemboli are too small to be detected. An embolus that is 1–2 mm can cause a devastating neurological deficit. Others abut on an endothelial surface and are difficult to separate from that surface. A particle of 1–2 mm is often beyond the resolution of echocardiography. The other major reason for failure is that thrombosis and embolism are dynamic processes. When a thrombus leaves the heart to go to the brain, echocardiography may not show a thrombus within the heart if performed soon after the clinical event. Later, the thrombus may reform.

TEE also yields important information about the proximal aorta, a region not imaged by TTE. TEE is important in all patients in whom TTE suggests, but does not adequately define, the cardiac pathology and in all patients in whom other studies (cerebrovascular, hematological, and other cardiac investigations) do not show the cause of brain embolism and brain ischemia. Radionuclide testing, including gated blood pool imaging (multigated acquisition scans), may also be helpful in selected patients, as might other cardiac imaging techniques.[377] Platelet scintigraphy is sometimes helpful in defining the presence of cardiac thrombi.[378] TEE, and CTA can effectively show aortic plaques as discussed in the Aorta section above.

Advanced CT and MRI technology can now show thrombi within the atria and atrial appendages and within the verntricles.[379-384] Dual-energy CT[381] and CTA[381,383,384] can show thrombi when these lesions are not well shown by TEE. Cardiac MRI is now more often used than in the past and shows promise in detecting thrombi and cardiac wall abnormalities.[379,380]

The extracranial and intracranial arteries should be studied to define potential arterial donor sources of embolism, provide information about blockage of recipient arteries by emboli, or both. The four most common and effective means of studying the brachiocephalic arteries are by MRA, CTA, ultrasound, and cerebral catheter-dye angiography. Brain imaging always should accompany the vascular studies to show the location, severity, and distribution of related brain ischemia. These diagnostic tests and their use in diagnosing large artery lesions in the anterior and posterior circulations have been extensively reviewed in Chapters 4, 7, and 8.

Hematological studies are also important in the evaluation of patients suspected of having brain embolism. Why does a patient with a chronic lesion, such as an aortic protruding atheroma, atrial fibrillation, or ICA stenosis develop a super-imposed thrombus at a given time? In many patients, the explanation lies in activation of platelets, the coagulation system, or both.[385] The two processes, an intimal–endothelial lesion and heightened coagulation, interact to explain the thromboembolic event. Various conditions affect the coagulation system. Coexisting infection, cancer, dehydration, congenital or acquired hypercoagulability (i.e., in patients with resistance to activated protein C or decreased antithrombin III activity) can activate the coagulation cascade that, in the presence of a suitable lesion, can lead to thrombus formation and embolism. Coagulation studies should be an integral part of the evaluation of patients with suspected brain embolism and those with potential sources of embolism who have not, as yet, had clinical events. Hematological evaluations are described in Chapter 4.

Treatment of patients with brain embolism

The goals of treatment are minimization of brain ischemic injury caused by brain embolism and prevention of acute recurrent embolism. Strategies for accomplishing this fall into four broad categories: (1) reperfusion of the brain region rendered ischemic by the embolus; (2) acute anticoagulation to prevent propagation and further embolization of thromboemboli; (3) making the brain more resistant to ischemia, allowing survival of nerve cells despite ischemia; (4) managing complications of embolic infarction such as brain edema and brain hemorrhage.[385] Treatment is discussed in great detail in Chaper 6 and will only be briefly summarized here. Herein we will discuss general strategies. In general embolic materials are more easily thrombolysed than clots formed in situ because they are not at first attached to the underlying recipient site arteries.

Reperfusion

The most important predictor of recovery from brain embolism is whether or not brain tissue rendered ischemic by an embolus blocking a recipient artery is reperfused with blood before irreversible damage occurs, and how quickly reperfusion develops. Reperfusion occurs in two different complementary ways: recanalization of the occluded artery when an embolus moves distally, either spontaneously or after treatment, and augmentation of blood flow through collateral circulation sufficient to restore adequate nutrition to ischemic tissue.

Opening of blocked recipient arteries

Angiographic opacification of cervico-cranial arteries soon after onset of brain ischemic symptoms shows that the intracranial arteries in a very high percentage of patients are occluded when angiography is performed within 6–8 hours of symptom onset.[40,41,386,387] Clinical and angiographic studies proved that emboli often passed distally from their initial resting place within recipient arteries.[13,14,43,44,388] In some patients passage of emboli is accompanied by dramatic clinical recovery.[13,14] When angiograms were performed 48 hours or more after neurological symptom onset in patients in the Harvard Stroke Registry, emboli had mostly passed and were not visible angiographically.[11,389] TCD can effectively show opening and reocclusion of embolic brain artery occlusions.[2]

Acute studies using MRI protocols that include MRA and diffusion-weighted images have clearly shown that patients rarely develop progressive brain infarction when arteries have

already recanalized.[390-393] Angiographic and TCD studies of untreated patients and those treated with intravenous or intra-arterial thrombolytic agents also show clearly that patients whose arteries recanalize do much better than patients whose arteries remain occluded.[394-398] These studies also help with prediction of the likelihood of hemorrhage after thrombolysis.[393] The extent of brain infarction and clinical recovery also correlate with the length of time that the recipient artery remained occluded.[394-398] The location, extent ("clot burden"), and the duration of arterial occlusion are the most important determinants of outcome.

Chemical or mechanical thrombolysis and clot removal

Opening of occluded arteries can be accomplished chemically by administering drugs that lyse clots, or mechanically using devices that extract thromboemboli. Thrombolytic drugs can be given either intravenously or intra-arterially. Each has advantages and disadvantages. Intravenous therapy can be given quickly and needs no special training. The amount of thrombolytic agent that reaches large obstructed arteries is however more limited than intra-arterial infusion of drug which delivers the drug locally within the obstructing clot. Intra-arterial therapy requires a trained interventionalist. Angiography is ordinarily required before, during, and after intra-arterial treatment. This delays treatment. The major advantage of intra-arterial therapy is that the interventionalist can physically manipulate the clot, a process that facilitates thrombolysis, and can retrieve clots mechanically. Angioplasty/stenting can also be performed during the same procedure if necessary, for example in a patient with an intra-arterial embolus arising from a very stenotic carotid artery in the neck. After lysing or extracting the intracranial embolus, the ICA could be stented. Usually less drug is used during intra-arterial therapy and the rate of hemorrhagic complications is lower than with intravenous therapy. Another strategy employed is to begin with intravenous treatment. MRI studies including MRA, or CT and CTA are then performed.[399,400] If the artery does not recanalize and the patient does not improve then angiography with intra-arterial therapy is given. Stroke thrombolysis is discussed in detail in Chapter 6.

Mechanical removal of thromboemboli can be used as an adjunct to chemical thrombolysis or pursued when there are absolute or relative contraindications for thrombolysis and thromboemboli are present. A variety of different types of instruments can be used to mechanically remove thrombi: suction techniques, snares, nets, corkscrew retrievers, or direct angioplasty or stenting.[401,402] Laser energy ("endovascular photoacoustic recanalization (EPAR)") can be used to emulsify and suction thrombi.[403] Mechanical removal of thrombi has some theoretical advantages over chemical thrombolysis. Chemical thrombolysis, whether intravenous or intra-arterial takes time. Recanalization can take 1–2 hours to accomplish after drug infusion.[16,76] Thrombi can be extracted solely mechanically or mechanical disruption could facilitate pharmacological thrombolysis by fragmenting the non-thrombotic components of the thrombus and increasing the surface area contact with the thrombolytic drugs. Mechanical thrombolysis should pose less of a threat for bleeding since systemic or local fibrinolytics would not be used and so there would be no decreased coagulability. Mechanical clot removal could be pursued in patients who are presently excluded from chemical thrombolysis; for example, those who have had a recent procedure and those already treated with anticoagulants. Stent retrievers open the artery and effect recanalization while capturing and retrieving the occlusive thrombus. The major limitation of mechanical clot removal is the need for a trained and experienced interventionalist who has familiarity and experience with the device used.

Selection of patients for thrombolysis or mechanical clot removal depends on assessing the benefit–risk ratio of treatment. The three key elements in the decision are: (1) whether an artery is occluded and where and how extensive is the clot; (2) the extent of brain already infarcted; and (3) the brain still at risk for further infarction. If there is a vascular occlusion, little or no infarction, and a sizable important area of brain at risk for further ischemic damage, then every attempt should be made to open the arterial occlusion. The presence of good collateral circulation also is important since this makes successful reperfusion more likely. The longer that the occlusion has been present the more likely that ischemic damage has included blood vessels within the ischemic zone, and so the more likely that reperfusion could be associated with bleeding and/or edema. Thrombi that have been in an artery for a long period are usually harder to lyse and extract than very recent emboli. Chapter 4 discusses the imaging techniques – MRI, DWI, MRA and MR perfusion, CT, CTA, and CT perfusion, and extracranial and transcranial ultrasound that can define the brain region infarcted, the vascular occlusion, and the region still at risk of further damage. Recommendations for thrombolysis in acute stroke are noted in Box 6.8.

Randomized trials discussed in Chapter 6 have now conclusively shown the effectiveness of aggressive interventional endovascular treatment of ischemic stroke patients diagnosed using modern brain and vascular imaging technology. In these studies most patients were given IV thrombolytics, and stent retrievers were used to retrieve clots that remained occlusive. These studies proved that patients carefully selected using advanced brain and vascular imaging had better outcomes by applying interventional techniques that opened occluded brain-supplying arteries than controls treated only with standard intravenous thrombolysis.

ML is a 46-year-old woman who suddenly developed aphasia and weakness of the right hand. She had a chronic myocardiopathy and during the preceding months reported increasing dyspnea and pedal edema. Examination 3.5 hours after onset of the neurological symptoms showed slight right-hand clumsiness and occasional word errors. She made reading, writing, and spelling errors. MR studies performed 4 hours after onset showed an occluded left MCA on MRA, a small elliptical zone of abnormal diffusion on DWI, and a normal T2-weighted and FLAIR MRI scan. TCD after intravenous recombinant tissue plasminogen activator showed reperfusion in the MCA territory. MRI and MRA studies were repeated 18 hours after

thrombolysis. The MCA obstruction had improved, but there was still a residual filling defect. The infarct was seen on T2-weighted MRI and DWI but had not expanded. Perfusion imaging showed a defect larger than the infarct. On a later study, the MCA completely recanalized and the perfusion deficit cleared. The infarct remained the same but her examination returned to normal, except for minor loss of dexterity with her right hand when she played the piano.

The timing of thrombolysis is important if brain tissue is to be saved. Time = brain. Experimental studies in animals show that after 3 hours, irreversible brain ischemia (infarction) has already developed. However, salvageability of ischemic brain tissue varies considerably from patient to patient. Sometimes ischemic but salvageable brain tissue persists for many hours. This hypoperfused tissue has inadequate blood supply to function but is not irreversibly damaged. Stunned brain and ischemic penumbra are terms used for ischemic non-functioning brain that is not yet infarcted. The major danger of thrombolysis and of spontaneous reperfusion is that reperfusion of damaged vessels in the ischemic zone could cause major bleeding. Ideally, the decision on whether to pursue thrombolysis or other means of reperfusion, such as angioplasty, should rest on the presence of viable salvageable penumbral tissue and the extent of brain that is already infarcted, not on the time that has expired since symptom onset. The extent of infarction determines the risk of treatment; the presence and size of penumbral, stunned tissue determines the potential benefit of thrombolysis that accomplishes reperfusion. The MR techniques of diffusion-weighted and perfusion MR scans performed with echo-planer equipment, when coupled with MRA, give clinicians a quantitative estimate of these factors.

The case of ML illustrates the power of this imaging tool. Despite the fact that over 4 hours had transpired after symptom onset, the imaging showed that there was considerable potential benefit of trying to recanalize the recipient artery and much risk of leaving the clot where it was. Had the artery not recanalized after intravenous treatment, we would have performed an arteriogram and attempted to remove the clot by intra-arterial thrombolysis and/or mechanical means.

Clinicians should estimate the extent of normal, infarcted and stunned brain supplied by the occluded artery by using brain imaging (CT and T2-weighted MRI scans), vascular studies (CTA, MRA, TCD, angiography), and neurological examination. If the patient has a severe neurological deficit and a large infarct is present on brain scans, then much of the brain is infarcted and there is little to gain by thrombolysis, which carries a substantial risk of hemorrhage in this circumstance. If the patient has a severe neurological deficit and brain scans are normal, however, then there could be considerable stunned, salvageable brain, which could be restored to function if thrombolysis were successful.

Augmenting brain blood flow and "neuroprotection"

Different medical strategies are available to try to improve circulation to brain regions rendered ischemic by a brain embolus. Optimal management of blood pressure, blood volume, and cardiac output can improve blood flow to the ischemic region. Cerebral blood flow increases with rising blood pressure until the pressure becomes very high, approaching the malignant range. During the acute period of brain ischemia, it is unwise to lower the systemic pressure unless it is extremely high; for example, above 200/120 torr.

In some patients with low blood pressure, elevation of blood pressure with phenylephrine, ephedrine or other catecholaminergic drugs might augment brain circulation. Blood volume also affects perfusion pressure and blood flow. Some patients who cannot eat normally will become dehydrated and relatively hemoconcentrated. Other factors – such as vomiting, restrictions on eating because of concern for aspiration, or simply the rush of diagnostic testing occupying patients at mealtimes – all contribute to reduced fluid intake during the early hours and days after the onset of brain embolism. It is best to keep blood volume, especially plasma volume, high. Fluids must often be given intravenously or by nasogastric or stomach tubes. Care, however, must be taken to avoid fluid overload and the complications of cardiac failure and brain edema. Careful monitoring of cardiac and cerebral function should accompany attempts to increase fluid volume.[56]

Many patients with brain embolism also have cardiac dysfunction. A strong pump helps maximize cerebral blood flow. Attention to cardiac rhythm and pump function is important, especially during the acute, fragile period of brain ischemia after embolism. Cardiac output can sometimes be improved by the use of digitalis or vasodilators, use of pacemakers or medications to treat slow rhythms and heart block, adjustment of already prescribed drugs such as digitalis and diuretics, correction of abnormal serum K^+ and Ca^{2+} levels, and control of tachyrhythmias. Cardiac-ejection fractions and output can be monitored by echocardiography.

Clinicians and researchers have explored the use of drugs that have the potential to make the brain more resistant to ischemia. This type of therapy is usually called neuroprotective treatment. Neuroprotective therapy attempts to ameliorate the cellular metabolic consequences of ischemic injury. Unfortunately all agents studied in randomized trials in humans have failed to show efficacy. However trials and studies have not been optimal. Neuroprotection is discussed at length in Chapter 6. Perhaps in the future, agents will be found that ameliorate the effects of brain ischemia.

Antithrombotic treatment

Heparin and heparin-like compounds are often prescribed to treat patients with acute thromboembolism. The posited purpose of heparinization is to prevent propagation of thrombi and breakoff of the tail of existing thrombi and so prevent further embolization. As far as is known, heparin does not lyse existing thrombi, although cardiac clots often disappear during heparin treatment. The arguments used to recommend acute heparinization are twofold: preventing further activity in the

embolus already present intracranially and preventing further clot formation in the original donor source region where the thrombus developed. Heparin is also often used after thrombolysis to maintain arterial patency. The newer oral anticoagulants now in use (the direct thrombin inhibitor dabigatran and the factor Xa inhibitors – apixaban, rivaroxaban, and edoxaban) all work quickly within hours and so could be used acutely instead of heparins.

Once an embolus has reached an intracranial artery recipient site it most often fragments at some point in time and does not usually accrue further clot material. The embolus that has already occurred is not the main focus of anticoagulant treatment. The decision on whether or not to prescribe heparin or a newer oral anticoagulant acutely to prevent the next thromboembolic stroke should depend on weighing the risk of acute re-embolization versus the risk of hemorrhage related to anticoagulant therapy. The risk of further acute thrombus formation and embolization depends primarily on the nature of the cardiac, aortic, and arterial source of the original thromboembolus.

In patients with cardiac lesions that carry high rates of re-embolization e.g., mitral stenosis with atrial fibrillation, atrial fibrillation with atrial thrombi or large left atria, and, acute myocardial infarction with mural thrombi, then acute anticoagulation is probably warranted. In patients with cardiac sources that have a low risk of acute re-embolization, such as chronic atrial fibrillation or mitral annulus calcification, anticoagulants can be withheld during the acute period.

Acute carotid and vertebral artery occlusions in the neck are important sources of intra-arterial embolism. When a thrombus first forms in a region of atherostenosis, the clot is not well organized and does not adhere to the arterial wall. The thrombus often extends and new thrombus forms especially since flow is reduced above the thrombus. With time, probably 3–4 weeks, the thrombus becomes well organized and adherent and further thrombus formation seems not to develop. Also during these weeks collateral circulation develops and stabilizes. An argument can be made to use anticoagulants during the 3–6 week period during which further thrombus development and embolization is a concern.

The other aspect of the decision regarding acute anticoagulation relates to the risk of bleeding into the brain or other organs. The major risks factors are: hypertension, the presence of potential bleeding lesions – e.g., peptic ulcer disease or hemorrhagic colitis – and the extent of brain infarction. If the patient has a large brain infarct then the risk of brain hemorrhage after acute anticoagulation is higher than when there is no brain infarct or a small brain infarct.

Reintroduction of anticoagulation in patients who have had an intracerebral hemorrhage while taking anticoagulants is a special problem.[404,405] The decision concerning if and when to restart anticoagulants depends on the risk of embolization from the donor source (atrial fibrillation, prosthetic heart valves, etc.) and the risk of further intracranial bleeding. Studies seem to show that the risk of embolization while anticoagulants are stopped is less than predicted and the risk of hemorrhage if anticoagulants are reintroduced is also less than expected.[404,405] We suggest waiting a week or 10 days when the risk of re-embolization is low.

Managing brain edema and mass effect

Brain edema also is an early occurrence in patients with embolic strokes. Ischemic edema can be intracellular (so-called cytotoxic edema or dry edema) or exist mostly in the extracellular spaces and connective tissue (vasogenic edema or wet edema).[406] Brain edema that lies in the interstices outside of cells might be posited to respond to osmotic diuretics such as hypertonic saline, mannitol and glycerol, or to corticosteroids. However, studies have shown that these agents are not very effective in series of stroke patients with large brain infarcts or hemorrhages. Most edema is probably within cells and indicates that the cells are sick. Restitution of the normal metabolic functions of these cells is likely to be more therapeutic than so-called anti-edema agents. There are some individuals, mostly young patients, who quickly develop extensive vasogenic, extracellular brain edema with the consequences of increased intracranial pressure and displacement and herniations of brain compartments. In these patients a therapeutic trial of osmotic agents and/or corticosteroids is warranted since the situation is often desperate.

In some patients with massive brain swelling and increased intracranial pressure, removal of the skull overlying the side of the infarct (hemicraniectomy) can be life-saving but patients are sometimes left with severe neurological residual deficits. Surprisingly some patients make extraordinary recoveries after hemicraniectomies and survive with very little neurological deficit.

Chronic prophylactic treatment to prevent re-embolization

Almost immediately, physicians caring for patients with brain embolism must think of preventing the next embolus. The three strategies used for prophylaxis are: (1) removal of the donor source of embolism whenever possible; (2) modification of risk factors that relate to disease at the donor site; and (3) modification of coagulation functions to prevent the formation of new thromboemboli. Some donor-site lesions can be corrected, or at least ameliorated surgically, or by using interventional radiological techniques. Cardiac valve lesions; cardiac tumors; atrial septal defects; PFOs; and protruding, mobile, large aortic atheromas can be treated surgically. Newer interventional techniques may permit effective interventional percutaneous treatment of PFO and aortic atheromas. Carotid and vertebral artery lesions can be corrected surgically (endarterectomy) or by stenting and angioplasty. Many patients with cardiac, aortic, and cerebrovascular donor site lesions have modifiable risk factors, such as

smoking, hyperlipidemia, hypertension, inactive sedentary lifestyle, and obesity. Counseling and medical treatment of these risk factors is an important part of the care of patients with brain embolism.

Manipulation of coagulation to prevent future thromboemboli is a strategy applicable to most patients with brain embolism. Embolic particles are diverse. White platelet thrombi, red erythrocyte–fibrin thrombi, cholesterol crystals, calcified particles from arteries and valves, myxomatous tissue, bacteria in patients with infective endocarditis, and bland fibrous vegetations in patients with non-infective endocarditis are the most important substances. Medical prophylactic treatment against re-entry of these particles into the circulation depends much on the "stuff" in the emboli rather than the source of the materials.[1,4,55] It's the bird rather than the location of the nest that is important.[55] For example, the most effective prophylaxis for prevention of embolization in patients with bacterial endocarditis is effective antibiotic sterilization of the bacterial vegetations. Cholesterol crystals, calcific particles, bacterial vegetation, and myxomatous emboli do not, as far as is known, respond to treatment with anticoagulants or drugs that modify platelet function.

The two types of medicinal agents most often used to prevent thromboemboli are standard anticoagulants (heparin, low-molecular-weight heparins, heparinoids, warfarin compounds and thrombin and Xa inhibitors) and agents that alter platelet adhesion, aggregation, and secretion, such as aspirin, ticlopidine, clopidogrel, dipyridamole, cilostazole and omega-3 fish oils. Chapter 6 contains a detailed discussion of the use of these compounds. White platelet–fibrin thrombi are posited to form on irregular surfaces in fast-moving bloodstreams in widely patent arteries and cavities. Red erythrocyte–fibrin thrombi, on the other hand, tend to form in regions of stasis, such as leg veins, dilatated cardiac atria, severely stenotic arteries, and so forth. At times, both white and red thrombi coexist because activated platelets are a stimulus for activation of the coagulation cascade and subsequent red-clot formation. We choose anticoagulant treatment for prophylaxis in patients who have lesions that promote red-clot formation and in patients whose imaging studies show thrombi. We continue anticoagulation as long as the situation that promotes red clots persists. These situations include persistent atrial fibrillation, myocardial aneurysm, prosthetic valves, and stenotic extracranial arteries. In patients with acute occlusive thrombi superimposed on preocclusive atherostenosis, we continue anticoagulants only for a short time (6–12 weeks), during which thrombi organize and no longer propagate or form fresh tails that embolize. During this time, collateral circulation has usually become maximal. Sometimes, lesions that caused the original thrombosis later improve (e.g., arterial dissections, regressing atheromas, or corrected cardiac right-to-left shunts), so anticoagulation can be stopped and replaced with antiplatelet drugs.

We use agents that alter platelet functions for patients with lesions posited to predispose to formation of white platelet–fibrin thrombi. Irregular non-stenosing atherosclerotic plaques and irregular, but non-stenotic valve surfaces are the most common situations. In patients who can tolerate aspirin, we usually prescribe 325 mg of coated aspirin daily or aspirin with modified-release dipyridamole. Cilostazole, and clopidogrel are other antiplatelet agents that are often prescribed. High fibrinogen levels increase whole blood viscosity and platelet aggregability and predispose to red clot formation. Drugs that lower fibrinogen levels are prescribed. In some situations, in which both red and white clots are likely to form, a combination of platelet antiaggregants and coumadin might be more effective than either agent alone.

Embolic materials that originate outside of the vascular system

Some embolic materials that enter the systemic and brain circulations do not originate in the heart, aorta, or cervico-cranial arteries and are not composed of blood elements or thrombi. Because the situations and nature of the emboli is so different from the much more common intravascular emboli, we discuss the major features of these emboli at the end of this chapter. The types of particles are diverse as are the clinical syndromes and circumstances of brain embolization. Fat and gas bubbles cause microembolism to many small brain capillaries and arterioles causing an encephalopathy-type syndrome while tumor and foreign body emboli usually block single discrete arteries causing strokes.

Fat embolism

Fat embolism occurs most often after serious physical trauma that causes bone fractures. The frequency, clinical and laboratory features, and circumstances of the fat embolism syndrome have been extensively described.[3,407-411] The syndrome consists of a triad of respiratory distress, decreased alertness, and a petechial rash developing 24–48 hours after an injury. Table 10.5 lists the major findings in patients with the fat

Table 10.5 Fat embolism

Major clinical features

Dyspnea and respiratory distress
Decreased alertness and cognitive function
Petechiae

Other findings

Fever
Tachycardia
Retinal infarcts
Jaundice

Laboratory and imaging

Anemia
Thrombocytopenia
Hypoxia
Abnormal chest x-ray
Fat globules and lipid in the urine
Microembolism during transcranial Doppler monitoring
Fat emboli visible during transesophageal echocardiography
MRI showing multiple infarcts and small hemorrhages

embolism syndrome. Fat embolism is most often found after blunt physical trauma with fractured bones but can occur after cardiac surgery and in patients who have bone infarctions. In patients with injuries, the long bones and pelvis are most often involved especially the femurs. The fat embolism syndrome is unusual in children and in patients with fractures limited to the upper extremities.[407] Often the cause is multiple fractures resulting from vehicular acccidents. Investigators retrospectively reviewed 10 years experience of the fat embolism syndrome found at one trauma center and found 27 instances among 3026 patients (0.9%) with long-bone fractures.[408] Occasionally the fat embolism syndrome develops after cardiac surgery when the atria or ventricles are entered.[412,413] The mechanism of fat embolism after open heart surgery is unclear but fat from the sternotomy or epicardial fat may directly enter the systemic circulation. Cardiotomy suction tubes draining the pericardium during cardioplumonary bypass contain variable quantities of fat globules.

Fat embolism has also been reported in patients with sickle cell anemia (homozygous S-S and those who have S-C disease).[413–416] In sickle cell disease patients, the fat originates from bone and bone marrow infarcts. Bone and joint pain and crisis may precede fat embolism in some patients. Fat embolism has also been described after therapeutic procedures that use lipid substances to form stable drugs for injection. Lipiodol has been used to mix with anticancer drugs that are fat soluble to form stable covalent conjugates. This mixture is then injected into an artery feeding a tumor; for example, in the liver. Fat embolism has been described after such therapeutic procedures.[418] In one report, the clinical findings included dyspnea and decreased alertness. Hypoxemia preceded or accompanied stupor. MRI showed multiple focal abnormalities mostly in borderzone regions. The neurological signs were severe but transient and cleared completely within weeks. None of the three reported patients had cardiac shunts demonstrable by echocardiography.[418] Fat emboli can occasionally be introduced during placement of pumps designed to release pharmaceutical agents into the cerebrospinal fluid.[419] Parenteral nutrition containing high lipid content occasionally is infused into a cervico-cranial artery when a catheter is misplaced into an artery rather than a vein.

The fat embolism syndrome usually develops after a delay of a few hours up to a few days after trauma. In one series of 14 patients, all of whom had traumatic injuries with long bone fractures, the latency of onset of signs of fat embolism after trauma ranged from 12 to 72 hours (mean 41 hours).[408] At times the clinical manifestations of fat embolism can be delayed for as long as 5 days.[406] Most patients have symptom onset between 24 and 72 hours after injury.

The major clinical manifestations of the fat embolism syndrome are dyspnea, tachypnea, fever, tachycardia, petechiae and neurological dysfunction.[411] Jaundice can also occur. Neurological symptoms and signs may precede or follow respiratory distress and are characterized as confusion with delirium often followed by a decrease in the level of consciousness. Neurological symptoms and signs are present in greater than 80% of patients. Most often patients develop an encephalopathy characterized by restlessness, agitation, confusion,

poor memory, and decreased alertness. This state often passes into stupor or coma. Seizures are common at onset or early during the course of illness. Seizures can be focal or generalized. Focal neurological signs are also common and include hemiparesis, conjugate eye deviation, aphasia and visual field abnormalities. Motor abnormalities including increased tone in the lower extremities, Babinski signs, and decerebrate rigidity are often found. Focal neurological signs were noted in 33% of patients in one series.[411] Some patients have scotomas and other visual abnormalities related to retinal dysfunction caused by fat embolism.

Pulmonary symptoms develop shortly after or concurrent with the neurological symptoms. Dyspnea and tachypnea are prominent and patients may become cyanotic. Tachycardia, high fever, and circulatory collapse also occur; hypotension is often related to blood loss, hypoxemia, and hypovolemia. Renal failure can develop. The pulmonary emboli can result in increased resistance in the pulmonary artery bed and increased pressures in the right side of the heart. In patients with a PFO the pulmonary hypertension may promote extensive right-to-left passage of fat emboli through the PFO.

An important clue to the presence of fat microemboli is the presence on physical examination of petechiae. Petechiae are found in 50–75% of patients with the fat embolism syndrome. They are most often found in the lower palpebral conjunctivae and the skin of the neck, shoulder, and the axillary folds.[1,407,410] Another important clinical clue is the appearance of fat emboli within the arteries of the eye. Microinfarcts are sometimes visible in the optic fundus especially in the perimacular regions. Small hemorrhages sometimes with white pale centers are also found. Fat globules can sometimes be seen within retinal arteries. Papilledema is occasionally found.

Laboratory tests are often helpful in diagnosis. Many patients develop abnormal chest x-rays. Fine stippling and fluffy lung infiltrates are common and are seen diffusely through the lung fields. Most patients have a drop in hemoglobin and Hct due to traumatic loss of blood and hemolysis. Thrombocytopenia, and prolonged prothrombin and activated partial thromboplastin times are common and are attributed to a consumptive coagulopathy. Frank disseminated intravascular coagulation may also occur. TCD monitoring of patients with long bone fractures can document fat emboli.[420,421] Brain imaging may show small hemorrhages, brain edema, and focal infarcts usually manifested by regions of gyral enhancement on CT or MRI scans. CT scans are most often normal but may show areas of hypodensity and small hemorrhages. MRI is much more sensitive and often shows abnormalities within the white matter and in borderzone regions.[422] FLAIR and contrast-enhanced images are particularly helpful in showing microinfarcts.[422] Figure 10.21 is an MRI FLAIR image that shows many small brain infarcts due to fat embolism in a patient who became stuporous after a leg fracture. Magnetic resonance spectroscopy (MRS) can also be used to identify the presence of fat.[419] In one reported patient who had fat embolism develop after a femoral fracture, MRS performed 35 hours after the onset of coma showed the presence of long-chain

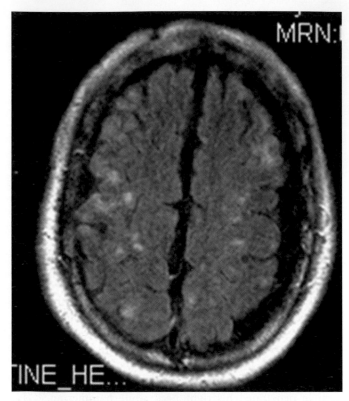

Figure 10.21 MRI FLAIR image showing multiple small infarcts in a patient with fat embolism after a leg fracture.

lipid resonance in high quantities in the periventricular white matter and occipital cerebral cortices of the patient with no associated lactate resonance. The lipid gradually disappeared on subsequent examinations.[419]

Lipid globules are sometimes found in the urine when fat stains are used. Skin, renal, and muscle biopsies may show fat globules within small skin, muscle, and renal vessels and in renal glomeruli. Cryostat frozen sections of blood also can show the presence of neutral fat; neutral fat is most often found in patients with hypoxemia and a partial pressure of arterial carbon dioxide ($PaCO_2$) of less than 60 mmHg. Hypoxemia is very common in patients with the fat embolism syndrome. One of the most effective and specific tests for fat embolism is bronchopulmonary lavage.[420,423] The technique involves microscopic examination of cells recovered by lavage and stained with a specific stain for neutral fat; for example, using oil Red O dye.

The mortality rate in patients with the fat embolism syndrome is quite high (as much as 50%) although the mortality rate has declined over time.[1,407,408] When coma, severe blood loss, hypotension, high fever, and disseminated intravascular coagulation (DIC) are present the mortality rate remains substantial. Necropsy of the brain of patients dying with the fat embolism syndrome shows many small ball or ring-shaped, and perivascular hemorrhages, brain edema, and regions of microinfarction.[424] Stains for fat reveal fat globules within hemorrhagic lesions and in small vessels throughout the brain. Small hemorrhages, edema, and hyaline membranes are often found in the lungs. Fat globules are also often visible in renal glomeruli, myocardium, liver, pancreas, spleen, and gastrointestinal mucosa.

Treatment of patients with the fat embolism syndrome has not been formally studied in therapeutic trials. Supportive care including oxygen administration often with assisted respiration and fluid and blood replacement is very important. Corticosteroids, heparin, and intravenous administration of 5% alcohol solutions have all been tried but their effectiveness has not been well studied. Heparin has been used in patients with consumptive coagulopathies and also because of its posited lipolytic effect. Alcohol is also believed to have a lipolytic capability. Among these treatments, corticosteroids administration has been most frequently used.

Air embolism

Gas bubbles occasionally enter the systemic circulation and cause air embolism to the brain and other organs. The sources of air are quite diverse. Most often air is introduced iatrogenically during procedures and surgery. Air embolism can follow endoscopy laparoscopy and surgery on the gastrointestinal tract,[1,425–428] spontaneous pneumothorax and procedures and surgery in the thorax involving the lungs,[425,429] pneumoorbitography, perineal and peritoneal air insufflation, pneumoarthrography, and surgery on the heart, neck, brain, and axilla.[425] Atrial-esophageal fistulas are another source of air entry into the vascular system. Air can also enter the cranium after fractures involving the cribiform plate and the paranasal sinuses[430] and after surgery on the sinuses. Venous and arterial catheterization and cardiopulmonary bypass are common causes of air embolism.[431,432] Air can also be introduced during home infusion therapy.[433] Less often air embolism follows penetrating traumatic injuries to the thorax, lungs, or major blood vessels. Air introduction into the vascular system is quite common during cesarean deliveries.[434] Precordial Doppler can demonstrate some air embolism in about half of all cesarean deliveries.[434,435]

Another important and quite different circumstance that leads to air embolism is in relation to scuba diving and rapid ascents after descents into deep water.[436,437] During diving accidents, air becomes trapped in the alveoli of the lungs due to partial bronchial occlusion from mucous plugs and failure to exhale. Because the volume of a gas varies inversely with pressure (Boyle's law), pressurized air bubbles in the lungs increase dramatically in volume as the diver ascends and the ambient surrounding pressure falls.[438] The rapid expansion of air in the lungs causes entry of air into the pulmonary arterial and venous outflow systems.[438] Gas bubbles pass through the lung vasculature or through a PFO into the systemic circulation. Similar to the situation in fat embolism, many small particles enter the circulation and block the microvasculature. The frequency of PFO in divers with clinical decompression syndromes is higher than expected by chance.

Introduction of a large quantity of air into the venous system can result in sudden blockage of the pulmonary artery and right ventricular outflow tract with resultant cardiac arrhythmia and sudden death or circulatory collapse.[438]

Dyspnea, cyanosis, chest pain, restlessness and a feeling of impending death can develop. When small amounts of air are released into the venous system filtering by the pulmonary vessels protects the coronary and brain circulations. Lung edema can result from air in the lungs especially when there is an increase in pulmonary artery pressure. Air can also stimulate the release of various thromboplastins, surfactants, and cytokines that cause lung injury and coagulopathy.

Air bubbles in arteries supplying the brain cause an immediate but transient block in blood flow. Air quickly moves through the capilllary bed into the venules and dissipates.[1,438] The gas bubbles cause arterial vasoconstriction followed by dilatation and stasis of blood flow.[438]

Symptoms and signs of brain gas embolism have been studied most thoroughly in individuals who have had diving-related incidents.[436,437,439] These occur during scuba diving and have been well studied in naval personnel who escape too quickly from submerged submarines.[439] Loss of consciousness often develops suddenly after the diver emerges onto the surface of the water. Dizziness, chest discomfort, paresthesias, weakness, blurred vision, nausea, and headache are the most common symptoms and may precede the loss of consciousness. Seizures and focal neurological signs, especially related to dysfunction of the brainstem and cerebellum are also quite common.[436,437,439]

Discrete focal collections of gas and multiple focal air collections are sometimes found in the brain on cranial CT examination.[440,441] Brain edema with compression of the ventricular system is another common and important finding on brain imaging examinations. DWI imaging using MRI can also show scatered areas of brain infarction. TCD is quite sensitive for detection of air microemboli.[440,441] Treatment has usually consisted of inhalation of 100% oxygen as well as the use of hyperbaric recompression chambers.[432,436]

Tumor embolism

Occasionally major arteries supplying the brain are occluded by tumor emboli. This occurs when a neoplasm directly erodes into a cervical artery, or a pulmonary vein, or when a tumor erodes into a systemic vein, embolizes to the heart, and then passes through a cardiac septal abnormality to enter the systemic circulation. The most frequent tumors that embolize are primary pulmonary neoplasms or tumors that have metastasized to the lungs.[442] Brain embolism has sometimes occurred after lung surgery for cancer. Necropsy has usually shown tumor invasion of pulmonary veins or invasion of the left atrium.[443] Surgical manipulation of the lungs in patients with lung tumors can promote systemic embolization of the tumor. Although most often the clinical syndrome is that of a stroke, embolism to other systemic organs also occurs. Tumor emboli can also pass through a PFO or another cardiac septal defect. Tumor emboli have also been reported in patients with thyroid and other neck cancers that eroded into neck arteries.[443]

Foreign body embolism

Occasionally foreign bodies enter the systemic vascular system and embolize to the brain. Foreign bodies that embolize to the brain must either enter the lungs and pulmonary veins, enter directly into the left side of the heart itself, enter the right side of the heart and traverse a defect in the cardiac septum, or penetrate the cervico-cranial arteries that supply the brain. Bullets and pellets may penetrate the skin and land in the heart.[444] Shotgun pellets have been reported to puncture a carotid artery in the neck and become visible on cranial CT scans causing brain embolic infarction.[445,446] Langenbach et al. described the case of a 52-year-old man in whom a small metal particle penetrated his right neck while hammering.[447] He soon developed a severe left hemiplegia. Plain skull films showed a 2 × 7 mm metal-dense particle to the right of the pituitary fossa. CT showed a large right middle cerebral artery territory infarct and angiography showed that the metal fragment was blocking the middle cerebral artery.[447] Figure 10.22 is a CT scan that shows a shotgun pellet proximal to a large middle cerebral artery territitory infarct and Figure 10.23 contains arteriograms of the same patient that show 2 mm-sized pellets blocking the intracranial carotid and middle cerebral arteries. These pellets originated from the heart in a patient who was shot in the chest during an argument.[444] One reason that echocardiograms often fail to show an embolic source is the very small size of potentially devastating thromboemboli. Foreign bodies for a variety of reasons can gain entry into the heart and embolize to systemic arteries and the brain.[448–450]

Retinal and brain arteries can become blocked by foreign particles in patients who mash drugs manufactured for oral use

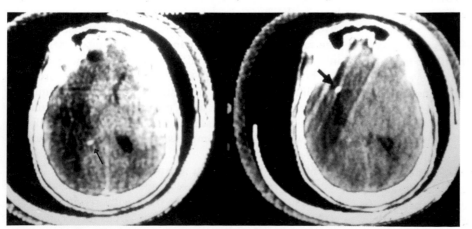

Figure 10.22 CT scans showing a large MCA territory infarct on the right of the scans (black open arrowheads). Black arrows point to the pieces of shotgun pellet seen within the brain images. From Kase CS, White R, Vinson TL, Eichelberger RP. Shotgun pellet embolism to the middle cerebral artery. *Neurology* 1981;31:458–461 with permission.

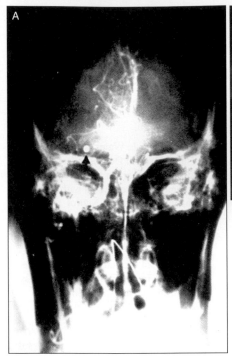

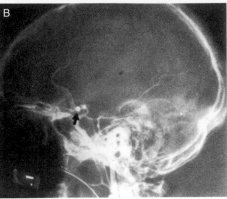

Figure 10.23 Carotid arteriograms: (A) anteroposterior and (B) lateral view showing two pieces of buckshot (black arrows) blocking the MCA. From Kase CS, White R, Vinson TL, Eichelberger RP. Shotgun pellet embolism to the middle cerebral artery. *Neurology* 1981;31:458–461 with permission.

and inject the drugs intravenously.[451–455] The most frequently reported particles are talc and methylcellulose that are used to bind drugs to maintain them in pill form. The particles first block lung vessels. Pulmonary vascular obliteration causes pulmonary hypertension and arteriovenous shunting develops in the lungs allowing the particles to enter the pulmonary veins and then the systemic circulation.[451,452] Talc and cornstarch emboli can be seen in the retinal arteries of some of these drug abusers.[453] Strokes have also been described in patients who have injected drugs directly into neck arteries.[455]

This chapter has reviewed the roles of the three leading actors in the drama of brain embolism – the recipient artery, the matter that embolized, and the source of the matter. We emphasize that the matter that represents the embolus is the most important focus for treatment both acutely and prophylactically.

References

1. Caplan LR. Embolic particles. In LR Caplan, W Manning (eds), *Brain Embolism*. New York: Informa Healthcare, 2006, pp 259–275.

2. Molina C, Alexandrov A. Transcranial Doppler ultrasound. In LR Caplan, W Manning (eds), *Brain Embolism*. New York: Informa Healthcare, 2006, pp 113–128.

3. Caplan LR. Brain embolism, revisited. *Neurology* 1993;43:1281–1287.

4. Caplan LR. Brain embolism. In LR Caplan, JW Hurst, M Chimowitz (eds), *Clinical Neurocardiology*. New York: Marcel Dekker, 1999, pp 35–185.

5. Markus HS. Transcranial Doppler detection of circulating cerebral emboli, a review. *Stroke* 1993;24:1246–1250.

6. Sliwka U, Job F-P, Wissuwa D, et al. Occurrence of transcranial Doppler high-intensity transient signals in patients with potential cardiac sources of embolism, a prospective study. *Stroke* 1995;26:2067–2070.

7. Daffertshofer M, Ries S, Schminke U, Hennerici M. High-intensity transient signals in patients with cerebral ischemia. *Stroke* 1996;27:1844–1849.

8. Sliwka U, Lingnau A, Stohlmann W-D, et al. Prevalence and time course of microembolic signals in patients with acute strokes, a prospective study. *Stroke* 1997;28:358–363.

9. Babikian VL, Caplan LR. Brain embolism is a dynamic process with variable characteristics. *Neurology* 2000;54:797–801.

10. Caplan LR. Recipient artery. In LR Caplan, W Manning (eds), *Brain Embolism*. New York: Informa Healthcare, 2006, pp 31–59.

11. Mohr JP, Caplan LR, Melski JW, et al. The Harvard Cooperative Stroke Registry: A prospective registry. *Neurology* 1978;29:754–762.

12. Caplan LR, Hier DB, D'Cruz I. Cerebral embolism in the Michael Reese Stroke Registry. *Stroke* 1983;14:530–536.

13. Mohr JP, Gautier JC, Hier DB, Stein RW. Middle cerebral artery. In HJM Barnett, JP Mohr, BM Stein, FM Yatsu (eds), *Stroke, Pathophysiology, Diagnosis, and Management*, Vol **1**. New York: Churchill Livingstone, 1986, pp 377–450.

14. Minematsu K, Yamaguchi T, Omae T. "Spectacular shrinking deficit": Rapid recovery from a major hemispheric syndrome by migration of an embolus. *Neurology* 1992;42:157–162.

15. Bogousslavsky J, van Melle G, Regli F. The Lausanne Stroke Registry: Analysis of 1000 consecutive patients with first stroke. *Stroke* 1988;19:1083–1092.

16. Gacs G, Merei FT, Bodosi M. Balloon catheter as a model of cerebral emboli in humans. *Stroke* 1982;13:39–42.

17. Helgason C. Cardioembolic stroke topography and pathogenesis.

Cerebrovasc Brain Metab Rev 1992;**4**:28–58.

18. Caplan LR. *Vertebrobasilar Ischemia and Hemorrhage: Clinical Findings, Diagnosis, and Management of Posterior Circulation Disease*. Cambridge: Cambridge University Press, 2015.

19. Caplan LR. Top of the basilar syndrome: Selected clinical aspects. *Neurology* 1980;**30**:72–79.

20. Mehler MF. The rostral basilar artery syndrome: Diagnosis, etiology, prognosis. *Neurology* 1989;**39**:9–16.

21. Caplan LR. Cerebellar infarcts: Key features. *Rev Neurol Dis* 2005;**2**:51–60.

22. Lodder J, Krijne-Kubat B, Broekman J. Cerebral hemorrhagic infarction at autopsy: Cardiac embolic cause and the relationship to the cause of death. *Stroke* 1986;**17**:626–629.

23. Hart RG, Easton JD. Hemorrhagic infarcts. *Stroke* 1986;**17**:586–589.

24. Timsit SG, Sacco RL, Mohr JP, et al. Brain infarction severity differs according to cardiac or arterial embolic source. *Neurology* 1993;**43**:728–733.

25. Bladin CF. *Seizures After Stroke*. Melbourne: University of Melbourne, 1997. Thesis.

26. Kittner SJ, Sharkness CM, Price TR, et al. Infarcts with a cardiac source of embolism in the NINCDS Stroke Data Bank: Historical features. *Neurology* 1990;**40**:281–284.

27. Hinton RC, Kistler JP, Fallon JR, Friedlich AL, Fisher CM. Influence of etiology of atrial fibrillation on incidence of systemic embolism. *Am J Card* 1977;**40**:509–513.

28. Abboud H, Labreuche J, Gongora-Riverra F, et al. Prevalence and determinants of subdiaphragmatic visceral infarction in patients with fatal stroke. *Stroke* 2007;**38**:1442–1446.

29. Ringelstein EB, Koschorke S, Holling A, et al. Computed tomographic patterns of proven embolic brain infarctions. *Ann Neurol* 1989;**26**:759–765.

30. Viehman JA, Saver JL, Liebeskind DS, et al. Utility of urinalysis in discriminating cardioembolic stroke mechanism. *Arch Neurol* 2007;**64**:667–670.

31. Slaoui T, Klein IF, Guidoux C, et al. Prevalence of subdiaphragmatic visceral infarction in cardioembolic stroke. *Neurology* 2010;**74**:1030–1032.

32. Ringelstein EB, Koschorke S, Holling A, et al. Computed tomographic patterns of proven embolic brain infarctions. *Ann Neurol* 1989;**26**:759–765.

33. Fisher CM, Adams R. Observations on brain embolism with special reference to the mechanism of hemorrhagic infarction. *J Neuropathol Exp Neurol* 1951;**10**:92–93.

34. Fisher CM, Adams RD. Observations on brain embolism with special reference to hemorrhagic infarction. In AJ Furlan (ed), *The Heart and Stroke*. London: Springer, 1987 pp 17–36.

35. Yamaguchi T, Minematsu K, Choki JI, Ikeda M. Clinical and neuroradiological analysis of thrombotic and embolic cerebral infarction. *Jpn Circ J* 1984;**48**:50–58.

36. Okada Y, Yamaguchi T, Minematsu K, et al. Hemorrhagic transformation in cerebral embolism. *Stroke* 1989;**20**:598–603.

37. Pessin MS, Estol C, Lafranchise F, Caplan LR. Safety of anticoagulation after hemorrhagic infarction. *Neurology* 1993;**43**:1298–1303.

38. Chaves CJ, Pessin MS, Caplan LR, et al. Cerebellar hemorrhagic infarction. *Neurology* 1996;**46**:346–349.

39. Garcia J, Ho K-L, Caccamo DV. Intracerebral hemorrhage: Pathology of selected topics. In CS Kase, LR Caplan (eds), *Intracerebral Hemorrhage*. Boston: Butterworth–Heinemann, 1994, pp 45–72.

40. Fieschi C, Argentino C, Lenzi G, et al. Clinical and instrumental evaluation of patients with ischemic stroke within the first six hours. *J Neurol Sci* 1989;**91**:311–322.

41. del Zoppo GJ, Poeck K, Pessin MS, et al. Recombinant tissue plasminogen activator in acute thrombotic and embolic stroke. *Ann Neurol* 1992;**32**:78–86.

42. Wolpert SM, Bruckmann H, Greenlee R, Wechsler L, Pessin MS, del Zoppo GJ. Neuroradiologic evaluation of patients with acute stroke treated with recombinant tissue plasminogen activator. The rt-PA Acute Stroke Study Group. *AJNR Am J Neuroradiol* 1993;**14**:3–13.

43. Dalal P, Shah P, Sheth S, et al. Cerebral embolism: Angiographic observations on spontaneous clot lysis. *Lancet* 1965;**1**:61–64.

44. Liebeskind A, Chinichian A, Schechter M. The moving embolus seen during cerebral angiography. *Stroke* 1971;**2**:440–443.

45. Caplan LR, Allam GJ, Teal PA. The moving embolus. *J Neurimag* 1993;**3**:195–197.

46. Sharma VK, Tsivgoulis G, Lao AY, Alexandrov AV. Role of transcranial Doppler ultrasonography in evaluation of patients with cerebrovascular disease. *Curr Neurol Neurosci Rep* 2007;**7**:8–20.

47. Thomassen L, Waje-Andreassen U, Naess H, et al. Doppler ultrasound and clinical findings in patients with acute ischemic stroke treated with thrombolysis. *Eur J Neurol* 2005;**12**:462–465.

48. Molina CA, Alexandrov AV, Demchuk AM, et al. Improving the predictive accuracy of recanalization on stroke outcome in patients treated with tissue plasminogen activator. *Stroke* 2004;**35**:151–156.

49. Askevold ET, Naess H, Thomassen L. Predictors of recanalization after intravenous thrombolysis in acute ischemic stroke. *J Stroke Cerebrovasc Dis* 2007;**16**:21–24.

50. Georgiadis D, Lindner A, Manz M, et al. Intracranial microembolic signals in 500 patients with potential cardiac or carotid embolic source and in normal controls. *Stroke* 1997;**28**:1203–1207.

51. Cho K-H, Kim JS, Kwon SU, Cho A-H, Kang D-W. Significance of susceptibility vessel sign on T2*-weighted gradient echo imaging for identification of stroke subtypes. *Stroke* 2005;**36**:2379–2383.

52. Kimura K, Iguchi V, Shibazaki K, Watanabe M, Iwanga T, Aoki J. M1 susceptiblity vessel sign on T2* as a strong predictor for no early recanalization after IV – t-PA in acute ischemic stroke. *Stroke* 2009;**40**:3130–3132.

53. Yamamoto N, Satomi J, Tada Y, et al. Two-layered susceptibility vessel sign on 3-Tesla T2*-weighted imaging is a predictive biomarker of stroke subtype. *Stroke* 2015;**46**:269–271.

54. Liebeskind DS, Sanossian N, Yong WH, et al. CT and MRI early vessel signs reflect clot composition in acute stroke. *Stroke* 2011;**42**:1237–1243.

55. Caplan LR. Of birds and nests and brain emboli. *Rev Neurol* 1991;**147**:265–273.

56. Caplan LR, Manning W. Cardiac sources of embolism: The usual suspects. In LR Caplan, W Manning (eds), *Brain Embolism*. New York: Informa Healthcare, 2006, pp 129–159.

57. Manning W. Cardiac sources of embolism: Pathophysiology and

identification. In LR Caplan, W Manning (eds), *Brain Embolism.* New York: Informa Healthcare, 2006, pp 161–186.

58. Virchow R. *Gesammelte Abhandlungen zur Wissenschaftlichenmedtezin.* Frankfurt: Meidinger Sohn, 1856, pp 219–732.

59. Harker LA, Slichter SL. Studies of platelet and fibrinogen kinetics in patients with prosthetic heart valves. *N Engl J Med* 1970;**283**:1302–1305.

60. Baumgartner HR, Haudenschild C. Adhesion of platelets to subendothelium. *Ann N Y Acad Sci* 1972;**201**:22–36.

61. Gustafsson C, Blomback M, Britton M, et al. Coagulation factors and the increased risk of stroke in nonvalvular atrial fibrillation. *Stroke* 1990;**21**:47–51.

62. Kumagai K, Fukunami M, Ohmori M, et al. Increased intracardiovascular clotting in patients with chronic atrial fibrillation. *J Am Coll Cardiol* 1990;**16**:377–380.

63. Hanna JP, Furlan AJ. Cardiac disease and embolic sources. In LR Caplan (ed), *Brain Ischemia.* London: Springer, 1995, pp 299–315.

64. Goldman ME, Pearce LA, Hart RG. Pathophysiologic correlates of thromboembolism in nonvalvular atrial fibrillation: I. Reduced flow velocity in the left atrial appendage (The Stroke Prevention in Atrial Fibrillation (SPAF-III) Study). *J Am Soc Echocardiogr* 1999;**12**:1080–1087.

65. Wolf PA, Dawber TR, Thomas HE, Kannel WB. Epidemiologic assessment of chronic atrial fibrillation and risk of stroke: The Framingham Study. *Neurology* 1978;**28**:973–977.

66. Wolf PA, Abbott RD, Kannel WB. Atrial fibrillation: A major contribution to stroke in the elderly. The Framingham Study. *Arch Intern Med* 1987;**147**:1561–1564.

67. Cairns JA, Connolly SJ. Nonrheumatic atrial fibrillation. Risk of stroke and role of antithrombotic therapy. *Circulation* 1991;**84**:469–481.

68. Dunn M, Alexander J, DeSilva R, Hildner F. Antithrombotic therapy in atrial fibrillation. *Chest* 1989;**95**:S118–S127.

69. The Stroke Prevention in Atrial Fibrillation Investigators. Predictors of thromboembolism in atrial fibrillation: 1. Clinical features of patients at risk. *Ann Intern Med* 1992;**116**:1–5.

70. Atrial Fibrillation Investigators. Risk factors for stroke and efficacy of antithrombotic therapy in atrial fibrillation: Analysis of pooled data from five randomized controlled trials. *Arch Intern Med* 1994;**154**:1449–1457.

71. Caplan LR, D'Cruz I, Hier DB, et al. Atrial size, atrial fibrillation, and stroke. *Ann Neurol* 1986;**19**:158–161.

72. Stroke Prevention in Atrial Fibrillation Investigators. Predictors of thromboembolism in atrial fibrillation: II. Echocardiographic features of patients at risk. *Ann Intern Med* 1992;**116**:6–12.

73. DiPasquale G, Urbinati S, Pinelli G. New echocardiographic markers of embolic risk in atrial fibrillation. *Cerebrovasc Dis* 1995;**5**:315–322.

74. Vernhorst P, Kamp O, Visser CA, Verheught FWA. Left atrial appendage flow velocity assessment using transesophageal echocardiography in nonrheumatic atrial fibrillation and systemic embolism. *Am J Cardiol* 1993;**71**:192–196.

75. Garcia-Fernandez MA, Torrecilla EG, San Roman D, et al. Left atrial appendage Doppler flow patterns: Implications of thrombus formation. *Am Heart J* 1992;**124**:955–965.

76. Beppu S, Nimura Y, Sakakibara H. Smoke-like echo in the left atrial cavity in mitral valve disease: Its features and significance. *J Am Coll Cardiol* 1985;**6**:744–749.

77. Merino A, Hauptman P, Badiman L, et al. Echocardiographic "smoke" is produced by an interaction of erythrocytes and plasma proteins modulated by shear forces. *J Am Coll Cardiol* 1992;**20**:1661–1668.

78. Black IW, Stewart WJ. The role of echocardiography in the evaluation of cardiac sources of embolism. *Echocardiography* 1993;**10**:429–439.

79. Chimowitz MI, DeGeorgia MA, Poole RM, et al. Left atrial spontaneous echo contrast is highly associated with previous stroke in patients with atrial fibrillation or mitral stenosis. *Stroke* 1993;**24**:1015–1019.

80. Warraich HJ, Gandhavadi M, Manning WJ. Mechanical discordance of the left atrium and appendage. *Stroke* 2014;**45**:1481–1484.

81. Manning WJ, Silverman DI, Gordon SPF, Krumholz HM, Douglas PS. Cardioversion from atrial fibrillation without prolonged anticoagulation with use of transesophageal echocardiography to exclude the presence of atrial thrombi. *N Engl J Med* 1993;**328**:750–756.

82. Stroke Prevention in Atrial Fibrillation Investigators Committee on Echocardiography. Transesophageal echocardiographic correlates of thromboembolism in high-risk patients with nonvalvular atrial fibrillation. *Ann Intern Med* 1998;**128**:639–647.

83. Weigner MJ, Thomas LR, Patel U, et al. Transesophageal-echocardiography-facilitated early cardioversion from atrial fibrillation: Short-term safety and impact on maintenance of sinus rhythm at 1 year. *Am J Med* 2001;**110**:694–702.

84. Klein AL, Grimm RA, Murray RD, et al. Use of transesophageal echocardiography to guide cardioversion in patients with atrial fibrillation. *N Engl J Med* 2001;**344**:1411–1420.

85. Stoddard MF, Dawkins PR, Prince CR, Ammash NM. Left atrial appendage thrombus is not uncommon in patients with acute atrial fibrillation and a recent embolic event: A transesophageal echocardiographic study. *J Am Coll Cardiol* 1995;**25**:452–459.

86. Manning WJ, Silverman DI, Waksmonski CA, Oettgen P, Douglas PS. Prevalence of residual left atrial thrombi in patients presenting with acute thromboembolism and newly recognized atrial fibrillation. *Arch Intern Med* 1995;**155**:2193–2197.

87. Kishore A, Vail A, Majid A, et al. Detection of atrial fibrillation after ischemic stroke or transient ischemic attack: A systematic review and meta-analysis. *Stroke* 2014;**45**:520–526.

88. Kamel H. Heart-rhythm monitoring for evaluation of cryptogenic stroke. *N Engl J Med* 2014;**370**:2532–2533.

89. Sanna T, Diener H-C, Passman RS, et al. for the CRYSTAL AF Investigators. Cryptogenic stroke and underlying atrial fibrillation. *N Engl J Med* 2014;**370**:2478–2486.

90. Gladstone DJ, Spring M, Dorian P, et al. for the EMBRACE Investigators. Atrial fibrillation in patients with cryptogenic stroke. *N Engl J Med* 2014;**370**:2467–2477.

91. Hoshino T, Nagao T, Shiga T, et al. Prolonged QTc interval predicts poststroke paroxysmal atrial fibrillation. *Stroke* 2015;**46**:71–76.

92. Mair J. Biochemistry of B-type natriuretic peptide – where are we now? *Clin Chem Lab Med* 2008;**46**:1507–1514.

93. Braunwald E. Biomarkers in heart failure. *N Engl J Med* 2008;**358**:2148–2159.

94. Patton KK, Ellinor PT, Heckbert SR, et al. N-terminal pro-B-type naturetic peptide is a major predictor of the development of atrial fibrillation: The Cardiovascular Health Study. *Circulation* 2009;**120**:1768–17774.

95. Boston Area Anticoagulation Trial for Atrial Fibrillation Investigators. The effect of low-dose warfarin on the risk of stroke in patients with nonrheumatic atrial fibrillation. *N Engl J Med* 1990;**323**:1505–1511.

96. EAFT Study Group. Silent brain infarction in nonrheumatic atrial fibrillation. *Neurology* 1996;**46**:159–165.

97. EAFT (European Atrial Fibrillation Trial) Study Group. Secondary prevention in non-rheumatic atrial fibrillation after transient ischaemic attack or minor stroke. *Lancet* 1993;**342**:1255–1262.

98. Petersen P, Godtfredsen J, Boysen G, et al. Placebo-controlled, randomized trial of warfarin and aspirin for prevention of thromboembolic complications in chronic atrial fibrillation: The Copenhagen AFASAK Study. *Lancet* 1989;**1**:175–179.

99. Stroke Prevention in Atrial Fibrillation Investigators. The Stroke Prevention In Atrial Fibrillation Study: Final results. *Circulation* 1991;**84**:527–539.

100. Stroke Prevention in Atrial Fibrillation Investigators. Adjusted-dose warfarin versus low-intensity, fixed-dose warfarin plus aspirin for high-risk patients with atrial fibrillation: Stroke Prevention in Atrial Fibrillation III randomised clinical trial. *Lancet* 1996;**348**:633–638.

101. Stroke Prevention in Atrial Fibrillation Investigators. Prospective identification of patients with nonvalvular atrial fibrillation at low risk of stroke during treatment with aspirin: Stroke Prevention in Atrial Fibrillation III Study. *Circulation* 1997;**96**(Suppl):1–281(abst).

102. Albers G. Atrial fibrillation and stroke. Three new studies, three remaining questions. *Arch Intern Med* 1994;**154**:1443–1448.

103. Samsa GP, Matchar DB, Goldstein LB, et al. Quality of anticoagulation management among patients with atrial fibrillation: Results of a review of medical records from two communities. *Arch Intern Med* 2000;**160**:967–973.

104. Chiquette E, Amato MG, Bussey HI. Comparison of an anticoagulation clinic with usual medical care: Anticoagulation control, patient outcomes, and health care costs. *Arch Intern Med* 1998;**158**:1641–1647.

105. Kucher N, Connolly S, Beckman JA, et al. International normalized ratio increase before warfarin-associated hemorrhage: Brief and subtle. *Arch Intern Med* 2004;**164**:2176–2179.

106. Rash A, Downes T, Portner R, et al. A randomized controlled trial of warfarin vs. aspirin for stroke prevention in octogenarians with atrial fibrillation (WASPO). *Age Ageing* 2007;**36**:151–156.

107. Mant J, Hobbs FD, Fletcher K, et al. Warfarin versus aspirin for stroke prevention in an elderly community population with atrial fibrillation (The Birmingham Atrial Fibrillation Treatment of the Aged Study, BAFTA): A randomized controlled trial. *Lancet* 2007;**370**:493–503.

108. Di Nisio M, Middeldorp S, Buller HR. Direct thrombin inhibitors. *Engl J Med* 2005;**353**:1028–1040.

109. Yeh CH, Fredenburgh JC, Weitz JI. Oral direct factor Xa inhibitors. *Circ Res* 2012;**111**:1069–1078.

110. Connolly SJ, Ezekowitz MD, Yusuf S, et al. Dabigatran versus warfarin in patients with atrial fibrillation. *N Engl J Med* 2009;**361**:1139–1151.

111. Connolly SJ, Eikelboom J, Joyner C, et al. Apixaban in patients with atrial fibrillation. *N Engl J Med* 2011;**364**:806–817.

112. Granger CB, Alexander JH, McMurray JJ, et al. Apixaban versus warfarin in patients with atrial fibrillation. *N Engl J Med* 2011;**365**:981–992.

113. Patel MR, Mahaffey KW, Garg J, et al. Rivaroxaban versus warfarin in nonvalvular atrial fibrillation. *N Engl J Med* 2011;**365**:883–891.

114. Giugliano RP, Ruff CT, Braunwald E, et al. Edoxaban versus warfarin in patients with atrial fibrillation. *N Engl J Med* 2013;**369**:2093–2104.

115. Cameron C, Coyle D, Richter D, et al. Systematic review and network meta-analysis comparing antithrombotic agents for the prevention of stroke and major bleeding in patients with atrial fibrillation. *BMJ Open* 2014;**4**:e004301.

116. Sherman DG. Stroke prevention in atrial fibrillation. Pharmacological rate vs. rhythm control. *Stroke* 2007;**38**(part 2):615–617.

117. Roy D, Talajic M, Nattel S, et al. for the Atrial Fibrillation and Congestive Heart Failure Investigators. Rhythm control versus rate control for atrial fibrillation and heart failure. *N Engl J Med* 2008;**358**:2667–2677.

118. Gillinov AM. Advances in surgical treatment of atrial fibrillation. *Stroke* 2007;**38** (part 2): 618–623.

119. Tung R, Buch E, Shivkumar K. Catheter ablation of atrial fibrillation. *Circulation* 2012;**126**:223–229.

120. Reddy VY, Doshi SK, Sievert H, et al. on behalf of the PROTECT AF Investigators. Percutaneous left atrial appendage closure for stroke prophylaxis in patients with atrial fibrillation. *Circulation* 2013;**127**:720–729.

121. Swaans MJ, Post MC, Rensing BJWM, Boersma LVA. Ablation for atrial fibrillation in combination with left atrial appendage closure: First results of a feasibility study. *J Am Heart Assoc* 2012;**1**:e002212.

122. Onalan O, Crystal E. Left atrial appendage exclusion for stroke prevention in patients with nonrheumatic atrial fibrillation. *Stroke* 2007;**38** (part 2):624–630.

123. Syed TM, Halperin JL. Left atrial appendage closure for stroke prevention in atrial fibrillation: State of the art and current challenges. *Nat Clin Pract Neurol* 2007;**4**:428–435.

124. Maisel WH. Left atrial appendage occlusion – closure or just the beginning. *N Engl J Med* 2009;**360**:2601–2603.

125. Rubenstein JJ, Schulman CL, Yurchak PM, et al. Clinical spectrum of the sick sinus syndrome. *Circulation* 1972;**46**:5–13.

126. Fairfax AJ, Lambert CD, Leatham A. Systemic embolism in chronic sinoatrial disorder. *N Engl J Med* 1976;**295**:190–192.

127. Lown B. Electrical reversion of cardiac arrhythmias. *Br Heart J* 1967;**29**:469–489.

128. Orencia AJ, Hammill SC, Whisnant JP. Sinus node dysfunction and ischemic stroke. *Heart Dis Stroke* 1994;**3**:91–94.

129. Phillips SJ, Whisnant JP, O'Fallon WM, Frye RL. Prevalence of cardiovascular disease and diabetes mellitus in residents of Rochester,

Minnesota. *Mayo Clin Proc* 1990;**65**:344–359.

130. Radford DJ, Julian DG. Sick sinus syndrome. Experience of a cardiac pacemaker clinic. *BMJ* 1974;**3**:504–507.

131. Rosenqvist M, Vallin H, Edhag O. Clinical and electrophysiologic course of sinus node disease: Five-year follow-up study. *Am Heart J* 1985;**109**:513–522.

132. Bathen J, Sparr S, Rokseth R. Embolism in sinoatrial disease. *Acta Med Scand* 1978;**203**:7–11.

133. Cerebral Embolism Task Force. Cardiogenic brain embolism. *Arch Neurol* 1986;**43**:71–84.

134. Stein PD, Sabbah HN, Pitha JV. Continuing disease process of calcific aortic stenosis. *Am J Cardiol* 1977;**39**:159–163.

135. Casella L, Abelmann WH, Ellis LB. Patients with mitral stenosis and systemic emboli. *Arch Int Med* 1964;**114**:773–781.

136. Weiss S, Davis D. Rheumatic heart disease: III. Embolic manifestations. *Am Heart J* 1933;**9**:45–52

137. Wallach JB, Lukash L, Angrist AA. An interpretation of the incidence of mitral thrombi in the left auricle and appendage with particular reference to mitral commissurotomy. *Am Heart J* 1953;**45**:252–254.

138. Bannister RB. Risk of deferring valvotomy in patients with moderate mitral stenosis. *Lancet* 1960;**2**:329–332.

139. Szekely P. Systemic embolism and anticoagulant prophylaxis in rheumatic heart disease. *BMJ* 1964;**1**:1209–1212.

140. Keen G, Leveaux VM. Prognosis of cerebral embolism in rheumatic heart disease. *BMJ* 1958;**2**:91–92.

141. Coulshed N, Epstein EJ, McKendrick CS, et al. Systemic embolism in mitral valve disease. *BMJ* 1970;**32**:26–34.

142. Daley R, Mattingly TW, Holt CL, et al. Systemic arterial embolism in rheumatic heart disease. *Am Heart J* 1951;**42**:566–581.

143. Fleming HA, Bailey SM. Mitral valve disease, systemic embolism and anticoagulants. *Postgrad Med J* 1971;**47**:599–604.

144. Carabello BA, Crawford FA. Valvular heart disease. *N Engl J Med* 1997;**337**:32–41.

145. Soulie P, Caramanian M, Soulie J, Bader JL, Colcher E. Les embolies calcaires des atteintes orificielles calcifees du coeur gauche. *Arch Mal Coeur Vaiss* 1969;**12**:1657–1684.

146. Holley KE, Bahn RC, McGoon DC, Mankin HT. Spontaneous calcific embolization associated with calcific aortic stenosis. *Circulation* 1963;**27**:197–202.

147. Klues HG, Maron BJ, Dollar AL, Roberts WC. Diversity of structural mitral valve alterations in hypertrophic cardiomyopathy. *Circulation* 1992;**85**:1651–1660.

148. Hardarson T, De la Calzada CS, Curiel R, Goodwin JF. Prognosis and mortality of hypertrophic obstructive cardiomyopathy. *Lancet* 1973;1462–1467.

149. Glancy DL, O'Brien KP, Gold HK, Epstein SE. Atrial fibrillation in patients with idiopathic hypertrophic subaortic stenosis. *Brit Heart J* 1970;**32**:652–659.

150. Tajik AJ, Giuliani ER, Frye RL, et al. Mitral valve and/or annulus calcification assoiated with hypertrophic subaortic stenosis (IHSS). *Circulation* 1972;**16**(Suppl II):228.

151. Barlow JB, Bosman CK. Aneurysmal protrusion of posterior leaflets of the mitral valve. An auscultatory-electrocardiographic syndrome. *Am Heart J* 1966;**71**:166–178.

152. Lauzier S, Barnett HJM. Cerebral ischemia with mitral valve prolapse and mitral annular calcification. In AJ Furlan (ed), *The Heart and Stroke: Exploring Mutual Cerebrovascular and Cardiovascular Issues.* London: Springer, 1987, pp 63–100.

153. Markiewicz W, Stoner J, London E, et al. Mitral valve prolapse in one hundred presumably healthy young females. *Circulation* 1976;**53**:464–473.

154. Cheitlin MD, Byrd RC. Prolapsed mitral valve: The commonest valve disease? *Curr Probl Cardiol* 1984;**8**:3–53.

155. Ranganatham N, Silver MD, Robinson T, et al. Angiographic–morphological correlation in patients with severe mitral regurgitation due to prolapse of the posterior mitral valve leaflet. *Circulation* 1973;**48**:514–518.

156. Kostuk WJ, Boughner DR, Barnett HJM, Silver MD. Strokes: A complication of mitral-leaflet prolapse? *Lancet* 1977;**2**:313–316.

157. Marks AR, Choong CY, Sanfillipo AJ, et al. Identification of high-risk and low-risk subgroups of patients with mitral-valve prolapse. *N Engl J Med* 1989;**320**:1031–1036.

158. Nishimura RA, McGoon MD, Shub C, et al. Echocardiographically documented mitral-valve prolapse: Long term follow-up of 237 patients. *N Engl J Med* 1985;**313**:1305–1309.

159. Barnett HJM. Transient cerebral ischemia: Pathogenesis, prognosis, and management. *Ann Royal Coll Phys Surg Can* 1974;**7**:153–173.

160. Barnett HJM, Jones MW, Boughner DR, Kostuk WJ. Cerebral ischemic events associated with prolapsing mitral valve. *Arch Neurol* 1976;**33**:777–782.

161. Barnett HJM, Boughner DR, Taylor DW, et al. Further evidence relating mitral-valve prolapse to cerebral ischemic events. *N Engl J Med* 1980;**302**:139–144.

162. Aronow WS, Koenigsberg M, Kronzon I, Gutstein H. Association of mitral annular calcium with new thromboembolic stroke and cardiac events at 39-month follow-up in elderly patients. *Am J Cardiol* 1990;**65**:1511–1512.

163. Benjamin EJ, Plehn JF, D'Agostino RB, et al. Mitral annular calcification and the risk of stroke in an elderly cohort. *N Engl J Med* 1992;**327**:374–379.

164. Korn D, DeSanctis R, Sell S. Massive calcification of the mitral valve, a clinicopathological study of fourteen cases. *N Engl J Med* 1962;**267**:900–909.

165. DeBono D, Warlow C. Mitral annulus calcification and cerebral or retinal ischemia. *Lancet* 1979;**2**:383–385.

166. Benjamin EJ, Plehn JF, D'Agostino RB, et al. Mitral annular calcification and the risk of stroke in an elderly cohort. *N Engl J Med* 1992;**327**:374–379.

167. Kizer J, Wiebers DO, Whisnant JP, et al. Mitral annular calcification, aortic valve sclerosis, and incident stroke in adults free of clinical cardiovascular disease. The Strong Heart Study. *Stroke* 2005;**36**:2533–2537.

168. Pomerance A. Pathological and clinical study of calcification of the mitral valve ring. *J Clin Pathol* 1970;**23**:354–361.

169. Stein JH, Soble JS. Thrombus associated with mitral valve calcification. A possible mechanism

for embolic stroke. *Stroke* 1995;**26**:1697–1699.

170. Barnett HJM. Stroke by cause. Some common, some exotic, some controversial. *Stroke* 2005;**36**:2523–2525.

171. Adler Y, Shohat-Zabarski R, Vaturi M, et al. Association between mitral annular calcium and aortic atheroma as detected by transesophageal echocardiographic study. *Am J Cardiol* 1998;**81**:784–786.

172. Vongpatanasin W, Hillis D, Lange RA. Prosthetic heart valves. *N Engl J Med* 1996;**335**:407–416.

173. Edmunds LH Jr. Thromboembolic complications of current cardiac valvular prostheses. *Ann Thor Surg* 1982;**34**:96–106.

174. Metzdorff MT, Grunkemeier GL, Pinson CW, Starr A. Thrombosis of mechanical cardiac valves: A qualitative comparison of the silastic ball valve and the tilting disc valve. *J Am Coll Cardiol* 1984;**4**:50–53.

175. Harker LA, Slichter SL. Studies of platelet and fibrinogen kinetics in patients with prosthetic heart valves. *N Engl J Med* 1970;**283**:1302–1305.

176. Silber H, Khan SS, Matloff JM, et al. The St. Jude valve: Thrombolysis as the first line of therapy for cardiac valve thrombosis. *Circulation* 1993;**87**:30–37.

177. Vitale N, Renzulli A, Cerasuolo F, et al. Prosthetic valve obstruction: Thrombolysis versus operation. *Ann Thorac Surg* 1994;**57**:365–370.

178. Cannegieter SC, Rosendaal FR, Briet E. Thromboembolic and bleeding complications in patients with mechanical heart valve prostheses. *Circulation* 1994;**89**:635–641.

179. Cohn LH, Mudge GH, Pratter F, Collins JJ Jr. Five to eight-year follow-up of patients undergoing porcine heart-valve replacement. *N Engl J Med* 1981;**304**:258–262.

180. Osler W. Gulstonian lectures on malignant endocarditis. *Lancet* 1885;**1**:459–465.

181. Jones HR, Siekert RG, Geraci J. Neurologic manifestations of bacterial endocarditis. *Ann Intern Med* 1969;**71**:21–28.

182. Salgado AV, Furlan AJ, Keys TF, et al. Neurologic complications of endocarditis: A 12-year experience. *Neurology* 1989;**39**:173–178.

183. Hart RG, Foster JW, Luther MF, Kanter MC. Stroke in infective endocarditis. *Stroke* 1990;**21**:695–700.

184. Kanter MC, Hart RG. Neurologic complications of infective endocarditis. *Neurology* 1991;**41**:1015–1020.

185. Keyser DL, Biller J, Coffman TT, Adams HP. Neurologic complications of late prosthetic valve endocarditis. *Stroke* 1990;**21**:472–475.

186. Matsushita K, Kuriyama Y, Sawada T, et al. Hemorrhagic and ischemic cerebrovascular complications of active infective endocarditis of native valve. *Eur Neurol* 1993;**33**:267–274.

187. Pruitt AA, Rubin RH, Karchmer AW, Duncan GW. Neurological complications of bacterial endocarditis. *Medicine* 1978;**57**:329–43.

188. Steckelberg JM, Murphy JG, Ballard D, et al. Emboli in infective endocarditis: The prognostic value of echocardiography. *Ann Intern Med* 1991;**114**:635–640.

189. Tunkel AR, Mandell GL. Infecting microorganisms. In D Kay, (ed.), *Infective Endocarditis*. New York: Raven Press, 1992, pp 85–97.

190. Garvey GJ, Neu HC. Infective endocarditis – an evolving disease. A review of endocarditis at the Columbia-Presbyterian Medical Center, 1968–1973. *Medicine* 1978;**57**:105–127.

191. Jaffe WM, Morgan DE, Pearlman AS, Otto CM. Infective endocarditis, 1983–1988: Echocardiographic findings and factors influencing morbidity and mortality. *J Am Coll Cardol* 1990:**15**:1227–1233.

192. Rohmann S, Erbel R, Gorge G, et al. Clinical relevance of vegetation localization by transesophageal echocardiography in infective endocarditis. *Eur Heart J* 1992;**12**:446–452.

193. Shively BK, Gurule FT, Roldan CA, Leggett JH, Schiller NB. Diagnostic value of transesophageal compared with transthoracic echocardiography in infective endocarditis. *J Am Coll Cardiol* 1991;**18**:391–397.

194. Sanfilippo AJ, Picard MH, Newell JB, et al. Echocardiographic assessment of patients with infectious endocarditis: Prediction of risk for complications. *J Am Coll Cardiol* 1991;**18**:1191–1199.

195. Hart RG, Kagan-Hallet K, Joerns S. Mechanisms of intracranial hemorrhage in infective endocarditis. *Stroke* 1987;**18**:1048–1056.

196. Masuda J, Yutani C, Waki R, et al. Histopathological analysis of the mechanisms of intracranial hemorrhage complicating infective endocarditis. *Stroke* 1992;**23**:843–850.

197. Klein I, Iung B, Wolff M, et al. Silent T2* cerebral microbleeds. A potential new imaging clue in infective endocarditis. *Neurology* 2007;**68**:2043.

198. Nandigam K. Silent T2* cerebral microbleeds: A potential new imaging clue in infective endocarditis. *Neurology* 2008;**70**:323–324.

199. Morawetz RB, Karp RB. Evolution and resolution of intracranial bacterial (mycotic) aneurysms. *Neurosurgery* 1984;**15**:43–49.

200. Moskowitz MA, Rosenbaum AE, Tyler HR. Angiographically monitored resolution of cerebral mycotic aneurysms. *Neurology* 1974;**24**:1103–1108.

201. Bingham WF. Treatment of mycotic intracranial aneurysms. *J Neurosurg* 1977;**46**:428–437.

202. Bertorini TE, Laster RE, Thompson BF, Gelfand M. Magnetic resonance imaging of the brain in bacterial endocarditis. *Arch Intern Med* 1989;**149**:815–817.

203. Libman E, Sacks B. A hitherto undescribed form of valvular and mural endocarditis. *Arch Intern Med* 1924;**33**:701–737.

204. Klemperer P, Pollack AD, Baehr G. Pathology of disseminated lupus erythematosus. *Arch Pathol* 1941;**32**:569–631.

205. Baehr G, Klemperer P, Schifrin A. A diffuse disease of the peripheral circulation usually associated with lupus erythematosus and endocarditis. *Trans Assoc Am Physicians* 1935;**50**:139–155.

206. Gross L. The cardiac lesions in Libman–Sacks disease, with a consideration of its relationship to acute diffuse lupus erythematosus. *Am J Pathol* 1940;**16**:375–407.

207. Roldan CA, Shively B, Crawford MH. An echocardiographic study of valvular heart disease associated with systemic lupus erythematosus. *N Engl J Med* 1996;**335**:1424–1430.

208. Moyssakis I, Tektonidou MG, Vassilios V, et al. Libman–Sacks endocarditis in systemic lupus erythematosus: Prevalence,

associations, and evolution. *Am J Med* 2007;**120**:636–642.

209. Barbut D, Borer J, Gharavi A, et al. Prevalence of anticardiolipin antibody in isolated mitral or aortic regurgitation, or both, and possible relation to cerebral ischemic events. *Am J Cardiol* 1992;**70**:901–905.

210. Barbut D, Borer J, Wallerson D, et al. Anticardiolipin antibody and stroke: Possible relation of valvular heart disease and embolic events. *Cardiology* 1991;**79**:99–109.

211. Antiphospholipid Antibodies in Stroke Study Group. Clinical and laboratory findings in patients with antiphospholipid antibodies and cerebral ischemia. *Stroke* 1990;**21**:1268–1273.

212. Amico L, Caplan LR, Thomas C. Cerebrovascular complications of mucinous cancer. *Neurology* 1989;**39**:522–526.

213. Reagan TJ, Okazaki H. The thrombotic syndrome associated with carcinoma. *Arch Neurol* 1974;**31**:390–395.

214. Edoute Y, Haim N, Rinkevich D, Brenner B, Reisner SA. Cardiac valvular vegetations in cancer patients: A prospective echocardiographic study of 200 patients. *Am J Med* 1997;**102**:252–258.

215. Connolly HM, Crary JL, McGoon MD, et al. Valvular heart disease associated with Fenflurmine-phentermine. *N Engl J Med* 1997;**337**:581–588.

216. Yamamoto M, Uesugi T, Nakayama T. Dopamine agonists and cardiac valvulopathy in Parkinson's disease: A case control study. *Neurology* 2006;**67**:1225–1229.

217. Lambl VA. Papillare exkreszenzen an der semilunar-klappe der aorta. *Wien Med Wochenscshr* 1856;**6**:244–247.

218. Magarey FR. On the mode of formation of Lambl's excrescences and their relation to chronic thickening of the mitral valve. *J Pathol Bacteriol* 1949;**61**:203–208.

219. Roldan CA, Shively BK, Crawford MH. Valve excrescences: Prevalence, evolution and risk for embolism. *J Am Coll Cardiol* 1997;**30**:1308–1314.

220. Freedberg RS, Goodkin GM, Perez JL, et al. Valve strands are strongly associated with systemic embolization: A transesophageal echocardiographic study. *J Am Coll Cardiol* 1995;**26**:1709–1712.

221. Roberts JK, Omarali I, Di Tullio MR, et al. Valvular strands and cerebral ischemia. Effect of demographics and strand characteristics. *Stroke* 1997;**28**:2185–2188.

222. Cohen A, Tzourio C, Chauvel C, et al. Mitral valve strands and the risk of ischemic stroke in elderly patients. *Stroke* 1997;**28**:1574–1578.

223. Lee RJ, Bartzokis T, Yeoh TK, et al. Enhanced detection of intracardiac sources of cerebral emboli by transesophageal echocardiography. *Stroke* 1991;**22**:734–739.

224. Nighoghossian N, Derex L, Loire R, et al. Giant Lambl excrescences. An unusual source of cerebral embolism. *Arch Neurol* 1997;**54**:41–44.

225. Vaitkus PT, Berlin JA, Schwartz JS, Barnathan ES. Stroke complicating acute myocardial infarction: A meta-analysis of risk modification by anticoagulation and thrombolytic therapy. *Arch Intern Med* 1992;**152**:2020–2024.

226. Konrad MS, Coffey CE, Coffey KS, et al. Myocardial infarction and stroke. *Neurology* 1984;**34**:1403–1409.

227. Chiarella F, Santoro E, Domenicucci S, et al. on behalf of the GISSI-3 Investigators. Predischarge two-dimensional echocardiographic evaluation of left ventricular thrombosis after acute myocardial infarction in the GISSI-3 study. *Am J Cardiol* 1998;**81**:822–827.

228. Meltzer RS, Visser CA, Fuster V. Intracardiac thrombi and systemic embolization. *Ann Intern Med* 1986;**104**:689–698.

229. Visser CA, Kan G, Meltzer RS, et al. Embolic potential of left ventricular thrombi after myocardial infarction: A two-dimensional echocardiographic study of 119 patients. *J Am Coll Cardiol* 1985;**5**:1276–1280.

230. Kouvaras G, Chronopoulas G, Soufras G, et al. The effects of long term antithrombotic treatment on left ventricular thrombi in patients after an acute myocardial infarction. *Am Heart J* 1990;**119**:73–78.

231. Asinger RW, Mikell FL, Elsperger J, Hodges M. Incidence of left-ventricular thrombosis after acute transmural myocardial infarction. Serial evaluation by two-dimensional echocardiography. *N Engl J Med* 1981;**305**:297–302.

232. Nihoyannopoulos P, Smith GC, Maseri A, Foale RA. The natural history of left ventricular thrombus in myocardial infarction: A rationale in support of masterly inactivity. *J Am Coll Cardiol* 1989;**14**:903–911.

233. Greaves SC, Zhi G, Lee RT, et al. Incidence and natural history of left ventricular thrombus following anterior wall acute myocardial infarction. *Am J Cardiol* 1997;**80**:442–448.

234. Keren A, Goldberg S, Gottlieb S, et al. Natural history of left ventricular thrombi: Their appearance and resolution in the posthospitalization period of acute myocardial infarction. *J Am Coll Cardiol* 1990;**15**:790–800.

235. Domenicucci S, Chiarella F, Bellotti P, et al. Long-term prospective assessment of left ventricular thrombus in anterior wall acute myocardial infarction and implications for a rational approach to embolic risk. *Am J Cardiol* 1999;**83**:519–524.

236. Lapeyre AC III, Steele PM, Kazmier FJ, et al. Systemic embolism in chronic left ventricular aneurysm: Incidence and the role of anticoagulation. *J Am Coll Cardiol* 1985;**6**:534–538.

237. Anticoagulants in acute myocardial infarction: Results of a cooperative clinical trial. *JAMA* 1973;**225**:724–729.

238. Faxon DP, Ryan TJ, Davis KB, et al. Prognostic significance of angiographically documented left ventricular aneurysm from the coronary artery surgery study (CASS). *Am J Cardiol* 1982;**50**:157–164.

239. Reeder GS, Lengyei M, Tajik AJ, et al. Mural thrombus in left ventricular aneurysm. Incidence, role of angiography, and relation between anticoagulation and embolism. *Mayo Clin Proc* 1981;**56**:77–81.

240. Loh E, Sutton M, Wun C-C, et al. Ventricular dysfunction and the risk of stroke after myocardial infarction. *N Engl J Med* 1997;**336**:251–257.

241. Stratton JR, Lighty GW, Pearlman AS, Ritchie JL. Detection of left ventricular thrombus by two-dimensional echocardiography: Sensitivity, specificity, and causes of uncertainty. *Circulation* 1982;**66**:156–166.

242. Ports TA, Cogan J, Schiller NB, Rapaport E. Echocardiography of left ventricular masses. *Circulation* 1978;**58**:528–536.

243. Chen C, Koschyk D, Hamm C, et al. Usefulness of transesophageal echocardiography in identifying small

left ventricular apical thrombus. *J Am Coll Cardiol* 1993;**21**:208–215.

244. Oppenheimer SM, Lima J. Neurology and the heart. *J Neurol Neurosurg Psychiatry* 1998;**64**:289–297.

245. Wong C, Marwick TH. Obesity cardiomyopathy: Diagnosis and therapeutic implications. *Nature Clin Practice Cardiovasc Med.* 2007;**4**:480–489.

246. Grabowski A, Kilian J, Strank C, Cieslinski G, Meyding-Lamade U. Takotsubo cardiomyopathy – a rare cause of cardioembolic stroke. *Cerebrovasc Dis* 2007;**24**:146–148.

247. Ziegelstein RC. Acute emotional stress and cardiac arrhythmias. *JAMA* 2007;**298**:324–329.

248. Wold LE, Lie JT. Cardiac myxomas: A clinicopathologic profile. *Am J Pathol* 1980;**101**:219–240.

249. Reynen K. Cardiac myxomas. *N Engl J Med* 1995;**333**:1610–1617.

250. Blondeau P. Primary cardiac tumors: French study of 533 cases. *Thorac Cardiovasc Surg* 1990;**38** (Suppl 2):192–195.

251. Lee VH, Connolly HM, Brown Jr RD. Central nervous system manifestations of cardiac myxoma. *Arch Neurol* 2007;**64**:1115–1120.

252. Sandok BA, von Estorff I, Giuliani ER. Subsequent neurological events in patients with atrial myxoma. *Ann Neurol* 1980;**8**:305–307.

253. Edwards FH, Hale D, Cohen A, et al. Primary cardiac valve tumors. *Ann Thorac Surg* 1991;**52**:1127–1131.

254. Giannesini C, Kubis N, N'Guyen A, et al. Cardiac papillary fibroelastoma: A rare cause of ischemic stroke in the young. *Cerebrovasc Dis* 1999;**9**:45–49.

255. Brown RD, Khandheria BK, Edwards WD. Cardiac papillary fibroelastoma: A treatable cause of transient ischemic attack and ischemic stroke detected by transesophageal echocardiography. *Mayo Clin Proc* 1995;**70**:863–868.

256. Klarich KW, Enriquez-Sarano M, Gura GM, et al. Papillary fibroelastoma: Echocardiographic characteristics for diagnosis and pathologic correlation. *J Am Coll Cardiol* 1997;**30**:784–90.

257. Gagliardi R, Franken R, Protti G. Cardiac papillary fibroelastoma and stroke in a young man – etiology and treatment. *Cerebrovasc Dis* 2008;185–187.

258. Azarbal B, Tobis J. Interatrial communications, stroke, and migraine headache. *Appl Neurol* 2005;**1**:22–36.

259. Hagen PT, Scholz DG, Edwards WD. Incidence and size of patent foramen ovale during the first 10 decades of life: An autopsy study of 965 normal hearts. *Mayo Clin Proc* 1984;**59**:17–20.

260. Lechat PH, Mas JL, Lascault G, et al. Prevalence of patent foramen ovale in patients with stroke. *N Engl J Med* 1988;**318**:1148–1152.

261. Di Tullio M, Sacco RL, Gopal A, et al. Patent foramen ovale as a risk factor for cryptogenic stroke. *Ann Intern Med* 1992;**117**:461–465.

262. Petty GW, Khanderia BK, Chu C-P, et al. Patent foramen ovale in patients with cerebral infarction. A transesophageal echocardiographic study. *Arch Neurol* 1997;**54**:819–822.

263. Gautier JC, Durr A, Koussa S, et al. Paradoxical cerebral embolism with a patent foramen ovale. A report of 29 patients. *Cerebrovasc Dis* 1991;**1**:193–202.

264. Venketasubramanian N, Sacco RL, Di Tullio M, et al. Vascular distribution of paradoxical emboli by transcranial Doppler. *Neurology* 1993;**43**:1533–1535.

265. Kim BJ, Kim N-Y, Kang D-W, Kim JS, Kwon SU. Provoked right-to-left shunt in patent foramen ovale associates with ischemic stroke in posterior circulation. *Stroke* 2014;**45**:3707–3710.

266. Konstantinides S, Kasper W, Geibel A, et al. Detection of left-to-right shunt in atrial septal defect by negative contrast echocardiography: A comparison of transthoracic and transesophageal approach. *Am Heart J* 1993;**126**:909–917.

267. Hamann GF, Schatzer-Klotz D, Frohlig G, et al. Femoral injection of echo contrast medium may increase the sensitivity of testing for a patent foramen ovale. *Neurology* 1998;**50**:1423–1428.

268. Hausmann D, Mügge A, Daniel WG. Identification of patent foramen ovale permitting paradoxic embolism. *J Am Coll Cardiol* 1995;**26**:1030–1038.

269. Homma S, Tullio MR, Sacco RL, et al. Characteristics of patent foramen ovale associated with cryptogenic stroke: A biplane transesophageal echocardiographic study. *Stroke* 1994;**25**:582–586.

270. Chimowitz MI, Nemec JJ, Marwick TH, et al. Transcranial Doppler ultrasound identifies patients with right-to-left cardiac or pulmonary shunts. *Neurology* 1991;**41**:1902–1904.

271. Albert A, Muller HR, Hetzel A. Optimized transcranial Doppler technique for the diagnosis of cardiac right-to-left shunts. *J Neuroimaging* 1997;**7**:159–163.

272. Di Tullio M, Sacco RL, Venketasubramanian N, et al. Comparison of diagnostic techniques for the detection of a patent foramen ovale in stroke patients. *Stroke* 1993;**24**:1020–1024.

273. Mohrs OK, Petersen SE, Erkapic D, et al. Diagnosis of patent foramen ovale using contrast-enhanced dynamic MRI: A pilot study. *AJR Am J Roetgenol* 2005;**184**:234–240.

274. Ilercil A, Meisner JS, Vijayaraman P, et al. Clinical significance of fossa ovalis membrane aneurysm in adults with cardioembolic cerebral ischemia. *Am J Cardiol* 1997;**80**:96–99.

275. Belkin RN, Hurwitz BJ, Kislo J. Atrial septal aneurysm: Association with cerebrovascular and peripheral embolic events. *Stroke* 1987;**18**:856–862.

276. Schneider B, Hanrath P, Vogel P, Meinertz T. Improved morphologic characterization of atrial septal aneurysm by transesophageal echocardiography: Relation to cerebrovascular events. *J Am Coll Cardiol* 1990;**16**:1000–1009.

277. Burger AJ, Sherman HB, Charlamb MJ. Low incidence of embolic strokes with atrial septal aneurysms: A prospective, long-term study. *Am Heart J* 2000;**139**:149–152.

278. Agmon Y, Khandheria BK, Meissner I, et al. Frequency of atrial septal aneurysms in patients with cerebral ischemic events. *Circulation* 1999;**99**:1942–1944.

279. Zabalgoitia-Reyes M, Herrera C, Gandhi DK, et al. A possible mechanism for neurologic ischemic events in patients with atrial septal aneurysm. *Am J Cardiol* 1990;**66**:761–764.

280. Berthet K, Lavergne T, Cohen A, et al. Significant association of atrial vulnerability with atrial septal abnormalities in young patients with ischemic stroke of unknown cause. *Stroke* 2000;**31**:398–403.

281. Silver MD, Dorsey JS. Aneurysms of the septum primum in adults. *Arch Pathol Lab Med* 1978;**102**:62–65.

282. Cabanes L, Mas JL, Cohen A, et al. Atrial septal aneurysm and patent foramen ovale as risk factors for cryptogenic stroke in patients less than 55 years of age. A study using transesophageal echocardiography. *Stroke* 1993;**24**:1865–1873.

283. Hanna JP, Sun JP, Furlan AJ, et al. Patent foramen ovale and brain infarct. Echocardiographic predictors, recurrence, and prevention. *Stroke* 1994;**25**:782–786.

284. Ay H, Buonanno FS, Abraham S, et al. An electrocardiographic criterion for diagnosis of patent foramen ovale associated with ischemic stroke. *Stroke* 1998;**29**:1393–1397.

285. Bogousslavsky J, Garazi S, Jeanrenaud X, et al. Stroke recurrence in patients with patent foramen ovale: The Lausanne study. *Neurology* 1996;**46**:1301–1305.

286. French Study Group on Patent Foramen Ovale and Atrial Septal Aneurysm. Recurrent cerebrovascular events in patients with patent foramen ovale or atrial septal aneurysms and cryptogenic stroke or TIA. *Am Heart J* 1995;**130**:1083–1088.

287. Devuyst G, Bogousslavsky J, Ruchat P, et al. Prognosis after stroke followed by surgical closure of patent foramen ovale: A prospective follow-up study with brain MRI and simultaneous transesophageal and transcranial Doppler ultrasound. *Neurology* 1996;**47**:1162–1166.

288. Kim D, Saver JL. Patent foramen ovale and stroke: What we do and don't know. *Rev Neurol Dis* 2005;**2**:1–7.

289. Bridges ND, Hellensbrand W, Catson L, et al. Transcatheter closure of patent foramen ovale after presumed paradoxical embolism. *Circulation* 1992;**86**:1902–1908.

290. Li Y, Zhou K, Hua Y, et al. Amplatzer occluder versus Cardioseal/Starflex occluder: A meta-analysis of the efficacy and safety of transcatheter occlusion for patent foramen ovale and atrial septal defect. *Cardiol Young* 2013;**23**:582–596.

291. Carroll JD, Saver JL, Thaler DE, et al. for the RESPECT Investigators. Closure of patent foramen ovale versus medical therapy after cryptogenic stroke. *N Engl J Med* 2013;**368**:1092–1100.

292. Meier B, Kalesan B, Mattle HP, et al. for the PC Trial Investigators. Percutaneous closure of patent foramen ovale in cryptogenic embolism. *N Engl J Med* 2013;**368**:1083–1091.

293. Furlan AJ, Reisman M, Joseph Massaro J, et al. for the CLOSURE I Investigators. Closure or medical therapy for cryptogenic stroke with patent foramen ovale. *N Engl J Med* 2012;**366**:991–999.

294. Kent DM, Ruthazer R, Weimar C, et al. An index to identify stroke-related vs. incidental patent foramen ovale in cryptogenic stroke. *Neurology* 2013;**81**:619–625.

295. Thaler DE, Ruthazer R, Weimar C, et al. Recurrent stroke predictors differ in medically treated patients with pathogenic vs. other PFOs. *Neurology* 2014;**83**:221–226.

296. Bogousslavsky J, Cachin C, Regli F, et al. Cardiac sources of embolism and cerebral infarction. Clinical consequences and vascular concomitants. *Neurology* 1991;**41**:855–859.

297. Tunick PA, Kronzon I. Protruding atherosclerotic plaque in the aortic arch of patients with systemic embolization: A new finding seen by transesophageal echocardiography. *Am Heart J* 1990;**120**:658–660.

298. Tunick PA, Culliford AT, Lamparello PJ, Kronzon I. Atheromatosis of the aortic arch as an occult source of multiple systemic emboli. *Ann Intern Med* 1991;**114**:391–392.

299. Tunick PA, Perez JL, Kronzon I. Protruding atheromas in the thoracic aorta and systemic embolization. *Ann Intern Med* 1991;**115**:423–427.

300. Amarenco P, Duyckaerts C, Tzourio C, et al. The prevalence of ulcerated plaques in the aortic arch in patients with stroke. *N Engl J Med* 1992;**326**:221–225.

301. Amarenco P, Cohen A, Baudrimont M, Bousser M-G. Transesophageal echocardiographic detection of aortic arch disease in patients with cerebral infarction. *Stroke* 1992;**23**:1005–1009.

302. Tobler HG, Edwards JE. Frequency and location of atherosclerotic plaques in the ascending aorta. *J Thor Cardiovasc Surg* 1988;**96**:304–306.

303. Bruns JL, Segel DP, Adler S. Control of cholesterol embolism by discontinuation of anticoagulant therapy. *Am J Med Sci* 1978;**275**:105–108.

304. French Study of Aortic Plaques in Stroke Group. Atherosclerotic disease of the aortic arch as a risk factor for recurrent ischemic stroke. *N Engl J Med* 1996;**334**:1216–1221.

305. Mitusch R, Doherty C, Wucherpfennig H, et al. Vascular events during follow-up in patients with aortic arch atherosclerosis. *Stroke* 1997;**28**:36–39.

306. Amarenco P, Cohen A. Update on imaging aortic atherosclerosis. *Adv Neurol* 2003;**92**:75–89.

307. Vaduganathan V, Ewton A, Nagueh SF, et al. Pathologic correlates of aortic plaques, thrombi and mobile "aortic debris" imaged in vivo with transesophageal echocardiography *J Am Coll Cardiol* 1997;**30**:357–363.

308. Weinberger J, Azhar S, Danisi F, Hayes R, Goldman M. A new noninvasive technique for imaging atherosclerotic plaque in the aortic arch of stroke patients by transcutaneous real-time B-mode ultrasonography. *Stroke* 1998;**29**:673–676.

309. Schwammenthal A, Schwammenthal Y, Tanne D, et al. Transcutaneous detection of aortic arch atheromas by suprasternal harmonic imaging. *J Am Coll Cardiol* 2002;**39**:1127–1132.

310. Kutz SM, Lee VS, Tunick PA, et al. Atheromas of the thoracic aorta: A comparison of transesophageal echocardiography and breath-hold gadolinium enhanced 3-dimensional magnetic resonance angiography. *J Am Soc Echocardiogr* 1999;**12**:853–858.

311. Barkhausen J, Ebert W, Heyer C, Debatin JF, Weinmann H-J. Detection of atherosclerotic plaque with gadofluorine-enhanced magnetic resonance imaging. *Circulation* 2003;**108**:605–609.

312. Harloff A, Dudler P, Frydrychowicz A, et al. Reliability of aortic MRI at 3 Tesla in patients with cryptogenic stroke. *J Neurol Neurosurg Psychiatry* 2007;**79**:540–546.

313. Chatzikonstantinou A, Krissak R, Fluchter S, et al. CT angiography of the aorta is superior to transesophageal echocardiography for determining stroke subtypes in patients with cryptogenic stroke. *Cerebrovasc Dis* 2012;**33**:322–328.

314. Wehrum T, Kams M, Strecker C, et al. Prevalence of potential retrograde embolization pathways in the proximal descending aorta in stroke

patients. *Cerebrovas Dis* 2014;**38**:410–417.

315. Yamashiro K, Funabe S, Tanaka R, et al. Primary aortic sarcoma. *Neurology* 2015;**84**:755–756.

316. Blackshear JL, Jahangir A, Oldenberg WA, Safford RE. Digital embolization from plaque-related thrombus in the thoracic aorta: Identification with transesophageal echocardiography and resolution with warfarin therapy. *Mayo Clin Proc* 1993;**68**:268–272.

317. Freedberg RS, Tunick PA. Culliform AT, Tatelbaum RJ, Kronzon I. Disappearance of a large intraaortic mass in a patient with prior systemic embolization. *Am Heart J* 1993;**125**:1445–1447.

318. Fine MJ, Kapoor W, Falanga V. Cholesterol crystal embolization: A review of 221 cases in the English literature. *Angiology* 1987;**38**:769–784.

319. Hausmann D, Gulba D, Bargheer, et al. Successful thrombolysis of an aortic-arch thrombus in a patient after mesenteric embolism. *N Engl J Med* 1992;**327**:500–501.

320. Belden JR, Caplan LR, Bojar RM, Payne DD, Blachman P. Treatment of multiple cerebral emboli from an ulcerated, thrombogenic ascending aorta with aortectomy and graft replacement. *Neurology* 1997;**49**:621–622.

321. Amarenco P, Davis S, Jones EF, et al. for the Aortic Arch Related Cerebral Hazard Trial Investigators. Clopidogrel plus aspirin versus warfarin in patients with stroke and aortic arch plaques. *Stroke* 2014;**45**:1248–1257.

322. Slogoff S, Girgis KZ, Keats AS. Etiologic factors in neuropsychiatric complications associated with cardiopulmonary bypass. *Anesth Analg* 1982;**61**:903–911.

323. Gilman S. Neurological complications of open heart surgery. *Ann Neurol* 1990;**28**:475–476.

324. Shaw PJ, Bates D, Cartledge NEF. Early neurological complications of coronary artery bypass surgery. *BMJ* 1985;**391**:1384–1387.

325. Breuer AC, Furlan AJ, Hanson MR, et al. Central nervous system complications of coronary artery bypass graft surgery: Prospective analysis of 421 patients. *Stroke* 1983;**14**:682–687.

326. Coffey CE, Massey EW, Roberts KB, et al. Natural history of cerebral complication of coronary artery bypass graft surgery. *Neurology* 1983;**33**:1416–1421.

327. Feeney DM, Gonzalez A, Law WA. Amphetamine, haloperidol and experience interact to affect the rate of recovery after motor cortex injury. *Science* 1982;**217**:855–857.

328. Houda DA, Feeney DM. Haloperidol blocks amphetamine induced recovery of binocular depth perception of the bilateral visual cortex abilities in the cat. *Proc West Pharmacol Soc* 1985;**28**:209–211.

329. Sila C. Neuroimaging of cerebral infarction associated with coronary revascularization. *AJNR Am J Neuroradiol* 1991;**12**:817–818.

330. Moody DM, Bell MA, Challa VR, et al. Brain microemboli during cardiac surgery or aortography. *Ann Neurol* 1990;**28**:477–486.

331. Pugsley W, Klinger L, Paschalis C, et al. The impact of microemboli during cardiopulmonary bypass on neuropsychological functioning. *Stroke* 1994;**25**:1393–1399.

332. Barbut D, Caplan LR. Brain complications of cardiac surgery. *Curr Probl Cardiol* 1997;**22**:445–476.

333. Barbut D, Lo Y, Gold JP, et al. Impact of embolization during coronary artery bypass grafting on outcome and length of stay. *Ann Thor Surg* 1997;**63**:998–1002.

334. Clark RE, Brillman J, Davis DA, et al. Microemboli during coronary artery bypass grafting: Genesis and effect on outcome. *J Thorac Cardiovasc Surg* 1995;**25**:1393–1399.

335. Tufo HM, Ostfeld AM, Shekelle R. Central nervous system dysfunction following open-heart surgery. *JAMA* 1970;**212**:1333–1340.

336. Stockard JJ, Bickford RG, Schauble JF. Pressure-dependent cerebral ischemia during cardiopulmonary bypass. *Neurology* 1973;**23**:521–529.

337. Gold JP, Charlson ME, Williams-Russo P, et al. Improvement of outcomes after coronary artery bypass: A randomized trial comparing intraoperative high vs. low mean arterial pressure. *J Thorac Cardiovasc Surg* 1995;**110**:1302–1314.

338. Gottesmann RF, Hillis AE, Grega MA, et al. Early postoperative cognitive dysfunction and blood pressure during coronary artery bypass graft operation. *Arch Neurol* 2007;**64**:1111–1114.

339. Dubinsky RM, Lai SM. Mortality from combined carotid endarterectomy and coronary artery bypass surgery in the US. *Neurology* 2007;**68**:195–197.

340. Breslau PJ, Fell G, Ivey TD, et al. Carotid arterial disease in patients undergoing coronary artery bypass operations. *J Thorac Cardiovasc Surg* 1981;**82**:765–767.

341. Turnipseed WD, Berkhoff HA, Belzer FO. Postoperative stroke in cardiac and peripheral vascular disease. *Ann Surg* 1980;**192**:365–368.

342. Chimowitz M. Neurological complications of cardiac surgery. In LR Caplan, JW Hurst, M Chimowitz (eds), *Clinical Neurocardiology*. New York: Marcel Dekker, 1999, pp 226–257.

343. Furlan A, Craciun A. Risk of stroke during coronary artery bypass graft surgery in patients with internal carotid artery disease documented by angiography. *Stroke* 1985;**16**:797–799.

344. Von Reutern G, Hetzel A, Birnbaum D, et al. Transcranial Doppler ultrasound during cardiopulmonary bypass in patients with internal carotid artery disease documented by angiography. *Stroke* 1988;**19**:674–680.

345. Hise JH, Nipper MN, Schnitker JC. Stroke associated with coronary artery bypass surgery. *AJNR Am J Neuroradiol* 1991;**12**:811–814.

346. Barbut D, Gold JP. Aortic atheromatosis and risks of cerebral embolization. *J Cardiothorac Vasc Anesth* 1996;**10**:24–30.

347. Blauth CI, Cosgrove DM, Webb BW, et al. Atheroembolism from the ascending aorta. An emerging problem in cardiac surgery. *J Thorac Cardiovasc Surg* 1992;**103**:1104–1112.

348. Masuda J, Yutani C, Ogata J, et al. Atheromatous embolism to the brain: A clinicopathologic analysis of 15 autopsy cases. *Neurology* 1994;**44**:1231–1237.

349. Katz ES, Tunick PA, Rusinek H, et al. Protruding aortic atheromas predict stroke in elderly patients undergoing cardiopulmonary bypass: Experience with intraoperative transesophageal echocardiography. *J Am Coll Cardiol* 1992;**20**:70–77.

350. Mills NL, Everson CT. Atherosclerosis of the ascending aorta and coronary artery bypass. Pathology, clinical correlates and operative management. *J Thorac Cardiovasc Surg* 1991;**102**:546–553.

351. Yao FSF, Barbut D, Hager DN, et al. Detection of aortic emboli by transesophageal echocardiography during coronary artery bypass surgery. *J Cardiothorac Vasc Anesth* 1996;**10**:314–317.

352. Gardner TJ, Horneffer PJ, Manolio TA, et al. Stroke following coronary artery bypass grafting: A ten-year study. *Ann Thorac Surg* 1985;**40**:574–581.

353. Caplan LR. Translating what is known about neurological complications of coronary artery bypass graft surgery into action (Editorial). *Arch Neurol* 2009;**66**:1062–1064.

354. Warehag TH, Davila-Roman VG, Barzilai B, et al. Management of the severely atherosclerotic aorta during cardiac operations. *J Thorac Cardiovasc Surg* 1992;**103**:453–462.

355. Barbut D, Yao FS, Hager DN, et al. Comparison of transcranial Doppler ultrasonography and transesophageal echocardiography during coronary artery bypass surgery. *Stroke* 1996;**27**:87–90.

356. Dittrich R, Ringelstein EB. Occurrence and clinical impact of microembolic signals during or after cardiosurgical procedures. *Stroke* 2008;**39**:503–511.

357. Marshall WG, Barzilai B, Kouchoukos NT, et al. Intraoperative ultrasonic imaging of the ascending aorta. *Ann Thorac Surg* 1989;**48**:339–344.

358. Borowicz I, Goldsborough M, Selnes O, McKann G. Neuropsychologic change after cardiac surgery. A critical review. *J Cardiothorac Vasc Anesth* 1996;**10**:105–111.

359. Barbut D, Hinton R, Szatrowski TP, et al. Cerebral emboli detected during bypass surgery are associated with clamp removal. *Stroke* 1994;**25**:2398–2402.

360. Hammon J, Stump D, Kon N, et al. Risk factors and solutions for the development of neurobehavioral changes after coronary artery bypass grafting. *Ann Thorac Surg* 1997;**63**:1613–1618.

361. Hanson MR, Hamid MA, Tomsak RL, Chou SS, Leigh RJ. Selective saccadic palsy caused by pontine lesions: Clinical, physiological, and pathological correlations. *Ann Neurol* 1986;**20**:209–217.

362. Tomsak RL, Volpe BT, Stahl JS, Leigh RJ. Saccadic palsy after cardiac surgery: Visual disability and rehabilitation. *Ann NY Acad Sci* 2002;**956**:430–433.

363. Eggers SDZ, Moster ML, Cranmer K. Selective saccadic palsy after cardiac surgery. *Neurology* 2008;**70**:318–320.

364. Solomon D, Ramat S, Tomsak RL, et al. Saccadic palsy after cardiac surgery: Characteristics and pathogenesis. *Ann Neurol* 2007;**63**:355–365.

365. van Dijk D, Spoor M, Hijman R, et al. for the Octopus Study Group. Cognitive and cardiac outcomes 5 years after off-pump vs. on-pump coronary artery bypass graft surgery. *JAMA* 2007;**297**:701–708.

366. Duncan A, Rumbaugh C, Caplan LR. Cerebral embolic disease, a complication of carotid aneurysms. *Radiology* 1979;**133**:379–384.

367. Fisher M, Davidson R, Marcus E. Transient focal cortical ischemia as a presenting manifestation of unruptured cerebral aneurysms. *Ann Neurol* 1980;**8**:367–372.

368. Pessin MS, Chimowitz MI, Levine SR, et al. Stroke in patients with fusiform vertebrobasilar aneurysms. *Neurology* 1989;**39**:16–21.

369. Caplan LR, Stein R, Patel D, et al. Intraluminal clot of the carotid artery detected radiographically. *Neurology* 1984;**34**:1175–1181.

370. Perloff JK. Congenital mitral stenosis, cor triatriatum, congenital pulmonary vein stenosis. In JK Perloff, Marelli AJ (eds), *The Clinical Recognition of Congenital Heart Disease*. Philadelphia: W B Saunders, 1987, pp 169–171.

371. Manning WJ, Weintraub, RM, Waksmonski, CA, et al. Accuracy of transesophageal echocardiography for identifying left atrial thrombi. A prospective, intraoperative study. *Ann Intern Med* 1995;**123**:817–822.

372. Fatkin D, Scalia G, Jacobs N, et al. Accuracy of biplane transesophageal echocardiography in detecting left atrial thrombus. *Am J Cardiol* 1996;**77**:321–323.

373. Pearson AC, Labovitz AJ, Tatineni S, Gomez CR. Superiority of transesophageal echocardiography in detecting cardiac source of embolism in patients with cerebral ischemia of uncertain etiology. *J Am Coll Cardiol* 1991;**17**:66–72.

374. DeRook FA, Comess KA, Albers GW, Popp RL. Transesophageal echocardiography in the evaluation of stroke. *Ann Intern Med* 1992;**117**:922–932.

375. Daniel WG, Mugge A. Transesophageal echocardiography. *N Engl J Med* 1995;**332**:1268–1279.

376. Horowitz DR, Tuhrim S, Weinberger J, et al. Transesophageal echocardiography: Diagnostic and clinical applications in the evaluation of the stroke patient. *J Stroke Cerebrovasc Dis* 1997;**6**:332–336.

377. Johnson LL, Pohost GM. Nuclear cardiology. In RC Schlant, RW Alexander (eds), *Hurst's The Heart*, 8th ed. New York: McGraw-Hill, 1994, pp 2281–2323.

378. Ezekowiz MD, Wilson DA, Smith EO, et al. Comparison of indium-111 platelet scintigraphy and two-dimensional echocardiography in the diagnosis of left ventricular thrombi. *N Engl J Med* 1982;**306**:1509–1513.

379. Daccarett M, McGann CJ, Akoum NW, MacLeod R, Marrouche NF. MRI of the left atrium: Predicting clinical outcomes in patients with atrial fibrillation. *Exp Rev Cardiovasc Ther* 2011;**9**:105–111.

380. Baher A, Mowla A, Kodali S, et al. Cardiac MRI improves identification of etiology of acute ischemic stroke. *Cerebrovasc Dis* 2014;**37**:277–284.

381. Hur J, Kim YJ, Lee HJ, et al. Left atrial appendage thrombi in stroke patients: Detection with two-phase cardiac CT angiography versus transesophageal echocardiography. *Radiology* 2009;**251**:683–690.

382. Hur J, Kim YJ, Lee HJ, et al. Cardioembolic stroke: Dual-energy cardiac CT for differentiation of left atrial appendage thrombus and circulatory stasis. *Radiology* 2012;**263**:688–695.

383. Romero J, Husain SA, Kelesidis I, Sanz J, Medina HM, Garcia MJ. Detection of left atrial appendage thrombus by cardiac computed tomography in patients with atrial fibrillation: A meta-analysis. *Circ Cardiovasc Imaging* 2013;**6**:185–194.

384. Romero J, Cao JJ, Garcia MJ, Taub CC. Cardiac imaging for assessment of left atrial appendage stasis and thrombosis. *Nat Rev Cardiol* 2014;**11**:470–480.

385. Caplan LR, Feinberg WM, Fisher MJ, del Zoppo GJ. The blood. In LR Caplan (ed), *Brain Ischemia. Basic Concepts and Clinical Relevance*. London: Springer, 1995, pp 83–126.

386. Caplan LR. Treatment of the acute embolic event. In LR Caplan,

W Manning (eds), *Brain Embolism*. New York: Informa Healthcare, 2006, pp 277–288.

387. Furlan A, Higashida R, Wechsler L, et al. Intraarterial prourokinase for acute ischemic stroke. The PROACT II Study: A randomized controlled trial. Prolyse in acute cerebral thromboembolism. *JAMA* 1999;**282**:2003–2011.

388. Fisher CM, Perlman A. The nonsudden onset of cerebral embolism. *Neurology* 1967;**17**:1025–1032.

389. Melski J, Caplan LR, Mohr JP, Geer D, Bleich H. Modeling the diagnosis of stroke at two hospitals. MD Computing 1989;**6**:157–163.

390. Staroselskaya I, Chaves C, Silver B, et al. Relationship between magnetic resonance arterial patency and perfusion-diffusion mismatch in acute ischemic stroke and its potential clinical use. *Arch Neurol* 2001;**58**:1069–1074.

391. Derex L, Nighoghossian N, Hermier M, Adeleine P, Froment JC, Trouillas P. Early detection of cerebral arterial occlusion on magnetic resonance angiography: Predictive value of the baseline NIHSS score and impact on neurological outcome. *Cerebrovasc Dis* 2002;**13**:225–229.

392. Parsons MW, Barber PA, Chalk J, et al. Diffusion- and perfusion-weighted response to thrombolysis in stroke. *Ann Neurol* 2002;**51**:28–37.

393. Campbell BC, Christensen S, Parsons MW, et al. for the EPITHET and DEFUSE Investigators. Advanced imaging improves prediction of hemorrhage after stroke thrombolysis. *Ann Neurol* 2013;**73**:510–519.

394. Pessin MS, del Zoppo GJ, Furlan AJ. *Thrombolytic treatment in acute stroke: Review and Update of Selected Topics in Cerebrovascular Disease. 19th Princeton Conference, 1994.* Boston: Butterworth–Heinemann, 1995, pp 409–418.

395. Caplan LR. *Caplan's Stroke, a Clinical Approach.* Boston, Butterworth–Heinemann, 2000, pp 124–130.

396. Caplan LR. Thrombolysis 2004: The good, the bad, and the ugly. *Rev Neurol Dis* 2004;**1**:16–26.

397. Christoforidis G, Mohammad Y, Bourekas E, Slivka A. Initial severity of angiographic occlusion predicts subsequent volume of cerebral infarction following intra-arterial thrombolysis in acute ischemic stroke. *Neurology* 2004;**62** (Suppl 5): A449.

398. Toni D, Fiorelli M, Zanette EM, et al. Early spontaneous improvement and deterioration of ischemic stroke patients: A serial study with transcranial Doppler ultrasonography. *Stroke* 1998;**29**:1144–1148.

399. Lewandowski C, Frankel M, Tomsick T, et al. Combined intravenous and intraarterial r-tPA versus intra-arterial therapy of acute ischemic stroke: Emergency Management of Stroke (EMS) Bridging Trial. *Stroke* 1999;**30**:2598–2605.

400. IMS Study Investigators. Combined intravenous and intra-arterial recanalization for acute ischemic stroke: The Interventional Management of Stroke Study. *Stroke* 2004;**35**:904–912.

401. Hausegger K, Hauser M, Kau T. Mechanical thrombectomy with stent retrievers in acute ischemic stroke. *Cardiovasc Intervent Radiol* 2014;**37**:863–74.

402. Ciccone A, Valvassori L. Endovascular treatment for acute ischemic stroke. *N Engl J Med* 2013;**368**:2433–2434.

403. Berlis A, Lutsep H, Barnwell S. Mechanical thrombolysis in acute ischemic stroke with endovascular photoacoustic recanalization. *Stroke* 2004;**35**:1112–1116.

404. Hacke W. The dilemma of reinstituting anticoagulation for patients with cardioembolic sources and intracranial hemorrhage: How wide is the strait between Skylla and Karybdis? *Arch Neurol* 2000;**57**:1682–1684.

405. Phan TG, Koh M, Wijdicks EF. Safety of discontinuation of anticoagulation in patients with intracranial hemorrhage at high thromboembolic risk. *Arch Neurol* 2000;**57**:1710–1713.

406. O'Brien MD. Ischemic cerebral edema in brain ischemia. In LR Caplan (ed.), *Basic Concepts and Clinical Relevance*, London: Springer-Verlag, 1995, pp 43–50.

407. Parisi DM, Koval K, Egol K. Fat embolism syndrome. *Am J Orthop (Belle Mead NJ)* 2002;**31**:507–512.

408. Bulger E, Smith DG, Maier RV, Jurkovich G. Fat embolism syndrome. A 10-year review. *Arch Surg* 1997;**132**:435–439.

409. Sevitt S. *Fat Embolism*. London: Butterworth & Co., 1962.

410. Dines DE, Burgher LW, Okazaki H. The clinical and pathological correlation of fat embolism syndrome. *Mayo Clin Proc* 1975;**50**:407–411.

411. Jacobson DM, Terrence CF, Reinmuth OM. The neurologic manifestations of fat embolism. *Neurology* 1986;**36**:847–851.

412. Hill JD, Aguilar MJ, Baranco AP, Gerbode F. Neuropathological manifestations of cardiac surgery. *Ann Thorac Surg* 1969;**7**:409–517.

413. Ghatal NR, Sinnenberg RJ, DeBlois GG. Cerebral fat embolism following cardiac surgery. *Stroke* 1983;**14**:619–621.

414. Charache S, Page DL. Infarction of bone marrow in sickle cell disorders. *Ann Intern Med* 1967;**67**:1195–1200.

415. Vichinsky E, Williams K, Das M, et al. Pulmonary fat embolism: A distinct cause of severe acute chest syndrome in sickle cell anemia. *Blood* 1994;**83**:3107–3112.

416. Shelley WM, Curtis EM. Bone marrow and fat embolism in sickle cell anemia and sickle cell-hemoglobin C disease. *Bull Johns Hopkins Hosp* 1958;**103**:8–25.

417. Chmel H, Bertles J. Hemoglobin S/C disease in a pregnant woman with crisis and fat embolization syndrome. *Am J Med* 1975;**58**:563–566.

418. Yoo KM, Yoo BG, Kim KS, Lee SU, Han BH. Cerebral lipiodol embolism during transcatheter arterial chemoembolization. *Neurology* 2004;**63**:181–183.

419. Qian Y, Ances BM, Pruitt A, Choi B, Moonis G. Intracranial fat embolization due to baclofen pump. *Neurology* 2005;**64**:919.

420. Simon A, Ulmer JL, Strottman JM. Contrast-enhanced MR imaging of cerebral fat embolism: Case report and review of the literature. *AJNR* 2003;**24**:97–101.

421. Forteza AM, Rabinstein A, Koch S, et al. Endovascular closure of a patent foramen ovale in the fat embolism syndrome. Changes in the embolic pattern as detected by transcranial Doppler. *Arch Neurol* 2002;**59**:455–459.

422. Forteza AM, Koch S, Romano JG, et al. Transcranial Doppler detection of fat emboli. *Stroke* 1999;**30**:2687–2691.

423. Guillevin R, Vallee JN, Demeret S, et al. Cerebral fat embolism: Usefulness of magnetic resonance spectroscopy. *Ann Neurol* 2005;**57**:434–439.

424. Chastre J, Fagon J-Y, Soler P, et al. Bronchoalveolar lavage for rapid

diagnosis of the fat embolism syndrome in trauma patients. *Ann Intern Med* 1990;**113**:583–588.

425. Godeau B, Schaeffer A, Bachir D, et al. Bronchoalveolar lavage in adult sickle cell patients with acute chest syndrome: Value for diagnostic assessment of fat embolism. *Am J Resp Care Med* 1996;**153**:1691–1696.

426. Kamenar E, Burger PC. Cerebral fat embolism: A neuropathological study of a microembolic state. *Stroke* 1980;**11**:477–484.

427. Menkin M, Schwartzman RJ. Cerebral air embolism. Report of five cases and review of the literature. *Arch Neurol* 1977;**34**:169–170.

428. Valentino R, Hilbert G, Vargas F, Gruson D. Computed tomographic scan of massive cerebral air embolism. *Lancet* 2003;**361**:1848.

429. Demaerel P, Gevers A-M, De Brueker Y, Sunaert S, Wilms G. Stroke caused by cerebral air embolism during endoscopy. *Gastrointest Endosc* 2003;**1**:134–135.

430. Weber M-A, Fiebach JB, Lichy MP, Schwark C, Grau A. Bilateral cerebral air embolism. *J Neurol* 2003;**250**:1115–1117.

431. Hodics T, Linfante I. Cerebral air embolism. *Neurology* 2003;**60**:112.

432. Hertz JA, Schinco MA, Frykberg ER. Extensive pneumocranium. *J Trauma* 2002;**52**:188.

433. Laskey AL, Dyer C, Tobias JD. Venous air embolism during home infusion therapy. *Pediatrics* 2002;**109**:e15.

434. Gei AF, Vadhera, Hankins GDV. Embolism during pregnancy: Thrombus, air, and amniotic fluid. *Anesthesiol Clin North America* 2003;**21**:165–182.

435. Malinow AM, Naulty JS, Hunt CO, et al. Precordial ultrasonic monitoring during cesarean delivery. *Anesthesiology* 1987;**66**:816–819.

436. Spencer MP, Campbell SD. Development of bubbles in venous and arterial blood during hyperbaric decompression. *Bull Mason Clin* 1968;**22**:26–32.

437. Gillen HW. Symptomatology of cerebral gas embolism. *Neurology* 1968;**18**:507–512.

438. van Hulst RA, Klein J, Lachman B. Gas embolism: Pathophysiology and treatment. *Clin Physiol Funct Imaging* 2003;**23**:237–246.

439. Cantais E, Louge P, Suppini A, Foster PP, Palmier B. Right-to-left shunt and risk of decompression illness with cochleovestibular and cerebral symptoms in divers: Case control study in 101 consecutive dive accidents. *Crit Care Med* 2003;**31**:84–88.

440. Jeon S-B, Kim JS, Lee DK, Kang D-W, Kwon SU. Clinicoradiological characteristics of cerebral air embolism. *Cerebrovasc Dis* 2007;**23**:459–462.

441. Yeh T, Austin EH, Sehic A, Edmonds HL. Rapid recognition and treatment of cerebral air embolism: The role of neuroimaging. *J Thor Cardiovasc Surg* 2003;**126**:589–591.

442. Lefkovitz NW, Roessman U, Kori S. Major cerebral infarction from tumor embolus. *Stroke* 1986;**17**:555–557.

443. Banerjee AK, Chopra JS. Cerebral embolism from a thyroid carcinoma. *Arch Neurol* 1972;**27**:186–187.

444. Kase CS, White R, Vinson TL, Eichelberger RP. Shotgun pellet embolus to the middle cerebral artery. *Neurology* 1981;**31**:458–461.

445. Yaari R, Ahmadi J, Chang GY. Cerebral shotgun pellet embolism. *Neurology* 2000;**54**:1487.

446. Duncan I, Fourie PA. Embolization of a bullet in the internal carotid artery. *AJR Am J Roentgenol* 2002;**178**:1572–1573.

447. Langenbach M, Leopold H-C, Hennerici M. Neck trauma with embolization of the middle cerebral artery by a metal splinter. *Neurology* 1990;**40**:552–553.

448. Dato GMA, Arsianian A, Di Marzio P, Filosso PL, Ruffini E. Posttraumatic and iatrogenic foreign bodies in the heart: Report of fourteen cases and review of the literature. *J Thor Cardiovascular Surg* 2003;**126**:408–414.

449. Crie JS, Hajar R, Folger G. Umbilical catheter masquerading at echocardiography as a left atrial mass. *Clin Cardiol* 1989;**12**:728–730.

450. Mattox KL, Beall AC, Ennix CL, DeBakey ME. Intravascular migratory bullets. *Am J Surg* 1979;**137**:192–195.

451. Caplan LR, Thomas C, Banks G. Central nervous system complications of "Ts and blues" addiction. *Neurology* 1982;**32**:623–628.

452. Caplan LR, Hier DB, Banks G. Current concepts of cerebrovascular disease – stroke: Stroke and drug abuse. *Stroke* 1982;**27**:869–73.

453. Atlee W. Talc and cornstarch emboli in the eyes of drug abusers. *JAMA* 1972;**219**:49–51.

454. Mizutami T, Lewis R, Gonatas N. Medial medullary syndrome in a drug abuser. *Arch Neurol* 1980;**37**:425–428.

455. Chillar RK, Jackson AL, Alaan L. Hemiplegia after intracarotid injection of methylphenidate. *Arch Neurol* 1982;**39**:598–599.

Hypoxic–ischemic encephalopathy, cardiac arrest, and cardiac encephalopathy

Louis R Caplan and Michael DeGeorgia

Introduction

The brain is particularly vulnerable to any major decrease in its blood, oxygen, or fuel supply. Patients with hypotension or hypoxia often present to their physicians or the emergency room because of brain dysfunction. Most often, decreased brain perfusion is caused by cardiac disease, either cardiac arrest, or cardiac arrhythmia or pump failure often caused by an acute myocardial infarction. Shock and hyopovolemia also decrease whole brain perfusion. Because circulatory failure usually leads to hypoventilation, and hypoxia soon causes diminished cardiac function, hypoxia and hypoperfusion are usually combined. The general term hypoxic-ischemic encephalopathy reflects the dual nature of the central nervous system stress. Pulmonary embolism is another acute disorder that causes hypotension and diminished blood oxygenation. In some patients, decreased cerebral perfusion is caused by acute blood loss or hypovolemia.

The effects of hypoxic-ischemic brain injury can be devastating for patients and their families. Some conditions, such as hanging, drowning, and carbon monoxide poisoning, result mostly in hypoxic brain injury. The nature and extent of brain injury depend on several factors: the severity, timing, and duration of the circulatory arrest and oxygen deprivation as well as the underlying cause. Patients can present with a broad spectrum of signs and symptoms. Care must be optimized at each point along the continuum to improve survival and neurological outcomes. This requires a team effort among all providers, including neurologists who are often called upon to determine the diagnosis and prognosis of brain injury and provide guidance in the intensive care unit. Neurologists are also often called to evaluate patients without obvious brain injury but with cognitive and behavioral abnormalities. Some of these patients, with heart failure, have syndromes of cardiac encephalopathy. These are often not recognized especially when they develop in the setting of critical illness. A thorough understanding of the underlying pathophysiology of cardiac encephalopathy along with a high index of suspicion is needed for accurate diagnosis and treatment.

Pathophysiology of the brain injury

Normal brain metabolism has several unique features including limited intrinsic stores of high-energy phosphate compounds and a high metabolic demand. The brain is critically dependent upon a continuous blood-borne supply of oxygen and glucose to meet that demand. Oxygen delivery is the product of cerebral blood flow (CBF) and arterial oxygen content. CBF is governed by the Hagen–Poiseuille equation, correlating directly with cerebral perfusion pressure (CPP), the difference between mean arterial pressure (MAP) and intracranial pressure (ICP), and vessel radius and inversely with blood viscosity and vessel length. Cardiac output also correlates directly with CBF, independent of blood pressure. Arterial oxygen content includes the total amount of oxygen carried in the blood, both the oxygen bound to hemoglobin and the oxygen dissolved in plasma (proportional to the partial pressure of oxygen). The oxygen that is dissolved in plasma diffuses into brain tissue according to the oxygen pressure gradient between the end capillaries and the cells.

When glucose is transported into the cell, it is converted anaerobically to pyruvate. Pyruvate is metabolized aerobically in the mitochondria to generate energy, adenosine triphosphate (ATP), needed to meet the metabolic demands of the cell. Reduced delivery of oxygen and substrates uncouples oxidative phosphorylation, reduces ATP production, and disrupts ionic pump function. Intracellular levels of sodium rise while potassium levels drop causing depolarization of neurons.[1] Voltage-gated calcium channels are opened by depolarization, allowing for the rapid influx of calcium and release of excitotoxic amino acids such as glutamate.[2] The excess glutamate binds N-methyl-D-aspartate (NMDA) and α-amino-3-hydroxy-5-methyl-4-isoxazolepropionic acid (AMPA) receptors on the post-synaptic membranes, causing depolarization of the post-synaptic neuron and propagating a wave of depolarization furthering the ischemic cascade. The excess intracellular sodium leads to osmotic swelling of nerve cells (cytotoxic edema).

The flood of calcium influx also results in activation of phospholipases and proteases that degrade cell membranes, and endonucleases that cause DNA cleavage.[3,4] Excess calcium also enters the mitochondria resulting in opening of the permeability transition pore on the inner mitochondrial membrane. This leads to loss of membrane potential, mitochondrial osmotic swelling, release of cytochrome c and the initiation of apoptosis, and creation of reactive oxygen species.[5,6] These events are followed by an influx of circulating inflammatory cells and proinflammatory mediators such as cytokines and chemokines and activation of matrix matalloproteinases (MMPs),[7] breakdown of the blood–brain barrier, and further inflammatory cell recruitment and inflammation.

Caplan's Stroke: A Clinical Approach, 5th Edition, ed. Louis R Caplan. Published by Cambridge University Press. © Cambridge University Press, 2016.

Paradoxically, restoration of blood flow may cause additional damage (reperfusion injury). Initially there is a reactive hyperemia, a result of loss of cerebral autoregulation, followed by profound hypoperfusion (no-reflow phenomenon) or microcirculatory impairment from sludging of white blood cells and platelets along capillary walls and swelling of endothelial cells and astrocytic end-feet.[8,9]

Any condition that leads to an abrupt reduction in CBF can trigger this devastating cascade. Such conditions include those associated with a drop in CPP (either from systemic hypotension, raised ICP, or both), narrowing of the vessel radius, or increase in blood viscosity. In patients with cardiac arrest, of course, it is a sudden ventricular arrhythmia that leads to the immediate loss of cardiac output, systemic blood pressure, CPP, and CBF. This is accompanied by sudden respiratory failure and reduced partial pressure of oxygen (hypoxemia). The combination of the two culminates in the dual nature of **ischemic-hypoxic brain injury**. Patients with hemodynamic impairment, often combined with severe large artery stenosis or occlusion, tend to develop ischemic injury in the so called borderzone areas between vascular territories. Conditions that suddenly lead to hypoxemia alone (e.g., asphyxia associated with hanging, drowning, or carbon monoxide poisoning) cause predominantly **hypoxic brain injury**. In most cases, this injury is less severe because of preserved cerebral perfusion, substrate delivery, and toxin removal. Some patients with hypoxemia develop secondary circulatory arrest. This combination results in a much greater burden of damage. Profound anemia can also, in theory, reduce arterial oxygen content and lead to **anemic-hypoxic brain injury**, and poisoning of the oxidative enzymes within the neuronal mitochondria (e.g., cyanide poisoning) resulting in **histotoxic-hypoxic brain injury**.[10,11]

Hypoxic-ischemic brain injury

Cardiac arrest

Patient 1

AR, a 51 year-old man with hypertension and diabetes mellitus was found unresponsive at home. His wife initiated cardiopulmonary resuscitation (CPR). When the paramedics arrived, the rhythm of the electrocardiogram (ECG) was ventricular fibrillation. Return of spontaneous circulation was achieved after approximately 20 minutes. At the hospital, therapeutic hypothermia was induced, targeting a core temperature of 33°C. He was mechanically ventilated and sedated with a propofol infusion. Shivering was suppressed with an atracurium infusion. After 24 hours, he was slowly rewarmed. Atracurium was discontinued when the patient's core temperature reached 35°C. He was maintained, however, on the propofol infusion together with intermittent boluses of intravenous fentanyl because of coughing on the endotracheal tube. At 48 hours, he was normothermic. A neurological consultation was requested to determine prognosis.

Overview

Out-of-hospital cardiac arrest affects up to 325 000 people in the United States each year.[12] An additional 200 000 have cardiac arrest in the hospital.[13] The resulting brain injury is a major cause of mortality and morbidity. Over the last decade, research into the pathophysiology of hypoxic-ischemic brain injury and cardiac arrest have resulted in a better understanding of the full and complex clinical picture. This includes not only the direct brain injury but also the subsequent myocardial stunning,[14,15] sepsis-like systemic proinflammatory response,[16] and systemic ischemic/reperfusion syndrome that collectively is referred to as the "post-cardiac arrest syndrome."[17] The term "post-cardiac arrest encephalopathy" encompasses the full spectrum of the neurological sequelae of cardiac arrest including disorders of arousal and consciousness, delirium, and syndromes associated with ischemic strokes.

For out-of-hospital cardiac arrest, the most common initial rhythm is ventricular tachycardia or ventricular fibrillation. These "shockable" rhythms quickly degenerate to asystole over the course of several minutes; as a result, the majority of cardiac arrest patients have asystole or pulseless electric activity when first examined by emergency medical services.[18] The proportion of cardiac arrests due to ventricular fibrillation may be decreasing over time,[19] a decline that has been attributed, in part, to the widespread use of β-blockers.[20] Outcomes are generally better with "shockable rhythms" than "non-shockable" rhythms but early defibrillation is critical; with each passing minute of untreated ventricular fibrillation, the likelihood of survival is reduced by 7–10%.[21] More than 80% of instances of ventricular fibrillation are caused by ischemic heart disease.[22,23] Dilated non-ischemic and hypertrophic cardiomyopathies account for the second largest number of cardiac arrests, whereas other cardiac disorders such as congenital heart disease and underlying genetically determined ion channel anomalies account for less than 10%.[24] The reported outcomes of out-of-hospital cardiac arrest vary considerably, but overall survival to hospital discharge rates is about 10%.[25] Survival rates are increasing in part because of more frequent bystander CPR.[26,27] Patients having in-hospital cardiac arrest often have multiple comorbidities and the cause of the arrest is usually multifactorial including non-ischemic cardiomyopathy, pulmonary embolism, bleeding, sepsis, and lung disease. For in-hospital cardiac arrests, "non-shockable" rhythms predominate: pulseless electrical activity, 41%; asystole, 32%; ventricular fibrillation, 16%; ventricular tachycardia, 11%.[28] The average survival to hospital discharge rate following in-hospital cardiac arrest is around 18%.[13,29]

In the 2010 American Heart Association (AHA) Guidelines for Cardiopulmonary Resuscitation (CPR) and Emergency Cardiovascular Care (ECC), several changes were introduced aimed at achieving better outcomes. Because interruptions in chest compressions reduce survival, a change in the CPR sequence from the traditional Airway-Breathing-Circulation (A-B-C) to Circulation-Airway-Breathing (C-A-B) was recommended. Finally, a greater emphasis was placed on post-cardiac arrest care.[30] Following return of spontaneous circulation, post-resuscitation treatment strategies have evolved to specifically target the different mechanisms of cardiac arrest and hypoxic-ischemic brain injury.

Immediate post-resuscitation treatment strategies

Coronary angiography and revascularization

The most common cause of ventricular tachycardia or ventricular fibrillation cardiac arrest is myocardial ischemia. The rationale of immediate coronary angiography and revascularization is that early revascularization may minimize myocardial necrosis, reduce the likelihood of arrhythmias, increase cardiac output, and augment cerebral blood flow. However, while non-cardiac arrest patients with ST-elevation infarctions clearly benefit from revascularization, because patients with cardiac arrest were excluded from most acute myocardial infarction trials, it remains unclear whether these patients, after resuscitation, would similarly benefit. Several non-randomized observational studies showed a survival benefit from early angiography/coronary intervention compared with no or delayed angiography.[31,32] 2015 guidelines advocate early coronary angiography for patients with ST elevation on a post-resuscitation 12-lead ECG. However, because the absence of ST elevation does not exclude the presence of critical coronary lesions, many advocate that all patients resuscitated after cardiac arrest should undergo early coronary angiography if there is no obvious noncardiac cause of the cardiac arrest.[33,34]

Targeted temperature management

Several animal models of global ischemia have shown profound protection of selectively vulnerable neurons with hypothermia.[35–38] This has been consistently confirmed in larger animal models of cardiac arrest.[39–41] The benefit of hypothermia has many explanations. While hypothermia reduces the cerebral metabolic rate and thus oxygen demand, this probably is not the primary mechanism of neuroprotection associated with mild or moderate hypothermia. More importantly, hypothermia reduces neuronal depolarization[42] and both the amount and rate of excitatory amino acid release.[42–44] Hypothermia also decreases intracellular calcium dependent kinase activity[45] and inhibits many of the steps leading to reperfusion injury by decreasing free radical production, endothelial adhesion molecule expression and leukocyte invasion, and apoptosis.[46–48] And hypothermia reduces MMP activity and damage to the blood–brain barrier.[49] Hypothermia improves outcomes in animal models by reducing the extent of the primary ischemic damage, attenuating reperfusion injury, and maintaining vascular integrity.

In 2002, two pivotal randomized clinical trials showed that moderate therapeutic hypothermia (32–34°C) could ameliorate brain injury, reduce mortality, and significantly improve neurological outcomes among survivors of cardiac arrest from shockable rhythms. In the European Multicenter Trial, conducted by the Hypothermia After Cardiac Arrest Study group, 55% of cooled patients had a good outcome at 6 months compared with 39% of normothermic control patients.[50] The second study, from Australia, found that 49% of cooled patients had good neurological outcomes compared with 26% of controls.[51] Cooling of comatose patients after out-of-hospital ventricular fibrillation arrest was given a level I recommendation in the 2010

AHA Guidelines for CPR and ECC.[52] A more recently published larger randomized trial, the Target Temperature Management (TTM) trial questioned the benefit of moderate hypothermia.[53] In this trial a total of 939 patients were randomly assigned to receive a targeted temperature of 33°C or 36°C. In contrast to the earlier studies, the TTM trial included patients with all initial cardiac rhythms, not just shockable rhythms. At 6 months there was no significant difference in mortality or neurological function. There was a nonsignificant trend toward more adverse events in the 33°C group compared with the 36°C group and at day 3 of hospitalization, more patients in the 33°C group required vasopressors or inotropes compared with those in the 36°C group. Because of differences in patient populations, it is difficult to compare these trials. For many patients strict normothermia (preventing fever) or slight hypothermia (36°C) may be just as effective as moderate levels of hypothermia. Some patients with more severe hypoxic-ischemic damage may still benefit from deeper levels of hypothermia (33°C) with the caveat that with lower temperatures, the therapeutic index may become narrower and complications can offset the benefit. Intra-arrest hypothermia, begun ultra-early in the ischemic cascade, may provide a significant benefit while minimizing risk.[54] More studies are needed to determine the true value of hypothermia after cardiac arrest, appropriate temperature targets, timing and duration of therapy, and methods for cooling.

Goal-directed hemodynamic optimization

Patients are often hemodynamically unstable in the immediate post-arrest phase as a result of increased catecholamines and myocardial stunning. This manifests as decreased cardiac output, hypotension, and tachycardia.[55] Hypotension after cardiac arrest correlates with poor outcome.[56] In some observational studies, higher blood pressures after cardiac arrest were associated with better outcomes.[57–60] While this may seem intuitive, in the immediate post-resuscitation period, standard management protocols have aimed at keeping the MAP greater than 65 mmHg, a level that secures coronary perfusion. Because cerebral autoregulation is either impaired or shifted to the right immediately after cardiac arrest,[61] this pressure may be too low to secure adequate brain perfusion especially in patients with the "no reflow phenomenon."[62] Sterz, and colleagues, in a reproducible canine cardiac arrest model, showed that induced hypertension was associated with better neurological outcomes and less histopathological damage.[63] Combining this with hypothermia resulted in even better outcomes.[64] Early hemodynamic optimization has been shown to improve survival in other critically ill populations, most notably in patients with sepsis,[65] and similar strategies instead may be beneficial after cardiac arrest. Hemodynamic optimization can be achieved with intravenous fluid administration combined with vasopressor (norepinephrine), inotropic (dobutamine), and inodilator (milrinone) agents. Using this strategy, Sunde and colleagues showed improved outcomes after cardiac arrest.[66] Gaieski and colleagues also combined early goal-directed hemodynamic optimization (targeting a MAP between

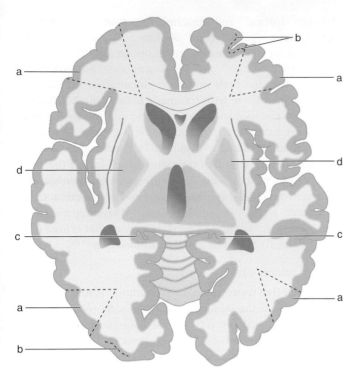

Figure 11.1 Drawing of a horizontal section of the cerebrum showing common patterns of hypoxic-ischemic brain damage. a. Borderzone infarct between anterior and middle cerebral arteries and between middle and posterior cerebral arteries. b. Zones of laminar necrosis within the cerebral cortex. c. Hippocampal necrosis. d. Necrosis of the nerve cells within the globus pallidus and putamen. Adapted from Caplan LR, Hurst JW, Chimowitz MI. *Clinical Neurocardiology*. New York: Marcel Dekker, 1999.

80 mmHg and 100 mmHg) with hypothermia and showed a trend towards improved survival.[67] Tagami et al. reported better neurological outcomes after the combination of all three strategies – early revascularization, hypothermia, and hemodynamic optimization – when compared with standard therapy.[68] Further studies are needed.

Neurological sequelae

Anatomy of hypoxic-ischemic brain injury

Neuronal susceptibility to hypoxic-ischemic injury varies throughout the brain. The most vulnerable neurons are those in the cerebral cortex, especially layers III, V, and VI. These layers are the main targets for corticocortical and thalamocortical afferents and are important for arousal and consciousness. Also vulnerable are neurons in the CA1 zone of the hippocampus, the amygdaloid nucleus, and anterior, dorsomedial, and pulvinar thalamic nuclei, caudate, putamen, globus pallidus, certain brainstem nuclei such as periaqueductal nuclei and the pars reticulata of the substantia nigra, and Purkinje cells in the cerebellar cortex.[69–71] This selective vulnerability may be due to higher metabolic demand and denser concentration of receptors for excitatory amino acids, thus a greater susceptibility to excitotoxicity. The induction of certain enzyme systems, such as heat shock proteins or c-fos or c-jun gene products, may also contribute to selective vulnerability.[72] Ischemic neurons do not necessarily die immediately but

often within days of reperfusion; this delayed cell death is particularly true for CA1 zone hippocampal neurons.[73] Selective vulnerability, arterial anatomy, and differential responses to hypoxia and ischemia explain the various patterns of brain injury (Figure 11.1).

Clinical manifestations of hypoxic-ischemic brain injury

Neurologists are typically called upon to evaluate patients *after* the cardiac arrest, resuscitation, and immediate post-resuscitation treatment. Clinical manifestations of post-cardiac arrest encephalopathy vary greatly and depend on the severity and anatomy of the hypoxic-ischemic brain injury and the effectiveness of the immediate resuscitation and post-resuscitation treatment. There can be a broad spectrum of signs and symptoms with disorders of arousal and consciousness being the most prominent. All patients are initially comatose. With time, patients who improve often ascend through several stages of increasing awareness beginning with spontaneous eye opening, followed by a vegetative state in which they are poorly responsive to environmental stimuli, followed by increasing voluntary behavior and a minimally conscious state. Patients can "plateau" at each stage or can continue on to full recovery depending on the extent of their injury. This pathway can also be characterized by agitation, restlessness, confusion, and delirium. Finally, once alert and oriented, other specific neurological syndromes are found that reflect damage to specific brain areas, especially the borderzone areas.

Coma

Consciousness is maintained by the continuous stimulation of the cerebral cortex by neurons within the brainstem tegmentum. The core areas for arousal, the ascending reticular activating system, consist of glutaminergic and cholinergic neurons in the dorsal tegmentum of the pons and midbrain.[74,75] These neurons activate the central thalamus (mainly the intralaminar nuclei) and basal forebrain. The central thalamus and basal forebrain subsequently activate the cortex through glutaminergic and cholinergic projections. The brainstem norepinephrine system also contributes to arousal by modulating the cortex, thalamic intralaminar nuclei, and basal forebrain.[76,77] Coma results from dysfunction of corticothalamic activity either directly from bihemispheric loss of cortical neuronal function or indirectly from damage to the ascending reticular activating system in the brainstem or thalamus.

Comatose patients are unresponsive, even when vigorously stimulated. Different patterns are observed depending on the extent of bihemispheric damage versus brainstem damage. In patients with bihemispheric damage, brainstem functions are intact. The pupils are usually reactive to light, symmetric, and of normal size. The eyes often rove from side to side or are deviated upward. Often, the doll's eye maneuver results in easily elicitable movements, indicating lack of cortical inhibition of the vestibulo-ocular reflex. There may be spontaneous movements of the limbs. Patients with preservation of the corticospinal tracts often have abducting movements of the

arms or forearms and limb withdrawal from pinch away from the site of stimulation. In the legs, there is flexion. Those with damage to the corticospinal tracts have stereotypical adduction and flexion movements of the arms to pinch, irrespective of the site of stimulation. In the legs, there is extension and internal rotation.[78] Major asymmetries of motor function usually mean asymmetric brain damage.

Some patients with bihemispheric damage keep their mouths open while others clamp their jaws shut and "bulldog" down on tubes or throat sticks placed in their mouths, making it difficult to see the pharynx or assess the gag reflex. They often spontaneously blink, yawn, sneeze, cough, hiccup, protrude their tongue, lick their lips, sigh, and swallow. These spontaneous mouth, face, and tongue movements are mediated through brainstem structures, and like roving eye movements, indicate that the brainstem is functioning.

Conversely, in patients with brainstem damage, the pupils are often not reactive to light, asymmetric in size, or are very large or small. The eyes remain midline and do not move horizontally or vertically to doll's-eyes maneuvers or to ice-water irrigation of the ears. Other brainstem reflexes (corneal at the pontine level and cough/gag at the medullary level) may be absent. The motor exam may show abnormal extensor responses in the upper extremities with adduction and internal rotation of the shoulder and pronation of the forearm. Most patients require endotracheal intubation and mechanical ventilation because of poor airway control, abnormal respirations, or both. Abnormal respiratory patterns may have localizing value: central neurogenic hyperventilation from lesions of the pons or midbrain, cluster (Biot's) breathing from lesions of the pons, ataxic breathing from lesions in the medulla. Some patients develop a dystonic rigid state that stems from severe damage to deep subcortical basal ganglionic areas and white matter tracts, usually with relative preservation of the cerebral cortex. Prolonged partial ischemia, especially in the young, can damage the basal ganglia, particularly the globus pallidus. Strangulation and carbon monoxide poisoning produce a similar insult, in which hypoxemia antedates and overshadows circulatory compromise.[79]

Coma is a self-limiting state. Patients either worsen until they fulfill neurological criteria for brain death (with absent brainstem reflexes and spontaneous breathing) or they improve within a few weeks and begin their ascent into a vegetative state.

Vegetative state

The first stage of recovery from coma is spontaneous eye opening followed by a vegetative state, that is patients have preserved vegetative nervous functions with generally intact sleep-wake cycles, respiration, digestion, and thermoregulation. While patients also have intermittent wakefulness, they show no indication of self or environmental awareness. They show no evidence of language comprehension or expression, or purposeful or voluntary responses to stimuli.[60,80] This vegetative state may be transitional on the path to recovery of consciousness or may be prolonged; some patients plateau at this stage. Necropsy examinations in such patients have shown

extensive cortical and thalamic necrosis and multiple microinfarcts.[81,82] The term *persistent vegetative state* was introduced for when the condition lasts, somewhat arbitrarily, for more than 30 days[83] and *permanent vegetative state* (PVS) for when there has been no improvement after three months (or one year in those with traumatic brain injury).[84] Because recovery of consciousness can occur within the first year or later, many have suggested that the term PVS be abandoned altogether and replaced with simply "VS" adding the cause of the injury and the length of time since onset, factors that seem to correlate with outcome.[85] Recently, *unresponsive wakefulness syndrome (UWS)* has been suggested as a more accurate and neutral term.[86] Recent functional MRI studies showing some preservation of mental imagery suggest that at least some patients with PVS may be *functionally locked in*.[87,88]

Minimally conscious state

The next level of recovery on the continuum from coma to full consciousness is the *minimally conscious state (MCS)*, defined as "a condition of severely altered consciousness in which minimal but definite behavioral evidence of self or environmental awareness is demonstrated."[89] Patients may follow simple commands, make yes or no responses, verbalize, and pursue visually moving objects. These responses can be intermittent, fluctuating, and subtle, making it hard to differentiate from the vegetative state. Those in MCS, usually have a better prognosis than those in PVS.[90] Pathology in patients in MCS has shown similar but less severe injury patterns as those in a vegetative state; sufficient neurons survive and connect between brainstem, thalamus, and cortex to support some level of behavioral responsiveness.[91]

Neuroimaging of hypoxic-ischemic brain injury

Brain computed tomography (CT) and magnetic resonance imaging (MRI) have become essential tools in the diagnosis, management, and prognostication of patients with hypoxic-ischemic brain injury. Brain CT is usually deceptively normal immediately after cardiac arrest. Subtle cortical hyperdensity can be confused with subarachnoid hemorrhage (pseudosubarachnoid hemorrhage).[92,93] After 48 hours, there are often signs of cytotoxic edema including effacement of sulci, loss of differentiation between cortical gray matter and underlying white matter, blurring of the insular ribbon, and loss of distinction of the margins of the deep gray nuclei (particularly the lenticular nucleus). In severe cases, the CT scan may display reversal of the gray and white matter densities with relatively increased attenuation of the thalami, brainstem, and cerebellum (so called "reversal sign").[94] Borderzone infarcts may not appear until after 24–48 hours (Figure 11.2).

MRI is more sensitive than CT for hypoxic-ischemic injury and cortical laminar necrosis. Cytotoxic edema in the cortical ribbon is responsible for the hyperintense signals seen on diffusion-weighted imaging (DWI) and the corresponding low apparent diffusion coefficient (ADC) values.[95] Accumulation of denatured proteins may cause hyperintense signals on T1-weighted sequences that can be confused with hemorrhage.[96] On fluid-attenuated inversion recovery

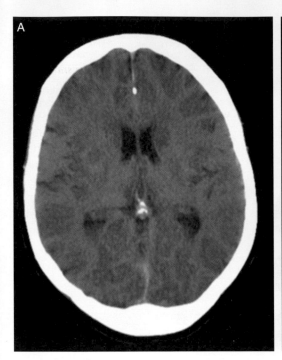 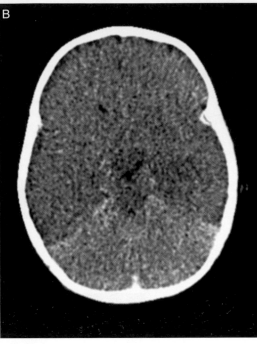

Figure 11.2 Changes of severe hypoxic-ischemic brain injury on brain CT scan. (A) Multiple areas of decreased attenuation in a gyri-fom distribution. (B) Diffuse cerebral edema with effacement of the cortical sulci, loss of distinction of gray–white matter junction, slit-like lateral ventricles and increased attenuation in the cerebellum ("reversal sign").

(FLAIR) sequences, damaged cortical areas usually become hyperintense after a month.[97] While all areas of the cortex may be affected, the perirolandic and occipital cortex are often involved to a greater extent than other regions, perhaps because of greater metabolic requirements. Although the hippocampi in the mesial temporal lobes are believed to be most susceptible to anoxia, radiological evidence of damage to these structures is seen much less commonly than are lesions in the perirolandic and occipital regions. Evidence of damage to the hippocampus may appear as a delayed manifestation of brain injury.[98] Changes in the deep gray nuclei are also seen in most cases of severe hypoxic-ischemic injury including bilateral thalami, lenticular nuclei, and caudate nuclei. The optimal time to image patients after cardiac arrest with MRI is between days 3 and 5.[99]

Prognostication after cardiac arrest

Accurate prognostication is critical to help families make decisions. Decreasing mortality has made prognostication of functional recovery even more important. Predicting outcome after cardiac arrest is complex and depends on many pre-arrest, intra-arrest, and post-arrest factors. For many years neurologists turned to the landmark paper by Levy and colleagues in 1985 to guide prognostication.[100] This early study had inconsistent definitions, limited statistical power, and had the problem of the self-fulfilling prophecy – when poor neurological outcomes are caused by decisions to withdraw or withhold therapy based on the *perception* of a poor neurological prognosis. In 2006, The American Academy of Neurology (AAN) Practice Parameter on Predicting Outcome in Comatose Survivors after Cardiopulmonary Resuscitation developed guidelines to assist in prognostication[101] (Figure 11.3). Because

hypothermia can alter the natural history of recovery, and along with use of sedative and paralytic agents the optimal timing of assessment of clinical features, these guidelines should be applied with greater caution in comatose survivors of cardiac arrest treated with hypothermia.[102] A validated tool for evaluation of in-hospital cardiac arrest patients is helpful in predicting outcomes; it is based on the Get-With-The-Guidelines Resuscitation registry of more than 40 000 patients – the Cardiac Arrest Survival Postresuscitation In-hospital (CASPRI) score.[28] Prognostication is best made based on the clinical examination complemented by electrophysiologic tests, biomarkers, and results of neuroimaging.

Clinical examination

The brainstem examination plays a central role in the assessment of comatose patients after cardiac arrest. Because the brainstem is more resistant to hypoxic–ischemic injury than the cerebral cortex, absence of brainstem reflexes suggests that the cortex must also be severely damaged. At 72 hours, absent pupillary or corneal reflexes predict a poor outcome with 100% specificity or a 0% false positive rate.[100,103,104] Most studies in the post hypothermia era confirm this high specificity.[105–107] However, in at least one study, the corneal reflex could not be used to reliably discriminate those with poor outcomes in cooled patients; an absent corneal reflex in cooled patients was associated with a false positive rate of 5%.[108] The best motor response to noxious stimulation is also very predictive of outcome. At 72 hours, absent motor or extensor responses predict poor outcomes, like absent brainstem reflexes, with essentially zero false-positives.[100,109,110] In patients treated with hypothermia, the motor exam may be less reliable, possibly because of the lingering effects of sedative and paralytic

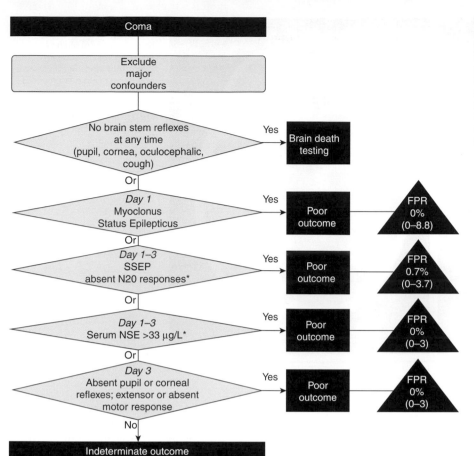

Figure 11.3 The AAN Practice Parameters for determining the neurological prognosis of patients resuscitated from cardiac arrest. FPR, false-positive rate; NSE, Neuron Specific Enolase; SSEP, somatosensory evoked potential. From Wijdicks EF, Hijdra A, Young GB, Bassetti CL, Wiebe S. Practice parameter: Prediction of outcome in comatose survivors after cardiopulmonary resuscitation (an evidence-based review): Report of the Quality Standards Subcommittee of the American Academy of Neurology. *Neurology* 2006;67:203–210 with permission.

medications, with false positive rates ranging from 11% to 24%.[105,107,111] To make reliable prognostic assessments, it is best to rely on examinations performed 72 hours after rewarming and ensure that all sedation has been discontinued for at least 12 hours.

Generalized multifocal myoclonus involving the face, trunk, and extremities often occurs during the first 24 hours after cardiac arrest. Electroencephalography (EEG) in these patients is variable but often displays bursts of generalized spikes or a burst suppression pattern. Patients with continued myoclonus usually have extensive damage to the cerebral cortex, especially the hippocampus and calcarine cortices as well as the basal ganglia, thalamus, cerebellum, and brainstem nuclei.[112] While there may be some overlap, this condition differs from post-anoxic status epilepticus of cortical origin. The abnormal movements should also not be confused with post-hypoxic myoclonus described by Lance and Adams that is characterized by arrhythmic fine or coarse muscle jerking, markedly exaggerated when the limbs are used and often triggered by startle.[113] Generalized multifocal myoclonus is almost always associated with a dismal prognosis[104,114] even in the setting of hypothermia.[105,107]

Electrophysiological testing

EEG has been extensively studied following cardiac arrest.[115] Poor outcome has been associated with certain malignant patterns such as generalized suppression (<20 μV), burst-suppression pattern with generalized epileptiform activity, and generalized periodic complexes on a flat background.[116] According to the AAN practice parameter, the false positive rate for predicting poor outcomes when using these malignant EEG patterns is 3%.[101] Good outcome has been associated with EEG reactivity and variability.[117,118] Post-anoxic status epilepticus has almost always been associated with a dismal prognosis after cardiac arrest.[119] Whether status epilepticus is as ominous in patients treated with hypothermia is less certain.[120] A subset of patients with status but with preserved brainstem reflexes, cortical somatosensory evoked potentials (SSEP), and reactive EEG backgrounds may still achieve good outcome[121] as can some of those with status evolving from a continuous EEG pattern (as opposed to a burst-suppression pattern).[122] Post-anoxic status epilepticus has also been reported to be *more prevalent* in patients treated with hypothermia plausibly because patients are surviving longer to develop it.[121,123,124] Finally, seizure activity, by inhibiting normal brain function, may make patients look worse than they actually are.[106]

Using SSEP, bilateral absence of N20 responses recorded 1–3 days after cardiac arrest is highly associated with a poor outcome (false-positive rate 0.7%).[101] The *presence* of the N20 cortical response is much less predictive.[125] The value of SSEPs in patients treated with hypothermia is probably similar[107,126]

although some studies have shown it to be less predictive.[127] Long-latency potentials (for example P300 and "mismatched negativity"), which evaluate the functional integrity of cortico-cortical and thalamocortical circuits, may also be useful in predicting recovery from coma.[128,129]

Biochemical markers of injury

Neuron specific enolase (NSE) is an isoenzyme of enolase produced in central and peripheral neurons (and in tumors of neuroectodermal origin). A key glycolytic enzyme when released into the blood, NSE is the most validated biochemical marker for prognosis after cardiac arrest. According to the AAN practice parameter, "Serum NSE levels >33 μg/L at days 1–3 post CPR accurately predict poor outcome."[101,104] Several studies have evaluated serum biochemical markers after cardiac arrest in the setting of induced hypothermia. The data are mixed with some showing a similar predictive value[106,130–132] and others showing reduced predictive value.[108,133,134] Unfortunately, differences in laboratory assays and different time points of sampling make comparisons between studies difficult. Greater standardization and larger studies are needed.

Recently, serum levels of tau protein have also been shown to be highly predictive of functional outcome at 6 months after cardiac arrest.[135]

Neuroimaging

Neuroimaging is emerging as a powerful tool for predicting outcome after cardiac arrest. Loss of distinction between gray and white matter on brain CT has been reported to be predictive of death (specifically a gray–white matter Hounsfield unit ratio of less than 1.18).[94,136] Sulcal effacement also correlates with poor outcome.[137] Extensive cortical signal on DWI or FLAIR MRI sequences are strongly associated with poor outcome.[138–140] Figure 11.4 shows an MRI in a patient with poor outcome. Changes in the brainstem and white matter are also associated with poor likelihood of recovery.[140] Most patients who regain consciousness have normal cortical structures though some may have mild to moderate changes on DWI or FLAIR. In one study, half of good-outcome patients even had abnormalities in the deep gray nuclei. None of the patients with moderate to severe cortical abnormalities awoke from coma.[99] In a prospective quantitative brain MRI study of comatose post-cardiac arrest survivors, Wijman et al. showed that those with more than 10% of brain volume less than 650×10^{-6} mm^2/second on the ADC map did not regain consciousness. Using this approach, the MRI was more predictive of outcome than the neurological examination.[141] Assessment of the integrity of white matter tracts using quantitative diffusion tensor imaging has been shown to be very predictive of one-year outcomes.[142]

Patient 1 (continued)

On examination, AR was comatose (though he had still been receiving propofol and fentanyl as late as that morning). His pupils were small but reactive to light. His corneal reflexes were absent. To noxious stimulation, he had flexion of his upper extremities and no movement of his lower extremities. The initial brain CT scan done at the time of the arrest was normal.

Even without hypothermia, prognostication after cardiac arrest should be delayed until 72 hours. This is especially the case in the setting of hypothermia because of the effect of cooling on the pharmacokinetics, metabolism, and clearance of medications, including sedative drugs and neuromuscular blocking agents. In the setting of hypothermia clinical parameters such as the corneal reflex and best motor response are less reliable in predicting outcome. It was recommended that all sedation be stopped.

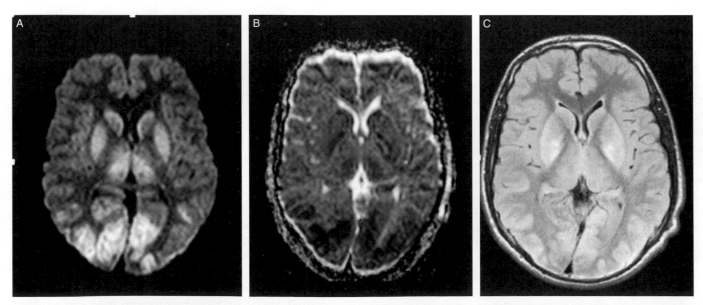

Figure 11.4 Changes of severe hypoxic-ischemic brain injury on MRI. (A) Axial DWI MRI scan demonstrating bilateral symmetrical hyperintensity within the basal ganglia, thalami, and occipital lobes consistent with cortical laminar necrosis. Corresponding (B) axial ADC MRI and (C) FLAIR MRI sequences.

He was examined again after another 48 hours. His pupils were reactive and corneal reflexes were present. To noxious stimulation, he grimaced and had brisk withdrawal of his upper extremities and flexion of his lower extremities. MR imaging done on day 5 revealed no areas of restricted diffusion. Examination at day 7 found him to be opening his eyes and though not following commands, he appeared to be tracking the examiner and spontaneously moving all limbs.

According to the AAN Practice Parameters, this patient's predicted outcome was "indeterminate." After discussing the results of the clinical exam and neuroimaging findings with his family, they opted to continue, and so supportive medical care was continued. At 3 months, AR was doing well with only minor cognitive deficits.

Borderzone infarcts and hemodynamic impairment

Patient 2

LB, a 63 year-old man, suddenly became agitated and restless and seemed confused. He had entered the hospital 2 days earlier for abdominal pain, fever, and possible sepsis. Neurologic examination showed an agitated, restless man. He could not say where he was; he could not give any account of the previous few days. He recalled none of the 3 objects told to him 3 minutes before, and could not even remember that he had been given objects to recall. He spoke normally and could repeat and understand spoken language. He could write but not read. He also could not identify objects in his environment by sight and saw only parts of pictures shown to him. When the same objects were placed in his hands, he correctly named them. There were no abnormalities of motor, reflex, or somatosensory function. Gait was normal but he held his hands outstretched when he walked, as if feeling for objects and walls.

Overview

Areas between vascular territories, borderzones, are especially vulnerable to hypoperfusion due to their distance from the main arterial supply. There are three such borderzones in the brain: (1) the *anterior borderzone*, around the superior frontal sulcus, lies in between the anterior cerebral artery (ACA) and middle cerebral artery (MCA) territories; (2) the *posterior borderzone*, the parieto-temporal or parieto-occipital area, lies in between the MCA and posterior cerebral artery (PCA) supply; and (3) the *internal borderzone*, the white matter of the centrum semiovale and corona radiata, lies in between the deep and superficial perforators of the MCA. There is also a borderzone in the thoracolumbar area of the spinal cord as this segment is perfused almost entirely by the single artery of Adamkiewicz that originates between the ninth thoracic and second lumbar segment (this vascular anatomy is detailed further in Chapter 16).

That systemic hypotension can cause borderzone infarcts has been well described[143–146] and confirmed in primate studies.[147] While such borderzone infarcts can occur following cardiac arrest, they are not very common. They are not typically seen in conjunction with extensive cortical laminar necrosis on neuroimaging. Borderzone infarcts occur more in instances of hypoperfusion *without* hypoxemia (as in the setting of carotid occlusion or critical stenosis together with hypotension), whereas laminar necrosis results more from severe hypoperfusion *with* hypoxemia.[148] Other factors that can contribute to impaired cerebral perfusion and borderzone ischemia are decreased cardiac output (e.g., cardiomyopathy with reduced ejection fraction) and increased blood viscosity (e.g., high fibrinogen or hematocrit).

Embolism can also lead to borderzone ischemia. Hypoperfusion and embolism are often considered to be mechanistically and topographically distinct. Caplan and Hennerici emphasized that the two mechanisms are interdependent; there is a synergistic interaction between hypoperfusion, intra-arterial embolism, and large artery stenosis.[149] Decreased blood flow in a potential embolic source, the heart or a narrowed neck or intracranial artery, promotes local thrombus formation. A recently formed thrombus does not adhere to the endothelium and readily fragments and embolizes. When antegrade blood flow is diminished, the force of the flowing blood is insufficient to propel the emboli through the vascular system. Reduced cerebral perfusion from proximal arterial stenosis or poor cardiac output limits the "washout" of distal microemboli that then lodge in anatomical borderzones. Multiple embolic occlusions in the microvascular bed can also further impair perfusion.[149] This mechanism may be more important for cortical borderzone infarcts than for deep borderzone infarcts.[150]

Neurologic sequelae

The clinical findings reflect the anatomy of the borderzones.[146] Lesions in the *posterior borderzone* often disconnect the preserved calcarine visual cortex in the occipital lobe from the more anterior centers that control eye movements. Patients with *posterior borderzone* ischemia initially may develop a period of blindness that rapidly improves but leaves a Balint's syndrome.[151–154] Patients act as if they cannot see, but often ironically notice small details. The features of Balint's syndrome are:

1. *Asimultagnosia*: Patients see things piecemeal; they do not see all the objects in their field of vision at one time and may notice only parts of objects. To test for this, physicians should ask patients to count the number of people or objects in a picture, ask patients to read a paragraph aloud to determine whether they omit words or phrases, and show patients multiple objects held up together for verbal identification.

2. *Optical ataxia*: Patients cannot coordinate hand and eye movements and point erratically at objects. To test for this, physicians should ask patients to touch specific parts of a picture or the crossing point of Xs on a page. Physicians should ask patients to trace, first with one hand and then the other, a complex drawing constructed by the examiner.

3. *Apraxia of gaze*: Patients are unable to gaze directly where desired. Physicians should ask patients to look at an object held to the side, look at the examiner's nose, and then

repeat the same task. Physicians should also note how patients explore a picture.

Visual abnormalities can be more severe in either the left or right visual field. Bilateral PCA territory strokes can also lead to Balint's syndrome. Occasionally, patients with Alzheimer's disease or Creutzfeldt–Jakob disease, or a degenerative condition dubbed "posterior cortical atrophy,"[155] have features of Balint's syndrome although the symptoms develop gradually and insidiously rather than abruptly.

The hippocampal formations are especially sensitive to lack of nutrients. After severe hypoperfusion, some patients become unable to recall recent events and cannot form new lasting memories. This amnesic state clinically resembles Korsakoff's syndrome and is caused by the selective vulnerability of the hippocampus and adjacent medial temporal lobe structures to hypoxic-ischemic insults.[69,70,156–159] Active memory testing is required to identify and quantify the memory loss. Physicians should give patients a ten-fact story, three objects, or three pictures, emphasizing that they will later be asked to recall the information. Patients should be asked to repeat the items to be certain that they have been registered. Later, patients should be asked to recite the items to be recalled. Memory dysfunction and agitation from bilateral PCA-territory infarcts are discussed further in Chapter 8.

When hypotension is more severe, lesions can spread to the *anterior borderzones* and may extend like a triangle toward the ventricle.[160,161] The areas of the motor homunculus most affected are those related to the shoulder, arm, and thigh. The face area in the central portion of the MCA territory and the foot area in the center of the ACA territory are usually spared. The distribution of weakness has been referred to as "man in a barrel."[151,162] Patients present with weakness initially involving the upper limbs that may be later confined to just the hands and forearms or to the shoulders. Superficial sensation is intact but there may be cortical sensory loss in the fingers. In addition, *anterior borderzone* ischemia in the dominant hemisphere often results in a transcortical aphasia. At times, because of asymmetric vascular occlusive disease, the signs can be asymmetric with unilateral or asymmetric arm paralysis and conjugate-eye deviation toward the side of the larger lesion. Stupor results from extensive bilateral borderzone ischemia. Some patients, especially those with pre-existing occlusive disease of the vertebral arteries, may have borderzone cerebellar infarcts, mostly between the main supply of the three major circumferential cerebellar arteries.

Occasionally, patients recover from coma following cardiac arrest without obvious cerebral damage but instead have paraplegia related to hypoxic-ischemic damage to the spinal cord, typically in the area of the thoracolumbar borderzone area.[156,163] The cervical spinal cord is usually not involved, so that the arms are normal despite severe weakness of the legs. The damage involves mostly the anterior portion of the spinal cord, which is fed by the anterior spinal artery. The anterior horn motor neurons and the pyramidal tracts are included, but usually the posterior columns are spared. The resulting syndrome is a flaccid paralysis of both lower limbs. Spasticity often develops later. Control of urination and defecation is often lost

and there may be a sensory level to pain and temperature on the trunk. Position and vibration sense and touch are usually preserved. Atrophy and fasciculations often develop in the thighs and legs. Spinal cord infarction is a rare but important consequence of cardiac arrest or prolonged hypotension. In some patients, it may not be recognized because the cerebral findings are so prominent.

Patient 2 (continued)

LB had abnormalities in three major spheres – memory, vision, and behavior. These findings indicate bilateral dysfunction of the posterior portions of the cerebral hemispheres. Embolization to the rostral basilar artery, causing bilateral temporo-occipital lobe infarcts in the PCA territory, could cause these findings. Alternatively, an unrecognized episode of prolonged hypotension might have led to hypoperfusion in the posterior borderzone between the MCA and PCA territories. Distal-field infarction most often affects the posterior hemispheres, possibly because they are the regions farthest from the heart.

A brain CT scan showed small but definite approximately symmetric hypodensities in the posterior parietal regions with sparing of the medial calcarine cortex and temporal lobes. ECG showed evidence for an acute myocardial infarction and echocardiography showed a reduced left ventricular contractility with an estimated ejection fraction of 20–25%. LB had a relatively slight insult and recuperated well with time.

Primarily hypoxic brain injury

Hanging

Patient 3

CW, A 27-year-old man, attempted suicide by hanging. He was found by his girlfriend who managed to cut the rope and call 911. She had last seen him 30 minutes before. She reported that his feet were touching the floor when she found him hanging in the closet. The ambulance arrived 5 minutes after being called. The patient was found on the floor with gasping, stertorous respirations. He was comatose and pupils were fixed and dilated. Motor exam showed only a flicker of movement to noxious stimulation. The Glasgow Coma Scale (GCS) score was 3. His systolic blood pressure was 130/80 mmHg and ECG showed sinus tachycardia of 120 beats/min. Strangulation marks were observed on his neck and bilateral conjunctival hemorrhages were detected. He was immediately intubated and ventilated with 100% oxygen. After 15 minutes, pupillary responses to light returned. He started having some spontaneous movements of his limbs. The cervical spine was stabilized with a rigid neck collar and he was admitted to the neurological intensive care unit.

Overview

Hanging has become the second most common cause of suicide in the United States after firearms.[164] The exact mechanism of brain injury from hanging remains debated but depends on the height from which the body is dropped. In judicial

hangings the subject is dropped from a distance equal to or greater than their height. This results in a fracture of the neural arch of C2 (a so called "hangman's fracture"), spinal cord injury, asphyxiation, and death. In suicide attempts, the drop height is usually less. The main mechanism of injury is thought to be neck compression resulting in jugular venous and carotid arterial obstruction combined with hypoxemia from airway obstruction. Cardiac inhibition secondary to vagal nerve stimulation has also been posited to play a role.[165] Hanging leads predominantly to a hypoxic form of brain injury, the severity of which depends on the duration, degree, and acuity of the insult and whether or not there is secondary cardiac arrest.[166] Neurons are somewhat more tolerant of hypoxia than ischemia.[167]

Neurologic sequelae

Neurologic outcome depends on the severity of brain damage which correlates with duration of hanging; hanging time of less than 5 minutes generally predicts a good outcome.[168] Longer durations increase the risk of cardiac arrest, which itself is associated with more severe brain damage and a worse prognosis. Clinically, almost all patients are initially comatose. The admission neurologic examination is not a reliable predictor of long-term outcome.[169,170] Only evidence of anoxia on admission brain CT scan has been shown to be independently associated with poor outcome.[171] Hyperintense signals on diffusion-weighted MRI may be seen in the posterior thalami and posterior parietal cortex.[10] MRI in cases of hypoxic injury may also be normal if obtained early after the event.[172] While patients with hanging and cardiac arrest usually have a poor prognosis,[168] many without cardiac arrest can achieve good outcomes.[10] In one study over a 10-year period, the overall mortality rate was 9.5%. The discharge status for most survivors was favorable with 91% having no or temporary disability.[171] For patients arriving in coma after hanging, aggressive treatment is warranted. Some have advocated induced hypothermia based on the results of several small studies that have shown a benefit.[173–175]

Patient 3 (continued)

> CW's neck CT showed no evidence of cervical fracture. Throughout the night he became more agitated and required light sedation with propofol. By the following morning he followed simple commands and moved all limbs. Brain MRI showed no areas of restricted diffusion. MRA and MRI with fat saturation technique showed no evidence for arterial dissection. Sedation was stopped after the MRI and later that afternoon, approximately 16 hours after the event, he was extubated. He had no focal neurologic deficits.

The initial neurologic examination and GCS score do not correlate well with long-term functional outcome. Therefore, the default approach is to initiate aggressive resuscitation and treatment in every patient admitted with signs of life regardless of the duration of hanging.

Drowning

Overview

Drowning is the fifth leading cause of accidental deaths in the United States.[176] The incidence follows a bimodal age pattern: the first peak is in young children under 5 years of age who are left unattended near swimming pools or in bathtubs and the second is among 15–25-year olds, especially males, in natural bodies of water.[177] Alcohol is a contributing factor in more than half of the cases.[176] In 2005, a new definition and classification scheme was introduced to facilitate greater consistency in reporting. For survivors, the term "non-fatal drowning" is preferred over "near-drowning."[178] With submersion, water is aspirated into the lungs and quickly leads to tissue and brain hypoxia and loss of consciousness. Upper airway obstruction from laryngospasm also causes hypoxemia. This is followed by tachycardia, bradycardia, pulseless electrical activity, and asystole.[179] The timing of this sequence ranges from seconds to minutes though rarely (e.g., in icy water) it may be extended to hours.[180] The incidence of cervical spine injury in drowning victims is very low (0.009%) and unless there is an obvious associated factor such as diving, signs of trauma, or alcohol intoxication, routine spinal stabilization is not recommended.[181] With the 2010 AHA Guidelines for CPR and ECC, CPR now begins with chest compressions in a C-A-B sequence. However, with drowning, given the hypoxic nature of the arrest, rescuers should revert to the traditional A-B-C approach; those with respiratory arrest only usually respond after a few artificial breaths are given.[182] A classification system of six grades was developed to help guide management after drowning; higher numbers indicate greater severity.[183] All patients with grades 3–6 generally require admission to the intensive care unit for management and close monitoring.

Neurologic sequelae

Neurological outcome mainly depends on the severity of brain injury, which usually correlates with duration of submersion. In those with submersion times of less than 5 minutes, 90% will have a good outcome. For submersion times longer than 10 minutes, only about 10% will have a good outcome.[180,184] In contrast to cardiogenic cardiac arrest and hanging, submersion, when it occurs in cold water, can provide significant neuroprotection. Cases of remarkable neurologic recoveries after non-fatal drowning in ice water have been reported[185,186] and several small studies of therapeutic hypothermia have shown improved outcomes.[182,187] As in cardiogenic cardiac arrest, MRI can be useful in prognostication when abnormal. In children, evidence of basal ganglia injury, cortical injury, and edema is associated with a poor outcome.[188] A normal MRI does not always mean a good outcome; in one study, a normal MRI was only 50% predictive of good outcome.[189] In the ICU, management is mainly focused on optimizing pulmonary function while attempting to minimize secondary brain injury.[190] Aspiration of water damages the lung alveoli and results in washout of surfactant, pulmonary edema,

decreased lung compliance, and atelectasis. Management is similar to that of acute respiratory distress syndrome (ARDS).[191] Adequate oxygenation may require the use of extracorporeal membrane oxygenation.[10]

Carbon monoxide poisoning

Overview

Carbon monoxide (CO) poisoning is the most common cause of poisoning morbidity and mortality in the United States.[192] Carbon monoxide is a tasteless, odorless, and non-irritating, highly toxic gas that is a by-product of the incomplete combustion of hydrocarbons in motor vehicle engines and heating units. Carbon monoxide gas binds strongly with heme containing compounds. It binds to hemoglobin leading to the formation of carboxyhemoglobin (COHb); the affinity of hemoglobin for CO is 200 times greater than its affinity for oxygen and CO easily displaces oxygen from hemoglobin.[193] The arterial oxygen content of the blood decreases, causing tissue hypoxia. To make matters worse, the dissociation curve of the remaining bound oxygen shifts to the left further decreasing the amount of the oxygen released. CO causes tissue hypoxia, ischemia and secondary injury through multiple mechanisms.

CO binds to cytochrome C oxidase, interrupting mitochondrial respiration with subsequent tissue acidosis and production of reactive oxygen species.[194] It causes lipid peroxidation and deposition of peroxynitrate in blood vessel endothelium causing vascular damage.[195] CO also depresses cardiac function through a variety of ways, including binding to myoglobin. Many patients develop reduced cardiac output and hypotension as a result.[196] In the brain, CO binds to heme iron-rich areas including the globus pallidus and pars reticulata of the substantia nigra causing direct damage. Thus, the toxicity from CO poisoning is due to tissue hypoxia and ischemia along with direct CO-mediated neuronal damage and demyelination.

Neurologic sequelae

Patients with acute CO poisoning may initially be asymptomatic. Symptoms, when they occur, are often non-specific including mild headache, dizziness, nausea, visual disturbances, and confusion. Patients can develop chest pain, tachycardia and tachypnea. Ongoing neuronal damage may result in seizures, coma, or death.[192] Some patients recover from the acute event with minor or no deficits only to develop a delayed encephalopathy days to weeks later with recurrence of neurological and psychiatric symptoms.[197] Often this manifests as delayed parkinsonian symptoms, usually the akinetic-rigid type that responds poorly to medical treatment.[198] Plum and colleagues described delayed progressive deterioration after a single hypoxic insult in which patients initially awakened from coma only to develop apathy, restlessness, confusion, rigidity and ataxia days later. Necropsy showed extensive white matter demyelination in the cerebral hemispheres.[199] This delayed deterioration can also occur in other causes of hypoxic brain damage. Reduction of arylsulfatase-A activity to less than 50%

of normal was found in 2 reports of delayed deterioration.[200,201] Arylsulfatase-A is a lysosomal enzyme active in the lipid metabolism of myelin. In the presence of local tissue acidosis, this enzyme deficiency could make patients vulnerable to demyelination. Delayed leukoencephalopathy has also been reported after heroin inhalation (so called "smoking the dragon").[202]

Other neurologic sequelae of CO poisoning include impaired memory, attention, visual spatial skills, and mental processing speed. Impaired executive function is often observed after frontal lobe damage, and impaired visuospatial abilities following parietal lobe damage.[203] Personality changes and psychosis are described.[204,205] Brain CT and MRI following CO poisoning typically show lesions of the globus pallidus but other lesions have also been described in the putamen,[206] caudate nucleus,[206] thalamus,[207] and substantia nigra.[208] CO poisoning results in lesions in the cerebellar white matter[209] and subcortical and periventricular white matter.[210] The extent of the globus pallidus and white matter lesions have been reported to predict neurological outcome following CO poisoning.[211,212] In the long term, patients may develop cortical, corpus callosum,[213] fornix,[214] and hippocampal atrophy.[204]

In patients with suspected CO poisoning, 100% oxygen is the mainstay of treatment and should be given immediately by mask. Treatment should not be based on the carboxyhemoglobin (COHb) levels, which do not correlate well with clinical severity. The goal is to increase the partial pressure of oxygen levels, decrease the half-life of CO, and facilitate its dissociation from hemoglobin. Hyperbaric oxygen therapy (HBO) is 100% oxygen at 2–3 times the atmospheric pressure at sea level. Usually HBO at 2.5–3.0 ATA for 90–120 minutes has often been used for patients with more severe neurologic symptoms.[215] The efficacy of hyperbaric versus normobaric oxygen in the treatment of acute and delayed symptoms remains controversial.[216]

Critical care management of the brain injury

Basic critical care

Regardless of the underlying mechanism of brain injury, attentive and meticulous critical care management is a key factor in achieving the best possible outcome. There has been considerable evolution in the management of critically ill patients over the last decade including the establishment of standardized post-resuscitation protocols that cover basic critical care and neurocritical care.[217,218] Most patients are intubated at the time of arrest because of respiratory failure but often remain intubated because of poor airway control. Impaired oxygenation is also common from aspiration, atelectasis, or pulmonary edema. Both hypoxemia and hyperoxemia have been associated with a poor outcome after cardiac arrest.[188] The fraction of inspired oxygen (FiO_2) should be adjusted to maintain an oxyhemoglobin saturation greater than 94%. A "protective ventilator strategy," extrapolated from patients with ARDS, is used targeting tidal volumes less than 6 ml/kg and sufficient

positive end expiratory pressure (PEEP) to prevent alveolar collapse while maintaining low plateau pressures.[219] Excessively high PEEP levels should be avoided as they may decrease cerebral venous outflow, cardiac output, and blood pressure and result in impaired cerebral perfusion. Patients should be ventilated to maintain a normal $PaCO_2$; hyperventilation should be avoided because it can result in cerebral vasoconstriction and reduced CBF. Every attempt should be made to minimize sedation. Minimizing sedation, including daily sedation interruption trials, are associated with a shorter duration of mechanical ventilation and a shorter intensive care unit length of stay.[220,221] When sedation is needed, non-benzodiazepine sedatives (such as propofol or dexmedetomidine) are recommended.[222] Deep sedation with benzodiazepines (such as midazolam or lorazepam) has been linked with increased delirium and worse long-term cognitive outcomes.[223]

Early nutritional support is important in critically ill patients, but recent randomized, controlled trials have not shown an unequivocal benefit with full-replacement feeding. We recommend starting hypocaloric gastric feeding, along with providing micronutrients, during the first week of critical illness. Electrolytes must be monitored closely and a hypoosmolar state, which can contribute to cerebral edema in patients with brain injury, avoided. Hyperglycemia is also common in critically ill patients and has emerged as an unfavorable prognostic indicator in hypoxic-ischemic brain injury, traumatic brain injury, ischemic and hemorrhagic stroke.[224–227] This recognition initially promoted much enthusiasm for tight glycemic control by intravenous insulin infusions,[228–230] but more recent studies have challenged this approach. A meta-analysis of studies found that tight glycemic control did not reduce mortality compared with standard glucose management and was associated with a markedly increased risk of hypoglycemia.[231] Tight glycemic control has a potential adverse effect on cerebral metabolism, resulting in low extracellular glucose and markers of brain energy crisis (elevated lactate–pyruvate ratios and glutamate levels).[230,232,233] A target glucose level of 140–180 mg/dl is recommended. Fever, akin to hyperglycemia, causes secondary neuronal injury and worse outcomes;[234] as such, in the intensive care unit, the target temperature for patients with acute central nervous system injury of any etiology should be normothermia (36.5–37.0°C). Comatose patients are at high risk for venous thromboembolism and should receive anticoagulant thromboprophylaxis with low-molecular-weight heparin or low-dose unfractionated heparin.[235]

Neurocritical care

Seizure activity should be treated promptly with anticonvulsants. The clinician should also be vigilant for non-convulsive status epilepticus detected only by continuous EEG monitoring. This is especially true for patients who are sedated and pharmacologically paralyzed. First-line medications for treatment include levetiracetam and lacosamide.[236] For myoclonic seizures, valproic acid and clonazepam are both effective.[237–239] Recently, levetiracetam has been shown to also be effective in post-hypoxic-ischemic myoclonus.[240] Review all of the patient's medications and stop any that may hinder recovery. These include centrally acting medications such as clonidine, neuroleptics and other dopamine receptor antagonists, benzodiazepines, and some anticonvulsants (phenytoin and phenobarbital).[241] Some medications have been shown to increase arousal and a trial may be warranted in selected patients. Specifically, dopaminergic agonists such as amantadine, levodopa, bromocriptine, or apomorphine enhance striatal background activity and enhance arousal and improve outcomes.[242,243] Fluoxetine, a selective serotonin reuptake inhibitor, has been posited to stimulate the pyramidal cells of the motor cortex and thereby improve motor recovery.[244] Zolpidem, an agonist of a subset of gamma-aminobutyric acid (A) (GABA-A) receptors, has also been shown to increase arousal at least in some patients with diffuse brain injury.[245,246] The mechanism of action of zolpidem is thought to be from inhibition of the globus pallidus interna, which normally inhibits thalamocortical firing, and so leads to enhanced cortical activity.[247] Deep brain stimulation (DBS) also has been used to directly activate the central thalamic outflow.[248,249]

Cardiac encephalopathy

Patient 4

A 67-year-old woman ML, entered the hospital in severe congestive heart failure. She was known to have severe aortic and mitral valve disease and had lower extremity edema, ascites, and pleural effusions. She was vigorously treated with diuretics, bed rest, and thoracentesis and her congestive heart failure greatly improved. As her heart failure improved, her husband and family noted a marked personality change. Usually outgoing, friendly, and talkative, now she became very quiet, uninterested, apathetic, and inert. She denied any feelings of discouragement or depression. She seemed not to heed questions. Her replies were usually one or two words – yes, no, or single-word – that were usually correct. Her motor, sensory, visual, and reflex examinations were normal except that she had bilateral Babinski signs. Brain CT scan was read as showing "cerebral atrophy" because of increased CSF in the sulci. After lumbar punctures that removed CSF, she returned to her former self and her plantar responses became flexor.

Overview

An estimated 5.1 million Americans develop heart failure. By 2030, the prevalence is expected to increase 25% because of the aging population.[250] Heart failure can lead to an encephalopathy that is both poorly understood and widely under recognized. The pathophysiology is complex and multifactorial. First, a decreased cardiac output and blood pressure results in decreased cerebral perfusion pressure and cerebral blood flow.[251] Second, poor diastolic emptying of the right atrium results in increased venous hydrostatic pressure that is transmitted to the dural venous sinuses and veins within the cranial

cavity leading to increased ICP. This further compromises cerebral perfusion pressure. Increased venous pressure also results in impaired CSF absorption with fluid accumulating in the cisterns around the brain, in the subarachnoid spaces, and sometimes within the cerebral ventricles. The mechanism of the CSF effusions is similar to pleural and peritoneal effusions. Like these systemic effusions, improvement in congestive heart failure does not always lead to absorption of the fluid and drainage of the fluid is often needed for its removal. Third, left heart failure is often associated with pulmonary edema and hypoxemia. Through these mechanisms, acute decompensation of cardiac pump function can lead to hypoxic-ischemic brain injury and encephalopathy. Compounding this encephalopathy is concomitant electrolyte and acid-base abnormalities and impaired clearance of medications from right-sided heart failure and liver and kidney dysfunction.[252,253] Cardiac drugs such as amiodarone and digitalis can also have neurological side effects. Finally, there is increasing evidence of autonomic nervous system dysfunction in heart failure, which may also play a role in the encephalopathy.[254,255]

Neurologic sequelae

Symptoms include dizziness, light-headedness, confusion, difficulty concentrating, and impaired executive function.[255] Clinically, cardiac encephalopathy is often initially indistinguishable from that found in patients with liver or renal failure. Symptoms tend to fluctuate from minute to minute and hour to hour. Patients may have asterixis and diffuse slowing of rhythms on EEG. A subset of patients develops a clinical picture similar to that found in hydrocephalus. ML's symptoms and signs provide an example of this clinical picture. The major features are apathy and abulia, a lack of motivation and initiative. Abulic patients have severely reduced spontaneous behavior. They seem content to sit or lie about without doing much. They show little or no interest in television, reading, listening to the radio, conversations, or any other activity. The quantity of spontaneous speech is reduced. When asked questions or urged to perform tasks, abulic patients often fail to respond or do so only after a long delay. When the examiner repeats questions or directions, patients often say that they had heard the request the first time, but just couldn't get started to reply or act. Responses when they are forthcoming are generally short, laconic, and terse. Patients don't persist with familiar tasks, such as naming 10 zoo animals or 10 articles of clothing, and counting backward from 20 to 1. Intellectual functions including memory, language, and ability to draw and copy are usually preserved, although these functions take longer than usual to perform and require frequent prodding to complete. Patients remain alert despite their inactivity and slowness in contrast to other encephalopathies that are invariably accompanied by drowsiness and later stupor. Friends and family describe abulic patients as "bumps on a log" or "couch potatoes." The cause is most likely from the retention of CSF within the intracranial cavity that may appear outside the brain (external hydrocephalus) or in the ventricular system (internal hydrocephalus). Because the extra CSF causes widening of the

sulci, the brain may appear "atrophic" on CT scan. Lumbar puncture and CSF drainage may be followed by clinical improvement and normalization of the "brain atrophy" on CT scan.

In the long term, patients with severe chronic heart failure have a higher frequency of cognitive abnormalities including impairments in memory, measures of attention, reasoning, and concept formation.[256–258] They also have depression.[259–263] Performance on neuropsychologic testing correlates directly with cardiac index[264] and studies before and after cardiac transplantation have shown dramatic improvement in cognitive functioning with the new heart.[264] Chronic heart failure has also been linked with wide-spread structural changes on brain MRI including smaller gray and white matter volumes, silent brain infarcts, and increased white matter hyperintensities.[265–268] White matter hyperintensities are thought to stem directly from ischemic-related injury, including axonal loss, rarefaction of myelin, gliosis, spongiosis, and fiber loss.[269]

Conclusions

Hypoxic-ischemic brain injury following cardiac arrest can be devastating. Usually caused by ischemic heart disease, cardiac arrest most often occurs in the community in patients without a known history of heart disease. Patients who have cardiac arrest in hospitals usually have multiple comorbidities. To improve survival and neurological outcomes after cardiac arrest, care must be optimized at each point along the continuum. It requires a team effort among all providers beginning with a rapid emergency response, bystander CPR, and rapid defibrillation followed by immediate postresuscitation care including early coronary angiography and revascularization, targeted temperature management, and hemodynamic optimization. Neurologists are often called upon to prognosticate and provide guidance after the arrest. Accurate prognostication is crucial and based on a careful consideration of pre-arrest, intra-arrest, and post-arrest factors along with the clinical examination and the results of electrophysiological tests, biomarkers, and neuroimaging studies.

Hanging, drowning, and carbon monoxide poisoning cause primarily hypoxic brain injury. Outcome after hanging depends mainly on the hanging duration and the presence of concomitant cardiac arrest. Because many patients can achieve good outcomes, aggressive treatment is warranted. Similarly, outcome after drowning depends on submersion duration, presence of cardiac arrest, and the extent of pulmonary damage. CO poisoning typically affects the globus pallidus and substantia nigra and can be associated with both acute and delayed neurological and psychiatric manifestations. Normobaric and potentially hyperbaric oxygen is the mainstay of treatment. For all types of severe brain injury, meticulous critical care management is a key factor in achieving the best possible outcome.

Many patients with heart failure develop neurological dysfunction and an encephalopathy that shares many clinical features with other metabolic encephalopathies. The causes are multiple and the pathophysiology complex. Some patients

377

develop a syndrome that resembles that seen with normal pressure hydrocephalus, characterized by apathy and abulia. In the long term, patients with chronic heart failure develop a range of cognitive abnormalities and structural changes on brain MRI including smaller gray and white matter volumes, scattered infarcts, and white matter hyperintensities.

References

1. Hansen AJ. Effect of anoxia on ion distribution in the brain. *Physiol Rev.* 1985;**65**(1):101–148.

2. Choi DW. Calcium-mediated neurotoxicity: Relationship to specific channel types and role in ischemic damage. *Trends Neurosci.* 1988;**11**(10):465–469.

3. Hossmann KA. Pathophysiological basis of translational stroke research. *Folia Neuropathol.* 2009;**47**(3):213–227.

4. Kristian T, Siesjo BK. Calcium in ischemic cell death. *Stroke.* 1998;**29**(3):705–718.

5. Starkov AA, Chinopoulos C, Fiskum G. Mitochondrial calcium and oxidative stress as mediators of ischemic brain injury. *Cell Calcium.* 2004;**36**(3–4):257–264.

6. Sanderson TH, Reynolds CA, Kumar R, Przyklenk K, Huttemann M. Molecular mechanisms of ischemia-reperfusion injury in brain: Pivotal role of the mitochondrial membrane potential in reactive oxygen species generation. *Mol Neurobiol.* 2013;**47**(1):9–23.

7. Wang Q, Tang XN, Yenari MA. The inflammatory response in stroke. *J Neuroimmunol.* 2007;**184**(1–2): 53–68.

8. Ames A, 3rd, Wright RL, Kowada M, Thurston JM, Majno G. Cerebral ischemia. II. The no-reflow phenomenon. *Am J Pathol.* 1968;**52**(2):437–453.

9. Fischer EG, Ames A, 3rd, Hedley-Whyte ET, O'Gorman S. Reassessment of cerebral capillary changes in acute global ischemia and their relationship to the "no-reflow phenomenon". *Stroke.* 1977;**8**(1):36–39.

10. Singhal AB, Topcuoglu MA, Koroshetz WJ. Diffusion MRI in three types of anoxic encephalopathy. *J Neurol Sci.* 2002; **196** (1–2): 37–40.

11. Brierley JB. Experimental hypoxic brain damage. *J Clin Pathol Suppl (R Coll Pathol).* 1977;**11**:181–187.

12. Nichol G, Thomas E, Callaway CW, et al. Regional variation in out-of-hospital cardiac arrest incidence and outcome. *JAMA.* 2008;**300**(12):1423–1431.

13. Morrison LJ, Neumar RW, Zimmerman JL, et al. Strategies for improving survival after in-hospital cardiac arrest in the United States: 2013 consensus recommendations: A consensus statement from the American Heart Association. *Circulation.* 2013;**127**(14):1538–1563.

14. Chang WT, Ma MH, Chien KL, et al. Postresuscitation myocardial dysfunction: Correlated factors and prognostic implications. *Intensive Care Med.* 2007;**33**(1):88–95.

15. Ruiz-Bailen M, Aguayo de Hoyos E, Ruiz-Navarro S, et al. Reversible myocardial dysfunction after cardiopulmonary resuscitation. *Resuscitation.* 2005;**66**(2):175–181.

16. Adrie C, Adib-Conquy M, Laurent I, et al. Successful cardiopulmonary resuscitation after cardiac arrest as a "sepsis-like" syndrome. *Circulation.* 2002;**106**(5):562–568.

17. Nolan JP, Neumar RW, Adrie C, et al. Post-cardiac arrest syndrome: Epidemiology, pathophysiology, treatment, and prognostication. A Scientific Statement from the International Liaison Committee on Resuscitation; the American Heart Association Emergency Cardiovascular Care Committee; the Council on Cardiovascular Surgery and Anesthesia; the Council on Cardiopulmonary, Perioperative, and Critical Care; the Council on Clinical Cardiology; the Council on Stroke. *Resuscitation.* 2008;**79**(3):350–379.

18. Teodorescu C, Reinier K, Dervan C, et al. Factors associated with pulseless electric activity versus ventricular fibrillation: The Oregon sudden unexpected death study. *Circulation.* 2010;**122**(21):2116–2122.

19. Cobb LA, Fahrenbruch CE, Olsufka M, Copass MK. Changing incidence of out-of-hospital ventricular fibrillation, 1980–2000. *JAMA.* 2002;**288**(23):3008–3013.

20. Youngquist ST, Kaji AH, Niemann JT. Beta-blocker use and the changing epidemiology of out-of-hospital cardiac arrest rhythms. *Resuscitation.* 2008;**76**(3):376–380.

21. Cummins RO, Ornato JP, Thies WH, Pepe PE. Improving survival from sudden cardiac arrest: The "chain of survival" concept. A statement for health professionals from the Advanced Cardiac Life Support Subcommittee and the Emergency Cardiac Care Committee, American Heart Association. *Circulation.* 1991;**83**(5):1832–1847.

22. Huikuri HV, Castellanos A, Myerburg RJ. Sudden death due to cardiac arrhythmias. *N Engl J Med.* 2001;**345**(20):1473–1482.

23. Berdowski J, Berg RA, Tijssen JG, Koster RW. Global incidences of out-of-hospital cardiac arrest and survival rates: Systematic review of 67 prospective studies. *Resuscitation.* 2010;**81**(11):1479–1487.

24. Rubart M, Zipes DP. Mechanisms of sudden cardiac death. *J Clin Invest.* 2005;**115**(9):2305–2315.

25. Go AS, Mozaffarian D, Roger VL, et al. Heart disease and stroke statistics – 2013 update: A report from the American Heart Association. *Circulation.* 2013;**127**(1):e6–e245.

26. Hollenberg J, Herlitz J, Lindqvist J, et al. Improved survival after out-of-hospital cardiac arrest is associated with an increase in proportion of emergency crew–witnessed cases and bystander cardiopulmonary resuscitation. *Circulation.* 2008;**118**(4):389–396.

27. Adielsson A, Hollenberg J, Karlsson T, et al. Increase in survival and bystander CPR in out-of-hospital shockable arrhythmia: Bystander CPR and female gender are predictors of improved outcome. Experiences from Sweden in an 18-year perspective. *Heart.* 2011;**97**(17):1391–1396.

28. Chan PS, Spertus JA, Krumholz HM, et al. A validated prediction tool for initial survivors of in-hospital cardiac arrest. *Arch Intern Med.* 2012;**172**(12):947–953.

29. Merchant RM, Yang L, Becker LB, et al. Incidence of treated cardiac arrest in hospitalized patients in the United States. *Crit Care Med.* 2011;**39**(11):2401–2406.

30. Field JM, Hazinski MF, Sayre MR, et al. Part 1: Executive summary: 2010 American Heart Association Guidelines for Cardiopulmonary Resuscitation and Emergency Cardiovascular Care. *Circulation.* 2010;**122**(18 Suppl 3): S640–656.

31. Spaulding CM, Joly LM, Rosenberg A, et al. Immediate coronary angiography

in survivors of out-of-hospital cardiac arrest. *N Engl J Med.* 1997;**336**(23):1629–1633.

32. Radsel P, Knafelj R, Kocjancic S, Noc M. Angiographic characteristics of coronary disease and postresuscitation electrocardiograms in patients with aborted cardiac arrest outside a hospital. *Am J Cardiol.* 2011;**108**(5):634–638.

33. Nolan JP, Lyon RM, Sasson C, et al. Advances in the hospital management of patients following an out of hospital cardiac arrest. *Heart.* 2012;**98**(16):1201–1206.

34. Sideris G, Voicu S, Dillinger JG, et al. Value of post-resuscitation electrocardiogram in the diagnosis of acute myocardial infarction in out-of-hospital cardiac arrest patients. *Resuscitation.* 2011;**82**(9):1148–1153.

35. Busto R, Dietrich WD, Globus MY, Ginsberg MD. Postischemic moderate hypothermia inhibits CA1 hippocampal ischemic neuronal injury. *Neurosci Lett.* 1989;**101**(3):299–304.

36. Buchan A, Pulsinelli WA. Hypothermia but not the N-methyl-D-aspartate antagonist, MK-801, attenuates neuronal damage in gerbils subjected to transient global ischemia. *J Neurosci.* 1990;**10**(1):311–316.

37. Colbourne F, Grooms SY, Zukin RS, Buchan AM, Bennett MV. Hypothermia rescues hippocampal CA1 neurons and attenuates down-regulation of the AMPA receptor GluR2 subunit after forebrain ischemia. *Proc Natl Acad Sci USA.* 2003;**100**(5):2906–2910.

38. Chopp M, Chen H, Dereski MO, Garcia JH. Mild hypothermic intervention after graded ischemic stress in rats. *Stroke.* 1991;**22**(1):37–43.

39. Leonov Y, Sterz F, Safar P, et al. Mild cerebral hypothermia during and after cardiac arrest improves neurologic outcome in dogs. *J Cereb Blood Flow Metab.* 1990;**10**(1):57–70.

40. Sterz F, Safar P, Tisherman S, Radovsky A, Kuboyama K, Oku K. Mild hypothermic cardiopulmonary resuscitation improves outcome after prolonged cardiac arrest in dogs. *Crit Care Med.* 1991;**19**(3):379–389.

41. Nozari A, Safar P, Stezoski SW, et al. Mild hypothermia during prolonged cardiopulmonary cerebral resuscitation increases conscious survival in dogs. *Crit Care Med.* 2004;**32**(10):2110–2116.

42. Sick TJ, Xu G, Perez-Pinzon MA. Mild hypothermia improves recovery of cortical extracellular potassium ion activity and excitability after middle cerebral artery occlusion in the rat. *Stroke.* 1999;**30**(11):2416–2421; discussion 2422.

43. Erecinska M, Thoresen M, Silver IA. Effects of hypothermia on energy metabolism in Mammalian central nervous system. *J Cereb Blood Flow Metab.* 2003;**23**(5):513–530.

44. Busto R, Globus MY, Dietrich WD, Martinez E, Valdes I, Ginsberg MD. Effect of mild hypothermia on ischemia-induced release of neurotransmitters and free fatty acids in rat brain. *Stroke.* 1989;**20**(7):904–910.

45. Harada K, Maekawa T, Tsuruta R, et al. Hypothermia inhibits translocation of CaM kinase II and PKC-alpha, beta, gamma isoforms and fodrin proteolysis in rat brain synaptosome during ischemia-reperfusion. *J Neurosci Res.* 2002;**67**(5):664–669.

46. Globus MY, Alonso O, Dietrich WD, Busto R, Ginsberg MD. Glutamate release and free radical production following brain injury: Effects of posttraumatic hypothermia. *J Neurochem.* 1995;**65**(4):1704–1711.

47. Zheng Z, Yenari MA. Post-ischemic inflammation: Molecular mechanisms and therapeutic implications. *Neurol Res.* 2004;**26**(8):884–892.

48. Fukuda H, Tomimatsu T, Watanabe N, et al. Post-ischemic hypothermia blocks caspase-3 activation in the newborn rat brain after hypoxia-ischemia. *Brain Res.* 2001;**910**(1–2):187–191.

49. Hamann GF, Burggraf D, Martens HK, et al. Mild to moderate hypothermia prevents microvascular basal lamina antigen loss in experimental focal cerebral ischemia. *Stroke.* 2004;**35**(3):764–769.

50. Group. HaCAS. Mild therapeutic hypothermia to improve the neurologic outcome after cardiac arrest. *N Engl J Med.* 2002;**346**(8):549–556.

51. Bernard SA, Gray TW, Buist MD, et al. Treatment of comatose survivors of out-of-hospital cardiac arrest with induced hypothermia. *N Engl J Med.* 2002;**346**(8):557–563.

52. Peberdy MA, Callaway CW, Neumar RW, et al. Part 9: Post-cardiac arrest care: 2010 American Heart Association Guidelines for Cardiopulmonary Resuscitation and Emergency Cardiovascular Care. *Circulation.* 2010;**122**(18 Suppl 3): S768–786.

53. Nielsen N, Wetterslev J, Cronberg T, et al. Targeted temperature management at 33° C versus 36° C after cardiac arrest. *N Engl J Med.* 2013;**369**(23):2197–2206.

54. Castren M, Nordberg P, Svensson L, et al. Intra-arrest transnasal evaporative cooling: A randomized, prehospital, multicenter study (PRINCE: Pre-ROSC IntraNasal Cooling Effectiveness). *Circulation.* 2010;**122**(7):729–736.

55. Laurent I, Monchi M, Chiche JD, et al. Reversible myocardial dysfunction in survivors of out-of-hospital cardiac arrest. *J Am Coll Cardiol.* 2002;**40**(12):2110–2116.

56. Kilgannon JH, Roberts BW, Reihl LR, et al. Early arterial hypotension is common in the post-cardiac arrest syndrome and associated with increased in-hospital mortality. *Resuscitation.* 2008;**79**(3):410–416.

57. Spivey WH AN, Safar P, et al. Correlation of blood pressure with mortality and neurologic recovery in comatose postresuscitation patients (abstract). *Ann Emerg Med.* 1991;**20**:453.

58. Martin DR PD, Brown CG, et al. Relation between initial post-resuscitation systolic blood pressure and neurologic outcome following cardiac arrest (abstract). *Ann Emerg Med.* 1993;**22**:206.

59. Mullner M SF, Binder M, Hellwagner K, Meron G, Herkner H, Laggner A. Arterial blood pressure after human cardiac arrest and neurologic recovery. *Stroke.* 1996;**27**:59–62.

60. Beylin ME, Perman SM, Abella BS, et al. Higher mean arterial pressure with or without vasoactive agents is associated with increased survival and better neurological outcomes in comatose survivors of cardiac arrest. *Intensive Care Med.* 2013;**39**(11):1981–1988.

61. Nishizawa H, Kudoh I. Cerebral autoregulation is impaired in patients resuscitated after cardiac arrest. *Acta Anaesthesiol Scan.* 1996;**40**:1149–1153.

62. Sundgreen C LF, Herzog TM, Knudsen GM, Boesgaard S, Aldershvie J. Autoregulation of cerebral blood flow in patients resuscitated from cardiac arrest. *Stroke.* 2001;**32**:128–132.

63. Sterz F, Leonov Y, Safar P, Radovsky A, Tisherman S, Oku K. Hypertension with or without hemodilution after cardiac arrest in dogs. *Stroke.* 1990;**21**:1178–1184.

64. Safar P, Xiao F, Radovsky A, et al. Improved cerebral resuscitation from cardiac arrest in dogs with mild hypothermia plus blood flow promotion. *Stroke.* 1996. 1996;**27**:105–113.

65. Dellinger RP, Carlet JM, Masur H, et al. Surviving Sepsis Campaign guidelines for management of severe sepsis and septic shock. *Crit Care Med.* 2004;**32**(3):858–873.

66. Sunde K, Dunlop O, Rostrup M, Sandberg M, Sjoholm H, Jacobsen D. Determination of prognosis after cardiac arrest may be more difficult after introduction of therapeutic hypothermia. *Resuscitation.* 2006;**69**(1):29–32.

67. Gaieski DF, Band RA, Abella BS, et al. Early goal-directed hemodynamic optimization combined with therapeutic hypothermia in comatose survivors of out-of-hospital cardiac arrest. *Resuscitation.* 2009;**80**(4):418–424.

68. Tagami T, Hirata K, Takeshige T, et al. Implementation of the fifth link of the chain of survival concept for out-of-hospital cardiac arrest. *Circulation.* 2012;**126**(5):589–597.

69. Caplan LR. Cardiac arrest and other hypoxic ischemic insults. In Caplan LR, Hurst JW, Chimowitz M, eds. *Clinical Neurocardiology.* New York: Marcel Dekker; 1999, 1–34.

70. Adams JH, Brierley JB, Connor RC, Treip CS. The effects of systemic hypotension upon the human brain. Clinical and neuropathological observations in 11 cases. *Brain.* 1966;**89**(2):235–268.

71. Smith ML, Auer RN, Siesjo BK. The density and distribution of ischemic brain injury in the rat following 2–10 min of forebrain ischemia. *Acta Neuropathol.* 1984;**64**(4):319–332.

72. Takemoto O, Tomimoto H, Yanagihara T. Induction of c-fos and c-jun gene products and heat shock protein after brief and prolonged cerebral ischemia in gerbils. *Stroke.* 1995;**26**(9):1639–1648.

73. Bottiger BW, Schmitz B, Wiessner C, Vogel P, Hossmann KA. Neuronal stress response and neuronal cell damage after cardiocirculatory arrest in rats. *J Cereb Blood Flow Metab.* 1998;**18**(10):1077–1087.

74. Steriade M, Glenn LL. Neocortical and caudate projections of intralaminar thalamic neurons and their synaptic excitation from midbrain reticular core. *J Neurophysiol.* 1982;**48**(2):352–371.

75. Parvizi J, Damasio A. Consciousness and the brainstem. *Cognition.* 2001;**79**(1–2):135–160.

76. Berridge CW. Noradrenergic modulation of arousal. *Brain Res Rev.* 2008;**58**(1):1–17.

77. Vogt BA, Hof PR, Friedman DP, Sikes RW, Vogt LJ. Norepinephrinergic afferents and cytology of the macaque monkey midline, mediodorsal, and intralaminar thalamic nuclei. *Brain Struct Funct.* 2008;**212**(6):465–479.

78. Fisher CM. The neurological examination of the comatose patient. *Acta Neurol Scand.* 1969;**45**:Suppl 36:31–56.

79. Dooling EC, Richardson EP, Jr. Delayed encephalopathy after strangling. *Arch Neurol.* 1976;**33**(3):196–199.

80. Jennett B, Plum F. Persistent vegetative state after brain damage. A syndrome in search of a name. *Lancet.* 1972;**1**(7753):734–737.

81. Adams JH, Graham DI, Jennett B. The neuropathology of the vegetative state after an acute brain insult. *Brain.* 2000;**123**(Pt 7):1327–1338.

82. Dougherty JH, Jr., Rawlinson DG, Levy DE, Plum F. Hypoxic-ischemic brain injury and the vegetative state: Clinical and neuropathologic correlation. *Neurology.* 1981;**31**(8):991–997.

83. Jennett B, Plum F. Persistent vegetative state after brain damage. *RN.* 1972;**35**(10):ICU1–4.

84. Multi-Society Task Force on PVS. Medical aspects of the persistent vegetative state (2). *N Engl J Med.* 1994;**330**(22):1572–1579.

85. Giacino JT, Kalmar K. Diagnostic and prognostic guidelines for the vegetative and minimally conscious states. *Neuropsychol Rehabil.* 2005;**15**(3–4):166–174.

86. Laureys S, Celesia GG, Cohadon F, et al. Unresponsive wakefulness syndrome: A new name for the vegetative state or apallic syndrome. *BMC Med.* 2010;**8**:68.

87. Bardin JC, Fins JJ, Katz DI, et al. Dissociations between behavioural and functional magnetic resonance imaging-based evaluations of cognitive function after brain injury. *Brain.* 2011;**134**(3):769–782.

88. Monti MM, Vanhaudenhuyse A, Coleman MR, et al. Willful modulation of brain activity in disorders of consciousness. *N Engl J Med.* 2010;**362**(7):579–589.

89. Giacino JT, Ashwal S, Childs N, et al. The minimally conscious state: Definition and diagnostic criteria. *Neurology.* 2002;**58**(3):349–353.

90. Luaute J, Maucort-Boulch D, Tell L, et al. Long-term outcomes of chronic minimally conscious and vegetative states. *Neurology.* 2010;**75**(3):246–252.

91. Jennett B, Adams JH, Murray LS, Graham DI. Neuropathology in vegetative and severely disabled patients after head injury. *Neurology.* 2001;**56**(4):486–490.

92. Given CA, 2nd, Burdette JH, Elster AD, Williams DW, 3rd. Pseudo-subarachnoid hemorrhage: A potential imaging pitfall associated with diffuse cerebral edema. *AJNR Am J Neuroradiol.* 2003;**24**(2):254–256.

93. Phan TG, Wijdicks EF, Worrell GA, Fulgham JR. False subarachnoid hemorrhage in anoxic encephalopathy with brain swelling. *J Neuroimaging.* 2000;**10**(4):236–238.

94. Han BK, Towbin RB, De Courten-Myers G, McLaurin RL, Ball WS, Jr. Reversal sign on CT: Effect of anoxic/ischemic cerebral injury in children. *AJNR Am J Neuroradiol.* 1989;**10**(6):1191–1198.

95. Lovblad KO, Wetzel SG, Somon T, et al. Diffusion-weighted MRI in cortical ischaemia. *Neuroradiology.* 2004;**46**(3):175–182.

96. Siskas N, Lefkopoulos A, Ioannidis I, Charitandi A, Dimitriadis AS. Cortical laminar necrosis in brain infarcts: Serial MRI. *Neuroradiology.* 2003;**45**(5):283–288.

97. Komiyama M, Nakajima H, Nishikawa M, Yasui T. Serial MR observation of cortical laminar necrosis caused by brain infarction. *Neuroradiology.* 1998;**40**(12):771–777.

98. Wanko M, Garavelli M, Bernardi F, Niehaus TA, Frauenheim T, Elstner M. A global investigation of excited state surfaces within time-dependent density-functional response theory. *J Chem Phys.* 2004;**120**(4):1674–1692.

99. Mlynash M, Campbell DM, Leproust EM, et al. Temporal and spatial profile of brain diffusion-weighted MRI after cardiac arrest. *Stroke.* 2010;**41**(8):1665–1672.

100. Levy DE, Caronna JJ, Singer BH, Lapinski RH, Frydman H, Plum F. Predicting outcome from hypoxic-ischemic coma. *JAMA.* 1985;**253**(10):1420–1426.

101. Wijdicks EF, Hijdra A, Young GB, Bassetti CL, Wiebe S. Practice parameter: Prediction of outcome in comatose survivors after cardiopulmonary resuscitation (an evidence-based review): Report of the Quality Standards Subcommittee of

the American Academy of Neurology. *Neurology*. 2006;**67**(2):203–210.

102. De Georgia M, Raad M. Prognosis of coma after cardiac arrest in the era of hypothermia. *Continuum (Minneap Minn)*. 2012;**18**(3):515–531.

103. Randomized clinical study of thiopental loading in comatose survivors of cardiac arrest. Brain Resuscitation Clinical Trial I Study Group. *N Engl J Med*. 1986;**314**(7):397–403.

104. Zandbergen EG, Hijdra A, Koelman JH, et al. Prediction of poor outcome within the first 3 days of postanoxic coma. *Neurology*. 2006;**66**(1):62–68.

105. Al Thenayan E, Savard M, Sharpe M, Norton L, Young B. Predictors of poor neurologic outcome after induced mild hypothermia following cardiac arrest. *Neurology*. 2008;**71**(19):1535–1537.

106. Cronberg T, Rundgren M, Westhall E, et al. Neuron-specific enolase correlates with other prognostic markers after cardiac arrest. *Neurology*. 2011;**77**(7):623–630.

107. Rossetti AO, Oddo M, Logroscino G, Kaplan PW. Prognostication after cardiac arrest and hypothermia: A prospective study. *Ann Neurol*. 2010;**67**(3):301–307.

108. Samaniego EA, Mlynash M, Caulfield AF, Eyngorn I, Wijman CA. Sedation confounds outcome prediction in cardiac arrest survivors treated with hypothermia. *Neurocrit Care*. 2011;**15**(1):113–119.

109. Edgren E, Hedstrand U, Kelsey S, Sutton-Tyrrell K, Safar P. Assessment of neurological prognosis in comatose survivors of cardiac arrest. BRCT I Study Group. *Lancet*. 1994;**343**(8905):1055–1059.

110. Lee YC, Phan TG, Jolley DJ, Castley HC, Ingram DA, Reutens DC. Accuracy of clinical signs, SEP, and EEG in predicting outcome of hypoxic coma: A meta-analysis. *Neurology*. 2010;**74**(7):572–580.

111. Schefold JC, Storm C, Kruger A, Ploner CJ, Hasper D. The Glasgow Coma Score is a predictor of good outcome in cardiac arrest patients treated with therapeutic hypothermia. *Resuscitation*. 2009;**80**(6):658–661.

112. Young GB, Gilbert JJ, Zochodne DW. The significance of myoclonic status epilepticus in postanoxic coma. *Neurology*. 1990;**40**(12):1843–1848.

113. Lance JW, Adams RD. The syndrome of intention or action myoclonus as a sequel to hypoxic encephalopathy. *Brain*. 1963;**86**:111–136.

114. Celesia GG, Grigg MM, Ross E. Generalized status myoclonicus in acute anoxic and toxic-metabolic encephalopathies. *Arch Neurol*. 1988;**45**(7):781–784.

115. Young GB. The EEG in coma. *J Clin Neurophysiol*. 2000;**17**(5):473–485.

116. Scollo-Lavizzari G, Bassetti C. Prognostic value of EEG in post-anoxic coma after cardiac arrest. *Eur Neurol*. 1987;**26**(3):161–170.

117. Snyder BD, Hauser WA, Loewenson RB, Leppik IE, Ramirez-Lassepas M, Gumnit RJ. Neurologic prognosis after cardiopulmonary arrest: III. Seizure activity. *Neurology*. 1980;**30**(12):1292–1297.

118. Rossetti AO, Urbano LA, Delodder F, Kaplan PW, Oddo M. Prognostic value of continuous EEG monitoring during therapeutic hypothermia after cardiac arrest. *Crit Care*. 2010;**14**(5):R173.

119. Wijdicks EF, Parisi JE, Sharbrough FW. Prognostic value of myoclonus status in comatose survivors of cardiac arrest. *Ann Neurol*. 1994;**35**(2):239–243.

120. Rossetti AO, Logroscino G, Liaudet L, et al. Status epilepticus: An independent outcome predictor after cerebral anoxia. *Neurology*. 2007;**69**(3):255–260.

121. Rossetti AO, Oddo M, Liaudet L, Kaplan PW. Predictors of awakening from postanoxic status epilepticus after therapeutic hypothermia. *Neurology*. 2009;**72**(8):744–749.

122. Rundgren M, Westhall E, Cronberg T, Rosen I, Friberg H. Continuous amplitude-integrated electroencephalogram predicts outcome in hypothermia-treated cardiac arrest patients. *Crit Care Med*. 2010;**38**(9):1838–1844.

123. Abend NS, Topjian A, Ichord R, et al. Electroencephalographic monitoring during hypothermia after pediatric cardiac arrest. *Neurology*. 2009;**72**(22):1931–1940.

124. Legriel S, Bruneel F, Sediri H, et al. Early EEG monitoring for detecting postanoxic status epilepticus during therapeutic hypothermia: A pilot study. *Neurocrit Care*. 2009;**11**(3):338–344.

125. Robinson LR, Micklesen PJ, Tirschwell DL, Lew HL. Predictive value of somatosensory evoked potentials for awakening from coma. *Crit Care Med*. 2003;**31**(3):960–967.

126. Bouwes A, Binnekade JM, Zandstra DF, et al. Somatosensory evoked potentials during mild hypothermia after cardiopulmonary resuscitation. *Neurology*. 2009;**73**(18):1457–1461.

127. Leithner C, Ploner CJ, Hasper D, Storm C. Does hypothermia influence the predictive value of bilateral absent N20 after cardiac arrest? *Neurology*. 2010;**74**(12):965–969.

128. Kane NM, Butler SR, Simpson T. Coma outcome prediction using event-related potentials: P(3) and mismatch negativity. *Audiol Neurootol*. 2000; **5**(3–4):186–191.

129. Young GB, Wang JT, Connolly JF. Prognostic determination in anoxic–ischemic and traumatic encephalopathies. *J Clin Neurophysiol*. 2004;**21**(5):379–390.

130. Rundgren M, Karlsson T, Nielsen N, Cronberg T, Johnsson P, Friberg H. Neuron specific enolase and S-100B as predictors of outcome after cardiac arrest and induced hypothermia. *Resuscitation*. 2009;**80**(7):784–789.

131. Shinozaki K, Oda S, Sadahiro T, et al. Serum S-100B is superior to neuron-specific enolase as an early prognostic biomarker for neurological outcome following cardiopulmonary resuscitation. *Resuscitation*. 2009;**80**(8):870–875.

132. Oksanen T, Tiainen M, Skrifvars MB, et al. Predictive power of serum NSE and OHCA score regarding 6-month neurologic outcome after out-of-hospital ventricular fibrillation and therapeutic hypothermia. *Resuscitation*. 2009;**80**(2):165–170.

133. Fugate JE, Wijdicks EF, Mandrekar J, et al. Predictors of neurologic outcome in hypothermia after cardiac arrest. *Ann Neurol*. 2010;**68**(6):907–914.

134. Steffen IG, Hasper D, Ploner CJ, et al. Mild therapeutic hypothermia alters neuron specific enolase as an outcome predictor after resuscitation: 97 prospective hypothermia patients compared to 133 historical non-hypothermia patients. *Crit Care*. 2010;**14**(2):R69.

135. Randall J, Mortberg E, Provuncher GK, et al. Tau proteins in serum predict neurological outcome after hypoxic brain injury from cardiac arrest: Results of a pilot study. *Resuscitation*. 2013;**84**(3):351–356.

136. Torbey MT, Selim M, Knorr J, Bigelow C, Recht L. Quantitative analysis of the loss of distinction between gray and white matter in comatose patients

after cardiac arrest. *Stroke.* 2000;**31**(9):2163–2167.

137. Inamasu J, Miyatake S, Suzuki M, et al. Early CT signs in out-of-hospital cardiac arrest survivors: Temporal profile and prognostic significance. *Resuscitation.* 2010;**81**(5):534–538.

138. Wijdicks EF, Campeau NG, Miller GM. MR imaging in comatose survivors of cardiac resuscitation. *AJNR Am J Neuroradiol.* 2001;**22**(8):1561–1565.

139. Jarnum H, Knutsson L, Rundgren M, et al. Diffusion and perfusion MRI of the brain in comatose patients treated with mild hypothermia after cardiac arrest: A prospective observational study. *Resuscitation.* 2009;**80**(4):425–430.

140. Els T, Kassubek J, Kubalek R, Klisch J. Diffusion-weighted MRI during early global cerebral hypoxia: A predictor for clinical outcome? *Acta Neurol Scand.* 2004;**110**(6):361–367.

141. Wijman CA, Mlynash M, Caulfield AF, et al. Prognostic value of brain diffusion-weighted imaging after cardiac arrest. *Ann Neurol.* 2009;**65**(4):394–402.

142. Luyt CE, Galanaud D, Perlbarg V, et al. Diffusion tensor imaging to predict long-term outcome after cardiac arrest: A bicentric pilot study. *Anesthesiology.* 2012;**117**(6):1311–1321.

143. Bogousslavsky J, Regli F. Unilateral watershed cerebral infarcts. *Neurology.* 1986;**36**(3):373–377.

144. Chaves CJ, Silver B, Schlaug G, Dashe J, Caplan LR, Warach S. Diffusion- and perfusion-weighted MRI patterns in borderzone infarcts. *Stroke.* 2000;**31**(5):1090–1096.

145. Adams JH, Brierley JB, Connor RC, Treip CS. The effects of systemic hypotension upon the human brain. Clinical and neuropathological observations in 11 cases. *Brain.* 1966;**89**(2):235–268.

146. Howard R, Trend P, Russell RW. Clinical features of ischemia in cerebral arterial border zones after periods of reduced cerebral blood flow. *Arch Neurol.* 1987;**44**(9):934–940.

147. Brierley JB, Excell BJ. The effects of profound systemic hypotension upon the brain of M. rhesus: Physiological and pathological observations. *Brain.* 1966;**89**(2):269–298.

148. Rabinstein A, Resnick A. Hypoxic-ischemic brain damage. In Rabinstein A, Resnick A, eds. *Practical Neuroimaging in Stroke: A Case-Based Approach.* Philadelphia: Saunders Elsevier; 2009, 1–17.

149. Caplan LR, Hennerici M. Impaired clearance of emboli (washout) is an important link between hypoperfusion, embolism, and ischemic stroke. *Arch Neurol.* 1998;**55**(11):1475–1482.

150. Moustafa RR, Izquierdo-Garcia D, Jones PS, et al. Watershed infarcts in transient ischemic attack/minor stroke with > or = 50% carotid stenosis: Hemodynamic or embolic? *Stroke.* 2010;**41**(7):1410–1416.

151. Mohr JP. Neurological complications of cardiac valvular disease and cardiac surgery including systemic hypotension. In Vinken PJ, Bruyn GW, eds. *Handbook of Clinical Neurology, vol 38. Neurological Manifestations of Systemic Disease.* Amsterdam: North Holland Publishing; 1979, 143–171.

152. Balint R. Seelenlahmung des Schauens, optische Ataxie, raumliche Storung der Aufmerksamkeit. *Z Psychiatr Neurol* 1909;**25**:51–81.

153. Tyler HR. *Cerebral Disturbance of Vision in Neuro-Ophthalmology*, Vol **4**. St. Louis: Mosby, 1968.

154. Hecaen H, De Ajuriaguerra J. Balint's syndrome (psychic paralysis of visual fixation) and its minor forms. *Brain.* 1954;**77**(3):373–400.

155. Benson DF, Davis RJ, Snyder BD. Posterior cortical atrophy. *Arch Neurol.* 1988;**45**(7):789–793.

156. Caronna JJ, Finklestein S. Neurological syndromes after cardiac arrest. *Stroke.* 1978;**9**(5):517–520.

157. Volpe BT, Hirst W. The characterization of an amnesic syndrome following hypoxic ischemic injury. *Arch Neurol.* 1983;**40**(7):436–440.

158. Cummings JL, Tomiyasu U, Read S, Benson DF. Amnesia with hippocampal lesions after cardiopulmonary arrest. *Neurology.* 1984;**34**(5):679–681.

159. Petito CK, Feldmann E, Pulsinelli WA, Plum F. Delayed hippocampal damage in humans following cardiorespiratory arrest. *Neurology.* 1987;**37**(8):1281–1286.

160. Zulch K. On the circulatory disturbances in the borderline zones of the cerebral and spinal vessels Paper presented at: *Proceedings of the Second International Congress on Neuropathology* 1955; Amsterdam.

161. Romanul F, Abramowicz A. Changes in brain and pial vessels in arterial border zones. *Arch Neurol* 1974;**11**:40–65.

162. Sage JI, Van Uitert RL. Man-in-the-barrel syndrome. *Neurology.* 1986;**36**(8):1102–1103.

163. Silver JR, Buxton PH. Spinal stroke. *Brain.* 1974;**97**(3):539–550.

164. Karch DL, Logan J, McDaniel D, Parks S, Pate lN. Surveillance for violent deaths – National Violent Death Reporting System, 16 States, 2009. *MMWR Surveill Summ.* 2012;**61**:1–43.

165. Clement R, Redpath M, Sauvageau A. Mechanism of death in hanging: A historical review of the evolution of pathophysiological hypotheses. *J Forensic Sci.*2010;**55**(5):1268–1271.

166. Miyamoto O, Auer RN. Hypoxia, hyperoxia, ischemia, and brain necrosis. *Neurology.* 2000;**54**(2):362–371.

167. Ames A, 3rd, Nesbett FB. Pathophysiology of ischemic cell death: I. Time of onset of irreversible damage; importance of the different components of the ischemic insult. *Stroke.* 1983;**14**(2):219–226.

168. Matsuyama T, Okuchi K, Seki T, Murao Y. Prognostic factors in hanging injuries. *Am J Emerg Med.* 2004;**22**(3):207–210.

169. Hanna SJ. A study of 13 cases of near-hanging presenting to an accident and emergency department. *Injury.* 2004;**35**(3):253–256.

170. Vander Krol L, Wolfe R. The emergency department management of near-hanging victims. *J Emerg Med.* 1994;**12**(3):285–292.

171. Salim A, Martin M, Sangthong B, Brown C, Rhee P, Demetriades D. Near-hanging injuries: A 10-year experience. *Injury.* 2006;**37**(5):435–439.

172. Hald JK, Brunberg JA, Dublin AB, Wootton-Gorges SL. Delayed diffusion-weighted MR abnormality in a patient with an extensive acute cerebral hypoxic injury. *Acta Radiol.* 2003;**44**(3):343–346.

173. Borgquist O, Friberg H. Therapeutic hypothermia for comatose survivors after near-hanging-a retrospective analysis. *Resuscitation.* 2009;**80**(2):210–212.

174. Legriel S, Bouyon A, Nekhili N, et al. Therapeutic hypothermia for coma after cardiorespiratory arrest caused by hanging. *Resuscitation.* 2005;**67**(1):143–144.

175. Baldursdottir S, Sigvaldason K, Karason S, Valsson F, Sigurdsson GH. Induced hypothermia in comatose survivors of asphyxia: A case series of 14 consecutive cases. *Acta Anaesthesiol Scand.* 2010;**54**(7):821–826.

176. Centers for Disease Control and Prevention. Available from http://www.cdc.gov/injury/wisqars. Accessed (cited 2014, June 16).

177. DeNicola LK, Falk JL, Swanson ME, Gayle MO, Kissoon N. Submersion injuries in children and adults. *Crit Care Clin.* 1997;**13**(3):477–502.

178. van Beeck EF, Branche CM, Szpilman D, Modell JH, Bierens JJ. A new definition of drowning: Towards documentation and prevention of a global public health problem. *Bull World Health Organ.* 2005;**83**(11):853–856.

179. Orlowski JP, Abulleil MM, Phillips JM. The hemodynamic and cardiovascular effects of near-drowning in hypotonic, isotonic, or hypertonic solutions. *Ann Emerg Med.* 1989;**18**(10):1044–1049.

180. Tipton MJ, Golden FS. A proposed decision-making guide for the search, rescue and resuscitation of submersion (head under) victims based on expert opinion. *Resuscitation.* 2011;**82**(7):819–824.

181. Handley AJ. Drowning. *BMJ.* 2014;**348**:g1734.

182. Vanden Hoek TL, Morrison LJ, Shuster M, et al. Part 12: Cardiac arrest in special situations: 2010 American Heart Association Guidelines for Cardiopulmonary Resuscitation and Emergency Cardiovascular Care. *Circulation.* 2010;**122**(18 Suppl 3):S829–861.

183. Szpilman D. Near-drowning and drowning classification: A proposal to stratify mortality based on the analysis of 1,831 cases. *Chest.* 1997;**112**(3):660–665.

184. Manolios N, Mackie I. Drowning and near-drowning on Australian beaches patrolled by life-savers: A 10-year study, 1973–1983. *Med J Aust.* 1988;**148**(4):165–167, 170–161.

185. Chochinov AH, Baydock BM, Bristow GK, Giesbrecht GG. Recovery of a 62-year-old man from prolonged cold water submersion. *Ann Emerg Med.* 1998;**31**(1):127–131.

186. Siebke H, Rod T, Breivik H, Link B. Survival after 40 minutes; submersion without cerebral sequelae. *Lancet.* 1975;**1**(7919):1275–1277.

187. Guenther U, Varelmann D, Putensen C, Wrigge H. Extended therapeutic hypothermia for several days during extracorporeal membrane-oxygenation after drowning and cardiac arrest. Two cases of survival with no neurological sequelae. *Resuscitation.* 2009;**80**(3):379–381.

188. Kilgannon JH, Jones AE, Parrillo JE, et al. Relationship between supranormal oxygen tension and outcome after resuscitation from cardiac arrest. *Circulation.* 2011;**123**(23):2717–2722.

189. Christophe C, Fonteyne C, Ziereisen F, et al. Value of MR imaging of the brain in children with hypoxic coma. *AJNR Am J Neuroradiol.* 2002;**23**(4):716–723.

190. Topjian AA, Berg RA, Bierens JJ, et al. Brain resuscitation in the drowning victim. *Neurocrit Care.* 2012;**17**(3):441–467.

191. Eggink WF, Bruining HA. Respiratory distress syndrome caused by near- or secondary drowning and treatment by positive end-expiratory pressure ventilation. *Neth J Med.* 1977;**20**(4–5):162–167.

192. Weaver LK. Carbon monoxide poisoning. *Crit Care Clin.* 1999;**15**(2):297–317.

193. Hardy KR, Thom SR. Pathophysiology and treatment of carbon monoxide poisoning. *J Toxicol Clin Toxicol.* 1994;**32**(6):613–629.

194. Miro O, Casademont J, Barrientos A, Urbano-Marquez A, Cardellach F. Mitochondrial cytochrome c oxidase inhibition during acute carbon monoxide poisoning. *Pharmacol Toxicol.* 1998;**82**(4):199–202.

195. Thom SR. Carbon monoxide-mediated brain lipid peroxidation in the rat. *J Appl Physiol.* 1990;**68**(3):997–1003.

196. Kalay N, Ozdogru I, Cetinkaya Y, et al. Cardiovascular effects of carbon monoxide poisoning. *Am J Cardiol.* 2007;**99**(3):322–324.

197. Lou M, Jing CH, Selim MH, Caplan LR, Ding MP. Delayed substantia nigra damage and leukoencephalopathy after hypoxic-ischemic injury. *J Neurol Sci.* 2009;**277**(1–2):147–149.

198. Scott BL, Jankovic J. Delayed-onset progressive movement disorders after static brain lesions. *Neurology.* 1996;**46**(1):68–74.

199. Plum F, Posner JB, Hain RF. Delayed neurological deterioration after anoxia. *Arch Intern Med.* 1962;**110**:18–25.

200. Weinberger LM, Schmidley JW, Schafer IA, Raghavan S. Delayed postanoxic demyelination and arylsulfatase-A pseudodeficiency. *Neurology.* 1994;**44**(1):152–154.

201. Gottfried JA, Mayer SA, Shungu DC, Chang Y, Duyn JH. Delayed posthypoxic demyelination. Association with arylsulfatase A deficiency and lactic acidosis on proton MR spectroscopy. *Neurology.* 1997;**49**(5):1400–1404.

202. Kriegstein AR, Shungu DC, Millar WS, et al. Leukoencephalopathy and raised brain lactate from heroin vapor inhalation ("chasing the dragon"). *Neurology.* 1999;**53**(8):1765–1773.

203. Parkinson RB, Hopkins RO, Cleavinger HB, et al. White matter hyperintensities and neuropsychological outcome following carbon monoxide poisoning. *Neurology.* 2002;**58**(10):1525–1532.

204. Gale SD, Hopkins RO, Weaver LK, Bigler ED, Booth EJ, Blatter DD. MRI, quantitative MRI, SPECT, and neuropsychological findings following carbon monoxide poisoning. *Brain Inj.* 1999;**13**(4):229–243.

205. Min SK. A brain syndrome associated with delayed neuropsychiatric sequelae following acute carbon monoxide intoxication. *Acta Psychiatr Scand.* 1986;**73**(1):80–86.

206. Ferrier D, Wallace CJ, Fletcher WA, Fong TC. Magnetic resonance features in carbon monoxide poisoning. *Can Assoc Radiol J.* 1994;**45**(6):466–468.

207. Tuchman RF, Moser FG, Moshe SL. Carbon monoxide poisoning: Bilateral lesions in the thalamus on MR imaging of the brain. *Pediatr Radiol.* 1990;**20**(6):478–479.

208. Kawanami T, Kato T, Kurita K, Sasaki H. The pallidoreticular pattern of brain damage on MRI in a patient with carbon monoxide poisoning. *J Neurol Neurosurg Psychiatry.* 1998;**64**(2):282.

209. Mascalchi M, Petruzzi P, Zampa V. MRI of cerebellar white matter damage due to carbon monoxide poisoning: Case report. *Neuroradiology.* 1996;**38** Suppl 1:S73–S74.

210. O'Donnell P, Buxton PJ, Pitkin A, Jarvis LJ. The magnetic resonance imaging appearances of the brain in acute carbon monoxide poisoning. *Clin Radiol.* 2000;**55**(4):273–280.

211. Vieregge P, Klostermann W, Blumm RG, Borgis KJ. Carbon monoxide

poisoning: Clinical, neurophysiological, and brain imaging observations in acute disease and follow-up. *J Neurol.* 1989;**236**(8):478–481.

212. Pracyk JB, Stolp BW, Fife CE, Gray L, Piantadosi CA. Brain computerized tomography after hyperbaric oxygen therapy for carbon monoxide poisoning. *Undersea Hyperb Med.* 1995;**22**(1):1–7.

213. Porter SS, Hopkins RO, Weaver LK, Bigler ED, Blatter DD. Corpus callosum atrophy and neuropsychological outcome following carbon monoxide poisoning. *Arch Clin Neuropsychol.* 2002;**17**(2):195–204.

214. Kesler SR, Hopkins RO, Blatter DD, Edge-Booth H, Bigler ED. Verbal memory deficits associated with fornix atrophy in carbon monoxide poisoning. *J Int Neuropsychol Soc.* 2001;**7**(5):640–646.

215. Prockop LD, Chichkova RI. Carbon monoxide intoxication: An updated review. *J Neurol Sci.* 2007;**262**(1–2):122–130.

216. Stoller KP. Hyperbaric oxygen and carbon monoxide poisoning: A critical review. *Neurol Res.* 2007;**29**(2):146–155.

217. Sunde K, Pytte M, Jacobsen D, et al. Implementation of a standardised treatment protocol for post resuscitation care after out-of-hospital cardiac arrest. *Resuscitation.* 2007;**73**(1):29–39.

218. Rittenberger JC, Guyette FX, Tisherman SA, DeVita MA, Alvarez RJ, Callaway CW. Outcomes of a hospital-wide plan to improve care of comatose survivors of cardiac arrest. *Resuscitation.* 2008;**79**(2):198–204.

219. Oba Y, Salzman GA. Ventilation with lower tidal volumes as compared with traditional tidal volumes for acute lung injury. *N Engl J Med.* 2000;**343**(11):813; author reply 813–814.

220. Kress JP, Pohlman AS, O'Connor MF, Hall JB. Daily interruption of sedative infusions in critically ill patients undergoing mechanical ventilation. *N Engl J Med.* 2000;**342**(20):1471–1477.

221. Girard TD, Kress JP, Fuchs BD, et al. Efficacy and safety of a paired sedation and ventilator weaning protocol for mechanically ventilated patients in intensive care (Awakening and Breathing Controlled trial): A randomised controlled trial. *Lancet.* 2008;**371**(9607):126–134.

222. Barr J, Fraser GL, Puntillo K, et al. Clinical practice guidelines for the management of pain, agitation, and delirium in adult patients in the intensive care unit. *Crit Care Med.* 2013;**41**(1):263–306.

223. Ruokonen E, Parviainen I, Jakob SM, et al. Dexmedetomidine versus propofol/midazolam for long-term sedation during mechanical ventilation. *Intensive Care Med.* 2009;**35**(2):282–290.

224. Rovlias A, Kotsou S. The influence of hyperglycemia on neurological outcome in patients with severe head injury. *Neurosurgery.* 2000;**46**(2):335–342; discussion 342–333.

225. Charpentier C, Audibert G, Guillemin F, et al. Multivariate analysis of predictors of cerebral vasospasm occurrence after aneurysmal subarachnoid hemorrhage. *Stroke.* 1999;**30**(7):1402–1408.

226. Badjatia N, Topcuoglu MA, Buonanno FS, et al. Relationship between hyperglycemia and symptomatic vasospasm after subarachnoid hemorrhage. *Crit Care Med.* 2005;**33**(7):1603–1609.

227. Dorhout Mees SM, van Dijk GW, Algra A, Kempink DR, Rinkel GJ. Glucose levels and outcome after subarachnoid hemorrhage. *Neurology.* 2003;**61**(8):1132–1133.

228. van den Berghe G, Wouters P, Weekers F, et al. Intensive insulin therapy in critically ill patients. *N Engl J Med.* 2001;**345**(19):1359–1367.

229. Van den Berghe G, Schoonheydt K, Becx P, Bruyninckx F, Wouters PJ. Insulin therapy protects the central and peripheral nervous system of intensive care patients. *Neurology.* 2005;**64**(8):1348–1353.

230. Vespa P, Boonyaputthikul R, McArthur DL, et al. Intensive insulin therapy reduces microdialysis glucose values without altering glucose utilization or improving the lactate/pyruvate ratio after traumatic brain injury. *Crit Care Med.* 2006;**34**(3):850–856.

231. Wiener RS, Wiener DC, Larson RJ. Benefits and risks of tight glucose control in critically ill adults: A meta-analysis. *JAMA.* 2008;**300**(8):933–944.

232. Oddo M, Schmidt JM, Carrera E, et al. Impact of tight glycemic control on cerebral glucose metabolism after severe brain injury: A microdialysis study. *Crit Care Med.* 2008;**36**(12):3233–3238.

233. Zetterling M, Hillered L, Enblad P, Karlsson T, Ronne-Engstrom E. Relation between brain interstitial and systemic glucose concentrations after subarachnoid hemorrhage. *J Neurosurg.* 2011;**115**(1):66–74.

234. Hajat C, Hajat S, Sharma P. Effects of poststroke pyrexia on stroke outcome: A meta-analysis of studies in patients. *Stroke.* 2000;**31**(2):410–414.

235. Guyatt GH, Akl EA, Crowther M, Gutterman DD, Schuunemann HJ. Executive summary: Antithrombotic Therapy and Prevention of Thrombosis, 9th ed: American College of Chest Physicians Evidence-Based Clinical Practice Guidelines. *Chest.* 2012;**141**(2 Suppl):7S–47S.

236. Claassen J, Silbergleit R, Weingart SD, Smith WS. Emergency neurological life support: Status epilepticus. *Neurocrit Care.* 2012;**17** Suppl 1:S73–S78.

237. Frucht S, Fahn S. The clinical spectrum of posthypoxic myoclonus. *Mov Disord.* 2000;**15** Suppl 1:2–7.

238. Wheless JW, Sankar R. Treatment strategies for myoclonic seizures and epilepsy syndromes with myoclonic seizures. *Epilepsia.* 2003;**44** Suppl 11:27–37.

239. Dijk JM, Tijssen MA. Management of patients with myoclonus: Available therapies and the need for an evidence-based approach. *Lancet Neurol.* 2010;**9**(10):1028–1036.

240. Muslu B, Kiklci O, Horasani E, Dikmen B. Dramatic effect of leveracetam on posthypoxic myoclonus: Difficult weaning from mechanical ventilation. *Clin Neuropharmacol.* 2009;**32**(4):236.

241. Goldstein LB. Common drugs may influence motor recovery after stroke. The Sygen In Acute Stroke Study Investigators. *Neurology.* 1995;**45**(5):865–871.

242. Meythaler JM, Brunner RC, Johnson A, Novack TA. Amantadine to improve neurorecovery in traumatic brain injury-associated diffuse axonal injury: A pilot double-blind randomized trial. *J Head Trauma Rehabil.* 2002;**17**(4):300–313.

243. Giacino JT, Whyte J, Bagiella E, et al. Placebo-controlled trial of amantadine for severe traumatic brain injury. *N Engl J Med.* 2012;**366**(9):819–826.

244. Pariente J, Loubinoux I, Carel C, et al. Fluoxetine modulates motor performance and cerebral activation of patients recovering from stroke. *Ann Neurol.* 2001;**50**(6):718–729.

245. Clauss RP, van der Merwe CE, Nel HW. Arousal from a semi-comatose state on zolpidem. *S Afr Med J.* 2001;**91**(10):788–789.

246. Brefel-Courbon C, Payoux P, Ory F, et al. Clinical and imaging evidence of zolpidem effect in hypoxic encephalopathy. *Ann Neurol.* 2007;**62**(1):102–105.

247. Schiff ND, Posner JB. Another "Awakenings". *Ann Neurol.* 2007;**62**(1):5–7.

248. Schiff ND, Fins JJ. Deep brain stimulation and cognition: Moving from animal to patient. *Curr Opin Neurol.* 2007;**20**(6):638–642.

249. Schiff ND. Central thalamic deep-brain stimulation in the severely injured brain: Rationale and proposed mechanisms of action. *Ann N Y Acad Sci.* 2009;**1157**:101–116.

250. Heidenreich PA, Albert NM, Allen LA, et al. Forecasting the impact of heart failure in the United States: A policy statement from the American Heart Association. *Circ Heart Fail.* 2013;**6**(3):606–619.

251. Choi BR, Kim JS, Yang YJ, et al. Factors associated with decreased cerebral blood flow in congestive heart failure secondary to idiopathic dilated cardiomyopathy. *Am J Cardiol.* 2006;**97**(9):1365–1369.

252. Caplan LR. Cardiac encephalopathy and congestive heart failure: A hypothesis about the relationship. *Neurology.* 2006;**66**(1):99–101.

253. Caplan LR. Encephalopathies and neurological effects of drugs used in cardiac patients. In Caplan LR, Hurst JW, Chimowitz MI, eds. *Clinical Neurocardiology.* New York: Marcel Dekker; 1999, 186–225.

254. Cohn JN, Levine TB, Olivari MT, et al. Plasma norepinephrine as a guide to prognosis in patients with chronic congestive heart failure. *N Engl J Med.* 1984;**311**(13):819–823.

255. Woo MA, Kumar R, Macey PM, Fonarow GC, Harper RM. Brain injury in autonomic, emotional, and cognitive regulatory areas in patients with heart failure. *J Card Fail.* 2009;**15**(3):214–223.

256. Garcia CA, Tweedy JR, Blass JP. Underdiagnosis of cognitive impairment in a rehabilitation setting. *J Am Geriatr Soc.* 1984;**32**(5):339–342.

257. Schall RR, Petrucci RJ, Brozena SC, Cavarocchi NC, Jessup M. Cognitive function in patients with symptomatic dilated cardiomyopathy before and after cardiac transplantation. *J Am Coll Cardiol.* 1989;**14**(7):1666–1672.

258. Bornstein RA, Starling RC, Myerowitz PD, Haas GJ. Neuropsychological function in patients with end-stage heart failure before and after cardiac transplantation. *Acta Neurol Scand.* 1995;**91**(4):260–265.

259. Friedmann E, Thomas SA, Liu F, Morton PG, Chapa D, Gottlieb SS. Relationship of depression, anxiety, and social isolation to chronic heart failure outpatient mortality. *Am Heart J.* 2006;**152**(5):940–948.

260. Jiang W, Alexander J, Christopher E, et al. Relationship of depression to increased risk of mortality and rehospitalization in patients with congestive heart failure. *Arch Intern Med.* 2001;**161**(15):1849–1856.

261. Koenig HG. Depression in hospitalized older patients with congestive heart failure. *Gen Hosp Psychiatry.* 1998;**20**(1):29–43.

262. Havranek EP, Ware MG, Lowes BD. Prevalence of depression in congestive heart failure. *Am J Cardiol.* 1999;**84**(3):348–350.

263. Freedland KE, Rich MW, Skala JA, Carney RM, Davila-Roman VG, Jaffe AS. Prevalence of depression in hospitalized patients with congestive heart failure. *Psychosom Med.* 2003;**65**(1):119–128.

264. Zuccala G, Cattel C, Manes-Gravina E, Di Niro MG, Cocchi A, Bernabei R. Left ventricular dysfunction: A clue to cognitive impairment in older patients with heart failure. *J Neurol Neurosurg Psychiatry.* 1997;**63**(4):509–512.

265. Kumar R, Woo MA, Macey PM, Fonarow GC, Hamilton MA, Harper RM. Brain axonal and myelin evaluation in heart failure. *J Neurol Sci.* 2011;**307**(1–2):106–113.

266. Vogels RL, van der Flier WM, van Harten B, et al. Brain magnetic resonance imaging abnormalities in patients with heart failure. *Eur J Heart Fail.* 2007;**9**(10):1003–1009.

267. Siachos T, Vanbakel A, Feldman DS, Uber W, Simpson KN, Pereira NL. Silent strokes in patients with heart failure. *J Card Fail.* 2005;**11**(7):485–489.

268. Russo C, Jin Z, Homma S, et al. Subclinical left ventricular dysfunction and silent cerebrovascular disease: The Cardiovascular Abnormalities and Brain Lesions (CABL) Study. *Circulation.* 2013;**128**(10):1105–1111.

269. Fazekas F, Kleinert R, Offenbacher H, et al. Pathologic correlates of incidental MRI white matter signal hyperintensities. *Neurology.* 1993;**43**(9):1683–1689.

Non-atherosclerotic vasculopathies

Louis R Caplan and José Biller

Many different non-atherosclerotic vascular diseases cause brain ischemia. Some of these conditions also cause ocular ischemia and intracranial hemorrhage. Some have been well characterized, whereas information about pathogenesis and clinical features for others is meager. Herein, we discuss the most frequent and important conditions. Some are also discussed in other chapters. The topic is so diverse that we can only include brief relatively concise descriptions that contain the most important information along with reference citations. *Uncommon Causes of Stroke*, third edition, offers much more detailed descriptions of many of these conditions.[1]

Arterial dissections[1–56]

Dissection of extracranial arteries was once considered rare. Reports of Fisher, Ojemann, and colleagues in the 1970s clarified the clinical and radiological features in patients with dissection of the internal carotid artery (ICA).[2,3] Increased awareness of the clinical symptoms and signs, and the advent of safe and rapid non-invasive vascular imaging has led to more frequent diagnosis of arterial dissections of brain-supplying arteries.[4–6] The extracranial ICA is the most commonly affected artery and is usually involved in its pharyngeal and distal extracranial segments well above the ICA origin. This location is unusual for atherosclerosis, which almost invariably affects the internal carotid origin or the carotid siphon. Dissections of the extracranial vertebral artery (ECVA) affect the vessel in its distal segment between its emergence from the vertebral column and its dural penetration, or in the first segment of the artery above the vertebral artery (VA) origin but before entrance into the transverse foramina.[5–9] The pharyngeal ICA and the first and third segments of the ECVA are more mobile and less firmly anchored than the origins and the intracranial penetration sites of these arteries. Dissections often involve loops and redundant portions of the extracranial arteries.[10]

Most dissections involve some trauma, stretch, or mechanical stress. Trauma may be severe but can be trivial (e.g., twisting the neck to avoid a falling tree branch, lunging for a Ping-Pong ball, or turning the neck abruptly while backing up a car or skiing). Many examples of so-called spontaneous dissections are triggered by minor trauma that is forgotten or deemed inconsequential by the patient. Congenital or acquired abnormalities of the connective tissue elements in the media or elastica of the arteries and edema of the arterial wall can promote dissection. Marfan's syndrome, cystic medial necrosis, fibromuscular dysplasia (FMD), Ehlers–Danlos type 4 syndrome, Loeys–Dietz syndrome, osteogenesis imperfecta type 1, and migraine are disorders found more often than expected in patients with arterial dissections.[5,6] Table 12.1 lists the situations and conditions that have been associated with arterial dissections. Skeletal, ocular, and skin abnormalities indicative of abnormal connective tissue are found in many patients with cervical artery dissections.[11] Ultrastructural connective tissue abnormalities of collagen and extracellular matrix are sometimes found in the skin of patients with extracranial arterial dissections.[12,13] Plasma levels of matrix metalloproteinase-2 (MMP-2) are higher in patients with cervical artery dissections than controls especially in patients with recurrent dissections.[14]

A tear within the arterial wall leads to bleeding. Blood often dissects within the media along the longitudinal course of the artery. Dissection in the plane between the media and adventitia sometimes causes aneurysmal out-pouching of the artery. Dissections also produce an intimal tear, allowing the intramural hematoma to reenter the lumen (Figure 12.1). The expanded arterial wall may encroach on the lumen. Thrombus is often present within the lumen as a result of reentry of the intramural hematoma or because of stasis of blood flow caused by luminal compromise. The intramural expansion probably also stimulates the endothelium to release factors promoting thrombosis. The luminal clot is usually only loosely adherent to the intima and can readily embolize distally. In the weeks and months after dissection, the intramural blood is absorbed, and the lumen usually returns to its normal size. Aneurysmal pouches may remain as a residue of the healed lesion.

Carotid artery dissections in the neck[1–23,25]

Often in carotid artery dissection, the most impressive feature is pain. Ipsilateral throbbing headache and sharp pain locally in the neck, jaw, pharynx, or face are often noted, separating dissection from ordinary atherosclerotic occlusion.[4,5,15–18] The sympathetic fibers traveling along the wall of the ICA are usually disturbed, leading to an ipsilateral partial Horner's syndrome characterized by ptosis and miosis. Facial sweat function is preserved because the sympathetic innervation of the sweat glands travels along the external carotid artery (ECA).

Caplan's Stroke: A Clinical Approach, 5th Edition, ed. Louis R Caplan. Published by Cambridge University Press. © Cambridge University Press, 2016.

Table 12.1 Disorders associated with cervical artery dissection

Major and minor cervical trauma

Various sporting and recreational activities
　　Football
　　Rugby
　　Basketball
　　Ice hockey
　　Softball
　　Tennis
　　Golf
　　Skiing
　　Cycling
　　Swimming
　　Calisthenics
　　Archery
　　Yoga
　　Gymnastics
　　Driving
　　Martial arts (karate, judo, tae kwon do)
　　Horse riding
　　Diving
　　Roller coaster
　　Bungee jumping
　　Others

Arterial hypertension

Oral contraceptives

Migraine

Fibromuscular dysplasia

Ultrastructural connective tissue abnormalities

Vascular Ehlers–Danlos type IV

Pseudoxanthoma elasticum

Marfan's syndrome

Turner's syndrome

Williams' syndrome

Arterial tortuosity syndrome

Hereditary hemochromatosis

Osteogenesis imperfecta type I

α_1-antitrypsin deficiency

Homocystinuria

677T genotype *MTHFR*

Hyperhomocysteinemia

Cystic medial necrosis of intracranial vessels

Styloid process length

ICAM-1 E4690 K gene polymorphism

Autosomal dominant polycystic kidney disease

Infections

Moyamoya disease

Table 12.1 (cont.)

Lentiginosis

Coils, kinks, loops (especially if bilateral)

Adapted from Giossi A, Ritelli M, Costa P, et al: Connective tissue anomalies in patients with spontaneous cervical artery dissection. *Neurology* 2014;83:2032–2037.

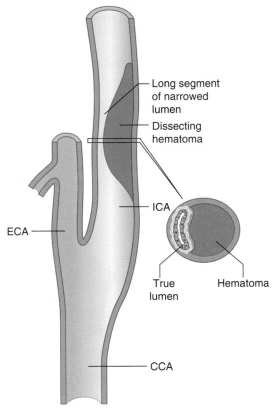

Figure 12.1 Cartoon showing dissection of the internal carotid artery. The inset is a cross-section view showing the hematoma and the luminal compromise. CCA, common carotid artery; ECA, external carotid artery; ICA, internal carotid artery.

Transient ischemic attacks (TIAs) are common and may involve the ipsilateral eye and brain. The spells often occur in rapid succession over hours or a few days leading Fisher to coin the term *carotid allegro*.[2] Some patients with ICA dissection have visual scintillations and bright sparkles resembling migraine, even though many have had no personal or family history of migraine. Some patients hear a pulsatile noise in the head or ear. TIAs are probably caused by luminal compromise with distal hypoperfusion, but most patients with severe strokes have evidence of embolization of clot to the middle cerebral artery (MCA) from thrombus at the site of the dissection. When the ICA dissection extends to the carotid siphon, ischemic optic neuropathy can develop as a result of decreased perfusion of arteries supplying the optic nerve.[19] If a stroke develops, it usually occurs soon after the ICA dissection but may occur during the days and weeks after the event. Late stroke is rare but has been reported after traumatic ICA

dissection.[20] At times, dissections cause sequential symptoms during days to weeks. Pain may first develop in the neck and persist for days and subside. The pain may recur days or even weeks later and be accompanied by TIAs or strokes. Undoubtedly, the initial tear extended and more intramural bleeding developed when the symptoms worsened. At times, both carotid arteries and even the VAs are dissected at the same time.

Ultrasound testing can suggest the presence of a dissection. B-mode ultrasound can show tapering of the ICA lumen beginning well above the ICA origin, an irregular membrane crossing the lumen, and even demonstration of true and false lumens.[21,22] Continuous wave (CW) Doppler can show a typical pattern characterized by a high-amplitude signal with markedly reduced systolic Doppler frequencies and alternating flow directions over the region of luminal narrowing.[23] This Doppler signal probably results from abnormal vessel wall pulsations and some bidirectional movement of the blood column. Duplex scans of the VAs in the neck can also suggest dissection.[24] Typical findings are increased arterial diameter, decreased pulsatility, intravascular abnormal echoes, and hemodynamic evidence of decreased flow. Color Doppler flow imaging can also show the regions of dissection within the neck. In patients with extracranial ICA dissections, transcranial Doppler (TCD) may show diminished intracranial velocities in the ICA siphon and MCA. When this occurs in young patients without risk factors for atherosclerosis or embolism with normal ICA bifurcations in the neck, the diagnosis of dissection is likely.

Diagnosis of arterial dissection has traditionally been made by standard catheter cerebral angiography. Figure 12.2 is a cartoon that illustrates various arteriographic features of carotid dissections. Figure 12.3 is a montage of angiograms in patients with extracranial ICA dissections. The most common angiographic finding is a string sign (see Figure 12.3A), consisting of a long, narrow column of contrast material that begins distal to the carotid bifurcation and can extend to the base of the skull.[2,3] There may also be total occlusion of the ICA. This occlusion differs from the typical atherosclerotic occlusion; ICA occlusions caused by dissection usually begin more than 2 cm distal to the origin of the ICA, spare the carotid sinus, and have a gradually tapering segment that ends in the occlusion. There may also be localized aneurysmal sacs or outpouchings both proximal and distal along a narrowed, normal, or unusually dilatated portion of the artery (see Figure 12.3B and C). Computed tomography (CT) and magnetic resonance imaging (MRI) taken as axial cross-sections through the area of dissection can show the intramural bleeding and mural expansion and can confirm the diagnosis of dissection. Figure 12.4 is an MRI cross-section that shows a bilateral traumatic ICA dissection. Figure 7.9C also shows a fat-saturated MRI examination of a carotid artery dissection.

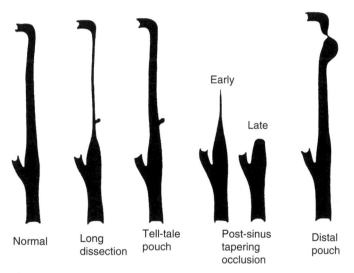

Figure 12.2 Drawings of various abnormal carotid arteriograms in patients with carotid-artery dissection. From Fisher CM, Ojemann RG, Robertson GH. *Spontaneous dissection of cervicocerebral arteries. Can J Neurol Sci* 1978;5:9–19 with permission.

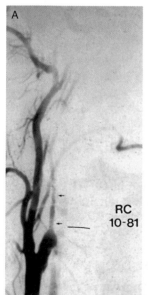
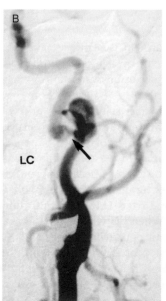
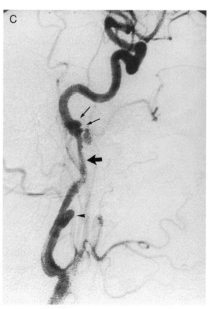

Figure 12.3 Montage of carotid artery angiograms in patients with extracranial ICA dissections. (A) Abrupt change in diameter of the internal carotid artery with a long string-like narrowing (small black arrows). (B) Aneurysmal dilatation of a tortuous carotid artery with an acute dissection. The large black arrow points to a region of narrowing. (C) Long carotid-artery dissection with regions of narrowing and aneurysmal pouches. The arrowhead points to an aneurysmal dilatation at the proximal end of the dissection. The lower black arrow points to a region of narrowing of the artery and the double black arrows point to an irregular aneurysmal dilatation more distally in the pharyngeal portion of the artery.

Magnetic resonance angiography (MRA) (Figure 7.9A and B) and computed tomography angiography (CTA) can also show typical abnormalities in patients with dissections.

ICA dissection, especially with pharyngeal segment aneurysm formation, can also lead to dysfunction of the lower cranial nerves at the skull base. Dysgeusia, Horner's syndrome, and weakness and atrophy of the tongue are the most common

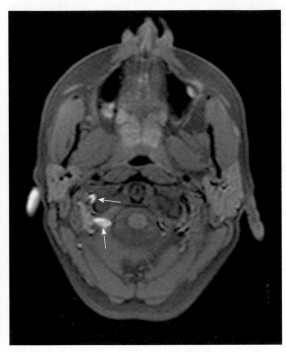

Figure 12.4 Axial cross-section, T1-weighted, fat-saturated image of a patient with an extracranial ICA dissection. The white hyperintensity is seen at two sites as the artery curves (white arrows). The dark flow void represents the arterial lumen and the high-intensity bright areas represent intramural hematoma.

cranial-nerve signs. Tongue weakness and atrophy are caused by compression and ischemia of the hypoglossal nerve as it lies adjacent to the carotid sheath. At times, the IX, X, XI, and XII cranial nerves are involved.[25]

Vertebral artery dissections in the neck[24–38]

ECVA dissections were first recognized in patients who had neck trauma or chiropractic manipulation.[15,26–28] VA injuries have also been reported in patients who manipulate their own necks[29,30] or have maintained their necks in a fixed position for some time.[28,31–34] ECVA dissections also occur after surgery and resuscitation presumably because of sustained neck postures in patients who are anesthetized or unresponsive.[35] These lesions most often involve the distal extracranial (third segment) of the VA. Figure 12.5 is a montage of angiograms in patients with ECVA dissections. Spontaneous ECVA dissections clinically and radiologically mimic those related to trauma.[5–9] Pain in the posterior neck or occiput and generalized headache are common.

Pain often precedes neurological symptoms by hours, days, and, rarely, weeks. Some patients with ECVA dissections have only neck pain and do not develop neurological symptoms or signs. TIAs most often include dizziness, diplopia, veering, staggering, and dysarthria. TIAs are less common in ECVA dissections than ICA dissections. Infarcts usually cause signs that begin suddenly. The most common patterns of ischemic brain damage are cerebellar infarction in posterior inferior cerebellar artery (PICA) distribution and lateral medullary infarction.[28] As in extracranial ICA dissections, infarcts are invariably explained by embolization of fresh thrombus to the ICVA. Occasionally, dissections extend or begin intracranially. Sometimes, emboli reach the superior cerebellar arteries (SCAs), basilar artery, or posterior cerebral arteries (PCAs). ECVA dissections can also cause cervical root pain.[36,37] Aneurysmal dilatation of the ECVA adjacent to nerve roots

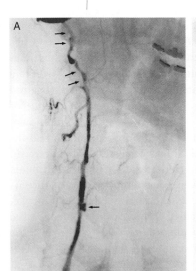
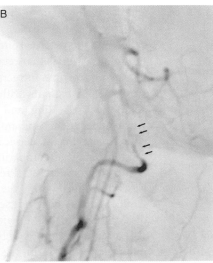
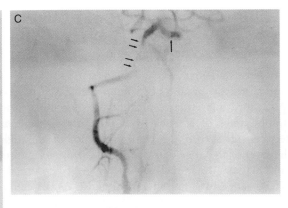

Figure 12.5 A montage of ECVA dissections. (A) Vertebral angiogram-lateral view. A long vertebral artery dissection showing regions of irregular narrowing (top arrows) and an aneurysmal pouch (lower arrow). (B) Vertebral angiogram, lateral view. Dissection in the distal extracranial vertebral artery with narrowing and near occlusion of the artery (black arrows). Flow above the dissection is severely compromised. (C) Vertebral angiogram, anteroposterior view. The distal ECVA is narrowed and flow is compromised (small black arrows). Dye refluxes into the contralateral ICVA (long black arrow at right of figure).

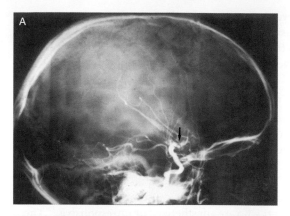

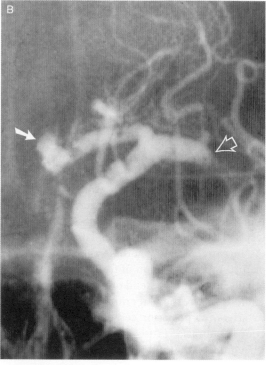

Figure 12.6 Intracranial ICA dissection in a child. (A) Carotid angiogram, lateral view. The black arrow points to the dissection within the intracranial ICA. (B) A magnified close-up view shows the dissection. The closed white arrow on the left shows that the MCA is occluded and the open arrow on the right of the picture points to an occluded anterior cerebral artery.

may cause radicular pain and can lead to radicular distribution motor, sensory, and reflex abnormalities.[36,37] Occasionally, spinal cord infarction results because of hypoperfusion in the supply zones of arteries from the ECVA that nourish the cervical spinal cord.[37,38] Diminished flow in the high neck at the level of the atlas detected by CW Doppler and decreased flow in the intracranial VA shown by transcranial Doppler (TCD) suggest the presence of distal ECVA dissections.

Intracranial dissections[39–44]

Many patients with extracranial ICA and VA dissections have headache, pain, and TIAs without lasting neurological deficits. Intracranial dissection is less common but has been considered more serious and almost invariably associated with severe deficits or death unless the dissection had a limited extent.

Intracranial dissections can cause infarction, subarachnoid bleeding, or mass effects.[5,28,39–44] When the dissections are between the media and the intima, luminal narrowing and local hypoperfusion usually occur and lead to infarction in the regions of supply. In the anterior circulation, the supraclinoid ICA and main stem of the MCA are most often involved.[39,41,43] Figure 12.6 is an arteriogram of an intracranial ICA dissection that extends into the MCA and anterior cerebral artery (ACA). In the posterior circulation, the intracranial vertebral arteries (ICVAs) and basilar artery are most often affected.[5,28,40] The PCAs are occasionally involved.[44] Intracranial dissections were considered in the past to always be devastating or fatal, but modern technology has led to increased recognition of patients with intracranial dissections who have only minor signs. When dissections extend between the media and the adventitia, aneurysms and tears through the adventitia may lead to subarachnoid hemorrhage (SAH), which can be repeated. At times, dissections lead to prominent aneurysmal masses, which can present as space-taking lesions that compress adjacent cranial nerves or brain parenchyma.

Management of arterial dissections[46–56]

Occasionally, patients have chronic dissections with aneurysms and multifocal regions of dissection of various ages.[5,28,40] These patients usually have abnormal arterial media and elastic membranes and the arteries show healing intramural hematomas and tears of different ages. One of us (LRC) has cared for two such patients, one with recurrent SAH and the other with recurrent posterior-circulation TIAs and strokes.[40] In the latter patient, thrombus was visible within each bilateral ICVA-dissecting aneurysm, and symptoms stopped after treatment with warfarin and aspirin combined. Some patients with chronic or recurrent dissections have FMD.[45] When intracranial arteries are involved, hemorrhage and local mass effect can be prominent.

Most extracranial dissections heal spontaneously with time. Their location high in the neck usually makes surgical repair difficult or impossible. When complete occlusion has occurred, the arteries often do not recanalize and remain occluded. Arteries that retain some residual lumen invariably heal and normalize. Intracranial dissections have been repaired surgically in patients with SAH, although the incidence of spontaneous healing and recurrent bleeding is unknown. Antiplatelet agents and anticoagulants are considered reasonable treatments of cervical artery dissection. However, no randomized trial comparing the efficacy of these treatments is currently available.[46] Prevention of embolization of thrombus at or shortly after the dissection should prevent stroke. Anticoagulants have not seemed to increase the extent of the dissections, which is a major theoretical concern. Because the risk of embolization is only during the acute period, heparin followed by warfarin has been advocated by experienced clinicians while trying to maximize cerebral blood flow (CBF) during the acute period to augment collateral circulation. Newer anticoagulants (direct thrombin and factor Xa inhibitors) theoretically could be used instead of warfarin and

preliminary experience among 149 patients indicates that they can be used effectively and safely in patients with dissections.[47]

Healing of dissections can be monitored using MRI, MRA,[48] CTA,[49] and ultrasound. Anticoagulants are often stopped after 6 weeks in patients with dissected arteries that remain occluded, or often continued in patients with patent arteries until luminal stenosis improves to the point that flow is not significantly obstructed. Patients are monitored using ultrasound or MRA. When arterial blood flow is improved, patients are then switched to drugs that modify platelet function, such as aspirin, clopidogrel, cilostazole, or aspirin in combination with extended-release dipyridamole.[50] Aspirin is the most commonly used agent in antiplatelet-naïve patients. Observational studies suggest that thrombolytic therapy with intravenous tissue plasminogen activator (tPA) is reasonably safe in the treatment of patients in whom a cervical artery dissection is associated with an acute ischemic stroke of less than 4.5 hours duration.[51,52]

Although stents have also been used to treat patients who have ICA dissections in the neck,[53–56] the indications for such stenting are very limited. When dissected arteries are open they almost invariably heal and become widely patent with time. The only indications for angioplasty and stenting are as part of an intra-arterial approach to lysing MCA intra-arterial emboli arising from ICA dissections when the ICA is occluded or nearly occluded,[54] and in patients with continued hypoperfusion, a rare occurrence.[55]

Dissections within the anterior circulation are also discussed in Chapter 7 and posterior circulation dissections are also covered in Chapter 8.

Fibromuscular dysplasia[52–68]

First recognized in the renal arteries, FMD is known to affect many other systemic arteries, including cervical and intracranial arteries.[57,58] It is a non-atherosclerotic, non-inflammatory, multifocal arterial disease that can involve any or all of the three layers of the arterial wall. In the cerebral circulation, it is reported in only 0.6% of non-selected consecutive cerebral arteriograms.[59,60] No data exist on its true incidence in patients evaluated for stroke. This blood vessel abnormality is most often described in middle-aged women.[60] Bilateral ICA involvement is common (86%); abnormalities usually involve the pharyngeal portion of the artery and extend from the level of C1 proximally 7–8 cm, with sparing of the carotid bifurcation and the intracranial carotid artery. Twenty percent of patients have coexistent FMD in the vertebral arteries in the neck.[60]

The most common form of FMD affects the media. Constricting bands composed of fibrous dysplastic tissue and proliferating smooth-muscle cells in the media alternate with areas of luminal dilatation related to medial thinning and disruption of the elastic membrane.[61,62] These abnormalities produce the characteristic string-of-beads appearance on arteriography (Figure 12.7A and B). Hypertrophy of fibrous tissues in the adventitia or intima can cause segmental areas of stenosis. Portions of involved arteries can become dilated often irregularly (Figure 12.7C). Occasionally, patients have band-like shelves or diaphragms within greatly enlarged carotid bulbs in the neck; superimposed thrombi sometimes develop in these "mega-bulbs."[63] Some patients with fibrous septa have had typical string-of-beads abnormalities in the pharyngeal

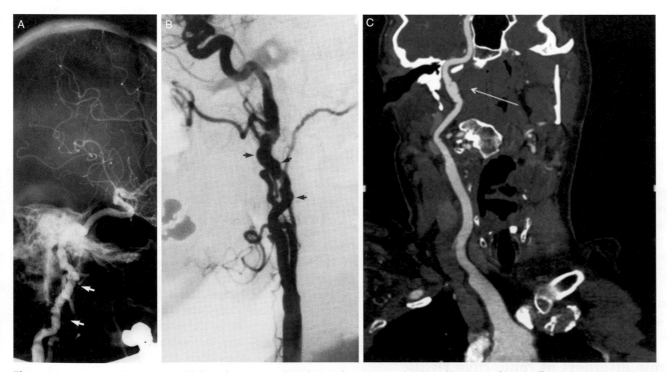

Figure 12.7 Fibromuscular dysplasia. (A) Carotid arteriogram, lateral view, showing typical sausage-like, string-of-beads effect (white arrows). (B) Carotid angiogram, subtraction lateral view. Contractile areas are shown with black arrows. (C) CTA anteroposterior view showing irregularly dilated segment of the ICA in the rostral pharynx (white arrow).

carotid arteries on angiography but some have not had other obvious changes characteristic of FMD.[63] FMD is probably not a single disease but may be a general term for a variety of different conditions that affect the arterial walls.

Although most FMD vascular lesions are asymptomatic, this vascular abnormality can cause brain ischemia. FMD can be accompanied by outpouchings and aneurysms of the extracranial and intracranial arteries.[57,64] In 1 series of 37 patients with FMD, 19 patients had a total of 25 aneurysms.[64] The diagnosis of FMD is occasionally made at the time of evaluating SAH. In the US Registry for FMD, the frequency of SAH among 447 patients was 1.1%.[65] FMD also predisposes patients to arterial dissections with related stroke syndromes. In other patients, FMD affecting an artery appropriate to explain the brain imaging and clinical findings is the only abnormality uncovered. The lumen is not often severely compromised. The mechanism of the distal ischemia in this circumstance is unknown. Functional changes in vessel contraction (vasoconstriction) could lead to distal hypoperfusion. Vasoconstriction can cause reversible constrictions.

Altered blood flow with stasis could lead to thrombus formation and distal intra-arterial embolism. Any medium-sized muscular intracranial artery can be affected. The most prominent clinical features are TIAs and strokes of minor or moderate severity. Fatal or severe strokes are unusual. Headache, pulsatile tinnitus, syncope, cervical bruits, and Horner's syndrome are also frequent accompanying manifestations. The frequency of neurologic events in the US Registry for FMD was as follows: 13.4% of patients had a hemispheric TIA, 5.2% had amaurosis fugax, 12.1% had a cervical artery dissection, and 9.8% had suffered a stroke.[65]

Most research and clinical interest have been directed at atherosclerotic disease of the intima and subintima of arteries. Little is known about the other portions of the arterial wall. Clearly, disease of the artery walls can lead to altered contractility, dilatation with aneurysm formation, and tears with intramural hematomas. FMD is pathologically heterogenous and may occur as a result of various etiologies that share abnormalities of connective tissue. The collagen, elastic tissue, and extracellular matrix can be involved. Knowledge of these disorders of vascular connective tissue is rudimentary.

Angioplasty, often with stenting, has been used to dilate arteries harboring FMD lesions.[66,67] In a series of patients with stroke presumably caused by FMD, the recurrence rate was quite low even without therapy.[61] Insufficient data are available to warrant rational therapeutic suggestions. Antiplatelet therapy is the mainstay of therapy for carotid or vertebral FMD, and we rarely recommend surgical or endovascular therapy.[68] Calcium-channel blockers are often prescribed to prevent vasoconstriction. If the patient is hypertensive, the renal arteries should be studied. When FMD is found on angiography, CTA, MRA, or standard arteriography is warranted to exclude associated intracranial aneurysms.

Heritable disorders of connective tissue[69–94]

Disorders of connective tissue are a group of hereditary disorders that are usually recognizable in childhood and

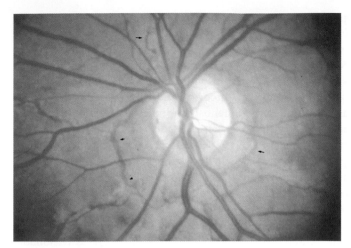

Figure 12.8 Angioid streaks (small black arrows) in the retina in a patient with pseudoxanthoma elasticum. Courtesy of Dr Thomas Hedges III.

involve the skin, vascular system, and skeletal tissues. The full spectrum of these disorders is still unraveling and little in-depth analysis has been made of the neurologic and cerebrovascular features.

Pseudoxanthoma elasticum (PXE), also referred to as Gronblad–Strandberg disease, has an estimated prevalence of approximately 1 in 160 000 and has both autosomal dominant and recessive hereditary patterns.[69,70] The genetic defect has now been mapped to the *ABCC6* gene on chromosome 16p13.1.[71,72] The *ABCC6* gene belongs to the ABC (ATP-binding cassette) transmembrane transporter family of proteins. Genetic studies have identified about 60 mutations as well as large deletions in the gene.[72] The most easily recognized abnormalities are skin changes.[71–74] The skin of the face, neck, axilla, antecubital, inguinal, and periumbilical regions first becomes thickened and grooved. Yellowish papules and plaques are seen in these areas and also on the mucosa of the lips, palate, buccal area, vagina, and rectum. Later, the skin becomes lax and redundant. Angioid streaks, which are reddish-brown or gray, radiate from the optic disk and are usually wider than veins. Figure 12.8 is a fundus photograph that shows angioid streaks in a patient with PXE. Another fundoscopic finding seen in some patients with PXE is a speckled, yellowish mottling of the posterior pole of the retina temporal to the macula. This appearance has been dubbed "peau d'orange" because it resembles the skin of an orange.

The abnormality of connective and elastic tissue causes tortuosity of vessels, premature vascular calcification, intimal thickening, microaneurysms, and fusiform aneurysms. Gastrointestinal bleeding is common and is a result of the vascular abnormalities.[73] Premature occlusive vascular disease affects the coronary, peripheral limb, retinal, and cerebral arteries. Degenerative vascular changes begin with fragmentation and calcification of the internal elastic lamina and are followed by extensive intimal and medial calcification.[73] Cardiac manifestations relate to premature coronary artery disease, and endocardial abnormalities. Coronary artery disease with resulting angina pectoris, myocardial infarction, and sudden death are common and may occur at quite a young

age.[70,71] Some patients have an ischemic cardiomyopathy. Histological examination of coronary artery specimens in patients with PXE show loss of elastic tissue, fragmentation of the internal elastic membrane, and calcifications between the intima and media.[71] Abnormalities in the elastic tissue of the endocardium can produce thickened mitral valves, mitral annular calcification, and mitral stenosis in patients with PXE. The abnormal mitral valve can show fragmentation, coiling, and disruption of collagen bundles.

The arteries of the aortic arch and intracranial arteries are involved. Some patients with PXE show tortuosity and ectasia of the neck arteries on angiography. One patient had occlusion of both ICAs at the skull base and a carotid-cavernous fistula.[75] Hypertension and mitral valve prolapse (MVP) are common,[70] and SAH and intracerebral hemorrhage (ICH) occur. The cerebrovascular lesions most often consist of lacunar infarcts and white matter ischemia of the microangiopathic Binswanger type. Cortical infarcts are less common. Many of the cerebrovascular complications relate to the hypertension that often accompanies PXE.

Ehlers–Danlos syndrome describes a group of clinically and genetically heterogeneous conditions that share defects in collagen.[76] The skin is hyperextensible and easily bruised, and the joints show hypermobility and excessive scarring after an injury. Over 80% of Ehlers–Danlos syndrome patients have types I, II, or III, but most individuals with cerebrovascular complications have type IV, which occurs in 1 in 50 000–500 000 individuals.[77] Cardiac and cerebrovascular lesions are common and include mitral and tricuspid valve prolapse, septal defects, and dilatation of the aortic root and pulmonary arteries.[78] Easy bruising, regions of translucent skin, intestinal and vascular rupture, and rupture of a gravid uterus are common non-neurological features. The most important and frequent cerebrovascular complications are carotid-cavernous fistulas, and arterial dissections.[76,79–81]

Extracranial and intracranial aneurysms have also been reported, including several individuals with multiple intracranial aneurysms.[82,83] The ICA is the most common site of aneurysm formation, typically in the cavernous sinus or just as it emerges from the sinus. Rupture of various systemic and cerebral vessels leads to frequent bleeding and SAH. Angiography and angioplasty have a high rate of complications and extreme caution should be exercised in choosing these procedures in Ehlers–Danlos syndrome patients.[76] Surgery is also difficult because the arteries are friable and difficult to suture.

Marfan's syndrome is a hereditary disorder that is probably more common than other hereditary disorders and occurs in approximately 4–6 per 100 000 individuals.[84] The condition is inherited as a dominant trait, being sporadic in less than one-quarter of individuals. A gene defect is located in the long arm of chromosome 15, in which a mutation in the *FBN1* gene that encodes fibrillin-1 was first reported in 1991.[85,86] Since then, more than 600 mutations were identified, most of them causing Marfanoid or fragments of the Marfan's syndrome phenotype.[85]

Marfan's syndrome is a connective tissue disorder associated with extensive and generalized malformation of organs and systems.[84] The skeleton is disproportionately arranged and unstable, the eyes often have subluxation of the lenses and are myopic; a cystic disease of the lungs can be present.[85] Defective formation of cardiac valves and blood vessels underlies the more serious occurrences in Marfan's syndrome. The vascular abnormalities relate to abnormal collagen and elastin. The phenotype of long limbs, pectus chest deformity, arachnodactyly, and joint laxity is easily recognizable. Subluxation of the lens occurs in more than one-half of the patients, and ophthalmological examination is helpful in diagnosis. The diameter of the aortic root is invariably enlarged, and aortic regurgitation and mitral valve prolapse are common. Aortic aneurysms and dissections are very frequent clinical problems in patients with Marfan's syndrome.

Most of the cerebrovascular events in patients with Marfan's syndrome relate to the cardiac and aortic manifestations of the condition. A few patients with carotid and vertebral artery dissections have been reported.[86,88] Whether or not there is also a predisposition for intracranial aneurysms in Marfan's syndrome patients has been debated with some data favoring a relationship,[89] and others arguing that the frequency is no higher than in the general population.[90] There does not appear to be an excess frequency of SAH in patients with Marfan's syndrome.[91]

The Loeys–Dietz syndrome (type 1A, 1B, 2A, 2B, 3, and 4) is an autosomal dominantly inherited syndrome consisting of various bony and connective tissue abnormalities and a predilection for aortic and arterial aneurysms and dissections.[92–94] Like Marfan's syndrome there are often long limbs and fingers and lax joints. Widely spaced eyes, cleft palate or bifid uvula, scoliosis, and indented or protruding chest wall are other common features. Gradual weakening and stretching of the dura mater can cause nerve root irritation and leg pains. Congenital heart abnormalities especially patent ductus arteriosus and atrial septal defects are also often found. This condition is caused by a mutation in the genes encoding transforming growth factor beta receptor (*TGFBR 1* or *TGFBR 2*).

Dilatative arteriopathy (dolichoectasia)[95–117]

Patients with dilatative arteriopathy have elongated, ectatic, tortuous intracranial arteries.[95,96] Dilatation can be so severe that portions of the artery become a fusiform aneurysm. Approximately one patient in eight who has brain imaging has some increase in the length and diameter of intracranial arteries.[95–98] This abnormality can be found in children and often involves multiple arteries.[95,99–103] Hereditary factors probably play an important role, especially in the young. In one reported family, three brothers had large fusiform basilar artery aneurysms and alpha-glucosidase deficiency.[101] In an 11-year-old girl who died from a ruptured dolichoectatic basilar artery aneurysm, necropsy showed that the artery had large gaps in the internal elastic lamina with only short segments of

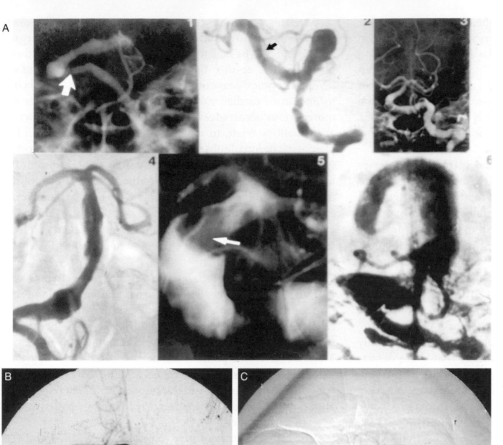

Figure 12.9 Dolichoectatic vertebrobasilar arteries. (A) Montage of vertebrobasilar fusiform aneurysms in six patients. Patient 1 (upper left) has marked tortuosity and ectasia of the basilar artery with a proximal atheromatous stenosis (white arrow); patient 2 has a filling defect (black arrow) representing thrombus in the midbasilar artery; patient 3 has a very tortuous left vertebral and basilar artery; patient 4 shows irregular plaques in a dilated basilar artery; patient 5 has a markedly dilated basilar artery with a filling defect (white arrow) representing thrombus. The apparent lower filling defect is an artifact representing an aerated sinus. Patient 6 has a very dilated ectatic artery with poor filling of the distal segment and non-filling of the PCAs because of reduced antegrade flow. From Pessin MS, Chimowitz MI, Levine SR, et al. Stroke in patients with fusiform vertebrobasilar aneurysms. *Neurology* 1989;39:16–21. (B) Vertebral angiogram, anteroposterior view. The basilar artery is extremely dilatated and the distal portion and its branches are poorly opacified. (C) Very irregular ectatic basilar artery with extensive atheromatous plaques. The branches of the rostral basilar artery are not well opacified because of reduced antegrade blood flow.

elastica remaining in some regions.[100] Pathological examination in other young patients with dolichoectasia has shown deficiencies in the muscularis and internal elastic lamina with irregular thickness of the media, multiple gaps in the internal elastica, and regions of fibrosis. At times, the intima is thickened, and there is severe elastic tissue degeneration and an increase in the vasa vasorum. Dolichoectasia is also prominent in children with Fabry's disease, sickle cell disease, and AIDS, and it occurs in patients with Ehlers–Danlos syndrome.[95] Patients with dilatative arteriopathy also have a high frequency of enlarged aortic diameters and lacunar infarcts due to penetrating artery disease.[104,105]

The most frequent location is in the posterior fossa where the basilar artery or one or both VAs are involved.[96,106–110] Figure 12.9A shows a montage of dye-contrast cerebral arteriograms of six patients with vertebrobasilar dolichoectatic arteries. Figure 12.9B and C shows ectatic basilar arteries with poor antegrade blood flow. The dolichoectatic anomaly is often recognized on CT as curvilinear, calcified channels that usually cross the cerebellopontine angle.[106,108] The MCAs are also often involved, and some patients have dolichoectatic abnormalities in both the anterior and posterior circulations.

Extensive atherosclerotic plaques, often with calcification, encroachment on the lumen, and thrombus formation, are often found at necropsy. On microscopic examination, there are often fibrotic changes in the vessel wall with reduced muscularis and attenuated, fragmented, or absent elastica.[96,111] Clinically, the most common symptoms are caused by brain ischemia. Mass effect with compression or displacement of cranial nerves or brain parenchyma is also common. The aneurysmally dilatated arteries can compress the medullary pyramids[112] and cerebral peduncles and may indent and

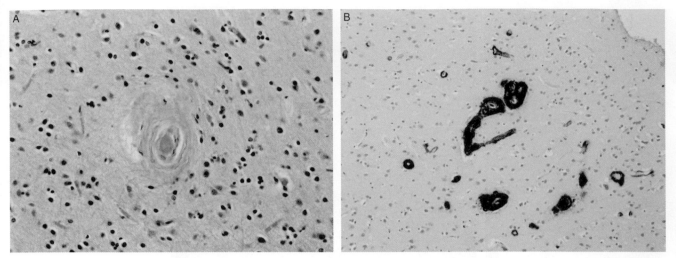

Figure 12.10 (A) Photomicrograph of the cerebral cortex, hematoxylin-eosin stain showing splitting of the amyloid-laden wall of a small artery. (B) Photomicrograph of the cerebral cortex immunostained for beta-amyloid with a hematoxylin counterstain. Amyloid is seen in many small vessels. Courtesy of Dr Steven Greenberg. A black and white version of this figure will appear in some formats. For the color version, please refer to the plate section.

deform the basis pontis. Some patients have had hydrocephalus, possibly related to the effects of the dolichoectatic aneurysms on the IIIrd ventricle.

Ischemia is most often found in the distribution of penetrating arteries to the brainstem and basal ganglia. Ischemia is related to the effects of the condition in the parent arteries on the branches. Plaques or clot may obliterate or obscure the orifices of branches or can embolize into the branches. Angiography may show thrombi within dolichoectatic aneurysms.[106,113] In other patients, distortion and elongation of the branches may reduce blood flow without obliteration of the branch ostia or lumens. Occasionally, clot within the aneurysms can embolize to the larger distal branches.[106,113,114] Rupture of these aneurysms with resulting subarachnoid bleeding is unusual but does occur.[106,111,113]

CT, CTA, MRI, and MRA usually suffice to identify the aneurysmally dilatated ectatic arteries and may suggest the presence of clot within the vessels.[115] TCD is helpful in diagnosis and may show reduced mean-flow velocities with relatively preserved peak-flow velocities.[116] Blood flow may be to and fro within the dilatated artery, causing reduced antegrade flow. The reduced antegrade flow may lead to poor opacification on MRA, falsely suggesting occlusion of the dolichoectatic artery. CTA and standard angiography are able to image the artery in this circumstance. In patients with recurrent ischemia and thrombi within the dolichoectatic arteries, warfarin may prevent strokes. Intravenous thrombolytic agents also have been used in patients with large thrombi within dolichoectatic arteries.[113] Agents that modify platelet function have not been studied in patients with dilatative arteriopathy. The vascular abnormality often increases with time and there is a relatively high frequency of strokes despite present therapy.[117]

Cerebral amyloid angiopathy[118–153]

Cerebral amyloid angiopathy (CAA), also called congophilic angiopathy, is also discussed in Chapter 14 because the major

clinical feature is recurrent lobar ICH. The disorder is characterized by thickening of the walls of small- and medium-sized arteries by an amorphous eosinophilic-staining material with a smudged appearance on light microscopy.[118,119] The walls of some amyloid-laden vessels appear to be split (Figure 12.10A). The material within the vessel wall shows a yellow-green birefringence when stained with Congo red and viewed under a polarizing microscope – hence the term *congophilic*. Figure 12.10B is a photomicrograph of the cerebral cortex stained for beta-amyloid in a patient with CAA. The abnormalities usually involve many arteries, especially those in the leptomeninges and cerebral cortex. The brainstem, basal gray nuclei, hippocampi, and subcortical white matter are spared.[118] The amyloid deposition is most prevalent in the parietal and occipital lobes, but ICH is also often frontal and central, and can be cerebellar.[119–124] Affected arteries, especially those in the leptomeninges, have a distinctive double-barrel lumen with amyloid found in the outer or inner media.[118]

The most common clinical syndromes recognized are ICH, usually multiple and subcortical lobar, SAH, and age-related cognitive decline.[118–125] MRI T2* susceptibility-weighted echo-planar images often show multiple, small, old hemorrhages in patients with CAA who present with a stroke. These small accumulations of hemosiderin-laden cells are usually referred to as "microbleeds." These microbleeds are common and their amount and location does predict a risk of further brain hemorrhage.[126,127] Figure 12.11A shows an echo-planar image of a patient with a recent amyloid angiopathy-related brain hemorrhage, as well as multiple old regions of bleeding. The smaller regions of susceptibility have often been labeled "microbleeds." Figure 12.11B shows an echo-planar image of a man who presented with transient aphasia whose images show many cortical microbleeds.

Some patients with CAA develop superficial hemorrhages along the convexal portions of the cerebral hemispheres.[127,128]

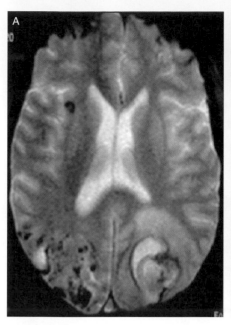 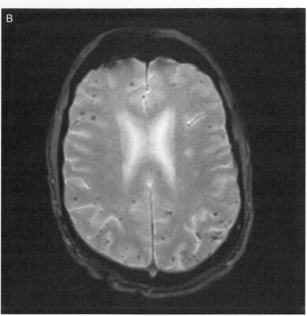

Figure 12.11 (A) Gradient-echo MRI images of a man with a recent left occipital-parietal intracerebral hemorrhage. Multiple old hemorrhages (black regions) are shown. Courtesy of Drs Charlotte Cordonnier and Didier Leys, and published in Caplan LR, Bogousslavsky J. *Uncommon Causes of Stroke*, 2nd ed. Cambridge: Cambridge University Press, 2008. (B) Gradient-echo MRI images of a 68-year-old man who presented with transient aphasia. Images show many lobar microbleeds diagnostic of cerebral amyloid angiopathy. Courtesy of Dr Steven Greenberg.

These small localized hemorrhages are found within the sulci. They are explained by the observation that many of the amyloid-laden vessels lie within the subarachnoid space. Patients may present with headache but often, also report localized sensory symptoms in a limb or hemicorpus. The explanation for the hemisensory symptoms is unclear. These superficial convexal hemorrhages are never caused by aneurysmal bleeding but are also found in patients with the reversible cerebral vasoconstriction syndrome (RCVS) and with cerebral venous occlusions. Superficial hemosiderosis is another relatively common finding in patients with CAA and is explained by repeated subarchnoid hemorrhages.[120–132] The subarachnoid bleeding is almost never accompanied by a sudden "thunderclap" headache. If headache occurs it is usually slight and the syndrome is dominated by hemisensory symptoms and signs.

Senile plaques containing amyloid and Alzheimer's changes are also prevalent in brains of patients harboring CAA. Some patients with CAA are demented or develop intellectual deterioration with time caused by multiple strokes and Alzheimer's pathology.[119] Both APOE2 and APOE4 play a role in facilitating the deposition of amyloid in cerebral blood vessels, and APOEΣ2 seems to increase the likelihood of ICH in patients with CAA.[133,134] ICH is especially common in APOE2 carriers after head trauma or use of antithrombotic agents.[135]

Early studies noted that scattered small infarcts were also prevalent in brains of patients with amyloid-related ICH.[121–123] TIAs can occur.[128,136] Some patients with CAA have multiple infarcts and a prominent leukoencephalopathy with periventricular, subcortical, and corona radiata lucency on CT and hyperintense signal abnormalities on MRI.[124,137–140] The clinical picture is that of Binswanger's disease. In fact, CAA may be an important, often unrecognized, cause of this chronic ischemic microangiopathy.

The cause of CAA is unknown. Familial CAA has been identified, especially in Icelandic, Dutch, and German families, and is usually inherited as an autosomal-dominant trait with high penetrance.[101] The Icelandic variety has been attributed to abnormal metabolism of a gamma-trace protein.[119,141,142]

At times, there are prominent inflammatory changes in relation to the amyloid-staining arteries, and there have been reports and reviews of patients who had CAA and granulomatous arteritis.[118,143–149] This entity has been referred to as Aβ-related angiitis.[147,149] Breakage of amyloid-containing vessels with release of Aβ amyloid into the subarachnoid space may induce an immunological response that causes an angiitis. Patients with this condition often have headache, cognitive and behavioral abnormalities, seizures, and focal neurological signs.[143–149] The CSF contains a modest pleocytosis and increase in protein content. Some patients have responded clinically to corticosteroids and immunosuppressants.

Although it was once considered that drainage of CAA-related hematomas might be hazardous, data show that surgical results are not different from other causes of ICH.[150,151] Reducing the systemic blood pressure to the lowest levels tolerated is a strategy often used to reduce the frequency of ICH. Advances in recognition and understanding the pathogenesis of CAA and biomarkers should lead to more specific therapeutic strategies.[152,153]

Vasculitis and other possibly inflammatory vascular disorders[154–399]

Arteritis (angiitis) is mentioned as a cause of stroke in the differential diagnosis of nearly every medical student, non-neurologist, and some neurologists. (Tables 12.2 and 12.3) Although often considered, documented arteritis is a rare

Table 12.2 Strokes and cerebral arteritis

Infectious vasculitides
  Bacterial
  Fungal
  Parasitic
  Spirochetal
  Viral
  Rickettsial
  Mycobacterial

Necrotizing vasculitides
  P-ANCA granulomatosis with polyangitis
  Classic polyarteritis nodosa
  Microscopic polyangiitis
  Allergic angiitis and granulomatosis (Churg–Strauss)
  Necrotizing systemic vasculitis-overlap syndrome
  Lymphomatoid granulomatosis

Vasculitides associated with collagen vascular diseases
  Systemic lupus erythematosus
  Rheumatoid arthritis
  Scleroderma
  Sjögren's syndrome

Vasculitides associated with other systemic diseases
  Behçet's disease
  Ulcerative colitis
  Sarcoidosis
  Relapsing polychondritis
  Kohlmeier–Degos disease

Giant cell arteritides
  Temporal arteritis
  Takayasu's arteritis

Hypersensitivity vasculitides
  Henoch–Schönlein purpura
  Drug-induced vasculitides
  Chemical vasculitides
  Essential mixed cryoglobulinemia

Miscellaneous
  Vasculitis associated with neoplasia
  Vasculitis associated with radiation
  Cogan's syndrome
  Dermatomyositis-polymyositis
  X-linked lymphoproliferative syndrome
  Thromboangiitis obliterans (Buerger's disease)
  Kawasaki disease

Primary angiitis of the central nervous system (PACNS)

Table 12.3 Strokes and miscellaneous infections

Cat-scratch disease

Mycoplasma pneumoniae

Coxsackie 9 virus

Parvovirus or B19 virus

California encephalitis virus

Mumps paramyxovirus

Hepatitis C virus

Enteroviruses

Cytomegalovirus

West Nile virus

Viral hemorrhagic fevers

Rickettsiaceae

Malaria

Leptospirosis

Typhoid fever

Gnasthoma spinigerium

Free living amebae

Sparganosis

Lemierre syndrome

Sphenoid sinusitis

Post-streptococcal glomerulonephritis

Infective endocarditis

Sepsis

Parasitic diseases (Chagas' disease)

AIDS or other immune disorders

Acute meningitis

Acute encephalitides

Subacute meningoencephalitides

cause of stroke. Most often, central nervous system (CNS) vasculitis presents as an encephalopathy with headache, seizures, decreased alertness, and cognitive and behavioral abnormalities, often with multifocal signs. Recognition of those rare instances in which arteritis is caused by a specific microbial infection is critical for effective treatment. Patients with allergic hypersensitivity and systemic vasculitis may respond to corticosteroids or other treatments used to control systemic autoimmune diseases.

Arteritis caused by infections[154–230]

Infectious vasculitides affecting the cerebral vasculature may cause ischemic or hemorrhagic cerebral complications and are predominantly bacterial, viral, or fungal in nature. Opportunistic CNS infections may also complicate immune-suppressive treatment of rheumatic diseases. Almost all species of bacteria or fungi can cause infective endocarditis. Endocarditis may also be caused by rickettsia and *Brucella* species.

Bacterial and fungal infections[154–186]

In patients with acute bacterial meningitis (e.g., pneumococcal or meningococcal), the pial arteries and veins are often

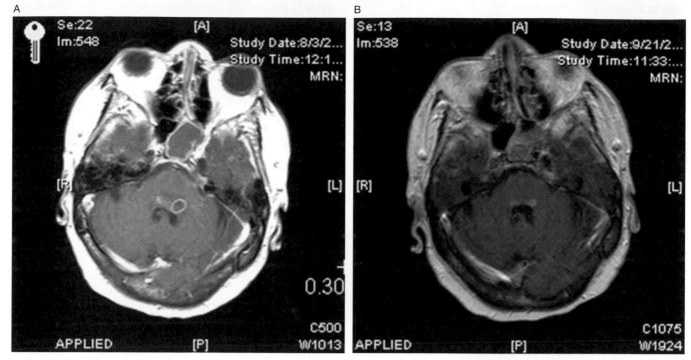

Figure 12.12 *Listeria rhombencephalitis.* (A) T1-weighted MRI after gadolinium enhancement showing ring-enhancing lesions in the pons adjacent to the floor of the IVth ventricle. (B) T1-weighted, gadolinium-enhanced MRI taken a month later after penicillin treatment. From Silvestri N, Ajani Z, Savitz S, Caplan LR. A 73-year-old woman with an acute illness causing fever and cranial nerve abnormalities. *Rev Neurol Dis* 2006;3:29–30,35–37. Figures reprinted with permission from MedReviews LLC. All rights reserved.

surrounded by pus. Vascular occlusions and strokes may complicate the clinical picture, which is invariably dominated by headache, fever, stiff neck, and decreased alertness. Brain infarction develops in about 15–20% of adults with bacterial meningitis, typically pneumococcal meningitis.[154–156] Purulent bacterial meningitis may also be complicated by intracranial vasospasm, arterial stenosis, and aneurysms. Occasionally spinal cord and brainstem infarction occur during meningococcal meningitis.[157,158] Hemorrhagic stroke is an uncommon complication of bacterial meningitis.

Listeria monocytogenes may produce a characteristic inflammatory disorder involving predominantly the medulla and pontine tegmentum.[159–162] Multiple, lower cranial-nerve palsies and vestibular and oculomotor signs develop. Figure 12.12 shows MRI scans from a patient with *Listeria rhombencephalitis* treated with penicillin.[162] At times, the onset of symptoms is abrupt and subsequent necropsy shows an arteritis with multiple infarcts as well as focal encephalitis. The cerebrospinal fluid (CSF) shows a pleocytosis.[159–162] Occasionally, patients with *cat-scratch disease*,[163] a disorder known to be caused by *Bartonella henselae*, have presented with an acute focal neurological deficit associated with intracranial stenoses and arteritis.[164]

In patients with *syphilis*, the spirochete probably invades cerebral arteries at the time of the meningitis of secondary lues. Meningovascular syphilis results in and is characterized by apoplectic attacks of hemiplegia, headache, seizures, and modest CSF lymphomononuclear pleocytosis, with elevated CSF protein and normal or low CSF glucose level.[165] Arteries may appear stenotic on vascular imaging.[166,167] The serology is

always positive in patients with meningovascular syphilis. The spinal arterial circulation can also be affected. All forms of syphilis are more common and severe in patients with AIDS.[165,168]

Lyme borreliosis mimics syphilis in many ways. Meningitis, multiple cranial-nerve palsies, and root- and peripheral-nerve syndromes predominate.[169–172] Lyme carditis can cause heart block and other cardiac arrhythmias; strokes have been described but rarely.[173–175] Strokes are much less common than peripheral nerve and root sensory symptoms and the syndrome of headache, fatigue, and difficulty concentrating. The CSF is invariably abnormal and specific antibodies to *Borrelia* are present in the blood and CSF.[175]

Chronic basal meningitis, usually caused by *tuberculosis*[176–180] or particular fungi (i.e., *Cryptococcus, Histoplasma,* and *Coccidioides*),[181–183] is often complicated by inflammation of the arteries within the exudate. Neurotuberculosis affects predominantly the basilar meninges. Predisposing conditions include alcoholism, substance abuse, corticosteroid use, and HIV infection. The proximal MCA and arteries in the posterior perforated substance are most often involved. The exudate surrounds the arteries, producing thickening and inflammation of the walls of the arteries. Infarcts in the basal ganglia and midbrain result and can develop even after sterilization of the microbial agent. Tuberculous meningitis results in modest lymphocytic and mononuclear pleocytosis, elevated protein content, and depressed glucose levels. CSF smears demonstrate Mycobacterium tuberculosis in 10–20% of cases. CSF polymerase chain reaction (PCR) is quite useful in the diagnosis of tuberculous meningitis (sensitivity 48–90%; specificity 100%).

Transplant recipients are at high risk for CSF infections, particularly fungal.

The fungi *Aspergillus*[184,185] and *Mucor*,[186] cause a necrotizing arteritis with regions of brain infarction and necrosis. *Mucor* is usually spread from the paranasal sinuses,[186] and *Aspergillus* reaches the cerebral circulation by hematogenous spread usually without meningitis.[184,185] *Aspergillus* infections are especially common in patients who take corticosteroids or who are immunosuppressed, and *Mucor* is common in patients with diabetic ketoacidosis and those in renal failure. Rhinocerebral mucormycosis may cause cavernous sinus and internal carotid artery thrombosis. Intracranial aspergillosis may cause SAH due to ruptured mycotic aneurysms or septic arteritis. Disseminated candidiasis may cause mycotic aneurysms, brain infarction, SAH, and cerebral vasculitis. Coccidioidal meningitis may result in vessel thrombosis. Cryptococcosis seldom involves the intracranial vessels.

Viral infections[188-211]

Viruses may be responsible for many cases of vasculitis that are now considered idiopathic. Hepatitis-B surface antigen, immunoglobulin, and complement are found in the vessel walls of patients with polyarteritis nodosa who have hepatitis-B antigenemia.[187] The **varicella-zoster virus** (VZV) is also known to directly invade CNS vessels, sometimes without causing much visible inflammatory reaction.[188,189] Viruses can cause vasculitis by direct invasion or by triggering an immune response to components of vessels.[189] Alternatively, immune-complex deposition can injure arteries and cause inflammation. Evidence of VZV infection by PCR analysis of biopsy or necropsy material may be found in patients with the typical clinical findings of polyarteritis nodosa.[189]

VZV is the most well known and best documented of the viral arteritides. The most common clinical vascular syndrome is delayed brain infarction, usually causing hemiplegia contralateral to herpes zoster ophthalmicus.[190-192] The symptoms begin days to weeks (range 6–18 weeks) after onset of the painful rash.[190,191,193] Infarcts are usually hemispheral and cause hemiparesis, hemisensory loss, and aphasia, or right-hemispheric types of cognitive and behavioral changes. Usually, the infarct is ipsilateral to the rash. However, VZV angiopathy can occur without a rash.[193] Angiography has shown occlusion of the carotid siphon, MCA, or ACA, and sometimes stenosis of these arteries.[190-192] Small arteries are also very often involved and may become occluded.[193] At times, TIAs may precede the stroke but most often the onset is abrupt and the neurological signs develop immediately. Some patients have an accompanying encephalitis. Recurrent ischemia and multiple infarcts have been reported. The mortality has been estimated at approximately 25%. This mortality rate is higher than comparable-sized infarcts caused by atherosclerosis.[191] The CSF usually shows a slight pleocytosis and immunoglobulins (Ig) and IgG indices may be elevated.[190,191] Rarely, the rash involves other divisions of the Vth cranial nerve (maxillary or mandibular) and can occur in the back of the neck and upper cervical dermatomes.[194-196]

The PCA and vertebrobasilar territory are occasionally involved.[194-196]

Postvaricella arteriopathy and brain infarction have now been studied extensively in children.[197-200] The course and progression of the arteriopathy was studied in 27 children who had serial vascular imaging.[200] They had chickenpox at age 1.0–10.4 (median 4.4 years) and had their first episode of brain ischemia 4–47 weeks later (median 17 weeks).[200] Arterial imaging abnormalities most often involved the supraclinoid ICA, the M1 and M2 segments of the MCA, and the A1 segment of the ACA. Single regions of focal ring-like stenosis and longer segments of stenosis and multifocal narrowings were found. Brain infarcts were predominantly deep in the basal ganglia, internal capsule, and thalamus. In some patients stenosis was maximal on the initial studies, but often later progressed to involve previously uninvolved arteries. The vascular abnormalities improved or completely regressed during follow-up during 6–79 months. Brain ischemic episodes recurred, either acutely or during the 1–33 weeks after symptom onset, often with progression of abnormalities on vascular imaging.[200]

At necropsy, patients with VZV arteritis may show inflamed necrotic arteries, granulomatous changes,[188-190] or occluded arteries with scant inflammation. Doyle and colleagues were able to recognize virions that were characteristic of VZV in the nuclei and cytoplasm of smooth-muscle cells in the involved arteries.[192] Amplification of VZV viral DNA by PCR was obtained in the left anterior, middle, and posterior cerebral arteries of a patient who developed left-cerebral hemisphere infarction after left herpes zoster ophthalmicus.[201] Presumably, the virus spread from the infected gasserian ganglion through trigeminovascular connections to the proximal portions of the ipsilateral MCA and ACA.[201] Trigeminovascular projections also go from V1 to the SCA, and the upper cervical ganglia probably project to the ICVAs, basilar artery, and the anterior inferior cerebellar artery (AICA) and SCA.[202] Spread to the intima can activate the endothelium to release factors promoting thrombosis. As in other virus diseases, inflammation is not always visible under the microscope.

Patients with **human immunodeficiency virus** (HIV) infection have an increased frequency of stroke.[203-207] The mechanisms of stroke in AIDS patients vary. Some strokes are caused by infective or marantic endocarditis, hypercoagulability provoked by chronic infection, concomitant drug abuse, infection with agents that can cause arteritis, such as syphilis, VZV, fungi, and other opportunistic infections, or hyperlipidemia and accelerated atherosclerosis due to use of protease inhibitors.[203-207] Children with AIDS may have a dilatative arteriopathy with fusiform aneurysms involving the intracranial arteries.[208] SAH may develop.

Strokes have been described in cat-scratch disease (*Bartonella henselae*), Mycoplasma pneumonia infection, coxsackie 9 virus, parvovirus or B19 virus, California encephalitis virus, mumps paramyxovirus, hepatitis C virus, enteroviruses, cytomegalovirus, VZV, HIV, and a variety of hemorrhagic fevers.

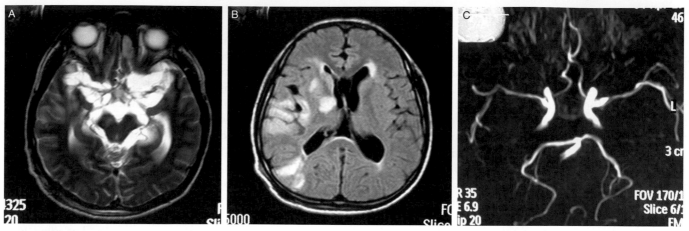

Figure 12.13 Cerebral infarction in patient with cysticercotic angiitis. (A) T2-weighted MRI shows huge subarachnoid racemose cysts in the sylvian fissures engulfing both middle cerebral arteries. (B) MRI FLAIR scan shows recent infarction in the territory of the right middle cerebral artery. (C) MRA shows stenosis of the MCAs bilaterally. Courtesy of Dr Julio Lama, Guayaquil, Ecuador; from Del Bruto OH. Stroke and vasculitis in patients with cysticercosis. In Caplan LR, Bogousslavsky J. *Uncommon Causes of Stroke*, 2nd ed. Cambridge: Cambridge University Press, 2008, pp 53–58 with permission.

Kawasaki disease is an acute disorder occurring predominantly in children that is posited to be caused by an as yet unidentified infectious agent.[209] It causes vasculopathies mostly in the form of coronary artery aneurysm and the aorta. The carotid arteries are sometimes also often involved.[209–211]

Parasitic infections[212–230]

Cysticercosis may be associated with endarteritis and strokes.[212–220] Cysticercosis is caused by infection with the larvae (*cysticerci*) of *Taenia solium*, the pork tapeworm. Parasitic cysts containing cysticerci lodge within brain parenchyma in the subarachnoid space and within the brain ventricles. Stroke occurs predominantly in the subarachnoid form of the disease.[212–217] Meningitic inflammation can spread to the major basal intracranial arteries, leading to an endarteritis and brain infarction. Subcortical small infarcts and large cortical–subcortical infarcts may occur. The most common vessels involved are the MCAs, PCAs, and the ACAs, but the basilar artery may also be affected.[217,218] Figure 12.13 shows a severe instance of subarachnoid cysticercosis that compromises the MCAs bilaterally. In one study, among 28 patients with subarachnoid cysticercosis who had cerebral angiography, 15 patients (53%) had angiographic evidence of arteritits.[218] A clinical stroke syndrome was present in 12 of these patients, and 8 patients had brain infarcts on MRI.[218] When patients with arterial narrowing caused by cysticercosis are followed sequentially using TCD, sometimes the stenosis improves with time.[219] Precipitation of brain infarction after praziquantel therapy has also been reported.[220] Destruction of the cysticercotic cysts within the subarachnoid space may cause an inflammatory response, which can cause or exacerbate an endarteritis.[212,220]

Plasmodium falciparum is the most frequent parasitic infection of the CNS. Cerebral malaria is characterized by coma and convulsions after a prodromal period of fever and headache.[221] Parasitized red blood cells distend capillaries and venules and lead to intracranial hypertension, brain edema, and petechial hemorrhages throughout the brain. Subarachnoid hemorrhage has also been reported.[222] In children, convulsions and hemiparesis are relatively common. Angiography and TCD in children with hemiparesis often shows focal stenosis of the basal intracranial arteries.[223,224]

Trypanosoma cruzi infection causes a disorder called *Chagas disease*, which is common in Brazil, Paraguay, and other parts of South America.[225] *T. cruzi* parasites are transmitted to humans by large bedbugs that deposit feces on the mucous membranes or scraped skin while they bite. When individuals rub the bite wound, the parasites enter the bloodstream. Cardiac involvement (cardiac dilatations, arrhythmias, and conduction abnormalities) is present in over 90% of patients. Intestinal (megaesophagus, megacolon) involvement is also common. The clinical presentation is that of a dilatated cardiomyopathy. The cardiac disorder is caused by involvement of the autonomic nervous system innervation of the heart rather than direct attack by the parasites. Strokes are relatively common in patients with Chagas disease and are mainly due to embolism from the heart.[225–230] Heart failure, mural thrombi, left ventricular apical aneurysms, and cardiac arrhythmias provide sources of brain emboli in Chagas disease.[230] Rarely, cerebral vasculitis in patients with AIDS has been associated with trypanosomiasis-related necrotizing encephalitis.

Large artery cerebrovascular occlusions have been found in association with meningoencephalitis caused by free-living amebae. Sparganosis is an infection with the migratory larvae of cestodes of the genus *Spirometra*; rare cases of sparganosis-induced cerebral vasculitis have been reported. Unilateral or bilateral carotid occlusion can also complicate necrotizing fasciitis of the lateral parapharyngeal space. A purulent thrombophlebitis of the jugular vein (Lemierre's syndrome) may develop. Atypical cases of Lemierre's syndrome have been reported in association with carotid artery thrombosis. Rarely, a sphenoid sinusitis has been associated with basilar artery vasculitis.

Systemic vasculitides, including collagen vascular diseases[187,231–290]

Systemic vasculitis syndromes can be conveniently divided into polyarteritis nodosa, allergic angiitis and granulomatosis (Churg–Strauss syndrome), hypersensitivity vasculitis, P-ANCA granulomatosis with polyangiitis, and overlap syndromes sharing features of other subtypes.[187,231–237] All of these syndromes have in common multi-system involvement.

Polyarteritis nodosa (PAN) affects small- and medium-sized arteries, especially at branch points.[235–239] Infiltration of polymorphonuclear leukocytes and monocytes is followed by intimal proliferation, fibrinoid necrosis, and thrombosis of arteries. The most common neurological signs probably relate to mononeuritis multiplex. CNS involvement occurs in 20–40% of patients and the onset occurs usually after systemic symptoms and signs and neuropathy.[232,238,239] Some patients have a diffuse encephalopathy and others have focal or multi-focal abnormalities. Occasionally, hemispheral, spinal cord, cerebellar and brainstem infarcts occur. When strokes occur, it is usually late in the illness. Hypertension is common in patients with PAN, and is responsible for many of the ischemic infarcts and hemorrhages. We have not seen or known of a report of PAN presenting initially as a stroke syndrome.

Patients with *Churg–Strauss syndrome* invariably have pulmonary involvement, including asthma, and eosinophilia.[232,240–243] A history of previous allergic disorders usually exists. The lesions tend to involve smaller vessels, especially capillaries and venules.[232,240–245] Encephalopathy and peripheral neuritis are common, but strokes are extremely rare.

The *hypersensitivity vasculitides* are a group of conditions in which the cause is usually known and a major finding is a rash, often with palpable purpuric skin lesions, especially on the legs. Some are drug induced, postinfectious, or related to known foreign antigens (e.g., serum sickness). Mixed cryoglobulinemia and *Henoch–Schönlein purpura* are other forms of hypersensitivity vasculitis. Neurological involvement is not prominent in patients with the various hypersensitivity vasculitis syndromes, and when it occurs, neuropathies, plexopathies, and encephalopathies predominate.[232,245] Strokes occur but rarely and most often are explained by bleeding related to systemic purpura.[246–248]

Wegener's granulomatosis – now often referred to as P-ANCA granulomatosis with polyangiitis is a necrotizing, often fatal, granulomatous vasculitis that involves chiefly the lungs, sinuses, upper respiratory tract, and kidneys.[232,249] Orbital involvement, palsies of extraocular muscles, and retinal and optic nerve ischemia are often reported.[250–253] Brain infarcts and cerebral arteritis are occasionally described.[254,255] The diagnosis can be made by biopsy and by detection of antineutrophilic cytoplasmic antibody and is treatable with cyclophosphamide and other immune suppressants.[256]

Systemic lupus erythematosus (SLE) is a multi-system autoimmune connective tissue disorder associated with hypercoagulability, endothelial dysfunction, cardiac embolic sources, and an increased risk of arterial hypertension.

Nervous system findings are quite common in patients with SLE.[257,258] Headaches that often share features with migraine, seizures, psychosis with decreased cognition, chorea, and mononeuropathies and polyneuropathies are important features of SLE.[257] The usual assumption has been that vasculitis underlies these diverse neurological syndromes. Necropsy and clinical studies, however, indicate that true arteritis is not a common cause of the CNS findings.[259,260] In a necropsy study, Johnson and Richardson found scant evidence of inflammation of brain arteries.[259]

Sudden-onset neurological signs do occur in patients with SLE and can be a prominent clinical feature. MRI often shows discrete focal lesions in patients with SLE usually in the absence of a clinical history of stroke.[260,261] The infarcts are of diverse causes. Small vessel vasculopathy with small deep infarcts and hemorrhages are usually caused by hypertension, which accompanies the renal disease of SLE. Cortical and cortical–subcortical infarcts are most often caused by abnormalities of coagulation and cardiac-origin embolism. Angiography often shows occlusion of intracranial artery branches.[262]

Hematological abnormalities are extremely common in SLE. The presence of lupus anticoagulant (LA) and antiphospholipid antibodies often correlates with clinical hypercoagulability, characterized by miscarriages, recurrent thrombophlebitis, and strokes.[263] Thrombocytopenia and other platelet abnormalities are also common, as is reduced prostacyclin activity.[264] In a 1988 clinicopathological study of 50 patients dying with SLE, a syndrome clinically resembling thrombotic thrombocytopenic purpura (TTP) developed in 14 patients (28%).[260] Seven of these 14 patients had platelet-thrombi occluding their capillaries and arteries, segmental subendothelial hyalin deposits, and arteriolar microaneurysms at necropsy – findings typical for TTP.[260] In this same study, vasculitis was not seen in the brain or spinal cord in any of the 50 patients.

Echocardiography in patients with SLE shows a high frequency of valvular disease, especially Libman–Sacks endocarditis.[265] Other heart lesions are also common. In their clinicopathological study, Devinsky et al. found that 25 of 50 patients had cardiac lesions that were potential sources of brain emboli.[260] These included Libman–Sacks vegetations (8 patients), acute and chronic mitral valvulitis (12 patients), marantic endocarditis (2 patients), and bacterial endocarditis (1 patient). Two patients had mural thrombi – one in the left atrium and one in the left ventricle.[260] Endocarditis in SLE is discussed in more detail in Chapter 10. Myocarditis is also a feature of SLE. Evaluation of patients with SLE who have focal neurological signs or focal lesions on MRI should include thorough hematological and cardiac evaluation.

Thrombotic thrombocytopenic purpura (TTP) is characterized clinically by fever, renal failure, thrombocytopenia, and microangiopathic hemolytic anemia.[266–269] Abnormalities of the metabolic pathway of von Willebrand factor (vWF), particularly of its cleaving protease, are thought to be important in the pathogenesis of TTP.[266] Platelet-rich thrombi fill arterioles and capillaries, causing microinfarcts within the brain. Transient focal neurological signs, which improve quickly,

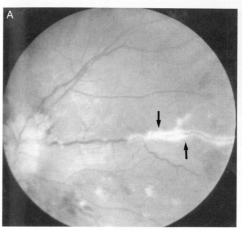
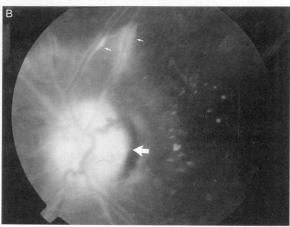

Figure 12.14 Retinal fundus photographs of patients with sarcoidosis illustrating periphlebitis. (A) Extensive focal perivenous sheathing (black arrows). From Forbes CD, Jackson WF. *A Color Atlas and Text of Clinical Medicine.* London: Mosby, 1993 with permission. (B) Perivenous sheathing is prominent, involving the veins at the top of the fundus photograph (small white arrows). The optic disc is pale and atrophic (large white arrow). Courtesy of Dr Larry Frohman, University of New Jersey School of Medicine, New Jersey, NJ.

and a more diffuse encephalopathy are common clinical features. Some reports note that neurological deficits occasionally persist, and occlusions of large intracranial arteries and their branches are sometimes found.[266,270,271] Brain hemorrhages have also been reported.[272] Some patients with TTP develop an encephalopathy associated with headache, seizures, and visual loss, accompanied by reversible brain-imaging abnormalities predominantly located in the posterior portions of the cerebral hemispheres.[272] This reversible posterior leukoencephalopathy syndrome is related to altered renal function and probably represents a "capillary leak" syndrome that is potentially reversible.[273] Modern neuroimaging might show in the future that strokes are rather common in TTP, but are usually minor and non-disabling. Some drugs, including ticlopidine and clopidogrel, are reported to cause TTP.[274–276] Plasma exchange can be an effective treatment, so this condition is important to recognize.[277]

Severe *rheumatoid arthritis (RA)* can be complicated by neuropathies, meningitis, and rheumatoid dural nodules. True arteritis with fibrinoid necrosis is occasionally seen and can cause an encephalopathy or multifocal small infarcts.[232,278–281] In patients with active RA, levels of fibrinogen, fibrinogen turnover, and fibrin degradation products are increased.[278–282] Also, high titers of circulating rheumatoid factor can cause a hyperviscosity syndrome.[283] Undoubtedly, these serological changes contribute to brain infarcts in patients with RA.

Patients with **Sjögren's syndrome** often have a neuropathy, especially involving the trigeminal nerves.[284] These patients also often have cognitive and behavioral abnormalities.[285,286] In a neuroimaging study of 38 patients with Sjögren's syndrome, 8 patients had focal neurological deficits – most often hemiparesis, aphasia, and ataxia, as well as other cognitive and behavioral abnormalities.[286] MRI in this study showed CNS abnormalities in 75% of patients, most often in the white matter. Occasionally, discrete cortical lesions were seen that resembled infarcts.[286] Vasculitis has been found at necropsy in patients with Sjögren's syndrome, but many of the lesions clinically and on MRI resemble multiple sclerosis, and are likely due to demyelination rather than brain infarcts.[286,287]

Headache is common in patients with **systemic sclerosis (scleroderma).** Occasionally, brain infarcts and SAH are reported.[288–290] Hypertension is common in scleroderma, and some of the neurovascular symptoms are probably caused by high blood pressure and reversible vasoconstriction.

Sarcoidosis[291–299]

Sarcoidosis causes a variety of CNS manifestations, including intraparenchymatous granulomas, meningitis, and myelopathy.[291–293] Sarcoidosis occasionally causes a cerebral vasculitis almost invariably accompanied by a CSF pleocytosis. The vasculitic form of sarcoidosis primarily affects the eyes, meninges, and cerebral arteries and veins. Retinal inflammatory changes are also often present.[294–297] The cerebrovascular abnormalities probably represent spread of inflammatory cells from the meninges through Virchow–Robin spaces to the smaller pial vessels. Veins are predominantly affected, so the vascular lesion is probably most accurately classified as a phlebitis or venulitis.[298] Periphlebitis can be noted on ophthalmoscopic examination. The retinal lesions are characterized by a yellowish-white focal or diffuse sheathing of retinal veins. Figure 12.14 shows fundus photographs that illustrate the periphlebitis. Hard exudates, sometimes termed *taches de bougie* because of their resemblance to candle-wax drippings, are often related to the periphlebitis and can leave white chorioretinal scars.[295,299]

TIAs, strokes, and evidence of meningeal, hypothalamic, and pituitary dysfunction are the clinical features of angiitic neurosarcoidosis, a disorder that can also affect the spinal cord, peripheral nervous system, and muscle. The periphlebitis and meningitis often respond to corticosteroids when given in substantial doses and over long periods (e.g., 60 mg of prednisone daily for 3–6 months or more). Immunosuppressant drugs, such as immuran, cyclosporine, and methotrexate, have been used with success in some patients.

Relapsing polychondritis[300]

Cerebral arteritis has been described in relapsing polychondritis, a rare disorder of cartilage characterized by auricular, nasal, and laryngotracheal chondritis, producing a saddle nose and

floppy ear deformities. Vasculitis may affect small, medium, and large vessels. Cardiovascular involvement is present in up to half of the patients. Aortic regurgitation is a frequent complication. Neurological involvement occurs in 3% of patients and includes meningoencephalitis, seizures, strokes, SAH, dementia, cerebellar and cranial nerve involvement. Corticosteroids may be effective in some patients.[300]

Giant cell (temporal) arteritis[301–309]

Giant cell arteritis usually affects older men and women.[301–303] Although the branches of the ECA, especially the superficial temporal and occipital arteries, are most frequently involved, the ICA, ECVA, subclavian, coronary, femoral, and even intracranial arteries can be affected.[302–305] Blindness is caused by granulomatous arteritis in the arteries supplying the optic nerve and retina.[301,303] The lesions most often causing strokes are located in the distal extracranial ICAs as they enter the carotid siphon and in the distal ECVAs.[305,306] Rarely, patients have been described with encephalopathy and multifocal neurological signs who have the findings of temporal arteritis in pial and brain arteries.[307] Occasional patients present with vascular dementia.[308]

Temporal arteritis usually presents as a systemic illness. Patients often develop headaches that differ from past headaches. Headaches are not pulsatile and are accompanied by aching in the proximal muscles, low-grade fever, weight loss, malaise, fatigue, and jaw claudication. Jaw claudication results from ischemia of the masseter muscles supplied by branches of the ECAs. The superficial temporal arteries may be tender, cord-like, and non-pulsatile, and the scalp may be diffusely tender. The best-known and most feared complication is loss of vision. An ischemic optic neuropathy results from occlusion of the short posterior ciliary arteries. Additionally, occlusion of the central retinal artery can lead to an ischemic retina. If vision loss occurs, it is usually severe. Involvement of one eye is often followed by involvement of the other.[302,303] Cerebral infarction occurs less often than ischemic optic neuropathy, and is more likely to involve the vertebrobasilar circulation. Infarction of the occipital cortex can cause cortical blindness. Cerebellar infarction and spinal cord ischemia have been reported. Laboratory findings that may be of help are an elevated erythrocyte sedimentation rate (ESR), elevated CRP, elevated fibrinogen levels, slight anemia, and an elevated leukocyte count.[302] Temporal arteritis may be present with a normal erythrocyte sedimentation rate. Color duplex ultrasonography of the superficial temporal arteries and their major branches may show stenoses, occlusions, or a diagnostic hypoechoic halo around the perfused lumen of the arteries.[309] Biopsy of the temporal artery is the most secure manner to make the diagnosis. Angiography with opacification of the ECA branches and the intracranial circulation can be suggestive. If possible, one should choose to biopsy a smaller scalp branch of the superficial temporal artery. It is best to biopsy a segment of artery identified as abnormal by palpation, ultrasonography, or angiography. A long segment of the artery is taken to avoid possible skip lesions, but the major portion of this artery is preserved. It is important to look for the general features of temporal arteritis in elderly patients with stroke. Stroke, however, is rarely the first manifestation of temporal arteritis.

Treatment with prednisone (60–80 mg/day) is begun before biopsy in patients with clinically probable temporal arteritis. In such patients, rapid relief of headache and other systemic symptoms usually occurs. Steroids are tapered by titrating the dose against the symptoms and the erythrocyte sedimentation rate. Treatment does not reverse established central or ocular ischemia but helps prevent further involvement of blood vessels.

Primary angiitis of the central nervous system[310–318]

In some patients, arteritis is limited to the CNS. This syndrome of primary angiitis of the CNS (PACNS), also called granulomatous angiitis and giant cell granulomatous angiitis of the CNS, is rare and can be difficult to diagnose.[310,311] Any age can be affected (mean age is approximately 49 years) and males predominate (nearly 2 to 1).[310,312] The disorder can be acute, with symptoms developing within a few weeks, or it can evolve during a period of months to years.[312,313] Usually, the clinical picture is that of a diffuse or multifocal encephalopathy.[310–316] Cognitive and behavioral changes are found in more than 60% of patients and headache, asymmetric motor signs, somnolence, and seizures are common findings.[312–315] Occasionally, TIAs or sudden strokes are described.[310–313] A myelopathy may also be present.[312,313] Focal signs may occur at onset, but more often step-like worsening punctuates the course of a progressive multifocal encephalopathy. The ESR is elevated in approximately two-thirds of patients, but other serological and systemic tests are not helpful.[312] The CSF usually has a slight-to-moderate lymphocytic pleocytosis, and the CSF protein is usually high (80%), often higher than 100 mg/dL.[312]

CT and MRI may show small or large focal lesions, usually infarcts, but small hematomas and hemorrhagic infarcts have also been noted.[312,317] In approximately one-half of the patients, angiography is abnormal and shows segmental narrowing and sausage-shaped dilatation of arteries ("beading").[312,317,318] In some patients, angiography is completely normal or shows non-specific abnormalities.[316,317] Segmental vascular narrowing is also found in patients who abuse drugs and in reversible vasoconstriction syndromes (RCVS), so this angiographic finding is not specific for arteritis. In fact, RCVS is many times more common than PACNS. Figure 12.15 shows a patient who had a RCVS and illustrates vascular narrowing and dilatation that is often misdiagnosed by radiologists as representing an arteritis.

Biopsy or necropsy shows a segmental, necrotizing granulomatous vasculitis affecting mostly the leptomeningeal, cortical, and spinal vessels. Any size artery or vein can be involved, but usually vessels 200–500 μm in diameter are most affected. In some patients, granulomatous changes have been predominantly venular.[312,313] The intima and adventitia of arteries are infiltrated with lymphocytes, giant cells, and granulomas.

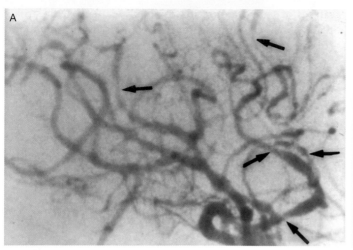
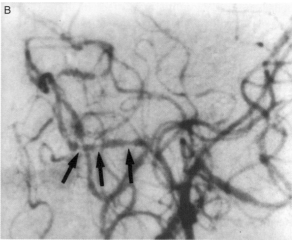

Figure 12.15 Carotid artery angiograms, intracranial magnified views from a patient with a reversible vasoconstriction syndrome. The black arrows point to focal regions of narrowing of arterial branches. Sausage-like dilatations are also present.

Granulomas can extend into the adjacent brain parenchyma. Specific diagnosis is important because treatment with prednisone and immunosuppressant agents, such as cyclophosphamide, may allow recovery from a disease that is nearly always fatal when untreated.[310,312,315] Biopsy should be pursued in patients with multifocal lesions and encephalopathy, especially if they have a CSF pleocytosis and a high-protein content. Moore urges biopsy of the non-dominant hemisphere, especially the tip of the temporal lobe, choosing tissue that contains a longitudinally oriented surface vessel.[315]

Takayasu's arteritis[319-335]

Takayasu's arteritis, also known as *pulseless disease*, is a chronic panarteritis localized to the aorta and its proximal branches (aortic arch or its branches, the ascending thoracic aorta, the abdominal aorta, or the entire aorta). Takayasu's arteritis was originally described in young Japanese girls and women.[319,320] The condition is well known in other countries, but is still uncommon in North America.[321] Although girls and women are predominantly affected, often at young ages, in India middle aged men develop a similar clinical picture.[322] Some patients have a prodromal phase of malaise, fever, and night sweats, and laboratory analysis reveals anemia and an increased sedimentation rate. Later, severe occlusive disease of the aortic arch and its branches develops, often leading to absent neck and limb pulses.[320-324]

Surprisingly, strokes or focal neurological signs are not the predominant clinical feature. Headache, dizziness, syncope, and visual blurring are more common. In some patients, neurological function is well preserved despite striking radiological signs of occlusion of vessels at their origin from the aortic arch.[325] Occlusions, stenosis, luminal irregularities, and ectasia or aneurysm formation are found. The most common sites of involvement are the midportion of the left CCA, left and right subclavian arteries, and the midportion of the innominate artery.[326-328] The inflammatory process involves the media and adventitia, which are infiltrated with plasma cells, lymphocytes, and histiocytes.[326-329] During the inflammatory stage, elastic fibers and smooth muscle cells are destroyed. After the inflammatory stage subsides, fibrosis replaces the damaged portions of the arterial intima, media, and adventitia.[329] The intracranial arteries,[330] heart, and heart valves are sometimes involved.[322,331]

The diagnosis of Takayasu's arteritis can often be made by ultrasonography. Duplex scans invariably show bilateral involvement in the proximal portions of the CCAs, consisting of long segments of concentric thickening of the arterial walls.[332] The subclavian artery lesions are also readily shown by ultrasonography.[332] Ultrasound can also be used to monitor the lesions and their response to treatment.

Arm and leg claudication is commonly related to the subclavian, aortic, and iliofemoral disease. Hypertension is present in more than one-half of the patients and may be difficult to control. The chronic proximal occlusive disease often leads to retinal microaneurysms and arteriovenous anastomoses. Vision loss can result from chronic eye ischemia.[333] The proximal occlusive disease leads to extensive collateral circulation. Hypertension and increased flow through collateral channels can cause SAHs and ICHs similar to that found in the moyamoya syndrome. Corticosteroids, immunosuppressive therapy, angioplasty, and surgical bypass treatment[329,334] have all been used. Corticosteroids (prednisone 30 mg/day initially, then tapered to 5–10 mg/day maintenance) may prevent or diminish vascular complications.[319,329,335]

Thromboangiitis obliterans (Buerger's disease)[336]

Thromboangiitis obliterans (Buerger's disease) is characterized by distal arterial occlusive disease of the limbs, with or without recurrent superficial thrombophlebitis, occurring mainly in adult men smokers in the fourth or fifth decades of life. Immunologic studies implicate a hypersensitivity reaction directed against arterial antigens. Cessation of tobacco products is critical.[336]

Behçet's disease[337–350]

Behçet's disease is a relapsing, remitting illness first described by a Turkish dermatologist who recognized the triad of oral ulcers, genital ulcers, and uveitis.[337,338] The disease is most often found in Turkey, Saudi Arabia, Mediterranean countries, and Japan but does occur in North America, Europe, and worldwide. Behçet's disease is important for neurologists to recognize. The predominant clinical systemic findings are aphthous ulcers in the mouth and genital tissues, uveitis, synovitis, other skin findings (e.g., folliculitis and erythema nodosum), ulcerative lesions in the bowel mucosa (especially the colon), and thrombophlebitis.[339–341] The disorder affects mostly young adults in their twenties. The male–female ratio ranges from 2 to 1 to 4 to 1.[338–343] Neurological involvement probably occurs in approximately 6–10% of patients. Among a large series containing 323 patients with Behçet's disease followed in a clinic in Turkey, only 46 patients were referred because of headache and neurological signs and only 17 patients (5.3%) had neurological abnormalities.[339]

The most common neurological syndromes are: (1) a meningoencephalitis form, in which headache is the major symptom; (2) an encephalitic form, with gradually evolving multifocal signs; (3) strokes, characterized by relatively acute-onset focal signs; and (4) headache, with papilledema caused by dural venous sinus thrombosis.[333,339–349] Characteristically, the neurological signs occur during attacks with remissions between, a course that closely mimics multiple sclerosis. CT and MRI show that the most frequent sites of involvement are the pons and midbrain, followed by the basal ganglia and thalamus. The lesions most often are small foci that have high signals on T2-weighted MRI images and are isointense or hypointense on T1-weighted images.[342,343] Some lesions are large. The brainstem lesions often do not conform to arterial territories and are larger than those found in arteritis.[340] The spinal cord is also often involved clinically and by MRI. The lesions often contain hemosiderin, and the distribution in gray and white matter separates the lesions from those found in multiple sclerosis. Usually, angiography does not show arterial abnormalities.

The CSF is almost always abnormal, including pleocytosis, high-protein content, and increased levels of immunoglobulins, that are produced intrathecally.[350] The CSF pressure is sometimes elevated. The levels of oligoclonal bands of IgA and IgM correlate well with neurological disease activity and are useful to follow. At necropsy, there often is a diffuse meningoencephalitis with perivascular lymphocytic cuffing predominantly around veins, venules, and capillaries, with occasional arterial involvement.[345,346] The dural sinuses and large veins may be occluded.[337,344,347,349] Thromboses of leg veins and even the vena cava are important systemic features, and the pathology is predominantly venous. The brain shows areas of necrosis, demyelination, and scarring, especially in the rostral brainstem, internal capsule, and basal ganglia, as well as in the spinal cord. The lesions probably represent focal hemorrhagic venous infarcts and areas of encephalitic change. Corticosteroids may suppress ocular and brain symptoms.[344]

Cogan's syndrome[351–356]

David Cogan described a syndrome of non-syphilitic interstitial keratitis with vestibulo-auditory dysfunction.[351] The condition is probably an autoimmune vasculitic disorder that affects young adults. The earliest symptoms are photophobia, reduced vision, and redness of the eyes.[352–354] An interstitial keratitis is found on ophthalmological examination, occasionally with uveitis. Blindness can result from corneal opacification. Tinnitus, reduced hearing, vertigo, and ataxia appear before, during, or after eye abnormalities.[352,354] Microscopic study shows a vasculitis of small- and medium-sized arteries. Some patients have fever, and the aortic valve and bowel may be involved.[352,353] The aorta is occasionally involved, causing aortitis and aortic aneurysm formation.[352,355] Some patients have an accompanying meningo-encephalitis,[352] intracranial vascular regions of constriction and dilatation and ectasia have been reported but are quite rare in Cogan's syndrome.[352,356]

Eales's disease[357–365]

Eales described an ocular condition characterized by abnormal retinal vessels and recurrent vitreous hemorrhages.[357,358] The condition that Eales described is probably not a specific disease entity, but is a retinopathy found in a variety of vascular retinal conditions.[358,359] Eales-type retinopathy affects mostly young men and is most common in the Middle East and India. Visual symptoms include specks, floaters, cobwebs, curtains, and blurred vision.[360] The visual symptoms are caused by retinal periphlebitis, non-perfusion of retinal capillaries, and vitreous hemorrhages.[358–360] Some patients have extensive retinal revascularization and fibrovascular proliferation.[358]

Ophthalmological examination shows prominent sheathing of veins and arteries, flame-shaped retinal hemorrhages, and vitreous hemorrhages. Although the symptoms usually begin in one eye, both eyes are invariably involved. The macular arteries are relatively spared, so that central vision is often preserved.[359] A vasculitis affecting both retinal arteries and veins causes the eye findings. Sometimes, the uvea is also involved.

CNS involvement has been described in the form of meningitis, focal infarcts, and vascular occlusions.[358,361–365] In one patient, a left cerebral infarct was caused by MCA occlusion.[362] Spinal cord involvement has also been reported.[364] Usually, there are no systemic symptoms or characteristic laboratory abnormalities, although the CSF may show a pleocytosis.[362] Diagnosis is made on the basis of the characteristic ophthalmoscopic abnormalities.

Microangiopathy of the brain, ear, and retina[366–373]

An unusual, but distinct, occlusive vascular disorder was called *microangiopathy of the brain and retina* by Susac and colleagues.[366–369] Although this condition (also called **Susac's syndrome** and retinocochleocerebral vasculopathy[370]) resembles granulomatous angiitis in some ways, there are important differences. In microangiopathy of the brain and retina, there

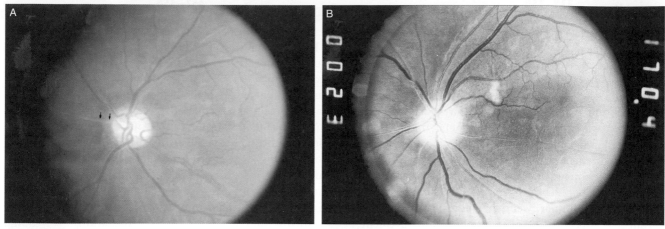

Figure 12.16 Retinal fundus photographs of a patient with microangiopathy of the brain and retina. (A) Small black arrows point to a white occluded retinal artery. The other arteries are also attenuated. The larger vessels are veins. The optic disc is very pale and atrophic. (B) The other eye shows many occluded and attenuated retinal arteries. Fluffy exudates and pale regions of retina are also shown. The optic disc is chalky white. The patient was blind because of the retinal arterial disease. Courtesy of Dr Thomas Hedges III.

is always obliteration of large retinal arteries, causing gradual, severe, bilateral visual loss.[366–373] The retinal vascular abnormalities are easily seen through the ophthalmoscope. Some retinal arteries are amputated, whereas others are severely narrowed or attenuated and light streaking characterizes their thickened arterial walls. Figure 12.16 shows photographs of the ocular fundus in a patient with this condition. Tinnitus and hearing loss are also prominent.

The most important clinical neurological signs are cognitive and behavioral abnormalities, bilateral motor weakness with pyramidal signs, and cerebellar dysfunction. MRI often shows small increased signal foci on T2-weighted brain imaging, located in both gray and white matter but usually involving the corpus callosum.[369] The condition affects mostly young women in their second to fourth decade and it usually progresses stepwise or gradually. The CSF protein is high, sometimes more than 1 g/dL, but usually there is no major pleocytosis. Brain biopsy has shown obliteration of small arteries without prominent inflammation or granulomas, as well as multiple microinfarcts.[366–373] Some patients with this condition have improved at least temporarily after corticosteroids and immunosuppressive therapy.[373]

Other oculocerebral arteriopathies[374–386]

Acute posterior, multifocal, placoid-pigment epitheliopathy was first described by J Donald Gass as an ophthalmological syndrome rather than a specific entity, that was characterized by "multiple cream-colored placoid lesions" located in the posterior pole at the level of the pigment epithelium and choroid.[374–376] It is an acute chorioretinal condition that usually develops in young adults often after a flu-like febrile illness.[374–378] Both eyes are usually affected simultaneously but sometimes sequentially. Symptoms include visual blurring, distortion, and scotomas. The optic fundus shows multiple, well-circumscribed, gray–white flat lesions at the level of the retinal pigment epithelium. Vision usually returns to normal after several weeks. Occasionally, however, patients develop

progressive disease with significant loss of vision.[378] A choroidal vasculitis is the posited cause. Headache, CSF pleocytosis, optic neuritis, and strokes have been reported.[374–381] Cerebral angiography sometimes shows an arteritis.[378] In one patient, brain histopathology showed focal granulomatous inflammation of medium-sized arteries.[382]

Vogt–Koyanagi–Harada syndrome is an important differential diagnostic consideration in patients with ocular inflammatory lesions. The disorder is often called uveo-meningo-encephalitis. Patients with this syndrome may have premature whitening of the hair and eyelashes, alopecia, vitiligo, iridocyclitis, choroiditis, and loss of hearing.[383] They may also have meningeal signs and a CSF pleocytosis.[383–386] An adhesive arachnoiditis develops and explains many of the symptoms. Fluorescein angiography shows leakage from retinal vessels. Papilledema and increased intracranial pressure can occur. Some patients have had prominent neurological signs but whether these were a manifestation of vascular inflammation is not clear. The clinical findings are similar to Behçet's disease except for the absence of dermatological abnormalities. Usually, the disorder remits after 6–12 months, but there may be recurrences.

We have seen a number of patients during the years with ocular inflammatory disorders with vascular abnormalities that involve the iris, aqueous and vitreous humors and the retina who also have had CSF pleocytosis, headache, neurological signs, and MRI lesions that could represent infarcts. These patients did not have illnesses that correspond to the commonly recognized oculocerebral vasculopathies. Many other arteriopathies probably exist that have a predilection for the eye and nervous system, among other organ involvement.

Sneddon's syndrome[387–394]

Sneddon's syndrome is characterized by livedo reticularis, and recurrent strokes. This syndrome is often found in young patients without risk factors for stroke.[387–391] The most

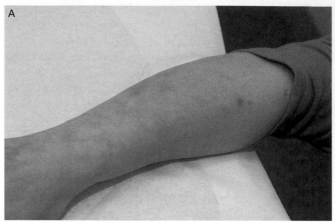 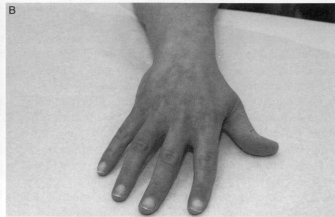

Figure 12.17 Photographs of the (A) arm and (B) hand of a patient with Sneddon's syndrome showing livedo reticularis.

important and diagnostic clinical feature is livedo reticularis, a bluish-gray mottling of the skin that usually involves the trunk and all limbs (Figure 12.17). The cutaneous findings are obvious by simply looking at the skin with the patient undressed. A cold environment makes the skin abnormality more obvious. Usually, the hands and feet are cold and peripheral pulses are reduced. Hand angiography may show dramatic occlusions of digital arteries with areas of narrowing and dilatation.[391] Skin biopsy may show distinctive abnormalities. Small- to medium-sized arteries at the border between the dermis and subcutis show early inflammatory lesions followed by subendothelial proliferation and later, fibrosis.[391]

We have also seen many patients with irregular grayish areas of irregular mottling of the skin especially in the thighs and proximal arms and trunk whose findings would not qualify for livedo reticularis who have had otherwise unexplained penetrating artery-related brain infarcts. Others have had migraine, and we wonder if their skin vascular abnormalities could be a window into a more generalized endotheliopathy or vascular contractile disorder that includes the blood vessels in the brain.

The neurological findings in patients with Sneddon's syndrome are explained by multiple acute-onset strokes. CT and MRI often show multiple infarcts in the cerebral cortex and white matter.[387,389–391] Cerebral angiography often shows branch occlusions of intracranial arteries.[388,392] At times, the disorder is familial.[393] Some patients with Sneddon's syndrome have antiphospholipid antibodies.[387,394] Valvular cardiac abnormalities are also relatively common in patients with Sneddon's syndrome, and some of the brain infarcts may be caused by cardiac-origin embolism.[389,393,394]

The skin vasculature may provide a clue to the small vessels within the eye and brain. It is essential to examine stroke patients undressed to ensure inspection of the trunk and extremities for skin abnormalities.

Kohlmeier–Degos syndrome[395–399]

Kohlmeier–Degos syndrome, also called malignant atrophic papulosis, is an unusual vascular occlusive disorder with characteristic skin changes.[395,396] The condition can begin at any

age and has been described in children.[396] The skin lesions begin as small, yellow-pink raised lesions, usually on the trunk and arms.[395–398] The central part of the skin lesions becomes atrophic and looks porcelain-white, flat, and depressed, and each lesion is surrounded by a raised pink zone, often with telangiectasis.[397] Small- and medium-sized arteries in the skin undergo a progressive fibrosis with infarcts of the skin.[395–399] Skin biopsy shows fibrous proliferation between the intima and internal elastica with rare inflammatory changes.[397–399] The bowel is also commonly involved, causing ulcers, decreased motility, bowel dilatation, and, often, perforation.[395–399] Although the vessels in other visceral organs are often involved at necropsy, systemic symptoms are usually limited to the skin and gut.

CNS symptoms occur in approximately one-fifth of patients with Kohlmeier–Degos syndrome.[397] Strokes do occur. Brain imaging shows infarcts and small hemorrhages. Angiography may show occlusion and beading of distal branches of intracranial arteries.[397] Neuropathological examination shows hyalinization or fibrous proliferation between the endothelium and internal elastic membrane, often with superimposed thrombosis.[395–399] Inflammatory abnormalities are slight or absent. Occasionally, SAH and dural sinus thrombosis are present.[397,399] At times, strokes precede skin and bowel involvement. Kohlmeier–Degos syndrome is often fatal, but some patients may have remissions.[399]

Vasculopathy in drug abusers[400–425]

Drug abuse has become an important cause of stroke in adolescents and young adults. ICH caused by drugs is considered in Chapter 14 and is most often caused by amphetamines and cocaine.[400] Ischemic stroke usually relates to one of five different situations: (1) heroin addiction; (2) amphetamine abuse; (3) abuse of drugs synthesized for oral use; (4) infection as a complication of an addictive lifestyle; and (5) cocaine use.

Heroin addiction[400–407]

Strokes in heroin addicts are most often ischemic and may be cerebral or spinal. Stroke frequently follows the reintroduction

of intravenous heroin after a period of abstinence.[401–405] Brain ischemia may directly follow the heroin injection but is more often delayed by 6–24 hours. Heroin addicts also often have serological and systemic abnormalities, including eosinophilia, elevated immune globulins and gamma globulins, false-positive serology, Coombs-positive hemolysis, and lymph-node hypertrophy.[404] Increased binding of serum globulins by morphine has been found in rabbits with implanted morphine pellets. In some narcotic addicts, morphine also binds gamma globulins.[406] Illicitly available heroin is often adulterated with a host of fillers and foreign substances. These observations make it likely that immune-complex deposition or other hyperimmune mechanisms underlie the strokes in patients who are chronically exposed to many recurrently introduced antigens.[404] Definitive immunological or pathological studies of strokes in heroin addicts are wanting.

Amphetamine use[407,408]

A number of amphetamine-like substances are used or abused, including dextroamphetamine, methamphetamine, methylphenidate, ephedrine, and pseudoephedrine.[401] More recently synthetic amphetamine-containing preparations have become available on the streets and are widely used and abused such as Ecstasy, Speed and Base, and Ice. Stimulation is the commonest reason for abuse, while weight-loss preparations and some cold remedies also often had contained amphetamine-like substances. Brain hemorrhages are more common after methamphetamine abuse than brain ischemia. Infarcts are sometimes seen at necropsy but a clinical ischemic stroke is unusual. Hemorrhages usually develop soon after amphetamine use and are caused by the sudden elevation in blood pressure induced by the surge of catecholamines.[400] Hypertension is likely an idiosyncratic reaction to phenylpropanolamine in some individuals.

In some patients with amphetamine abuse, necrotizing angiitis has been shown pathologically. The lesions resemble polyarteritis nodosa and can affect the brain and other viscera.[407] In experimental animals[408] and humans[409] who have taken amphetamines orally or intravenously, angiography shows segmental changes in intracerebral arteries with prominent beading. Patients with SAH or ICH after amphetamine abuse have a relatively low frequency of harboring aneurysms and vascular malformations that are the source of intracranial bleeding.[400]

Abuse of drugs synthesized for oral use[410–414]

A different pattern of disease affects patients who inject intravenous drugs that have been designed for oral use; methylphenidate (Ritalin) and pentazocine (Talwin) with pyribenzamine are the best-documented drugs. These compounds contain talc, microcrystalline cellulose, and other fillers that are used to maintain the chemicals in pill form. Addicts mash the pills, dissolve them in tap water, and inject them intravenously or even directly into the carotid artery.[410] Particles of drugs and fillers still remain in the fluid injected and are trapped by the lung arterioles and small arteries, causing an obliterative arteritis.[410,411] Pulmonary arteriovenous shunts develop and passage through these shunts is probably responsible for crystals that reach the brain and eyes of addicts.[410–412] Strokes and seizures usually follow quickly after intravenous injection. Deep, small cerebral arteries, such as the lenticulostriate[410] and anterior spinal arteries, are most often affected.[413] Talc particles may be seen within the retinal vessels on ophthalmoscopy.[414]

Infection as a complication of an addictive lifestyle

Drug abusers seldom follow strict sterile precautions. Hepatitis, AIDS, infective endocarditis, and fungal infections are common complications of their habit and lifestyle. Endocarditis can cause embolic strokes. Fungal infections, especially *Nocardia* and *Aspergillus*, can cause focal necrotic infarcts or brain abscesses.[181,183,184]

Cocaine use[415–425]

Cocaine use has become the most common cause of drug-related strokes. Cocaine use is rampant. In a 1990 study among 214 patients aged 15–44 years admitted to the San Francisco General Hospital during a 10-year period, 34% were drug users and cocaine was the predominant drug used.[415] Cocaine is snorted or injected as cocaine hydrochloride or is smoked as the free-base alkaloidal form, usually called crack cocaine.[401,405,416–418] Crack cocaine is made by mixing aqueous cocaine hydrochloride with ammonia and sometimes baking soda. The free-base cocaine is usually smoked after the cocaine has become alkalinized and precipitated. Crack cocaine induces a more rapid increase in blood levels than cocaine hydrochloride and produces a more rapid high than does snorted or injected cocaine hydrochloride. Its use is associated with a higher frequency of brain infarcts.[401,405,419] The strokes usually begin shortly after cocaine use, irrespective of the portal of entry (snorted, inhaled, or injected). Brain infarcts have a predilection for the brainstem.[420] Spinal cord infarcts also have been reported to develop soon after cocaine use.[421] The mechanism of ischemia is unknown but vasoconstriction related to cocaine itself or its metabolites is the major posited mechanism. Bowel and myocardial ischemia and an eosinophilic myocarditis are also found after chronic cocaine abuse.[401,422] Many patients drink alcohol while using cocaine. There appears to be a synergism between cocaine and ethanol.[401,422] Cocaine is metabolized in the presence of ethanol to cocaethylene, which binds more powerfully than cocaine itself to monoamine transporter proteins.[401,423]

Vasoconstriction, increased platelet aggregation, and apparent vasculitis are posited as potential causes of stroke in cocaine users. Arterial constrictions (predominantly MCAs and PCAs (focal and diffuse)) were found on MRA studies taken 20 minutes after intravenous cocaine administration in healthy subjects who had previously used cocaine but were not addicts.[424]

Cocaine use is also associated with SAHs and ICHs.[400,401,425] For unclear reasons, there is a higher incidence of aneurysms and

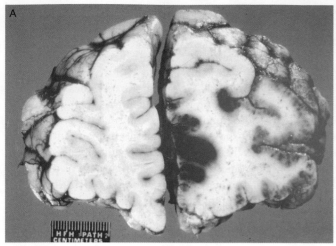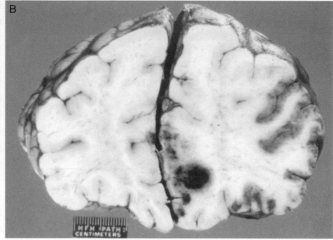

Figure 12.18 Brain specimens at necropsy in a patient who died after crack cocaine use. Multiple brain hemorrhages and brain edema are shown. Courtesy of Dr Steven Levine.

vascular malformations in cocaine-related hemorrhages than in hemorrhages after amphetamines.[390,400] Angiography should be performed unless the cocaine-related hemorrhage is in a characteristic location for hypertensive ICH. Cocaine also enhances vasospasm after aneurysmal SAH.[401] Cocaine users can also develop a picture that resembles hypertensive encephalopathy with multiple hemorrhages and brain edema. Figure 12.18 is a brain specimen that illustrates hypertensive encephalopathy with hemorrhages after cocaine use.

Migraine and vasoconstriction syndromes[426–464]

Vascular headaches are among the most common disorders treated by physicians and neurologists. Migraine is prevalent at all ages, including young children and the elderly. Although migraine most likely begins with a discharge within the brain, vasoconstriction is an important part of the migraine syndrome.[426–428] A genetic tendency for migraine also predisposes patients to a number of neurologic syndromes in which reversible vasoconstriction plays an important role.[426–428] During migraine attacks, angiography, cerebral blood flow (CBF) studies, and TCD have clearly shown changes in intracranial vessel diameter, flow velocities, and CBF.[428] Reversible vasoconstriction has been shown to be an important cause of organ ischemia, especially in the coronary circulation and in the brain after subarachnoid bleeding. Migraine is a clinical diagnosis usually applied when there is a past history and family history of pulsating, usually unilateral headaches, with or without characteristic visual, somatosensory, or other migraine accompaniments and followed by nausea and vomiting. Although vasoconstriction and vasodilatation have been shown to occur during migraine attacks, not all vasoconstriction occurs in patients with migraine.

Neuroimaging in patients with migraine shows a more frequent-than-expected incidence of brain infarcts.[426,429] Migraine-related strokes have been the subject of a number of reports and case series.[426,428,430–433] Retrospective and prospective studies report an increased risk of ischemic stroke especially among migraineurs with aura.[434,435] A meta-analysis of several observational studies showed a twofold risk of ischemic stroke in patients with migraine and a threefold risk if migraine was accompanied with aura.[436] Stroke is especially common in young women who have migraine with aura for 12 or more years.[437]

Infarction can be caused by prolonged intense vasoconstriction,[426,427,438] causing permanent ischemia or thrombosis of arteries. Intense vasoconstriction can impede flow, promoting thrombosis; platelets are activated during migraine, and the vasoconstrictive process itself may stimulate the endothelium to release factors that promote thrombosis. Investigations on stroke within the PCA and basilar-artery territories in patients with migraine have shown that some patients develop thrombi within the basilar artery and the PCA.[428,432,439]

Migrainous accompaniments can precede, accompany, or follow headache and can occur in the absence of headache. Transient vasoconstriction accounts for many examples of temporary spells of neurologic dysfunction in the elderly,[440–442] including transient global amnesia.[426,428,443,444] Fisher[440,441] and Caplan[428] have attempted to distinguish migraine accompaniments from atherosclerotic ischemia by analyzing the clinical features (Table 12.4). To complicate matters, atherosclerotic lesions in the coronary arteries of humans and in the extracranial and retinal arteries of experimental animals seem to predispose them to superimposed vasoconstriction. Thus, vasoconstriction can complicate atherostenosis. TCD shows promise in identification of vasoconstriction by showing high velocities that change with time and various pharmacological treatments.

Call, Fleming, and colleagues called attention to a syndrome currently called **reversible cerebral vasoconstriction syndrome (RCVS)**.[427,445] RCVS most often affects young women, especially during the puerperium, but also occurs at menopause and is found at all ages. When it occurs after childbirth, the syndrome has been called postpartum angiopathy.[446] The onset is often with a severe thunderclap

Table 12.4 Migraine accompaniments versus atherosclerotic ischemia

Migraine	Atherosclerotic ischemia
Sensory modalities involved sequentially (e.g., vision, tactile, speech)	Modalities involved together (e.g., visual, somatosensory, and aphasic abnormalities noted at same time)
Within each modality, first symptoms are "positive" (e.g., visual brightness, shining, somatosensory paresthesias)	Usually negative symptoms (e.g., loss of vision, numbness)
Symptoms gradually progress within each modality; vision loss gradually affects field; paresthesias move from one finger to hand to body – often takes 20 min to travel fully	Visual field or body involved at once without spread
Within each modality, positive followed by negative (e.g., brightness leaves scotoma in its wake; paresthesias followed by numbness)	Usually negative effects only
One modality clears before the next is involved	Modalities are involved simultaneously
Headache most often follows after neurological symptoms have cleared	Headache accompanies persistent deficits or is absent
Attacks usually last 15–30 min (average, 20 min)	Attacks last usually about 1–2 min, often ≤5 min
Different attacks involve different sides and vascular territories	Attacks always involve the same vascular territory
Spells may occur over years and often begin in the 20–40-years of age span	Attacks occur during a span usually limited to days, weeks, or months; most patients are 50 years of age
Stroke risk factors often absent	Stroke risk factors present
Women predominate over men	Men predominate over women except after the menopausal years

headache.[447,448] Some patients have developed this syndrome after carotid endarterectomy.[449] The use of serotonin reuptake inhibitors prescribed for depression and cannabis, especially when smoked in a binge, can provoke the syndrome.[448,450] A more comprehensive list of conditions associated with RCVS are highlighted in Table 12.5.

Recurrent headache, focal neurological signs, and occasionally seizures are the predominant symptoms. Vasoconstriction involves many large, medium, and small-sized brain-supplying arteries. The clinical findings include severe headache, decreased alertness, seizures, and changing multifocal neurological signs. Brain edema and death can occur. Brain imaging may show focal subarachnoid blood on the surface of the brain,[448,451] and in adjacent sulci and small regions of abnormality on FLAIR-MRI representing small infarcts. Angiography shows sausage-shaped focal regions of vasodilatation and multifocal regions of vascular narrowing. Figure 12.15 shows angiographic abnormalities in a patient with RCVS. TCD shows high velocities in many intracranial arteries. At times the initial vascular imaging studies are normal and only become abnormal after a few days or a week.[448] There have been no therapeutic trials that have clearly defined optimal treatment and most patients recover within weeks or a few months. Corticosteroids, calcium-channel blockers (e.g., nimodipine, nicardipine), antiepileptic drugs (AEDs), intravenous magnesium, and treatments for increased intracranial pressure have been used to treat this disorder. In the experience of one of us (LRC) treatment early after symptom onset with verapamil has proven very effective in relieving symptoms and preventing major brain damage. Some evidence indicates that corticosteroid treatment is not effective and may be harmful. Its use is not recommended.[450–453] Many of the patients have had a history of migraine.

Two other important clinical syndromes that include migraine-like headache and neurologic signs are the Bartleson and SMART syndromes.[426] The syndrome of transient headache and neurological deficits with cerebrospinal fluid lymphocytosis (HaNDL syndrome) also referred to as Bartleson's syndrome[454] or pseudomigraine syndrome with temporary neurologic symptoms and lymphocytic pleocytosis (PMP syndrome) is characterized by attacks resembling migrainous auras that occur in a flurry and are accompanied by prominent headache and cerebrospinal fluid pleocytosis.[454–456] The CSF contains a lymphocytic predominant pleocytosis (>100 cells) and an elevated protein content. Many patients have recurrent aphasia sometimes associated with visual blurring or scotomata and with right limb sensory or motor dysfunction. Papilledema and CN VI palsy may also occur. The attacks are relatively stereotyped in individual patients and always involve either the left or right cerebral hemisphere in each attack. The attacks last between 15 and 60 minutes. Attacks may occur more than once a day and cluster during a period of 3–6 weeks. The condition may represent a primary migraine disorder with an inflammatory etiology but other possibilities include a viral meningovascular infection or some other undefined aseptic meningitis. In one patient the syndrome followed Herpesvirus 6 infection.[457] Diagnosis of HaNDL is challenging and requires careful exclusion of alternative diagnoses. The clinical course of HaNDL syndrome is typically self-limited, and lasts usually from 4 to 12 weeks. Treatment is symptomatic. Calcium-channel blockers, especially verapamil, and acetazolamide may be useful.

Stroke-like migraine attacks after radiation therapy (SMART) is a relatively new syndrome in which stroke-like migraine attacks occur as a late consequence of brain

Table 12.5 Conditions associated with the RCVS

Pregnancy and puerperium	Exposure to drugs and blood products	Miscellaneous
Early puerperium	Pseudoephedrine	Unruptured intracranial aneurysms
Late pregnancy	Ephedrine	Post-carotid endarterectomy
Pre-eclampsia	Ergotamine tartrate	Cervical artery dissections
Eclampsia	Methylergonovine	Hypercalcemia
Delayed postpartum eclampsia	Bromocriptine	Acute intermittent porphyria
	Lisuride	Pheochromocytoma
	Triptans	Bronchial carcinoid tumor
	Isometheptene	Head trauma
	Cocaine	Neurosurgical procedures
	SSRIs	Spinal subdural hematoma
	Methylenedioxymethamphetamine (Ecstasy)	Cerebrospinal fluid hypotension
	Amphetamines	Autonomic dysreflexia
	Marijuana	
	LSD	
	Tacrolimus	
	Cyclophosphamide	
	Erythropoietin	
	Intravenous immunoglobulin	
	Interferon alpha	
	Red blood cell transfusions	
	Binge drinking	
	Ginseng	
	Nicotine patches	

irradiation.[426,458,459] Attacks may begin years after radiation. The migraine-like events consist of prolonged, but usually reversible, neurological dysfunction that may persist for several weeks. Headaches are often but not always preceded by aura. MRI may show diffuse cortical enhancement that resolves. No pattern to date has been found that associates the dose of radiation, tumor type, or specific chemotherapeutic agents with the occurrence of this syndrome.[426,458-461]

ICH occasionally complicates a severe migraine attack.[426,462-464] Intense vasoconstriction leads to ischemia of a local brain region with edema and ischemia of the small vessels perfused by the constricted artery. When vasoconstriction abates, blood flow to the region is augmented and the reperfusion can cause hemorrhage from the damaged arteries and arterioles.[426,462-464] The mechanism is the same as that found in hemorrhage after carotid endarterectomy and in reperfusion after brain embolization.[464]

Preeclampsia/eclampsia[465-474]

Preeclampsia/eclampsia is a very important, serious, often life- and brain-threatening disorder of pregnancy and the early postpartum period that, like RCVS, includes cerebral vasoconstriction.[446,465-468] Preeclampsia is characterized by increased blood pressure over the usual base-line value and often proteinuria, hyperreflexia, and restlessness. If a seizure then occurs, the condition is called eclampsia. Severe preeclampsia and eclampsia can develop during the first days and weeks after delivery.

Although magnesium sulfate has been shown to prevent seizures it is not a very effective agent to reduce the hypertension and the blood pressure must be reduced. Brain hemorrhage, brain infarction, renal and liver failure, and the HELLP syndrome (hemolysis, elevated liver function tests, and low platelets) are important complications of inadequately treated preeclampsia and eclampsia. Vascular imaging testing in patients with eclampsia often shows reversible vasoconstriction identical to that found in non-pregnant women with the Call–Fleming syndrome discussed and illustrated above.[446,465-469]

One complication of eclampsia is the *posterior reversible encephalopathy syndrome (PRES)*.[470-474] The syndrome is characterized by agitation and restlessness, confusion, seizures, and visual dysfunction that includes visual hallucinations, hemianopia, visual neglect, and cortical blindness. Brain imaging most often shows white matter hyperintensities maximal in the occipital and posterior temporal white matter but sparing the paramedian occipital striate regions. Figure 12.19 shows CT and MRI scans in a patient with PRES. This syndrome is likely a capillary leak syndrome related to endothelial dysfunction and increased body fluid volumes. Many different conditions, including preeclampsia and eclampsia, are associated with the syndrome including: hypertensive encephalopathy, immunosuppressive drugs including cyclosporine and tacrolimus, pheochromocytoma, acute glomerulonephritis, and acute endocrinopathies (Table 12.6). Many are accompanied by increased blood pressure, proteinuria, and tissue edema. Experience has

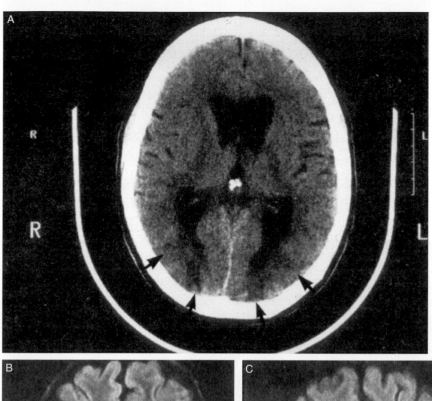

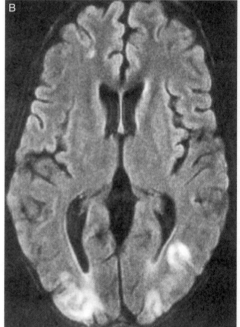
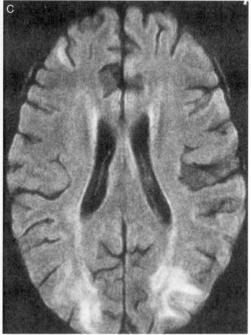

Figure 12.19 Posterior reversible leukoencephalopathy. (A) CT scan showing hypodensity in the occipital lobes. (B) and (C) T2-weighted MRI scans of same patient showing bilateral occipital temporal hyperintensities.

shown that the cortex as well as white matter are often involved, that the abnormalities can be frontal, brainstem, cerebellar, and diffuse and are not always limited to the posterior cerebral hemispheres, and in some patients irreversible tissue damage develops, especially if the blood pressure elevations and edema are not treated rapidly and effectively.[474]

Moyamoya syndrome[475–492]

Moyamoya, although sometimes referred to as a disease, is probably better thought of as a syndrome defined by a characteristic angiographic appearance.[475] The intracranial ICAs undergo progressive tapering and progressive occlusion at their intracranial bifurcations (the so-called T-portion of the ICAs). Basal penetrating branches of the ICAs, ACAs, and MCAs enlarge to provide collateral circulation. These vessels form large prominent anastomosing channels, basal telangiectasias, which appear on angiograms as a "cloud of smoke". These arteries are especially prominent because of the paucity of MCA sylvian branches. The appearance of these basal telangiectasias led Japanese clinicians to use the non-medical term moyamoya, which colloquially means "something is hazy, vague or indescribable, like 'a puff of smoke drifting in the

Table 12.6 Disorders associated with PRES

Hypertensive encephalopathy

Toxemia of pregnancy

- Preeclampsia/eclampsia

Acute/chronic renal disease

Pheochromocytoma, primary aldosteronism, Cushing disease

Post-transplantation

- Bone marrow

Infection/sepsis

- Systemic inflammatory response syndrome
- Multiorgan dysfunction syndrome

Autoimmune disease

- SLE
- Scleroderma
- P-ANCA granulomatosis with polyangiitis
- Polyarteritis nodosa

Post-cancer chemotherapy

- Cytarabine
- Cisplatin
- L-asparaginase
- Gemcitabine
- Tiazofurin
- Bevacizumab (avastin)
- Bortezomib
- Vincristine
- Kinase inhibitor BAY 34–9006
- Intrathecal chemotherapy
- Combination chemotherapy

Miscellaneous

- Hypomagnesemia
- Hypercalcemia/hypocalcemia
- Hypocholesterolemia
- Guillain–Barré syndrome
- Acute intermittent porphyria
- Cocaine, amphetamines, over-the-counter stimulants (ephedrine, pseudoephedrine)
- Dialysis/erythropoietin
- Triple H therapy
- Blood transfusion
- Tumor lysis syndrome
- Hydrogen peroxide
- Dimethyl sulfide stem cells
- Thermal injury
- Scorpion envenomation

Immunosuppressive drugs

- Cyclosporine
- Tacrolimus
- Sirolimus

Table 12.6 (cont.)

Other drugs

- Interferon alpha
- Interleukin
- Tumor necrosis factor antagonist (Kastrup)
- Antiretroviral Rx (HIV)
- Granulocyte-stimulating factor
- Intravenous immunoglobulin

air'."[475–477] Although first described in Japan, the condition has been reported worldwide.[475,477–480]

Necropsy studies, although few, have shown severe vascular occlusive abnormalities characterized by endothelial hyperplasia and fibrosis, with intimal thickening and abnormalities of the internal elastic lamina.[481] In contrast, the intracerebral perforating arteries show microaneurysm formation, lipohyalinosis, focal fibrin deposition, and thinning of the elastic laminas and arterial walls.[482] These changes in the perforating arteries are probably the result of greatly increased flow through these small vessels.[475–477,482] The vessels do not show inflammatory abnormalities.

In 1991, Ikeda studied the extracranial arteries of 13 Japanese patients with spontaneous occlusions of the circle of Willis at necropsy who met the research definition of moyamoya syndrome.[483] Extracranial arteries showed the same intimal lesions as the intracranial arteries. Characteristically, the proximal pulmonary arteries had fibrous nodular intimal thickening without inflammatory abnormalities.[483] Five discrete moyamoya disease syndromes (MYMY1–5) have been described.[484] Moyamoya vascular abnormalities have been found in a variety of situations (Table 12.7) and can be found in young women, especially those who smoke cigarettes and take oral contraceptives.[481] A variety of different conditions can probably cause intimal changes, which lead to fibrosis and luminal narrowing.[484]

Classical childhood-onset moyamoya disease is much more common in girls and women than in boys and men. Clinically, the disorder has a bimodal distribution, presenting most often in children younger than 15 years and in adults in their 3rd–5th decades of life. Children usually present with transient episodes of hemiparesis or other focal neurological signs often precipitated by physical exercise or hyperventilation. Several of our own young patients have had intermittent choreoathetosis. Other patients have sudden-onset deficits, such as hemiplegia, or the gradual development of intellectual deterioration. Headaches and seizures are common.[475–477] These symptoms are often accompanied by CT and MRI evidence of infarction and CBF studies that show regions of hypoperfusion. The abnormal vasculature is often visible on MRI.

Adults, in contrast, usually present with brain hemorrhages, typically in the thalamus, basal ganglia, or deep white matter. These hemorrhages are the result of degenerative changes (aneurysmal dilatation and thinning) in the

Table 12.7 Disorders associated with moyamoya syndrome

Neonatal anoxia	Marfan's syndrome
Head trauma	Turner's syndrome
Basilar meningitis (TB), leptospirosis	Williams' syndrome
Post-radiation vasculopathy	Prader–Willi syndrome
Neurofibromatosis type 1	Alagille's syndrome
Tuberous sclerosis complex	Apert's syndrome
Sturge–Weber syndrome	Down's syndrome
Phakomatosis pigmentovascularis type IIIB	Grange's syndrome
Pseudoxanthoma elasticum	Atherosclerotic disease
Hypomelanosis of Ito	Hypertension
Sickle cell anemia	Use of oral contraceptives
β-Thalassemia	Drug abuse (cocaine, etc.)
Fanconi anemia	Fibromuscular dysplasia (FMD)
Aplastic anemia	Cerebral dissecting and saccular aneurysms
Hereditary spherocytosis	Arteriovenous malformations
Protein C deficiency	Cavernous malformations
Protein S deficiency	Homocystinuria
Antiphospholipid antibody syndrome	Type 1 glycogenosis
Thrombotic thrombocytopenic purpura	Primary oxalosis
Factor XII deficiency	Polyarteritis nodosa
Brain tumors	Sjögren's syndrome
Parasellar tumors	Hirschprung disease
Wilms' tumor	Coarctation of the aorta
Sarcoidosis	Renal artery stenosis
Systemic lupus erythematosus	Hyperthyroidism
Sneddon's syndrome	Graves' disease
Microcephalic osteodysplastic primodial dwarfism type II	

anastomotic basal vessels that are overtaxed and cannot accommodate the volume of blood needed for perfusion. At times, the hemorrhages are subarachnoid and intraventricular. Some patients with moyamoya syndrome develop aneurysms involving arteries of the circle of Willis, especially the anterior cerebral-anterior communicating artery region and the basilar artery.[485,487] Angiography shows progressive changes that may be asymmetric initially but always involve the intracranial ICAs bilaterally and usually also involve the proximal portions of the MCAs and ACAs. As the intracranial arteries narrow, collaterals develop involving the basal penetrating arteries, orbital vessels (so-called ethmoidal moyamoya), and vessels over the vault derived from transdural anastomoses from the meningeal and superficial temporal arteries.[475–477] Figure 12.20 shows digital subtraction angiograms from a patient with moyamoya. Later, the telangiectasias may regress and become less prominent. Suzuki and others have staged the severity of disease by the angiographic findings.[476,477]

Some patients with moyamoya syndrome stabilize clinically, often after they have developed disabilities. The best treatment is not known.[478] A variety of different surgical revascularization procedures have been used. These usually involve anastomosing the superficial temporal artery to the MCA or placing the superficial temporal and middle meningeal arteries adjacent to the pia, or placing vascularized connective tissue elements and muscle on the surface of the pia matter.[487–490] The surgical revascularization created is often called synangiosis. Angiography after surgical revascularization shows improved collateral blood flow.[485,487–490] It is hoped that revascularization might prevent further ischemia and hemorrhage, but no systematic randomized therapeutic trials have investigated the effectiveness of revascularization procedures.

A strong association was recently established between moyamoya disease and polymorphisms of the Ring finger 213 (*RNF213*) gene on chromosome 17q25-ter.[491] The most common polymorphism seen in patients with moyamoya disease is the p.R4810K polymorphism of the *RNF213* gene. About one-third of patients who have the p.R4810K polymorphism of the *RNF213* gene develop moyamoya disease.[492] Until now most of the genetic studies have been performed on Asian populations. Identification of the genetic defect may greatly aid research on this heretofore very puzzling disorder.

Hematological disorders, including abnormalities of coagulation, viscosity, and serum constituents[493–577]

Since the 1980s, knowledge of blood constituents and their function in the coagulation process has dramatically advanced and research and knowledge are still expanding. Brain ischemia and hemorrhage can develop as a direct result of hematological abnormalities rather than from primary diseases of the blood vessels.[491,492] In other patients with endothelial lesions in the aorta, heart, and blood vessels, activation of coagulation functions causes thrombi to form on the abnormal endothelial surfaces and often precipitates strokes. In turn, occlusion of arteries increases coagulation factors. The endothelia, blood vessels, and circulating blood are so intricately interwoven that it is often difficult to know which changes are primary and cause the disorder and which are secondary to the occlusive vascular process. Hematological conditions are discussed

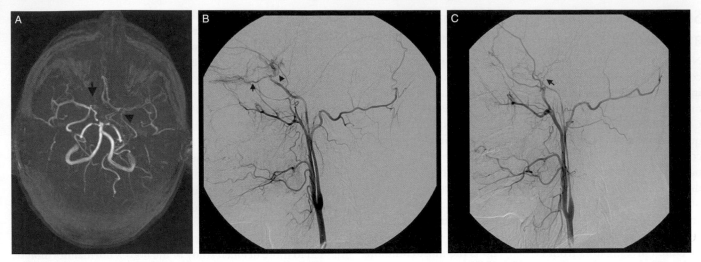

Figure 12.20 A 23-year-old woman with moyamoya syndrome. (A) MR angiography shows occlusion of the distal right internal carotid artery with dilatated lenticulostriate collaterals (puff of smoke, arrow) with a small left internal carotid artery that is occluded in the cavernous portion (arrowhead). There is poor flow in the left middle cerebral artery via collaterals. (B) Catheter digital-subtraction, right-common-carotid artery angiogram shows a large, right ophthalmic artery (arrow), occlusion of the terminal internal carotid artery with dilatated lenticulostriate collaterals (arrowhead). (C) Left common-carotid angiogram shows a small, collapsed, left internal carotid artery with distal occlusion (arrow) and no filling of the left middle and anterior cerebral arteries.

in Chapters 4 and 6 regarding laboratory diagnosis and treatment. Only a brief cataloging of these disorders is presented here.

Cellular abnormalities[493–513]

Abnormalities in the formed cellular constituents of the blood may be quantitative or qualitative. Polycythemia has long been known to increase blood viscosity, decrease CBF, and increase thrombosis. Severe anemia is also associated with increased coagulability and can predispose to venous sinus thrombosis.

Sickle cell disease and sickle cell hemoglobin C disease are examples of qualitative red blood cell abnormalities that affect blood flow. Sickle cell disease is associated with occlusive changes in large intracranial arteries and small penetrating vessels.[493–498] Subcortical, cortical, and borderzone infarcts are often found on CT and MRI. Angiography has shown intracranial occlusions of the major basal arteries. The walls of intracranial arteries are thickened, and intimal and subintimal proliferation occurs. Arteries in patients with sickle cell disease may become dilated and ectatic even in childhood.[499] Occasionally, veins and dural sinuses thrombose.[500] TCD offers a non-invasive method for detecting velocity changes related to intracranial large artery narrowing and allows monitoring of patients with sickle cell disease.[493,494,501,502] Blood transfusions for children whose TCD blood-flow velocities in the ICAs or MCAs or both exceed 200 cm per second have been shown in a trial to prevent stroke from developing.[494]

Paroxysmal nocturnal hemoglobinuria (PNH) is characterized by a qualitative abnormality of red blood cells that leads to hemolysis and life-threatening thrombotic episodes.[503–505] This condition is known to be caused by a mutation in hematopoietic stem cells that leads to clones of blood cells that are deficient in surface proteins that are normally attached to cell membranes. Neutropenia and thrombocytopenia are also common. The incidence of thrombosis reaches about 30% by 8 years after diagnosis and increases to nearly 50% after 15 years.[504,505] Cerebrovascular events are an important contributor to morbidity and mortality. The cranial veins and arteries are the second most important site of thrombosis secondary only to hepatic vein thromboses.[504,505] Cerebral venous and dural sinus thromboses are the most common clinical neurological manifestations. Systemic and intracranial hemorrhages can result from the thrombocytopenia, which may be severe.

Increased platelet counts, especially those higher than 1 million, are also associated with hypercoagulability. The thrombocytosis can be primary, so-called essential *thrombocythemia*, and can be associated with other myeloproliferation, or, less often, can be secondary to systemic disease. Essential thrombocythemia is associated with strokes and digital occlusions.[506–510] The lack of correlation between the platelet count and the thrombotic complications has led to the assumption that there are also qualitative abnormalities of platelet function.[491,506–508] In some patients, increased coagulability has been attributed to increased adhesion and aggregation of platelets (so-called sticky platelets) in the absence of thrombocytosis.[507,508,511–513] Thrombocytopenia caused by a variety of different conditions can lead to important brain and systemic bleeding.

Leukemia is complicated occasionally by brain hemorrhages and microinfarcts. When the white blood cell count is high (increased leukocrit), the white blood cells can pack capillaries, leading to microinfarcts and vascular rupture with small brain hemorrhages. Larger brain hemorrhages and SAHs are most often related to thrombocytopenia caused by replacement of the bone marrow with leukocyte precursors.

Serological abnormalities: hypercoagulability and bleeding[514–551]

Normally, natural inhibitors of coagulation circulate to discourage spontaneous blood clotting. The best known of these inhibitors, antithrombin and proteins C and S, can be deficient on a hereditary basis or be reduced by disease.[491,492,514] Congenital deficiency of antithrombin may be quantitative or qualitative and is most often an autosomal-dominant condition.[491,514,515] Reduced synthesis of antithrombin, as in patients with liver disease or renal loss in the nephrotic syndrome, can lead to acquired deficiencies. Inherited deficiencies of proteins C and S can also contribute to or cause increased coagulability.[491,492,514,516] An inherited coagulation deficit referred to as resistance to activated protein C was described by Dutch investigators from Leiden, and is the most common cause of abnormal protein C activity.[517,518] In most instances, resistance to activated protein C is caused by a point mutation in the gene that encodes for coagulation factor V.[518] The presence of this mutation, called factor V Leiden, is accompanied by a threefold to fivefold increase in the frequency of venous thromboembolism in the lower extremities[519] and an increased frequency of cerebral venous and dural sinus thrombosis. Factor V Leiden is the most common genetic disorder that leads to hypercoagulability.

The second most common genetic mutation that leads to a prothrombic state is a mutation in the gene encoding prothrombin.[520] This mutation involves a transition from guanine to adenine at position 20210 in the sequence of the 3' untranslated region of the prothrombin gene.[520] The frequency of cerebral and peripheral venous thrombosis is greatly increased in carriers of the prothrombin gene mutation, especially if they also take oral contraceptive pills.[521,522] Genetic analysis is warranted in patients with unexplained hypercoagulability, especially those with cerebral venous thrombosis and recurrent peripheral venous thromboembolism. Most often, clotting is venous, but arterial occlusions have also been described.

Systemic and inherited conditions can alter the levels of the serine protease coagulation factors. The best known of these disorders is hemophilia, which causes bleeding into the joints, skin, and cranium. Some patients with chronically increased concentrations of factor VIII, have frequent episodes of venous thrombosis, spontaneous abortion, and ischemic strokes.[523,524] In others, factor VIII levels are high, probably as an epiphenomenon to the initial thromboembolic event.

Some patients with infectious and inflammatory diseases, such as Crohn's disease and ulcerative colitis, have increased factor VIII levels as a result of serological changes induced by the primary disease.[525–528] Venous dural sinus occlusions, thrombophlebitis, and arterial occlusions may result. Hematological changes in inflammatory bowel disease are complex because elevated levels of factors V and VIII, reduced levels of antithrombin III, and quantitative and qualitative platelet abnormalities have all been described.[525,527]

Studies have also shown that infections of various types are often present in the days and weeks before stroke onset.[529,530]

Infections and various inflammatory disorders provoke an increase in acute phase reactants and white blood cells, fibrinogen, and coagulation factors V, VII, and VIII, which induce thrombosis in patients with pre-existing endothelial lesions.[531,532]

Cancers are also often associated with hypercoagulability.[533–535] Patients with mucinous adenocarcinomas can develop venous occlusions, large artery thrombi, and multiple small artery occlusions.[536] In some situations (e.g., during pregnancy, the puerperium, or use of oral contraceptives), the mechanism of hypercoagulability is not fully known. D-dimer levels are usually quite high in patients with cancer-related strokes indicating increased thrombus formation and high fibrin turnover.[537]

The advent of recombinant tissue plasminogen activator has led to more detailed study of the body's normal fibrinolytic activity and abnormalities of the fibrinolytic system.[538–540] Plasminogen deficiencies, dysfibrinogenemias, and abnormalities of tissue plasminogen activator and its inhibitors can cause an increased tendency toward both venous and arterial thrombosis.[538,541–544] Increased thrombosis is caused by a deficiency of plasminogen or increased inhibition of plasminogen activator by plasminogen inhibitor (PAI-1).[541–544] Thrombin and fibrinolytic activity can be monitored during acute stroke by measuring a number of substances.[538,545,546] For example, the levels of fibrinopeptide A correlate with thrombin activity, and the levels of cross-linked D-dimer, a breakdown product of fibrin polymer, are a useful index of fibrinolytic activity.[545,546]

Bleeding can also result from serological abnormalities. Acquired hemophilia is a condition seen most often in adults in whom factor VIII autoantibodies, usually of the IgG type develop and can cause life-threatening bleeding.[547,548] Acquired hemophilia may develop after pregnancy and after a variety of illnesses including cancer and collagen vascular disease. Patients show a prolonged aPTT that is not normalized by mixing their plasma with normal plasma because an inhibitor is preventing thromboplastin generation. Excess fibrinolytic activity can also cause bleeding and is most common after thrombolysis for myocardial or brain ischemia.

Von Willebrand disease is another condition that can occasionally be associated with intracranial as well as systemic bleeding. The condition is caused by a deficiency or altered function of von Willebrand factor, a plasma glycoprotein that is involved in platelet adherence and adhesion and that stabilizes blood coagulation factor VIII.[549–551] The disease has autosomal dominant and recessive inheritance. The von Willebrand-factor gene is located on chromosome 12. Bleeding is related to impaired platelet functions or reduced concentrations of factor VIII. Bleeding is often heavily menstrual or after wounds or surgeries.

Immunological abnormalities and abnormalities of blood flow[552–577]

Some patients develop circulating antibodies that react to various hematological and vascular components. Acquired

hemophilia was mentioned as an example. The best known and most common of these autoantibodies are the lupus anticoagulant (LA) and anticardiolipin antibodies. These substances react against phospholipids. Phospholipids are ubiquitous components of vascular structures and various blood constituents.

The presence of LA or anticardiolipins has been referred to as the antiphospholipid antibody (APLA) syndrome.[552] The LA (a misnomer because it is associated with increased coagulability, not bleeding) is a phospholipid antibody that interferes with the formation of the prothrombin activator.[552–554] In the laboratory, there is a prolonged activated partial thromboplastin time that does not correct when normal plasma is added, indicating the presence of an inhibitor of clotting rather than a deficiency of a needed component.[552–565] Some patients with LA have SLE but most do not.

When antiphospholipids of the IgG, IgM, or IgA classes are found in the absence of a known systemic illness, the disorder is referred to as a primary APLA syndrome.[551,554–560] Clinically, these patients have an increased incidence of spontaneous abortions, thrombophlebitis, pulmonary embolism, and large- and small-artery occlusions. In addition to the presence of LA or anticardiolipins or both, laboratory abnormalities include positive VDRL, thrombocytopenia, and antinuclear antibodies. Some patients have mitral and aortic valve abnormalities and ocular ischemia.[552,554,559,560] The cardiac lesions are identical to those described by Libman and Sacks and involve the valves as well as the endothelium of the heart. The mechanism of increased coagulability and valvular changes is not known, but these probably relate to immune-related endothelial and valve-surface injuries.[561–563] Patients with high-positive IgG and APLA have a high incidence of subsequent vascular occlusive lesions.[564,565] Anti-beta 2-glycoprotein I and antiphosphatidylserine antibodies seem to be better predictive of the tendency to thrombosis than other measured antibodies.[562,563] Antiphosphatidylserine antibodies form complexes with prothrombin.[563] Angiography in patients with APLA syndrome shows a high frequency of intracranial occlusive disease, atypical extracranial occlusive arterial disease, and venous and dural sinus occlusions.[566] Some patients with APLA have a Binswanger type leukoencephalopathy.

Disseminated intravascular coagulation (DIC) is a disorder that affects cellular and serological factors.[567–571] When a primary disorder leads to local or diffuse clotting, the coagulation cascade can be activated with generation of excess intravascular thrombin. The coagulation system then is further activated, fibrin is deposited into the microcirculation, hemostatic elements have a shortened survival, and the fibrinolytic system is activated.[567] The most common disorders inciting DIC are infections, obstetric and vascular emergencies, and cancer.[568,569] Head trauma, SAH, brain tumors, and vascular malformations can also cause DIC.[568,570,571] The laboratory findings include thrombocytopenia, reduced fibrinogen levels, prolongation of prothrombin time and partial thromboplastin time, and increased levels of fibrin split products. DIC can be associated with non-bacterial thrombotic endocarditis, especially in patients with cancer.[533,536,568,570,571] Neurological

findings are frequent and include an encephalopathy with multifocal signs and frank thrombotic and embolic infarcts. Bleeding can also occur.

Blood flow, especially in the brain microcirculation, depends heavily on the viscosity of the blood. *Blood viscosity* is most affected by the erythrocyte content of the blood and serum fibrinogen level.[572–574] Polycythemia and hyperfibrinogenemia can increase whole-blood viscosity and decrease CBF, especially in patients with cerebrovascular disease. High fibrinogen levels are an important risk factor for stroke and other large artery occlusive disease.[575] Less often, increased viscosity is caused by high levels of globulins (e.g., in Waldenström's macroglobulinemia or in other disorders with abnormal proteins or cryoglobulins, such as multiple myeloma).[576] Rarely, high levels of serum lipids cause significant hyperviscosity.[572,577]

Clinically, patients with hyperviscosity syndromes have an encephalopathy characterized by somnolence, stupor, headache, seizures, ataxia, and decreased vision.[572,576] A clue to the presence of hyperviscosity is the ophthalmoscopic appearance of the retina. Retinal veins are dilatated and tortuous and may show segmentations in the blood columns within retinal vessels. Serum viscosity is measured relative to water; the average normal level is approximately 1.8. Serum viscosity of 5 or 6 is usually associated with encephalopathy but lower levels may be important in patients with hypertensive microvasculopathy and atherosclerotic disease.

Neoplastic conditions[578–589]

Vasculopathies often precede, accompany or follow neoplasia, especially lymphoproliferative and myeloproliferative disorders. *Lymphomatoid granulomatosis* is an angiocentric lymphoproliferative condition predominantly affecting the lungs in which granulomatous nodules can involve brain arteries and veins and produce stroke-like deficits.[578–580] Lymphomatoid granulomatosis was found to be caused by an Epstein-Barr viral infection of B lymphocytes and is classified as an Epstein-Barr virus–associated form of lymphoproliferative disease.[580] The lung and brain regions of necrosis are presumably related to infarction caused by the cellular vascular infiltrate ("angiitis"). The most common extrapulmonary findings are in the skin and nervous system – each accounting for about a third of patients. The skin lesions usually consist of a raised erythematous rash and occasionally skin nodules, especially on the trunk. CNS lesions are more common than cranial or peripheral neuropathies and usually consist of focal and multifocal brain mass lesions.[578–581]

Lymphomas can present as a solely intravascular tumor. This entity, now called *intravascular lymphoma*, was previously called neoplastic angioendotheliosis.[581–587] Large pleomorphic mononuclear cells proliferate within the lumens of capillaries, venules, arterioles, and small arteries. The neoplastic intraluminal cells usually have a B-cell phenotype although they rarely are of T-cell or NK-cell origin.[582] The neoplastic cells occlude small arteries, leading to multiple microinfarcts. The disorder can be systemic, producing erythematous skin plaques and

417

patches, subcutaneous nodules, high sedimentation rates, fever, and renal failure. The disorder can affect the spinal cord.[588] Headache, multifocal neurologic signs, and a progressive course are typical. The brain lesions on MRI vary and range between white matter hyperintensity to large areas of signal abnormalities. Meningeal enhancement can occur and is explained by microinfarcts within the meninges or slow flow through meningeal blood vessels. Angiography is usually normal because the blood vessels involved are too small to be seen during angiograms.

Hodgkin's disease in the meninges often causes occlusions of meningeal arteries and veins, with hemorrhagic infarction in the underlying cerebral cortex. We have already commented in this chapter on leukemic blockage of small arteries and on the coagulopathies associated with cancer, especially of the mucinous adenocarcinoma type. A fatal necrotizing cerebral vasculitis resembling polyarteritis nodosa has been described in Purtillo syndrome or X-linked lymphoproliferative disese (XLP). The mechanism for this vasculitis is unclear. A diffuse CNS vasculopathy with dilation of intracranial vessels has been reported in patients with XLP syndrome complicated by CNS manifestations of Epstein–Barr virus infection.[589] Hypersensitivity vasculitis may also be observed with essential mixed cryoglobulinemia.

Some genetic disorders that cause strokes[590–661]

Many of the conditions already discussed in this chapter, such as hereditary disorders of connective tissue and the heredito-familial cerebral amyloid angiopathies, are known to be genetically determined. Many others are probably influenced by genetic predispositions. Dyslipoproteinemias, hemoglobino-pathies, diabetes, hypertension, and atherosclerosis are strongly governed by genetic factors. We close this chapter by briefly discussing a few other disorders with mendelian etiologies. This edition contains a full chapter on genetics and stroke and enlarges coverage of many of the entities discussed concisely herein. Knowledge of the genetic factors in stroke is growing rapidly.[590–594]

The *MELAS syndrome* (mitochondrial myopathy, encephalopathy, lactic acidosis, and stroke-like episodes) is one form of mitochondrial encephalomyopathy.[595–597] Seizures, migraine-like headaches, and intellectual deterioration are most prominent clinically.[598–600] Short stature and sensorineural hearing loss are also common features.[597] Constipation is common before and at onset of neurological symptoms. Affected patients often have acute-onset episodes of visual deterioration, hemiparesis, and ataxia, often with seizures. Lactic and pyruvic acid levels in the blood are often high and muscle biopsy shows ragged red fibers.[595–598] CT and MRI show discrete multifocal abnormalities that are most often in the parieto-occipital and temporal lobes.[599–603] These lesions affect the cortex and underlying white matter. These lesions are caused by ischemia, but the arteries supplying these zones are normal. They are probably explained by the metabolic abnormality characterized by decreased cytochrome oxidase activity within mitochondria, leading to energy failure. Basal ganglia calcifications are also prominent. The disorder is caused by a maternal mutation in mitochondrial DNA.[592,595] Other mitochondrial disorders are also often accompanied by white matter abnormalities on MRI that resemble infarcts.

Strokes, renal failure, painful limb dysesthesias, corneal opacities, and cutaneous angiokeratomas characterize *Fabry's disease*. The disorder is a sex-linked lysosomal storage disease. Most clinical cases involve homozygous men. Occasionally, heterozygous women are affected.[604–611] The diagnosis is suggested by finding the characteristic tiny, pinhead-size, dark-reddish purple nonpruritic papules that are located predominantly along the inner thighs, perineum, and near the umbilicus in a so-called bathing trunk distribution (Figure 12.21). Because of a deficiency of a lysosomal enzyme (alpha-galactosidase), trihexosyl ceramide, a sphingolipid, accumulates and causes a diffuse

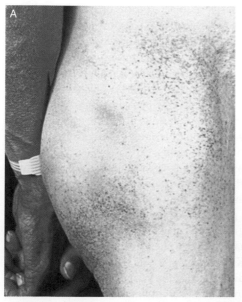
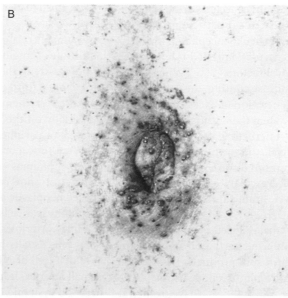

Figure 12.21 Angiokeratomas in Fabry's disease. (A) Photograph of the buttocks showing typical small lesions. (B) Periumbilical angiokeratomas. Courtesy of Dr Edward Kaye. A black and white version of this figure will appear in some formats. For the color version, please refer to the plate section.

vasculopathy.[604-609] The disease is often manifest in adolescent boys who have severe lower extremity pain especially during and after exercise and syncope related to a small fiber and autonomic neuropathy. Sweating is also diminished or absent, so that heat and exercise intolerance are common. The myocardium is also often involved, and the condition presents in some patients as a cardiomyopathy. Deafness is also common and may begin abruptly.

Multiple vascular occlusions and strokes are common. Strokes tend to be lacunar related to penetrating artery disease. Some patients have had dolichoectatic dilatated intracranial arteries.[604,605] Some strokes are cardioembolic related to the cardiomyopathy sometimes found in patients with Fabry's disease. Angiography often shows occlusion of branch arteries. The endothelium is infiltrated with the sphingolipid. Death is most often caused by renal failure unless dialysis is performed. Regular infusions of recombinant alpha-galactosidase A is able to clear endothelial deposits of globotriaosylceramide in the kidneys, skin, and endomyocardium and to reduce pain from autonomic neuropathy.[609,610] Young individuals with Fabry's disease and enzyme deficiency should receive infusions of the enzyme.[610]

Cerebral autosomal dominant arteriopathy with subcortical infarcts and leukoencephaly (CADASIL) is an important familial condition characterized by migraines with aura, multiple lacunar infarcts, and extensive white matter abnormalities.[612-617] The small arteries within the brain are thickened by eosinophilic, periodic acid-Schiff-positive granular deposits, which have not been characterized fully biochemically.[612,617,618] The substance within the arteries differs from amyloid. Skin biopsy, especially using electron microscopy, shows the same material within skin arteries. The clinical findings are strokes, progressive gait disorder, and frontal lobe-type subcortical dementia.[612-617] Mood disorders, especially depression, are also common. Migraines are a prominent symptom in some patients and in relatives of patients with this leukoencephalopathy. Uncommon clinical manifestations include seizures, intracerebral hemorrhages, deafness and parkinsonism.[619]

The MRI shows characteristic lesions.[612,620] White matter hyperintensities are sometimes found before clinical symptoms develop. The white matter abnormalities are common in the anterior temporal lobes, a location rare in hypertensive Binswanger leukoencephalopathy. CADASIL is caused by a mutation of the *Notch 3* gene on chromosome 19.[612,621] A somewhat similar microangiopathic familial disorder has also been described in Japan known as cerebral autosomal recessive arteriopathy with subcortical infarcts and leukoencephalopathy (CARASIL).[622,623] This condition affects predominantly young men and is characterized by a leukoencephalopathy, alopecia, and prominent low back pain, spondylosis deformans or disk herniation.[622,623] The small arteries are infiltrated by fibrous intimal proliferation and severe hyalinosis, with splitting of the intima and internal elastic membrane.[622,623] There are likely other genetically determined microangiopathies that involve deposition of different biochemical materials

into cerebral and systemic arteries that differ genetically from CADASIL.

Menkes disease (trichopoliodystrophy or kinky-hair disease) is an X-linked recessive condition in which mitochondrial dysfunction is caused by impaired intestinal absorption of copper.[624-627] The basic genetic defect is a mutation in *ATP7A*, a gene mapped to the long arm of the X-chromosome (Xq12-q13) that encodes a highly evolutionarily conserved P-type ATP protein (ATP7A) essential for the translocation of metal cations across cellular membranes.[624,626,627] The delivery of copper to cells requires transporters, one of which is deficient in patients with Menkes disease. The deficiency of copper leads to subnormal cytochrome oxidase function within mitochondria and widespread energy failure. The copper content of cultured fibroblasts, myotubes, and lymphocytes derived from patients with Menkes disease is several times greater than control cells.[624] The hair is abnormal and is course, stiff, and easily broken. Hypotonia, hypothermia, seizures, and failure to thrive are common.[624,625,628,629] Ragged red fibers may be seen on muscle biopsy. Electron microscopic studies of the brain can show abnormal mitochondria. MRI studies of the brain show rapidly developing cerebral atrophy and often small deep and cortical infarcts. Subdural hematomas are also common.[624] At necropsy, the brain contains multiple microinfarcts and intracranial branch arteries are often occluded. Most patients die in early childhood. Neonatal diagnosis is now possible and the early diagnosis provides an opportunity for early life copper supplementation.[630] Copper supplementation, using daily injections of copper-histidine, is the most promising treatment. Parenterally administered copper corrects the hepatic copper deficiency and restores serum copper and ceruloplasmin levels to normal.[624,630]

Patients with *neurofibromatosis type 1 (NF1)* are known to develop renal and systemic artery and cerebrovascular abnormalities. NF1 is due to a mutation on chromosome 17q11.2, the gene product being neurofibromin (a GTPase-activating enzyme).[631] Café-au-lait spots, peripheral neurofibromas, and Lisch nodules are the commonest clinical manifestations of NF1.[631] Aneurysms and arterial stenoses occur. Both ischemic stroke and subarachnoid hemorrhage are described.[573-576] Aneurysms can develop both in the neck and intracranially. The most frequent intracranial aneurysm site is within the ICAs as they emerge from the cavernous sinus just after the origins of the ophthalmic arteries.[631-634] A moyamoya picture can result from multiple occlusions of basal arteries. Hypertension may be caused by renal artery stenosis or pheochromocytomas, which occur at increased frequency in patients with this genetic condition.

Homocystinuria is probably the most common genetic disease that affects the brain vasculature and leads to premature atherosclerosis and strokes.[635,636] Severe hyperhomocysteinemia and homocystinuria is a genetic disorder first described in children and known to be associated with premature strokes, mental retardation, and a Marfan-like syndrome. Lesser degrees of hyperhomocysteinemia are associated with premature atherosclerosis.

Classic homocystinuria is caused by a hereditary deficiency of the enzyme cystathione-beta-synthase, an enzyme that is required for the conversion of methionine-derived homocysteine to cystathione. In humans, approximately 15–20 mmol/l of homocysteine is formed each day by demethylation of the amino acid methionine.[636] Homocysteine is subsequently metabolized by one of two pathways, either remethylation or transulfuration. In the remethylation process, homcysteine is remethylated to methionine in a reaction catalyzed by methionine synthase.[636] Vitamin B_{12} is an essential cofactor for methionine synthase, and N5-methyl-tetrahydrofolate is the methyl donor in this reaction. N5,N10-methylene-tetrahydrofolate reductase functions as the catalyst in this remethylation reaction.[636,637] Homocysteine can also be transulfurated when homocysteine condenses with serine to form cystathione, a reaction catalyzed by the vitamin B_6-dependent enzyme cystathione beta-synthase.[636–638] Cystathione is then hydrolyzed to cysteine, which in turn can be incorporated into glutathione or further metabolized to sulfate and excreted in the urine.[636,637,639]

Cystathione-beta-synthase deficiency is the most common genetic cause of severe hyperhomocysteinemia. The homozygous form of this disorder is called congenital homocystinuria and is associated with plasma homocysteine concentrations of up to 400 μmol/l during the fasting state.[636,637] This genetic disorder is rare (5 in 1 million births). Affected individuals have ectopic lenses, skeletal deformities, a Marfan-like habitus, and severe premature atherosclerosis. Typically, a clinical thromboembolic event in the form of strokes or myocardial infarcts occur before age 30 years.[640] A homozygous deficiency of N5,N10-methylene-tetrahydrofolate reductase, the enzyme involved in the B_{12}-dependent remethylation of homocysteine, can also cause severe hyperhomocysteinemia. Patients with this metabolic defect have an even worse prognosis than those with cystathione-beta-synthase deficiency.[636,637]

Less severe forms of hyperhomocysteinemia occur in heterozygotes with these enzyme deficiencies. Deficiencies in the cofactors folate and vitamins B_{12} and B_6, which are required for homocysteine metabolism, can also cause an elevated homocysteine level. In patients with nutritional deficiencies in these vitamin cofactors, prescribing these substances can reduce homocysteine levels. Increased levels of homocysteine also occur in patients being treated with methotrexate, theophylline, and phenytoin and in patients with: (1) renal insufficiency; (2) hyperthyroidism; (3) breast, pancreatic, and ovarian cancers; (4) lymphatic leukemia; and (5) pernicious anemia.[636,637] Cigarette smoking has also been associated with elevated homocysteine levels, presumably because of interference with the synthesis of pyridoxal phosphate.[641]

Elevated levels of homocysteine have been unequivocally related to strokes, premature atherosclerosis, myocardial infarction, and venous thromboembolism.[636,637,642,643] Evidence from more than 20 case-controlled studies that included more than 2000 individuals has validated the relationship between elevated homocysteine levels and accelerated atherosclerosis.[636,637] Patients with increased levels of homocysteine have more severe carotid artery disease than

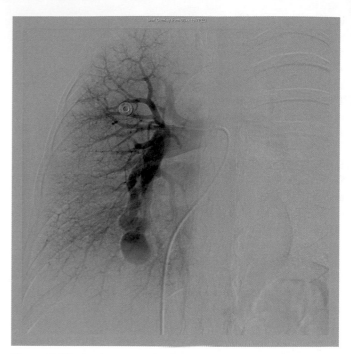

Figure 12.22 A pulmonary angiogram in a patient with hereditary hemorrhagic telangiectasia that shows a pulmonary arteriovenous fistula. This was the cause of a paradoxical embolus to the brain.

individuals with normal levels.[644] Experimental evidence shows that increased homocysteine levels injure the vascular endothelium. This injury leads to platelet activation and the formation of thrombi.[645,646] Homocysteine also stimulates vascular smooth muscle cells to proliferate.[647]

Progeria (Hutchinson–Gilford progeria syndrome) is a rare condition characterized by premature ageing beginning in very early life and ending in premature death.[648,649] Clinical manifestations involve the skin and appendages, joints, and blood vessels causing coronary and cerebrovascular disease during youth.[648] Progeric individuals have a characteristic facial and body appearance readily recognized during the first decade of life. Progeria can result from mutations of the *LMNA* gene coding for the nuclear membrane protein lamin A and from abnormal DNA repair. Progeria is most often caused by a mutation of the *LMNA* gene on chromosome 1q.[648–651] The *LMNA* gene encodes lamin A and C, filamentous structural proteins found in the nuclear lamina. In progeria, the *LMNA* mutation results in the accumulation of a lipid-modified (farnesylated) prelamin A (*progerin*), impairing nuclear membrane function.[648] Vascular occlusive large artery lesions in the neck and intracranially can appear in the first decade and mirror lesions found in atherosclerotic adults.

Hereditary hemorrhagic telangiectasia (Osler–Weber–Rendu disease) is a disorder characterized by frequent epistaxis, cutaneous and visceral telangiectasia with gastrointestinal bleeds, brain vascular malformations, and pulmonary arteriovenous fistulas (Figure 12.22).[652–655] Mutations on two genes, endoglin and activin receptor-like kinase 1, located on chromosomes 9 and 12, respectively, that encode proteins expressed predominantly on vascular endothelial cells relate

to the vascular abnormalities.[652,654] The telangiectasias are composed of dilatated postcapillary venules. With time venules become more dilatated and convoluted and are characterized by excessive layers of smooth muscle without elastic fibers.[652,654] Arterioles can also dilatate and communicate directly with venules without intervening capillaries. Hereditary hemorrhagic telangiectasia patients often have brain arteriovenous malformations and arteriovenous fistulas. The largest arteriovenous malformations occur in the lungs, liver, and brain. Paradoxical brain embolism can develop in patients with these pulmonary fistulas. Examination of patients with hereditary hemorrhagic telangiectasia nearly always shows telangiectasias on the lips, nasal mucosa, and mucosal surfaces in the mouth.

The *COL4A1 mutation syndrome* has recently been characterized as a familial syndrome of fragile blood vessels with a susceptibility to intracranial hemorrhage.[618,656–659] Different mutations in the *COL4A1* gene that encodes the alpha 1 chain of type IV collagen are implicated. Type IV collagen is an essential component of basement membranes. In mice, *COL4A1* mutants have frequent perinatal hemorrhages and have structurally abnormal basement membranes in brain, eyes, and kidneys.[656,657]

Infantile hemiparesis with congenital porencephaly and perinatal hemorrhages are probably related to brain hemorrhages in utero or perinatally. The clinical picture is characterized by a susceptibility to intracerebral and subarachnoid hemorrhages after trauma and during anticoagulation. The retinal blood vessels are tortuous and white matter hyperintensities are common. The *COL4A1* mutation syndrome shares with CADASIL a predilection for involvement of small intracranial blood vessels but the tendency for hemorrhage and vascular fragility is unique.[618,656–659] There are likely other hereditary causes of vascular-related chronic white matter pathology that are as yet not well characterized. One condition was described in children who develop progressive cognitive and motor signs and brain imaging shows extensive white matter gliosis and cyst formation and calcifications in the basal ganglia, cerebellar nuclei and deep white matter.[660] On microscopy angiomatous-like changes in small penetrating arteries was found.[27a] Similar findings have now been described in a 44-year-old woman.[661]

References

1. Caplan LR (ed): *Uncommon Causes of Stroke*, 2nd ed. Cambridge: Cambridge University Press, 2008.

2. Ojemann RG, Fisher CM, Rich JC: Spontaneous dissecting aneurysms of the internal carotid artery. *Stroke* 1972;**3**:434–440.

3. Fisher CM, Ojemann RG, Roberson GH: Spontaneous dissection of cervicocerebral arteries. *Can J Neurol Sci* 1978;**5**:9–19.

4. Baumgartner RW, Bogousslavsky J, Caso V, Paciaroni M (eds): *Handbook on Cerebral Artery Dissection*. Basel: Karger, 2005.

5. Caplan LR: Dissections of brain-supplying arteries. *Nat Clin Pract Neurol* 2008;**4**:34–42.

6. Debette S, Leys D: Cervical-artery dissections: Predisposing factors, diagnosis, and outcome. *Lancet Neurol* 2009;**8**:668–678.

7. Caplan LR, Zarins C, Hemmatti M: Spontaneous dissection of the extracranial vertebral artery. *Stroke* 1985;**16**:1030–1038.

8. Mokri B, Houser OW, Sandok BA, Piepgras DG: Spontaneous dissection of the vertebral arteries. *Neurology* 1988;**38**:880–885.

9. Caplan LR, Tettenborn B: Vertebrobasilar occlusive disease: Review of selected aspects: I. Spontaneous dissection of extracranial and intracranial posterior circulation arteries. *Cerebrovasc Dis* 1992;**2**:256–265.

10. Barbour PJ, Castaldo JE, Rae-Grant AD, et al: Internal carotid artery redundancy is significantly associated with dissection. *Stroke* 1994;**25**:1201–1206.

11. Giossi A, Ritelli M, Costa P, et al: Connective tissue anomalies in patients with spontaneous cervical artery dissection. *Neurology* 2014;**83**:2032–2037.

12. Brandt T, Hausser I, Orberk E, et al: Ultrastructural connective tissue abnormalities in patients with spontaneous cervicocerebral artery dissections. *Ann Neurol* 1998;**44**:281–285.

13. Arnold M, Fischer U, Nedeltchev K: Carotid artery dissection and sports. *Kardiovaskuläre Medizin* 2009;**12**:209–213.

14. Guillon B, Peynet J, Bertrand M, et al: Do extracellular-matrix-regulating enzymes play a role in cervical artery dissections? *Cerebrovasc Dis* 2007;**23**:299–303.

15. Hart RG, Easton JD: Dissection of cervical and cerebral arteries. In Barnett HJM (ed): *Neurologic Clinics*, vol **1**. Philadelphia: Saunders, 1983, pp 155–182.

16. Friedman WA, Day AL, Quisling RG, et al: Cervical carotid dissecting aneurysms. *Neurosurgery* 1980;**7**:207–214.

17. Silbert PL, Mokri B, Schievink WI: Headache and neck pain in spontaneous internal carotid and vertebral artery dissection. *Neurology* 1995;**45**:1517–1522.

18. Bogousslavsky J, Despland PA, Regli F: Spontaneous carotid dissection with acute stroke. *Arch Neurol* 1987;**44**:137–140.

19. Biousse V, Schaison M, Touboul P-J, et al: Ischemic optic neuropathy associated with internal carotid artery dissection. *Arch Neurol* 1998;**55**:715–719.

20. Pozzali E, Giuliani G, Poppi M, Faenza A: Blunt traumatic carotid dissection with delayed symptoms. *Stroke* 1989;**20**:412–416.

21. Sturzenegger M: Ultrasound findings in spontaneous carotid artery dissection: The value of duplex sonography. *Arch Neurol* 1991;**48**:1057–1063.

22. Alecu C, Fortrat JO, Ducrocq X, et al: Duplex scanning diagnosis of internal carotid artery dissections. *Cerebrovasc Dis* 2007;**23**:441–447.

23. Hennerici M, Steinke W, Rautenberg W: High-resistance Doppler flow pattern in extracranial ICA dissection. *Arch Neurol* 1989;**46**:670–672.

24. Touboul PJ, Mas JL, Bousser M-G, Laplane D: Duplex scanning in extracranial vertebral artery dissection. *Stroke* 1987;**18**:116–121.

25. Caplan LR, Gonzalez, RG, Buonanno, FS: Case 18–2012: A 35-year-old man

with neck pain, hoarseness, and dysphagia. *N Engl J Med* 2012;**366**:2306–2313.

26. Krueger BR, Okazaki H: Vertebral-basilar distribution infarction following chiropractic cervical manipulation. *Mayo Clin Proc* 1980;**55**:322–332.

27. Sherman DG, Hart RG, Easton JD: Abrupt change in head position and cerebral infarction. *Stroke* 1981;**12**:2–6.

28. Caplan LR: *Posterior circulation disease: Clinical Findings, Diagnosis, and Management*. Boston: Blackwell Science, 1996.

29. Cook JW, Sanstead JK: Wallenberg's syndrome following self-induced manipulation. *Neurology* 1991;**41**:1695–1696.

30. Rothrock JF, Hesselink JR, Teacher TM: Vertebral artery occlusion and stroke from cervical self-manipulation. *Neurology* 1991;**41**:1696–1697.

31. Tramo MJ, Hainline B, Petito F, et al: Vertebral artery injury and cerebellar stroke while swimming: Case report. *Stroke* 1985;**16**:1039–1042.

32. Hope EE, Bodensteiner JB, Barnes P: Cerebral infarction related to neck position in an adolescent. *Pediatrics* 1983;**72**:335–337.

33. Bostrom K, Liliequist B: Primary dissecting aneurysm of the extracranial part of the internal carotid and vertebral arteries. *Neurology* 1967;**17**:179–186.

34. Grossman FI, Davis KR: Positional occlusion of the vertebral artery: A rare cause of embolic stroke. *Neuroradiology* 1982;**23**:227–230.

35. Tettenborn B, Caplan LR, Sloan MA, et al: Postoperative brainstem and cerebellar infarcts. *Neurology* 1993;**43**:471–477.

36. Giroud M, Gras P, Dumas R, Becker F: Spontaneous vertebral artery dissection initially revealed by a pain in one upper arm. *Stroke* 1993;**24**:480–481.

37. Dubard T, Pouchot J, Lamy C, et al: Upper limb peripheral motor deficits due to extracranial vertebral artery dissection. *Cerebrovasc Dis* 1994;**4**:88–91.

38. Goldsmith P, Rowe D, Jager R, Kapoor R: Focal vertebral artery dissection causing Brown–Séquard syndrome. *J Neurol Neurosurg Psychiatry* 1998;**64**:416–417.

39. Yonas H, Agamanolis D, Takaoka Y, White RJ: Dissecting intracranial aneurysms. *Surg Neurol* 1977;**8**:407–415.

40. Caplan LR, Baquis G, Pessin MS, et al: Dissection of the intracranial vertebral artery. *Neurology* 1988;**38**:868–879.

41. Anson J, Crowell RM: Cervicocranial arterial dissection. *Neurosurg* 1991;**29**:89–96.

42. O'Connell B, Towfighi J, Brennan R, et al: Dissecting aneurysms of head and neck. *Neurology* 1985;**35**:993–997.

43. Chaves C, Estol C, Esnaola MM, et al: Spontaneous intracranial internal carotid artery dissection. *Arch Neurol* 2002;**59**:977–981.

44. Caplan LR, Estol CJ, Massaro AR: Dissection of the posterior cerebral arteries. *Arch Neurol* 2005;**62**:1138–1143.

45. de Bray JM, Marc G, Pautot G, et al: Fibromuscular dysplasia may herald symptomatic recurrence of cervical artery dissection. *Cerebrovasc Dis* 2007;**23**:448–452.

46. Schievink WI: The treatment of spontaneous carotid and vertebral artery dissections. *Curr Opin Carotid* 2000;**15**:316–321.

47. Caprio FZ, Bernstein RA, Alberts MJ, et al: Efficacy and safety of novel oral anticoagulants in patients with cervical artery dissections. *Cerebrovasc Dis* 2014;**38**:247–253.

48. Kasner SE, Hankins LL, Bratina P, Morganstern LB: Magnetic resonance angiography demonstrates vascular healing of carotid and vertebral artery dissections. *Stroke* 1997;**28**:1993–1997.

49. Leclerc X, Lucas C, Godefroy O, et al: Helical CT for the follow-up of cervical internal carotid artery dissections. *AJNR Am J Neuroradiol* 1998;**19**:831–837.

50. Engelter ST, Brandt T, Debette S, et al: Antiplatelets versus anticoagulation in cervical artery dissection. Cervical Artery Dissection in Ischemic Stroke Patients 5(CADISP) Study Group. *Stroke* 2007;**38**:2605–2611.

51. Georgiadis D, Lanczik O, Schwab S, et al: IV thrombolysis in patients with acute stroke due to spontaneous carotid dissection. *Neurology* 2005;**64**:1612–1614.

52. Biller J, Sacco R, Albuquerque FC, et al: Cervical arterial dissections and association with cervical manipulative therapy: A statement for healthcare professionals from the American Heart Association/American Stroke Association. *Stroke* 2014;**45**:3155–3174.

53. Kadkhodayan Y, Jeck DT, Moran CJ, et al: Angioplasty and stenting in carotid artery dissection with or without associated pseudoaneurysm. *AJNR Am J Neuroradiol* 2005;**26**:2328–2335.

54. Lavallee PC, Mazighi M, Saint-Maurice J-P, et al: Stent-assisted endovascular thrombolysis versus intravenous thrombolysis in internal carotid artery dissection with tandem internal carotid and middle cerebral artery occlusion. *Stroke* 2007;**38**:2270–2274.

55. Ansari SA, Thompson BG, Gemmete JJ, Gandhi D: Endovascular treatment of distal cervical and intracranial dissections with the neuroform stent. *Neurosurgery* 2008;**62**:636–646.

56. Janjua N, Qureshi AI, Kirmani J, Pullicino P: Stent-supported angioplasty for acute stroke caused by carotid dissection. *Neurocrit Care* 2006;**4**:47–53.

57. Caplan LR: Fibromuscular dysplasia. In Caplan LR (ed): *Uncommon Causes of Stroke*, 2nd ed. Cambridge: Cambridge University Press, 2008, pp 491–495.

58. Slovut DP, Olin JW: Fibromuscular dysplasia. *N Engl J Med* 2004;**350**:1862–1871.

59. So EL, Toole JF, Dalal P, et al: Cephalic fibromuscular dysplasia in 32 patients. *Arch Neurol* 1981;**38**:619–622.

60. Corrin LS, Sandok BA, Houser OW: Cerebral ischemic events in patients with carotid artery fibromuscular dysplasia. *Arch Neurol* 1981;**38**:616–618.

61. Sandok BA: Fibromuscular dysplasia of the internal carotid artery. *Neurol Clin* 1983;**1**:17–26.

62. Luscher TF, Lie JT, Stanson AW, et al: Arterial fibromuscular dysplasia. *Mayo Clin Proc* 1987;**62**:931–952.

63. Kubis N, von Langsdorrff D, Petitjean C, et al: Thrombotic carotid megabulb: Fibromuscular dysplasia, septae, and ischemic stroke. *Neurology* 1999;**52**:883–886.

64. Mettinger K, Ericson K: Fibromuscular dysplasia and the brain. *Stroke* 1982;**13**:46–52.

65. Olin JW, Froehlich J, Gux, et al: The United States Registry for Fibromuscular Dysplasia: Results in the first 447 patients. *Circulation* 2012;**125**:3182–3190.

66. Finsterer J, Strassegger J, Haymerle A, Hagmuller G: Bilateral stenting and asymptomatic internal carotid artery stenosis due to fibromuscular dysplasia. *J Neurol Neurosurg Psychiatry* 2000;**69**:683–686.

67. Assadian A, Senekowitsch C, Assadian O, et al: Combined open and endovascular stent grafting of internal carotid artery fibromuscular dysplasia: Long-term results. *Eur J Vasc Endovasc Surg* 2005;**29**:345–349.

68. Olin JW, Gornik HL, Bacharach JM, Biller J, et al: Fibromusclar dysplasia: State of the science and critical unanswered questions. A Scientific Statement from the American Heart Association. *Circulation* 2014;**129**:1048–1078.

69. Pessin MS, Chung C-S: Eales disease and Gröenblad-Strandberg disease (pseudoxanthoma elasticum). In Bogousslavsky J, Caplan LR (eds): *Stroke Syndromes.* Cambridge: Cambridge University Press, 1995, pp 443–447.

70. Lebwohl MG, Distefano D, Prioleau PG, et al: Pseudoxanthoma elasticum and mitral-valve prolapse. *N Engl J Med* 1982;**307**:228–231.

71. Caplan LR, Chung C-S: Pseudoxanthoma elasticum. In Caplan LR (ed): *Uncommon Causes of Stroke,* 2nd ed. Cambridge: Cambridge University Press, 2008, pp 135–138.

72. Laube S, Moss C: Pseudoxanthoma elasticum. *Arch Dis Child* 2005;**90**:754–756.

73. Strole WE, Margolis R: Case records of the Massachusetts General Hospital: Case 10–1983. *N Engl J Med* 1983;**308**:579–585.

74. Altman LK, Fialkow PJ, Parker F, et al: Pseudoxanthoma elasticum: An underdiagnosed genetically heterogenous disorder with protean manifestations. *Arch Intern Med* 1974;**134**:1048–1054.

75. Rios-Montenegro E, Behrens MM, Hoyt WF: Pseudoxanthoma elasticum: Association with bilateral carotid rete mirabile and unilateral carotid-cavernous sinus fistula. *Arch Neurol* 1972;**26**:151–155.

76. Roach ES: Ehlers–Danlos syndrome. In Caplan LR (ed): *Uncommon Causes of Stroke,* 2nd ed. Cambridge: Cambridge University Press, 2008, pp 139–144.

77. Byers PH: Ehlers–Danlos syndrome type IV: A genetic disorder in many guises. *J Invest Dermatol* 1995;**105**:311–313.

78. Leier CV, Call TD, Fulkerson PK, Wooley CF: The spectrum of cardiac defects in the Ehlers–Danlos syndrome types I and III. *Ann Intern Med* 1980;**92**:171–178.

79. Pretorius ME, Butler IJ: Neurologic manifestations of Ehlers–Danlos syndrome. *Neurology* 1983;**33**:1087–1089.

80. Lach B, Nair SG, Russell NA, Benoit BG: Spontaneous carotid-cavernous fistula and multiple arterial dissections in type IV Ehlers–Danlos syndrome. *J Neurosurg* 1987;**66**:462–467.

81. Sareli AE, Janssen WJ, Sterman D, et al: What's the connection? *N Engl J Med* 2008;**358**:626–632.

82. North KN, Whiteman DAH, Pepin MG, Byers PH: Cerebrovascular complications in Ehlers–Danlos syndrome type IV. *Ann Neurol* 1995;**38**:960–964.

83. Schievink WI, Limburg M, Oorthuys JW, et al: Cerebrovascular disease in Ehlers–Danlos syndrome type IV. *Stroke* 1990;**21**:626–632.

84. Schievink WI, Parisi JE, Piepgras DG, Michels VV: Intracranial aneurysms in Marfan's syndrome: An autopsy study. *Neurosurgery* 1997;**41**:866–870.

85. Conway JE, Hutchins GM, Tamargo RJ: Marfan syndrome is not associated with intracranial aneurysms. *Stroke* 1999;**30**:1632–1636.

86. Pyeritz RE: The Marfan syndrome. *Annu Rev Med* 2000;**51**:481–510.

87. Cunha L: Marfan's syndrome. In Caplan LR (ed): *Uncommon Causes of Stroke,* 2nd ed. Cambridge: Cambridge University Press, 2008, pp 131–134.

88. Kainulainen K, Pulkkinen L, Savolainen A, et al: Location on chromosome 15 of the gene defect causing Marfan syndrome. *N Engl J Med* 1990;**323**:935–939.

89. Schievink WI, Björnsson J, Piepgras DG: Coexistence of fibromuscular dysplasia and cystic medial necrosis in a patient with Marfan's syndrome and bilateral carotid artery dissections. *Stroke* 1994;**12**:2492–2496.

90. Youl BD, Coutellier A, Dubois B, et al: Three cases of spontaneous extracranial vertebral artery dissection. *Stroke* 1990;**4**:618–625.

91. van den Berg JS, Limburg M, Hennekam RC: Is Marfan syndrome associated with symptomatic intracranial aneurysms? *Stroke* 1996;**27**:10–12.

92. Loeys BL, Chen J, Neptune ER, et al: A syndrome of altered cardiovascular, craniofacial, neurocognitive and skeletal development caused by mutations in *TGFBR1* or *TGFBR2*. *Nat Genet* 2005;**37**:275–281.

93. Loeys BL, Schwarze U, Holm T, et al: Aneurysm syndromes caused by mutations in the TGF-beta receptor. *N Engl J Med* 2006;**355**:788–798.

94. LeMaire SA, Pannu H, Tran-Fadulu V, et al: Severe aortic and arterial aneurysms associated with *TGFBR2* mutation. *Nat Clin Pract Cardiovasc Med* 2007;**4**:167–171.

95. Savitz S, Caplan LR: Dilatative arteriopathy (dolichoectasia). In Caplan LR (ed): *Uncommon Causes of Stroke,* 2nd ed. Cambridge: Cambridge University Press, 2008, pp 479–482.

96. Lou M, Caplan LR: Vertebrobasilar dilatative arteriopathy (dolichoectasia). *Ann NY Acad Sci* 2010;**1184**:121–133.

97. Smoker WR, Price MJ, Keyes WD, et al: High-resolution computed tomography of the basilar artery: 1. Normal size and position. *AJNR Am J Neuroradiol* 1986;**7**:55–60.

98. Pico F, Labreuche J, Cohen A, et al: Intracranial arterial dolichoectasia is associated with enlarged descending thoracic aorta. *Neurology* 2004;**63**:2016–2021.

99. Read D, Esiri MM: Fusiform basilar artery aneurysm in a child. *Neurology* 1979;**29**:1045–1049.

100. Hirsch CS, Roessmann U: Arterial dysplasia with ruptured basilar artery aneurysm: Report of a case. *Hum Pathol* 1975;**6**:749–758.

101. Makos MM, McComb RD, Hart MN, Bennett DR: Alpha-glucosidase deficiency and basilar artery aneurysm: Report of a sibship. *Ann Neurol* 1987;**22**:629–633.

102. Schwartz A, Rautenberg W, Hennerici M: Dolichoectatic intracranial arteries: Review of selected aspects. *Cerebrovasc Dis* 1993;**3**:273–279.

103. Caplan LR: Dilatative arteriopathy (dolichoectasia): What is known and not known. *Ann Neurol* 2005;**57**:469–471.

104. Pico F, Labreuche J, Touboul PJ, Amarenco P: Intracranial arterial dolichoectasia and its relation with atherosclerosis and stroke subtype. *Neurology* 2003;**61**:1736–1742.

105. Pico F, Labreuche J, Touboul PJ, et al: Intracranial arterial dolichoectasia

and small-vessel disease in stroke patients. *Ann Neurol* 2005;**57**:472–479.

106. Pessin MS, Chimowitz MI, Levine SR, et al: Stroke in patients with fusiform vertebrobasilar aneurysms. *Neurology* 1989;**39**:16–21.

107. Moseley IF, Holland IM: Ectasia of the basilar artery: The breadth of the clinical spectrum and the diagnostic value of computed tomography. *Neuroradiology* 1979;**18**:83–91.

108. Little JR, St Louis P, Weinstein M, et al: Giant fusiform aneurysms of the cerebral arteries. *Stroke* 1981;**12**:183–188.

109. Echiverri HC, Rubino FA, Gupta SR, Gujrati M: Fusiform aneurysm of the vertebrobasilar arterial system. *Stroke* 1989;**20**:1741–1747.

110. Nishizaki T, Tamaki N, Takeda N, et al: Dolichoectatic basilar artery: A review of 23 cases. *Stroke* 1986;**17**:1277–1281.

111. Shokunbi MT, Vinters HV, Kaufmann JC: Fusiform intracranial aneurysms: Clinicopathologic features. *Surg Neurol* 1988;**29**:263–270.

112. Savitz SI, Ronthal M, Caplan LR: Vertebral artery compression of the medulla. *Arch Neurol* 2006;**63**:234–241.

113. DeGeorgia M, Belden J, Pao L, et al: Thrombus in vertebrobasilar dolichoectatic artery treated with intravenous urokinase. *Cerebrovasc Dis* 1999;**9**:28–33.

114. Cohen MM, Hemalatha CP, D'Addario RT, Goldman HW: Embolism from a fusiform middle cerebral artery aneurysm. *Stroke* 1980;**11**:158–161.

115. Aichner FT, Felber SR, Birhamer GG, Posch A: Magnetic resonance imaging and magnetic resonance angiography of vertebrobasilar dolichoectasia. *Cerebrovasc Dis* 1993;**3**:280–284.

116. Hennerici M, Rautenberg W, Schwartz A: Trans-cranial Doppler ultrasound for the assessment of intracranial arterial flow velocity: II. *Evaluation of intracranial arterial disease. Surg Neurol* 1987;**27**:523–532.

117. Passero S, Rossi S: Natural history of vertebrobasilar dolichoectasia. *Neurology* 2008;**70**:66–72.

118. Vinters HV: Cerebral amyloid angiopathy: A critical review. *Stroke* 1987;**18**:311–324.

119. Cordonnier C, Leys D: Cerebral amyloid angiopathies. In Caplan LR (ed): *Uncommon Causes of Stroke*, 2nd ed. Cambridge: Cambridge University Press, 2008, pp 455–464.

120. Vinters HV, Gilbert JJ: Cerebral amyloid angiopathy: Incidence and complications in the aging brain: II. The distribution of amyloid vascular changes. *Stroke* 1983;**14**:924–928.

121. Okazaki H, Reagan TJ, Campbell RJ: Clinicopathological studies of primary cerebral amyloid angiopathy. *Mayo Clin Proc* 1979;**54**:22–31.

122. Cosgrove G, Leblanc R, Meagher-Villemure K, et al: Cerebral amyloid angiopathy. *Neurology* 1985;**34**:625–631.

123. Gilbert JJ, Vinters HV: Cerebral amyloid angiopathy: Incidence and complications in the aging brain: I. Cerebral hemorrhage. *Stroke* 1983;**14**:915–923.

124. Kase CS: Cerebral amyloid angiopathy. In Kase CS, Caplan LR (eds): *Intracerebral Hemorrhage.* Boston: Butterworth–Heinemann, 1994, pp 179–200.

125. Viswanathan A, Greenberg SM: Cerebral amyloid angiopathy in the elderly. *Ann Neurol* 2011;**70**:871–880.

126. Greenberg SM, Eng JA, Ning M, et al: Hemorrhage burden predicts recurrent intracerebral hemorrhage after lobar hemorrhage. *Stroke* 2004;**35**:1415–1420.

127. Greenberg SM, Finklestein SP, Schaefer PW: Petechial hemorrhages accompanying lobar hemorrhage: Detection by gradient-echo MRI. *Neurology* 1996;**46**:1751–1754.

128. Kumar S, Goddeau RP, Selim MH, et al. Atraumatic convexal subarachnoid hemorrhage: Clinical presentation, imaging patterns, and etiologies. *Neurology* 2010;**74**:893–899.

129. Beitzke M, Gattringer T, Enzinger C, Wagner G, Niederkorn K, Fazekas F: Clinical presentation and long term prognosis in patients with nontraumatic convexal subarachnoid hemorrhage. *Stroke* 2011;**42**:3055–3060.

130. Linn J, Herms J, Bruckmann H, Fesl G, Freilinger T, Wiesmann M: Subarachnoid hemosiderosis and superficial cortical hemosiderosis in cerebral amyloid angiopathy. *AJNR Am J Neuroradiol* 2008;**29**:184–186.

131. Linn J, Halpin A, Demaerel P, et al: Prevalence of superficial siderosis in patients with cerebral amyloid angiopathy. *Neurology* 2010;**74**:1346–1350.

132. Shoamanesh A, Martinez-Ramirez S, Oliveira-Filho J, et al: Interrelationship of superficial siderosis and microbleeds in cerebral amyloid angiopathy. *Neurology* 2014;**83**:1838–1843.

133. Greenberg SM, Hyman BT: Cerebral amyloid angiopathy and apolipoprotein E: Bad news for the good allele? *Ann Neurol* 1997;**41**:701–702.

134. O'Donnell HC, Rosand J, Knudsen KA, et al: Apolipoprotein E genotype and the risk of recurrent lobar intracerebral hemorrhage. *N Engl J Med* 2000;**342**:240–245.

135. McCarron MO, Nicoll JA, Ironside JW, et al: Cerebral amyloid angiopathy-related hemorrhage. I. Interaction of APOE ε2 with putative clinical risk factors. *Stroke* 1999;**30**:1643–1646.

136. Smith DB, Hitchcock M, Philpott PJ: Cerebral amyloid angiopathy presenting as transient ischemic attacks: Case report. *J Neurosurg* 1985;**63**:963–964.

137. Gray F, Dubas F, Roullet E, Escourolle R: Leukoencephalopathy in diffuse hemorrhagic cerebral amyloid angiopathy. *Ann Neurol* 1985;**18**:54–59.

138. Loes DJ, Biller J, Yuh WTC, et al: Leukoencephalopathy in cerebral amyloid angiopathy: MR imaging in four cases. *AJNR Am J Neuroradiol* 1990;**11**:485–488.

139. DeWitt LD, Louis DN: Case records of the Massachusetts General Hospital: Case 27–1991. *N Engl J Med* 1991;**325**:42–54.

140. Greenberg SM, Vonsattel JPG, Stakes JW, et al: The clinical spectrum of cerebral amyloid angiopathy: Presentations without lobar hemorrhage. *Neurology* 1993;**43**:2073–2079.

141. Grubb A, Jensson O, Gudmundsson G, et al: Abnormal metabolism of Y-trace alkaline microprotein: The basic defect in hereditary cerebral hemorrhage with amyloidosis. *N Engl J Med* 1984;**311**:1547–1549.

142. Stefansson K, Antel JP, Ojer J, et al: Autosomal dominant cerebrovascular amyloidosis: Properties of peripheral blood lymphocytes. *Ann Neurol* 1980;**7**:436–440.

143. Fountain NB, Eberhard DA: Primary angiitis of the central nervous system

associated with cerebral amyloid angiopathy: Report of two cases and review of the literature. *Neurology* 1996;**46**:190–197.

144. Caplan LR: Case records of the Massachusetts General Hospital. Case 10–2000. *N Engl J Med* 2000;**342**:957–964.

145. Eng JA, Frosch MP, Choi K, et al: Clinical manifestations of cerebral amyloid angiopathy-related inflammation. *Ann Neurol* 2004;**55**:250–256.

146. Marotti JD, Savitz SI, Kim W-K, et al: Cerebral amyloid angiitis progressing to generalized angiitis and leucoencephalitis. *Neuropathol Appl Neurobiol* 2007;**33**:1–5.

147. Scolding NJ, Joseph F, Kirby PA, et al: Aβ-related angiitis: Primary angiitis of the central nervous system associated with cerebral amyloid angiopathy. *Brain* 2005;**128**:500–515.

148. Chung KK, Anderson NE, Hutchinson D, Syneck B, Barbar PA: Cerebral amyloid angiopathy related inflammation: Three case reports and a review. *J Neurol Neurosurg Psychiatry* 2011;**82**:20–26.

149. Salvarani C, Hunder GG, Morris JM, Brown RD Jr, Christianson T, Giannini C: Aβ-related angiitis: comparison with CAA without inflammation and primary CNS vasculitis. *Neurology* 2013;**81**:1596–1603.

150. Greene GM, Godersky JC, Biller J, et al: Surgical experience with intracerebral hemorrhage secondary to cerebral amyloid angiopathy. *Stroke* 1990;**21**:170.

151. Izumihara A, Ishihara T, Iwamoto N, et al: Postoperative outcome of 37 patients with lobar intracerebral hemorrhage related to cerebral amyloid angiopathy. *Stroke* 1999;**30**:29–33.

152. Greenberg SM: Cerebral amyloid angiopathy. Prospects for clinical diagnosis and treatment. *Neurology* 1998;**51**:690–694.

153. Greenberg SM, Salman RA-S, Biessels GJ, et al: Outcome markers for clinical trials in cerebral amyloid angiopathy. *Lancet Neurol* 2014;**13**:419–428.

154. van de Beek D, de Gans J, Spanjaard L, et al: Clinical features and prognostic factors in adults with bacterial meningitis. *N Engl J Med* 2004;**351**:1849–1859.

155. van de Beek D, de Gans J, Tunkel AR, et al: Community-acquired bacterial meningitis in adults. *N Engl J Med* 2006;**354**:44–53.

156. Bentley P, Quadri F, Wild EJ, et al: Vasculitic presentation of staphylococcal meningitis. *Arch Neurol* 2007;**64**:1788–1789.

157. O'Farrell R, Thornton J, Brennan P, et al: Spinal cord infarction and tetraplegia – Rare complications of meningococcal meningitis. *Br J Anesth* 2000;**84**:514–517.

158. van de Beek D, Patel R, Wijdicks EFM: Meningococcal meningitis with brainstem infarction. *Arch Neurol* 2007;**64**:1350–1351.

159. Weinstein AJ, Schianone WA, Furlan AJ: *Listeria* rhomboencephalitis. *Arch Neurol* 1982;**39**:514–516.

160. Brown RH, Sobel RA: Case records of the Massachusetts General Hospital. *N Engl J Med* 1989;**321**:739–750.

161. Frayne J, Gates P: *Listeria* rhomboencephalitis. *Clin Exp Neurol* 1987;**24**:175–179.

162. Silvestri N, Ajani Z, Savitz S, Caplan LR: A 73-year-old woman with an acute illness causing fever and cranial nerve abnormalities. *Rev Neurol Dis* 2006; **3**:29–30, 35–37.

163. Windsor JJ: Cat-scratch disease: Epidemiology, aetiology and treatment. *Br J Biomed Sci* 2001;**58**:101–110.

164. Selby G, Walker GL: Cerebral arteritis in cat-scratch disease. *Neurology* 1979;**29**:1413–1418.

165. Davis LE, Graham GD: Neurosyphilis and stroke. In Caplan LR (ed): *Uncommon Causes of Stroke*, 2nd ed. Cambridge: Cambridge University Press, 2008, pp 35–40.

166. Flint AC, Liberato BB, Anziska Y, et al: Meningovascular syphilis as a cause of basilar artery stenosis. *Neurology* 2005;**64**:391–392.

167. Gaa J, Weidauer S, Sitzer M, et al: Cerebral vasculitis due to treponema pallidum infection: MRI and MRA findings. *Eur Radiol* 2004;**14**:746–747.

168. Golden MR, Marra CM, Holmes KK: Update on syphilis: Resurgence of an old problem. *JAMA* 2003;**290**:1510–1514.

169. Rahn DW, Malawista SE: Lyme disease: Recommendations for diagnosis and treatment. *Ann Intern Med* 1991;**114**:472–481.

170. Steere AC, Sikand VK: The presenting manifestations of Lyme disease and the outcomes of treatment. *N Engl J Med* 2003;**348**:2472–2474.

171. Halperin JJ, Luft BJ, Anand AK, et al: Lyme neuroboreliosis: Central nervous system manifestations. *Neurology* 1989;**39**:753–759.

172. Pachner AR, Duray P, Steere AC: Cerebral nervous system manifestations of Lyme disease. *Arch Neurol* 1989;**46**:790–795.

173. Uldry PA, Regli F, Bogousslavsky J: Cerebral angiopathy and recurrent strokes following Borrelia burgdorferi infection. *J Neurol Neurosurg Psychiatry* 1987;**50**:1703–1704.

174. Schmiedel J, Gahn G, von Kummer R, Reichmann H: Cerebral vasculitis with multiple infarcts caused by Lyme disease. *Cerebrovasc Dis* 2004;**17**:79–81.

175. Halperin JJ: Stroke in Lyme disease. In Caplan LR (ed): *Uncommon Causes of Stroke*, 2nd ed. Cambridge: Cambridge University Press, 2008, pp 59–66.

176. Katrak SM: Vasculitis and stroke due to tuberculosis. In Caplan LR (ed): *Uncommon Causes of Stroke*, 2nd ed. Cambridge: Cambridge University Press, 2008, pp 41–46.

177. Leiguarda R, Berthier M, Starkstein S, et al: Ischemic infarction in 25 children with tuberculous meningitis. *Stroke* 1988;**19**:200–204.

178. Katrak SM, Shembalkar PK, Bijwe SR, Bhandarkar LD: The clinical, radiological and pathological profile of tuberculous meningitis in patients with and without human deficiency virus infection. *J Neurol Sci* 2000;**181**:118–126.

179. Bernaerts A, Vanhoenacker FM, Parizel PM, et al: Tuberculosis of the central nervous system: overview of neuroradiological findings. *Eur Radiol* 2003;**13**:1876–1890.

180. Chan KH, Cheung RT, Lee R, et al: Cerebral infarcts complicating tuberculous meningitis. *Cerebrovasc Dis* 2005;**19**:391–395.

181. Hier DB, Caplan LR: Stroke due to fungal infections. In Caplan LR (ed): *Uncommon Causes of Stroke*, 2nd ed. Cambridge: Cambridge University Press, 2008, pp 47–52.

182. Kobayashi RM, Coil M, Niwayama G, Trauner D: Cerebral vasculitis in coccidioidal meningitis. *Ann Neurol* 1977;**1**:281–284.

183. Walsh TJ, Hier DB, Caplan LR: Fungal infection of the central nervous system: Comparative analysis of the risk factors and clinical signs in 57 patients. *Neurology* 1985;**35**:1654–1657.

184. Walsh TJ, Hier DB, Caplan LR: Aspergillosis of the central nervous system: Clinicopathological analysis of 17 patients. *Ann Neurol* 1985;**18**:574–582.

185. Kleinschmidt-DeMasters BK: Central nervous system aspergillosis: A 20 year retrospective series. *Hum Pathol* 2002;**33**:116–124.

186. Rangel-Guerra R, Martinez HR, Saenz C, et al: Rhinocerebral and systemic mucormycosis. Clinical experience in 36 cases. *J Neurol Sci* 1996;**143**:19–30.

187. Moore PM, Cupps TR: Neurologic complications of vasculitis. *Ann Neurol* 1983;**14**:155–167.

188. Bischof M, Baumgartner RW: Varicella-zoster and other virus-related cerebral vasculopathy. In Caplan LR (ed): *Uncommon Causes of Stroke*, 2nd ed. Cambridge: Cambridge University Press, 2008, pp 17–26.

189. Gilden DH, Kleinschmidt-DeMasters BK, Wellish M, et al: Varicella-zoster virus, a cause of waxing and waning vasculitis: The *New England Journal of Medicine* case 5–1995 revisited. *Neurology* 1996;**47**:1441–1446.

190. Bourdette DN, Rosenberg NL, Yatsu FM: Herpes zoster ophthalmicus and delayed ipsilateral cerebral infarction. *Neurology* 1983;**33**:1428–1432.

191. Hilt DC, Buchholz D, Krumholz A, et al: Herpes zoster ophthalmicus and delayed contralateral hemiparesis caused by cerebral angiitis: Diagnosis and management approaches. *Ann Neurol* 1983;**14**:543–553.

192. Doyle PW, Gibson G, Dolman C: Herpes zoster ophthalmicus with contralateral hemiplegia: Identification of cause. *Ann Neurol* 1983;**14**:84–85.

193. Nagel MA, Cohrs RJ, Mahalingam R, et al: The varicella zoster virus vasculopathies. Clinical, CSF, imaging and virologic features. *Neurology* 2008;**70**:853–860.

194. Powers JM: Herpes zoster maxillaris with delayed occipital infarction. *J Clin Neuroophthalmol* 1986;**2**:113–115.

195. Snow BJ, Simcock JP: Brainstem infarction following cervical herpes zoster. *Neurology* 1988;**38**:1331.

196. Ross MH, Abend WK, Schwartz RB, Samuels MA: A case of C2 herpes zoster with delayed bilateral pontine infarction. *Neurology* 1991;**41**:1685–1686.

197. Caekebeke JFV, Peters ACB, Vandvik B, et al: Cerebral vasculopathy associated with primary varicella infection. *Arch Neurol* 1990;**47**:1033–1035.

198. Askalan R, Laughlin S, Mayank S, et al: Chickenpox and stroke in childhood: A study of frequency and causation. *Stroke* 2001;**32**:1257–1262.

199. Hausler MG, Ramaekers VT, Reul J, et al: Early and late onset manifestations of cerebral vasculitis related to varicella zoster. *Neuropediatrics* 1998;**29**:202–207.

200. Lanthier S, Armstrong D, Domi T, deVeber G: Post-varicella arteriopathy of childhood. *Neurology* 2005;**64**:660–663.

201. Melanson M, Chalk C, Georgevich L, et al: Varicella-zoster virus DNA in CSF and arteries in delayed contralateral hemiplegia: Evidence for viral invasion of cerebral arteries. *Neurology* 1996;**47**:569–570.

202. Saito K, Moskowitz MA: Contributions from the upper cervical dorsal roots and trigeminal ganglia to the feline circle of Willis. *Stroke* 1989;**20**:524–526.

203. Pinto AN: AIDS and cerebrovascular disease. *Stroke* 1996;**27**:538–543.

204. Gillams AR, Allen E, Hrieb K, et al: Cerebral infarction in patients with AIDS. *AJNR Am J Neuroradiol* 1997;**18**:1581–1585.

205. Cole John W, Pinto AN, Hebel JR, et al: Acquired immunodeficiency syndrome and the risk of stroke. *Stroke* 2004;**35**:51–56.

206. Berger JR: AIDS and stroke risk. *Lancet Neurol* 2004;**3**:206–207.

207. Fritz V, Bryer A: Stroke in persons infected with HIV. In Caplan LR (ed): *Uncommon Causes of Stroke*, 2nd ed. Cambridge: Cambridge University Press, 2008, pp 93–100.

208. Dubrovsky T, Curless R, Scott G, et al: Cerebral aneurysmal arteriopathy in childhood AIDS. *Neurology* 1998;**51**:560–565.

209. Lipton J, Rivkin MJ: Kawasaki disease: Cerebrovascular and neurologic complications. In Caplan LR (ed): *Uncommon Causes of Stroke*, 2nd ed.

Cambridge: Cambridge University Press, 2008, pp 81–86.

210. Amano S, Hazama F, Hamashima Y: Pathology of Kawasaki disease: II. Distribution and incidence of the vascular lesions. *Jpn Circ J* 1979;**43**:741–748.

211. Amano S, Hazama F, Kubagawa H, et al: General pathology of Kawasaki disease. On the morphological alterations corresponding to the clinical manifestations. *Acta Pathol Jpn* 1980;**30**:681–694.

212. Del Bruto OH: Stroke and vasculitis in patients with cysticercosis. In Caplan LR (ed): *Uncommon Causes of Stroke*, 2nd ed. Cambridge: Cambridge University Press, 2008, pp 53–58.

213. García HH, Del Brutto OH: Neurocysticercosis: Updated concepts about an old disease. *Lancet Neurol* 2005;**4**:653–661.

214. Escobar A, Weidenheim KM: The pathology of neurocysticercosis. In Singh G, Prabhakar S (eds): *Taenia Solium Cysticercosis. From Basic to Clinical Science*. Wallingford, Oxon, UK: CAB International, 2002, pp 289–305.

215. Caplan LR: How to manage patients with neurocysticercosis. *Eur Neurol* 1997;**37**:124–131.

216. Rodriguez-Carbajal J, del Brutto OH, Penagos P, et al: Occlusion of the middle cerebral artery due to cysticercotic angiitis. *Stroke* 1989;**20**:1095–1099.

217. Monteiro L, Almeida-Pinto J, Leite I, et al: Cerebral cysticercus arteritis: Five angiographic cases. *Cerebrovasc Dis* 1994;**4**:125–133.

218. Barinagarrementaria F, Cantu C: Frequency of cerebral arteritis in subarachnoid cysticercosis. An angiographic study. *Stroke* 1998;**29**:123–125.

219. Cantu C, Villarreal J, Soto JL, Barinagarrementaria F: Cerebral cysticercotic arteriits: Detection and follow-up by transcranial Doppler. *Cerebrovasc Dis* 1998;**8**:2–7.

220. Bang OY, Heo JH, Choi SA, Kim DI: Large cerebral infarction during praziquantel therapy in neurocysticercosis. *Stroke* 1997;**28**:211–213.

221. Newton CR, Warrell DA: Neurological manifestations of falciparum malaria. *Ann Neurol* 1998;**43**:695–702.

222. Gall C, Spuler A, Fraunberger P: Subarachnoid hemorrhage in a patient with cerebral malaria. *N Engl J Med* 1999 **341**:611–613.

223. Omanga U, Ntihinyurwa M, Shako D, Mashako M: Les hemiplegies au cours de l'acces pernicieux a *Plasmodium falciparum* de l'enfant. *Ann Pediatr (Paris)* 1983;**30**:294–296.

224. Newton CR, Marsh K, Peshu N, Kirkham FJ: Perturbations of cerebral hemodynamics in Kenyan children with cerebral malaria. *Pediatr Neurol* 1996;**15**:41–49.

225. Massaro AR: Cerebrovascular problems in Chagas disease. In Caplan LR (ed): *Uncommon Causes of Stroke*, 2nd ed. Cambridge: Cambridge University Press, 2008, pp 87–92.

226. Carod-Artal FJ, Vargas AP, Melo M, Horan TA: American trypanosomiasis (Chagas' disease): An unrecognised cause of stroke. *J Neurol Neurosurg Psychiatry* 2003;**74**:516–518.

227. Carod-Artal FJ, Vargas AP, Horan TA, Nunes LG: Chagasic cardiomyopathy is independently associated with ischemic stroke in Chagas disease. *Stroke* 2005;**36**:965–970.

228. Leon-Sarmiento FE, Mendoza E, Torres-Hillera M, et al: Trypanosoma cruzi-associated cerebrovascular disease: A case-control study in Eastern Colombia. *J Neurol Sci* 2004;**217**:61–64.

229. Oliveira-Filho J, Viana LC, Vieira de Melo RM, et al: Chagas disease is an independent risk factor for stroke: Baseline characteristics of a Chagas disease cohort. *Stroke* 2005;**36**:2015–2017.

230. Carod-Artal FJ, Gascon J: Chagas disease and stroke. *Lancet Neurol* 2010;**9**:533–542.

231. Fauci AS, Haynes BF, Katz P: The spectrum of vasculitis: Clinical, pathologic, immunologic and therapeutic considerations. *Ann Intern Med* 1978;**89**:660–676.

232. Moore PM, Richardson B: Neurology of the vasculitides and connective tissue disease. *J Neurol Neurosurg Psychiatry* 1998;**65**:10–22.

233. Scott DG: Classification and treatment of systemic vasculitis. *Br J Rheumatol* 1988;**27**:251–257.

234. Moore PM, Fauci AS: Neurologic manifestations of systemic vasculitis: A retrospective and prospective study of the clinico-pathologic features and responses to therapy in 25 patients. *Am J Med* 1981;**71**:517–524.

235. Kissel JT, Rammohan KW: Pathology and therapy of nervous system vasculitis. *Clin Neuropharmacol* 1991;**14**:28–48.

236. Moore PM, Richardson B: Neurology of the vasculitides and connective tissue diseases. *J Neurol Neurosurg Psychiatry* 1998;**65**:10–22.

237. Villringer A, Moore PM: Vasculitides and other nonatherosclerotic vasculopathies of the nervous system. In Brandt T, Caplan LR, Dichgans J, et al. (eds): *Neurological Disorders.* San Diego: Academic Press, 1996, pp 305–327.

238. Reichhart MD, Meuli R, Bogousslavsky J: Microscopic polyangiitis (MPA) and polyarteritis nodosa (PAN). In Caplan LR (ed): *Uncommon Causes of Stroke*, 2nd ed. Cambridge: Cambridge University Press, 2008, pp 311–330.

239. Caplan LR, Hedley-White ET: Case records of the Massachusetts General Hospital: Case 5–1995. *N Engl J Med* 1995;**332**:452–459.

240. Mehdirrata M, Caplan LR: Churg–Strauss syndrome. In Caplan LR (ed): *Uncommon Causes of Stroke*, 2nd ed. Cambridge: Cambridge University Press, 2008, pp 331–334.

241. Churg J, Strauss L: Allergic granulomatosis, allergic angiitis, and periarteritis nodosa. *Am J Pathol* 1951;**27**:277–301.

242. Chumbley LC, Harrison EG, DeRemee RA: Allergic granulomatosis and angiitis (Churg–Strauss syndrome): Report and analysis of 30 cases. *Mayo Clin Proc* 1977;**52**:477–484.

243. Sehgal M, Swanson JW, DeRemee RA, Colby TV: Neurologic manifestations of Churg–Strauss syndrome. *Mayo Clin Proc* 1995;**70**:337–341.

244. Hauser SL, Shahani B, Hedley-White ET: Case records of the Massachusetts General Hospital: Case 38–1990. *N Engl J Med* 1990;**323**:812–822.

245. Jennette JC, Falk RJ: Small-vessel vasculitis. *N Engl J Med* 1997;**337**:1512–1523.

246. Savitz S, Caplan LR: Cerebrovascular complications of Henoch– Schönlein purpura. In Caplan LR (ed): *Uncommon Causes of Stroke*, 2nd ed. Cambridge: Cambridge University Press, 2008, pp 309–310.

247. Chiaretti A, Caresta E, Piastra M, et al: Cerebral hemorrhage in Henoch–Schönlein syndrome. *Childs Nerv Syst* 2002;**18**:365–367.

248. Eun SH, Kim SJ, Cho DS, et al: Cerebral vasculitis in Henoch–Schönlein purpura: MRI and MRA findings, treated with plasmapharesis alone. *Pediatr Int* 2003;**45**:484–487.

249. Fauci AS, Haynes BF, Katz P, Wolff SM: Wegener's granulomatosis: Prospective clinical and therapeutic experience with 85 patients for 21 years. *Ann Intern Med* 1983;**98**:76–85.

250. Haynes BF, Fishman ML, Fauci AS, Wolff SM: The ocular manifestations of Wegener's granulomatosis: Fifteen years' experience and review of the literature. *Am J Med* 1977;**63**:131–141.

251. Lapresle J, Lasjaunias P: Cranial nerve ischemic arterial syndromes. *Brain* 1985;**109**:207–215.

252. Palaic M, Yeadon C, Moore S, Cashman N: Wegener's granulomatosis mimicking temporal arteritis. *Neurology* 1991;**41**:1694–1695.

253. Frohman LP, Lama P: Annual review of systemic diseases: 1995–1996, part 1. *J Neuroophthalmol* 1998;**18**:67–79.

254. Satoh J, Miyasaka N, Yamada T, et al: Extensive cerebral infarction due to involvement of both anterior cerebral arteries by Wegener's granulomatosis. *Ann Rheum Dis* 1988;**47**:606–611.

255. Provenzale JM, Allen NB: Wegener granulomatosis: CT and MR findings. *AJNR Am J Neuroradiol* 1996;**17**:785–792.

256. Nölle B, Specks U, Lüdemann J, et al: Anticytoplasmic autoantibodies: Their immunodiagnostic value in Wegener's granulomatosis. *Ann Intern Med* 1989;**111**:28–40.

257. Feinglass EJ, Arnett SC, Dorsch CA, et al: Neuropsychiatric manifestations of systemic lupus erythematosus: Diagnosis, clinical spectrum, and relationship to other features of the disease. *Medicine (Baltimore)* 1976;**55**:323–339.

258. Futrell N: Systemic lupus erythematosus. In Caplan LR (ed): *Uncommon Causes of Stroke*, 2nd ed. Cambridge: Cambridge University Press, 2008, pp 335–342.

259. Johnson RT, Richardson EP: The neurological manifestations of systemic lupus erythematosus: A clinical–pathological study of 24 cases and review of the literature. *Medicine (Baltimore)* 1968;**47**:337–369.

260. Devinsky O, Petito C, Alonso D: Clinical and neuropathological findings in systemic lupus erythematosus: The role of vasculitis, heart emboli, and thrombotic thrombocytopenic purpura. *Ann Neurol* 1988;**23**:380–384.

261. Alsen AM, Gabrulsen TO, McCune WJ: MR imaging of systemic lupus erythematosus involving the brain. *AJNR Am J Neuroradiol* 1985;**6**:197–201.

262. Trevor RF, Sondheimer FK, Fessel WJ, et al: Angiographic demonstration of major cerebral vessel occlusion in systemic lupus erythematosus. *Neuroradiology* 1972;**4**:202–207.

263. Hart R, Miller V, Coull B, et al: Cerebral infarction associated with lupus anticoagulants: Preliminary report. *Stroke* 1984;**15**:114–118.

264. McVerry BA, Machin SJ, Parry H, et al: Reduced prostacycline activity in systemic lupus erythematosus. *Ann Rheum Dis* 1980;**39**:524–525.

265. Galve E, Candell-Riera J, Pigrau C, et al: Prevalence, morphological types, and evaluation of cardiac valvular disease in systemic lupus erythematosus. *N Engl J Med* 1988;**319**:817–823.

266. Moncayo-Gaete J: Thrombotic thrombocytopenic purpura. In Caplan LR (ed): *Uncommon Causes of Stroke*, 2nd ed. Cambridge: Cambridge University Press, 2008, pp 301–308.

267. Petitt RM: Thrombotic thrombocytopenic purpura: A thirty year review. *Semin Thromb Hemost* 1980;**6**:350–355.

268. Kwaan HC: Clinicopathological features of thrombotic thrombocytopenic purpura. *Semin Hematol* 1987;**24**:71–81.

269. Silverstein A: Thrombotic thrombocytopenic purpura: The initial neurological manifestations. *Arch Neurol* 1968;**18**:358–362.

270. Rinkel G, Wijdicks E, Hene RJ: Stroke in relapsing thrombotic thrombocytopenic purpura. *Stroke* 1991;**22**:1087–1088.

271. Kelly PJ, McDonald CT, Neill GO, et al: Middle cerebral artery main stem thrombosis in two siblings with familial thrombocytopenic purpura. *Neurology* 1998;**50**:1157–1160.

272. Bakshi R, Shaikh ZA, Bates VE, Kinkel PR: Thrombotic thrombocytopenic purpura: Brain CT and MRI findings in 12 patients. *Neurology* 1999;**52**:1285–1288.

273. Hinchey J, Chaves C, Apignani B, et al: A reversible posterior leukoencephalopathy syndrome. *N Engl J Med* 1996;**334**:494–500.

274. Bennett CL, Weinberg PD, Rozenberg-Ben-Dror K, et al: Thrombotic thrombocytopenic purpura associated with ticlopidine. A review of 60 cases. *Ann Intern Med* 1998;**128**, 541–544.

275. Bennett CL, Connors JM, Carwile JM, et al: Thrombotic thrombocytopenic purpura associated with clopidogrel. *N Engl J Med* 2000;**342**:1773–1777.

276. Zakarija A, Bennett C: Drug-induced thrombotic microangiopathy. *Semin Thromb Hemost* 2005;**31**:681–690.

277. Shepard KV, Bukowski RM: The treatment of thrombotic thrombocytopenic purpura with exchange transfusions, plasma infusions and plasma exchange. *Semin Hematol* 1987;**24**:178–193.

278. Rubens E, Savitz S: Rheumatoid arthritis and cerebrovascular disease. In Caplan LR (ed): *Uncommon Causes of Stroke*, 2nd ed. Cambridge: Cambridge University Press, 2008, pp 343–346.

279. Ramos M, Mandybur TI: Cerebral vasculitis in rheumatoid arthritis. *Arch Neurol* 1975;**32**:271–275.

280. Watson P: Intracranial hemorrhage with vasculitis in rheumatoid arthritis. *Arch Neurol* 1979;**36**:58.

281. Watson P, Fekete J, Dick J: Central nervous system vasculitis in rheumatoid arthritis. *Can J Neurol Sci* 1977;**4**:269–271.

282. Takeda Y: Studies of the metabolism and distribution of fibrinogen in patients with rheumatoid arthritis. *J Lab Clin Med* 1967;**69**:624–633.

283. Jasin HE, LoSpalluto J, Ziff M: Rheumatoid hyperviscosity syndrome. *Am J Med* 1970;**49**:484–493.

284. Alexander EL, Provost TT, Stevens MB, Alexander GE: Neurologic complications of primary Sjögren's syndrome. *Medicine (Baltimore)* 1982;**61**:247–257.

285. Alexander GE, Provost TT, Stevens MB, Alexander EL: Sjögren syndrome: Central nervous system manifestations. *Neurology* 1981;**31**:1391–1396.

286. Alexander EL, Beall S, Gordon B, et al: Magnetic resonance imaging of cerebral lesions in patients with the Sjögren syndrome. *Ann Intern Med* 1988;**108**:815–823.

287. Alexander EL, Malinow K, Lijewski JE, et al: Primary Sjögren syndrome with central nervous system disease mimicking multiple sclerosis. *Ann Intern Med* 1986;**104**:323–330.

288. Rubens E: Scleroderma. In Caplan LR (ed): *Uncommon Causes of Stroke*, 2nd ed. Cambridge: Cambridge University Press, 2008, pp 429–431.

289. Estey E, Lieberman A, Pinto R, et al: Cerebral arteritis in scleroderma. *Stroke* 1979;**10**:595–597.

290. Pathak R, Gabor AJ: Scleroderma and central nervous system vasculitis. *Stroke* 1991;**22**:410–413.

291. Olugemo O, Stern BJ: Stroke and neurosarcoidosis. In Caplan LR (ed): *Uncommon Causes of Stroke, 2nd ed.* Cambridge: Cambridge University Press, 2008, pp 75–80.

292. Newman LS, Rose CS, Maier LA: Sarcoidosis. *N Engl J Med* 1997;**336**:1224–1234.

293. Scott TF: Neurosarcoidosis: Progress and clinical aspects. *Neurology* 1993;**43**:8–12.

294. Stern BJ, Krumholz A, Johns C, et al: Sarcoidosis and its neurological manifestations. *Arch Neurol* 1985;**42**:909–917.

295. Caplan LR, Corbett J, Goodwin J, et al: Neuro-ophthalmological signs in the angiitic form of neurosarcoidosis. *Neurology* 1983;**33**:1130–1135.

296. Meyer J, Foley J, Campagna-Pinto D: Granulomatous angiitis of the meninges in sarcoidosis. *Arch Neurol Psychiatry* 1953;**69**:587–600.

297. Alajouanine T, Bertrand J, Degos R, et al: Sarcoidose ganglionaire, cutanee et oculaire, avec atteinte secondaire diffuse, peripherique et centrale du système nerveux. *Rev Neurol (Paris)* 1958;**99**:421–447.

298. Urich H: Neurosarcoidosis or granulomatous angiitis: A problem of definition. *Mt Sinai J Med* 1977;**44**:718–725.

299. Karmi A: Ophthalmic changes in sarcoidosis. *Acta Ophthalmol* 1979;**141**(Suppl):1–94.

300. Stewart SS, Ashizawa T, Dudley Jr AW, et al: Cerebral vasculitis in relapsing poychondritis. *Neurology* 1988;**38**:150.

301. Thevathasan AW, Davis SM: Temporal arteritis. In Caplan LR (ed): *Uncommon Causes of Stroke*, 2nd ed. Cambridge: Cambridge University Press, 2008, pp 9–16.

302. Melson MR, Weyland CM, Newman NJ, Biousse V: The diagnosis of giant cell arteritis. *Rev Neurol Dis* 2007;**4**:128–142.

303. Goodwin J: Temporal arteritis. In Vinken P, Bruyn G (eds): *Handbook of Clinical Neurology*, vol **39**, part 2. Amsterdam: North Holland, 1980, pp 313–342.

304. Klein RG, Hunder GG, Stanson AW, et al: Large artery involvement in giant cell arteritis. *Ann Intern Med* 1975;**83**:806–812.

305. Wilkinson I, Russel R: Arteries of the head and neck in giant cell arteritis. *Arch Neurol* 1972;**27**:378–391.

306. Thielen KR, Wijdicks EFM, Nichols DA: Giant cell (temporal) arteritis: Involvement of the vertebral and internal carotid arteries. *Mayo Clin Proc* 1998;**73**:444–446.

307. Enzmann D, Scott WR: Intracranial involvement of giant-cell arteritis. *Neurology* 1977;**27**:794–797.

308. Casselli RJ: Giant cell (temporal) arteritis: A treatable cause of multi-infarct dementia. *Neurology* 1990;**40**:753–755.

309. Schmidt WA, Kraft HE, Vorpahl K, et al: Color Duplex ultrasonography in the diagnosis of temporal arteritis. *N Engl J Med* 1997;**337**:1336–1342.

310. Zuber M: Isolated angiitis of the central nervous system. In Caplan LR (ed): *Uncommon Causes of Stroke*, 2nd ed. Cambridge: Cambridge University Press, 2008, pp 1–8.

311. Salvarani C, Brown RD, Calamia KT, et al: Primary central nervous system vasculitis of 101 patients. *Ann Neurol* 2007;**62**:442–451.

312. Hankey GJ: Isolated angiitis/angiopathy of the central nervous system. *Cerebrovasc Dis* 1991;**1**:2–15.

313. Kolodny EH, Rebeiz JJ, Caviness VS, Richardson EP: Granulomatous angiitis of the central nervous system. *Arch Neurol* 1968;**19**:510–524.

314. Vollmer TL, Guarnaccia J, Harrington W, et al: Idiopathic granulomatous angiitis of the central nervous system. Diagnostic challenges. *Arch Neurol* 1993;**50**:925–930.

315. Moore PM: Diagnosis and management of isolated angiitis of the central nervous system. *Neurology* 1989;**39**:167–173.

316. Burger PC, Burch JG, Vogel FS: Granulomatous angiitis: An unusual etiology of stroke. *Stroke* 1977;**8**:29–35.

317. Harris KG, Tran DD, Sickels WJ, et al: Diagnosing intracranial vasculitis: The role of MR and angiography. *AJNR Am J Neuroradiol* 1994;**15**:317–330.

318. Alhalabi M, Moore PM: Serial angiography in isolated angiitis of the central nervous system. *Neurology* 1994;**44**:1221–1226.

319. Shinohara Y: Takayasu disease. In Caplan LR (ed): *Uncommon Causes of Stroke*, 2nd ed. Cambridge: Cambridge University Press, 2008, pp 27–32.

320. Shimizuki K, Sano K: Pulseless disease. *J Neuropathol Clin Neurol* 1951;**1**:37–47.

321. Ask-Upmark E: On the pulseless disease outside of Japan. *Acta Med Scand* 1954;**149**:161–178.

322. Subramanyan R, Joy J, Balakrishnan KG: Natural history of aortoarteritis (Takayasu's disease). *Circulation* 1989;**80**:429–437.

323. Lupi-Herrera E, Sanchez-Torres G, Marcushamer J, et al: Takayasu's arteritis: Clinical study of 107 cases. *Am Heart J* 1977;**93**:94–103.

324. Ishikawa K: Natural history and classification of occlusive thromboaortopathy (Takayasu's disease). *Circulation* 1978;**57**:27–35.

325. Sano K, Alga T, Saito I: Angiography in pulseless disease. *Radiology* 1970;**94**:69–74.

326. Hall S, Barr W, Lee JT, et al: Takayasu arteritis: A study of 32 North American patients. *Medicine (Baltimore)* 1985;**54**:89–99.

327. Hargraves RW, Spetzler RF: Takayasu's arteritis: Case report. *Barrow Neurol Inst Q* 1991;**7**:20–23.

328. Kerr GS, Hallahan CW, Giordano J, et al: Takayasu's arteritis. *Ann Intern Med* 1994;**120**:919–929.

329. Naritomi H: Takayasu's arteritis. In Bogousslavsky J, Caplan LR (eds): *Stroke Syndromes*. Cambridge: Cambridge University Press, 1995, pp 437–442.

330. Klos K, Flemming KD, Petty GW, Luthra HS: Takayasu's arteritis with arteriographic evidence of intracranial vessel involvement. *Neurology* 2003;**60**:1550–1551.

331. Talwar KK, Kumar K, Chopra P, et al: Cardiac involvement in nonspecific aortoarteritis (Takayasu's arteritis). *Am Heart J* 1991;**122**:1666–1670.

332. Sun Y, Yip P-K, Jeng J-S, et al: Ultrasonographic study and long-term follow-up of Takayasu's arteritis. *Stroke* 1996;**27**:2178–2182.

333. Ishikawa K, Uyama M, Asayama K: Occlusive thromboaortopathy (Takayasu's disease): Cervical occlusive stenosis, retinal artery pressure, retinal microaneurysms and prognosis. *Stroke* 1983;**14**:730–735.

334. Takagi A, Tada Y, Sato O, et al: Surgical treatment for Takayasu's arteritis: A long-term follow-up study. *J Cardiovasc Surg* 1989;**30**:553–558.

335. Fraga A, Mintz G, Valle L, Flores-Izquierdo G: Takayasu's arteritis: Frequency of systemic manifestations (study of 22 patients) and favorable response to maintenance steroid therapy with adrenocorticosteroids (12 patients). *Arthritis Rheum* 1972;**15**:617–624.

336. Biller J, Asconape J, Challa V, et al: A case for cerebral thromboangiitis obliterans. *Stroke* 1981;**12**:585–689.

337. Kumral E: Behçet's disease. In Caplan LR (ed): *Uncommon Causes of Stroke*, 2nd ed. Cambridge: Cambridge University Press, 2008, pp 67–74.

338. Chajek T, Fainaro M: Behçet's disease: Report of 41 cases and a review of the literature. *Medicine (Baltimore)* 1975;**54**:179–195.

339. Shimizu T, Ehrlich GE, Inaba G, et al: Behçet's disease (Behçet's syndrome). *Semin Arthritis Rheum* 1979;**8**:223–260.

340. Wechsler B, Davatchi F, Mizushima Y, et al: Criteria for diagnosis of Behçet's disease. *Lancet* 1990;**335**:1078–1080.

341. International Study Group for Behçet's Disease: Evaluation of diagnostic ("classification") criteria in Behçet's disease: Towards internationally agreed criteria. *Br J Rheum* 1992;**31**:299–308.

342. Serdaroglu P, Yazici H, Ozdemir C, et al: Neurologic involvement in Behçet's syndrome: A prospective study. *Arch Neurol* 1989;**46**:265–269.

343. Herskovitz S, Lipton RB, Lantos G: Neuro-Behçet's disease: CT and clinical correlates. *Neurology* 1988;**38**:1714–1720.

344. Bousser M-G, Wechsler B: Behçet's disease. In Bogousslavsky J, Caplan LR (eds): *Stroke Syndromes*. Cambridge: Cambridge University Press, 1995, pp 460–465.

345. Al Kawi MZ, Bohlega S, Banna M: MRI findings in neuro-Behçet's disease. *Neurology* 1991;**41**:405–408.

346. Banna M, El-Ramahi K: Neurologic involvement in Behçet's disease:

Imaging findings in 16 patients. *AJNR Am J Neuroradiol* 1991;**12**:791–796.

347. Pamir MN, Kansu T, Erbengi A, Zileli T: Papilledema in Behçet's syndrome. *Arch Neurol* 1981;**38**:643–645.

348. Bousser MG, Chiras J, Bories J, Castaigne P: Cerebral venous thrombosis: A review of 38 cases. *Stroke* 1985;**16**:199–213.

349. Wechsler B, Vidailhet M, Piette JC, et al: Cerebral venous thrombosis in Behçet's disease: Clinical study and long-term follow-up of 25 cases. *Neurology* 1992;**42**:614–618.

350. Sharief MK, Hentges R, Thomas E: Significance of CSF immunoglobulins in monitoring neurologic disease in Behçet's disease. *Neurology* 1991;**41**:1398–1401.

351. Cogan DG: Syndrome of nonsyphilitic interstitial keratitis and vestibulo-auditory symptoms. *Arch Ophthalmol* 1945;**33**:144–149.

352. Calvetti O, Biousse V: Cogan's syndrome. In Caplan LR (ed): *Uncommon Causes of Stroke*, 2nd ed. Cambridge: Cambridge University Press, 2008, pp 259–262.

353. Cheson BD, Bluming AZ, Alroy J: Cogan's syndrome: A systemic vasculitis. *Am J Med* 1976;**60**:549–555.

354. Peeters GJ, Pinckers AJ, Cremers CW, Hoefnagels WH: Atypical Cogan's syndrome: An autoimmune disease. *Ann Otol Rhinol Laryngol* 1986;**95**:173–175.

355. Romain PL, Aretz HT: Case records of the Massachusetts General Hospital: Case 6–1999. *N Engl J Med* 1999;**340**:635–641.

356. Albayram MS, Wityk R, Yousem DM, Zinreich SJ: The cerebral angiographic findings in Cogan syndrome. *AJNR Am J Neuroradiol* 2001;**22**:751–754.

357. Eales H: Case of retinal hemorrhage, associated with epistaxis and constipation. *Birmingham Med Rev* 1880;**9**:262–273.

358. Biousse V: Eales retinopathy. In Caplan LR (ed): *Uncommon Causes of Stroke*, 2nd ed. Cambridge: Cambridge University Press, 2008, pp 235–236.

359. Biswas J, Sharma T, Gopal L, et al: Eales disease – An update. *Surv Ophthalmol* 2002;**47**:197–214.

360. Miller NR: *Walsh and Hoyt's Clinical Neuroophthalmology*, vol **4**, 4th ed. Baltimore: Williams & Wilkins, 1991.

361. Raizman MB, Haas JJ: Case records of the Massachusetts General Hospital:

Case 4–1998. *N Engl J Med* 1998;**338**:313–319.

362. Gordon MF, Coyle PK, Golub B: Eales disease presenting as stroke in the young adult. *Ann Neurol* 1988;**24**:264–266.

363. Herson RN, Squier M: Retinal perivasculitis with neurological involvement. *J Neurol Sci* 1978;**36**:111–117.

364. Singhal BS, Dastur DK: Eales disease with neurological involvement. *J Neurol Sci* 1976; **27**:312–321, 323–345.

365. White RH: The etiology and neurological complications of retinal vasculitis. *Brain* 1961;**84**:262–273.

366. Susac J, Hardman J, Selhorst J: Microangiopathy of the brain and retina. *Neurology* 1979;**29**:313–316.

367. Susac JO: Susac's syndrome: The triad of microangiopathy of the brain and retina with hearing loss in young women. *Neurology* 1994;**44**:591–593.

368. Papo T, Biousse V, Lehoang P, et al: Susac syndrome. *Medicine (Baltimore)* 1998;**77**:3–11.

369. Henriques I, Bogousslavsky J, Caplan LR: Microangiopathy of the retina, inner ear, and brain: Susac's syndrome. In Caplan LR (ed): *Uncommon Causes of Stroke*, 2nd ed. Cambridge: Cambridge University Press, 2008, pp 247–254.

370. Petty G, Engel A, Younge BR, et al: Retinocochleocerebral vasculopathy. *Medicine (Baltimore)* 1998;**77**:122–140.

371. Coppeto J, Currie J, Monteiro M, et al: A syndrome of arterial-occlusive retinopathy and encephalopathy. *Am J Ophthalmol* 1984;**98**:189–202.

372. Swanson R, Mario L, Monteiro M, et al: A microangiopathic syndrome of encephalopathy, hearing loss and retinal artery occlusion. *Neurology* 1985;**35**(Suppl 1):145.

373. Bogousslavsky J, Gaio JM, Caplan LR, et al: Encephalopathy, deafness, and blindness in young women: A distinct retino-cochleo-cerebral arteriolopathy. *J Neurol Neurosurg Psychiatry* 1989;**52**:43–46.

374. Reichhart M: Acute posterior multifocal placoid pigment epitheliopathy (APMPPE). In Caplan LR (ed): *Uncommon Causes of Stroke*, 2nd ed. Cambridge: Cambridge University Press, 2008, pp 237–246.

375. Gass JDM: Acute posterior multifocal placoid pigment epitheliopathy. *Arch Ophthalmol* 1968;**80**:177–185.

376. Gass JD: Acute posterior multifocal placoid pigment epitheliopathy. *Retina* 2003;**23**:177–185.

377. Jones NP: Acute posterior multifocal placoid pigment epitheliopathy. *Br J Ophthalmol* 1995;**79**:384–389.

378. Comu S, Verstraeten T, Rinkoff JS, Busis NA: Neurological manifestations of acute posterior multifocal placoid pigment epitheliopathy. *Stroke* 1996;**27**:996–1001.

379. Smith CH, Savino PJ, Beck RW, et al: Acute posterior multifocal placoid pigment epitheliopathy and cerebral vasculitis. *Arch Neurol* 1983;**40**:48–50.

380. Weinstein JM, Bresnick GH, Bell CL, et al: Acute posterior multifocal placoid pigment epitheliopathy with cerebral vasculitis. *J Clin Neuroophthalmol* 1988;**8**:195–201.

381. Bewermeyer H, Nelles G, Huber M, et al: Pontine infarction in acute posterior multifocal placoid pigment epitheliopathy. *J Neurol* 1993;**241**:22–26.

382. Wilson CA, Choromokos EA, Sheppard R: Acute posterior multifocal placoid pigment epitheliopathy and cerebral vasculitis. *Arch Ophthalmol* 1988;**106**:796–800.

383. Manor RS: Vogt–Koyanagi–Harada syndrome and related diseases. In Vinken P, Bruyn G, Klawans H (eds): *Handbook of Clinical Neurology*, vol **34**, part 2. Amsterdam: North Holland, 1978, pp 513–544.

384. Andreoli CM, Foster CS: Vogt–Koyanagi–Harada disease. *Int Ophthalmol Clin* 2006;**46**:111–122.

385. Kato Y, Kurimura M, Yahata Y, et al: Vogt–Koyanagi–Harada's disease presenting polymorphonuclear pleocytosis in the cerebrospinal fluid at the early active stage. *Intern Med* 2006;**45**:779–781.

386. Khoury T, Gonzalez-Fernandez F, Munschauer 3rd FE, Ostrow P: A 47-year-old man with sudden onset of blindness, pleocytosis, and temporary hearing loss. Vogt–Koyanagi–Harada syndrome (Uveomeningoencephalitic syndrome). *Arch Pathol Lab Med* 2006;**130**:1070–1072.

387. De Reuck JL, De Bleecker JL: Sneddon's syndrome. In Caplan LR (ed): *Uncommon Causes of Stroke*, 2nd ed. Cambridge: Cambridge University Press, 2008, pp 405–412.

388. Sneddon B: Cerebro-vascular lesions and livedo reticularis. *Br J Dermatol* 1965;**77**:180–185.

389. Tourbah A, Piette JC, Iba-Zizen MT, et al: The natural course of cerebral lesions in Sneddon syndrome. *Arch Neurol* 1997;**54**:53–60.

390. Thomas DJ, Kirby JD, Britton KE, Galton DJ: Livedo reticularis and neurological lesions. *Br J Dermatol* 1982;**106**:711–712.

391. Rebollo M, Val JF, Garijo F, et al: Livedo reticularis and cerebrovascular lesions (Sneddon's syndrome). *Brain* 1983;**106**:965–979.

392. Stockhammer G, Felber SR, Zelger B, et al: Sneddon syndrome: Diagnosis by skin biopsy and MRI in 17 patients. *Stroke* 1993;**24**:685–690.

393. Pettee AD, Wasserman BA, Adams NL, et al: Familial Sneddon's syndrome: Clinical, hematologic, and radiographic findings in two brothers. *Neurology* 1994;**44**:399–405.

394. Levine SR, Langer SL, Albers JW, Welch KMA: Sneddon's syndrome: An antiphospholipid antibody syndrome? *Neurology* 1988;**38**:798–800.

395. Cornett O, Rosenbaum DH: Kohlmeier–Degos disease (malignant atrophic papulosis). In Caplan LR (ed): *Uncommon Causes of Stroke*, 2nd ed. Cambridge: Cambridge University Press, 2008, pp 377–380.

396. Caviness Jr VS, Sagar P, Israel EJ, et al: Case 38–2006: A 5-year-old boy with headache and abdominal pain. *N Engl J Med* 2006;**355**:2575–2584.

397. Petit WA, Soso MJ, Higman H: Degos disease: Neurologic complications and cerebral angiography. *Neurology* 1982;**32**:1305–1309.

398. Strole WE, Clark WH, Isselbacher KJ: Progressive arterial occlusive disease (Kohlmeier–Degos). *N Engl J Med* 1967;**276**:195–201.

399. Subbiah P, Wijdicks E, Muenter M, et al: Skin lesion with a fatal neurologic outcome (Degos' disease). *Neurology* 1996;**46**:636–640.

400. Caplan LR: Drugs. In Kase CS, Caplan LR (eds): *Intracerebral Hemorrhage*. Boston: Butterworth–Heinemann, 1994, pp 201–220.

401. Brust JC: Stroke and substance abuse. In Caplan LR (ed): *Uncommon Causes of Stroke*, 2nd ed. Cambridge: Cambridge University Press, 2008, pp 365–370.

402. Brust J, Richter R: Stroke associated with addiction to heroin. *J Neurol Neurosurg Psychiatry* 1978;**39**:194–199.

403. Woods B, Strewler G: Hemiparesis occurring six hours after intravenous heroin injection. *Neurology* 1972;**22**:863–866.

404. Caplan LR, Hier DB, Banks G: Current concepts in cerebrovascular disease – stroke: Stroke and drug abuse. *Stroke* 1982;**13**:869–872.

405. Brust JC: Stroke and drugs. In Vinker P, Bruyn G, Klawans H (eds): *Handbook of Clinical Neurology*, vol **11**. Amsterdam: Elsevier, 1989, pp 517–531.

406. Pearson J, Richter R: Addiction to opiates: Neurologic aspects. In Vinken P, Bruyn G (eds): *Handbook of Clinical Neurology*, vol **37**. Amsterdam: North Holland, 1979, pp 365–400.

407. Citron B, Halpern M, McCarron M, et al: Necrotizing angiitis associated with drug abuse. *N Engl J Med* 1970;**283**:1003–1011.

408. Rumbaugh C, Bergeron R, Gang H, et al: Cerebral vascular changes secondary to amphetamine abuse in the experimental animal. *Radiology* 1971;**101**:345–351.

409. Rumbaugh C, Bergeron R, Gang H, et al: Cerebral angiographic changes in the drug abuse patient. *Radiology* 1971;**101**:335–344.

410. Caplan LR, Thomas C, Banks G: Central nervous system complications of "T's and Blues" addiction. *Neurology* 1982;**32**:623–628.

411. Szwed JJ: Pulmonary angiothrombosis caused by "blue velvet" addiction. *Ann Intern Med* 1970;**73**:771–774.

412. Atlee W: Talc and cornstarch emboli in the eyes of drug abusers. *JAMA* 1972;**219**:49–51.

413. Mizutami T, Lewis R, Gonatas N: Medial medullary syndrome in a drug abuser. *Arch Neurol* 1980;**37**:425–428.

414. Schoenberger SD, Agarwal A: Talc retinopathy. *N Engl J Med* 2013;**368**:852.

415. Kaku D, Lowenstein DH: Emergence of recreational drug abuse as a major risk factor for stroke in young adults. *Ann Intern Med* 1990;**133**:821–827.

416. Levine SR, Welch KM: Cocaine and stroke: Current concepts of cardiovascular disease. *Stroke* 1988;**19**:779–783.

417. Daras M, Tuchman AJ, Marks S: Central nervous system infarction related to cocaine abuse. *Stroke* 1991;**22**:1320–1325.

418. Levine SR, Washington JM, Jefferson ME, et al: "Crack" cocaine-associated stroke. *Neurology* 1987;**37**:1849–1853.

419. Levine SR, Brust JC, Futrell N, et al: A comparative study of the cerebrovascular complications of cocaine-alkaloidal versus hydrochloride – a review. *Neurology* 1991;**41**:1173–1177.

420. Rowley HA, Lowenstein DH, Rowbotham MC, Simon RP: Thalamomesencephalic strokes after cocaine abuse. *Neurology* 1989;**39**:428–430.

421. Di Lazzaro, V, Restuccia D, Oliviero A, et al: Ischaemic myelopathy associated with cocaine: Clinical, neurophysiological, and neuroradiological features. *J Neurol Neurosurg Psychiatry* 1997;**63**:531–533.

422. Isner JM, Estes NA, Thompson PD, et al: Acute cardiac events temporally related to cocaine. *N Engl J Med* 1986;**315**:1438–1443.

423. Brust JCM: *Neurological Aspects of Substance Abuse*, 2nd ed. Boston: Butterworth–Heinemann, 2004.

424. Kaufman MJ, Levin JM, Ross MH, et al: Cocaine-induced cerebral vasoconstriction detected in humans with magnetic resonance angiography. *JAMA* 1998;**279**:376–380.

425. Nolte KB, Brass LM, Fletterick CF: Intracranial hemorrhage associated with cocaine abuse: A prospective study. *Neurology* 1996;**46**:1291–1296.

426. Savitz S, Caplan LR: Migraine and migraine-like conditions. In Caplan LR (ed): *Uncommon Causes of Stroke*, 2nd ed. Cambridge: Cambridge University Press, 2008, pp 529–531.

427. Singhal AB, Koroshetz WF, Caplan LR: Reversible cerebral vasoconstriction syndromes. In Caplan LR (ed): *Uncommon Causes of Stroke*, 2nd ed. Cambridge: Cambridge University Press, 2008, pp 505–514.

428. Caplan LR: *Migraine in Posterior Circulation Disease: Diagnosis, Clinical Findings, and Management*. Boston: Blackwell Science, 1996.

429. Kruit MC, van Buchem MA, Hofman PA, et al: Migraine as a risk factor for subclinical brain lesions. *JAMA* 2004;**291**:427–434.

430. Rothrock JF, Walicke P, Swendon M, et al: Migrainous stroke. *Arch Neurol* 1988;**45**:63–67.

431. Bogousslavsky J, Regli F, Van Melle G, et al: Migraine stroke. *Neurology* 1988;**38**:223–227.

432. Caplan LR: Migraine and vertebrobasilar ischemia. *Neurology* 1991;**41**:55–61.

433. Rothrock J, North J, Madden K, et al: Migraine and migrainous stroke: Risk factors and prognosis. *Neurology* 1993;**43**:2473–2476.

434. Henrich JB, Horwitz RI: A controlled study of ischemic stroke risk in migraine patients. *J Clin Epidemiol* 1989;**42**:773–780.

435. Stang PE, Carson AP, Rose KM, et al: Headache, cerebrovascular symptoms, and stroke: The Atherosclerosis Risk in Communities Study. *Neurology* 2005;**64**:1573–1577.

436. Etminan M, Takkouche B, Isorna FC, Samii A: Risk of ischaemic stroke in people with migraine: Systematic review and meta-analysis of observational studies. *BMJ* 2005;**330**:63.

437. Donaghy M, Chang CL, Poulter N: European Collaborators of The World Health Organisation Collaborative Study of Cardiovascular Disease and Steroid Hormone Contraception: Duration, frequency, recency, and type of migraine and the risk of ischaemic stroke in women of childbearing age. *J Neurol Neurosurg Psychiatry* 2002;**73**:747–750.

438. Solomon S, Lipton RB, Harris PY: Arterial stenosis in migraine: Spasm or arteriopathy? *Headache* 1990;**30**:52–61.

439. Pessin MS, Lathi ES, Cohen MB, et al: Clinical features and mechanisms of occipital infarction in the posterior cerebral artery territory. *Ann Neurol* 1987;**21**:290–299.

440. Fisher CM: Late-life migraine accompaniments as a cause of unexplained transient ischemic attacks. *Can J Neurol Sci* 1980;**7**:9–17.

441. Fisher CM: Late-life migraine accompaniments: Further experience. *Stroke* 1986;**17**:1033–1042.

442. Wijman CAC, Wolf PA, Kase CS, et al: Migrainous visual accompaniments are not rare in late life. The Framingham Study. *Stroke* 1998;**29**:1539–1543.

443. Caplan LR, Chedru F, Lhermitte F, Mayman C: Transient global amnesia and migraine. *Neurology* 1981;**31**:1167–1170.

444. Caplan LR: Transient global amnesia: Characteristic features and overview. In Markowitsch HJ (ed): *Transient Global Amnesia and Related Disorders*. Toronto: Hogrife and Huber, 1990, pp 15–27.

445. Call GK, Fleming MC, Sealfon S, et al: Reversible cerebral segmental vasoconstriction. *Stroke* 1988;**19**:1159–1170.

446. Bogousslavsky J, Despland PA, Regli F, Dubuis PY: Postpartum cerebral angiopathy: Reversible vasoconstriction assessed by transcranial Doppler ultrasound. *Eur Neurol* 1989;**29**:102–105.

447. Chen S-P, Fuh J-L, Lirng J-F, et al: Recurrent primary thunderclap headache and benign CNS angiopathy. *Neurology* 2006;**67**:2164–2169.

448. Ducros A, Boukobza M, Porcher R, et al: The clinical and radiological spectrum of reversible cerebral vasoconstriction syndrome. A prospective series of 67 patients. *Brain* 2007;**130**:3091–3101.

449. Lopez-Valdes E, Chang H-M, Pessin MS, Caplan LR: Cerebral vasoconstriction after carotid surgery. *Neurology* 1997;**49**:303–304.

450. Calabrese LH, Dodick DW, Schwedt TJ, et al: Narrative reviews: Reversible cerebral vasoconstriction syndrome. *Ann Intern Med.* 2007;**146**:34–44.

451. Moustafa RR, Allen CMC, Baron J-C: Call–Fleming syndrome associated with subarachnoid haemorrhage: Three new cases. *J Neurol Neurosurg Psychiatry* 2008;**79**:602–605.

452. Ducros A: Reversible cerebral vasoconstriction syndrome. *Lancet Neurol* 2012;**11**:906–917.

453. French KF, Hoesch RE, Allred J, et al: Repetitive use of intra-arterial verapamil in the treatment of reversible cerebral vasoconstriction syndrome. *J Clin Neurosci* 2012;**19**:174–76.

454. Bartleson JD, Swanson JW, Whisnant JP: A migrainous syndrome with cerebrospinal fluid pleocytosis. *Neurology* 1981;**31**:1257–1262.

455. Gomez-Aranda F, Canadillas F, Marti-Masso JF, et al: Pseudomigraine with temporary neurological symptoms and lymphocytic pleocytosis. A report of 50 cases. *Brain* 1997;**120**:1105–1113.

456. Martin-Balbuena S, Arpa-Gutierrez FJ: Pseudomigraine with cerebrospinal fluid pleocytosis or syndrome of headache, temporary neurological deficit and cerebrospinal fluid. A historical review. *Rev Neurol* 2007;**45**:624–630.

457. Emond H, Schnorf H, Poloni C, Vulliemoz S, Lalive PH: Syndrome of transient headache and neurological deficits with CSF lymphocytosis (HaNDL) associated with recent human herpesvirus-6 infection. *Cephalalgia.* 2009;**29**:487–491.

458. Black DF, Bartleson JD, Bell ML, Lachner DH: SMART: Stroke-like migraine attacks after radiation therapy. *Cephalgia* 2006;**26**:1137–1142.

459. Pruitt A, Dalmau J, Detre J, et al: Episodic neurologic dysfunction with migraine and reversible imaging findings after radiation. *Neurology* 2006;**67**:676–678.

460. Black DF, Morris JM, Lindell, EP, et al: Stroke-like migraine attacks after radiation therapy (SMART) syndrome is not always completely reversible: A case series. *Am J Neuroradiol* 2013;**36**:1–6.

461. Wang N, Prasad S: SMART syndrome. Stroke-like migraine attacks after radiation therapy. *Neurol Clin Pract* 2014;**1**:530–531.

462. Cole AJ, Aube M: Migraine with vasospasm and delayed intracerebral hemorrhage. *Arch Neurol* 1990;**47**:53–56.

463. Gautier JC, Majdalani A, Juillard JB, et al: Hemorragies cerebrales au cours de la migraine. *Rev Neurol (Paris)* 1993;**149**:407–410.

464. Caplan LR: Intracerebral hemorrhage revisited. *Neurology* 1988;**38**:624–627.

465. Digre K, Varner M, Caplan LR: Eclampsia and stroke during pregnancy and the puerperium. In Caplan LR (ed): *Uncommon Causes of Stroke*, 2nd ed. Cambridge: Cambridge University Press, 2008, pp 515–528.

466. Siderov E, Feng W, Caplan LR: Stroke in pregnant and postpartum women. *Expert Rev Cardiovasc Ther* 2011;**9**:1235–1247.

467. Edlow JA, Caplan LR, O'Brien K, Tibbles C: Diagnosis of acute neurological emergencies in pregnant and postpartum women. *Lancet Neurol* 2013;**12**:175–185.

468. Hoffmann M, Keiseb J, Moodley J, Corr P: Appropriate neurological evaluation

and multimodality magnetic resonance imaging in eclampsia. *Acta Neurol Scand* 2002;**106**:159–167.

469. Neudecker S, Stock K, Krasnianski M: Call–Fleming postpartum angiopathy in the puerperium: A reversible cerebral vasoconstriction syndrome. *Obstet Gynecol* 2006;**107**:446–449.

470. Duncan R, Hadley D, Bone I, et al: Blindness in eclampsia: CT and MR imaging. *J Neurol Neurosurg Psychiatry* 1998;**52**:899–902.

471. Easton JD, Mas J-L, Lamy C, et al: Severe preeclampsia/eclampsia: hypertensive encephalopathy of pregnancy? *Cerebrovasc Dis* 1998;**8**:53–58.

472. Hinchey J, Chaves C, Appignani B, et al: A reversible posterior leukoencephalopathy syndrome. *N Engl J Med* 1996;**334**:494–500.

473. Schwartz RB, Feske SK, Polak JF, et al: Preeclampsia-eclampsia: Clinical and neuroradiographic correlates and insights into the pathogenesis of hypertensive encephalopathy. *Radiology* 2000;**217**:371–376.

474. Hinchey JA: Reversible leukoencephalopathy syndrome: what have we learned in the past 10 years. *Arch Neurol* 2008;**65**:175–176.

475. Adams H, Davis P, Hennerici M: Moyamoya. In Caplan LR (ed): *Uncommon Causes of Stroke*, 2nd ed. Cambridge: Cambridge University Press, 2008, pp 465–478.

476. Suzuki J, Kodama N: Moyamoya disease – a review. *Stroke* 1983;**14**:104–109.

477. Suzuki J: *Moyamoya Disease*. Berlin: Springer, 1986.

478. Kuroda S, Hashimoto N, Yoshimoto T, et al: Radiological findings, clinical course, and outcome in aymptomatic moyamoya disease. *Stroke* 2007;**38**:1430–1435.

479. Chiu D, Shedden P, Bratina P, Grotta JC: Clinical features of moyamoya disease in the United States. *Stroke* 1998;**29**:1347–1351.

480. Taveras JM: Multiple progressive intracranial arterial occlusions: A syndrome of children and young adults. *AJR Am J Roentgenol* 1969;**106**:235–268.

481. Bruno A, Adams HOP, Bilbe J, et al: Cerebral infarction due to moyamoya disease in young adults. *Stroke* 1988;**19**:826–833.

482. Mauro AJ, Johnson ES, Chikos PM, Alvord EC: Lipohyalinosis and miliary microaneurysms causing cerebral hemorrhage in a patient with moyamoya. A clinicopathological study. *Stroke* 1980;**11**:405–412.

483. Ikeda E: Systemic vascular changes in spontaneous occlusion of the circle of Willis. *Stroke* 1991;**22**:1358–1362.

484. Southerland AM, Meschia JF, Worrall BB: Shared associations of nonatherosclerotic, large-vessel, cerebrovascular arteriopathies: Considering intracranial aneurysms, cervical artery dissection, moyamoya disease and fibromuscular dysplasia. *Curr Opin Neurol* 2013;**26**:13–28.

485. Ueki K, Meyer FB, Mellinger JF: Moyamoya disease: The disorder and surgical treatment. *Mayo Clin Proc* 1994;**69**:749–757.

486. Herreman F, Nathal E, Yasui N, Yonekawa Y: Intracranial aneurysms in moyamoya disease: Report of ten cases and review of the literature. *Cerebrovasc Dis* 1994;**4**:329–336.

487. Robertson RL, Burrows PE, Barnes PD, et al: Angiographic changes after pial synangiosis in childhood moyamoya disease. *AJNR Am J Neuroradiol* 1997;**18**:837–845.

488. Houkin K, Kamiyama H, Abe H, et al: Surgical therapy for adult moyamoya disease. Can surgical revascularization prevent the recurrence of intracerebral hemorrhage? *Stroke* 1996;**27**:1342–1346.

489. Smith ER, Scott RM: Surgical management of moyamoya syndrome. *Skull Base* 2005;**15**:15–26.

490. Scott RM, Smith ER: Moyamoya disease and moyamoya syndrome. *N Engl J Med* 2009;**360**:1226–1237.

491. Kamada F, Aoki Y, Narisawa A, et al: A genome-wide association study identifies *RNF213* as the first moyamoya disease gene. *J Hum Genet* 2011;**56**:34–40.

492. Liu W, Morito D, Takashima S, et al: Identification of *RNF213* as a susceptibility gene for moyamoya disease and its possible role in vascular development. *PLoS One*. 2011;**6**:e22542.

493. Hart RG, Kanter MC: Hematologic disorders and ischemic stroke: A selective review. *Stroke* 1990;**21**:1111–1121.

494. Markus HS, Hambley H: Neurology and the blood: Haematological abnormalities in ischaemic stroke. *J Neurol Neurosurg Psychiatry* 1998;**64**:150–159.

495. Adams RJ: Big strokes in small persons. *Arch Neurol* 2007;**64**:1567–1574.

496. Switzer JA, Hess DC, Nichols FT, Adams RJ: Pathophysiology and treatment of stroke in sickle-cell disease: Present and future. *Lancet* 2006;**5**:501–512.

497. Rothman SM, Fulling KH, Nelson JS: Sickle cell anemia and central nervous system infarction: A neuropathological study. *Ann Neurol* 1986;**20**:684–690.

498. Adams RJ, Nichols FT, McKie V, et al: Cerebral infarction in sickle cell anemia: mechanisms based on CT and MRI. *Neurology* 1988;**38**:1012–1017.

499. Steen RG, Langston JW, Ogg RJ, et al: Ectasia of the basilar artery in children with sickle cell disease: Relationship to hematocrit and psychometric measures. *J Stroke Cerebrovasc Dis* 1998;**7**:32–43.

500. Oguz M, Aksungur EH, Soyupak SK, Yildirim AU: Vein of Galen and sinus thrombosis with bilateral thalamic infarcts in sickle cell anemia: CT follow-up and angiographic demonstration. *Neuroradiology* 1994;**36**:155–156.

501. Adams RJ: TCD in sickle-cell disease: An important and useful test. *Pediatr Radiol* 2005;**35**:229–234.

502. Adams RJ, McKie VC, Hsu L, et al: Prevention of a first stroke by transfusions in children with sickle cell anemia and abnormal results on transcranial Doppler ultrasonography. *N Engl J Med* 1998;**339**:5–11.

503. Hillmen P, Lewis SM, Bessler M, et al: Natural history of paroxysmal nocturnal hemoglobinuria. *N Engl J Med* 1995;**333**:1253–1258.

504. Ziakas PD, Poulou LS, Rokas GI, et al: Thrombosis in paroxysmal nocturnal hemoglobinuria: Sites, risks, outcome. An overview. *J Thromb Haemost* 2007;**5**:642–645.

505. Poulou LS, Vakrinos G, Pomoni A, et al: Stroke in paroxysmal nocturnal haemoglobinuria: Patterns of disease and outcome. *Thromb Haemost* 2007;**98**:699–701.

506. Murphy S, Iland H, Rosenthal D, Laszlo J: Essential thrombocythemia: An interim report from the Polycythemia Vera Study Group. *Semin Hematol* 1986;**23**:177–182.

507. Jabaily J, Iland HJ, Laszlo J, et al: Neurologic manifestations of essential thrombocythemia. *Ann Intern Med* 1983;**99**:513–518.

508. Hehlmann R, Jahn M, Baumann B, Kopcke W: Essential thrombocythemia. Clinical characteristics and course of 61 cases. *Cancer* 1988;**61**:2487–2496.

509. Arboix A, Besses C, Acin P, et al: Ischemic stroke as the first manifestation of essential thrombocythemia. *Stroke* 1995;**26**:1463–1466.

510. Ogata J, Yonemura K, Kimura Y, et al: Cerebral infarction associated with thrombocythemia: An autopsy case study. *Cerebrovasc Dis* 2005;**19**:201–205.

511. Wu K: Platelet hyperaggregability and thrombosis in patients with thrombocythemia. *Ann Intern Med* 1978;**88**:7–11.

512. Al-Mefty O, Marano G, Rajaraman S, et al: Transient ischemic attacks due to increased platelet aggregation and adhesiveness. *J Neurosurg* 1979;**50**:449–453.

513. Trip MD, Cats VM, van Capelle FJL, Vreeken J: Platelet hyperreactivity and prognosis in survivors of myocardial infarction. *N Engl J Med* 1990;**322**:1549–1554.

514. Védy D, Schapira M, Angelillo-Scherrer A: Bleeding disorders and thrombophilia. In Caplan LR (ed): *Uncommon Causes of Stroke*, 2nd ed. Cambridge: Cambridge University Press, 2008, pp 283–300.

515. Thaler E, Lechner K: Antithrombin III deficiency and thromboembolism. *Clin Haematol* 1981;**10**:369–390.

516. Camerlingo M, Finazzi G, Casto L, et al: Inherited protein C deficiency and nonhemorrhagic arterial stroke in young adults. *Neurology* 1991;**41**:1371–1373.

517. Dahlback B, Carlsson M, Svensson PJ: Familial thrombophilia due to a previously unrecognized mechanism characterized by poor anticoagulant response to activated protein C: Prediction of a cofactor to activated protein C. *Proc Natl Acad Sci U S A* 1993;**90**:1004–1008.

518. Zoller B, Dahlback B: Linkage between inherited resistance to activated protein C and factor V gene mutation in venous thrombosis. *Lancet* 1994;**343**:1536–1538.

519. Ridker PM, Miletich JP, Stampfer MJ, et al: Factor V Leiden and risks of recurrent idiopathic venous thromboembolism. *Circulation* 1997;**95**:1777–1782.

520. Poort SR, Rosendaal FR, Reitsma PH, Bertina RM: A common genetic variation in the 3' untranslated region of the prothrombin gene is associated with elevated prothrombin levels and an increase in venous thrombosis. *Blood* 1996;**88**:3698–3703.

521. Huberfeld G, Kubis N, Lot G, et al: G20210A Prothrombin gene mutation in two siblings with cerebral venous thrombosis. *Neurology* 1998;**51**:316–317.

522. Martinelli I, Sacchi E, Landi G, et al: High risk of cerebral-vein thrombosis in carriers of a prothrombin-gene mutation and in users of oral contraceptives. *N Engl J Med* 1998;**338**:1793–1797.

523. Estol C, Pessin MS, DeWitt LD, Caplan LR: Stroke and increased factor VIII activity. *Neurology* 1989;**39**(suppl 1):1159.

524. Kosik KS, Furie B: Thrombotic stroke associated with elevated factor VIII. *Arch Neurol* 1980;**8**:435–437.

525. De Georgia MA, Rose DZ: Stroke in patients who have inflammatory bowel disease. In Caplan LR (ed): *Uncommon Causes of Stroke*, 2nd ed. Cambridge: Cambridge University Press, 2008, pp 381–386.

526. Talbot RW, Heppell J, Dozois RR, Beart RW: Vascular complications of inflammatory bowel disease. *Mayo Clin Proc* 1986;**61**:140–145.

527. Johns DR: Cerebrovascular complications of inflammatory bowel disease. *Am J Gastroenterol* 1991;**86**:367–370.

528. Sigsbee B, Rottenberg DA: Sagittal sinus thrombosis as a complication of regional enteritis. *Ann Neurol* 1978;**3**:450–452.

529. Grau A, Buggle F, Heindl S, et al: Recent infection as a risk factor for cerebrovascular ischemia. *Stroke* 1995;**26**:373–379.

530. Syrjanen J, Valtonen VV, Iivanainen M, et al: Preceding infection as an important risk factor for ischaemic brain infarction in young and middle aged patients. *BMJ* 1988;**296**:1156–1160.

531. Grau A, Buggle F, Steichen-Wiehn C, et al: Clinical and histochemical analysis in infection-associated stroke. *Stroke* 1995;**26**:1520–1526.

532. Grau A: Infection, inflammation, and cerebrovascular ischemia. *Neurology* 1997;**49**(suppl 4):S47–S51.

533. Leira R, Davalos A, Castillo J: Cancer and paraneoplastic strokes. In Caplan LR (ed): *Uncommon Causes of Stroke*, 2nd ed. Cambridge: Cambridge University Press, 2008, pp 371–376.

534. Sack GH, Levin J, Bell WR: Trousseau's syndrome and other manifestations of chronic disseminated coagulopathy in patients with neoplasms. *Medicine (Baltimore)* 1977;**56**:1–37.

535. Graus F, Rodgers LR, Posner JB: Cerebrovascular complications in patients with cancer. *Medicine (Baltimore)* 1985;**64**:16–35.

536. Amico L, Caplan LR, Thomas C: Cerebrovascular complications of mucinous cancers. *Neurology* 1989;**39**:523–526.

537. Kablau M, Michael G, Hennerici MG, Marc Fatar M, et al: Stroke and cancer: The importance of cancer-associated hypercoagulation as a possible stroke etiology. *Stroke* 2012;**43**:3029–3034.

538. Hajjar K, Francis CW: Fibrinolysis and thrombolysis. In Lichtman MA, Beutler E, Kipps TJ, Seligsohn U, Kaushansky K, Prchal JT (eds): *Williams Hematology*, 7th ed. New York: McGraw-Hill, 2006, pp 2089–2115.

539. Sloane MA: Thrombolysis and stroke – past and future. *Arch Neurol* 1986;**44**:748–768.

540. Del Zoppo GH, Zeumer H, Harker LA: Thrombolytic therapy in stroke: Possibilities and hazards. *Stroke* 1986;**17**:595–607.

541. Francis RB: Clinical disorders of fibrinolysis. *Blut* 1989;**59**:1–14.

542. Nilsson IM, Ljungner H, Tengborn L: Two different mechanisms in patients with venous thrombosis and defective fibrinolysis: Low concentrations of plasminogen activator or increased concentration of plasminogen activator inhibitor. *BMJ* 1985;**290**:1453–1456.

543. Collen D, Lijnen HR: The fibrinolytic system in man. *Crit Rev Oncol Hematol* 1986;**4**:249–301.

544. Nagayama T, Shinohara Y, Nagayama M, et al: Congenitally abnormal plasminogen in juvenile ischemic cerebrovascular disease. *Stroke* 1993;**24**:2104–2107.

545. Hunt FA, Rylatt DB, Hart R, Bundesen PG: Serum cross-linked fibrin (XDP) and fibrinogen/fibrin degradation products (FDP) in disorders associated with activation of the coagulation or fibrinolytic systems. *Br J Haematol* 1985;**60**:715–722.

546. Feinberg WM, Bruck DC, Ring ME, Corrigan JJ: Hemostatic markers in acute stroke. *Stroke* 1989;**20**:582–587.

547. Delgado J, Jimenez-Yuste V, Hernandez-Navarro F, Villar A: Acquired hemophilia. Review and meta-analysis focused on therapy and prognostic factors. *Br J Haematol* 2003;**121**:21–35.

548. Johansen RF, Sorensen B, Ingerslev J: Acquired haemophilia: Dynamic whole blood coagulation utilized to guide haemostatic therapy. *Haemophilia* 2006;**12**:190–197.

549. Ruggeri ZM, Zimmerman TS: von Willebrand factor and von Willebrand disease. *Blood* 1987;**70**:895–904.

550. Wilde JT: Von Willebrand disease. *Clin Med* 2007;**7**:629–632.

551. Nurden P, Nurden AT: Congenital disorders associated with platelet dysfunctions. *Thromb Haemost* 2008;**99**:253–263.

552. Roldan J, Brey RL: Antiphospholipid antibody syndrome. In Caplan LR (ed): *Uncommon Causes of Stroke*, 2nd ed. Cambridge: Cambridge University Press, 2008, pp 263–274.

553. Levine SR, Welch KMA: Cerebrovascular ischemia associated with lupus anticoagulant. *Stroke* 1987;**18**:257–263.

554. DeWitt LD, Caplan LR: Antiphospholipid antibodies and stroke. *AJNR Am J Neuroradiol* 1991;**12**:454–456.

555. Cervera R, Piette JC, Font J, et al: Antiphospholipid syndrome: Clinical and immunologic manifestations and patterns of disease expression in a cohort of 1,000 patients. *Arthritis Rheum* 2002;**46**:1019–1027.

556. Coull BM, Goodnight SH: Antiphospholipid antibodies, prethrombotic states, and stroke. *Stroke* 1990;**21**:1370–1374.

557. Levine SR, Kim S, Deegan MI, Welch KMA: Ischemic stroke associated with anticardiolipin antibodies. *Stroke* 1987;**18**:1101–1106.

558. Montalban J, Codina A, Ordi J, et al: Antiphospholipid antibodies in cerebral ischemia. *Stroke* 1991;**22**:750–753.

559. Pope JM, Canny CL, Bell DA: Cerebral ischemic events associated with endocarditis, retinal vascular disease, and lupus anticoagulant. *Am J Med* 1991;**90**:299–309.

560. Antiphospholipid Antibodies in Stroke Study (APASS) Group: Clinical and laboratory findings in patients with antiphospholipid antibodies and cerebral ischemia. *Stroke* 1990;**21**:1268–1273.

561. Lopez LR, Dier KJ, Lopez D, et al: Anti-beta 2-glycoprotein I and antiphosphatidylserine antibodies are predictors of arterial thrombosis in patients with antiphospholipid syndrome. *Am J Clin Pathol* 2004;**121**:142–149.

562. Atsumi T, Ieko M, Bertolaccini ML, et al: Association of autoantibodies against the phosphatidylserine-prothrombin complex with manifestations of the antiphospholipid syndrome and with the presense of lupus anticoagulant. *Arthritis Rheum* 2000;**43**:1982–1993.

563. Feldmann E, Levine SR: Cerebrovascular disease with antiphospholipid antibodies: Immune mechanisms, significance, and therapeutic options. *Ann Neurol* 1995;**37**(suppl 1):S114–S130.

564. Levine SR, Salowich-Palm L, Sawaya KL, et al: IgG anticardiolipin antibody titer 40 GPL and the risk of subsequent thrombo-occlusive events and death. A prospective cohort study. *Stroke* 1997;**28**:1660–1665.

565. Verro P, Levine SR, Tietjen GE: Cerebrovascular ischemic events with high positive anticardiolipin antibodies. *Stroke* 1998;**29**:2245–2253.

566. Provenzale JM, Barboriak DP, Allen NB, Ortel TL: Antiphospholipid antibodies: Findings at arteriography. *AJNR Am J Neuroradiol* 1998;**19**:611–616.

567. Bick RL: Disseminated intravascular coagulation and related syndromes: A clinical review. *Semin Thromb Hemost* 1988;**14**:299–338.

568. Wen PY, Sobel RA: Case records of the Massachusetts General Hospital: Case 36–1991. *N Engl J Med* 1991;**325**:714–726.

569. Colman RW, Rubin RN: Disseminated intravascular coagulation due to malignancy. *Semin Oncol* 1990;**17**:172–186.

570. Schwartzman RJ, Hill JB: Neurologic complications of disseminated intravascular coagulation. *Neurology* 1982;**32**:791–797.

571. Schwartzman RJ, Kumar M: Disseminated intravascular disease. In Caplan LR (ed): *Uncommon Causes of Stroke*, 2nd ed. Cambridge: Cambridge University Press, 2008, pp 275–282.

572. Dashe J: Hyperviscosity and stroke. In Caplan LR (ed): *Uncommon Causes of Stroke*, 2nd ed. Cambridge: Cambridge University Press, 2008, pp 347–356.

573. Grotta J, Ackerman R, Correia J, et al: Whole blood viscosity parameters and cerebral blood flow. *Stroke* 1982;**13**:296–301.

574. Coull BM, Beamer N, de Garmo P, et al: Chronic blood hyperviscosity in subjects with acute stroke, transient ischemic attack, and risk factors for stroke. *Stroke* 1991;**22**:162–168.

575. Ernst E, Resch KL: Fibrinogen as a cardiovascular risk factor: A meta-analysis and review of the literature. *Ann Intern Med* 1993;**118**:956–963.

576. Fahey JL, Barth WF, Solomon A: Serum hyperviscosity syndrome. *JAMA* 1965;**192**:464–467.

577. Rosenson RS, Baker AL, Chow M, Hay R: Hyperviscosity syndrome in a hypercholesterolemic patient with primary biliary cirrhosis. *Gastroenterology* 1990;**98**:1351–1357.

578. Fauci A, Haynes BF, Costa J, et al: Lymphatoid granulomatosis: Prospective clinical and therapeutic experience over 10 years. *N Engl J Med* 1982;**306**:68–74.

579. Hogan PJ, Greenberg MK, McCarty GE: Neurologic complications of lymphomatoid granulomatosis. *Neurology* 1981;**31**:619–620.

580. Hochberg EP, Gilman MD, Hasserjian RP: Case records of the Massachusetts General Hospital. Case 17–2006 – a 34-year-old man with cavitary lung lesions. *N Engl J Med* 2006;**354**:2485–2493.

581. Mizuno T, Takanashi Y, Onodera H, et al: A case of lymphomatoid granulomatosis/angiocentric immunoproliferative lesion with long clinical course and diffuse brain involvement. *J Neuro Sci* 2003;**213**:67–76.

582. Rubens EO: Intravascular lymphoma. In Caplan LR (ed): *Uncommon Causes of Stroke*, 2nd ed. Cambridge:

Cambridge University Press, 2008, pp 533–537.

583. Petito CK, Gottlieb GJ, Dougherty JH, Petito FA: Neoplastic angioendotheliosis: Ultrastructural study and review of the literature. *Ann Neurol* 1978;**3**:393–399.

584. Beal MF, Fisher CM: Neoplastic angioendotheliosis. *J Neurol Sci* 1982;**53**:359–375.

585. Reinglass JL, Miller J, Wissman S: Central nervous system angioendotheliosis. *Stroke* 1977;**8**:218–221.

586. Raroque HG, Mandler RN, Griffey MS, et al: Neoplastic angioendotheliomatosis. *Arch Neurol* 1990;**47**:929–930.

587. Glass J, Hochberg FH, Miller DC: Intravascular lymphomatosis – a systemic disease with neurologic manifestations. *Cancer* 1993;**71**:3156–3164.

588. Hamada K, Hamada T, Satoh M, et al: Two cases of neoplastic angioendotheliomatosis presenting with myelopathy. *Neurology* 1991;**41**:1139–1140.

589. Kanegane H, Ito Y, Ohshima K, et al: X-linked lymphoproliferative syndrome presenting with systemic lymphocytic vasculitis. *Am J Hematol* 2005;**78**:130–133.

590. Natowicz M, Kelley RI: Mendelian etiologies of stroke. *Ann Neurol* 1987;**22**:175–192.

591. Albert M: *Genetics of Cerebrovascular Disease*. Armonk, NY: Futura, 1999.

592. Alberts MJ: Genetics of cerebrovascular disease. *Stroke* 2004;**35**:342–344.

593. Meschia JF, Worrall BB: New advances in identifying genetic anomalies in stroke-prone probands. *Curr Neurol Neurosci Rep* 2004;**4**:420–426.

594. Hoy A, Leininger-Muller B, Poirier O, et al: Myeloperoxidase polymorphisms in brain infarction. Association with infarct size and functional outcome. *Atherosclerosis* 2003;**167**:223–230.

595. Hirt L: MELAS and other mitochondrial disorders. In Caplan LR (ed): *Uncommon Causes of Stroke*, 2nd ed. Cambridge: Cambridge University Press, 2008, pp 149–154.

596. Pavlakis SG, Phillips PC, DiMauro S, et al: Mitochondrial myopathy, encephalopathy, lactic acidosis, and stroke-like episodes: A distinctive clinical syndrome. *Ann Neurol* 1984;**16**:481–488.

597. Morgan-Hughes JA: Mitochondrial diseases. In Engel AG, Franzini-Armstrong C (eds): *Myology*, vol **2**, 2nd ed. New York: McGraw-Hill, 1994, pp 1610–1660.

598. Kuriyama M, Umezaki H, Fukuda Y, et al: Mitochondrial encephalomyopathy with lactate-pyruvate elevation and brain infarctions. *Neurology* 1984;**34**:72–77.

599. Allard JC, Tilak C, Carter AP: CT and MR of MELAS syndrome. *AJNR Am J Neuroradiol* 1988;**9**:1234–1238.

600. Koo B, Becker LE, Chuang S, et al: Mitochondrial encephalomyopathy, lactic acidosis, stroke like episodes (MELAS): Clinical, radiological, and genetic observations. *Ann Neurol* 1993;**34**:25–32.

601. Matthews PM, Tampieri D, Berkovic SF, et al: Magnetic resonance imaging shows specific abnormalities in the MELAS syndrome. *Neurology* 1991;**41**:1043–1046.

602. Clark JM, Marks MP, Adalsteinsson E, et al: MELAS: Clinical and pathological correlations with MRI, Xenon/CT, and MR spectroscopy. *Neurology* 1996;**46**:223–227.

603. Sue CM, Crimmins DS, Soo YS, et al: Neuroradiological features of six kindreds with MELAS tRNALeu A3243 G point mutation: Implications for pathogenesis. *J Neurol Neurosurg Psychiatry* 1998;**65**:233–240.

604. Mitsias P, Levine SR: Cerebrovascular complications of Fabry's disease. *Ann Neurol* 1996;**40**:8–17.

605. Mitsias P, Papamitsakis NIH, Amory CF, Levine SR: Cerebrovascular complications of Fabry disease. In Caplan LR (ed): *Uncommon Causes of Stroke*, 2nd ed. Cambridge: Cambridge University Press, 2008, pp 123–130.

606. Brady RO, Gal AE, Bradley RM, et al: Enzymatic defect in Fabry's disease: Ceramide trihexosidase deficiency. *N Engl J Med* 1967;**276**:1163–1167.

607. Dawson DM, Miller DC: Case records of the Massachusetts General Hospital: Case 2–1984. *N Engl J Med* 1984;**310**:106–114.

608. Kint JA: Fabry's disease: Alpha-galactosidase deficiency. *Science* 1970;**167**:1268–1269.

609. Eng CM, Guffon N, Wilcox WR, et al: Safety and efficacy of recombinant human alpha-galactosidase A – replacement therapy in Fabry's disease. *N Engl J Med* 2001;**5**:345:9–16.

610. Desnick RJ, Brady R, Barranger J, et al: Fabry disease, an under-recognized multi-systemic disorder: Expert recommendations for diagnosis, management, and enzyme replacement therapy. *Ann Intern Med* 2003;**138**:338–346.

611. Kolodny E, Fellgiebel A, Hilz MJ, et al: Cerebrovascular involvement in Fabry disease. Current status of knowledge. *Stroke* 2015;**46**:302–313.

612. Chabriat H, Bousser M-G: Cerebral autosomal dominant arteriopathy with subcortical infarcts and leukoencephalopathy (CADASIL). In Caplan LR (ed): *Uncommon Causes of Stroke*, 2nd ed. Cambridge: Cambridge University Press, 2008, pp 115–122.

613. Tournier-Lasserve E, Iba-Zizen M-T, Romero N, Bousser M-G: Autosomal dominant syndrome with stroke-like episodes and leukoencephalopathy. *Stroke* 1991;**22**:1297–1302.

614. Mas JL, Dilouya A, de Recondo J: A familial disorder with subcortical ischemic strokes, dementia, and leukoencephalopathy. *Neurology* 1992;**42**:1015–1019.

615. Hutchinson M, O'Riordan J, Javed M, et al: Familial hemiplegic migraine and autosomal dominant arteriopathy with leukoencephalopathy (CADASIL). *Ann Neurol* 1995;**38**:817–824.

616. Ragno M, Tournier-Lasserve E, Fiori MG, et al: An Italian kindred with cerebral autosomal dominant arteriopathy with subcortical infarcts and leukoencephalopathy (CADASIL). *Ann Neurol* 1995;**38**:231–236.

617. Dichgans M, Mayer M, Uttner I, et al: The phenotypic spectrum of CADASIL: Clinical findings in 102 cases. *Ann Neurol* 1998;**44**:731–739.

618. Caplan LR, Arenillas J, Cramer SC, et al: Stroke-related translational research (Review). *Arch Neurol* 2011;**68**:1110–1123.

619. Chabriat H, Joutel A, Dichgans M, et al: CADASIL. *Lancet Neurol* 2009;**8**:643–653.

620. Chabriat H, Levy C, Taillia H, et al: Patterns of MRI lesions in CADASIL. *Neurology* 1998;**51**:452–457.

621. Joutel A, Corpechot C, Ducros A, et al: Notch 3 mutations in CADASIL, a hereditary adult-onset condition causing stroke and dementia. *Nature* 1996;**383**:707–710.

622. Fukutake T, Hirayama K: Familial young-adult-onset arteriosclerotic leukoencephalopathy with alopecia and lumbago without arterial hypertension. *Eur Neurol* 1995;**35**:69–79.

623. Fukutake, T: Cerebral autosomal recessive arteriopathy with subcortical infarcts and leukoencephalopathy (CARASIL): From discovery to gene identification. *J Stroke Cerebrovasc Dis* 2011;**20**:85–93.

624. Menkes J: Menkes disease (kinky hair disease). In Caplan LR (ed): *Uncommon Causes of Stroke*, 2nd ed. Cambridge: Cambridge University Press, 2008, pp 225–230.

625. Menkes J, Alter M, Steigleder G, et al: A sex-linked recessive disorder with retardation of growth, peculiar hair and focal cerebral and cerebellar degeneration. *Pediatrics* 1962;**29**:764–779.

626. Moller JV, Juul B, Le Maire M: Structural organization, ion transport, and energy transduction of P-type ATP-ases. *Biochem Biophys Acta* 1996;**1286**:1–51.

627. Moller LB, Tumer Z, Lund C, et al: Similar splice-site mutations of the *ATP7A* gene lead to different phenotypes: Classical Menkes disease or occipital horn syndrome. *Am J Hum Genet* 2000;**66**:1211–1220.

628. Iannaccone ST, Rosenberg RN: Menkes disease. In Berg B (ed): *Principles of Child Neurology*. New York: McGraw-Hill, 1995, pp 473–475.

629. Morgello S, Peterson HD, Kahn LJ, Laufer H: Menkes kinky hair disease with "ragged red fibers." *Dev Med Child Neurol* 1988;**30**:812–816.

630. Kaler S, Holmes CS, Goldstein DS, et al: Neonatal diagnosis and treatment of Menkes disease. *N Engl J Med* 2008;**358**:605–614.

631. Nedeltchev N, Mattle HP: Cerebrovascular manifestations of neurofibromatosis. In Caplan LR (ed): *Uncommon Causes of Stroke*, 2nd ed. Cambridge: Cambridge University Press, 2008, pp 221–224.

632. Taboada D, Alonso A, Moreno J: Occlusion of the cerebral arteries in Recklinghausen's disease. *Neuroradiology* 1979;**18**:281–284.

633. Levinsohn PM, Mikhael MA, Rothman SM: Cerebrovascular changes in neurofibromatosis. *Dev Med Child Neurol* 1978;**20**:789–793.

634. Rizzo JF, Lessell S: Cerebrovascular abnormalities in neurofibromatosis type l. *Neurology* 1994;**44**:1000–1002.

635. Boers GH, Smals AG, Trijbels FJ, et al: Heterozygosity for homocystinuria in premature peripheral and cerebral occlusive disease. *N Engl J Med* 1985;**313**:709–715.

636. Welch GN, Loscalzo J: Homocysteine and atherothrombosis. *N Engl J Med* 1998;**338**:1042–1050.

637. Caplan LR, Hurst JW: Homocysteinemia and homocystinuria. In Caplan LR, Hurst JW, Chimowitz M (eds): *Clinical Neurocardiology*. New York: Marcel Dekker, 1999, pp 431–432.

638. Ueland PM, Refsum H, Stabler SP, et al: Total homocysteine in plasma or serum: methods and clinical applications. *Clin Chem* 1993;**39**:1764–1769.

639. Finkelstein JD, Martin JJ, Harris BJ: Methionine metabolism in mammals: The methionine-sparing effect of cystine. *J Biol Chem* 1988;**263**:11750–11754.

640. Mudd SH, Skovby F, Levy HL, et al: The natural history of homocystinuria due to cystathione-beta-synthase deficiency. *Am J Hum Genet* 1985;**37**:1–31.

641. Vermaak WJ, Ubbink JB, Barnard HC, et al: Vitamin B$_6$ nutrition status and cigarette smoking. *Am J Clin Nutr* 1990;**51**:1058–1061.

642. Clarke R, Daly L, Robinson K, et al: Hyperhomocysteinemia: An independent risk factor for vascular disease. *N Engl J Med* 1991;**324**:1149–1155.

643. Evers S, Koch H-G, Grotemeyer K-H, et al: Features, symptoms, and neurophysiological findings in stroke associated with hyperhomocysteinemia. *Arch Neurol* 1997;**54**:1276–1282.

644. Selhub J, Jacques PF, Bostom AG, et al: Association between plasma homocysteine concentrations and extracranial carotid-artery stenosis. *N Engl J Med* 1995;**332**:286–291.

645. Harker LA, Slichter SJ, Scott CR: Homocysteinemia: Vascular injury and arterial thrombosis. *N Engl J Med* 1974;**291**:537–543.

646. Harker LA, Ross R, Slichter SJ, Scott CR: Homocysteine-induced arteriosclerosis: The role of endothelial cell injury and platelet response in its genesis. *J Clin Invest* 1976;**58**:731–741.

647. Tsai J-C, Perrella MA, Yoshizumi M, et al: Promotion of vascular smooth muscle cell growth by homocysteine: A link to atherosclerosis. *Proc Natl Acad Sci U S A* 1994;**91**:6369–6373.

648. Roach ES, Anselm I, Rosman NP, Caplan LR: Progeria. In Caplan LR (ed): *Uncommon Causes of Stroke*, 2nd ed. Cambridge: Cambridge University Press, 2008, pp 145–148.

649. Merideth MA, Gordon LB, Clauss S, et al: Phenotype and course of Hutchinson–Gilford progeria syndrome. *N Engl J Med* 2008;**358**:592–604.

650. Delgado Luengo W, Rojas Martinez A, Ortiz Lopez R, et al: Del(1)(q23) in a patient with Hutchinson–Gilford progeria. *Am J Med Genet* 2002;**113**:298–301.

651. McClintock D, Gordon LB, Djabali K: Hutchinson–Gilford progeria mutant lamin A primarily targets human vascular cells as detected by an anti-lamin A G608 G antibody. *Proc Natl Acad Sci U S A* 2006;**103**:2154–2159.

652. Zuber M: Hereditary hemorrhagic telangiectasia (Osler–Weber–Rendu disease). In Caplan LR (ed): *Uncommon Causes of Stroke*, 2nd ed. Cambridge: Cambridge University Press, 2008, pp 109–114.

653. Osler W: On a family form of recurring epistaxis, associated with multiple telengiectases of the skin and mucous membranes. *John Hopkins Hosp Bull* 1901;**12**:333–337.

654. Peery WH: Clinical spectrum of hereditary haemorrhagic telengiectasia (Osler–Weber–Rendu disease). *Am J Med* 1987;**82**:989–997.

655. Guttmacher AE, Marchuk DA, White RI: Hereditary hemorrhagic telangiectasia. *N Engl J Med* 1995;**333**:918–924.

656. Gould DB, Phalan FC, Breedveld GJ, et al: Mutations in *COL4A1* cause perinatal cerebral hemorrhage and porencephaly. *Science* 2005;**308**:1167–1171.

657. Gould DB, Phalan FC, van Mil SE, et al: Role of *COL4A1* in small vessel

disease and hemorrhagic stroke. *N Engl J Med* 2006;**354**:1489–1496.

658. Vahedi K, Boukobza M, Massin P, et al: Clinical and brain MRI follow-up study of a family with *COL4A1* mutation. *Neurology* 2007;**69**:1564–1568.

659. Meschia JF, Rosand J: Fragile vessels. Handle with care. *Neurology* 2007;**69**:1560–1561.

660. Labrune P, Lacroix C, Goutieres F, et al: Extensive brain calcifications, leukodystrophy, and formation of parenchymal cysts: A new progressive disorder due to diffuse cerebral microangiopathy. *Neurology* 1996;**46**:1297–1301.

661. Corboy JR, Gault J, Kleinschmidt-Demasters BK: An adult case of leukoencephalopathy with intracranial calcifications and cysts. *Neurology* 2006;**67**:1890–1892.

Subarachnoid hemorrhage, aneurysms, and vascular malformations

Tudor Jovin and Louis R Caplan

Intracranial hemorrhages involve the brain parenchyma or subarachnoid space, or both. Approximately 20% of all strokes are hemorrhagic, with subarachnoid hemorrhage (SAH) and intracerebral hemorrhage (ICH) accounting for about 10%. SAH occurs when a blood vessel near the brain surface leaks, causing extravasation of blood into the subarachnoid space. Apart from head injury SAH is most often caused by rupture of a saccular aneurysm. Less common causes include, use of illicit drugs, especially amphetamines and cocaine, amyloid angiopathy, hemorrhage from an arteriovenous malformation (AVM) or dural arteriovenous fistula, rupture of an artery near the pial surface due to hypertension, bleeding into an ischemic stroke, dural venous sinus thrombosis, and bleeding disorders. Dolichoectatic aneurysms and dissecting aneurysms can also rupture, causing SAH. These lesions are discussed and illustrated in Chapter 12.

Symptoms depend on the rapidity and duration of the bleeding and the volume of blood. Rupture of an arterial aneurysm causes the abrupt introduction of blood under arterial pressure into the subarachnoid space. This abruptly increases intracranial pressure and leads to transient cessation of activity, severe headache, and vomiting. Slower leakage of blood does not increase intracranial pressure as rapidly. Blood in the subarachnoid space acts as a meningeal irritant and incites headache, photophobia, and stiff neck. Confusion, seizures, restlessness, and transient or persistent decreased levels of consciousness are common in patients with SAH and are caused by the increased intracranial pressure, and meningeal irritation.

Aneurysms

Ruptured saccular aneurysms are a common and serious medical problem. According to necropsy and angiography series, about 5–6% of individuals have intracranial aneurysms.[1,2] The prevalence of aneurysms is low during the first two decades of life and increases steadily after the third decade.[1] The frequency of SAH from ruptured saccular aneurysms is relatively low, estimated at between 6 and 11 per 100 000 persons per year, or about 1 per 10 000.[3–8] The relatively low rupture-to-prevalence rate shows that most aneurysms do not rupture. Several prospective studies have addressed the risk of rupture of never symptomatic intracranial aneurysms and have identified size, location, and shape of the aneurysm as strong predictors of rupture.[9–11] According to a large such study a prospective international study of unruptured intracranial aneurysms, in patients with no history of SAH, the 5-year cumulative rate of rupture of aneurysms located in the internal carotid artery, anterior communicating artery, anterior cerebral artery, or middle cerebral artery is zero for aneurysms under 7 mm, 2.6% for 7–12 mm, 14.5% for 13–24 mm, and 40% for 25 mm or more.[12,13] For same size aneurysms in the posterior circulation and posterior communicating artery rates are higher at 2.5%, 14.5%, 18.4%, and 50%, respectively.

Overall, ruptured aneurysms are more common in women and smokers. Although ruptured aneurysms are more common in men younger than 40 years, women prevail after age 40.[12] The average age at rupture is approximately 50 years.[4]

Once an aneurysm ruptures, death or severe long-term disability often results. Among 100 typical patients with SAH caused by ruptured aneurysms, about 33 will die before receiving medical attention. Another 20 will die while in the hospital or will remain incapacitated from the original hemorrhage. Seventeen patients who survive the initial hemorrhage will deteriorate later, with eight patients recovering and nine patients left with severe neurological sequelae.[13] Only 30 of the original 100 patients will do well, surviving without major disability. If the ruptured aneurysm remains surgically untreated and the patient does not have recurrent hemorrhage during the first 6 months, approximately 3% of the remaining patients will rebleed each year.[14] Even among patients admitted to the hospital in good condition, the overall prognosis is poor especially in patients presenting with significant neurological impairment. In one series, 29% of these patients died and only 55% made a good recovery at 90 days.[15] A delay often occurs in referring patients with SAH to neurological and neurosurgical centers for treatment. In one series among 150 consecutive patients with aneurysmal SAH, only 36% were referred within 48 hours.[16] The median time to referral was 3.6 days. Tragically, delayed diagnosis by physicians and logistic and policy issues accounted for more than 70% of the delays.[16]

Locations, familial occurrence, and pathogenesis

Saccular aneurysms typically develop at arterial bifurcations (see Figure 2.35). Aneurysms are especially likely to be found at

bifurcations that have a hypoplastic small branch and bifurcations with a sharp acute angle.[17] Approximately 90% of aneurysms involve anterior circulation arteries.[4,18] Common sites in the anterior circulation include: (1) the junction between the anterior communicating artery (AComA) and the anterior cerebral artery (ACA); (2) bifurcation of the middle cerebral artery (MCA); and (3) the internal carotid artery (ICA) junction with the ophthalmic artery, posterior communicating artery (PComA), anterior choroidal artery (AChA), and MCAs.[4] In the posterior circulation, the apex of the basilar artery and the intracranial vertebral artery, especially at the origins of the posterior inferior cerebellar arteries (PICAs), are the most common sites.[4,18]

Multiple aneurysms are present in approximately 14–24% of patients and are more common in women.[2,5,19] In patients with multiple aneurysms, 2 are present in 77%, 3 in 15%, and 4 or more in 8%.[5] Saccular aneurysms are known to be more common in patients with polycystic kidney disease, coarctation of the aorta, Ehlers–Danlos syndrome (especially type IV), fibromuscular dysplasia, pseudoxanthoma elasticum, and Marfan's syndrome.

The familial occurrence of intracranial aneurysms is well known.[20–22] Approximately 7–20% of patients with a ruptured aneurysm have a first- or second-degree relative with an intracranial aneurysm, and, among first-degree relatives of a patient who has had a ruptured aneurysm, the risk of having a ruptured intracranial aneurysm is about four times higher than in the general population.[2,5,20–22] Late teenage and adult first-degree relatives in families where two or more first-degree relatives have been shown to have a cerebral aneurysm should be screened with magnetic resonance angiography (MRA) or computed tomography angiography (CTA) for the presence of aneurysms. Since aneurysms can develop later, they probably should later be screened again, although the optimal interval between screenings is not clear. Preliminary studies are beginning to show some genetic associations in patients with familial and sporadic saccular aneurysms.[23–28] Variations in or near the proteoglycan versican gene likely play a role in susceptibility to intracranial aneurysm formation.[27]

No completely satisfactory explanation of the origin, growth, and rupture of saccular aneurysms exists. Intracerebral arteries are normally composed of an outer collagenous adventitia, a prominent muscular media, an internal elastic lamina, and an intima lined by endothelial cells. An external elastic lamina does not exist. Intracranial arteries are more susceptible than extracranial arteries to aneurysm formation because intracranially, the arterial walls are thin, there is less elastin, an external elastic lamina is not present, and arteries that are located within the subarachnoid space lack surrounding supporting tissue. Various theories cite congenital and genetic abnormalities that cause defects in the arterial media, hypertensive and atherosclerotic degenerative changes in the vessel walls, inflammatory proliferative arteritis, and focal degeneration of the internal elastic lamina. Some investigators emphasize that aneurysms form because of congenital defects in the media of arteries. The most common defect in the arterial media is a localized loss of muscular elements. These focal deficits

are often located at arterial bifurcations. Some patients with intracranial aneurysms have reduced production of type III collagen.[29]

Ferguson proposed a theory of aneurysm development and growth that we find plausible and attractive.[30] He suggested that cerebral aneurysms result from mechanically induced degeneration of arteries. Maximal hemodynamic stress occurs at the apices and bifurcations of arteries. Imbalance between the strength of an artery at a particular bifurcation and the hemodynamic stresses applied to it cause degeneration of the internal elastic lamina and aneurysmal outpouching. Turbulent flow in and around aneurysms produces vibration in vessel walls, further weakening the vessel's structural integrity and allowing aneurysm growth.[30] The observation that aneurysms tend to form at sites of increased flow-feeding AVMs and in arteries that provide collateral blood flow supports the contention that increased pressure and flow contribute to aneurysm formation. Stress on the vessel wall increases as aneurysms become thinner, the radius of the aneurysm enlarges, or the intra-aneurysmal pressure increases because of elevated blood pressure. When the wall stress exceeds the wall strength, aneurysms rupture.

Aneurysms may rupture at any time, but especially when blood pressure or blood flow is increased. Rupture often occurs during strenuous activity, such as weight lifting, exercise, coition, defecation, and heavy work. Many aneurysms, however, bleed during relatively inactive periods. One-third of the aneurysms in the Cooperative Study of Intracranial Aneurysms and Subarachnoid Hemorrhage ruptured while patients were asleep, and another one-third ruptured during ordinary daily activities.[12,13,31] Size plays a major role; up to a point, the larger the aneurysm, the more likely it is to rupture. In different autopsy series, the critical size for rupture has varied from 7 to 10 mm.[32–34] Aneurysms larger than 10 mm in diameter are more likely to rupture during follow-up than smaller aneurysms.[2]

Aneurysms larger than 2.5 cm in size are usually referred to as giant aneurysms. The notion that they rarely rupture and produce SAH is not correct. Drake reported that 33% of giant aneurysms present with bleeding and another 10% have a history of remote hemorrhage.[35] Giant aneurysms often contain thrombi within their arterial lumens.

Once an intracranial aneurysm has ruptured, the course is often stormy and the outcome poor. It is estimated that among the 28 000 patients with ruptured aneurysms each year in the United States and Canada, 7000 are misdiagnosed, never referred, or referred too late for definitive therapy.[16,36] The greatest impact improving morbidity and mortality from SAH is not through the efforts of neurologists or neurosurgeons, but rather through early recognition of SAH by primary care physicians and emergency room physicians.[37,38] Diagnosed early, these patients can be referred while still relatively intact to centers with appropriate neurological, neurosurgical, neuroradiological, and neuroanesthetic capabilities. Neurological/neurosurgical intensive care units are especially important for definitive treatment of patients with ruptured aneurysms and their complications.

Clinical findings

A 32-year-old woman, PN, came to the emergency ward because of a headache that had been unremitting for 48 hours. She had migraine headaches as an adolescent. One month ago, she awakened at night with moderately severe headache and vomiting. After the headache persisted for 3 days, she consulted her physician, who diagnosed her with the flu. Although she had no fever, she felt too ill to do her daily chores and stayed in bed for a week, after which the headache gradually cleared. Two days ago, she developed a severe headache that came on suddenly. She was taking heavy trash cans out for garbage collection when the pain struck her in the left temple and top of the head and quickly spread to her neck and back. Her knees buckled with the pain and she vomited. She stumbled into the house and was in bed and rather sleepy when her husband returned from work and insisted that she go to the hospital.

Headache

Intracranial saccular aneurysms often present with a warning leak or so-called sentinel hemorrhage – a minute disruption in the aneurysmal wall results in bleeding that lasts only seconds, spilling blood into the subarachnoid space under high pressure. The patient has sudden, severe headaches, often occipital or nuchal in location, and constant. The headache usually resolves in 48 hours but can last longer. It is best distinguished from migraine by its rapidity of onset and longer duration. Only seconds elapse before it reaches maximum intensity. Vomiting and cessation of activity (e.g., the knees buckling in patient PN) and decrease in alertness often accompany the headache. Migraine headaches, on the other hand, are usually more throbbing and build in intensity over minutes or hours. Nausea and vomiting usually develop after migraine headache has been present for a while. Sentinel headaches usually last from days to a week, during which time patients are seldom able to continue normal activities. Sentinel hemorrhages are often misdiagnosed as migraine, flu, hypertensive encephalopathy, aseptic meningitis, cervical neck strain, or even gastroenteritis.[37,38] Headache, restlessness, and vomiting are often falsely attributed to food poisoning or an acute gastrointestinal disorder.

In patient PN, the headache that she had one month before her episode was probably a warning leak. The duration was too long for migraine, and inability to carry out daily activities should have alerted her physician to evaluate her further. In the Michael Reese Stroke Registry and the University of Illinois Stroke Registry, 31% of patients with SAH had sentinel headaches.[39] In the Danish Aneurysm Study, a warning leak was present in 166 of 1076 patients (15.4%).[35] In 99 of the 166 patients (59.6%) with warning leaks, the headache episode was evaluated by a doctor but misdiagnosed.[40] Ostergaard estimated that as many as 50–60% of patients with SAH have headache or other warning signs before presenting with major bleeds.[41] In patients with headaches of acute onset, the index of suspicion for SAH should be high and the threshold for lumbar puncture (LP) low.[37,38] In patients with sudden, severe headache without focal neurological signs, the only absolute contraindications to LP are no back or no needle. If series of LPs for headache contain only

taps positive for blood, then too few LPs are being performed, and sentinel hemorrhages are being missed.

PN's headache that began 2 days before her episode is typical of that found in SAH. Sudden onset with rapid radiation, especially to the neck and back or sciatic region, suggests meningeal irritation. The focal asymmetric headache is a fairly reliable sign that the bleeding lesion was on the left side – the site of the head pain.

Neurological symptoms and signs

Examination of PN in the emergency room showed a restless but sleepy woman with a stiff neck. The left eyelid drooped. When the lid was lifted, the left eye rested down and out. The left pupil was dilated and unreactive to light. Plantar responses were bilaterally extensor.

Aneurysms may present by compressing adjacent brain tissue or cranial nerves. Giant aneurysms are particularly likely to cause focal symptoms and signs related to mass effect. Giant MCA aneurysms can cause seizures, hemiparesis, or dysphasia. The third nerve can be compressed by aneurysms that occur at the intracranial ICA and PCA junction (often referred to as *posterior communicating artery aneurysms* (PComA)) or by superior cerebellar artery (SCA) aneurysms. A giant SCA aneurysm can cause contralateral hemiplegia (Weber's syndrome) by compressing the pyramidal tracts in the midbrain. Figure 13.1 shows a large aneurysm compressing the cerebral

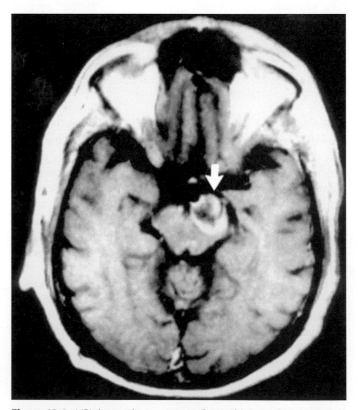

Figure 13.1 MRI shows a large aneurysm (large white arrow) compressing the cerebral peduncle on one side associated with a IIIrd-nerve palsy and contralateral hemiparesis (Weber's syndrome). From Winn WR, Richardson AE, Jane JA. The long-term prognosis in untreated cerebral aneurysms: I. The incidence of late hemorrhage in cerebral aneurysms – A 10 year evaluation of 364 patients. *Ann Neurol* 1977;1:358–370 with permission.

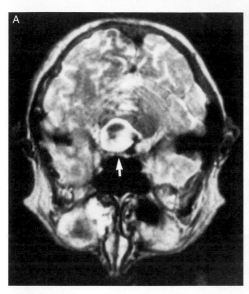

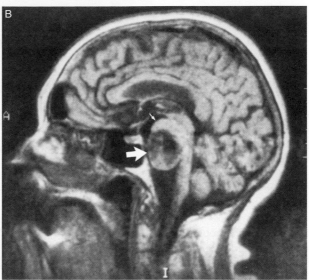

Figure 13.2 (A) T2-weighted MRI; white arrow points to large basilar artery aneurysm containing heterogeneous signals representing thrombus formation. (B) Sagittal MRI showing aneurysm with clot (large white arrow) compressing the pons (small white arrow).

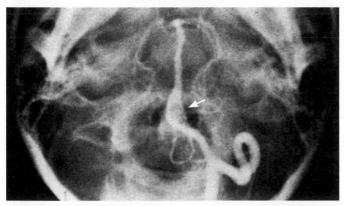

Figure 13.3 Vertebral arteriogram, intracranial Towns view; arrow points to a filling defect in a dissecting aneurysm, representing thrombus.

peduncle on one side. An isolated VIth-nerve paresis can be caused by mass effect. In the cavernous sinus, an aneurysm may compress the VIth, IVth, or IIIrd cranial nerves, producing ophthalmoplegia. Basilar bifurcation aneurysms that point forward can mimic pituitary tumors and cause visual field defects and hypopituitarism. Basilar bifurcation aneurysms that point vertically can cause an amnesic syndrome combined with IIIrd-nerve paresis, bulbar signs, and quadriparesis.[18,42] In PN, the right IIIrd-nerve palsy suggested a right PComA aneurysm.

Occasionally, aneurysms present with transient neurological deficits. These transient ischemic attacks may be secondary to ischemia or seizures. Stewart and colleagues reported short, recurrent, stereotyped episodes in three patients with ischemia and in a fourth patient with transient spells secondary to partial complex seizures.[43] Cranial computed tomography (CT) scans, LP, and electroencephalograms were normal. No cardiac source of embolism could be identified. Cerebral arteriography showed aneurysms in appropriate locations to explain the symptoms in all cases. Thrombi may form within aneurysms, dislodge, and then embolize distally, causing stroke. Fisher and colleagues reported seven patients who had episodes of transient focal brain ischemia.[44] All had saccular aneurysms in arteries that

would explain the symptoms and no other embolic source. Thrombosis within the aneurysmal sac had embolized distally. Sutherland et al. confirmed this thromboembolic hypothesis, by showing deposition of platelets within giant aneurysms.[45] In three of the six patients in their series with active platelet deposition, episodes of recurrent transient neurological dysfunction occurred. Identification of aneurysms presenting in this manner is another indication for performing vascular imaging in patients with recurrent transient neurological deficits, particularly those in whom no cardiac source has been identified and in patients younger than 45 years of age. Magnetic resonance imaging (MRI) scans also often show heterogeneous signals, indicating thrombi within aneurysms. In the MRI scans shown in Figure 13.2A and B, a basilar artery aneurysm contains heterogeneous signals, indicating thrombus; this large aneurysm compressed the pons. Figure 13.3 is an angiogram that shows a filling defect caused by thrombus within an aneurysm.

Patients with SAH usually report sudden-onset constant headaches that reach maximal intensity within seconds. Nausea, vomiting, stiff neck, and transient loss of consciousness are common accompaniments. The patient is often quite agitated and restless. The headache is of such note that the patient is sometimes later able to describe in minute detail the circumstances surrounding the episode. SAH is rarely present without headache. Occasionally, we have cared for patients in whom the initial manifestation of the subarachnoid bleed was neck pain or backache with sciatic radiation. Patients may not report headache if they have confusion, lethargy, aphasia, or amnesia for the event.

Transient loss of consciousness is caused by the sudden increase of intracranial pressure (ICP) that occurs as arterial blood suddenly enters the subarachnoid space. The increased ICP, dissection of blood into the optic-nerve sheath, and increased pressure in central retinal veins can cause retinal hemorrhages, usually subhyaloid in location (Terson's syndrome). These hemorrhages appear as large red masses of blood spreading outward from the optic disk into the retina.

Table 13.1 Focal signs in patients with aneurysmal rupture

1. Leg weakness, confusion, and bilateral Babinski's signs in patients with AComA aneurysms

2. Homonymous hemianopia in PCA aneurysms

3. Aphasia, hemiparesis, and anosognosia in MCA aneurysms

4. Monocular visual disturbances in ophthalmic artery aneurysms

Table 13.2 World Federation of Neurosurgeons Scale

Grade	Score on Glasgow Coma Scale	Motor deficit
1	15	No motor deficit
2	13–14	No motor deficit
3	13–14	Motor deficit
4	7–12	With or without motor deficit
5	3–6	With or without motor deficit

Table 13.3 Glasgow Coma Scale

Eyes open	
Spontaneous	4
To sound	3
To pain	2
Never	1
Best verbal response	
Oriented	5
Confused conversation	4
Inappropriate words	3
Incomprehensible sounds	2
None	1
Best motor response	
Obeys commands	6
Localize pain	5
Flexion (withdrawal)	4
Flexion (abnormal)	3
Extension	2
None	1
Total	**3–15**

Papilledema may develop later. Unilateral or bilateral VIth-nerve paresis is also common, and is a reflection of increased ICP. Some focal signs that suggest the sites of aneurysmal rupture have already been mentioned. Additional signs are noted in Table 13.1.

Because aneurysms that have previously bled may become adherent to the adjacent brain, recurrent rupture is often characterized by intracerebral and subarachnoid bleeding, so-called meningocerebral hemorrhage. Interhemispheric and callosal hematomas can be seen with rupture of ACoA and distal ACA aneurysms,[46] whereas sylvian or temporal lobe hematoma are typically associated with MCA bifurcation aneurysms. Frontal hematomas are associated with a variety of aneurysm locations.[47] Certain aneurysms, especially PCommA and posterior carotid wall may rupture into the subdural space causing subdural hematomas.

In clinical practice, the most widely used clinical severity scale is the Hunt and Hess scale.[48] In this classification patients who are asymptomatic or who have minimal headache are grade I. If they have moderate to severe headache but no neurological signs other than cranial nerve palsies they are grade II. If they are drowsy or confused or have slight focal deficits they become grade III. Severely compromised patients are grade IV (stupor, moderate to severe hemiparesis), or V (deep coma, decerebrate rigidity, moribund appearance).[48] The World Federation of Neurological Surgeons (WFNS) scale (Table 13.2) is also often used.[49] This scale is now preferred since it is based on the sum score of the Glasgow Coma Scale and the presence of focal neurological signs.[49,50]

The scale of Hunt and Hess is useful for predicting short- and long-term prognosis.[48] The higher the grade, the worse the prognosis. LRC classified patient PN's status as Hunt and Hess grade II. Other scales have traditionally been used to grade comatose patients. The most commonly used is the Glasgow Coma Scale (Table 13.3).[50–53] This scale was designed for prognosticating recovery in patients with severe head injury but has since been widely used to evaluate any patient with reduced consciousness. It included grading eye opening and best motor and verbal responses. More recently, Mayo Clinic physicians devised a new scale that includes eye movements, brainstem reflexes, aspects of motor behavior, and respiration and entitle their scale the Four Score Scale[53] (Table 13.4). This scale is likely more useful for neurologists than the Glasgow Coma Scale in grading coma of different etiologies. Since these scales are in relatively wide use, neurologists should become familiar with them.

Diagnostic testing

Cranial CT in PN was suboptimal because of motion. Diffuse opacification of the cortical gyri occurred, and blood was visible in the basal cisterns. LP revealed bloody fluid with an opening pressure of 420 mmHg. She was transferred to the neurological intensive care unit where she underwent placement of an external ventricular drain. She had frequent neurological assessment while at bed rest.

Table 13.4 Four Score Scale

Eye response

4. Eyelids open or opened; tracking or blinking to command

3. Eyelids open but not tracking

2. Eyelids closed but open to loud voice

1. Eyelids closed but open to pain

0. Eyelids remain closed with pain

Motor response

4. Thumbs up, fist or peace sign to command

3. Localizes to pain

2. Flexion response to pain

1. Extensor posturing

0. No response to pain or myoclonic status epilepticus

Brainstem reflexes

4. Pupil and corneal reflexes present

3. One pupil wide and fixed

2. Pupil or corneal reflexes absent

1. Both pupil and corneal reflexes absent

0. Absent pupil, corneal, and cough reflex

Respiration

4. Not intubated; regular breathing pattern

3. Not intubated; Cheyne–Stokes breathing

2. Not intubated; irregular breathing pattern

1. Breathes above ventilator rate

0. Breathes at ventilator rate or apnea

Total 0–16

Computed tomography

Cranial CT is most often the first diagnostic test in the evaluation of patients with suspected SAH. CT often verifies the presence of blood in the subarachnoid space and shows associated intraparenchymal blood.[54,55] The location of the blood often suggests the etiology and the site of the aneurysm that bled.[56] In patients with AComA aneurysms blood often pools in the subfrontal region at the base of the brain and extends into the frontal interhemispheric fissure and the pericallosal cistern.[46,51–53] Often there is an accompanying frontal lobe hematoma or a midline hematoma that extends through the lamina terminalis into the septum pellucidum. The bleeding often extends into the lateral ventricles.[46,51–53] A temporal-lobe hematoma or collection of blood in the sylvian fissure predominantly on one side suggests a MCA aneurysm. Figure 13.4 is a CT scan that shows blood in the subarachnoid space and basal cisterns with the major collection occurring in the left sylvian fissure region. This patient had a large ruptured left MCA aneurysm.

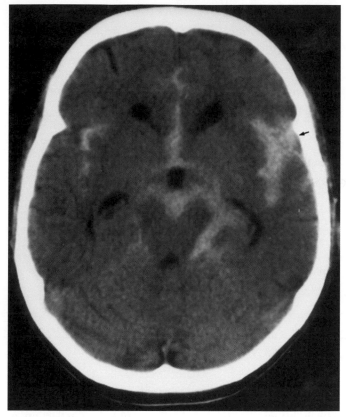

Figure 13.4 CT scan showing blood in the subarachnoid space and basal cisterns. The most blood is pooled in the left sylvian fissure (small black arrow). This patient had an aneurysm of the left MCA that is shown in Figure 13.7B.

Blood localized mostly in the perimesencephalic and prepontine cisterns with little in the supratentorial regions suggests a perimesencephalic (pre-truncal) hemorrhage usually not caused by bleeding from an aneurysm.[57–61] The presence of subarachnoid blood localized to the convexity sulci and fissures on one side is also not indicative of aneurysmal bleeding but suggests an unusual cause such as cerebral amyloid angiopathy, reversible cerebral vasoconstriction syndrome, dural sinus or venous occlusion, or focal arterial disease.[62–65]

CT may show a dilated ventricular system with hydrocephalus caused by disturbance of cerebrospinal fluid (CSF) dynamics by blood clogging the basal cisterns and pacchionian granulations. The amount of blood in the subarachnoid space has been used to predict the likelihood of development of arterial vasoconstriction and delayed brain ischemia.[66–69]

A normal CT scan does not exclude SAH; a normal scan occurs if the hemorrhage is small, especially if the scan is delayed 24–72 hours.[38,70] CTA can most often image intracranial aneurysms on the arteries of the circle of Willis.[71–73] In PN, SAH was confirmed by CT (Figure 13.5); the amount of blood was moderate and most of the blood was located in the basal cisterns, with more on the left side.

Magnetic resonance imaging

MRI is probably less sensitive than CT in showing acute subarachnoid blood. Vascular malformations, especially cavernous angiomas, however, are seen clearly on MRI as well-circumscribed structures with heterogeneous signals. MRA is

Table 13.5 Common spinal fluid findings in patients with SAH

1. Large numbers of red blood cells, without clearing of cells, between the first and last tubes

2. A faint pink color of supernatant fluid if examined within 4–5 hours of hemorrhage

3. A deep yellow (xanthochromic) color of the centrifuged supernatant fluid, secondary to breakdown of heme pigments; hemoglobin is first formed and is later transformed to bilirubin

4. Elevated protein

5. Pleocytosis, usually mononuclear

6. Increased pressure

7. Normal glucose

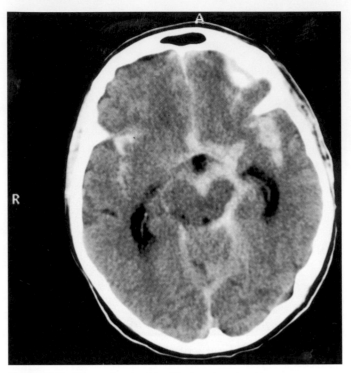

Figure 13.5 CT scan showing blood in the subarachnoid space, predominantly in the basal cisterns. There is more blood on the left side.

proving quite accurate in imaging aneurysms and showing the relationship of the aneurysm to adjacent brain structures. In one series, aneurysms as small as 3–4 mm were usually reliably detected by MRA, but some lesions (3/21 aneurysms) were missed.[74] Some arteries and aneurysms were not well imaged, and details were often insufficient for surgeons to define the neck and the extent of the aneurysms. Others have shown an acceptable aneurysm detection rate for MRA especially when contrast enhancement is performed.[75,76] CTA and MRA are now best used as screening tests for asymptomatic aneurysms in patients with a familial history of aneurysms or known risk factors such as polycystic kidney disease and fibromuscular arterial dysplasia. These techniques reliably show large aneurysms. They often do not show sufficient detail to guide surgical or interventional management of aneurysms that are shown.

Lumbar puncture

We advocate LP as a very important diagnostic step, especially if CT is normal and clinical suspicion of SAH is still present.[38,77,78] The usual spinal fluid findings are noted in Table 13.5.

The opening and closing pressures should be measured and noted. Some advocate waiting at least 6 and preferably 12 hours after headache onset to perform a lumbar puncture.[79] The rationale is that it takes that long for bilirubin to form and color the fluid yellow. Spinal fluid obtained after 72 hours may show only an elevated pressure, xanthochromia, and increased protein content. Spectrophotometry, by quantifying the amounts of hemoglobin and bilirubin, provides information regarding the approximate age of the hemorrhage.[77,80] However, spectrophotometric analysis of CSF shows only moderate specificity for the demonstration of subarachnoid hemorrhage.[81]

Controversy exists as to the advisability of LP in confirmed SAH. Some argue that sudden lowering of pressure may provoke bleeding. We advocate LP, even in CT-confirmed SAH. The initial LP gives a baseline pressure and quantification of the number of red blood cells. This information may be useful later if the patient deteriorates and a second hemorrhage is suspected. The level of CSF pressure is an important parameter to follow. Spinal tap also helps remove blood and CSF. Also, by lowering CSF pressure, spinal tap often relieves headache. Subsequent LPs help document the pressure and blood contents. Surgical complications are more common when the CSF pressure is greater than 180 mmHg at the time of surgical treatment of aneurysms.

Digital subtraction cerebral angiography

Following placement of an external ventricular drain, PN gradually became more alert and her headache waned. Digital subtraction cerebral angiography showing an 8-mm by 12-mm large irregular aneurysm at the junction of the left ICA and PComA (Figure 13.6) was performed within 24 hours of presentation. After review of the angiographic findings by the vascular neurosurgeon and the neuroendovascular surgeon the decision was made to proceed with immediate clipping of the aneurysm. Although the aneurysm was also favorable for coil embolization, the presence of a IIIrd nerve palsy along with the patient's young age and good clinical condition were important considerations that led to this treatment decision. Surgical clipping of the aneurysm was accomplished successfully the same day.

Cerebral angiography remains the definitive method for optimal characterization of the size and anatomical features of intracranial aneurysms. Arterial digital subtraction angiography is the preferred technique, allowing excellent arterial opacification and rapid filming with less dye. The increased use of interventional management of aneurysms has changed the approach to the timing of angiography. Since interventions are often performed emergently soon after SAH, early and definitive imaging of aneurysms and other etiologies is important in guiding treatment decisions and should be performed as soon

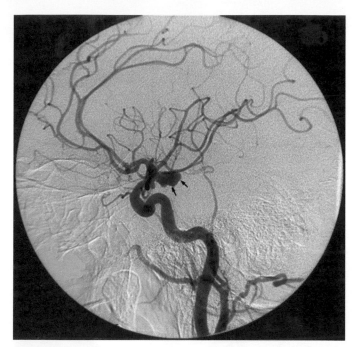

Figure 13.6 Large left PComA aneurysm (small black arrows), 8 × 12 mm in size. Courtesy of Galen Henderson, MD, and Rafael Linas, MD.

as possible. Figure 13.7 shows angiograms of aneurysms at the most common sites.

Because aneurysms may be multiple, all four intracranial arteries should be studied, with anteroposterior, lateral, and oblique views if needed. Table 13.6 lists observations concerning identification of the aneurysm that most likely bled when multiple aneurysms are identified. At times, despite well-documented SAH, no aneurysm is identified angiographically. The prognosis of these patients is usually better than when an aneurysm is shown, but the etiologies of such bleeds are diverse.[82,83] However, in cases with significant volume of blood in the basilar cisterns, particularly if it extends superior to the membrane of Liliquist, repeat delayed angiography is warranted to rule out an occult aneurysm.

Other diagnostic techniques

Transcranial Doppler (TCD) ultrasound is a useful technology for monitoring the intracranial circulation for vasoconstriction.[84–89] Serial TCD measurements of flow velocities in the basal arteries after moderate- and large-volume SAHs often show an increase in velocities during days 3–10 and maximum velocities between days 11 and 20. Time-averaged maximum velocities in the MCA greater than 140 cm/s accurately predict vascular narrowing at angiography. Velocities greater than 200 cm/s predict severe vasoconstriction.[84,86] Doppler-measured velocities in the MCA have an inverse relationship to vascular diameter.

Single-photon-emission computed tomography (SPECT) is also a useful test for monitoring the presence of vasoconstriction because of its ability to show regions of decreased cerebral blood flow (CBF). Regional hypoperfusion correlates well with vasoconstriction and delayed brain infarcts in patients with

SAH.[89,90] Xenon-enhanced CT scanning can also show and quantify regional blood flows.[91,92] Diffusion and perfusion MR scanning has the added capability of showing zones of infarction as well as underperfused regions.[93,94] These techniques and CT perfusion scanning are all potentially effective in monitoring SAH patients.

Differential diagnosis

Van Gijn and colleagues noted that a high proportion of patients with SAHs located predominantly in the perimesencephalic cisterns by CT had normal cerebral angiography.[57–60,95] Newer-generation CT scans and MRI have shown that these hemorrhages are often centered around the prepontine cistern. Because these hemorrhages are concentrated around the brainstem, Schievink, Wijdicks, and colleagues suggest that they be called pretruncal subarachnoid hemorrhages (truncus cerebri is another term for the brainstem), rather than perimesencephalic hemorrhages.[59,95] The clinical course in patients with pretruncal hemorrhage is different from aneurysmal SAH because few patients die, rebleed acutely, or develop delayed cerebral infarction or hydrocephalus.[59,95,96] The outcome is much more benign than in patients with aneurysms shown by angiography. The etiology of these hemorrhages around the brainstem is unknown, but a venous or capillary leak is often posited. In one patient with a pretruncal hemorrhage, a capillary telangiectasia was shown in the ventral pons by MRI.[97] Because SAH resulting from rupture of a posterior circulation aneurysm can also cause bleeding centered around the brainstem, an angiogram is always warranted in such patients. If the initial angiogram is technically adequate and negative, however, a repeat angiogram has a low yield of showing an aneurysm.

Patients with SAH and normal angiography have a variety of different etiologies.[82,83] We have seen a number of patients who had hemorrhage into the caudate nucleus with extension into the ventricular system, which simulates SAH clinically but CT or MRI would show the caudate and intraventricular blood.[98] AVMs may also involve the subependymal region and may bleed directly into the ventricles and CSF. Before the era of CT scans, these intraventricular hemorrhages and other brain hemorrhages may have accounted for some examples of SAH with normal arteriography. Cerebral amyloid angiopathy is an important, oft-neglected cause of bleeding into the subarachnoid space. Amyloid laden arteries are common along the pial surface of the brain. The differential diagnosis of subarachnoid blood is listed in Table 13.7.[99–105]

The possibility of an erroneous diagnosis of SAH should also be considered. Other conditions, such as tumor, infection, or traumatic LP, can mimic SAH. If the clinical picture is characterized by back pain, radicular signs, or myelopathic signs, we order a spinal MRI and perform studies seeking a spinal aneurysm, AVM, or spinal dural fistula (see Chapter 16). In situations in which vasoconstriction is prominent but no aneurysm is seen, we repeat angiography to better visualize the intracranial arteries after the clinical state improves.

Table 13.6 Identifying the aneurysm that most likely bled when multiple aneurysms are present

1. Largest aneurysm

2. Most irregularly shaped aneurysm

3. Aneurysm with the most associated focal spasm

4. Aneurysm in the vascular territory, explaining the focal signs

5. Aneurysm that best correlates with the collection of blood on CT

Complications of aneurysmal subarachnoid hemorrhage and their management

Management of patients with SAH is one of the most difficult problems in clinical medicine. The complications are myriad and management trends change almost yearly. Table 13.8 lists common complications of SAH during the acute and later periods. For ease of recall, we think of the nine H's: hypertension (systemic); hypertension (intracranial); heart failure and arrhythmia; hematoma; hemorrhage (rebleed); hypoperfusion (vasoconstriction); hydrocephalus; hypovolemia; and hyponatremia.

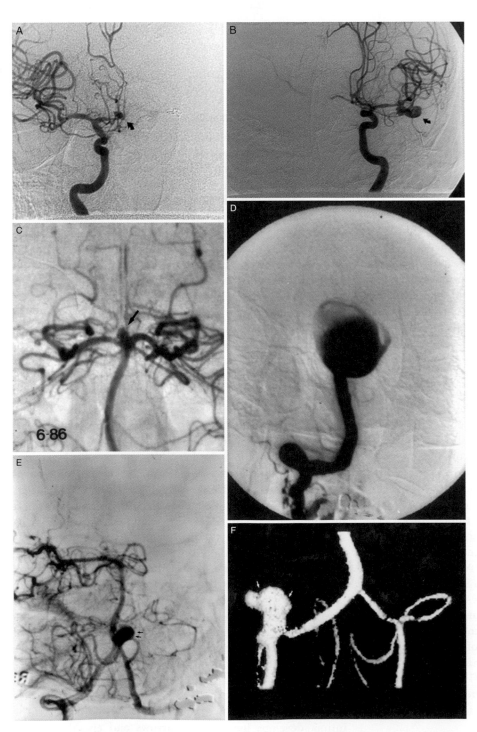

Figure 13.7 Angiograms showing aneurysms at other common sites. (A) AComA aneurysm (black arrow). (B) Large MCA aneurysm (black arrow). (C) Small basilar bifurcation aneurysm (black arrow). (D) Very large basilar bifurcation aneurysm. (E) Aneurysm (small black arrows) at the vertebral-basilar artery junction. (F) Aneurysm at the vertebral posterior–inferior cerebellar artery junction (small white arrows) shown on CTA. A and B, courtesy of Galen Henderson, MD, and Rafael Linas, MD.

Table 13.7 Entities to be considered in the differential diagnosis of SAH when no aneurysm has been found

1. SAH secondary to occult trauma
2. Blood dyscrasias and sickle cell disease
3. Non-visualized arteriovenous malformations or an unseen small aneurysm
4. Thrombosis of a ruptured aneurysm
5. Leakage from a small non-aneurysmal artery on the brain surface
6. Dural arteriovenous malformations
7. Spinal arteriovenous malformations
8. Cerebral venous and dural sinus occlusions
9. Intracranial arterial dissections
10. Cerebral amyloid angiopathy
11. Cocaine abuse
12. Pituitary apoplexy
13. Vasculitis (especially polyarteritis nodosa and Wegener's granulomatosis)

Table 13.8 Complications of SAH (the nine H's)

Early

1. Hypertension (intracranial)
2. Hypertension (systemic)
3. Heart failure and arrhythmia
4. Hematoma

Delayed

5. Hemorrhage (rebleed)
6. Hypoperfusion (vasospasm)
7. Hydrocephalus
8. Hypovolemia
9. Hyponatremia

Rebleeding (hemorrhage)

The most feared complication in patients with SAH is recurrent aneurysmal rupture. The initial bleed and rehemorrhage are major causes of death in patients with aneurysmal SAH. In one study that had a 45% (36/80) mortality, 64% (23/36) of deaths were attributable to the initial SAH and 8 of the remaining 13 deaths were caused by recurrent hemorrhages.[106] The mortality rate in patients who rebleed has been cited as about 50%.[106,107]

Rebleeding is heralded by sudden, abrupt, severe headache. Rebleeds tend to be both intraparenchymal and subarachnoid. The frequency of bleeding into the brain is higher than in the original aneurysm rupture. Signs include meningismus, focal neurological abnormalities associated with intraparenchymal hemorrhage, and often rapid development of coma. Among aneurysms that rebleed, approximately 20% do so in the first 2 weeks, 30% by the end of the first month, and 40% by the end of 6 months. Beyond 6 months, rerupture occurs at a rate of approximately 3% per year.[6,12] No infallible rules predict which patients will have recurrent hemorrhages.

Efforts are directed to reduce those factors that promote rebleeding. Patients are placed at bed rest with minimal stimuli. Pain is controlled with analgesics. Sedatives are used. Patients are kept from straining at stool by regular use of laxatives and stool softeners. These measures are attempts to avoid elevations in blood pressure, which could increase intra-aneurysmal pressure and increase the risk of rebleeding. Blood pressure is monitored, and medications are used to lower pressure when greater than in the 160/100 mmHg range. When feasible, early obliteration of the aneurysm by surgery or intravascular interventional measures is the best way to prevent a second bleed.

Delayed cerebral ischemia (vasoconstriction)

Second only to rebleeding as a cause of significant morbidity and mortality is vasoconstriction. Vasoconstriction is defined as abnormal narrowing of intracranial arteries and when it causes neurological deficits or brain infarcts evident on brain imaging, the clinical syndrome is referred to as delayed cerebral ischemia (DCI). The narrowing of intracranial arteries found in patients with SAH has customarily been called *vasospasm*. Purists argue that vasoconstriction is a more accurate designation because it is a structural term that does not imply duration or mechanism, whereas spasm usually refers to functional reversible changes that have a relatively short duration. The narrowing of arteries often persists, and chronic morphological changes develop in both experimental animals[108] and humans[109,110] with SAH. Therefore, vasospasm is an inaccurate designation.

The pathogenesis of vasoconstriction is not fully clarified but is probably related to the release of substances into the CSF from the subarachnoid blood and the interaction of these substances with the arteries in the subarachnoid space. Erythrocytes and their subsequent hemolysis are necessary for vasoconstriction to develop.[111,112] The most likely putative substance is oxyhemoglobin, which affects the function of platelet-derived growth factor which is released from platelets adherent to the arterial wall. Oxyhemoglobin also has an affect on endothelial factors, especially endothelial-derived relaxing factor, and components of the coagulation cascade, especially thrombin, plasmin, and fibrinogen.[112] The result of these interactions is abnormal contraction or failure of relaxation of arterial smooth muscle of the arteries bathed by the CSF.

Patients who die from SAH with vasoconstriction less than 3 weeks after the initial hemorrhage show necrosis of the media, whereas patients who live longer than 3 weeks show marked concentric intimal thickening, subendothelial fibrosis, and medial atrophy.[112–116] The adventitia shows adherent clot with inflammatory cell infiltrates and degeneration of perivascular nerve terminals.[112] The media shows smooth muscle contraction with varying degrees of fibrosis and necrosis. The intima develops longitudinal furrows and endothelial cells

often desquamate, necrose, and have abnormalities of inter-cellular tight junctions.[112]

SAH probably induces vasoconstriction that is then followed by arterial wall necrosis. Vasoconstriction usually has its onset 3–5 days after the hemorrhage. The peak timing for vasoconstriction is 5–9 days. Most vasoconstriction resolves after the second week.[112,117–119] Vasoconstriction also occurs postoperatively, probably because of the handling of arteries and, at times, is caused by intraoperative bleeding. Vasoconstriction has been detected arteriographically in 30–70% of SAH patients.[120] Approximately two-thirds of patients undergoing angiography during the second week after SAH show vasoconstriction.[102–112] Angiographic diagnosis is based on the narrowed appearance of the intracranial arteries. Severe vasoconstriction is characterized by a lumen smaller than 0.5 mm with delayed antegrade blood flow. Some arteries are diffusely narrowed, whereas others show focal constrictions. Among patients with subarachnoid hemorrhage, CTA and digital subtraction angiography have a very high correlation.[121] The absence of vasoconstriction on CTA has a negative predictive value of 95%.[121] Decreased blood flow as imaged by CT perfusion studies is also helpful in predicting the development of brain infarction.[122] Increased blood-flow velocities detected by TCD correlate well with angiographic vasoconstriction.[84,94,123] Only about one-half of the patients with arteriographically demonstrable vasoconstriction are symptomatic. This suggests that delayed cerebral ischemia also involves other mechanisms beyond reduction in blood flow due to arterial constriction.

Early signs of DCI include tachycardia, hypertension, electroencephalographic (EEG) abnormalities, and decreased level of consciousness.[124] Some patients, especially those with diffuse vasoconstriction, develop signs of diffuse brain dysfunction, including headache, stupor, and confusion. Focal neurological signs often accompany these global signs and depend on the arteries involved. Often, the most severe vasoconstriction is in the artery harboring the aneurysm or lying within the surrounding blood clot. Occasionally, maximal vasoconstriction occurs at a distance from the aneurysm. Patients with DCI due to MCA vasoconstriction develop hemiparesis, hemisensory loss, aphasia, anosognosia, and confusion. With ACA vasoconstriction, there may be weakness in one or both lower extremities, abulia, and apraxia. PCA-territory ischemia causes hemianopia and hemisensory loss. CT scans and MRI protocols of the brain provide confirmatory data, ruling out intraparenchymal hemorrhage and hydrocephalus as a cause of the delayed deterioration. Focal hypodensity representing infarction is often seen. SPECT, Xenon-enhanced CT scans, CT perfusion studies, and perfusion MRI can provide images of regions of decreased perfusion of brain supplied by the constricted arteries. There is likely to be genetic variability in the development of vasoconstriction and of delayed brain ischemia. A meta-analysis showed that patients with an E4 allele in the APOE genotype have a higher risk of delayed ischemia and poor outcome after SAH.[125]

The clinical, laboratory, and neuroimaging findings that correlate with the development of significant vasoconstriction

Table 13.9 Findings that correlate with development of cerebral vasoconstriction after SAH

1. Thick blood clots localized in subarachnoid cisterns and amount of subarachnoid blood

2. Arterial lumen size <0.5 mm, with low distal perfusion

3. Aneurysms located on circle of Willis

4. Decreased level of consciousness

5. Intraventricular blood

6. Elevated levels of brain natriuretic peptide

are noted in Table 13.9. The ideal treatment of DCI is prevention. Prevention has taken various directions, including early aneurysm clipping or coiling, volume expansion, clot removal or lysis, and prophylactic drug regimens.[112] Blood can be washed from the subarachnoid space during early surgery, and some authors report a low incidence of symptomatic vasospasm in those patients in whom postoperative CT scans showed removal of blood.[126,127] Another approach has been to use urokinase or, more commonly, tissue plasminogen-activator to lyse CSF clots after aneurysm clipping.[128,129] Placement of nicardipine prolonged-release implants within the basal cisterns in contact with the exposed blood vessels among 32 SAH patients decreased angiographic vasoconstriction (73% in control patients and 7% in those with implants) and delayed cerebral ischemia (47% controls vs. 14% of those with implants) in one randomized, double-blind study.[130]

Patients with vasoconstriction were often given "triple-H therapy," which consisted of hypervolemia, hypertension (often induced pharmacologically), and hemodilution, usually accomplished by volume expansion with colloids or crystalloids.[131–133] Elevation of arterial pressure pharmacologically is only advisable after aneurysms are clipped or when patients are hypotensive. Volume expansion, induced hypervolemia, hypertension, and hemodilution have no known effects on the vascular narrowing but are posited to help maintain CBF above ischemic thresholds by increasing cardiac output and improving blood rheology.[131–135] Hypervolemic therapy with aggressive volume expansion requires intensive care, and carries a substantial risk of complications.[119] The benefit of hypervolemia has been increasingly called into question and euvolemia rather than hypervolemia is currently the preferred treatment goal related to volume status.[136,137] A trial of hypervolemics concluded that: "Hypervolemic therapy resulted in increased cardiac filling pressures and fluid intake but did not increase CBF or blood volume compared with normovolemic therapy. Although careful fluid management to avoid hypovolemia may reduce the risk of delayed cerebral ischemia after SAH, prophylactic hypervolemia therapy is unlikely to confer an additional benefit."[136]

Since anemia is a risk factor for DCI and poor neurological outcome,[138,139] hemodilution is increasingly being abandoned as a prophylactic measure for DCI. Higher hemoglobin concentration may be beneficial in patients with DCI.[140,141] Blood transfusions may on occasion be necessary to achieve this goal.

Current guidelines suggest that "the use of packed red cell transfusions to treat anemia might be reasonable in patients with SAH who are at risk of cerebral ischemia. The optimal hemoglobin level is still to be determined."[142] Many neurologists and neurosurgeons advocate avoidance of hypotension, hyponatremia, hypovolemia, and when necessary administer normal saline boluses rather than aggressive volume expansion.[112] When this therapy fails to reverse the clinical syndrome, endovascular angioplasty (mechanical dilatation of the arteries in spasm by balloons) and/or intra-arterial infusions of vasodilators such as calcium-channel blockers or the less frequently used inotropic agents such as Milrinone have been shown to at least temporarily improve the degree of vasoconstriction.[5,79,107]

The results of preliminary British[143] and American[144] trials reported during the early 1980s suggested that nimodipine, a calcium-channel blocker, might decrease the incidence and severity of vasoconstriction and could improve outcome. Potential mechanisms of action of nimodipine, nicardipine, and other calcium-channel blockers include a decrease in vasoconstriction, improved blood flow by dilation of collateral arteries, neuronal protection by decreasing entry of calcium into cells, and improvement of blood rheology.[112] A number of trials have shown that nimodipine does improve outcome and decreases the frequency of delayed cerebral infarction.[145] A systematic review of 10 trials (including 2756 patients) of calcium-channel blockers in patients with SAH reported a 33% relative risk reduction in the frequency of ischemic neurological deficits and a 20% relative risk reduction in the development of infarcts on CT scans.[145] The relative risk reduction of poor outcome (death or dependence) was 16% and 10% for death alone.[145] Administration of nimodipine, nicardipine, and other calcium-channel-blocking agents can cause decreased blood pressure and renal function, especially when the drugs are given intravenously, so that blood pressure, urinary output, and renal function must be carefully monitored. Nimodipine is the drug of choice and is given 15–30 g/kg per hour intravenously or 30–90 mg enterally every 4 hours. More experience is needed concerning implantation of calcium-channel drugs into the CSF in sustained-release forms. The inotropic agent milrinone, a phosphodiesterase inhibitor was shown by Fraticelli and colleagues to be a potentially safe and effective treatment for cerebral vasoconstriction after SAH.[146] This agent increases cardiac output and in doing so increases CBF.[146]

Since 1989, patients with vasoconstriction shown angiographically who have accompanying neurological symptoms and/or signs, have been treated by neurointerventionalists with transluminal angioplasty using various catheter devices.[147–150] The technology is still evolving and often changes. Using new-generation compliant balloons, this technique is now safe and effective in reversing vasoconstriction. A calcium-channel blocker such as verapamil or nicardipine are often used as an adjunct to angioplasty or as stand alone treatment. Although infusion of these vasodilator agents do readily improve vessel caliber and downstream perfusion, the effect

may be temporary and repeat treatment is often required. The use of prophylactic angioplasty is not now recommended due to an unfavorable risk–benefit ratio.

It seems prudent to prevent hypovolemia by liberal use of fluids orally and intravenously in patients with SAH. Nimodipine is given intravenously or enterally for the first 10 days. In patients with vasoconstriction shown angiographically, normovolemia and maintenance of blood pressure should be pursued. This is best supervised in an intensive care unit, and, sometimes, measurement of pulmonary wedge pressures are needed for appropriate volume management although routine use of invasive volume status monitoring is currently not recommended. ICP monitoring is also often helpful in following the effects of osmotic diuretics, steroids, and fluid removal on ICP and CBF. TCD is used to monitor blood-flow velocities in the basal arteries and hemispheric blood flow. Diffusion- and perfusion-weighted MRI is also helpful in detecting and quantifying vasoconstriction-related regions of hypoperfusion. Small, often multiple regions of ischemia shown by diffusion-weighted imaging are surrounded by larger regions of decreased perfusion.[93] Angioplasty performed by a trained and experienced neurointerventionist is used when available in patients with symptomatic vasospasm who have not responded to medical therapy. Surgery or intra-arterial aneurysm embolization should be performed as early as possible when patients are in good condition.[5,129,151]

Supportive critical care medicine

Once the aneurysm is secure, meticulous critical care medicine is essential to achieving good outcomes. Emphasis is placed on initiating early nutrition with tight control of blood sugar, deep vein thrombosis prophylaxis as well as pain and agitation control to minimize elevations in ICP. Seizure prophylaxis is not routinely recommended. Although statins and magnesium were posited to improve outcomes in patients with SAH, recent studies have failed to show improved outcomes with the routine use of statins[152] or intravenous magnesium.[153]

Hydrocephalus

In addition to rebleeding and vasospasm, other complications can lead to deterioration of patients with ruptured aneurysms. Acute hydrocephalus is caused by alteration in normal CSF dynamics. CSF flow is blocked by blood in the cisterns around the brainstem and reabsorption is impaired when blood attaches to the pacchionian granulations. The syndrome can be recognized by increasing headache, lethargy, incontinence, and decreased spontaneity. Diagnosis is readily confirmed by non-contrast CT scans. In a large study of the timing of aneurysm surgery, the authors analyzed factors that predicted hydrocephalus among 3521 patients with SAH admitted within 3 days of bleeding.[154] The factors that increased the likelihood of hydrocephalus were older age, hypertension (by history, admission blood pressure, and postoperative measures), thick local or diffuse blood on CT, intraventricular hemorrhage, use of antifibrinolytic drugs, and reduced level of consciousness.[154] Patients with significant hydrocephalus will need ventricular

drainage using a catheter inserted into a lateral ventricle, although some can be effectively treated using serial lumbar taps or placement of a lumbar spinal subarachoid drain. In the months to years that follow SAH, normal-pressure hydrocephalus may develop as the arachnoid becomes fibrotic and adhesions prevent normal CSF flow.

Cardiac and pulmonary abnormalities

Cardiopulmonary complications occur often in patients with SAH. Careful surveillance for arrhythmias, heart failure, and myocardial infarction is required. We monitor cardiac rhythm, obtain baseline and follow-up ECGs, and cardiac enzymes, and carefully watch for clinical signs of congestive heart failure. SAHs can be accompanied by ECG abnormalities,[155,156] myocardial creatine kninase and troponin enzyme elevations mimicking myocardial infarction,[157,158] regional left ventricular wall motion abnormalities,[159] and arrhythmias.[156,160–162] The most striking ECG changes are so-called waterfall T waves, which are seen across the endocardium. ECG abnormalities include alterations in QRS configuration, Q-T interval prolongation, T-wave abnormalities, and S-T segment elevation or depression.[156]

Subendocardial hemorrhages and myofibrillary degeneration have been noted at necropsy after SAH and other strokes.[156,163,164] The pathological abnormalities of cardiac muscle cells has usually been referred to as myocytolysis. Striations within myocardial muscle cells are lost, and the cytoplasm often becomes hyalinized. Measurements show that some enzymes are lost from the muscle cells. The number of muscle cells decrease, but the sarcolemma, stroma, and nuclei usually remain. Lipofuchsin is found within myofibrils. Often, there is a coagulative type of myocytolysis in which cardiac muscle cells die in a hypercontracted state with early myofibrillar damage and anomalous irregular cross-band formation.[156,164] This type of pathological change has also been called myofibrillar degeneration and contraction band necrosis. Early calcium entry with calcifications are seen in regions of myocytolysis.[156,164]

Elevated circulating serum catecholamines or sympathetic discharges that originate from the hypothalamus and affect the myocardium may be responsible for these myocardial cell abnormalities.[156,164] SAH-related myocardial dysfunction is associated with increased blood pressure, high levels of brain naturetic peptide (BNP), increased heart rate and biological and ECG signs of myocardial injury and these signs are accompanied by elevated catecholamine levels.[165] Marked and rapid catecholamine release is already present on admission and is prevalent in those with signs of cardiac dysfunction.[165] Cardiac lesions probably represent excitotoxin-induced injury. Although ECG changes are common, myocardial infarction is rare.

When echocardiography was introduced into clinical care, some SAH patients were often found to have ballooning of the apex of the heart, a finding labeled takotsubo cardiomyopathy by the Japanese.[166–168] Takotsubo cardiomyopathy is characterized by reversible left ventricular apical ballooning in the absence of angiographically significant coronary artery stenosis. In Japanese, "tako-tsubo" is a term that refers to a "fishing pot for trapping octopus," and the left ventricle of a patient diagnosed with this condition resembles that particular shape. Some patients show apical-sparing variants (inverted takotsubo) in which the distal apex demonstrates preserved systolic function with isolated transient systolic dysfunction involving the midventricular segments and/or basal myocardial segments.[164,166] Takotsubo cardiomyopthy is usually transient in patients with SAH.[169,170]

Cardiac abnormalities are occasionally accompanied by clinical and necropsy evidence of pulmonary edema.[156,171–173] In one series of 178 fatal SAHs, 71% had necropsy evidence of pulmonary edema, recognized clinically in only 31%.[147] Pulmonary edema is neurogenic in origin. It is characterized by rapid onset, high protein in the edema fluid, and acutely elevated ICP. Weir suggested that pulmonary edema is caused by an acute rise in ICP, which triggers a massive autonomic discharge that results in increased cerebral perfusion and accumulation of fluid within the lungs and hypoxemia.[172] Patients with SAH-related pulmonary edema have lower circulating blood volumes then those who do not develop this complication.[173] Treatment of pulmonary edema is directed at lowering ICP and eliminating excess fluid. Intubation, controlled ventilation, positive end-expiratory pressure, osmotic and loop diuretics, and drainage of spinal fluid may be needed.

Fluid, electrolyte, and endocrine abnormalities

Less common, but still an important cause of neurological worsening, are fluid and electrolyte abnormalities.[174–177] Hyponatremia is the most common electrolyte imbalance in patients with aneurysmal SAH, occurring in 30–50% of patients.[177] Slight sodium and potassium shifts without clinical consequence are common. Hyponatremia is associated with a poor prognosis. Hydrocortisone or fludrocortisone given intravenously after surgery at a rate of 1200 mg/day overcomes excess naturesis and prevents hyponatremia.[177,178] In the past, hyponatremia has been attributed mainly to inappropriate secretion of antidiuretic hormone, but recently an increased importance has been attributed to the cerebral salt wasting syndrome as a coexisting etiological factor. Due to the multitude of contributing factors hyponatremia after SAH is not treated with fluid restriction but with free water restriction and mildly hypertonic fluids (1.5–2.0%). Vasopressin receptor agonists are also increasingly being used. Plasma concentration of atrial natriuretic factor is elevated and higher in patients with suprasellar and intraventricular blood.[179,180]

Neuroendocrine dysfunction can also follow SAH.[181] In one study among 21 patients screened, 9 (43%) had deficiency of at least one pituitary axis hormone.[182] In another analysis of pituitary function, 14 of 30 (47%) patients screened 12–24 months after aneurysmal SAH had isolated or combined deficiencies of neuroendocrine hormones.[183] Growth hormone deficiency was most common followed by low adrenocorticotrophin (ACTH) values. Weight gain often accompanied the growth hormone abnormalities. Aneurysms of the AComA most often were followed by neuroendocrine

dysfunction.[182,183] Hypoperfusion to the hypothalamic-pituitary blood supply is the posited mechanism that led to the endocrine abnormalities.

Other treatment considerations

Blood pressure control

Care must be taken in managing blood pressure. Elevated ICP causes an increase in venous pressure inside the cranium. To perfuse the brain, an arteriovenous pressure gradient must be maintained for systemic blood pressure to rise. Both too-high and too-low blood pressure can have adverse effects. Patients whose mean arterial pressure exceeds 130 mmHg or is lower than 70 mmHg have poorer outcomes than comparable patients with blood pressures between those two values.[184] The fundamental approach to blood pressure management in aneurysmal SAH takes into consideration whether the offending aneurysm has been treated or not. If the aneurysm is not secured, strict blood pressure control to mean arterial blood pressure values of less than 110 mmHg is advocated. Short acting and easily titratable agents such as intravenous calcium-channel blockers (nicardipine, clevedipine) are the agents of choice for this purpose and intravenous nitrates should be avoided due to their propensity to cause an increase in ICP. After the aneurysm is secured, blood pressure is liberalized and permissive hypertension is typically used to mitigate the effects of vasoconstriction.

If the blood pressure is not excessively high, we do not routinely lower it, especially if vasoconstriction is present. Nimodipine and nicardipine also lower blood pressure when used to treat or prophylax against vasoconstriction. No absolute levels of blood pressure to aim for exist; rather, the patient's clinical state should be observed to ensure that blood flow and cerebral perfusion are adequate.

Antifibrinolytic agents

Antifibrinolytic agents have been used in patients with SAH to prevent rebleeding.[142,185–187] The most frequently used antifibrinolytic drug was aminocaproic acid (Amicar), which was usually given in a dose of 24 g per day intravenously for 3 days, followed by oral administration for 3 weeks or until surgery. Kassell and colleagues reviewed the experience of the Cooperative Study of Intracranial Aneurysms and Subarachnoid Hemorrhage with respect to antifibrinolytic drugs.[188] Although Amicar decreased the rate of rebleeding, it did not improve morbidity or mortality. Vasoconstriction, thrombophlebitis with pulmonary embolism, and hydrocephalus were more common in patients given antifibrinolytic agents.[188] Although they may be useful in selected patients with high potential for rebleeding who for various reasons cannot undergo immediate treatment of the aneurysm, antifibrinolytic agents have too many adverse effects to be recommended for general use in patients with SAH.

Obliteration of aneurysms by microsurgical clipping or endovascular interventions

Obliteration of aneurysms is essential to prevent rebleeding. All agree that aneurysms should be ablated as soon as feasible after rupture. Debate, however, still surrounds the optimal means – surgical clipping or coiling through endovascular embolization in individual patients with various aneurysms.

During intracranial surgery, the patient is anesthetized using hypotensive anesthesia. The brain is made slack by using dehydrating agents and controlled removal of CSF, and the neurosurgeon uses a dissecting microscope to approach the aneurysm. Ideally, the aneurysm is clipped at its origin from the parent artery at its neck. If this is not possible, the aneurysm may be trapped between two clips and wrapped in supportive material, or the feeding arteries may be obliterated. During operations to obliterate aneurysms, rebleeding and ischemic infarction may occur. Infarction is secondary to arterial injury during retraction of the brain or from injury to penetrating arteries as aneurysms are approached and treated. Amnesic syndromes are common after surgery for AComA aneurysms, particularly if the aneurysms are trapped rather than ligated at their neck.[189,190] Trapping leads to disruption of the perforators that originate from the ACA and AComA, with resultant ischemia in the area of the anterior wall of the IIIrd ventricle and the orbital frontal lobes and basal forebrain nuclei.[189,190] Similar clinical deficits are often caused by vasoconstriction in patients with ruptured AComA aneurysms. Similarly, surgery on basilar artery bifurcation aneurysms can be followed by infarction in the paramedian midbrain and thalamus, causing a "top of the basilar syndrome."

Historically, surgery was often delayed until 10–14 days after the hemorrhage. This technically difficult surgery is easier to perform as the brain edema resolves and the clot and blood in the subarachnoid space are diminished. Rebleeding at the time of surgery is also minimized, because the thrombus surrounding the aneurysm is better organized. However, early surgery may afford a better outcome with regard to vasoconstriction. If blood clots can be removed from the subarachnoid space at the time of surgery, vasoconstriction may be less likely to occur although this concept still remains to be proven. If vasoconstriction develops after the aneurysm has been clipped, more hyperdynamic treatment may be undertaken without concerns about promoting rebleeding.

Although endovascular treatment of aneurysms has been known for more than 3 decades, it is only recently that the frequency of interventional intra-arterial treatment has equaled and even surpassed that of direct surgical management. Fedor Serbinenko, a Russian neurosurgeon was the first to popularize endovascular treatment of aneurysms. He used catheters with detachable latex balloons.[191] Guido Guglielmi and colleagues in 1991 reported their experience using a technique that involved electrolytic detachable platinum coils.[192,193] These coils (named Guglielmi detachable coils (GDCs)) were introduced into aneurysms through a microcatheter and detached from a stainless-steel microguidewire by an electrical current.[192,193] The techniques of coil embolization has greatly improved since then. By the middle of 2002, about 10 000 patients had had coiling used to obliterate aneurysms through an endovascular approach. About 1500 patients or more each month have endovascular treatment of their aneurysms.[194,195] Rare patients whose

aneurysms are coiled develop an inflammatory, hypersensitivity reaction to the metals used in the coils.[196] In these patients, transient ischemic symptoms and MRI (FLAIR) lesions develop in the hemisphere fed by the parent artery of the coiled aneurysm. Corticosteroids are effective in stopping the symptoms and reversing the MRI lesions. The mechanism of the syndrome is posited to be hypersensitivity to the nickel–titanium (nitinol) guidewire used when placing the coils.[196]

An international study whose results were published in 2005, the International Subarachnoid Aneurysm Trial (ISAT) compared clipping versus coiling of aneurysms.[197,198] Patients were included in the study if they had a SAH due to a ruptured aneurysm that was considered suitable for both neurosurgical clipping and endovascular treatment. The study group consisted of 1070 patients randomized to the surgical group and 1063 to coiling. These patients were derived from an initial 9559 patients with aneurysmal SAH, among whom 9% refused participation and 69% were excluded because their aneurysm was deemed unsuited to either coiling or surgery.[198] Rebleeding was slightly more common in the endovascular treated patients (7 vs. 2) during one-year period, and seizures were more frequent in the surgical group (44 vs. 27 discharge to one-year period).[197] This cohort was followed for 10.0–18.5 years after treatment.[199] Ten years after treatment, 674 (83%) of 809 patients allocated to endovascular coiling and 657 (79%) of 835 patients allocated to neurosurgical clipping were alive (odds ratio (OR) 1.35, 95% confidence interval (CI) 1.06–1.73). Among 1003 patients who returned questionnaires at 10 years, 435 (82%) patients treated with endovascular coiling and 370 (78%) patients who had clipping were independent. Patients in the endovascular treatment group were more likely to be alive and independent at 10 years than were patients in the neurosurgery group (OR 1.34, 95% CI 1.07–1.67). 33 patients had a recurrent subarachnoid hemorrhage more than 1 year after their initial hemorrhage (17 from the target aneurysm).[199]

Treatment outcomes depend heavily on the experience and skill of the individual performing the endovascular or surgical procedure, as well as patient selection. For both surgery and endovascular occlusion, larger aneurysm size is associated with an increased rate of complications and of incomplete occlusion. The size of the neck of an aneurysm has been a predictor of complete occlusion by coiling. A neck diameter of less than 5 mm and a ratio of neck diameter to largest aneurysm dimension of less than 0.5 are associated with better outcomes after coiling.[194,200]

Intravascular stents and balloons are occasionally used to exclude aneurysms from the circulation and to ensure patency of parent arteries.[201–204] When aneurysms have a wide neck, coils placed within an aneurysm can readily escape into the circulation. Intracranial stents designed to navigate tortuous intracranial vessels are now increasingly used in the treatment of wide-necked aneurysms. A stent is placed within the parent artery on the luminal side covering the neck of the aneurysm. A microcatheter is introduced through the cells of the stent into the aneurysm. Coils are then inserted through the microcatheter into the aneurysm, after which the microcatheter is removed. The stent prevents the coils from prolapsing into the parent artery. The use of stenting is typically avoided in the acute setting as it necessitates the use of dual antiplatelets, although in selected patients in whom other treatment modalities are considered higher risk, emergent use of stents can be achieved with reasonable safely. Flow diverting devices (stent type constructs with high density stent struts) have been developed that completely exclude aneurysms from the parent vessel and lead to thrombosis of the aneurysm and are increasingly replacing coil embolization procedures. Figure 13.8 shows a large cavernous carotid artery aneurysm that was treated with stent assisted coiling.

Location of the aneurysm is also very important. MCA and other bifurcation aneurysms are at times difficult to coil and surgical results in treating these aneurysms compared to endovascular modalities is better than at other loci.[194] Endovascular aneurysm bifurcation devices are actively being developed that are thought to overcome these limitations of endovascular aneurysm treatment. Posterior circulation aneurysms have a

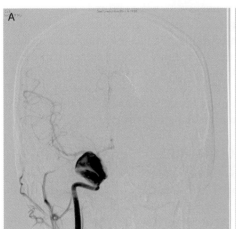
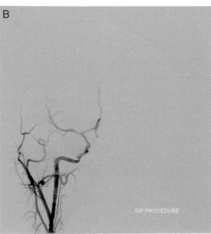
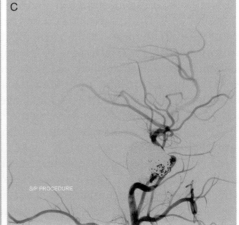

Figure 13.8 Carotid artery angiograms. (A) Anteroposterior view showing a large petrous carotid artery aneurysm. Anteroposterior (B) and lateral (C) view after coiling. A catheter was first placed in the aneurysm. A stent was then deployed internal to the catheter. Coils were then introduced into the aneurysm through the catheter. After coiling, the stent was removed. The stent covered the large neck of the aneurysm preventing the coils from entering the parent artery. Dr Ajith Thomas, Neurosurgery, Beth Israel Deaconess Medical Center, Boston, MA.

relatively high surgical morbidity and mortality and are best treated with coiling when feasible.[194] Cavernous carotid artery aneurysms rarely cause SAH or severe neurological morbidity,[205] are very difficult to treat surgically, and are best treated by endovascular techniques when they become symptomatic.

All other considerations being equal, there is a general consensus that if an aneurysm is suitable for endovascular treatment, this approach is preferred over craniotomy with neurosurgical management.

Mycotic aneurysms

Patients with bacterial endocarditis often develop cerebral aneurysms caused by bacterial embolization to the vasa vasorum of intracranial arteries. These so-called mycotic aneurysms usually do not develop in the basal arteries of the circle of Willis but favor branch arteries. Mycotic aneurysms are often multiple. Identical aneurysms develop in patients with cardiac myxomas.

These aneurysms may be identified after subarachnoid hemorrhage but many are found during evaluations for meningitis, embolic brain infarction, and encephalopathy in patients with infective endocarditis.[206] Some aneurysms identified by angiography resolve after effective antibiotic treatment.[206,207] In one series, 20 of 28 mycotic aneurysms were followed angiographically.[206] Ten aneurysms became smaller or disappeared, 10 were unchanged or enlarged – one with a fatal rupture. Seven mycotic aneurysms ruptured, resulting in two deaths and two with aphasia or cognitive impairment.[206] The authors suggested that single accessible aneurysms in medically stable patients be obliterated and that vascular imaging should be performed after medical treatment in patients in whom mycotic aneurysms had been shown earlier.[206] Surgical resection or endovascular obliteration should be considered when there is evidence of mycotic aneurysm rupture.

Treatment of unruptured aneurysms

Management of patients with unruptured aneurysms presents a challenging problem in benefit versus risk analysis.[33,34,208] Unruptured aneurysms are discovered as part of the evaluation of another ruptured aneurysm, during investigation of a mass lesion, or during evaluation of another neurological problem, such as ischemic vascular disease. Large aneurysms, symptoms, location within the posterior circulation, female sex, and age over 60 years increase the likelihood of aneurysm rupture.[209]

The operative mortality in patients with aneurysms and normal neurological function is quite low (≤1.6%).[210] Mortality after endovascular coiling of neurologically intact patients is even lower. One series compared outcomes of coiling and clipping of unruptured aneurysms. Among 130 patients – 68 treated surgically and 62 endovascularly – more treated surgically than by endovascular management had a change in Rankin scale of 2 or more (25% vs. 8%).[208] We recommend endovascular treatment or surgical therapy in selected patients with unruptured aneurysms.

The rate of aneurysm rupture is related to size. The International Study of Unruptured Intracranial Aneurysms showed that aneurysms of 10 mm or larger ruptured much more often than smaller aneurysms.[2] In other studies, the critical size for aneurysmal rupture has been 7–10 mm, 9 mm, and 8 mm.[32] The morbidity and mortality of surgery on unruptured aneurysms highly depends on age. In a meta-analysis that included 2460 patients (in 61 studies), the mortality of surgery was 2.6%, and the permanent morbidity was 10.9%.[211] In a study of 1172 patients operated on for newly diagnosed unruptured intracranial aneurysms, the combined surgery-related morbidity and mortality at one year was 6.5% for patients younger than 45 years, 14.4% for those between 45 and 64 years, and 32% for those older than 64 years.[2] We concur with Kassell and Drake that the data support the idea that aneurysms 5–10 mm in size bleed more often than smaller lesions,[36] and aneurysms larger than 10 mm probably rupture at an even higher rate.[2] In good-risk young patients, aneurysms larger than 5 mm should most often be obliterated. In light of the natural history data, one group advocates for the treatment of unruptured aneurysms in the case of: (1) symptomatic aneurysms (regardless of size); (2) incidental aneurysms larger than 5 mm of size in younger patients (<60 years of age); and (3) incidental aneurysms larger than 10 in nearly all patients younger than 70 years of age.[212]

An endovascular approach is preferred in posterior fossa aneurysms and in others that are suitable for coiling. Some unruptured aneurysms are likely more suitably treated surgically by neurosurgeons with extensive experience with aneurysm surgery. Lesions smaller than 5 mm should be followed up using vascular imaging. If these smaller aneurysms show growth, then endovascular or surgical therapy can be considered. CTA and MRA allow recognition and monitoring of unruptured aneurysms because patients can be studied non-invasively as outpatients. The decision with regard to surgery or interventional obliteration of unruptured aneurysms is complex, especially in older patients, and many factors must be carefully considered in each patient. Blood pressure control is important in patients with unruptured aneurysms.

Once a cerebral aneurysm has ruptured, the course is stormy, and the prognosis may be grim, even in the best of hands. To make a major impact on the morbidity and mortality of cerebral aneurysms, there must be early recognition of this serious disease, so that appropriate therapy can be undertaken while the patient is still in good condition. We stress the need for a high index of suspicion of SAH and a low threshold for use of LP and vascular imaging in suspected cases.

Vascular malformations

AVMs are the second most common cause of non-traumatic SAH. AVMs are one-tenth as common as aneurysms. In 1980, it was estimated that about 1000 new cases were identified every year in the United States.[213] Others have estimated the AVM detection rate at 1.1[214] and 1.27[215] per 100 000 person-years. Cerebral aneurysms have a peak incidence of rupture beyond age 30 years: while AVMs rupture more commonly in the second and third decades of life.[215,216] Hemorrhage from

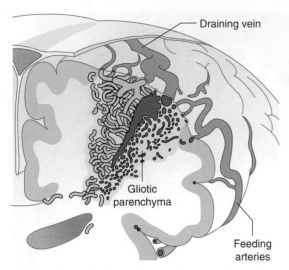

Figure 13.9 Drawing illustrating an unruptured, parietal-lobe arteriovenous malformation.

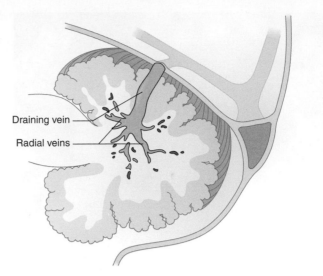

Figure 13.10 Drawing illustrating a cerebellar DVA (venous angioma).

an AVM is most often intraparenchymal and rarely just subarachnoid.

Classification and distribution

Vascular malformations, usually arise from the failure of normal development of embryonic vascular networks. Some malformations, such as some arteriovenous fistulas, especially dural AVMs, and some cavernous angiomas are acquired during life. Because dural arteriovenous fistulas represent different clinical problems, they are discussed separately at the end of this chapter. McCormick wrote extensively about his experience with vascular malformations and classified them into five subtypes based on the predominant vasculature.[18,217–221]

Arteriovenous malformations

AVMs contain arteries, arterialized veins, and veins. The size of the component vessels varies greatly, but the largest vessels are always venous. Sometimes the arterial supply is small and "cryptic." These lesions contain no recognizable normal capillary bed;[220] abnormal gliotic parenchyma usually is found between the component vessels. The small arteries within the malformation often have a deficient muscularis.[222] Thrombosis and inflammation are often found within AVMs. Arteriograms usually show shunting through the nidus directly from the arteries to the venous components of the malformations. Figure 13.9 is a drawing that illustrates the appearance of an unruptured AVM.

Lasjaunias and colleagues described a subtype of AVMs that they dubbed "cerebral proliferative angiopathy."[223] The distinctive feature of this condition is a large nidus made up of densely enhancing vascular spaces intermingled with normal parenchyma associated with a small volume of blood shunting to the venous drainage. These occur predominantly in young women who present with headaches, seizures, and ischemic symptoms and a low frequency of hemorrhage.[223] Angiogenesis may be a prominent feature of these large lesions.

Developmental venous anomalies

The most common type of vascular malformation found in the brain at necropsy were called venous angiomas by McCormick and colleagues;[217–221] they are composed of anomalous veins. There is no direct arterial input. These lesions are now most appropriately referred to as developmental venous anomalies (DVAs), rather than angiomas. They are composed of a group of anomalous veins usually separated by morphologically normal brain parenchyma and drain normal brain parcenchyma. One or more large central draining veins are usually conspicuous, and may be dilated into a varix or varices. The walls of the veins can become thick and hyalinized. These lesions do not opacify during the arterial phase of cerebral angiography. Figure 13.10 is a drawing that illustrates a DVA. Figure 13.11 shows a DVA within a brain specimen, and Figure 13.12 is an MRI that shows a DVA.

Cavernous angiomas

Cavernous angiomas consist of a relatively compact mass of sinusoidal vessels close together without intervening brain parenchyma. The lesions are well encapsulated, especially those that are superficial and large. Hyalinization and thickening of the component vessels, especially on the periphery of the angiomas, is common. These angiomas are not visualized well, if at all, on angiography because they have no direct arterial input. Cavernous malformations occur in a sporadic, non-hereditary form, in patients who tend to have a single isolated lesion, and in a familial form characterized by the presence of multiple lesions.[224–227] In the familial form, the number of lesions found increases with age. The familial form has been noted to occur with greater frequency in Hispanics. Mutations in the Krev interaction trapped 1 (*KRIT1*) gene have been identified as underlying the familial form of cerebral cavernous malformations.[227,228] The KRIT1 protein, the product of the *KRIT1* gene, is found in vascular endothelium, astrocytes, and pyramidal cells in adult brains.[227] Figure 13.13 is a drawing that illustrates the gross appearance of a cavernous angioma in

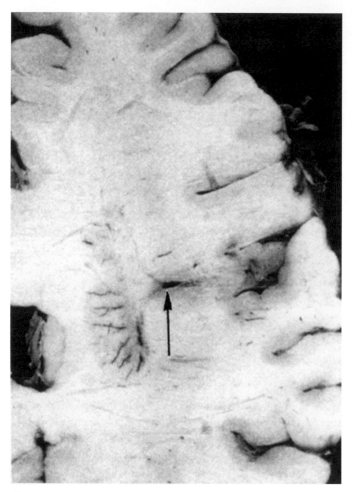

Figure 13.11 Brain specimen showing a venous malformation located mostly in the cerebral periventricular white matter. A radial array of dilated medullary veins drain into a dilated central vein (black arrow), which then drains toward the cerebral cortex. From Johnson PC, Wachser TM, Golfinos J, Spetzler RF. Definition and pathologic features. In Awad IA, Barrow DL (eds). *Cavernous Malformations*. Park Ridge, IL: American Association of Neurological Surgeons, 1993, pp 1–11 with permission.

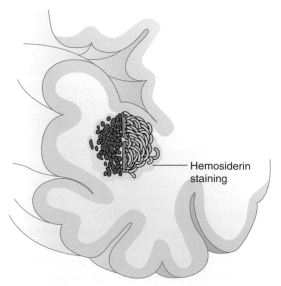

Figure 13.13 Drawing illustrating an unruptured cavernous malformation. There is no smooth muscle or intervening brain parenchyma within the interstices of the thin-walled vascular channels. Surrounding hemosiderin indicates prior bleeding.

Hemosiderin staining

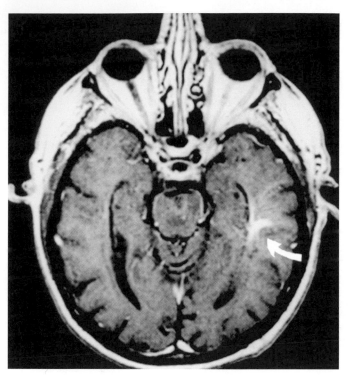

Figure 13.12 MRI showing a DVA located in temporal lobe. The *white arrow* points to an abnormal venous structure. From Caplan LR. Subarachnoid hemorrhage, aneurysms, and vascular malformations. In Caplan LR. *Posterior Circulation Disease: Clinical Findings, Diagnosis, and Management*. New York: Blackwell Science, 1996, pp 633–685, with permission of Blackwell Publishing Ltd.

the brain. Figures 13.14, 13.15, and 13.16 show cavernous angiomas in the temporal lobe, pons, and lateral ventricles.

Patients with DVAs have a much-higher-than-expected co-occurrence of cavernous angiomas, especially in the posterior fossa.[227] These two congenital lesions often occur close together, so that these lesions probably share etiological features during their development.[227,229,230] Cavernous angiomas are also known to develop after cranial irradiation.

Telangiectases

Telangiectases (also called *telangiectasias*) are small lesions in which the component capillaries are separated from each other by normal brain parenchyma. They appear as small, pink, spongy areas most often located in the pons. These lesions are not shown by angiography.

Pathogenesis of arteriovenous malformations

AVMs are composed of clusters of abnormal vessels comprised of arteries and veins of varying size. The arteries within the cluster are large, thin-walled vessels with poorly developed internal elastic lamina and media, whereas the arteries feeding this abnormality have hypertrophy of the media and endothelial thickening.[217] The hypertrophic media and endothelial thickening sometimes lead to thrombosis of feeding arteries. Deep AVMs are usually fed by penetrating arteries and drain into the deep venous system, whereas superficial cortical malformations usually drain into cortical veins.[222] In some patients, the afferent vessels of the malformation can become

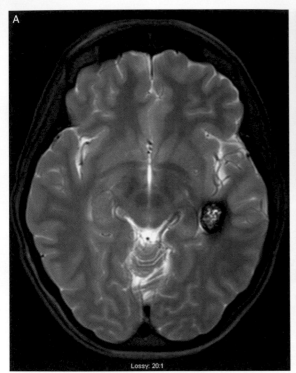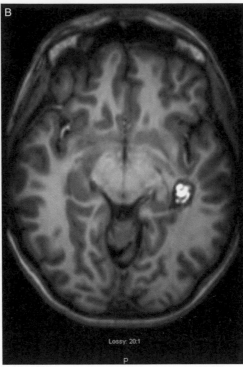

Figure 13.14 Temporal-lobe cavernous angioma shown in (A) gradient echo and (B) T1-weighted MRI images. Courtesy of Robert Hamill, MD.

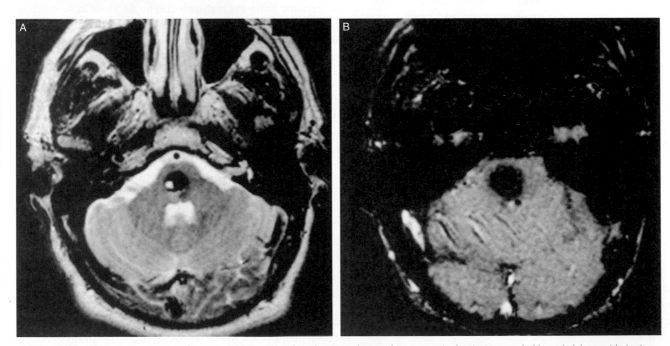

Figure 13.15 Cavernous angioma in the pons. (A) T2-weighted axial section shows white eccentric density surrounded by a dark hemosiderin ring. (B) Gradient-echo MRI section shows the hemosiderin ring around the lesion quite well. From Caplan LR. Subarachnoid hemorrhage, aneurysms, and vascular malformations. In Caplan LR. *Posterior Circulation Disease: Clinical Findings, Diagnosis, and Management*. New York: Blackwell Science, 1996, pp 633–685, with permission of Blackwell Publishing Ltd.

stenotic and even occluded.[231,232] Some patients with AVMs have diffuse occlusive arterial disease, despite the fact that they do not have atherosclerotic risk factors.[232] Blood circulates rapidly through the central core of AVMs and is quickly shunted into large, dilated, draining veins. The increased flow can promote the formation of aneurysms, and, occasionally,

aneurysms are found associated with AVMs, especially along major feeding arteries.[233,234] Aneurysms are explained by altered vascular hemodynamic factors involving the inflow channels. Occlusive changes can also be found in the draining venous channels and contribute to changes in pressures and flow within the malformations.[235,236]

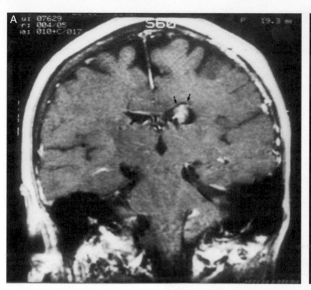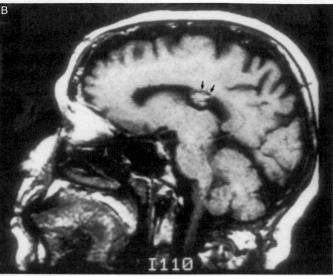

Figure 13.16 T2-weighted MRI images showing an intraventricular cavernoma. The lesion appears as a white hyperintensity (small black arrows) within the lateral ventricle.

Location of the various malformations

Any part of the brain and spinal cord can harbor a vascular malformation. Cavernous angiomas and AVMs are often larger than the other types of malformations and more commonly cause symptoms. Telangiectases are usually asymptomatic but can be a source of repeated small bleeds. Some extensive malformations extend from the cortical surface to abut on the ventricular surface. Cavernous angiomas can be limited to the brain, spinal cord, subarachnoid space, or dura, or they may involve more than one of these regions. Table 13.10 notes the locations of cavernous angiomas in one large series.[18,237] Bleeding from cavernous angiomas is predominantly into their capsules which are usually within brain parenchyma, but angiomas that abut on the ventricular or meningeal surface may also leak into the CSF.

AVMs can be predominantly within brain parenchyma or within the subarachnoid space, but most AVMs have parenchymatous and subarachnoid components, so bleeding can be intracerebral, subarachnoid, or meningocerebral. Table 13.11 notes the location of AVMs in three large series of patients.[18,238–241] The blood supply of large AVMs is usually extensive, originating from the anterior and posterior intracranial circulations, as well as from extracranial components.

AVMs are believed to arise in early fetal life as a result of the failure of primitive vessels to differentiate into normal arteries, veins, and capillaries. Despite their congenital origin, AVMs rarely produce symptoms during the first decade of life. The asymptomatic nature of lesions in early life is probably related to their small size and the inherent plasticity of the developing brain, which allows the function of one area of the brain to be assumed by another. AVMs often enlarge as individuals age. The feeding arteries and draining veins grow, and additional vasculature is recruited. Malformations enlarge for multiple reasons. Hook suggested that undifferentiated arteries and veins might not easily tolerate arterial pressure and therefore would enlarge.[242]

Small recurrent ICHs cause loss of brain substance as clot and necrotic brain are reabsorbed. The decrease in supporting tissue around malformations might allow growth of the vascular anomaly.[243] Decreased strength of supporting tissue may also be caused by pulsation of arteries, which can damage the surrounding brain.

Clinical symptoms and signs

As vascular malformations enlarge, symptoms are related to a number of mechanisms. Consider the following patient:

> At 15 years of age, AG began to have spells in which she saw sparkling lights off to her left. Some spells were followed by loss of consciousness and a generalized seizure. By age 21 years, she noted progressive loss of vision toward her left. Four years later during the first trimester of her first pregnancy while shopping, she fell to the ground with a severe headache, nausea, vomiting, and a stiff neck. Examination showed a left homonymous hemianopia.

The most frequent and dramatic presentation of vascular malformations is bleeding. Prior to modern brain imaging, intracerebral hemorrhage was the event that led to diagnosis of AVMs in about 50% of patients.[242] Now about two-thirds of AVMs are diagnosed before they have bled.[215] The immediate cause of bleeding in AVMs is not known, but probably relates to fragility of the abnormal vessels. Vessels on the cortical or ventricular surfaces are more prone to rupture, because they lack the support offered by the surrounding brain parenchyma. A first hemorrhage from an AVM usually occurs between the ages of 20 and 40 years of age.[244]

Symptoms and signs depend on the location of the hemorrhage. With CSF extension of blood, there are signs of meningeal irritation similar to those accompanying aneurysmal rupture.

Table 13.10 Distribution of cavernous angiomas

Distribution	No.	Percent
Supratentorial	455	74
Lobar	256	41
Frontal lobe	99	–
Temporal lobe	68	–
Parietal lobe	72	–
Occipital lobe	16	–
Deep	31	5
Basal ganglia	22	–
Thalamus	7	–
Hypothalamus	2	–
Ventricular	20	3
Lateral ventricles	13	–
Paraventricular	2	–
IIIrd ventricle	5	–
Extra-axial	4	0.5
Infratentorial	163	26
Cerebellum	28	4.5
Brainstem	82	13
Midbrain	20	–
Pons	43	–
Medulla	13	–
Pontomedullary	6	–
IVth ventricle	3	0.5
Cerebellopontine angle	6	1
Spinal cord	2	0.3
Unspecified	58	9

Data from Caplan LR. Subarachnoid hemorrhage, aneurysms, and vascular malformations. In Caplan LR (ed), *Posterior Circulation Disease: Clinical Findings, Diagnosis, and Management.* Boston: Blackwell Science, 1996, pp 633–685.

Table 13.11 Location of AVMs diagnosed during life

Location of AVMs	Perret and Nishioka[239] N (%)	Crawford et al.[240] N (%)	Graf et al.[241] N (%)
Frontal lobe	102 (23)	85 (21)	33 (25)
Temporal lobe	82 (18)	41 (10)	25 (19)
Parietal lobe	122 (27)	145 (36)	41 (30)
Occipital lobe	23 (5)	69 (17)	7 (5)
Brainstem	11 (2)		5 (4)
Cerebellum	21 (4)	36* (9)	6 (4.5)
Basal ganglia		27	14 (10)
Other	92 (20)		3 (2.5)
Total	**453**	**403**	**134**

* Brainstem and cerebellar lesions grouped together.
Data from Caplan LR. Subarachnoid hemorrhage, aneurysms, and vascular malformations. In Caplan LR (ed), *Posterior Circulation Disease: Clinical Findings, Diagnosis, and Management.* Boston: Blackwell Science, 1996, pp 633–685.

Progressive neurological symptoms occur in only about 8–11% of AVM patients.[215,246] In the past, progression has often been explained by "stealing" of blood away from normal tissue, but this mechanism has been difficult to establish. Venous hypertension and increased mass effect of the nidus of the AVM and occult bleedings are alternate explanations.[215,246]

Chronic headaches are also a frequent complaint in patients with AVMs. The headaches may be throbbing in nature, sometimes closely mimicking classic migraine. No good rules exist to distinguish ordinary migraine from migrainous headaches related to vascular malformations. Migraine-like accompaniments that are always stereotyped and occur on the same side or headaches always localized to the same side should lead doctors to suspect the possibility of an AVM. Even patients with unruptured AVMs can have increased ICP and papilledema.[247] The increased pressure may contribute to headaches.

In the brainstem, AVMs and cavernous angiomas may present with serious bleeding or gradually progressive neurological deficits. Depending on location, there may be cranial nerve, cerebellar, pyramidal, or sensory dysfunction. Some have a fluctuating course of neurological dysfunction, which can simulate multiple sclerosis.[18,227,248,249] Distinction between these two processes is now easily accomplished with modern brain imaging. With cavernous angiomas, the neurological dysfunction can be localized to one site, most often in the pons. CT or MRI usually shows a typical cavernoma as the site of prior bleeding.

AVMs rarely present with hydrocephalus. In such cases, the mass of blood vessels can compress the ventricular system, disrupting the normal flow of CSF. Aneurysms of the vein of Galen are the most common cause of this rare presentation. Prior small bleeds can also block absorption of CSF, leading to

Not all ruptures are symptomatic. Frequently, patients with no clinical history of hemorrhage show evidence of bleeding at surgery or necropsy. In one surgical series, 6 of 55 patients with AVMs had evidence of hemorrhage without recognized symptoms.[213]

In the years before the hemorrhage, AG had partial seizures with secondary generalization and progressive neurological signs. Seizures are the presenting feature in 15–53% of AVM patients.[215,245] Most are grand mal but partial and partial complex seizures are also common. Supratentorial cavernous angiomas often present because of seizures.

Table 13.12 Common presenting features in patients with AVMs

1. History of a seizure disorder or progressive neurological deficit

2. Throbbing headaches or migraine-like auras, or both, always localized to one side of the cranium

3. A patient in the second or third decade of life

4. Subarachnoid hemorrhage in a pregnant woman. AVMs may enlarge or bleed during pregnancy

5. Clinical signs and symptoms of intraparenchymal and subarachnoid blood

6. Cranial bruit

Table 13.13 Normal angiography in patients with hemorrhages that clinically suggest AVM as cause

1. Spontaneous thrombosis of the malformation may have occurred, representing a self-cure

2. With rupture, obliteration of the malformation may have occurred, representing another cure

3. Malformation may be a cavernous angioma or developmental venous anomaly, without a direct arterial feeder, and therefore not visualized on angiography

4. The bleeding could arise from a spinal-origin aneurysm or malformation

hydrocephalus. Rarely, patients with large AVMs can present because of a bruit that is audible to the patient or doctor. In children, large AVMs can produce enough shunting of blood to cause high-output congestive heart failure.

Spinal cord vascular malformations typically present with back pain, myelopathic symptoms, and root dysfunction. These lesions are discussed in Chapter 16. Because headache so often accompanies spinal AVM rupture, cerebral sources of hemorrhage are often sought, and the spinal origin can be missed. In one series, 80% of patients with spinal malformations had intracranial symptoms, including headache, mental status changes, loss of consciousness, papilledema, decreased vision, nystagmus, diplopia, seizures, VIth-nerve paresis, and oculomotor paresis.[250]

Diagnosis and imaging findings

The diagnosis of vascular malformations can often be suspected clinically. Common features are noted in Table 13.12.

Brain imaging in nearly all patients shows vascular malformations. MRI is able to define the lesions better than CT. Plain unenhanced CT scans can show serpiginous channels; these vessels are enhanced after intravenous contrast administration.[251] Brain atrophy and dilatation of ventricles adjacent to malformations may exist. Small calcifications may be seen within malformations. Sometimes, frank cysts are also found adjacent to AVMs.[252] If there has been a recent hemorrhage, these recent findings may be obscured by the intraparenchymal, subarachnoid, and intraventricular blood. Cavernomas are often missed on CT scans unless there has been recent bleeding. Developmental venous anomalies are seldom identifiable on CT scans.

MRI has vastly improved the diagnosis of vascular malformations. AVMs usually appear as a region of honeycomb-like spaces with flow voids that contrast with the surrounding brain tissue on T1-weighted and T2-weighted images. MRI gives useful information about the localization and topographic relationships between AVM vessels, nidus, and nervous structures, as well as showing past hemorrhage.[253–255] MRA gives some information about the arterial and venous components but is not as definitive as catheter angiography.

Cavernous angiomas usually appear as well-circumscribed, well-defined lesions, with a central core of mixed

heterogeneous signal intensity surrounded by a rim of signal void.[227,256–259] Figures 13.14 and 13.15 are MRIs that show this appearance. The heterogeneous center is caused by blood and blood metabolites in various stages of evolution, and the dark rim is caused by hemosiderin.

The typical MRI appearance of DVAs is a linear or globular hypointense region on T1-weighted images and hypo- or hyper-intensity on T2-weighted images.[260–262] DVAs can usually be seen to join deep and/or superficial veins.[262] Figure 13.12 illustrates the MRI findings in a patient with a DVA. Recent hemorrhages in all types of malformations have the same imaging characteristics as other causes of ICH. MRI can also be helpful by showing hemosiderin resulting from old hemorrhage in the lesions and adjacent meninges.

TCD is also useful in the initial diagnosis and monitoring of AVMs.[84,85] The increased flow to the AVMs is associated with increased flow velocities in arteries feeding the malformations.[266] At times, musical-type murmurs can be heard, and unusual unmodulated high- or middle-frequency bands are seen on the Doppler spectrum.[84] Abnormal collateralization and steal effects can be found with reduction of mean and peak flow velocities in some arteries.[84] Changes in velocities can be monitored during therapeutic embolization and after surgical or radiation therapy. Vasomotor reactivity to CO_2 inhalation also gives information about AVMs. Relatively normal vasomotor reactivity in arteries ipsilateral to AVMs suggests a high-pressure AVM with a high risk of bleeding, whereas abnormal vasomotor reactivity in ipsilateral and contralateral arteries is most often found in low-pressure AVMs that show hemodynamically-induced neurological signs.[226]

A detailed angiogram is needed to identify all possible arterial feeders when surgery is considered in patients. Angiographic features typical of AVMs include: (1) large feeding arteries; (2) a central tangle of vessels; (3) enlarged, tortuous draining veins; and (4) rapid arterial-to-venous shunting of blood. Some angiographic findings, such as large size, presence of multiple feeding arteries, and drainage into peripheral cortical veins, correlate with the development of progressive neurological signs that have been attributed by some to stealing of blood from normal vessels to the malformations.[264] Arteriography is occasionally normal in patients in whom clinical suspicion of an AVM is high. The explanations for this are noted in Table 13.13.

Table 13.14 Spetzler–Martin grading system for AVMs

Graded feature		Points
Size	Small (<3 cm)	1
	Medium (3–6 cm)	2
	Large (>6 cm)	3
Eloquence	Non-eloquent	0
	Eloquent	1
Venous drainage	Superficial only	0
	Deep	1

From Spetzler RF, Martin NA. A proposed grading system for arteriovenous malformations. *J Neurosurg* 1986;65:476–483.

Prognosis of the various malformations

Arteriovenous malformations

Features that have been identified to both predict the risk of bleeding from a known AVM and the risks associated with surgery are captured in the Spetzler–Martin scale noted in Table 13.14.[215,265–267] AVMs that have already bled have a higher risk of bleeding than those that have not as yet bled.[215] In the short term, the prognosis of ruptured AVMs is much better than that of aneurysms. The rebleeding rate is low – only about 6% during the first year,[268] and vasoconstriction occurs only rarely. Mortality from the first hemorrhage is relatively low (1.5–9.0%).[215] In the long term, however, the prognosis of AVMs is not as good. Estimates of recurrent hemorrhage during subsequent years vary from 1% in 4–7 years[243] to 2% per year after the first year.[268] With repeated hemorrhages, the morbidity and mortality rates increase.[264]

With each recurrent hemorrhage, the chances of additional hemorrhages increase.[243] In 1 large series of 137 patients with AVMs treated conservatively between 1942 and 1967, 10% died from AVMs, 24% were disabled, and only 40% were well at the time of the 1970 report;[268] 7 years later, only 19% of the initial group were well.[269,270] Because AVMs tend to occur in younger patients, the probability that recurrent hemorrhage with disability or death will occur is substantial. The authors of one study estimated that almost 50% of patients with recurrent hemorrhage will have some deterioration in working capacity or become an invalid during the 20–40 years after the first hemorrhage.[271] One study noted a better outcome for patients with hemorrhage from AVMs than prior reports. Among 119 AVM patients followed at Columbia Presbyterian Medical Center, 115 had a bleed as the presenting diagnostic event, and 27 of these patients had subsequent hemorrhages.[272] Four other patients had symptoms other than hemorrhage that prompted diagnosis, but had subsequent bleeds during follow-up. The incident hemorrhage resulted in no clinical deficit in 47%, and another 37% were independent in daily activities. During follow-up, 20 of 27 patients (74%) with more than 1 hemorrhage were still normal or independent.[272]

Parietal, central, and infratentorial malformations may be more likely to bleed than frontal, temporal, or occipital malformations.[270] Morbidity from hemorrhages depends on the location of the malformation. Occurrence in an "eloquent" brain region poses a higher risk for morbidity from a bleed, but also from surgical intervention. High arterial input pressures and restriction of venous outflow to only deep venous drainage are risk factors that increase the likelihood of hemorrhage in AVMs.[273]

Patients who present with seizures alone have a better prognosis than those that present with hemorrhage. Only a 25% chance exists of a clinically symptomatic hemorrhage in 15 years.[271] In one long-term series of patients with seizures, there was only a 12% mortality and an additional 16% overall disability.[268] A more conservative approach, prescribing only anticonvulsant therapy for patients with seizures alone, is reasonable. Seizures can be well controlled by anticonvulsants, and surgical removal of malformations often does not improve seizure control.[274] Patients presenting with progressive neurological deficits have a poor prognosis, but these patients also often have the largest malformations, which are difficult to treat.[264]

Data are not available regarding long-term prognosis in patients with asymptomatic AVMs. These lesions are usually discovered during the evaluation of other problems. Aminoff argued convincingly for conservative management of most unruptured AVMs.[274] AVMs that have not bled have a better prognosis than those lesions that have already bled. The ARUBA trial compared the outcomes in patients with unruptured AVMs that were managed medically (109 patients) versus surgically (114 patients).[275] The trial showed that at 33 month follow-up, medical management led to the primary outcome of stroke or death in 10.1% of patients as compared to 30.7% of patients in the surgical arm.[275] These findings of lower incidence of stroke or death with conservative management were mirrored by a study conducted in Scotland.[276] Among 204 Scottish patients aged 16 years or older who had unruptured brain AVMs, the use of conservative management compared with intervention was associated with better clinical outcomes for up to 12 years. Whether these disparities between intervention and conservative management will persist in the long-term remains to be seen.

Cavernomas

The most common presentation of cavernous angiomas is seizures, which occur in approximately one-half of the patients.[277] Focal deficits and hemorrhages are the next most common presentations. Although almost all cavernous malformations show some surrounding blood on MRI or when examined pathologically, clinically significant hemorrhage is not as common. Hemorrhage is more common in patients who have already bled than in patients whose lesions have never bled. Robinson and colleagues prospectively followed 76 cavernomas detected by MRI among 66 patients.[278] Only 1 hemorrhage occurred during a 26-month period, for a rate of 0.7% per lesion per year.[278] In another study, follow-up information was available for 122 patients with cavernous malformations.[279] Multiple lesions were present in one-fifth of these patients. Cavernomas were located in the brainstem (35%), basal ganglia and thalamus (17%), and cerebral

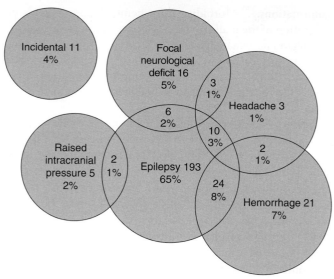

Figure 13.17 The clinical findings among 296 patients with supratentorial cavernous malformations. From Moran NF, Fish DR, Kitchen N, et al. Supratentorial cavernous haemangiomas and epilepsy: A review of the literature and case series. *J Neurol Neurosurg Psychiatry* 1999;66:561–568 with permission.

hemispheres (48%). In retrospect, 50% of the patients had one bleed, 7% had two hemorrhages, and 2% had had three bleeds.[279] The retrospective annual hemorrhage rate was 1.3%. Prospective follow-up of these patients for an average of 34 months showed a prospective annual rate of hemorrhage of only 0.6% for those lesions that had never previously bled. Patients with prior bleeds had a 4.5% per year rate of recurrent hemorrhage.[279] In this study, location of the cavernomas did not affect the rate of bleeding.[279] Hemorrhages are more common in women, especially if they are pregnant.[280] Hemorrhages are often difficult to document clinically or on MRI because part of the natural history of cavernous angiomas is slow oozing of blood into surrounding brain tissue, forming a hemosiderin-laden ring around the angioma.[280] Moran et al. performed a systematic review of the literature and analyzed the findings among supratentorial cavernous angiomas.[281] Figure 13.17 from this report diagrams the clinical manifestations among 296 patients and shows overlapping of symptoms. Seizures were by far the most common presentation, followed by hemorrhage and focal neurological deficits.[281] After diagnosis, only 6 patients developed a hemorrhage during a mean 5.6 years of follow-up, yielding a hemorrhage rate of 0.7% per year.[281]

Developmental venous anomalies

In the large majority of patients, venous malformations have a benign course.[282–284] Garner et al. observed 100 patients with DVAs, only one of whom had a hemorrhage.[282] Naff et al. followed 92 patients with DVAs for an average of 4.2 years.[284] The most common locations of the lesions were the frontal lobes (56%) and the cerebellum (27%). The most frequent presenting symptoms were headache (51%), focal neurological deficits (40%), and seizures (30%). The prevalence of headache and seizures decreased over time, even without treatment. Only 2 patients developed a symptomatic hemorrhage during follow-up, giving an annual risk of hemorrhage of 0.15%.[284]

Occasional patients with DVAs have recurrent brain edema or ischemia in regions drained by the anomalous veins.[285]

Treatment of vascular malformations

A 33-year-old, right-handed school teacher, BC, had occasional left-sided throbbing headaches while in college. At age 27 years, he had his first epileptic seizure, which began with a warm feeling in his right lip and tongue. The feeling rapidly spread to his hand, and then he lost consciousness. At age 33 years while shoveling snow, he developed a severe diffuse headache and vomited. On examination, he was restless and complained of headache, but had no abnormal neurological signs except a right extensor plantar response. LP showed blood-tinged CSF at a pressure of 210 mmHg. CT showed a thin layer of subarachnoid blood, and contrast injection opacified a large sylvian group of tortuous veins. Angiography revealed a large parasylvian central AVM fed primarily from the left MCA.

How should this patient be treated? In this case, the diagnosis of AVM is certain. The prodromal history of headaches and seizures was typical. The present bleed was subarachnoid, arising from the surface of the lesion. No intraparenchymal hematoma was evident, either clinically or by CT. The lesion was in an "eloquent" region that relates to his potential ability to communicate verbally and in writing. In this patient, surgery or embolization carries the risk of aphasia or right hemiparesis, each potentialy disabling. Because there were no important neurological signs, LRC chose to watch the patient during the next years to see the natural history of the lesion. If he had presented with an intracerebral hematoma and had aphasia and right hemiplegia, the situation would have been quite different and surgery might have been indicated.

Four therapeutic options are available that can be used in combination or alone to treat vascular malformations: (1) surgery; (2) interventional using embolization; (3) radiotherapy; and (4) a strictly medical approach. Embolization is only used for AVMs because the other lesions do not have important arterial feeders. Because venous anomalies are developmental abnormalities with a benign natural history, and resection carries a substantial risk of venous infarction, hemorrhage, and brain edema, lesions should be managed only medically.[284]

Surgery

A surgical approach is the oldest method of treatment. Initially, neurosurgeons ligated the major feeding arteries to the malformation. This method of treatment has been largely abandoned because of its failure to obliterate the lesion and the hazards inherent in the procedure. Stroke often occurs as blood flow to normal brain is interrupted. Malformations continue to draw blood from non-ligated, deep, inaccessible vessels.

Direct surgical excision of lesions has been improved with the use of the operating microscope. Lesions are meticulously approached, avoiding critical cerebral vessels and vital neurological structures. Operations may be performed using evoked response monitoring, so that the exact location of vital areas can be accurately determined. Dissection is done, if possible, in

the gliotic plane that surrounds the tangle of vessels, so that malformations can be removed en bloc.

Surgical excision can be carried out in most appropriate patients with a relatively low morbidity and mortality by very experienced and skilled neurosurgeons.[269,270] Castel and Kantor reviewed the results among 2425 AVM patients who had surgery.[286] Among these patients, postoperative mortality was 3.3% and postoperative permanent morbidity varied from 1.5% to 18.7% in different series.[286]

The major complications of surgical excision are loss of normal brain tissue, with additional loss of neurological function and bleeding. A phenomenon unique to obliteration of AVMs is so-called normal perfusion pressure breakthrough phenomenon.[287] This term is used to describe massive brain swelling and ICH occurring postoperatively caused by redirection of the large volume of blood that previously flowed into the malformation into the small vessels surrounding the malformation. These vessels are unable to handle the large volume of blood, and cerebral edema or hemorrhage can result.[287]

The advent of microsurgical techniques also makes it possible to remove deep-seated cavernous angiomas, including those in the brainstem. Surgical treatment of cavernomas is appropriate only for lesions that have caused intractable seizures and serious neurological signs or have re-bled.[227] Some cavernomas can be shelled out by experienced neurosurgeons who take advantage of the plane between the lesions and the normal brain.[227]

Endovascular treatment

Embolization of AVMs can be performed alone, before surgery, or at the time of surgery. Initially, small pellets were used to fill the abnormal vessels within the central nidus. Because flow to malformations is increased, pellets released into feeding arteries tend to travel to the malformations. There, they occlude the lumens of vessels, it is hoped, in sufficient quantity to thrombose the vascular malformation. The particle embolization technique, however, has many problems. Emboli rarely enter arteries with acute or right angles. Also, as vessels within malformations become occluded, flow to the malformations equals the flow to the normal brain and particles stray into the normal circulation, causing ischemia.

Modern-day embolization is accomplished with liquid embolic agents. These include ethylene vinyl alcohol (Onyx) and various kinds of "glues," rapidly setting tissue adhesives, such as isobutyl-2-cyanoacrylate, or n-butyl-cyanoacrylate that can then be administered.[288-291] These adhesives form clots in the segments of the lesion irrigated predominantly by that artery. Several feeding arteries are then injected. This technique often reduced the size of the lesion, but rarely obliterated the vascular malformation in the case of high grade lesions. Ethyl-vinyl alcohol copolymers, labeled Onyx, has now often been used as the embolization agent. In one series, among 350 patients treated with injection of Onyx into the nidus, 179 patients (51%) achieved complete obliteration of the AVM with only interventional treatment.[291]

Complications do develop during and after embolization with liquid embolic agents. These include: postembolization

hemorrhage related to altered blood flow, hemorrhage or ischemic stroke induced by the balloon catheter, gluing of the balloon catheter complex in place by the tissue adhesive, and occlusion of normal arteries by the plastic material. In addition, some substances, such as bucrylate, can be toxic to tissues and cause angionecrosis and escape into the extravascular spaces.[292]

Endovascular techniques are especially important in treating lesions that are not surgically accessible and as an adjunct to surgical removal. Newer imaging technology has clearly facilitated the use of various interventional techniques.

Radiotherapy

Attempts have been made to use radiotherapy to obliterate AVMs. High energy from conventional x-rays, gamma rays, or protons induces subendothelial deposition of collagen and hyaline substances, which narrow the lumen of small vessels and shrink the nidus of the malformation by progressive occlusion of vessels during the months after treatment. Newer techniques focus the radiation beam on small regions. An example is gamma knife, a system that uses a cobalt source to generate highly collimated gamma rays that converge on a focal point.[293] Modified linear accelerators can deliver radiation to a defined volume of tissue with good accuracy. Radiation necrosis occurs in approximately 9% of patients.[293] Approximately 40% of AVMs are obliterated in one year, 84% after 2 years, and 97% after 3 years.[294] Small volume, deep location, and plexiform angioarchitecture correlate with successful obliteration of AVMs by radiotherapy.[294,295] One study examined the effectiveness of single-stage stereotactic radiosurgery in patients with large (>10 cm^3) AVMs.[296] At 6 years after treatment 81% of AVM nidi were obliterated and the hemorrhage rate (2% per year) and the permanent adverse event rate was only 3% of patients.[296] The major disadvantage of radiation treatment of AVMs is that it may take months to years after treatment until the AVM is obliterated.[215] During this time the AVM is at risk of hemorrhage.

In a review of 3854 patients who had AVMs treated by radiotherapy, the average rate of permanent neurological deficits in these 16 series was about 6%.[215,297] Complications include radionecrosis of normal brain, hydrocephalus, immediate posttherapy seizures, loss of body temperature regulation, and possibly long-term cognitive-function deficits. Further data are needed before the frequency of these complications and the therapeutic use of focused radiotherapy in patients with AVMs is known. Focused radiotherapy is probably best reserved for small deep lesions not easily amenable to surgery that have bled.

Because cavernous angiomas have only been well defined since the advent of MRI, there is less information about the use of radiotherapy in treating cavernomas as compared to AVMs. Gamma knife radiosurgery aiming the treatment precisely at the lesions using a stereotaxic three-dimensional frame has made it possible to treat small, deep lesions in the brainstem, basal ganglia, and thalamus with preliminary success.[298]

Medical treatment

The most conservative therapeutic option for AVMs is a medical approach. Blood pressure is strictly controlled within the normal range. Anticoagulants and antiplatelet drugs are avoided. Because the rate of hemorrhage in pregnant women with AVMs is relatively high, we discuss the risk of pregnancy with fertile women and suggest appropriate contraception if desired.

Arteriovenous vascular malformations, if left untreated, are often hazardous. No one therapeutic option is entirely successful or without risk. Treatment of these malformations is often complicated by numerous feeding arteries, extensive size, or location within the brain parenchyma in areas vital to normal neurological function. Decisions regarding therapy must consider all of these factors.[299] Also important is the age of the patient and the mode of presentation. These two factors are major determinants of the natural history of the disease.

For the most common mode of presentation – hemorrhage in patients with AVMs – we most often recommend an aggressive approach, including surgery or surgery combined with embolization if the following criteria are met:

1. The patient is relatively young (<55 years and has a life expectancy of >15 years).
2. Recovery of neurological function after the hemorrhage is moderately good, so that a reasonable lifestyle can be anticipated.
3. The malformation is superficial in location and does not extensively involve vital neural structures – so-called eloquent brain.

Because the rate of early rebleeding is low unless high risk features such as intranidal aneurysms are present, we wait until the patient is in good medical condition before suggesting surgery. Because surgery can cause neurological signs, the presence of a remaining neurological deficit related to the bleeding is a factor favoring surgery, whereas postbleed return to complete normality argues against surgery.

We adopt a more conservative approach, using embolization and radiotherapy if available, or strictly medical management if the following criteria are met:

1. The patient is older than 60 years, and life expectancy is less than 10 years.
2. The deficit from the initial hemorrhage is severe.
3. The malformation is extensive and deep within the dominant hemisphere, in the brainstem or other vital eloquent areas.

We use these same criteria for patients who present with progressive neurological deficits. We treat patients who present with seizures medically. Anticonvulsants are given to control the seizures, blood pressure is regulated, and anticoagulants and antiplatelet drugs are avoided. If seizures remain intractable despite medical therapy, a more aggressive plan using surgical excision might be considered.

In asymptomatic patients, including those with only headache, we follow a conservative medical approach. Because the natural history of asymptomatic lesions is unknown, it is unwise to undertake therapy that may be more hazardous than the lesion itself. Furthermore, initial hemorrhages are rarely fatal; if a hemorrhage does occur, the opportunity for more aggressive therapy is then available.

Dural arteriovenous malformations

Dural arteriovenous malformations (DAVMs) are lesions that contain abnormal arteriovenous shunts within the leaflets of the dura mater, usually within or near the walls of dural venous sinuses.[18,300] The terms dural arteriovenous malformations and dural arteriovenous fistulas have often been used interchangeably. Figure 13.18 shows angiograms in a patient who has a DAVM with filling from arterial branches of the MCAs and external carotid arteries that drain into the superior sagittal sinus and torcula herophili. DAVMs have different etiologies, pathophysiologies, and clinical symptoms when compared with parenchymal and pial AVMs. DAVMs represent 10–15% of all AVMs.

DAVMs may drain only into dural sinuses or there may be prominent drainage into the cortical and deep venous systems. DAVMs with prominent cortical venous drainage have a higher incidence of bleeding than those without.[301,302] The

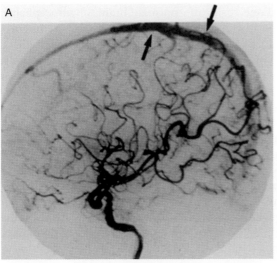
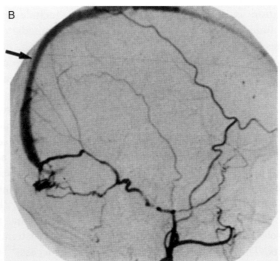

Figure 13.18 DAVM of the superior sagittal sinus and torcula. (A) Internal carotid artery angiogram. Lateral view shows that multiple branches of the MCA drain directly into the superior sagittal sinus (black arrows). (B) External carotid injection shows that internal maxillary branches also fill the sagittal sinus (black arrow). From Dion J. Dural arteriovenous malformations: Definition, classification, and diagnostic imaging. In Awad IA, Barrow DL (eds), *Dural Arteriovenous Malformations*. Park Ridge, IL: American Association of Neurological Surgeons, 1993, pp 1–19 with permission.

cause of most of the complications and symptoms and signs in patients with DAVMs is thought to be venous hypertension.[303,304] The two major mechanisms of increased pressure within the venous drainage system are: (1) increased blood flow through draining veins (e.g., related to increased arterial inputs); and (2) restriction or obstruction of the draining system, causing an increase in pressure in the tributary veins. Venous hypertension probably promotes cortical venous drainage and increases the risk of brain hemorrhage.

Some DAVMs are probably congenital, especially those that involve the vein of Galen. Retention of an embryonic median prosencephalic vein, which normally drains the choroid plexus of the fetus, is the explanation usually given for vein of Galen malformations.[305] When this vein persists, it becomes the sac for the aneurysmally enlarged vein of Galen. These lesions should probably be classified as AVMs rather than true DAVMs. Most DAVMs are probably acquired.[18,304] Well-documented instances exist of adult patients who had normal angiograms and later, angiography showed that DAVMs had formed, proving these lesions were acquired in these patients.[306] Trauma is undoubtedly an important cause in some patients. Hormonal factors may also be important because female hormones are known to influence placental and uterine vascular growth and increase angiomas at many body sites.

Dural sinus thrombosis, an important cause of DAVMS, is more common in women. Approximately twice as many women as men have the most common form of DAVM with drainage into the lateral sinuses.[307,308] DAVMs may first become symptomatic during pregnancy. Some DAVMs regress after delivery. Occlusion of a dural sinus is an important cause of DAVMs.[307,309] Houser and colleagues reported two patients in whom dural sinus thrombosis was documented years before development of DAVMs.[307] One patient had previous angiography because of transient bilateral limb weakness that showed sigmoid sinus occlusion but no fistula; a year later after the development of pulsatile tinnitus, a repeat angiogram showed a DAVM of the transverse sinus adjacent to the occluded sigmoid sinus. Another patient with a history of thrombophlebitis and thromboembolism developed headache, drowsiness, leg weakness, and papilledema. Angiography showed a transverse sinus occlusion. When he developed an increase in his symptoms, a repeat angiogram 2.5 years later showed a transverse sinus DAVM.[307] Thrombosis or stenosis within the draining dural sinus often causes enlargement of the DAVMs and augments venous hypertension. Trauma is a very important cause of dural fistula formation, especially in patients with carotid-cavernous fistulas.[309,310] Several reports document progressive obstruction and occlusion of dural sinuses in patients known to have DAVMs.[18,311]

The clinical problems that develop in patients with DAVMs, such as headaches, papilledema, hydrocephalus, and hemorrhages, are probably explained by venous hypertension.[311] The focal symptoms and signs that develop depend heavily on the location of the DAVMs and whether the lesions are solely dural or have a prominent drainage pattern into the brain's cortical and deep veins.[312] Hemorrhages are most often intraparenchymatous or subdural, but occasionally are subarachnoid. First hemorrhages from DAVMs have an approximate 30% mortality rate. An especially high mortality and severe disabling morbidity rate occurs in patients with hemorrhages from DAVMs who are taking anticoagulants. Venous infarcts, which are often hemorrhagic, and brain edema can also result from the venous hypertension. Seizures, headache, and signs of increased intracranial pressure develop, often with papilledema. Brain edema is an important sequel in some patients with DAVMs, especially those with venous hypertension and dural sinus occlusions.[18,313]

Pulsatile tinnitus is another frequent and annoying symptom. Some patients only have headaches, either generalized or localized to the side of the DAVM. We have seen several patients with DAVMs who had positionally sensitive headache with worsening in the supine position and improvement when sitting or standing.[18] The erect position may have allowed better venous drainage toward the heart.

The most common location of DAVMs is in relation to the lateral sinuses, involving the transverse or sigmoid portion of the lateral sinus. Lateral sinus malformations account for five eighths of DAVMs.[18,314] Potential feeding arteries to these lateral sinus fistulas include: (1) external carotid artery branches, such as the occipital, middle meningeal, accessory meningeal, and ascending pharyngeal arteries; (2) dural branches of the ICA, especially the meningohypophyseal trunk (the artery of Bernasconi and Casaneri); and (3) dural branches of the vertebral arteries, such as posterior meningeal, cerebellar falcine, and cervical muscular anastomotic arteries. Venous drainage of lateral sinus DAVMs can be into a normal transverse or sigmoid sinus, or the wall of the sinus may be irregular and partially or completely thrombosed.

Cavernous sinus fistulas are the next most common lesion and are found in approximately one eighth of patients with DAVMs.[314] These lesions are characterized by abnormal shunting of blood from the internal or external carotid arteries into the cavernous sinus. Blood often drains into the orbital veins, causing increased venous pressure in the eye and orbital contents leading to proptosis, chemosis caused by conjunctival edema, scleral injection, conjunctival hemorrhages, glaucoma, and papilledema.[310,315,316] These lesions can drain into the petrosal veins and sinuses and the basal vein of Rosenthal, and cause venous hypertension within the brainstem.[317,318] Trauma and rupture of infraclinoid carotid artery aneurysms into the cavernous sinus are important causes of these fistulas.

Tentorial-incisural DAVMs account for approximately one-twelfth of all DAVMs.[319] Less common locations include the cerebral convexity–sagittal sinus region, orbital–anterior falx region, sylvian–middle fossa region, and those that drain into the torcula herophili. Some DAVMs drain into deep structures, such as the vein of Galen, straight sinus, or dural venous structures in the posterior falx region. The vein of Galen is an unusual structure, both anatomically and embryologically. It is a bridge between the subarachnoid venous system and the dural straight sinus. The vein of Galen can be the site of shunting or can be recruited into the venous

drainage pattern in cases of high flow lesions or when distal outlets are stenosed or thrombosed. The two distinct types of vein of Galen malformations follow:[305]

1. A congenital lesion that develops in utero in which the arterial input is into a persistent medial prosencephalic vein, which can become aneurysmally dilatated. These patients present with congestive heart failure. These lesions are probably true AVMs and the dural sinuses are patent.

2. A DAVM in which the shunt is into the wall of the vein of Galen. These are acquired in adulthood usually in relation to dural sinus occlusions in a similar fashion to other DAVMs. True vein-of-Galen DAVMs presenting in adulthood are supplied from the middle meningeal and vertebral artery, PCA, and meningohypophyseal artery branches. Occasionally, a vein-of-Galen aneurysm can be associated with DAVMs.

DAVMs are difficult to diagnose without angiography. In our experience, the angiographic results often come as a surprise and were not suspected from the clinical or imaging data. CT does not show the DAVM but can show related abnormalities, such as hemorrhages, thrombosed sinuses, hydrocephalus, and dilatated pial veins or varices. Contrast enhancement aids recognition of the abnormal veins and thrombosed sinuses. Similarly, MRI may show the abnormal veins and sinuses, suggesting the diagnosis, but does not show the arterial input. Although MRI and MRA can undoubtedly be helpful in suggesting the diagnosis, catheter angiography using high-resolution digital arterial subtraction angiography is still needed to identify the arterial feeders and draining venous patterns.

The natural history of DAVMs is variable. Some close spontaneously. In others, symptoms are slight and include mostly headache and pulsatile tinnitus. The nature of the venous drainage pattern is considered by many to be important in predicting the prognosis.[18] Drainage into subarachnoid and parenchymal veins with retrograde flow away from the lesion seems to correlate with dural sinus outflow obstruction and venous hypertension.[235] This venous drainage pattern predicts an aggressive course, often with brain hemorrhages, intraventricular hemorrhages, subdural hemorrhages, and SAHs.[314] Scales that are based primarily on venous drainage patterns have been developed that predict risk of bleeding (Table 13.15).[320]

Endovascular treatment of DAVMs is rapidly changing.[321,322] The plethora of arterial feeders from multiple major arterial systems, and the small size of many of the feeders, especially pial arteries, can complicate the ability to cure the lesion with embolization. The advent of Onyx has enabled cure of some DAVMs through transarterial embolization.[323] In one study 41 of 50 (82%) of cranial dural fistulas had angiographic cures 5 months after tranarterial embolization using Onyx with and without other embolic agents.[323] Transvenous endovascular treatment is often very effective. In some patients, a combined approach using transarterial embolization, transvenous ablation, and microneurosurgery has been succsefully used.[322]

Surgical treatment of DAVMs is often quite difficult. Mullan emphasized that surgeons should attempt to obliterate the fistulous communication, which appears as "multiple watering can spouts into the sinus lumen."[324] Some fistulas drain into an isolated vein in the wall of a dural sinus. Effective obliteration involves occluding the vein flush with the external wall of the sinus.[324] Obliteration or ligation of feeders often does not result in effective ablation of the DAVMs because new feeders are recruited. Packing the sinus in the region of the fistula is usually effective but is difficult and requires considerable surgical experience. The high flow in DAVMs makes blood loss and a bloody surgical field important problems in effective ablation. A conservative non-surgical approach to DAVMs is probably best in fistulas that do not have prominent leptomeningeal venous drainage or variceal or aneurysmal abnormalities within the draining venous system.[325] Clinical observation, repeat neuroimaging, and angiography are advised for those patients not treated surgically.[325]

Modern neuroimaging technology greatly facilitates diagnosis and should allow physicians to learn more about the natural history of DAVMs and other craniocerebral vascular malformations. Modern technology facilitates logical treatment selection and monitoring.

Table 13.15 Cognard classification of dural arteriovenous fistulas (DAVFs)

- Type I: DAVF draining into a sinus, with a normal antegrade flow direction

- Type II: DAVF draining into a sinus. Insufficient antegrade venous drainage and reflux

  The insufficiency of the venous drainage may be due to stenosis or occlusion of the sinus draining moderate flow rate DAVF, or to a very high flow rate DAVF that cannot be drained by a normal or even enlarged sinus. Depending on the retrograde venous drainage, three subtypes are distinguished:
  - Type IIa: Retrograde venous drainage into sinus(es) only
  - Type IIb: Retrograde venous drainage into cortical vein(s) only
  - Type IIa±b: Retrograde venous drainage into sinus(es) and cortical vein(s)

- Type III: DAVFs draining directly into a cortical vein without venous ectasia

- Type IV: DAVFs draining into a cortical vein with a venous ectasia >5 mm in diameter and three times larger than the diameter of the draining vein

- Type V: DAVFs (intracranial) draining into spinal perimedullary veins

From Cognard C, Gobin YP, Pierot L, et al. Cerebral dural arteriovenous fistulas: Clinical and angiographic correlation with a revised classification of venous drainage. *Radiology* 1995;194:671–80 with permission.

References

1. Rinkel GJE, Djibuti M, Algra A, van Gijn J: Prevalence and risk of rupture of intracranial aneurysms. A systematic review. *Stroke* 1998;**29**:251–256.

2. International Study of Unruptured Intracranial Aneurysms Investigators: Unruptured intracranial aneurysms – risk of rupture and risks of surgical intervention. *N Engl J Med* 1998;**339**:1725–1733.

3. Mayberg MR, Batjer HH, Dacey R, et al: Guidelines for the management of aneurysmal subarachnoid hemorrhage. A statement for healthcare professionals from a special writing group of the Stroke Council, American Heart Association. *Stroke* 1994;**25**:2315–2328.

4. Weir B: *Aneurysms Affecting the Central Nervous System*. Baltimore: Williams & Wilkins, 1987.

5. Kaibara T, Heros RC: Aneurysms. In Caplan LR (ed): *Uncommon Causes of Stroke*, 2nd ed. Cambridge: Cambridge University Press, 2008, pp 171–179.

6. Parkarinen S: Incidence, etiology, and prognosis of primary subarachnoid hemorrhage: A study based on 589 cases diagnosed in a defined urban population during a defined period. *Acta Neurol Scand* 1967;**43**(suppl 29):1–128.

7. Phillips LH, Whisnant JP, O'Fallan W, et al: The unchanging pattern of subarachnoid hemorrhage in a community. *Neurology* 1980;**30**:1034–1040.

8. Ingall TJ, Whisnant JP, Wiebers DO, O'Fallon WM: Has there been a decline in subarachnoid hemorrhage mortality? *Stroke* 1989;**20**:718–724.

9. The UCAS Japan Investigators. The natural course of unruptured cerebral aneurysms in a Japanese cohort. *N Engl J Med* 2012;**366**:2474–2482.

10. Wiebers, DO, Whisnant, JP, Huston, J III, et al: Unruptured intracranial aneurysms: natural history, clinical outcome, and risks of surgical and endovascular treatment. *Lancet* 2003;**362**:103–110.

11. Korja M, Lehto H, Juvela S: Lifelong rupture risk of intracranial aneurysms depends on risk factors: a prospective Finnish Cohort Study. *Stroke* 2014;**45**:1958–1963.

12. Locksley HB: Report of the Cooperative Study of Intracranial Aneurysms and Subarachnoid Hemorrhage. Sec V, part I: Natural history of subarachnoid hemorrhage, intracranial aneurysms, and arteriovenous malformation-based on 6,368 cases in the cooperative study. *J Neurosurg* 1966;**25**:219–239.

13. Locksley HB: Report of the Cooperative Study of Intracranial Aneurysms and Subarachnoid Hemorrhage. Sec V, part II: Natural history of subarachnoid hemorrhage, intracranial aneurysms, and arteriovenous malformation. *J Neurosurg* 1966;**25**:321–368.

14. Heros RC, Kistler JP: Intracranial arterial aneurysms – an update. *Stroke* 1983;**14**:628–631.

15. Winn WR, Richardson AE, Jane JA: The long-term prognosis in untreated cerebral aneurysms: I. The incidence of late hemorrhage in cerebral aneurysms – a ten-year evaluation of 364 patients. *Ann Neurol* 1977;**1**:358–370.

16. Kassell NF, Kongable GL, Torner JC, et al: Delay in referral of patients with ruptured aneurysms to neurosurgical attention. *Stroke* 1985;**16**:587–590.

17. Bor ASE, Velthuis BK, Majoie CB, Rinkel GJE: Configuration of intracranial arteries and development of aneurysms. *Neurology* 2008;**70**:700–705.

18. Caplan LR: Subarachnoid hemorrhage, aneurysms, and vascular malformations. In Caplan LR (ed): *Posterior Circulation Disease: Clinical Findings, Diagnosis, and Management*. Boston: Blackwell, 1996, pp 633–685.

19. Suzuki J, Onuma T, Yoshimoto T: Results of early operations on cerebral aneurysms. *Surg Neurol* 1979;**11**:407–412.

20. Bromberg JE, Rinkel GJ, Algra A, et al: Familial subarachnoid hemorrhage: Distinctive features and patterns of inheritance. *Ann Neurol* 1995;**38**:929–934.

21. Raaymakers TW, Rinkel GJ, Ramos LM: Initial and follow-up screening for aneurysms in families with familial subarachnoid hemorrhage. *Neurology* 1998;**51**:1125–1130.

22. Schievink WI, Schaid DJ, Rogers HM, et al: On the inheritance of intracranial aneurysms. *Stroke* 1994;**25**:2028–2037.

23. Ruigrok YM, Rinkel GJE, Wijmenga C: Genetics of intracranial aneurysms. *Lancet Neurology* 2005;**4**:179–189.

24. Ruigrok YM, Seitz U, Wolterink S, et al: Association of polymorphisms and pairwise haplotypes in the elastin gene in Dutch patients with subarachnoid hemorrhage from non-familial aneurysms. *Stroke* 2004;**35**:2064–2068.

25. Ruigrok YM, Rinkel GJE: Genetics of intracranial aneurysms. *Stroke* 2008;**39**:1049–1055.

26. Nahed BV, Bydon M, Ozturk AK, et al: Genetics of intracranial aneurysms. *Neurosurgery* 2007;**60**:213–225.

27. Ruigrok YM, Rinkel GJE, Wijmenga C: The Versican gene and the risk of intracranial aneurysms. *Stroke* 2006;**37**:2372–2374.

28. Ruigrok YM, Wijmenga C, Rinkel GJE, et al: Genomewide linkage in a large Dutch family with intracranial aneurysms. *Stroke* 2008;**39**:1096–1102.

29. Van den Berg JSP, Limburg M, Pais G, et al: Some patients with intracranial aneurysms have a reduced type III/type I collagen ratio. *Neurology* 1997;**49**:1546–1551.

30. Ferguson GG: Physical factors in the initiation, growth, and rupture of human intracranial saccular aneurysms. *J Neurosurg* 1972;**37**:666–677.

31. Adams HP, Kassell N, Torner JC, et al: Early management of aneurysmal subarachnoid hemorrhage. *J Neurosurg* 1981;**54**:141–145.

32. Ferguson GG, Peerless SJ, Drake CG: Natural history of intracranial aneurysms. *N Engl J Med* 1981;**305**:99.

33. Caplan LR: Should intracranial aneurysms be treated before they rupture? *N Engl J Med* 1998; **339**:1774–1775.

34. Wiebers DO, Whisnant JP, O'Fallon WM: The natural history of unruptured intracranial aneurysms. *N Engl J Med* 1981;**304**:696–698.

35. Drake CG: Giant intracranial aneurysm: Experience with surgical treatment in 174 patients. In Carmel PW (ed): *Clinical Neurosurgery*. Baltimore: Williams & Wilkins, 1979, pp 12–95.

36. Kassell N, Drake CG: Review of the management of saccular aneurysms. In Barnett HJM (ed): *Neurological Clinics*, vol **1**. Philadelphia: Saunders, 1983, pp 73–86.

37. Adams HP, Jergenson DD, Kassell NF, Sahs AL: Pitfalls in the recognition of subarachnoid hemorrhage. *JAMA* 1980;**244**:794–796.

38. Edlow JA, Caplan LR: Avoiding pitfalls in the diagnosis of subarachnoid hemorrhage. *N Engl J Med* 2000;**342**:29–36.

39. Gorelick PB, Hier DB, Caplan LR, Langenberg P: Headache in acute cerebrovascular disease. *Neurology* 1986;**36**:1445–1450.

40. Hauerberg J, Andersen BB, Eskesen V, et al: Importance of the recognition of a warning leak as a sign of a ruptured intracranial aneurysm. *Acta Neurol Scand* 1971;**83**:61–64.

41. Ostergaard JR: Warning leak in subarachnoid haemorrhage. *BMJ* 1990;**301**:190–191.

42. Drake CG: The treatment of aneurysms of the posterior circulation. In Carmel PW (ed): *Clinical Neurosurgery*. Baltimore: Williams & Wilkins, 1979, pp 96–144.

43. Stewart RM, Samsom D, Diehl J, et al: Unruptured cerebral aneurysms presenting as recurrent transient neurological deficits. *Neurology* 1980;**30**:47–51.

44. Fisher M, Davidson RI, Marcus EM: Transient focal cerebral ischemia as a presenting manifestation of unruptured cerebral aneurysms. *Ann Neurol* 1980;**8**:367–372.

45. Sutherland GR, King ME, Peerless SJ, et al: Platelet interaction within giant intracranial aneurysms. *J Neurosurg* 1982;**56**:53–61.

46. Weisberg LA: Ruptured aneurysms of anterior cerebral or anterior communicating arteries. *Neurology* 1985;**35**:1562–1566.

47. Tokuda Y, Inagawa T, Katoh Y, Kumano K, Ohbayashi N, Yoshioka H: Intracerebral hematoma in patients with ruptured cerebral aneurysms. *Surg Neurol* 1995;**43**:272–277.

48. Hunt WE, Hess RM: Surgical risk as related to time of intervention in the repair of intracranial aneurysms. *J Neurosurg* 1968;**28**:14–20.

49. Drake CG, Hunt WE, Sano K, et al. Report of World Federation of Neurological Surgeons Committee on a Universal Subarachnoid Hemorrhage Grading Scale. *J Neurosurg* 1988;**68**:985–986.

50. van Heuven AW, Dorhout Mees SM, Algra A, Rinkel GJ: Validation of a prognostic subarachnoid hemorrhage grading scale derived directly from the Glasgow Coma Scale. *Stroke* 2008;**39**:1347–1348.

51. Teasdale G, Jennett B: Assessment of coma and impaired consciousness. A practical scale. *Lancet* 1974;**2**:81–84.

52. Teasdale G, Jennett B: Assessment and prognosis of coma after head injury. *Acta Neurochir (Wien)* 1976;**34**:45–55.

53. Wijdicks EFM: Clinical scales for comatose patients: The Glasgow Coma Scale in historical context and the new Four Score. *Rev Neurol Dis* 2006;**3**:109–117.

54. Weisberg L: Computed tomography in aneurysmal subarachnoid hemorrhage. *Neurology* 1979;**29**:802–808.

55. Liliequist B, Lindquist M: Computer tomography in the evaluation of subarachnoid hemorrhage. *Acta Radiol Diagn (Stockh)* 1980;**21**:327–331.

56. Van der Jagt M, Hasan D, Bijvoet HWC, et al: Validity of prediction of the site of ruptured intracranial aneurysm with CT. *Neurology* 1999;**52**:34–39.

57. Van Gijn J, van Dongen KJ, Vermeulan M, et al: Perimesencephalic hemorrhage: A nonaneurysmal and benign form of subarachnoid hemorrhage. *Neurology* 1985;**35**:483–487.

58. Rinkel GJ, Wijdicks E, Vermeulen M, et al: The clinical course of perimesencephalic nonaneurysmal subarachnoid hemorrhage. *Ann Neurol* 1991;**29**:463–468.

59. Schievink WI, Wijdicks EFM: Pretruncal subarachnoid hemorrhage: An anatomically correct description of the perimesencephalic subarachnoid hemorrhage. *Stroke* 1997;**28**:2572.

60. Van Gijn J, Rinkel JE: Subarachnoid hemorrhage syndromes. In Caplan LR, van Gijn J (eds), *Stroke Syndromes*, 3rd ed. Cambridge, Cambridge University Press, 2012, pp 534–541.

61. Kershenovich A, Rappaport ZH, Maimon S: Brain computed tomography angiographic scans as the sole diagnostic examination for excluding aneurysms in patients with perimesencephalic subarachnoid hemorrhage. *Neurosurgery* 2006;**59**:798–801.

62. Patel KC, Finelli PF: Non-aneurysmal convexity subarachnoid hemorrhage. *Neurocrit Care* 2006;**4**:229–233.

63. Spitzer C, Mull M, Rohde V, Kosinski CM: Non-traumatic cortical subarachnoid haemorrhage: Diagnostic work-up and aetiological background. *Neuroradiology* 2005;**47**:525–531.

64. Kumar S, Goddeau RP, Selim MH, et al: Atraumatic convexal subarachnoid hemorrhage: Clinical presentation, imaging patterns, and etiologies. *Neurology* 2010;**74**:893–899.

65. Nakajima M, Inatomi Y, Yonehara T, Hirano T, Ando Y: Nontraumatic convexal subarachnoid hemorrhage concomitant with acute ischemic stroke. *J Stroke Cerebrovasc Dis* 2014;**23**:1564–1570.

66. Fisher CM, Kistler JP, Davis JM: Relation of cerebral vasospasm to subarachnoid hemorrhage visualized by computed tomographic scanning. *Neurosurgery* 1980;**6**:1–9.

67. Kistler JP, Crowell RM, Davis KR, et al: The relation of cerebral vasospasm to the extent and location of subarachnoid blood visualized by CT scan: A prospective study. *Neurology* 1983;**33**:424–437.

68. Hijdra A, van Gijn J, Nagelkerke N, et al: Prediction of delayed cerebral ischemia, rebleeding, and outcome after aneurysmal subarachnoid hemorrhage. *Stroke* 1988;**19**:1250–1256.

69. Brouwers PJ, Dippel DW, Vermeulen M, et al: Amount of blood on computed tomography as an independent predictor after aneurysm rupture. *Stroke* 1993;**24**:809–814.

70. Sherlock M, Agha A, Thompson CJ: Aneurysmal subarachnoid hemorrhage. *N Engl J Med* 2006;**354**:1755–1757.

71. Alberico RA, Patel M, Casey S, et al: Evaluation of the circle of Willis with three-dimensional CT angiography in patients with suspected intracranial aneurysms. *AJNR Am J Neuroradiol* 1995;**16**:1571–1578.

72. Jayaraman MV, Mayo-Smith WW, Tung GA, et al: Detection of intracranial aneurysms: multi-detector row CT angiography compared with DSA. *Radiology* 2004;**230**:510–518.

73. Yoon DY, Lim KJ, Choi CS, et al: Detection and characterization of intracranial aneurysms with 16-channel multidetector row CT angiography: A prospective comparison of volume-rendered images and digital subtraction angiography. *AJNR Am J Neuroradiol* 2007;**28**:60–67.

74. Ross J, Masaryk T, Modic M, et al: Intracranial aneurysms: Evaluation by MR angiography. *AJNR Am J Neuroradiol* 1990;**11**:449–456.

75. Okahara M, Kiyosue H, Yamashita M, et al: Diagnostic accuracy of magnetic resonance angiography for cerebral aneurysms in correlation with 3D-digital subtraction angiographic images: A study of 133 aneurysms. *Stroke* 2002;**33**:1803–1808.

76. Unlu E, Cakir B, Gocer B, et al: The role of contrast-enhanced MR angiography in the assessment of recently ruptured intracranial aneurysms: A comparative study. *Neuroradiology* 2005;**47**:780–791.

77. Caplan LR, Flamm ES, Mohr JP, et al: Lumbar puncture and stroke. *Stroke* 1987;**18**:540A–544A.

78. Edlow JA: Diagnosis of subarachnoid hemorrhage. *Neurocrit Care* 2005;**2**:99–109.

79. Van Gign J, Kerr RS, Rinkel GJE: Subarachnoid haemorrhage. *Lancet* 2007;**369**:306–318.

80. Van der Meulen JP: Cerebrospinal fluid xanthochromia: An objective index. *Neurology* 1966;**16**:170–178.

81. Perry JJ, Sivilotti ML, Stiell IG, et al: Should spectrophotometry be used to identify xanthochromia in the cerebrospinal fluid of alert patients suspected of having subarachnoid hemorrhage? *Stroke* 2006;**37**:2467–2472.

82. Hayward RS: Subarachnoid hemorrhage of unknown etiology. *J Neurol Neurosurg Psychiatry* 1977;**40**:926–931.

83. Rinkel GJE, van Gijn J, Wijdicks EFM: Subarachnoid hemorrhage without detectable aneurysm: A review of the causes. *Stroke* 1993;**24**:1403–1409.

84. Caplan LR, Brass LM, DeWitt LD, et al: Transcranial Doppler ultrasound: Present status. *Neurology* 1990;**40**:696–700.

85. Sloan MA, Alexandrov AV, Tegeler CH, et al: Assessment: Transcranial Doppler ultrasonography: Report of the Therapeutics and Technology Assessment. Subcommittee of the American Academy of Neurology. *Neurology* 2004;**62**:1468–1481.

86. Harders AG, Gilsbach JM: Time course of blood velocity changes related to vasospasm in the circle of Willis measured by transcranial Doppler ultrasound. *J Neurosurg* 1987;**66**:718–728.

87. Sloan MA, Haley EC, Kassell NF, et al: Sensitivity and specificity of transcranial Doppler ultrasonography in the diagnosis of vasospasm following subarachnoid hemorrhage. *Neurology* 1989;**391**:1514–1518.

88. Sekhar L, Wechsler L, Yonas H, et al: Value of transcranial Doppler examination in the diagnosis of cerebral vasospasm after subarachnoid hemorrhage. *Neurosurgery* 1988;**22**:813–821.

89. Davis SM, Andrews JT, Lichtenstein M, et al: Correlations between cerebral arterial velocities, blood flow, and delayed ischemia after subarachnoid hemorrhage. *Stroke* 1992;**23**:492–497.

90. Davis S, Andrews J, Lichtenstein M, et al: A single-photon emission computed tomography study of hyperperfusion after subarachnoid hemorrhage. *Stroke* 1990;**21**:252–259.

91. Chieregato A, Sabia G, Tanfani A, et al: Xenon-CT and transcranial Doppler in poor-grade or complicated aneurysmatic subarachnoid hemorrhage patients undergoing aggressive management of intracranial hypertension. *Intensive Care Med* 2006;**32**:1143–1150.

92. Hillman J, Sturnegk P, Yonas H, et al: Bedside monitoring of CBF with xenon-CT and a mobile scanner: A novel method in neurointensive care. *Br J Neurosurg* 2005;**19**:395–401.

93. Rordorf G, Koroshetz WJ, Copen WA, et al: Diffusion- and perfusion-weighted imaging in vasospasm after subarachnoid hemorrhage. *Stroke* 1999;**30**:599–605.

94. Condette-Auliac S, Bracard S, Anxionnat R, et al: Vasospasm after subarachnoid hemorrhage: Interest in diffusion-weighted MR imaging. *Stroke* 2001;**32**:1818–1824.

95. Wijdicks EFM, Schievink W, Miller GM: Pretruncal subarachnoid hemorrhage. *Mayo Clin Proc* 1998;**73**:745–752.

96. Rinkel GJ, Wijdicks E, Vermeulen M, et al: Outcome in perimesencephalic (nonaneurysmal) subarachnoid hemorrhage: A follow-up study in 37 patients. *Neurology* 1990;**40**:1130–1132.

97. Wijdicks EFM, Schievink WI: Perimesencephalic nonaneurysmal subarachnoid hemorrhage: First hint of a cause? *Neurology* 1997;**49**:634–636.

98. Stein RW, Kase CS, Hier DB, et al: Caudate hemorrhage. *Neurology* 1984;**34**:1549–1554.

99. Hochberg F, Fisher CM, Roberson G: Subarachnoid hemorrhage caused by rupture of a small superficial artery. *Neurology* 1974;**24**:309–311.

100. Lasjaunias P, Chiu M, ter Brugge K, et al: Neurological manifestations of intracranial dural arteriovenous malformations. *J Neurosurg* 1986;**64**:724–730.

101. Chang R, Friedman DP: Isolated cortical venous thrombosis presenting as subarachnoid hemorrhage: A report of three cases. *AJNR Am J Neuroradiol* 2004;**25**:1676–1679.

102. Oppenheim C, Domigo V, Gauvrit JY, et al: Subarachnoid hemorrhage as the initial presentation of dural sinus thrombosis. *AJNR Am J Neuroradiol* 2005;**26**:614–617.

103. Ohshima T, Endo T, Nukui H, et al: Cerebral amyloid angiopathy as a cause of subarachnoid hemorrhage. *Stroke* 1990;**21**:480–483.

104. Thompson B, Burns A: Subarachnoid hemorrhages in vasculitis. *Am J Kidney Dis* 2003;**42**:582–585.

105. Fomin S, Patel S, Alcasid N, et al: Recurrent subarachnoid hemorrhage in a 17 year old with Wegener granulomatosis. *J Clin Rheumatol* 2006;**12**:212–213.

106. Broderick JP, Brott TG, Duldner JE, et al: Initial and recurrent bleeding are the major causes of death following subarachnoid hemorrhage. *Stroke* 1994;**25**:1342–1347.

107. Suarez JI, Tarr RW, Selman WR: Aneurysmal subarachnoid hemorrhage. *N Engl J Med* 2006;**354**:387–396.

108. Bambidakis NC, Selman WR: Subarachnoid hemorrhage. In Suarez JL (ed): *Critical Care Neurology and Neurosurgery*. Towata, NJ: Humana Press, 2004, pp 365–377.

109. Clower BR, Smith RR, Haining JL, Lockard J: Constrictive endarteropathy following experimental subarachnoid hemorrhage. *Stroke* 1981;**12**:501–508.

110. Smith RR, Clower BR, Grotendorst GM, et al: Arterial wall changes in early human vasospasm. *Neurosurgery* 1985;**16**:171–176.

111. Yamamoto Y, Smith RR, Bernanke DH: Accelerated nonmuscle contraction after subarachnoid hemorrhage: Culture and characterization of myofibroblasts from human cerebral arteries in vasospasm. *Neurosurgery* 1992;**30**:337–345.

112. Macdonald RL, Weir BKA: A review of hemoglobin and the pathogenesis of cerebral vasospasm. *Stroke* 1991;**22**:971–982.

113. Macdonald RL: Cerebral Vasospasm. In Welch KMA, Caplan LR, Reis DJ, et al. (eds): *Primer on Cerebrovascular Diseases*. San Diego: Academic Press, 1997, pp 490–497.

114. Hughes JT, Schianchi PM: Cerebral artery spasm: A histological study at necropsy of the blood vessels in cases of subarachnoid hemorrhage. *J Neurosurg* 1978;**48**:515–525.

115. Conway LW, McDonald LW: Structural changes of the intradural

469

arteries following subarachnoid hemorrhage. *J Neurosurg* 1972;**37**:715–723.

116. Wellum GR, Peterson JW, Zervas NT: The relevance of in vivo smooth muscle experiments to cerebral vasospasm. *Stroke* 1985;**16**:573–581.

117. Kassell NF, Sasaki T, Colohan AR, Nazar G: Cerebral vasospasm following aneurysmal subarachnoid hemorrhage. *Stroke* 1985;**16**:562–572.

118. Kwak R, Niizuma H, Ohi J, et al: Angiography study of cerebral vasospasm following rupture of intracranial aneurysms: I. Time of the appearance. *Surg Neurol* 1979;**11**:257–262.

119. Weir B, Grace M, Hansen J, et al: Time course of vasospasm in man. *J Neurosurg* 1978;**48**:173–178.

120. Heros RC, Zervas NT, Varsos V: Cerebral vasospasm after subarachnoid hemorrhage: An update. *Ann Neurol* 1983;**14**:599–608.

121. Chaudhary SR, Ko N, Dillon W, et al: Prospective evaluation of multidetector-row CT angiography for the diagnosis of vasospasm following subarachnoid hemorrhage: A comparison with digital subtraction angiography. *Cerebrovasc Dis* 2008;**25**:144–150.

122. Pham M, Johnson A, Bartsch AJ, et al: CT perfusion predicts secondary cerebral infarction after aneurismal subarachnoid hemorrhage. *Neurology* 2007;**69**:762–765.

123. Sviri GE, Feinsod M, Soustiel JF: Brain natriuretic peptide and cerebral vasospasm in subarachnoid hemorrhage: Clinical and TCD correlations. *Stroke* 2000;**31**:118–122.

124. Hop JW, Rinkel GJE, Algra A, van Gijn J: Initial loss of consciousness and risk of delayed cerebral ischemia after subarachnoid hemorrhage. *Stroke* 1999;**30**:2268–2271.

125. Lanterna LA, Ruigrok Y, Alexander S, et al: Meta-analysis of APOE genotype and subarachnoid hemorrhage. *Neurology* 2007;**69**:766–775.

126. Mizukami M, Kawase T, Usami T, et al: Prevention of vasospasm by early operation with removal of subarachnoid blood. *Neurosurgery* 1982;**10**:301–307.

127. Taneda M: Effect of early operation for ruptured aneurysm in prevention of delayed ischemic symptoms. *J Neurosurg* 1982;**5**:622–628.

128. Findlay JM, Kassell NF, Weir BKA, et al: A randomized trial of intraoperative, intracisternal tissue plasminogen activator for prevention of vasospasm. *Neurosurgery* 1995;**37**:168–178.

129. Sasaki T, Kodama N, Kawakami M, et al: Urokinase cisternal irrigation therapy of symptomatic vasospasm after aneurismal subarachnoid hemorrhage. *Stroke* 2000;**31**:1256–1262.

130. Barth M, Capelle H-H, Weidauer S, et al: Effect of nicardipine prolonged-release implants on cerebral vasospasm and clinical outcome after severe aneurismal subarachnoid hemorrhage. A prospective randomized double-blind phase II study. *Stroke* 2007;**38**:330–336.

131. Macdonald RL: Cerebral vasospasm. *Neurosurg Quarterly* 1995;**5**:73–97.

132. Kassell NF, Peerless SJ, Durward QJ, et al: Treatment of ischemic deficits from vasospasm with hypervolemia and induced arterial hypertension. *Neurosurgery* 1982;**11**:337–343.

133. Solomon RA, Fink ME, Lennihan L: Prophylactic volume expansion therapy for the prevention of delayed cerebral ischemia after early aneurysm surgery. *Arch Neurol* 1988;**45**:325–332.

134. Solomon RA, Post KD, McMurty JG: Depression of circulating blood volume in patients after subarachnoid hemorrhage: Implications for the management of symptomatic vasospasm. *Neurosurgery* 1984;**15**:354–361.

135. Wood JH, Simeone FA, Kron RE, et al: Rheological aspects of experimental hypervolemic hemodilution with low molecular weight dextran. *Neurosurgery* 1982;**11**:739–753.

136. Lennihan L, Mayer SA, Fink ME, et al. Effect of hypervolemic therapy on cerebral blood flow after subarachnoid hemorrhage: a randomized controlled trial. *Stroke* 2000;**31**:383–391.

137. Dankbaar JW, Slooter AJC, Rinkel GJE, van der Schaaf IC: Effect of different components of triple-H therapy on cerebral perfusion in patients with aneurysmal subarachnoid haemorrhage: a systematic review. *Critical Care* 2010;**14**:R23.

138. Naidech AM, Drescher J, Ault ML, Shaibani A, Batjer HH, Alberts MJ: Higher hemoglobin is associated with less cerebral infarction, poor outcome, and death after subarachnoid hemorrhage. *Neurosurgery* 2006;**59**:775–779.

139. Kramer AH, Gurka MJ, Nathan B, Dumont AS, Kassell NF, Bleck TP: Complications associated with anemia and blood transfusion in patients with aneurysmal subarachnoid hemorrhage. *Crit Care Med* 2008;**36**:2070–2075.

140. Naidech AM, Jovanovic B, Wartenberg KE, et al: Higher hemoglobin is associated with improved outcome after subarachnoid hemorrhage. *Crit Care Med* 2007;**35**:2383–2389.

141. Dhar R, Zazulia AR, Videen TO, et al. Red blood cell transfusion increases cerebral oxygen delivery in anemic patients with subarachnoid hemorrhage. *Stroke* 2009;**40**:3039–3044.

142. Connolly ES, Rabinstein AA, Carhuapoma JR, et al. on behalf of the American Heart Association Stroke Council, Council on Cardiovascular Radiology and Intervention, Council on Cardiovascular Nursing, Council on Cardiovascular Surgery and Anesthesia, and Council on Clinical Cardiology: Guidelines for the management of aneurysmal subarachnoid hemorrhage. A Guideline for healthcare professionals from the American Heart Association/ American Stroke Association. *Stroke* 2012;**43**:1711–1737.

143. Pickard JD, Murray GD, Illingworth R, et al: Effect of oral nimodipine in cerebral infarction and outcome after subarachnoid hemorrhage: British Aneurysm Nimodipine trial. *BMJ* 1981;**298**:636–642.

144. Allen GS: Cerebral arterial spasm: A controlled trial of nimodipine in subarachnoid hemorrhage patients – the Nimodipine Cerebral Arterial Spasm Study Group. *Stroke* 1983;**14**:122.

145. Feigin VL, Rinkel GJE, Algra A, et al: Calcium antagonists in patients with aneurysmal subarachnoid hemorrhage. A systematic review. *Neurology* 1998;**50**:876–883.

146. Fraticelli AT, Cholley BP, Losser M-R, et al: Milrinone for the treatment of cerebral vasospasm after aneurismal subarachnoid hemorrhage. *Stroke* 2008;**39**:893–898.

147. Higashida RT, Halbach VV, Cahan LD, et al: Transluminal angioplasty for treatment of intracranial arterial vasospasm. *J Neurosurg* 1989;**71**:648–653.

148. Hoh BL, Ogilvy CS: Endovascular treatment of cerebral vasospasm: Transluminal balloon angioplasty, intra-arterial papaverine, and intra-arterial nicardipine. *Neurosurg Clin N Am* 2005;**16**:501–516.

149. Brisman JL, Eskridge JM, Newell DW: Neurointerventional treatment of vasospasm. *Neurol Res* 2006;**28**:769–776.

150. Newell DW, Eskridge JM, Mayberg M, et al: Angioplasty for the treatment of symptomatic vasospasm following subarachnoid hemorrhage. *J Neurosurg* 1989;**91**:654–660.

151. Leroux PD, Winn HR: Timing of surgery and special features of ruptured anterior circulation aneurysms. In Welch KMA, Caplan LR, Reis DJ, et al. (eds): *Primer on Cerebrovascular Diseases.* San Diego: Academic Press, 1997, pp 450–454.

152. Kirkpatrick PJ, Turner CL, Smith C, Hutchinson PJ, Murray GD, STASH Collaborators: Simvastatin in aneurysmal subarachnoid hemorrhage (STASH): A multicenter randomized phase 3 trial. *Lancet Neurol* 2014;**13**:666–675.

153. Dorhout Mees SM, Algra A, Vandertop WP et al., MASH-2 Study Group: Magnesium for aneurysmal subarachnoid haemorrhage (MASH-2): A randomised placebo-controlled trial. *Lancet* 2012;**380**;44–49.

154. Graff-Radford NR, Torner J, Adams HP, Kassell NF: Factors associated with hydrocephalus after subarachnoid hemorrhage. *Arch Neurol* 1989;**46**:744–752.

155. Brouwers PJ, Wijdicks EF, Hasan D, et al: Serial electrocardiographic recording in aneurysmal sub-arachnoid hemorrhage. *Stroke* 1989;**20**:1162–1167.

156. Caplan LR, Hurst JW: Cardiac and cardiovascular findings in patients with nervous system diseases. In Caplan LR, Hurst JW, Chimowitz MI (eds): *Clinical Neurocardiology.* New York: Marcel Dekker, 1999, pp 298–312.

157. Fabinyi G, Hunt D, McKinley L: Myocardial creatine kinase isoenzyme in serum after subarachnoid hemorrhage. *J Neurol Neurosurg Psychiatry* 1977;**40**:818–820.

158. Ramappa P, Thatai D, Coplin W, et al: Cardiac troponin-I: A predictor of prognosis in subarachnoid hemorrhage. *Neurocrit Care* 2008;**8**:398–403.

159. Kothavale A, Banki NM, Kopelnik A, et al: Predictors of left ventricular regional wall motion abnormalities after subarachnoid hemorrhage. *Neurocrit Care* 2006;**4**:199–205.

160. Oppenheimer SM, Cechetto DF, Hachinski VC: Cerebrogenic cardiac arrhythmias. Cerebral electrocardiographic influences and their role in sudden death. *Arch Neurol* 1990;**47**:513–519.

161. Di Pasquale G, Pinelli G, Andreoli A, et al: Holter detection of cardiac arrhythmias in intracranial subarachnoid hemorrhage. *Am J Cardiol* 1987;**59**:596–600.

162. Di Pasquale G, Pinelli G, Andreoli A, et al: Torsade de pointes and ventricular flutter-fibrillation following spontaneous cerebral subarachnoid hemorrhage. *Int J Cardiol* 1988;**18**:163–172.

163. Kolin A, Norris JW: Myocardial damage from acute cerebral lesions. *Stroke* 1984;**15**:990–993.

164. Samuels MA: The brain–heart connection. *Circulation* 2007;**116**:77–84.

165. Salem R, Vallée F, Dépret F, et al: Subarachnoid hemorrhage induces an early and reversible cardiac injury associated with catecholamine release: One-week follow-up study *Critical Care* 2014;**18**:558–568.

166. Tsuchihashi K, Ueshima K, Uchida T, Ohmura N, Kimura K: Transient left ventricular apical ballooning without coronary artery stenosis: a novel heart syndrome mimicking acute myocardial infarction. Angina pectoris–myocardial infarction investigations in Japan. *J Am Coll Cardiol* 2001;**38**:11–18.

167. Kurisu S, Sato H, Kawagoe T, et al: Takotsubo-like left ventricular dysfunction with ST-segment elevation: A novel cardiac syndrome mimicking acute myocardial infarction. *Am Heart J* 2002;**143**:448–455.

168. Bybee KA, Kara T, Prasad A, et al: Systematic review: transient left ventricular apical ballooning: a syndrome that mimics ST-segment elevation myocardial infarction. *Ann Intern Med* 2004;**141**:858–865.

169. Hakeem A, Marks AD, Bhatti S, Chang SM: When the worst headache becomes the worst heartache! *Stroke* 2007;**38**:3292–3295.

170. Bybee KA, Prasad A: Stress-related cardiomyopathy syndromes. *Circulation* 2008;**118**:397–409.

171. Ciongoli AK, Poser CM: Pulmonary edema secondary to subarachnoid hemorrhage. *Neurology* 1972;**22**:867–870.

172. Weir BK: Pulmonary edema following fatal aneurysmal rupture. *J Neurosurg* 1978;**49**:502–507.

173. Hoff RG, Rinkel GJE, Verweij BH, Algra A, Kalkman CJ: Pulmonary edema and blood volume after aneurysmal subarachnoid hemorrhage: A prospreective observational study. *Critical Care* 2010;**14**;R43–R50.

174. Takaku A, Shindo K, Tanaki S, et al: Fluid and electrolyte disturbances in patients with intracranial aneurysms. *Surg Neurol* 1979;**11**:349–356.

175. Qureshi AI, Suri MF, Sung GY, et al: Prognostic significance of hypernatremia and hyponatremia among patients with aneurysmal subarachnoid hemorrhage. *Neurosurgery.* 2002;**50**:749–755.

176. Zheng B, Qiu Y, Jin H, et al: Predictive value of hyponatremia for poor outcome and cerebral infarction in high-grade aneurysmal subarachnoid haemorrhage patients. *J Neurol Neurosurg Psychiatry* 2011;**82**:213–217.

177. Rabinstein AA, Bruder N: Management of hyponatremia and volume contraction. *Neurocrit Care* 2011;**15**:354–360.

178. Katayama Y, Haraoka J, Hirabayashi H, et al: A randomized controlled trial of hydrocortisone against hyponatremia in patients with aneurismal subarachnoid hemorrhage. *Stroke* 2007;**38**:2373–2375.

179. Diringer MN, Lim JS, Kirsch JR, Hawley DF: Suprasellar and intraventricular blood predict elevated plasma atrial natriuretic factor in subarachnoid hemorrhage. *Stroke* 1991;**22**:572–581.

180. Wijdicks EFM, Ropper AH, Hunnicutt EJ, et al: Atrial natriuretic factor and salt wasting after aneurysmal subarchnoid hemorrhage. *Stroke* 1991;**22**:1519–1524.

181. Schneider HJ, Kreitschmann-Andermahr I, Ghiko E, et al: Hypothalamopituitary dysfunction following traumatic brain injury and aneurismal subarachnoid hemorrhage. A systemic review. *JAMA* 2007;**298**:1429–1438.

182. Kreitschmann-Andermahr I, Hoff C, Niggemeier S, et al: Pituitary deficiency following aneurismal

subarachnoid haemorrhage. *J Neurol Neurosurg Psychiatry* 2003;**74**:1133–1135.

183. Dimopoulou I, Kouyialis AT, Tzanella M, et al: High incidence of neuroendocrine dysfunction in long-term survivors of aneurismal subarachnoid hemorrhage. *Stroke* 2004;**35**:2884–2489.

184. Claasen J, Vu A, Kreiter KT, et al: Effect of acute physiologic derangements on outcome after subarachnoid hemorrhage. *Crit Care Med* 2004;**32**:832–838.

185. Adams HP: Current status of antifibrinolytic therapy for treatment of patients with aneurysmal subarachnoid hemorrhage. *Stroke* 1982;**13**:256–259.

186. Ramirez-Laseppas M: Antifibrinolytic therapy in subarachnoid hemorrhage caused by ruptured intracranial aneurysm. *Neurology* 1981;**31**:316–322.

187. Bederson JB, Connolly ES Jr, Batjer HH, et al:. Guidelines for the management of aneurysmal subarachnoid hemorrhage. A statement for healthcare professionals from a special writing group of the Stroke Council of the American Heart Association. *Stroke* 2009;**40**:994–1025.

188. Kassell N, Torner D, Adams H: Antifibrinolytic therapy in the acute period following aneurysmal subarachnoid hemorrhage. *J Neurosurg* 1984;**61**:225–230.

189. Garde A: Amnesia after operations on aneurysms of the anterior communicating artery. *Surg Neurol* 1982;**18**:46–49.

190. Damasio AR, Graff-Radford N, Eslinger P, et al: Amnesia following basal forebrain lesions. *Arch Neurol* 1985;**42**:263–271.

191. Serbinenko FA: Balloon catheterization and occlusion of major cerebral vessels. *J Neurosurg* 1974;**41**:125–145.

192. Guglielmi G, Vinuela F, Sepetka I, Macellari V: Electrothrombosis of saccular aneurysms via endovascular approach, part 1: Electrochemical basis, technique, and experimental results. *J Neurosurg* 1991;**75**:1–7.

193. Guglielmi G, Vinuela F, Dion J, Duckwiler G: Electrothrombosis of saccular aneurysms via endovascular approach, part 2: Preliminary clinical experience. *J Neurosurg* 1991;**75**:8–14.

194. Johnston SC, Higashida RT, Barrow DL, Caplan LR, et al: Recommendations for the endovascular treatment of intracranial aneurysms. A statement for health care professionals from the Committee on Cerebrovascular Imaging of the American Heart Association Council on Cardiovascular Radiology. *Stroke* 2002;**33**:2536–2544.

195. Hopkins LN, Lanzino G, Guterman LR: Treating nervous system vascular disorders through a "needle stick": Origins, evolution, and future of endovascular therapy. *Neurosurgery* 2001;**48**:463–475.

196. Lobotesis K, Mahady K, Ganesalingam J, et al: Coiling-associated delayed cerebral hypersensitivity: Is nickel the link? *Neurology* 2015;**84**:97–99.

197. Molyneux AJ, Kerr RSC, Yu L-M, et al: International Subarachnoid Aneurysm Trial (ISAT) of neurosurgical clipping versus endovascular coiling in 2143 patients with ruptured intracranial aneurysms: A randomized comparison of effects on survival, dependency, seizures, rebleeding, subgroups, and aneurysm occlusion. *Lancet* 2005;**366**:809–817.

198. Britz GW: ISAT trial: Coiling or clipping for intracranial aneurysms? *Lancet* 2005;**366**:783–785.

199. Molyneux AJ, Birks J, Clarke A, Sneade M, Kerr RSC: The durability of endovascular coiling versus neurosurgical clipping of ruptured cerebral aneurysms: 18 year follow-up of the UK cohort of the International Subarachnoid Aneurysm Trial (ISAT). *Lancet* 2015;**385**:691–697.

200. Debrun GM, Aletich VA, Kehrli P, et al: Selection of cerebral aneurysms for treatment using Guglielmi detachable coils: The preliminary University of Illinois at Chicago experience. *Neurosurgery* 1998;**43**:1281–1295.

201. Lanzino G, Wakhloo AK, Fessler RD, et al: Efficacy and current limitations of intravascular stents for intracranial internal carotid, vertebral, and basilar artery aneurysms. *J Neurosurg* 1999;**91**:538–546.

202. Greenberg E, Katz JM, Janardhan V, et al: Treatment of a giant vertebrobasilar artery aneurysm using stent grafts. Case report. *J Neurosurg* 2007;**107**:165–168.

203. Katsaridis V, Papagiannaki C, Violaris C: Placement of a Neuroform2 stent into the parent vessel by navigating it along the inner wall of the aneurysm sac: A technical case report. *Neuroradiology* 2007;**49**:57–59.

204. Pero G, Denegri F, Valvassori L, et al: Treatment of a middle cerebral artery giant aneurysm using a covered stent. Case report. *J Neurosurg* 2006;**104**:965–968.

205. Kupersmith MJ, Stiebel-Kalish H, Huna-Baron R, et al: Cavernous carotid aneurysms rarely cause subarachnoid hemorrhage or major neurological morbidity. *J Stroke Cerebrovasc Dis* 2002;**11**:9–14.

206. Brust JCM, Dickinson PCT, Hughes JEO, Holtzman RNN: The diagnosis and treatment of cerebral mycotic aneurysms. *Ann Neurol* 1990;**27**:238–246.

207. Moskowitz MA, Rosenbaum AE, Tyler HR: Angiographically monitored resolution of cerebral mycotic aneurysms. *Neurology* 1974;**24**:1103–1108.

208. Johnston SC, Wilson CB, Halbach VV, et al: Endovascular and surgical treatment of unruptured cerebral aneurysms: Comparison of risks. *Ann Neurol* 2000;**48**:11–19.

209. Wermer MJH, van der Schaaf IC, Algra A, Rinkel GJE: Risk of rupture of unruptured intracranial aneurysms in relation to patient and aneurysm characteristics. An updated meta-analysis. *Stroke* 2007;**38**:1404–1410.

210. Sundt TM, Whisnant JP: Subarachnoid hemorrhage from intracranial aneurysm. *N Engl J Med* 1978;**299**:116–122.

211. Raaymakers TWM, Rinkel GJE, Limburg M, Algra A: Mortality and morbidity of surgery for unruptured intracranial aneurysms. *A meta-analysis. Stroke* 1998;**29**:1531–1538.

212. Komotar RJ, Moccoj, Solomon RA: Guidelines for the surgical treatment of unruptured intracranial aneurysms. *Neurosurgery* 2008;**62**:183–193, discussion 193–194.

213. Stein BM, Wolpert SM: Arteriovenous malformations of the brain: I. Current concepts and treatment. *Arch Neurol* 1980;**37**:1–5.

214. Brown RD, Wiebers DO, Torner JC: Frequency of intracranial hemorrhage as a presenting symptom and subtype analysis: A population-based study of intracranial vascular malformations in Olmstead County, Minnesota. *J Neurosurg* 1996;**85**:29–32.

215. Hartmann A, Mast H, Choi JH, et al: Treatment of arteriovenous

malformations of the brain. *Curr Neurol Neurosci Rep* 2007;7:28–34.

216. Tonnis W, Schiefer W, Walter W: Signs and symptoms of supratentorial arteriovenous aneurysms. *J Neurosurg* 1953;15:471–480.

217. McCormick WF: The pathology of vascular ("arteriovenous") malformations. *J Neurosurg* 1966;24:807–816.

218. McCormick WF: Pathology of vascular malformations of the brain. In Wilson CB, Stein BM (eds): *Intracranial Arteriovenous Malformations: Current Neurosurgical Practice.* Baltimore: Williams & Wilkins, 1984, pp 44–63.

219. McCormick WF, Boulter TR: Vascular malformations ("angiomas") of the dura mater. *J Neurosurg* 1966;25:309–311.

220. McCormick WF: The pathology of angiomas. In Fein JM, Flamm ES (eds): *Cerebrovascular Surgery,* vol **IV.** New York: Springer, 1985, pp 1073–1095.

221. McCormick WF, Hardman JM, Boulter TR: Vascular malformations ("angiomas") of the brain, with special reference to those occurring in the posterior fossa. *J Neurosurg* 1968;28:241–251.

222. Arteriovenous Malformations Study Group: Arteriovenous malformations of the brain in adults. *N Engl J Med* 1999;340:1812–1818.

223. Lasjaunias PL, Landrieu P, Rodesch G, et al: Cerebral proliferative angiopathy. Clinical and angiographic description of an entity different from cerebral AVMs. *Stroke* 2008;39:878–885.

224. Rigamonti D, Hadley MN, Drayer BP, et al: Cerebral cavernous malformations: Incidence and familial occurrence. *N Engl J Med* 1988;319:343–347.

225. Savoiardo M, Strada L, Passerini A: Intracranial cavernous hemangiomas: Neuroradiologic review of 36 operated cases. *AJNR Am J Neuroradiol* 1983;4:945–950.

226. Mason I, Aase JM, Orrison WW, et al: Familial cavernous angiomas of the brain in an Hispanic family. *Neurology* 1988;38:324–326.

227. Metellus P, Kharkar S, Lin D, et al: Cavernous angiomas and developmental venous anomalies. In Caplan LR (ed): *Uncommon Causes of Stroke,* 2nd ed. Cambridge: Cambridge University Press, 2008, pp 189–219.

228. Denier C, Labauge P, Brunereau L, et al: Clinical features of cerebral cavernous malformations patients with *KRIT1* mutations. *Ann Neurol* 2004;55:213–220.

229. Wilms G, Bleus E, Demaerel P, et al: Simultaneous occurrence of developmental venous anomalies and cavernous angiomas. *AJNR Am J Neuroradiol* 1994;15:1247–1254.

230. Abe T, Singer RJ, Marks MP, et al: Coexistence of occult vascular malformations and developmental venous anomalies in the central nervous system: MR evaluation. *AJNR Am J Neuroradiol* 1998;19:51–57.

231. Omojola M, Fox A, Vinuela F, Debrun G: Stenosis of afferent vessels of intracranial arteriovenous malformations. *AJNR Am J Neuroradiol* 1985;6:791–793.

232. Mawad ME, Hilal SK, Michelson J, et al: Occlusive vascular disease associated with cerebral arteriovenous malformations. *Radiology* 1984;153:401–408.

233. Marks MP, Lane B, Steinberg GK, Snipes GJ: Intranidal aneurysms in cerebral arteriovenous malformations: Evaluation and endovascular treatment. *Radiology* 1992;183:355–360.

234. Kondziolka D, Nixon BJ, Lasjaunias P, et al: Cerebral arteriovenous malformations with associated arterial aneurysms: Hemodynamic and therapeutic considerations. *Can J Neurol Sci* 1988;15:130–134.

235. Miyasaka Y, Yada K, Ohwada T, et al: An analysis of the venous drainage system as an actor in hemorrhage from arteriovenous malformations. *J Neurosurg* 1992;76:239–243.

236. Vinuela F, Nombela L, Roach MR, et al: Stenotic and occlusive disease of the draining venous system of deep brain AVMs. *J Neurosurg* 1985;63:180–184.

237. Hsu FPK, Rigamonti D, Huhn SL: Epidemiology of cavernous malformations. In Awad IA, Barrows DL (eds): *Cavernous Malformations.* Park Ridge, IL: American Association of Neurological Surgeons, 1993, pp 13–23.

238. Kase CS: Aneurysms and vascular malformations. In Kase CS, Caplan LR (eds): *Intracerebral Hemorrhage.* Boston: Butterworth–Heinemann, 1995, pp 153–178.

239. Perret G, Nishioka H: Report on the Cooperative Study of Intracranial Aneurysms and Subarachnoid Hemorrhage. Section VI. Arteriovenous malformations. An analysis of 545 cases of cranio-cerebral arteriovenous malformations and fistulae reported to the Cooperative Study. *J Neurosurg* 1966;25:467–490.

240. Crawford PM, West CR, Chadwick DW, et al: Arteriovenous malformations of the brain: Natural history in unoperated patients. *J Neurol Neurosurg Psychiatry* 1986;49:1–10.

241. Graf CJ, Perret GE, Torner JC: Bleeding from cerebral arteriovenous malformations as part of their natural history. *J Neurosurg* 1983;58:331–337.

242. Hook C, Johanson C: Intracranial arteriovenous aneurysms: A follow-up study with particular attention to their growth. *Arch Neurol Psych* 1958;80:39–54.

243. Patterson JH, McKissock W: A clinical survey of intracranial angiomas with special reference to their mode of progression and surgical treatment: A report of 110 cases. *Brain* 1965;79:233–266.

244. Friedlander RM: Arteriovenous malformations of the brain. *N Engl J Med* 2007;356:2704–2712.

245. Hofmeister C, Stapf C, Hartman A, et al: Demographic, morphological, and clinical characteristics of 1289 patients with brain arteriovenous malformation. *Stroke* 2000;31:1307–1310.

246. Mast H, Mohr JP, Osipov A, et al: "Steal" is an unestablished mechanism for the clinical presentation of cerebral arteriovenous malformations. *Stroke* 1995;26:1215–1220.

247. Chimowitz MI, Little JR, Awad IA, et al: Intracranial hypertension associated with unruptured cerebral arteriovenous malformations. *Ann Neurol* 1990;27:474–479.

248. DeJong RN, Hicks SP: Vascular malformation of the brainstem: Report of a case with long duration and fluctuating course. *Neurology* 1980;30:995–997.

249. Stahl SM, Johnson KP, Malamud N: The clinical and pathological spectrum of brainstem vascular malformations. *Arch Neurol* 1980;37:25–29.

250. Caroscio JT, Brannan T, Budabin M, et al: Subarachnoid hemorrhage secondary to spinal arteriovenous

malformation and aneurysm. *Arch Neurol* 1980;**37**:101–103.

251. Jensen H, Klinge H, Lemke J, et al: Computerized tomography in vascular malformations of the brain. *Neurosurg Rev* 1980;**3**:119–127.

252. Daniels D, Houghton V, Williams A, et al: Arteriovenous malformation simulating a cyst on computed tomography. *Radiology* 1979;**133**:393–394.

253. Kaibara T, Heros RC: Arteriovenous malformations of the brain. In Caplan LR (ed): *Uncommon Causes of Stroke*, 2nd ed. Cambridge: Cambridge University Press, 2008.

254. Leblanc R, Levesque M, Comair Y, Ethier R: Magnetic resonance imaging of cerebral arteriovenous malformations. *Neurosurgery* 1987;**21**:15–20.

255. Smith HJ, Strother CM, Kikuchi Y, et al: MR imaging in the management of supratentorial intracranial AVMs. *AJR Am J Roentgen* 1988;**150**:1143–1153.

256. Rigamonti D, Drayer B, Johnson PC, et al: The MRI appearance of cavernous malformations (angiomas). *J Neurosurg* 1987;**67**:518–524.

257. Gomori JM, Grossman RI, Hackney DB, et al: Variable appearances of subacute intracranial hematomas on high-field spin-echo MR. *AJR Am J Roentgen* 1988;**150**:171–178.

258. Requena I, Arias M, Lopez-Iber L: Cavernomas of the central nervous system in clinical and neuroimaging manifestations in 47 patients. *J Neurol Neurosurg Psychiatry* 1991;**54**:590–594.

259. Perl J, Ross JS: Diagnostic imaging of cavernous malformations. In Awad IA, Barrow DL (eds): *Cavernous Malformations*. Park Ridge, IL: American Association of Neurological Surgeons, 1993, pp 37–48.

260. Hardjasudarma M: Cavernous and venous angiomas of the central nervous system. Neuroimaging and clinical controversies. *J Neuroimaging* 1991;**1**:191–196.

261. Rigamonti D, Spetzler RF, Drayer BP, et al: Appearance of venous malformations on magnetic resonance imaging. *J Neurosurg* 1988;**69**:535–539.

262. Lee C, Pennington MA, Kenney CM: MR evaluation of developmental venous anomalies: medullary venous anatomy of venous angiomas. *AJNR Am J Neuroradiol* 1996;**17**:61–70.

263. Diehl RR, Henkes H, Nahser H-C, et al: Blood flow velocity and vasomotor reactivity in patients with arteriovenous malformations. A transcranial Doppler study. *Stroke* 1994;**25**:1574–1580.

264. Marks M, Lane B, Steinberg G, Chang P: Vascular characteristics of intracerebral arteriovenous malformations in patients with clinical steal. *AJNR* 1991;**12**:489–496.

265. Stapf C, Mohr JP, Sciacca RR, et al: Incident hemorrhage risk of brain arteriovenous malformations located in the arterial borderzones. *Stroke* 2000;**31**:2365–2368.

266. Mast H, Young WL, Koennecke HC, et al: Risk of spontaneous hemorrhage after diagnosis of cerebral arteriovenous malformation. *Lancet* 1997;**350**:1065–1068.

267. Mansmann U, Meisel J, Brock M, et al: Factors associated with intracranial hemorrhage in cases of cerebral arteriovenous malformations. *Neurosurgery* 2000;**46**:272–279.

268. Drake CG: Arteriovenous malformations of the brain: The options for management. *N Engl J Med* 1983;**309**:308–310.

269. Heros RC, Tu Y-K: Is surgical therapy needed for unruptured arteriovenous malformations? *Neurology* 1987;**37**:279–286.

270. Drake CG: Cerebral arteriovenous malformations: Considerations for and experience with surgical treatment in 166 cases. *Clin Neurosurg* 1979;**26**:145–208.

271. Forster DMC, Steiner L, Hakanson S: Arteriovenous malformations of the brain: A long-term clinical study. *J Neurosurg* 1972;**37**:562–570.

272. Hartmann A, Mast H, Mohr JP, et al: Morbidity of intracranial hemorrhage in patients with cerebral arteriovenous malformation. *Stroke* 1998;**29**:931–934.

273. Duong DH, Young WL, Vang MC, et al: Feeding artery pressure and venous drainage pattern are primary determinants of hemorrhage from arteriovenous malformations. *Stroke* 1998;**29**:1167–1176.

274. Aminoff MJ: Treatment of unruptured cerebral arteriovenous malformations. *Neurology* 1987;**37**:815–819.

275. Mohr JP, Parides MK, Stapf SC, et al. for the International ARUBA Investigators: Medical management with or without interventional therapy for unruptured brain arteriovenous malformations (ARUBA): A multicentre, non-blinded, randomised trial. *Lancet* 2014;**383**:614–621.

276. Al-Shahi Salman R, White PM, Counsell CE, et al: Outcomes after conservative management or intervention for unruptured brain arteriovenous malformations. *JAMA* 2014;**311**:1661–1669.

277. Barrow DL: Classification and natural history of cerebral vascular malformations: Arteriovenous, cavernous, and venous. *J Stroke Cerebrovasc Dis* 1997;**6**:264–267.

278. Robinson JR, Awad IA, Little JR: Natural history of the cavernous angioma. *J Neurosurg* 1991;**75**:709–714.

279. Kondziolka D, Lundsford LD, Kestle JRW: The natural history of cerebral cavernous malformations. *J Neurosurg* 1995;**83**:820–824.

280. Robinson JR, Awad IA: Clinical spectrum and natural course. In Awad IA, Barrows DL (eds): *Cavernous Malformations*. Park Ridge, IL: American Association of Neurological Surgeons, 1993, pp 25–36.

281. Moran NF, Fish DR, Kitchen N, et al: Supratentorial cavernous haemangiomas and epilepsy: A review of the literature and case series. *J Neurol Neurosurg Psychiatry* 1999;**66**:561–568.

282. Garner TB, Curling OD Jr, Kelly DL Jr, et al: The natural history of intracranial venous angiomas. *J Neurosurg* 1991;**75**:715–722.

283. Rigamonti D, Spetzler RF, Medina M, et al: Cerebral venous malformations. *J Neurosurg* 1990;**73**:560–564.

284. Naff NJ, Wemmer J, Hoenig-Rigamonti K, Rigamonti DR: A longitudinal study of patients with venous malformations: Documentation of a negligible hemorrhage risk and benign natural history. *Neurology* 1998;**50**:1709–1714.

285. Ruiz DS, Yilmaz H, Gailloud P: Cerebral developmental anomalies: Current concepts. *Ann Neurol* 2009;**66**:271–283.

286. Castel JP, Kantor G: Postoperative morbidity and mortality after microsurgical exclusion of cerebral

arteriovenous malformations. Current data and analysis of recent literature. *Neurochiurgie* 2001;**47**:369–383.

287. Spetzler RF, Wilson CB, Weinstein P, et al: Normal perfusion pressure breakthrough theory. *Clin Neurosurg* 1978;**25**:651–672.

288. Fournier D, TerBrugge KG, Willinsky R, et al: Endovascular treatment of intracerebral arteriovenous malformations: Experience in 49 cases. *J Neurosurg* 1991;**75**:228–233.

289. Vinuela F, Fox AJ, Debrun G, et al: Progressive thrombosis of brain arteriovenous malformations after embolization with isobutyl-2-cyanoacrylate. *AJNR Am J Neuroradiol* 1983;**4**:959–966.

290. N-BCA Trialists: N-butyl cyanoacrylate embolization of cerebral arteriovenous malformations: Results of a prospective, multi-center trial. *AJNR Am J Neuroradiol* 2002;**23**:748–755.

291. Saatci I, Geyik S, Yavuz K, Cekirge HS: Endovascular treatment of brain arteriovenous malformations with prolonged intranidal Onyx injection technique: Long-term results in 350 consecutive patients with completed endovascular treatment course. *J Neurosurg* 2011;**115**:78–88.

292. Vinters HV, Lundie MJ, Kaufmann JC: Long-term pathological follow-up of cerebral arteriovenous malformations treated by embolization with buccylate. *N Engl J Med* 1986;**314**:477–483.

293. Lunsford LD, Flickinger J, Coffey RJ: Stereotactic gamma knife radiosurgery. Initial North American experience in 207 patients. *Arch Neurol* 1990;**47**:169–175.

294. Heros R, Korosue K: Radiation treatment of cerebral arteriovenous malformations. *N Engl J Med* 1990;**323**:127–129.

295. Meder JF, Oppenheim C, Blustajn J, et al: Cerebral arteriovenous malformations: The value of radiologic parameters in predicting response to radiosurgery. *AJNR Am J Neuroradiol* 1997;**18**:1473–1483.

296. Hanakita S, Koga T, Shin M, Igaki H, Saito N: Application of single-stage stereotactic radiosurgery for cerebral arteriovenous malformations >10 cm^3. *Stroke* 2014;**45**:3543–3548.

297. Hartmann A, Marx P, Schilling A, et al: Neurologic complications following radiosurgical treatment of brain arteriovenous malformations. *Cerebrovasc Dis* 2002;**13**:50.

298. Coffey RJ, Lunsford LD: Radiosurgery of cavernous malformations and other angiographically occult vascular malformations. In Awad IA, Barrow DL (eds): *Cavernous Malformations.* Park Ridge, IL: American Association of Neurological Surgeons, 1993, pp 187–200.

299. Ogilvy CS, Stieg PE, Awad I, et al: Recommendations for the management of intracranial arteriovenous malformations. A statement for healthcare professionals from a special writing group of the Stroke Council, American Stroke Association. *Circulation* 2001;**103**:2644–2657.

300. Dion J: Dural arteriovenous malformations: Definition, classification, and diagnostic imaging. In Awad IA, Barrow DL (eds): *Dural Arteriovenous Malformations.* Park Ridge, IL: American Association of Neurological Surgeons, 1993, pp 1–19.

301. Castaigne P, Bories J, Brunet P, et al: Les fistules arterio-veineuse meningees pures a drainage veineux cortical. *Rev Neurol (Paris)* 1976;**132**:169–181.

302. Gaston A, Chiras J, Bourbotte G, et al: Meningeal arteriovenous fistulae draining into cortical veins: 31 cases. *J Neuroradiol* 1984;**11**:161–177.

303. Bederson JB: Pathophysiology and animal models of dural arteriovenous malformations. In Awad IA, Barrow DL (eds): *Dural Arteriovenous Malformations.* Park Ridge, IL: American Association of Neurological Surgeons, 1993, pp 23–33.

304. Friedman AH: Etiologic factors in intracranial dural arteriovenous malformations. In Awad IA, Barrow DL (eds): *Dural Arteriovenous Malformations.* Park Ridge, IL: American Association of Neurological Surgeons, 1993, pp 35–47.

305. Raybaud CA, Hald JK, Strother CM, et al: Aneurysms of the vein of Galen. Angiographic study and morphogenetic considerations. *Neurochirurgie* 1987;**33**:302–314.

306. Hansen JH, Segaard I: Spontaneous regression of an extra- and intracranial arteriovenous malformation: Case report. *J Neurosurg* 1976;**45**:338–341.

307. Houser OW, Campbell JK, Campbell RJ: Arteriovenous malformation affecting the transverse dural venous sinus: An acquired lesion. *Mayo Clin Proc* 1979;**54**:651–661.

308. Fermand M, Reizine D, Melki JP, et al: Long term follow-up of 43 pure dural arteriovenous fistulae (AVF) of the lateral sinus. *Neuroradiology* 1987;**29**:348–353.

309. Chung SJ, Kim JS, Kim JC, et al: Intracranial dural arteriovenous fistulas: Analysis of 60 patients. *Cerebrovasc Dis* 2002;**13**:79–88.

310. Feiner L, Bennett J, Volpe NJ: Cavernous sinus fistulas: Carotid cavernous fistulas and dural arteriovenous malformations. *Curr Neurol Neurosci Rep* 2003;**3**:415–420.

311. Lasjaunias PL, Rodesch G: Lesion types, hemodynamics, and clinical spectrum. In Awad IA, Barrow DL (eds): *Dural Arteriovenous Malformations.* Park Ridge, IL: American Association of Neurological Surgeons, 1993, pp 49–79.

312. Awad IA, Little JR, Akrawi WP, et al: Intracranial dural arteriovenous malformations: Factors predisposing to an aggressive neurological course. *J Neurosurg* 1990;**72**:839–850.

313. Zeidman SM, Monsein LH, Arosarena O, et al: Reversability of white matter changes and dementia after treatment of dural fistulas. *AJNR Am J Neuroradiol* 1995;**16**:1080–1083.

314. Awad IA: Dural arteriovenous malformations with aggressive clinical course. In Awad IA, Barrow DL (eds): *Dural Arteriovenous Malformations.* Park Ridge, IL: American Association of Neurological Surgeons, 1993, pp 93–104.

315. Wecht DA, Awad IA: Carotid cavernous and other dural arteriovenous fistulas. In Welch KMA, Caplan LR, Reis DJ, et al. (eds): *Primer on Cerebrovascular Diseases.* San Diego: Academic Press, 1997, pp 541–548.

316. Purdy PD: Management of carotid cavernous fistula. In Batjer HH, Caplan LR, Friberg L, et al. (eds): *Cerebrovascular Disease.* Philadelphia: Lippincott–Raven, 1997, pp 1159–1168.

317. Takahashi S, Tomura N, Watarai J, et al: Dural arteriovenous fistula of the cavernous sinus with venous congestion of the brain stem: Report of two cases. *AJNR Am J Neuroradiol* 1999;**20**:886–888.

318. Halbach VV, Higashida RT, Hieshima GB, et al: Treatment of dural fistulas

475

involving the deep cerebral venous system. *AJNR Am J Neuroradiol* 1989;**10**:393–399.

319. Awad IA: Tentorial incisura and brain stem dural arteriovenous malformations. In Awad IA, Barrow DL (eds): *Dural Arteriovenous Malformations*. Park Ridge, IL: American Association of Neurological Surgeons, 1993, pp 131–146.

320. Cognard C, Gobin YP, Pierot L, et al: Cerebral dural arteriovenous fistulas: clinical and angiographic correlation with a revised classification of venous drainage. *Radiology* 1995;**194**:671–680.

321. Halbach VV, Higashida RT, Hieshima GB, et al: Transvenous embolization of dural fistulas involving the transverse and sigmoid sinuses. *AJNR Am J Neuroradiol* 1989;**10**:385–392.

322. Barnwell S: Endovascular therapy of dural arteriovenous malformations. In Awad IA, Barrow DL (eds): *Dural Arteriovenous Malformations*. Park Ridge, IL: American Association of Neurological Surgeons, 1993, pp 193–211.

323. Hu YC, Newman CB, Dashti SR, Albuquerque FC, McDougall GC: Cranial dural arteriovenous fistula: Transarterial Onyx embolization experience and technical nuances. *J Neurointerv Surg* 2011;**3**:5–13.

324. Mullan S: Surgical therapy: Indications and general principles. In Awad IA, Barrow DL (eds): *Dural Arteriovenous Malformations*. Park Ridge, IL: American Association of Neurological Surgeons, 1993, pp 213–229.

325. Awad IA, Barrow DL: Conceptual overview and management strategies. In Awad IA, Barrow DL (eds): *Dural Arteriovenous Malformations*. Park Ridge, IL: American Association of Neurological Surgeons, 1993, pp 131–241.

Intracerebral hemorrhage

Louis R Caplan and Carlos S Kase

Bleeding into the substance of the brain was recognized as a cause of stroke by Morgagni in 1761.[1] Cheyne wrote a treatise on apoplexy and coma in 1812, in which he included examples of intracerebral hemorrhage (ICH).[2] Clinicians of the nineteenth and twentieth centuries considered ICH invariably lethal. Post-mortem examples were usually studied because the tests available could not identify ICH during life. Clinicians correlated the clinical findings with the size and location of hemorrhages found in brains at necropsy. Gowers[3] and Osler,[4] writing at the turn of the twentieth century, included long and detailed chapters on the usual locations of ICH, and accompanying clinical signs and symptoms in their respective textbooks. In 1935, Aring and Merritt correlated the clinical and pathological findings among 245 patients with stroke who came to necropsy at the Boston City Hospital.[5] Aring and Merritt emphasized the features that separated hemorrhage from infarction. The major teachings emanating from these works are summarized in the following general rules:

1. ICH occurred at a younger age than brain infarction.
2. The major cause of ICH was hypertension, often severe.
3. Symptoms of ICH began abruptly.
4. Loss of consciousness was a nearly constant feature.
5. Headache always accompanied ICH, and was usually severe.
6. The most common locations for ICH were the putamen, internal capsule, thalamus, pons, and cerebellum.
7. ICH was invariably fatal or devastating, with few, if any, intact survivors.

This work, however, was published long before computed tomography (CT) scanning. Aring and Merritt's teachings evolved from correlation with fatal cases. Technology did not exist to diagnose less severe hemorrhages during life, especially if the lesions did not communicate with the cerebrospinal fluid (CSF). CT now allows accurate localization of small- and medium-sized hemorrhages. CT not only shows clinicians whether a lesion is a hemorrhage, but also accurately shows the location, size, spread within the brain, the presence and extent of drainage into the ventricles and spaces around the brain, and the presence of edema and mass effect. Magnetic resonance imaging (MRI), by its capability of showing the presence of hemosiderin, can help define whether lesions are old hemorrhages. Old infarcts and hemorrhages can look similar on CT. When the subject of ICH is reviewed in light of results with newer imaging techniques, the old rules are found to apply to larger hemorrhages, which account for only a small fraction of ICHs. We begin this chapter by reviewing the general rules and findings applicable to ICH at any site. We then review the etiologies of ICH and the findings in hemorrhages at their common locations in the brain.

Incidence and epidemiology

Approximately 10% of strokes are caused by ICH. The Pilot Stroke Data Bank (SDB),[6] the Michael Reese Stroke Registry (MRSR),[7] and the Harvard Stroke Registry (HSR)[8] found that approximately one stroke in 10 was caused by parenchymatous brain hemorrhage; the same figure was reached in studies of stroke at the Mayo Clinic in Rochester, Minnesota.[9,10] Populations that have a high frequency of hypertension, such as African-Americans and individuals of Chinese, Korean, Japanese, and Thai ancestry, have higher frequencies of ICH. ICH affects a wide age range, with many examples in the seventh, eighth, and ninth decades of life. Figure 14.1 displays the age and sex distribution of ICH in the HSR.[11] Although it is probably accurate to say that a higher percentage of strokes in patients younger than 40 years are hemorrhagic, ICH is also common during the later years of life.

Clinical course and accompanying symptoms

JT, a 44-year-old African-American school teacher, rushed to arrive at an important job interview. While being stressfully

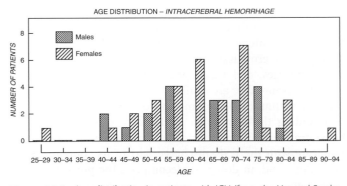

Figure 14.1 Age distribution in patients with ICH (from the Harvard Stroke Registry). From Caplan LR, Mohr JP. Intracerebral hemorrhage: An update. *Geriatrics* 1978;33:42–52 with permission.

Caplan's Stroke: A Clinical Approach, 5th Edition, ed. Louis R Caplan. Published by Cambridge University Press. © Cambridge University Press, 2016.

interrogated, he noted tingling in his left hand, which gradually spread to his arm. He excused himself to go to the bathroom, and then noted a similar feeling in his left leg. As he washed his hands, he realized his left hand and arm were clumsy and weak. He tripped on his left foot as he walked back. The interviewer was alarmed by slurring of words and a droop of the left face, which he noticed when JT returned. An ambulance was called. JT began to feel a headache over his right scalp. After 10 minutes, the emergency team arrived. JT could no longer move his left arm and leg, but seemed unaware and unconcerned with his handicap. He now had a severe headache and was sleepy. While being placed on a stretcher, he began to vomit. He had no history of hypertension or drug use. Blood pressure was 185/110 mmHg when he was first examined by the emergency room personnel.

The course of illness in this patient was the gradual accumulation of focal neurological signs, during a period of approximately 20 minutes. As the neurological symptoms and disability worsened, headache, decreased alertness, and vomiting developed.

ICH develops gradually. Bleeding into the brain tissues from small, deep, penetrating vessels is usually under arteriolar or capillary pressure. This situation contrasts with subarachnoid hemorrhage (SAH), in which arteries on the brain surface leak blood under systemic arterial pressure. Symptoms in patients with aneurysmal SAH begin instantaneously and consist of headache, decline in the level of consciousness, and vomiting. These symptoms are caused by sudden increase in intracranial pressure (ICP), resulting from blood rapidly disseminating through the CSF around the brain substance. In contrast, ICH develops gradually during minutes or sometimes hours.

Fisher examined serial sections of ICH studied at necropsy (Figure 14.2A and B).[12] At the center of the hematoma (labeled A in Figure 14.2) was a large mass of red blood cells. At the periphery (labeled B in the figure) were many of what he called fibrin globes, representing little caps of fibrinous material that plugged small vessels, which had broken and leaked during life. As ICH develops, pressure within the central core increases and compresses small vessels at the periphery of the hematoma. These peripheral arterioles and capillaries in turn break, and blood escapes, enlarging the lesion. The hematoma grows like a snowball rolling downhill, accumulating more snow on its outer circumference as it rolls. Figure 2.44 is a cartoon that illustrates the growth of a pontine hematoma. ICP rises as the lesion enlarges, and tissue pressure around the lesion also mounts. Eventually, an equilibrium is reached between the pressure within the hematoma and the pressure in the tissues surrounding the hematoma, and the bleeding stops. If the hematoma reaches the ventricle or brain surface, it may communicate with the CSF, discharge part of its contents at the same time, and, in doing so, decompress the pressure within the lesion.

Visualizing the pathology of the lesion and its development helps predict the pace of the symptoms. Bleeding is directly into brain parenchyma, rather than the CSF, as occurs in SAH. The brain is devoid of pain fibers, so the initial release of blood does not cause headache. Instead, blood disrupts the function

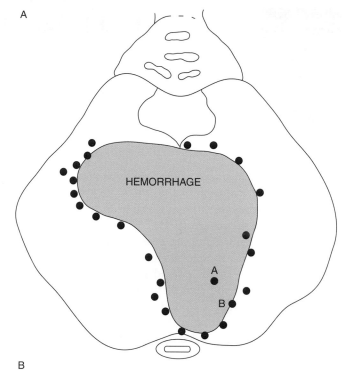

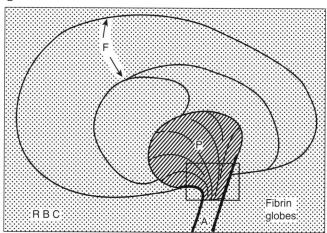

Figure 14.2 Miller Fisher's drawings of a necropsy specimen of a patient who died of a pontine hemorrhage. (A) Along the circumference of the hemorrhage dots mark the presence of fibrin globes that represent recently ruptured capillaries. (B) View of the fibrin globes that represent enlarged capillaries or arterioles – platelets are in the center and fibrin on the periphery. A = the main body of the hemorrhage; B = the outer edge of the hemorrhage; F = fibrin; P = a mass of platelets. From Fisher CM. Pathological observations in hypertensive cerebral hemorrhages. *J Neuropathol Exp Neurol* 1971;30:536–550 with permission.

of that particular local brain region. If the hematoma began in the left putamen, the patient might note right-limb weakness. As the hemorrhage grows during the next few minutes, the weakness becomes more severe. Sensory symptoms, loss of speech, and conjugate eye deviation to the side of the hemorrhage might ensue. In JT, the combination of sensory (tingling) and motor symptoms in the left side of his face, and left arm and leg, suggests a process in the deep structures of the right cerebral hemisphere, affecting the internal capsule region. If the hemorrhage grew to a size that increased ICP and distorted adjacent meningeal structures, the patient would develop

headache, vomiting, and reduced alertness. In JT, headaches, sleepiness, and vomiting started and evolved after he became hemiplegic and his lesion expanded. If the hematoma continued to grow, coma and death might result from compression of vital brain stem centers.

Sometimes, clinical symptoms and signs evolve over a period of days, rather than minutes or hours. Some of this evolution relates to edema formation surrounding the hematoma. Studies of patients with acute ICHs using sequential CT scans show that hematomas can, at times, expand dramatically during hours.[13–16] Repeat CT may show dramatic enlargement of hematoma mass and ventricular extension, developing within hours after the first CT scan. Invariably, clinical worsening was also present and was an indication for repeat scanning in some patients. In one study, 41 out of 204 patients with ICH had expansion of ICHs on repeat CT scans.[16] Expansion in this study was most often detected during the first 6 hours, but 5 out of 33 hematomas (15%) expanded between 6 and 12 hour scans, and 2 out of 34 hematomas (6%) enlarged between 12 and 24 hour scans.[16] Patients with ICH who have a bleeding diathesis are especially prone to hematomas that expand gradually and enlarge over periods of days.[17,18]

Analysis of the course of illness in 54 well-documented patients with ICH studied in the HSR showed that 37 had gradual development of symptoms during a period of minutes or a few hours.[11] In the 17 remaining patients, progression of symptoms did not seem to occur after the patients were first found by others. In many of this latter group, an accurate account of the earliest development of symptoms was not available because of aphasia, lack of awareness of the deficit, or stupor. A smooth, gradual worsening of function during minutes, followed by headache and vomiting, was the rule in larger lesions. Some patients who had stabilized during the first 24–48 hours, later developed progressively decreased alertness and increasing focal signs within 48–72 hours, probably caused by edema around the hematomas.

We find an early description of the gradual evolution of symptoms in a fatal case of ICH memorable.[19] This patient, seen in 1937, developed and evolved his hematoma while entirely under medical observation. He was sent to the hospital because of "malignant hypertension." While his history was taken, he noted weakness and dizziness. He stated that he noted numbness and tingling of the hands just before he left the admitting area, at which time his heart had been examined. He became extremely restless and apprehensive while his history was taken. He complained of inability to hear, difficulty in swallowing, and dyspnea. The patient was placed on the examining table, and his blood pressure was found to be 245 systolic and 170 diastolic. Under the eyes of several examiners, complete bilateral palsy of the VIth nerve developed; both pupils dilated, and the corneal reflexes disappeared. The patient was still able to talk, but with a typical bulbar speech, and he appeared almost completely deaf. His left leg became paretic, and rapid clonic movements were observed. Babinski's sign was present bilaterally. Within an hour, the patient was stuporous and his blood pressure had risen to 280 systolic and 170 diastolic. This rapidly progressive chain of events was most

unpleasant to witness and produced a depressing effect on the nurses and physicians.[19]

LRC had a similar experience during his first week as a medical intern at the Boston City Hospital. An elderly hypertensive Chinese man came to the emergency room with slight weakness of his right limbs. He spoke normally. He was placed on the danger list, and a porter and LRC pushed his stretcher through the underground hospital tunnels toward the ward. As we pushed the stretcher, his right limbs became weaker, and he stopped talking. Soon, his eyes and head deviated to the left, and LRC could not arouse him. By the time we reached the ward, he was comatose and decerebrate. He died within hours.

Like Kornyey and his colleagues,[19] LRC felt helpless watching brain function inexorably vanish. When a detailed history is possible, nearly all patients with ICH have had a gradual evolution of symptoms and signs – some more rapidly evolving than others.[20] When a hematoma expands by more than a third of its original volume, the prognosis becomes significantly worse for good survival. Recently physicians have sought ways to identify hematomas that have a high risk of enlarging. Heterogeneity of the density of a hematoma on CT scan implies different ages of growth. A major recent imaging advancement is recognition of the "spot sign," shown on CT angiography (CTA).[21] The spot sign is one or more small regions of contrast enhancement within an acute primary ICH that is visible on CTA source images and is separate from adjacent normal or abnormal blood vessels. It should not be present on pre-contrast images. It corresponds to sites of active, dynamic hemorrhage and is a signature of active bleeding in ICH. Patients with the spot sign have high risk of hematoma expansion.[22]

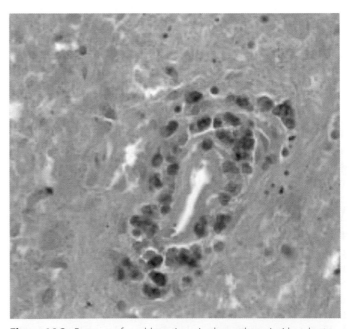

Figure 14.3 Remnant of an old pontine microhemorrhage, incidental autopsy finding in a 70-year-old woman. An elongated deep intracerbral artery with surrounding hemosiderin-laden macrophages. (hematoxylin/eosin stain). From Fiehler J. Cerebral microbleeds: Old leaks and new haemorrhages. *Int J Stroke* 2006;1:122–130 with permission. A black and white version of this figure will appear in some formats. For the color version, please refer to the plate section.

With time, macrophages surround the bleeding and phagocytize the blood. This is seen best in small bleeds often called microbleeds, which are visible on MRI images (Figure 14.3).

Headache

Headache was not an invariable symptom in the 60 HSR patients with ICH. Headache was described in only 17 patients (28%) near the outset of neurological symptoms.[11] Another 7 patients (12%) noted headache later. Twenty-four patients (40%) had no headache at any time during their ICH. The 12 stuporous or comatose patients (20%) could not provide data regarding headache.[11] Headache was much more frequent with larger lesions, and was often absent or minimal in patients with small lesions.

Among 289 patients with ICH studied at one Portuguese hospital, 165 patients (57%) had a headache near the onset of their ICHs.[23] Headache was most common in patients with lobar and cerebellar hematomas, locations near the meningeal surface, and was common in patients with meningeal signs.[23] Patients with small, deep hematomas almost never develop headache during their course of illness. In many patients, headache occurs as the hematoma enlarges and is accompanied by vomiting and decreased alertness.[20]

Decreased level of consciousness

Loss of consciousness accompanies only large hematomas and those found in the brainstem. Diminished alertness in patients with ICH is caused by mass effect and increased ICP, or direct involvement of the brainstem reticular activating system. In the HSR, 30 of 60 patients were alert when first seen. Fourteen patients (23%) were lethargic, and 16 patients (27%) were stuporous or comatose.[11] Decreased level of consciousness was the most important adverse prognostic sign among patients in the SDB who had ICH. Decreased level of consciousness has been found to be an important adverse prognostic sign in all studies of prognosis in patients with ICH.[20,24–26] All patients with ICH who had severely reduced levels of consciousness in the SDB died.[24] Early reduction of consciousness is not an invariable accompaniment of ICH. When it occurs, however, it has an ominous prognosis. The sleepiness that developed in JT was a serious finding and should have triggered urgent evaluation and treatment when he arrived at the hospital.

Vomiting

JT started to vomit while he was taken to the hospital, and continued to vomit in the emergency room. Vomiting is an especially important sign in patients with ICH. In ICH and SAH, vomiting is usually caused by increased ICP or local distortion of the IVth ventricle. Few patients with ischemic lesions within the cerebral hemispheres vomit, but nearly one-half of patients with hemispheral hemorrhages vomit. In the posterior circulation, vomiting usually reflects dysfunction of the vestibular nuclei, or the so-called vomiting center, in the floor of the IVth ventricle.[27] Vomiting occurs in approximately one-third of patients with occlusive posterior circulation disease and in more than one-half of patients with posterior circulation hemorrhages. Patients with cerebellar hemorrhage almost always vomit early in their clinical course.

Seizures

Seizures are not common during the acute phase of a stroke, but are slightly more frequent in ICH than other stroke types, except embolism.[8,20] Among three series of patients with spontaneous non-traumatic ICH, 12.5%,[28] 15.4%,[29] and 17%[30] of patients had seizures during their early course. Lobar hemorrhages situated near the gray–white junction of the cortex, and putaminal hemorrhages that undercut the cerebral cortex[31] are especially epileptogenic. When patients with subcortical large and expanding ICHs are monitored using continuous electroencephalographic (EEG) recordings, electrographic seizure discharges are often found.[32] Whether these discharges represent "non-convulsive seizures" and whether they affect outcome remains uncertain.[33] The effect on patient outcome by anticonvulsant treatment has not been clarified. At present LRC usually opts not to treat with anticonvulsants unless clinical seizures develop or there are unexplained episodes of transient loss of consciousness in an awake patient.

Other symptoms and signs

Neck stiffness is uncommon in putaminal hemorrhage,[31] but is often found in patients with caudate, thalamic, and cerebellar hemorrhages.[34,35] Fever is relatively common, but is often related to infectious complications, such as pulmonary and urinary tract infections. Subhyaloid retinal hemorrhages, common in SAH, are rare in ICH, unless the hematoma has developed rapidly and is large.[36] Cardiac arrhythmias and pulmonary edema develop in some patients with ICH, and are usually attributed to changes in ICP and catecholamine release, a similar pathogenesis to that used to explain cardiac findings in patients with SAH.[20]

Etiologies

Although aneurysms and vascular malformations are important causes of ICH, these vascular lesions are discussed in Chapter 13 and are not included here.

Hypertension

The most common cause of ICH is hypertension, but the blood pressure does not need to be elevated to malignant ranges. Many patients present to the hospital with ICH and have no prior history of hypertension, but have high blood pressure on admission. In this circumstance, it is difficult to know how much, if any, of the blood pressure elevation is secondary to raised ICP (the Cushing response), and what the level of blood pressure was before the bleed.

When hypertension first develops, the small arteries and capillaries are exposed to a high head of pressure and can leak. This situation is comparable to the hemodynamics found in patients with mitral valve stenosis. Left atrial failure develops

because of mitral valve obstruction. The left atrial failure causes increased pressure in the pulmonary veins. To perfuse the lungs, pulmonary artery pressure rises to maintain an arteriovenous pressure gradient. The pulmonary capillaries and arterioles are exposed to the increased head of pressure and break, causing hemoptysis. Later, small arteries and arterioles hypertrophy, protecting the capillary bed from high central pressure. Hemoptysis becomes less frequent when arterioles hypertrophy, but the heart bears the brunt of the increased arterial resistance. In this instance, right heart failure may develop. Similarly, increased arterial pressure, early in the course of development of systemic hypertension, causes arteriolar and capillary rupture. Later in the course of hypertension, degenerative changes in the form of lipohyalinosis and miliary Charcot-Bouchard aneurysms develop, caused by long-standing pressure elevations. ICH occurs when these and related degenerative abnormalities cause arterial and arteriolar rupture. The occurrence of ICH is biphasic, with patients presenting both at the onset of hypertension and later, after developing considerable wear and tear on penetrating brain arteries.[37,38]

Some hypertensive hemorrhages arise from degenerative changes, such as fibrinoid degeneration and microaneurysms, which develop in patients with hypertension. Cole and Yates examined the brains of 100 hypertensive patients and 100 normotensive controls.[39] All 13 patients with ICH had microaneurysms and were hypertensive. Among 63 patients with microaneurysms, 46 patients had hypertension recognized during life. The age distribution of microaneurysms in this study is also interesting. Among 21 hypertensive patients younger than 50 years, only 2 patients had microaneurysms, whereas 71% of hypertensive patients in the 65- to 69-year age range had microaneurysms.[39]

Rosenblum analyzed the morphology of microaneurysms and their parent vessels.[40] Some arteries bore early aneurysmal dilatations, whereas others had sclerosed aneurysms with flask-shaped collections of collagen joined to a small artery by a narrow neck. Microaneurysms are often surrounded by hemosiderin-laden macrophages, indicating previous leakage. Figure 14.3 shows a small elongated intracerebral artery surrounded by hemosiderin containing macrophages.[41] Hemosiderin is visible on gradient echo (susceptibility-weighted – T2*-weighted) MRI images as tiny "microbleeds."[41–43] Microaneurysms are most common in penetrating arteries that supply the basal ganglia, thalamus, pons and cerebellum, and arteries supplying the gray–white matter cortical junctions of the hemispheres. Figure 14.4 shows a section through a microaneurysm that was found associated with a hemorrhage in the pons.[44] The same arteries that bear microaneurysms also contain foci of lipohyalinosis and fibrinoid degeneration, which explains the dictum that hypertensive ICH has the same relative distribution as ischemic lacunes.

Fisher described the results from examination of serial sections of patients with ICH. Fibrin globes, meshes of platelets encircled by a thin layer of fibrin, protruded from ruptured sites and clearly marked vessels that had bled[12] (Figure 14.2).

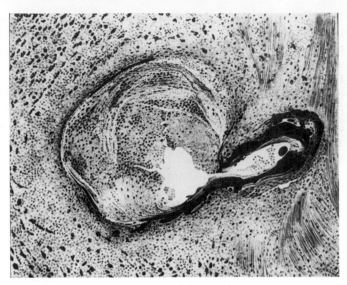

Figure 14.4 Section of a pontine microaneurysm stained with Hematoxylin and Eosin and Sudan III. The sac is partialy occluded by organizing blood clot. Recent hemorrhage is seen around the aneurysm. From Green FHK. Miliary aneurysms in the brain. *J Pathol Bacteriol* 1930;33:71–77 with permission.

A relationship between iris aneurysms and cerebral microaneurysms exists because rabbits with experimentally induced hypertension develop iris aneurysms approximately proportional to their development of cerebral microaneurysms.[45] Studies from Japan regarding surgical specimens of acute ICH show that penetrating arteries frequently break, but often not in relation to microaneurysms.[46,47] Degenerative lipohyalinotic changes were present in the broken and adjacent arteries. Degenerative changes caused by aging and hypertension can predispose to ICH, but it is not certain that microaneurysms always represent the bleeding lesion.[38,46,47]

Considerable evidence has accumulated that indicates that acute changes in blood pressure and blood flow can precipitate rupture of penetrating arteries in the absence of prior hypertension.[37,38] In a large necropsy study of patients who died from ICH, Bakemuka used heart weights to estimate the frequency of past hypertension; only 46% of fatal cases of spontaneous ICH had moderate to severe chronic hypertension or left ventricular hypertrophy.[48] Brott and colleagues reviewed the records of 154 patients with spontaneous ICH in Cincinnati, Ohio, during 1 year, to determine the frequency of hypertension.[49] Only 45% had a history of hypertension; another 12% without a history of hypertension had left ventricular hypertrophy. The authors judged that approximately 50% of cases were not attributable to chronic hypertension.[49]

In these two series,[48,49] the location of the hemorrhages, increased blood pressure on admission, and absence of other etiologies makes it highly probable that these hematomas were, in fact, satisfactorily classified as hypertensive ICH. Probably, hypertension was acute and led to bleeding from unprotected capillaries and arterioles. LRC's own observations and those of others have documented ICH in situations in which blood pressure probably increased abruptly.[37,38]

LRC's first experience with patients who had acute hypertension-related ICH was with patients who developed

ICH after exposure to severe cold weather.[50] While outdoors in temperatures below 10°F, 3 patients developed putaminal, thalamic, and cerebellar hematomas, respectively. One patient was in the midst of alcohol withdrawal, one was removing ice from his car window, and the third patient was waiting in line to pay rent. All had increased blood pressure on admission, but their pressures normalized soon thereafter. Immersion in cold is known to be a strong sympathetic nervous system stimulus. The cold-pressor test (immersion of hands in ice water) has been used clinically to induce transient hypertension, a phenomenon said to be more common in patients with essential hypertension.[51] Sympathetic stimulation caused by alcohol withdrawal and stress may have added to the effects of cold exposure in the patients that LRC reported.[50]

Dental procedures,[52,53] surgery directly involving or placing traction on the trigeminal nerve,[53,54] and stimulation of the trigeminal nerve[55] have also been associated with ICH. In one patient known to have been previously normotensive, dental pain after irrigation of the mouth was followed immediately by a fatal temporal lobe hemorrhage.[53] Blood pressure was elevated acutely. Necropsy showed no evidence of hypertensive vascular damage in any organ and no other cause of brain hemorrhage.[52] In a series of patients operated on intracranially for trigeminal neuralgia, hematomas developed at locations typical for hypertensive ICH.[54] Other procedures involving manipulation of the trigeminal nerve for treatment of trigeminal neuralgia have also been complicated by ICH.[38,56] Monitoring of blood pressure and heart rate during trigeminal stimulation often shows important fluctuations in blood pressure and pulse rate.[57,58] The blood vessels of the brains of animals and humans have important trigeminal innervation.[59,60]

ICH has often been associated with the use of illicit drugs, especially cocaine and methamphetamine, which are known to have sympatheticomimetic effects. We discuss drug-induced ICH in more detail later in this chapter because of its growing frequency as an important cause of stroke and ICH. Patients have also developed ICH after sudden augmentation of cerebral blood flow, either locally to one hemisphere, as in the circumstance of ICH after carotid endarterectomy,[61-63] or systemically, after correction of congenital heart defects or cardiac transplantation in the young.[64,65] ICH has also been reported to develop during recovery from migraine.[37,66,67] Intense vasoconstriction leads to diminished flow and, perhaps, ischemia to local blood vessels. Reperfusion then leads to ICH in the zone of prior vascular damage. A similar mechanism probably underlies most examples of hemorrhagic infarction caused by cerebral embolism.[68] This mechanism of brain hemorrhage is discussed in Chapter 10 on brain embolism.

Probably more important than the unusual circumstances just cited are events of everyday life that can raise blood pressure. Wilson was quite aware of this concept. He wrote in his neurology text, "Emotional experience, joy, anger, fear, or apprehension may disturb the action of the heart, trivial though the incident may be – an address at a public meeting, trouble with a cook, and so on."[69]

A patient of LRC's, LF, presented a vivid example of the possible interrelationship between daily activities and stresses, and the triggering of ICH. He was a retired university professor who came to ask his opinion about what he called a "strange stroke" he had a few years previously. Because he never had high blood pressure before or after the stroke, he was puzzled that his physicians attributed his condition to a hypertensive ICH. The events of his day are as follows:

> LF had an active teaching day, with more than the usual responsibilities. He hurried to finish his work so he could be on time for an engagement that night. His wife had symphony tickets. They planned to go with a couple (whom he considered to be unpleasant bores) to hear Mahler (whom he found tedious). He arrived late at the restaurant, and had a hurried and unpleasant meal. The two couples had to run to the symphony hall nearby to arrive in time to be seated, and they rushed to their seats in front. As he hustled toward his seat, he recalled thinking how wonderful it would have been to remain at work. He got to his seat in a sweat and noticed a gradually developing left hemiparesis.

LRC reviewed LF's CT and hospital records. A typical small right putaminal hemorrhage was present. His blood pressure was transiently elevated on admission, but soon normalized. Other patients, older men in LRC's experience, have developed ICH while straining during sex, often with younger women. Anger, and unusual straining while swimming laps or performing other exercises also have precipitated ICH in usually normotensive individuals.

Acute fluctuations in blood pressure and flow, and chronic degenerative changes are both important in the etiology of so-called hypertensive ICH. In either case, bleeding is into the territories of penetrating arteries. It is not known whether the size, location, and clinical picture differs in normotensive individuals who have an acute spike in blood pressure from those who have chronic hypertension.

In the case of JT, the patient described in the first portion of this chapter, he was hypertensive when first examined, but had no history of hypertension. Could the stressful interview have contributed to an acute blood pressure rise, or had he developed hypertension recently? His blood pressure stayed elevated during hospitalization, and he required antihypertensive treatment at the time of hospital discharge.

Older patients, often in their 70s or 80s, may present with ICH. Is this because of degenerative changes in these patients' arterial system? Does ICH occur because of coexistent amyloid angiopathy, which is recognized with increasing frequency when sought in elderly patients with lobar hemorrhages? Some older patients seem to develop ICH at relatively lower blood pressures than younger patients. Probably because of atrophy, symptoms of increased ICP, such as headache, vomiting, and reduced alertness, are less common in older patients, even with sizable lesions. This observation makes differentiation between hemorrhage and infarction more difficult in geriatric patients.

The usual loci of hypertensive ICH are shown in Table 14.1, which represents the actual distribution of lesion sites in a combined series of patients with ICH. Because hemorrhages

Table 14.1 Hypertensive ICH in the Michael Reese Stroke Registry and South Alabama cases

Anatomical site	Patients N (%)
Caudate nucleus	17 (9%)
Putamen and internal capsule	63 (32.5%)
Thalamus	43 (22%)
Lobar locations	38 (19.5%)
Cerebellum	14 (7%)
Pons	20 (10%)
Totals	**195 (100%)**

arise from deep penetrating arteries, they primarily affect brain regions nurtured by these vessels. In post-mortem analyses, an increasing number of patients dying of lobar brain hemorrhages are found to have unsuspected amyloid angiopathy. Rupture of fragile amyloid-containing arteries could be enhanced by raised arterial pressure.

Bleeding diathesis

A variety of coagulopathies can lead to bleeding into the brain substance, sometimes accompanied by systemic bleeding. Anticoagulation with heparin or warfarin accounts for an all-too-high percentage of this type of ICH and the frequency increased during the early years of the twenty-first century.[17,18,70,71] Considering the large number of patients treated with anticoagulants, the number that develop ICH is relatively small. Among a series of 1626 patients treated with long-term anticoagulants, 30 had ICH, of which two-thirds were fatal.[72] The most consistent risk factor for intracranial or systemic bleeding is prolongation of the international normalized ratio (INR) beyond the therapeutic range. Some hemorrhages occur even when the INR is in the therapeutic range.[17,18] As with other etiologies of ICH, hypertension aggravates the tendency to bleed intracranially. The three features that characterize anticoagulant-induced ICH as distinct from other causes are as follows:

1. Hemorrhage often develops gradually and insidiously during many hours, or even days (6/14 patients with anticoagulant-related ICH had an insidious clinical course).[17]
2. Hematoma growth is greater in patients with oral anticoagulant-related hemorrhage than in patients who had other spontaneous (that is non-traumatic, not associated with vascular malformations or aneurysms) causes. Among 303 ICH patients in one series, 21 had oral anticoagulant-related hemorrhages.[73] Baseline median ICH volume was greater in patients with oral anticoagulant-related hemorrhages compared to those with other spontaneous ICH causes (30.6 vs. 14.4 ml, $P = 0.03$).[73] Hemorrhage expansion (defined as >33% increase in ICH volume) occurred in 56% of patients with oral anticoagulant-related

hemorrhage compared to 26% of those who had other causes ($P = 0.006$).[73]

3. The cerebellum and cerebral lobes are involved more frequently than in hypertensive ICH.[17,18]
4. Oral anticoagulant-related hemorrhages have a high morbidity and mortality rate. In one series 15 of 24 patients died,[17,18] and only patients with smaller hematomas (<30-cc volume) had a favorable chance for survival; only one of 24 patients with ICH had bleeding elsewhere.[17,18] In another series 303 patients, the mortality was substantially higher in those with oral anticoagulant-related hemorrhage (62% vs. 17%, $P <0.001$).[73]

Anticoagulant-related ICH is a particularly difficult situation to treat because many patients take warfarin to prevent ischemic stroke. Patients with prosthetic heart valves, rheumatic mitral stenosis, or atrial fibrillation have a high risk for cerebral emboli without warfarin or other anticoagulant therapy. Especially when the indication for anticoagulants is strong and the early presenting symptoms are slight, treating physicians might not be inclined to reverse the bleeding using vitamin K, fresh frozen plasma, prothrombin complex concentrates, or recombinant factor VIIa. Some may choose to continue anticoagulant therapy after episodes of warfarin-related ICH. In our experience, this tactic is a mistake because many anticoagulant-related hemorrhages insidiously progress. Because of their size and location in the surgically accessible cerebellum and cerebral lobes, many eventually require lifesaving surgery.

The initial clinical diagnosis may also be difficult in the group on warfarin for stroke prophylaxis because the first reaction to the neurological symptoms is to predict that the patient had an ischemic stroke despite the treatment. I have found two useful axioms:

1. If a patient on anticoagulants develops neurological symptoms, the cause is anticoagulant-related hemorrhage until proven otherwise.
2. If anticoagulant (vitamin K antagonist) hemorrhage is verified, immediately give vitamin K, fresh frozen plasma, or prothrombin complex concentrates.

During the last decade newer oral anticoagulants that work through mechanisms other than vitamin K antagonism (direct thrombin inhibitors and factor Xa inhibitors) are gradually replacing heparin and warfarin. These agents, when compared to warfarin in patients with atrial fibrillation, were found to be equally or more effective in preventing new embolic strokes and had fewer instances of serious bleeding, especially less ICH.[74–78] There is too little information now available to know whether the location, size, and development of ICH will prove different with these newer anticoagulants compared to vitamin K antagonists. The management of hemorrhage after use of these agents will be discussed in the latter part of this chapter on treatment.

A common dilemma for clinicians is when to restart anticoagulants after an ICH or major systemic hemorrhage in

patients who require long-term anticoagulation (e.g., patients who have mechanical heart valves, atrial fibrillation with prior brain embolism).[79–84] The timing of re-instituting anticoagulants must be based on the situation in the individual patient. Some studies show that waiting 3 weeks or more after hemorrhage to restart led to fewer recurrent brain infarctions than expected.[79–81] In other patients restarting anticoagulation early (within 7–10 days) led to less recurrent hemorrhage than anticipated.[79,82] The treating clinician must weigh the risk of recurrent embolization (that is the benefit from anticoagulation) versus the risk of rebleeding. When the risk of rembolization is high and the risk of rebleeding low, then early reinstitution is recommended. When the risk of embolization is small (atrial fibrillation with normal left atrial size and no past brain infarcts) and the risk of rebleeding is substantial (poorly controlled hypertension) then a much longer delay, or using an antiplatelet rather than an anticoagulant seems prudent. Researchers used a Markov state transition decision model to compare the risk of anticoagulation after ICH in patients with deep hemorrhages (usually hypertensive) versus lobar hemorrhages (cerebral amyloid and/or hypertensive).[84] Anticoagulation of patients with lobar ICH had more risk and less potential gain than patients with deep hemorrhages (in whom hypertension could usually be controlled).[84]

Leukemia, hemophilia, thrombocytopenia, and disseminated intravascular coagulation are other important causes of ICH, although it is unusual in these disorders for bleeding to be confined only to the brain. Patients given recombinant tissue plasminogen activator (tPA) to treat coronary artery thrombosis sometimes develop ICH, most often in the cerebral lobes or cerebellum.[85] The frequency is low, but the brain hematomas can be devastating or fatal.[85] ICH also occurs after recombinant tPA infusion to treat occlusive cerebrovascular lesions.[86,87] In this circumstance, hematomas usually but not always develop within the region of brain infarction. In one analysis, among 312 tPA-treated patients, 20 developed symptomatic ICH.[87] Compared with placebo-treated patients, patients given tPA who developed brain hemorrhages were older, had more severe stroke neurological deficits, had higher serum glucose levels, and pretreatment brain imaging more often showed mass effect.[87] Saver calculated the number needed to harm: for every 100 patients treated with tPA, approximately one will become severely disabled or die as a result of tPA-related ICH.[86]

Drugs

A variety of commonly abused substances are known to cause ICH.[88–90] Alert clinicians should always think of the possibility of drug-related hemorrhage in young normotensive patients, in whom other causes of ICH, except trauma and arteriovenous malformations (AVMs), are rare. Best known are amphetamine ("speed") hemorrhages. Hemorrhage often develops within a few minutes of drug use. The most frequent presenting symptoms are headache, confusion, and seizures.[88,91,92] Despite large-volume ICHs, few focal signs are present in such patients. This phenomenon is perhaps explained by the frequent coexistence of brain edema, infarcts, and a diffuse vasculopathy, in addition to the focal ICH. In some patients, acute hypertension follows amphetamine use and can potentiate ICH. When first examined by physicians, most patients with amphetamine hemorrhage do not have signs of sympathetic overactivity, such as hypertension, tachycardia, or fever.[88–92]

Citron et al. studied 14 drug abusers, almost all admitting use of methamphetamine, among other drugs.[93] At necropsy, a fibrinoid necrosis of the media and intima of small- and medium-sized arteries existed, resembling polyarteritis nodosa.[93] Rumbaugh and colleagues studied the angiographic features of a group of methamphetamine abusers and noted beaded arteries with segmental constriction and dilatation of intracranial arteries.[94] In monkeys given intravenous amphetamines, angiography showed similar changes as found in human patients. Necropsy showed small brain hemorrhages, zones of infarction, microaneurysms, and a vasculitis similar to that described by Citron.[95] Recall that Fisher found prominent fibrinoid changes in small intracranial arteries and arterioles in patients who clinically had accelerated hypertension.[12,96] The rapid elevation in blood pressure may promote fibrinoid changes and even necrosis.

LRC reviewed 30 reported, well-documented examples of intracranial hemorrhage after amphetamine use.[88] Twenty-four patients were known drug abusers; some patients also used other drugs, and many often used alcohol along with amphetamines. Amphetamine, methamphetamine, and dextroamphetamine were the most frequently used other drugs. Seventeen individuals (57%) took oral amphetamines, 12 (40%) administered the drug intravenously, and one person inhaled amphetamine nasally. Amphetamine (14% of patients) and methamphetamine use were more often responsible for hemorrhage than dextroamphetamine (4%) use. The dose used was often unknown or unstated, but hemorrhage followed doses as small as 20 mg of oral amphetamine.[88,91] Age ranged from 19 years to 51 years, with an average age of 25.4 years.[88] In 23 individuals, the bleeding was intracerebral and most often lobar. In contrast to cocaine-related hemorrhage, only one of the 30 individuals (3%) had an underlying vascular lesion in the form of an aneurysm or AVM.[88,97] Amphetamine-related hemorrhage can be serious; 7 patients with hemorrhage died (23%), and 9 required surgical drainage (30%).[88] A potent solid form of D-methamphetamine base that can be smoked is available on the streets under the name ice. This form is more potent and rapid acting. The ice–amphetamine relation has the potential to prove similar to the crack-cocaine hydrochloride relationship in terms of complications and potency.

Angiography has often shown striking abnormalities in chronic amphetamine users and other patients with amphetamine-related ICH. Most common are segmental areas of constriction, irregularity, and occasionally fusiform dilatation.[88,91,92,98,99] The focal vascular abnormalities usually occur in superficial cortical arterial branches and are often referred to as beading. At times, the changes disappear on subsequent angiography.[98] These arteriographic changes have

been attributed to arteritis. Immunological phenomena are common in drug users.[88] Amphetamines are known to be potent vasoconstrictors. Vasoconstriction can become chronic and produce persistent morphological changes in the media of involved arteries. Segmental changes and beading in some amphetamine users are probably caused by pharmacological effects of the drugs used, and do not represent a true arteritis.

Since the early 1980s, cocaine has far surpassed amphetamines as a public health problem and cause of stroke and drug-related ICH. Cocaine hydrochloride is usually snorted nasally. During the 1980s, addicts turned to crack cocaine, a substance made by mixing aqueous cocaine hydrochloride with ammonia and sometimes baking soda. Crack cocaine is smoked or inhaled after the cocaine is mixed in the alkaline solution and is precipitated as alkaloidal cocaine. Crack cocaine is absorbed quickly, reaching the brain in less than 10 seconds.[88–90] Cocaine hydrochloride can be taken in a variety of ways-orally, vaginally, rectally, sublingually, nasally, and by subcutaneous, intramuscular, or intravenous injection. Cardiovascular effects begin immediately after use and consist of an increase in pulse, blood pressure, temperature, and metabolism. The pressor effects of cocaine are similar to those of amphetamine and are probably mediated through a peripheral catecholamine mechanism.[88–90,100,101]

In a 1994 text, LRC reviewed 45 examples of cocaine-related ICH.[88] The series included 28 men and 17 women, with ages ranging from 22 years to 57 years (average age, 33.6 years). Headache, focal neurological signs, and sudden loss of consciousness were the most frequent symptoms and usually began immediately or shortly after the episode of drug use.[88,101] Concurrent use of alcohol was common. ICH followed use of cocaine when taken by any route. Fifteen individuals used crack, 14 snorted cocaine nasally, and 11 injected the drug intravenously. The acute mortality was relatively high (14/45, 31%).[88]

The most common location of cocaine-related ICH was lobar (57%). In others, the bleeding often involved deep structures known as frequent sites of hypertensive ICH. These included one caudate, three thalamic, and eight putaminal hematomas. Of great interest and importance was the frequent presence of an underlying vascular lesion. Twelve patients had AVMs, three had aneurysms, and one had a glioma with recurrent hemorrhage.[88] Similarly, among 31 patients who developed SAH after cocaine use, 15 (48%) had aneurysms. Among 29 patients with adequate angiographic or necropsy study, or both, 25 (86%) had aneurysms.[88] Cocaine-related ICH has a high mortality and high frequency of underlying aneurysms and AVMs. Clearly, cocaine-related intracranial bleeding is an indication for angiography, especially when the bleeding is subarachnoid or lobar. Underlying vascular lesions are less common when the ICH is deep. Most authors have attributed cocaine-related hemorrhage to the sympatheticomimetic effects of the drug. In some reported cases, the blood pressure is high after admission (i.e., 240/140 mmHg, 220/110 mmHg, or 210/120 mmHg).[88] Some patients have had a hypertensive encephalopathy with multiple ICHs and brain edema. An example of these changes is shown in Figure 12.18.

Another drug known to have sympatheticomimetic capabilities is phencyclidine, known as PCP or angel dust, which has also been occasionally implicated as a cause of ICH[102,103] and hypertensive encephalopathy.[104] Two other hallucinogens, lysergic acid diethylamide (known as LSD) and mescaline, are also known to raise blood pressure and cause vasoconstriction. To our knowledge (LRC), however, no reports document ICH after use of these drugs.

More controversial is the issue of ICH after use of amphetamine-like drugs that are mostly used as anorexic agents to lose weight and in cough and cold remedies. These drugs were usually sold over the counter. The most commonly cited agent was phenylpropanolamine (PPA), which was often combined with an antihistamine and caffeine. PPA is primarily a partial alpha-adrenergic agonist and has little, if any, beta-adrenergic agonist activity.[105,106] PPA was used by individuals who developed ICH, but the numbers are relatively small, considering the frequency of use. Among 19 patients, only 4 were men.[88] Ten of the 19 patients were younger than 30 years old. In some, the PPA compounds were taken in high doses in suicidal attempts. Two patients had SAH only, and 17 patients had ICH (2 of which were multiple).[107,108] Twelve PPA-related hematomas were lobar, seven were putaminal-capsular, and two were thalamic.[88] Blood pressures recorded on initial examination were usually within the normal range, but some were high (i.e., 210/130 mmHg, 160/104 mmHg, and 210/110 mmHg). Kernan and colleagues compared the frequency of hemorrhagic stroke among 702 patients who had taken phenylpropanolamine in some form with 1376 controls.[106] No men reported the use of appetite suppressants in this analysis. For women, the adjusted odds ratio (OR) was 16.58 (95% confidence interval (CI) 1.51–182.21, $P = 0.02$) for the association between the use of appetite suppressants containing PPA and the risk of a hemorrhagic stroke. The OR for an association with cough or cold suppressants was much lower (1.23, 95% CI 0.68–2.24, $P = 0.49$).[105] The frequency of hemorrhage was most common when PPA was given shortly before the hemorrhage and when doses higher than 75 mg were consumed.[105]

Segmental vascular changes on angiography, similar to those found after amphetamine use, have been described.[109] In one patient, the angiographic changes cleared after abstinence from PPA for one month.[109] In four patients, histological analysis of tissue removed at surgical drainage of hematomas was available. Three patients had no indication of vascular lesion on light microscopy, but the fourth patient did have a necrotizing vasculitis.[110]

Examples of putative PPA-related hemorrhages are difficult to evaluate. In some cases, use of diet pills was surely incidental, and in other patients, multiple other drugs and risk factors coexisted.[88] In several patients, ICH occurred a few weeks postpartum, a time of vulnerability for spontaneous vascular complications. Although PPA has been shown to be associated with ICH in experimental animals[111] and humans,[88,107–112] reactions to PPA compounds are often idiosyncratic. A risk of ICH clearly exists for those who use PPA in a higher-than-suggested dose. Prior hypertension; additional

485

use of alcohol, coffee, or caffeine; concomitant use of mono-amine oxidase inhibitors; and use during the postpartum period increase the risk of hemorrhage after PPA ingestion. Phenylephrine has been associated with precipitating the reversible cerebral vasoconstriction syndrome (discussed in Chapter 12). Because it has sympatheticomimetic properties it has the potential to provoke ICH in some individuals.[113]

Occasionally, ICH develops after the intravenous use of drugs that are manufactured for oral consumption, such as pentazocine and pyribenzamine ("T's and blues") or methylphenidate.[88,114] Talc, methylcellulose crystals, and cornstarch obliterate the lung arterioles, allowing the injected particles to reach the systemic circulation after intravenous use. The damage to brain arterioles then predisposes users to develop ICH.[114]

Occasional examples of ICH have been described after the use of the phosphodiesterase inhibitors sildenafil (Viagra), vardenafil (Levitra), and tadalafil (Cialis) prescribed to enhance erectile function in men.[115–118] It is unclear if the ICH in these patients was attributable to the phosphodiesterase inhibitor alone or to physical effort involved during sexual intercourse, or to a combination of the agents and circulatory changes that occurred during coition.

Cerebral amyloid angiopathy

Congophilic or cerebral amyloid angiopathy (CAA) was recognized by Zenkevich as a potential cause of ICH,[119] but Jellinger is probably most responsible for bringing this disorder to the attention of the neurological community.[120,121] This condition is also discussed in Chapter 12.

Awareness of CAA and its clinical and imaging findings has led to recognition that an ever-increasing percentage of ICH, especially in the elderly, is related to CAA.[122,123] The disorder usually affects small arteries and arterioles in the leptomeninges and cerebral cortex; involved arteries are thickened by an acellular hyaline material that stains positively with periodic acid-Schiff stains, and has an apple-green birefringence under polarized light on Congo red stain.[124] Figure 12.10 shows a brain section that contains amyloid-staining arterioles. Sometimes, the vessel wall seems to be reduplicated or split. CAA predominantly affects persons older than 65 years, but some individuals show symptoms in their 50s. The frequency of finding CAA at necropsy increases in the eighth and ninth decades.[124] In some series of patients, a striking female predilection exists.[125,126] At necropsy, most patients have senile plaques, and many patients have been diagnosed clinically with Alzheimer's disease.

Amyloid-laden arteries are most often found in the occipital and parietal regions, less often in the other cerebral lobes; rarely, if ever, are these arteries found in the deep basal gray matter, brain stem, or cerebellum. Hemorrhages may be quite large and are often multiple.[126–129] Some patients have recurrent ICH or SAH in different lobar sites, a finding in an elderly person that is virtually diagnostic of CAA. At necropsy, small scattered cerebral infarcts and Alzheimer's-related changes are found, along with evidence of old slit-like lobar hemorrhages. Echo planar MRI scans may show many small old hemorrhages (Figure 12.11). Some patients have a Binswanger-like picture,

with chronic white matter gliosis and atrophy. Like anticoagulant-related hemorrhages, CAA-related hemorrhages may develop insidiously. Perhaps because of coexisting atrophy, increased intracranial pressure symptoms such as headache and vomiting, are less frequent than in younger patients with hypertensive or AVM-related hemorrhages.

Trauma

Trauma is an important cause of intracerebral bleeding. In some patients, a traumatic etiology is not clear from the history. We have seen several patients who were rendered aphasic or stuporous by head blows delivered by others and who could give no history of the trauma; assailants and others did not disclose their complicity. In other patients, retrograde amnesia developed after the head injury, and patients had no recollection of a fall or other injury. A search for superficial head bruises or lacerations is worthwhile when the etiology of ICH is not obvious. Traumatic ICH is most often accompanied by contusions in the basal frontal and temporal lobes, which may be multiple.[130] Occasionally, a late or delayed hemorrhage, referred to as a spät hemorrhage, develops into an area of traumatic brain edema when the local swelling subsides.[130,131]

Other causes and frequency of various etiologies

Brain tumors[132] and vasculitis and vasculopathies of various types[133] are occasionally complicated by ICH. Dural sinus and cerebral venous thrombosis is another important cause of ICH and is discussed in Chapter 15. Table 14.2 lists the frequencies of common etiologies among six large series of ICH patients.[134–141] Table 14.3 shows the frequency of various causes of ICH in a series of 200 Mexican patients younger than 40 years. This table illustrates the locations of hemorrhages in patients with these etiologies according to age.[142]

Signs and symptoms of intracerebral hemorrhage at common locations

Just as there are physicians who believe the introduction of chest x-rays made the stethoscope obsolete, some doctors believe that detailed knowledge of the findings on neurological examination of patients with central nervous system lesions is no longer necessary since the advent of CT and MRI scans. Because hemorrhages are so well imaged by CT, why bother to learn the physical findings? In the future, physicians will probably not have a pocket or portable CT or MRI to replace the examination of patients. Prognosis and treatment of ICH often depends on the locale of the hemorrhage. Particular locations (i.e., cerebral lobes, right putamen, and cerebellum) are relatively accessible to surgical drainage, whereas others (i.e., thalami and brainstem) are not accessible. Clinical distinction between ICH and superficial cerebral infarction caused by large vessel occlusive disease or cerebral embolism depends on localization of the lesion to deep (ICH) or superficial (infarct) location. Knowledge of findings in patients with hemorrhages at various locations teaches clinicians to search for tumors, abscesses, demyelinating lesions, and other disorders in the same locations in other patients.

Table 14.2 Causes of ICH in large series of patients

	Russell[135] (%)	Mutlu et al.[136] (%)	McCormick and Rosenfield[137] (%)	Schutz[138] (%)	Jellinger[139] (%)	Weisberg[140] (%)	Qureshi et al.[141] (%)
Hypertension	232(50)	135(60)	37(26)	140(56)	80(47)	197(66)	311(77)
Vasc malform	117(25)	50(22)	35(24)	30(12)	53(31)	28(9)	11(3)
Bleeding dis	36(8)	30(13)	28(20)	21(8)	5(3)	14(5)	8(2)
Tumor	9(2)	2(1)	13(9)	8(3)	12(7)	5(2)	–
Arteritis	13(3)	2(1)	5(3)	2(1)	2(1)	–	–
Other	38(8)	6(3)	14(10)	–	13(8)	2(1)	–
Unknown	16(4)	–	12(8)	49(20)	5(3)	50(17)	73(18)
Totals	**461**	**225**	**144**	**250**	**170**	**296**	**403**

Bleeding dis, bleeding disorder (including thrombolysis/anticoagulation); Vasc malform, vascular malformations including aneurysms.
Modified from Caplan LR, Kase CS. Mechanisms of intracerebral hemorrhage. In Kase CS, Caplan LR (eds), *Intracerebral Hemorrhage*. Boston: Butterworth–Heinemann, 1994, pp 95–98 with permission.

Table 14.3 Frequency of location of ICH by cause in patients younger than 40 years of age

Cause	Lobar (N = 110)	Ganglionic (N = 43)	Brainstem (N = 26)	Cerebellum (N = 10)	Ventrical (N = 8)	Mixed (N = 3)
Hypertension (N = 22)	2	**16**	3	0	0	1
AVM (N = 67)	**45**	7	6	**6**	3	0
Cav angioma (N = 32)	**15**	3	**11**	2	1	0
CVT (N = 10)	9	1	0	0	0	0
Drugs (N = 7)	3	4	0	0	0	0
Toxemia (N = 7)	3	4	0	0	0	0
Other (N = 14)	9	1	0	1	2	1
Unknown (N = 41)	24	7	6	1	2	1

AVM, arteriovenous malformation; Cav angioma, cavernous angioma; CVT, cerebral venous thrombosis; Ventrical, intraventricular; toxemia, preeclampsia and eclampsia.
From Ruiz-Sandoval JL, Cantu C, Barinagarrementeria F. Intracerebral hemorrhage in young people: Analysis of risk factors, locations, causes, and prognosis. *Stroke* 1999;30:537–541 with permission.

Historically, hemorrhages in the cerebellum, thalami, and caudate nucleus were recognized before cerebellar, thalamic, or caudate infarction. Awareness of the clinical syndromes associated with ICH in these locations made it possible to later recognize infarcts in these regions. For these and many other regions, it is still important for clinicians to know the common clinical syndromes in ICH and be able to localize clinically the lesion in most patients with intracranial hemorrhages.[143]

Keys to localization of ICH are as follows:

1. Motor signs – quadriparesis, hemiparesis, or no paresis
2. Pupillary function – asymmetry, size, and light reaction
3. Extraocular movements – supranuclear, nuclear, internuclear gaze palsies
4. Gait abnormalities – especially ataxia

Figure 14.5 **and** Table 14.4 summarize the usual abnormalities of these functions in patients with hemorrhages at the most common locations of ICH.

Hemorrhages of the lateral basal ganglia, putamen, and internal capsule

The most common location of hypertensive ICH is the lateral basal ganglionic capsular region.[141–145] These lesions have traditionally been referred to as putaminal hemorrhages because they most often begin in the putamen but the globus pallidus and capsular white matter are often also involved. Striatocapsular hemorrhage is a more accurate term. The usual findings include contralateral hemiparesis, contralateral hemisensory loss, and conjugate deviation of the eyes toward

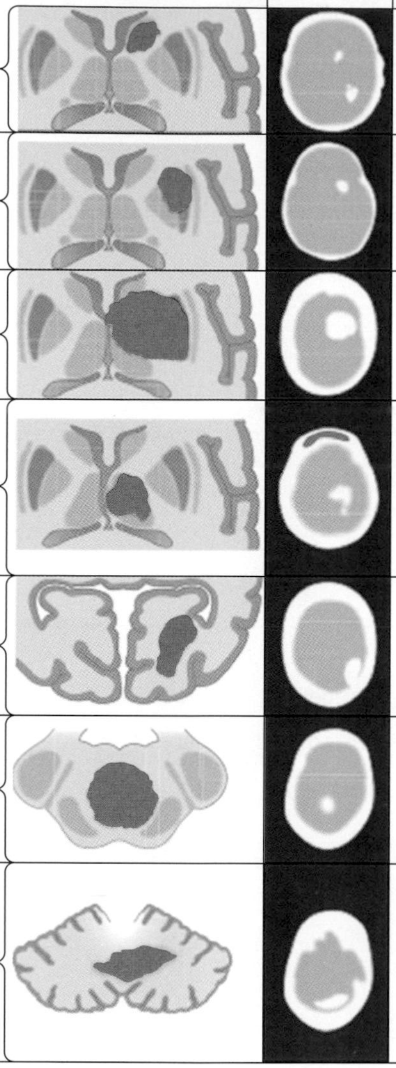

	Pathology	CT	Pupils	Eye movements	Motor and sensory deficits	Other
Caudate nucleus (blood in ventricle)			Sometimes ipsilaterally constricted	Conjugate deviation to side of lesion, slight ptosis	Contralateral hemiparesis, often transient	Headache, confusion
Putamen (small hemorrhage)			Normal	Conjugate deviation to side of lesion	Contralateral hemiparesis and hemisensory loss	Aphasia (if lesion on left side)
Putamen (large hemorrhage)			In presence of herniation, pupil dilated on side of lesion	Conjugate deviation to side of lesion	Contralateral hemiparesis and hemisensory loss	Decreased consciousness
Thalamus			Constricted, poorly reactive to light bilaterally	Both lids retracted. Eyes positioned downward and medially. Cannot look upward	Slight contralateral hemiparesis, but greater hemisensory loss	Aphasia (if lesion on left side)
Occipital lobar white matter			Normal	Normal	Mild, transient hemiparesis	Contralateral hemianopsia
Pons			Constricted, reactive to light	No horizontal movements. Vertical movements preserved	Quadriplegia	Coma
Cerebellum			Slight constriction on side of lesion	Slight deviation to opposite side. Movements toward side of lesion impaired, or sixth cranial nerve palsy	Ipsilateral limb ataxia. No hemiparesis	Gait ataxia, vomiting

Figure 14.5 Clinical manifestations related to site in ICH. Copyright 1986 CIBA Pharmaceutical Company, division of CIBA-GEIGY Corporation. Reprinted with permission from The Ciba Collection of Medical Illustrations, illustrated by Frank H Netter, MD. All rights reserved.

the side of the hematoma. The pupils are generally normal and gait is hemiparetic. Patients with a left putaminal hemorrhage usually have a non-fluent aphasia with relative preservation of ability to repeat spoken language. Right-sided lesions are associated with left visual neglect, motor impersistence, and constructional dyspraxia. These abnormalities of higher cortical function are probably caused by disconnection and undercutting of cortical zones, and are usually more transient than in patients with cortical infarcts of equal size. Some patients develop ipsilateral adventitious movements that the family or observers call "tremor;" these movements are probably caused by involvement of ipsilateral descending projections of the extrapyramidal system.

In patients with large putaminal hemorrhages, stupor increases as the lesion enlarges; the ipsilateral pupil at first becomes smaller, and later, larger than the opposite pupil; the ipsilateral plantar response becomes extensor; and a bilateral horizontal gaze palsy develops. The presence of any of these signs – ipsilateral Babinski's sign, abnormal ipsilateral pupil, or ipsilateral gaze paresis – has a grim prognosis.[11,24,144] These additional findings are caused by midline shift or compression of the rostral brain stem by the expanding hematoma. Figure 14.6 shows necropsy brain specimens of large putaminal hemorrhages.

The findings described so far are those found in patients with large hematomas, which involve the medial and most anterior portions of the posterior putamen, and the anterior two-thirds of the posterior limb of the internal capsule.[145–147] This location is the most common site for putaminal hemorrhage because it is supplied by the largest of the lateral lenticulostriate arteries. Some lesions affect the anterior limb of the internal capsule and anterior putamen and produce a milder, more transient hemiparesis without sensory abnormalities.[144–146] When hematomas are in the posterior third of the internal capsule and at the far posterior extreme of the putamen, sensory abnormalities predominate, with little or no hemiparesis. An inferior quadrantanopia or hemianopia may be present. Patients with lesions in the far posterior left putamen may

Table 14.4 Neurological signs in patients with ICHs at common sites

Location	Motor signs	Sensory loss	Hemianopia	Pupils	Eye movements	Other signs
Caudate	±Hemiparesis	No	No	Normal	Normal	Confusion, dysmemory
Putaminal small	Hemiparesis++	+	No	Normal	Normal	None
Large	Hemiparesis++++	++	++	*	Contralateral CGP	L–aphasia; R–left neglect, anosognosia
Thalamic	±Hemiparesis	++	±	Ipsilateral small, non-reactive	Eyes down or down and upward vertical gaze palsy	Confusion, decreased alertness; L–aphasia
Lobar frontal	±Hemiparesis	No	No	Normal	Normal	Abulia, L–aphasia
Parietal	±Hemiparesis	+	++	Normal	Normal	L–aphasia; R–left neglect, anosognosia
Temporal	No	No	+	Normal	Normal	L–aphasia
Occipital	No	No	++++	Normal	Normal	L–dyslexia
Pontine (large tegmentobasal)	Quadriparesis ++++; can be locked-in	±	No	Small, reactive	Bilateral horizontal gaze palsy	Coma
Cerebellar	No	No	No	Ipsilateral small	Ipsilateral VIth-nerve palsy or CGP	Gait ataxia; veering to one side

CGP, conjugate gaze palsy; L, left; R, right.
* When there is significant mass effect the ipsilateral pupil becomes at first small and then becomes large and non-reactive.

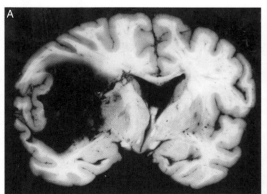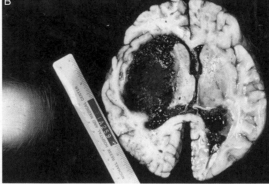

Figure 14.6 Large putaminal hemorrhages. (A) A coronal section of the brain at necropsy showing a large hemorrhage on the left of the figure. The insular cortex is displaced laterally and the basal ganglia are displaced medially. The hemorrhage has drained into the lateral ventricles. The midline is shifted to the right. (B) Axial section (in usual CT plane) of the brain at necropsy showing a very large putaminal hemorrhage that displaces the midline and drains into the lateral ventricles. From Caplan LR. Putaminal hemorrhage. In Kase CS, Caplan LR (eds), *Intracerebral Hemorrhage*. Boston: Butterworth–Heinemann, 1994, pp 309–327 with permission.

have fluent Wernicke-like aphasia because of undercutting of the temporal lobe or extension of the lesion into the temporal isthmus, giving the hematoma a hockey stick-like configuration. Figure 14.7 shows the anatomical distribution of lesions within the lateral basal ganglionic region on horizontal brain section. The most common and largest lesions affecting the anterior part of the posterior limb of the internal capsule are often referred to as the middle type, whereas the others are termed anterior or posterior types of putaminal hematomas.[144] Figure 14.8 shows drawings that illustrate various typical striatocapsular hemorrhages

Putaminal hemorrhages vary greatly in size. In 1 series of 24 patients,[31] the smallest hematoma volume was 20 mm^3, whereas the largest was 225 mm^3. Patients with small hematomas, as shown in Figure 14.9, have a good outcome. Larger hemorrhages are more likely to rupture into the ventricle, and have a much higher mortality than small putaminal hematomas.[31,144,145,148,149] Hematoma volume is the most important determinant of outcome.[149] Most often, bleeding extends along the anteroposterior axis of the brain, but some lesions are globoid, and others extend laterally toward the cortical surface along white matter tracts.[31,144,145] Analysis of

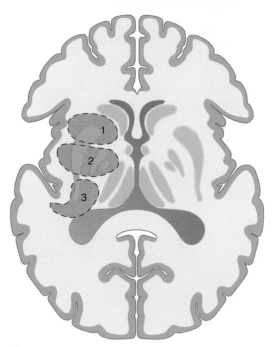

Figure 14.7 Drawing of an axial brain section showing, using circles, the loci of striatocapsular hemorrhages: 1. Anterior type involving the anterior putamen and the anterior limb of the internal capsule; 2. middle type involving the capsular genu and the globus pallidus and the middle of the putamen; and 3. posterior type involving the far posterior limb of the internal capsule and often affecting the optic radiations and spreading into the temporal lobe isthmus.

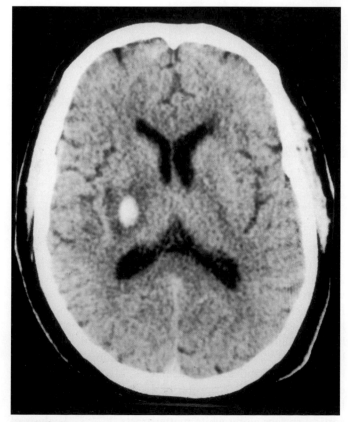

Figure 14.9 CT showing a small left putaminal hemorrhage.

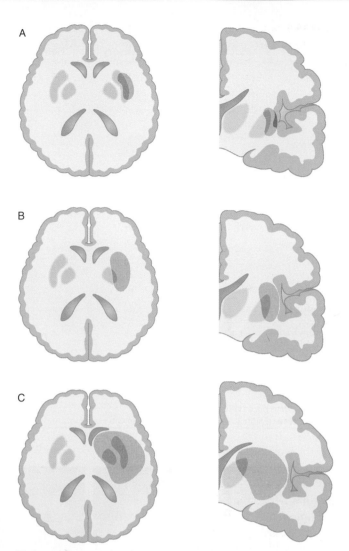

Figure 14.8 Examples of putaminal hemorrhages in axial and coronal sections. A. Hemorrhage within the boundaries of the putamen. B. Encroachment on the internal capsule. C. Hematoma expanding laterally and also medially where it compresses the lateral ventricle.

CT scans at the level of the body of the lateral ventricles can help prognosticate the likelihood of recovery from hemiplegia.[146] When the hematoma occupies CT-sections containing the bodies of the lateral ventricles, then the middle type of hematoma is usually present and hemiplegia is likely to persist. When this region is free of bleeding, hemiparesis is more often absent, slight, or transient.[146]

Before the advent of CT scanning, cerebral angiography was used to study and localize putaminal hemorrhages. Using microangiography, Mizukami and colleagues studied 60 post-mortem specimens from patients with ICH.[150] They identified the source of bleeding as lateral lenticulostrate arteries, analyzed the post-mortem displacement of these vessels, and correlated their findings with the angiographic anatomy in 100 other patients with autopsy or surgically confirmed ICH.[150] In large putaminal hemorrhages, the most lateral lenticulostrate arteries are displaced medially, increasing the distance between the most lateral lenticulostrate arteries and the insular artery. Anterior and posterior lesions have different patterns of displacement of lenticulostrate arteries.[150]

Since the mid-1980s, positron emission tomography and single-photon emission computed tomography have yielded insights into the clinical findings in patients with putaminal hemorrhage.[151] Anterior lesions show depression of frontal lobe function ipsilaterally, whereas posterior lesions more often affect the temporal and parietal lobes. The pattern of cortical depression helps predict aphasia type and recovery.[151]

Caudate hemorrhage

Hemorrhage into the caudate nucleus accounts for approximately 7% of ICH.[152–155] Hematomas at this site frequently discharge quickly into the adjacent lateral ventricle, or may spread laterally toward the internal capsule or inferiorly toward the hypothalamus. Figure 14.10 is a necropsy specimen of a caudate hemorrhage that emptied into the adjacent lateral ventricle. Early ventricular dilatation by blood probably accounts for the most common symptoms of caudate hemorrhage (headache, vomiting, decreased alertness, and stiff neck).[152–155] Some patients also are confused, disoriented, and have poor memory. The larger parenchymatous hematomas cause a contralateral hemiparesis, conjugate deviation of the eyes to the side of the lesion, conjugate gaze palsy to the opposite side, and an ipsilateral small pupil or Horner's syndrome.[152,154] Sensory findings are usually absent or minimal. The usual cause of caudate hemorrhage is hypertension, but AVMs are also common, especially in the young. Caudate hematomas have a better prognosis than comparable-sized putaminal hemorrhages.

Symptoms and signs of caudate hemorrhage closely mimic SAH, but the CT appearance of blood in the caudate and lateral ventricles is distinctive.

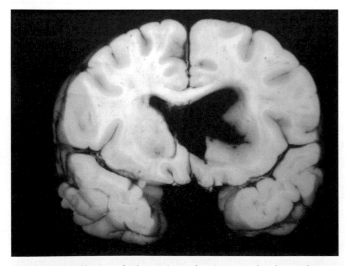

Figure 14.10 Necropsy brain specimen showing a caudate hemorrhage that extended into the adjacent lateral ventricle. From Caplan LR. Caudate hemorrhage. In Kase CS, Caplan LR (eds), *Intracerebral Hemorrhage*. Boston: Butterworth–Heinemann, 1994, pp 329–340 with permission. A black and white version of this figure will appear in some formats. For the color version, please refer to the plate section.

Thalamic hemorrhage

Neurological signs in patients with thalamic hemorrhages differ greatly depending on the size, location within the thalamus of the hematoma, and dissection into and pressure effects on the IIIrd ventricle and adjacent brain structures.[156,157] The largest hemorrhages are located in the ventrolateral and posteromedial portions of the thalamus in the territories of the thalamogeniculate and thalamic-subthalamic arteries.[157] Other hemorrhages are located anteriorly in the territory of the tuberothalamic (polar) arteries and dorsally in the territory of the lateral posterior choroidal arteries.[157]

Most thalamic hematomas are posterior and medial to the pyramidal-tract fibers in the internal capsule, so that contralateral sensory abnormalities are usually more prominent than contralateral hemiparesis. Some large thalamic hematomas dissect rostrally and involve the anterior portion of the posterior limb of the internal capsule, causing a hemiplegia. Sometimes, limbs contralateral to hematomas are slightly ataxic or have choreic movements. The contralateral hand may rest in a fisted or dystonic posture. The key neurological findings that separate thalamic from caudate or putaminal hemorrhages are the eye signs. Patients with caudate or putaminal hemorrhages who have abnormal eye movements have conjugate deviation of the eyes toward the side of the lesion and paresis of conjugate gaze to the opposite side. The characteristic oculomotor abnormalities in patients with thalamic hematomas are as follows:

1. Paralysis of upward gaze, often with one or both eyes resting downward.
2. Hyperconvergence of one or both eyes,[36,156,158] with a combination of these findings giving patients the appearance of peering downward and inward at the tip of their noses.
3. Ocular skewing, in which one eye rests below the other, with this divergence in vertical eye position remaining constant in gaze in all directions.
4. Eyes gazing the wrong way resting toward the opposite side.[36,156]
5. Disconjugate gaze, with limited abduction of one or both eyes not attributable to involvement of the VIth nerve (so-called pseudo VIth-nerve paresis),[156,159] a failure of ocular abduction caused by visual fixation from the adducted eye, and increased convergence vectors neutralizing abduction.

These oculomotor abnormalities are caused by direct extension of the hematoma to the diencephalic–mesencephalic junction or compression of the quadrigeminal plate region by the thalamic hematoma. In thalamic hemorrhage, the pupils are usually small and react poorly to light because of interruption of the afferent limb of the pupillary reflex arc.

Patients with large left thalamic hemorrhages may have an unusual aphasia.[156,160–162] After beginning a conversation almost normally, patients may lapse into a remarkable fluent aphasia, with many jargon or non-existent words and poor communication of ideas. In contrast to patients with Wernicke's aphasia, comprehension of spoken language is

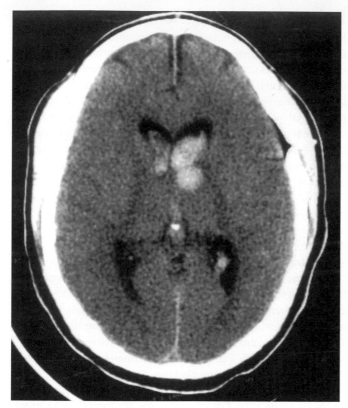

Figure 14.11 CT showing a small left anterior thalamic hematoma, which drained into the lateral ventricles; blood casts are seen within the ventricle.

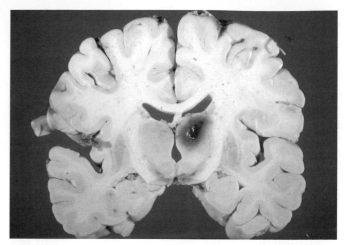

Figure 14.12 Necropsy specimen showing a small anterior thalamic hemorrhage. From Caplan LR. Thalamic hemorrhage. In Kase CS, Caplan LR (eds), *Intracerebral Hemorrhage*. Boston: Butterworth–Heinemann, 1994, pp 341–362 with permission. A black and white version of this figure will appear in some formats. For the color version, please refer to the plate section.

good. Patients with thalamic ICH may repeat and duplicate words or syllables at the ends of words in spoken and written language. Paraphasic errors and poor naming are also common. Patients with right thalamic hematomas often have left visual neglect, anosognosia, and visuospatial abnormalities.[156,163]

Decreased levels of alertness, consciousness, and hypersomnolence are common at the onset of thalamic hemorrhage because of involvement of the rostral reticular activating system. The prognosis for recovery from thalamic hemorrhages is not as good as caudate or putaminal hemorrhages of comparable size, but coma is not as dire a prognostic sign in thalamic lesions as it is in other supratentorial sites. Also, unlike putaminal hemorrhage, the severity of the deficit and mortality do not correlate with ventricular extension in patients with thalamic hematomas.[164] Figure 14.11 shows a CT scan from a patient with an anterior thalamic hematoma, which spread into the ventricles. She made an excellent recovery. Thalamic hemorrhages are not accessible surgically unless they extend far laterally. Most studies have not differentiated medial from lateral or posterior thalamic hematomas, although lesions at these various sites yield different clinical syndromes and have different prognoses for recovery.[156,157]

Since the mid 1980s it has been possible to distinguish syndromes related to small discrete hemorrhages in the thalamus using CT/MRI scanning.[156,157,165,166] The posterolateral type in the territory of the thalamogeniculate arteries are the most common and largest type of thalamic hematoma. These lesions often spill out of the thalamus laterally and may cause

motor paralysis by involving the internal capsule. Sensorimotor signs predominate, and pupillary and eye-movement abnormalities are slight or absent, unless the hematoma is quite large and spreads to or compresses the medial thalamus.[156,157] Anterior or anterolateral thalamic hematomas are in the distribution of the tuberothalamic (polar) artery. Figure 14.12 is a necropsy specimen showing an anterior thalamic hemorrhage. Behavioral abnormalities predominate, especially apathy and abulia.[156,157] Posteromedial hematomas are in the distribution of the thalamic–subthalamic thalamoperforating arteries; abnormalities of consciousness, pupillary function, and vertical gaze predominate. The hematoma often spreads to the IIIrd ventricle and can compress the diencephalic–mesencephalic junction and obstruct the IIIrd ventricle, causing hydrocephalus.[156] Oculomotor abnormalities found in patients with posteromedial hematomas may improve after ventricular drainage, indicating these abnormalities were caused by downward pressure on the midbrain.[167,168] Far posterior and dorsal lesions predominantly involve the pulvinar in the distribution of the posterior choroidal arteries; slight sensorimotor signs may be found but are usually transient, and aphasia and behavioral abnormalities are common.[157] Figure 14.13 shows a montage of CT and MRI scans of thalamic hemorrhages. Figure 14.14 shows MRI scans of a large thalamic hematoma that likely originated in the pulvinar region in a patient with a prior putaminal hemorrhage.

Lobar hemorrhages

ICH may develop beneath the region of the gray–white junction of the cerebral cortex. These subcortical hemorrhages usually spread in a linear direction along white matter pathways. When the hematomas absorb, linear cavities remain, giving the lesions the name slit hemorrhage. The lesions undercut cortex and often do not obey the strict divisions of cerebral lobes; hence, the term lobar hemorrhage actually is inaccurate. Nonetheless, we use this term because of its widespread acceptance. Undercutting of the cortex can be epileptogenic, causing repeated focal seizures of limited duration.[169–172]

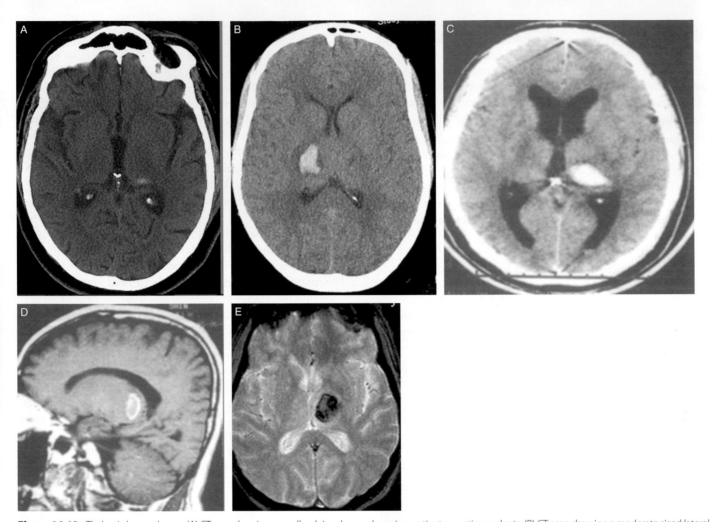

Figure 14.13 Thalamic hemorrhages. (A) CT scan showing a small pulvinar hemorrhage in a patient on anticoagulants. (B) CT scan showing a moderate sized lateral thalamic hemorrhage with surrounding edema. (C) CT showing a larger pulvinar hemorrhage. (D) MRI T1-weighted sagittal view of a pulvinar hemorrhage. From Chung C-S, Caplan LR, Han W, et al. Thalamic haemorrhage. *Brain* 1996;119:1873–1886 with permission of Oxford University Press. (E) GRE MRI image of a large thalamic hemorrhage.

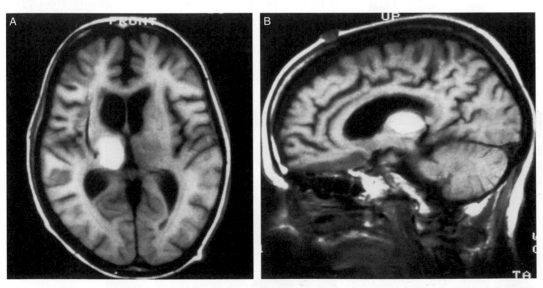

Figure 14.14 MRI T2-weighted axial (A) and sagittal (B) sections, showing a large right thalamic hematoma located in the pulvinar. A cavity related to an old slit putaminal hemorrhage is also visible in the axial section.

Subcortical hemorrhages are important to diagnose because the symptoms and signs are often erroneously attributed to cerebral infarction. Inappropriate therapy might be prescribed unless brain imaging shows the hematomas. Also, if subcortical hemorrhages are large, they are relatively superficial and are more accessible to surgical drainage than deeper hematomas. In the past, subcortical hemorrhages were rarely diagnosed antemortem, but CT and MRI greatly enhance

recognition of these lesions. Many lobar hemorrhages are caused by AVMs, cavernous angiomas, and amyloid angiopathy, each of which has a predilection for cortical and subcortical regions. Hypertension is also an important cause of lobar hematomas. The parietal and occipital lobes are affected more often than the frontal and parietal regions. Symptoms and signs depend on the lobes affected, as follows:[169–172]

1. Frontal hematomas: Far anterior lesions usually cause abulia. Patients appear apathetic and have reduced spontaneity, prolonged latency in responding, and short, terse replies. If the lesions extend deeply or toward the precentral gyrus, conjugate eye deviation toward the side of the hematoma and contralateral hemiparesis are found. Figure 14.15 shows a CT scan of a large recent left frontal hemorrhage.

2. Paracentral hematomas: Lesions near the central sulcus produce contralateral motor and sensory signs, sometimes with aphasia if the lesion is in the left hemisphere.

3. Parietal hemorrhages: Parietal hemorrhages are usually accompanied by contralateral hemisensory loss, with neglect of the contralateral visual field. The limbs contralateral to the hemorrhage are often uncoordinated. Aphasia and disorders of reading, writing, and arithmetic functions are present when the lesions involve the left inferior parietal lobule. Patients with right inferior parietal hematomas have defective drawing and copying and may have difficulty with visual-spatial functions.

4. Occipital hematomas: Occipital hemorrhages cause a severe contralateral hemianopia, often with slight contralateral hemisensory or motor signs and visual neglect.

5. Temporal-lobe lesions: Temporal-lobe lesions often cause agitation and delirium. Wernicke-type aphasia accompanies left temporal lesions. Temporal-lobe hematomas are particularly likely to swell and may cause herniation without preceding hemiparesis. Brainstem compression may develop insidiously, with deepening stupor. An ipsilaterally dilated pupil follows.

Figure 14.16 shows a montage of CT scans that contain lobar hemorrhages. Lobar hematomas are usually smaller in volume than deep lesions and have a lower mortality rate.[169–172] The functional outcome in patients with lobar ICH is also generally better than other forms of ICH. The diagnosis is often quite difficult without CT or MRI. Because of the higher incidence of vascular malformations and other bleeding lesions in patients with lobar hematomas, angiography is often indicated, especially in patients who are young and not hypertensive.[173]

Primary intraventricular hemorrhages

In some patients, the principal locus of bleeding is into the ventricular cavities.[174–177] Figure 14.17 is a post-mortem specimen of a primary intraventricular hemorrhage. Ventricular bleeding usually arises from small subependymal AVMs or cavernous angiomas, or from hemorrhage into the caudate nucleus just adjacent to the ventricles. The clinical syndrome closely mimics SAH, with sudden headache, stiff neck,

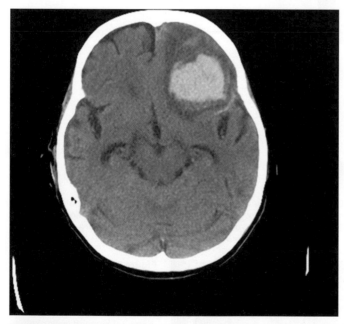

Figure 14.15 CT scan showing a large left frontal hematoma.

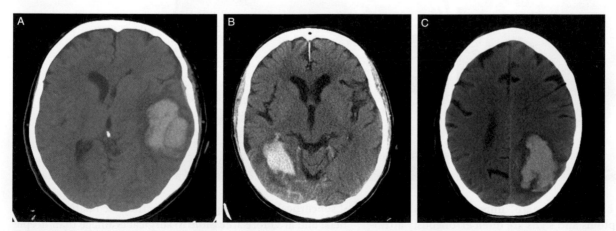

Figure 14.16 (A) CT scan showing a large left temporal lobar hematoma with compression of the ipsilateral lateral ventricle. (B) CT scan showing a smaller right posterior temporal lobar hematoma. (C) CT scan showing a large left occipito-parietal lobar hemorrhage with a surrounding rim of edema. Kindly submitted by Dr Qaioshu Wang.

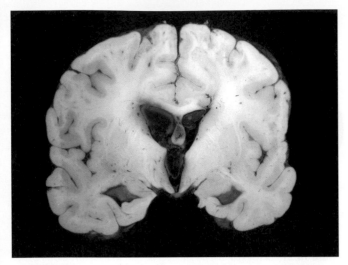

Figure 14.17 Necropsy specimen showing a primary intraventricular hemorrhage. From Caplan LR. Intraventricular hemorrhage. In Kase CS, Caplan LR (eds), *Intracerebral Hemorrhage*. Boston: Butterworth–Heinemann, 1994, pp 383–401 with permission. A black and white version of this figure will appear in some formats. For the color version, please refer to the plate section.

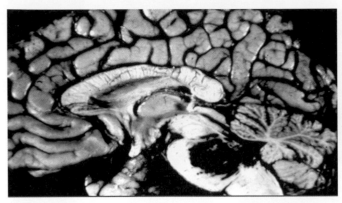

Figure 14.19 Sagittal section of a necropsy specimen that shows a very large middle of the pons hematoma which has destroyed the tegmentum and ruptured into the IVth ventricle. From Caplan LR. Pontine hemorrhage. In Kase CS, Caplan LR (eds), *Intracerebral Hemorrhage*. Boston: Butterworth–Heinemann, 1994, pp 403–423 with permission.

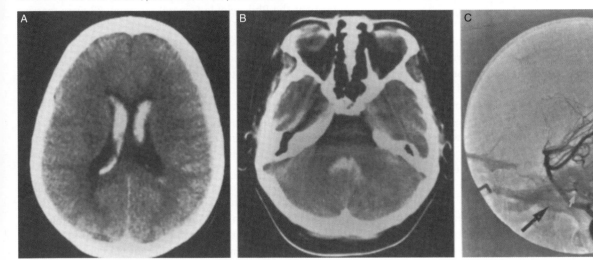

Figure 14.18 Intraventricular bleeding from a cerebellar AVM. (A) CT scan showing blood within the lateral ventricles. (B) CT scan of the posterior fossa showing blood within the IVth ventricle but not in the cerebellum. (C) Angiogram showing a large AVM that bled directly into the IVth ventricle. Long black arrow at the bottom left of the figure points to the basilar artery; small white arrow points to the posterior inferior cerebellar artery that feeds the malformation; the vertically oriented black arrow points to the superior cerebellar artery, which also feeds the AVM. From Caplan LR. Intraventricular hemorrhage. In Kase CS, Caplan LR (eds), *Intracerebral Hemorrhage*. Boston: Butterworth–Heinemann, 1994, pp 383–401 with permission.

vomiting, and lethargy. At times, bilateral, usually symmetric hyperreflexia and extensor plantar responses occur. Decreased consciousness is an almost invariable sign. CT shows blood distending the lateral ventricles and IIIrd ventricle, and some blood density within the subarachnoid space. In childhood, the most common cause is an AVM, which can destroy itself as it ruptures. Small angiomas may arise in the choroid plexus.[174] In adults, most intraventricular hemorrhages are caused by ventricular spread of primary hypertensive bleeds into periventricular structures.[174–177] Intraventricular hemorrhage, both primary and secondary to drainage of supratentorial brain parenchymatous hemorrhages has recently received increased attention because of the advent of stereotactic, hemostatic and thrombolytic treatments that can be effective in removing blood from the ventricles.[177–181] Figure 14.18 shows CT scans and an angiogram of a patient with a cerebellar arteriovenous malformation that bled directly into the IVth ventricle who presented as an intraventricular hemorrhage.

Pontine hemorrhage

Primary brain stem hemorrhages are located most often in the pons. Midbrain and medullary hemorrhages are rare and, when present, are usually caused by blood dyscrasias and vascular malformations.[182] Raised ICP, especially if it develops quickly, frequently causes secondary lesions, so-called Duret hemorrhages, in the median or paramedian zones of the thalamus, midbrain, and pons caused by stretching of paramedian vascular structures.[130,182–185] Primary pontine hemorrhages usually begin in the center of the pons at the tegmental-basal junction. Figure 14.19 is a sagittal section of a large pontine hematoma found at necropsy. These hematomas grow quickly and assume a round or oval shape, usually

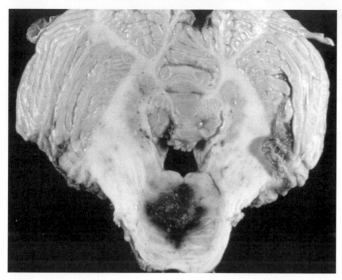

Figure 14.20 Cross-section of the pons and cerebellum showing a large middle of the pons hematoma, The lesion is limited to the pons and has not spread to the IVth ventricle. From Caplan LR. Pontine hemorrhage. In Kase CS, Caplan LR (eds), *Intracerebral Hemorrhage*. Boston: Butterworth–Heinemann, 1994, pp 403–423 with permission.

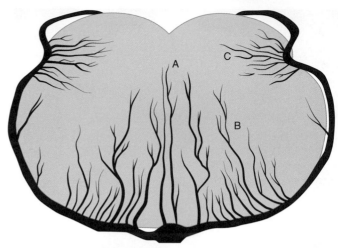

Figure 14.21 Drawing of the penetrating arteries to the pons showing the pattern of arterial supply. A. Midline large median arteries; B. paramedian penetrators; C. penetrating arteries into the lateral tegmentum of the pons.

destroying the center of the tegmentum and base of the pons. Blood may dissect rostrally into the midbrain, but rarely extends caudally into the medulla. Hematomas frequently dissect into the IVth ventricle. Figure 14.20 shows a large pontine hematoma. These large pontine hemorrhages arise from the larger median pontine penetrating vessels that originate from the basilar artery. Figure 14.21 shows various pontine arteries. Bleeding from these arteries causes various syndromes, depending on the location and size of the pontine hematomas. The largest hematomas come from arteries labeled A in the figure.

Signs accompanying large medial pontine hematomas include: (1) quadriparesis, often with limb stiffness and rigidity; (2) coma; (3) absent horizontal eye movements; (4) small but reactive pupils; and (5) rapid or irregular respirations.[182–184,186,187] Headache and vomiting occasionally occur. Some pontine hemorrhages develop gradually,[19] and early findings may be asymmetric. A hemiparesis is common early in the course. Deafness, dysarthria, facial numbness, asymmetric facial or limb weakness, and dizziness occasionally precede the development of coma. Some patients have twitching, shivering, or spasmodic movements of the limbs, usually culminating in decerebrate rigidity. Hyperthermia is sometimes noted. Vertical reflex eye movements are preserved unless the lesion extends rostrally into the midbrain. In some patients, the eyes spontaneously and repeatedly bob downward.[183] Massive pontine hemorrhages are invariably fatal, but not usually instantaneously. Death usually occurs 24–48 hours after onset. Survival for 7–10 days is not rare. Some patients with large medial pontine hematomas survive with quadriplegia.

MRI allows documentation of two other types of pontine hemorrhage (lateral tegmental pontine hematomas[183,184,188–193] and small basal hematomas).[183,184,194–198] These sites correspond to the usual distribution of penetrating pontine arteries (see Figure 14.21). In Silverstein's series of 50 necropsy-proven pontine hemorrhages found during autopsy at the Philadelphia General Hospital, 28 were massive central hematomas. Eleven were located in the lateral basis pontis, and 11 were tegmental.[187] Nakajima reported 24 patients with pontine hematomas who came to necropsy; among these, 21 patients had large central hematomas, 2 had bilateral tegmental lesions, and one had a unilateral basal-tegmental hematoma.[199] Undoubtedly, series of cases involving pontine hematomas identified by neuroimaging scans contain a higher frequency of unilateral basal, tegmental, and basal-tegmental lesions than older necropsy-based series.

Lateral basal hematomas can cause pure motor hemiparesis,[194,195] ataxic hemiparesis,[196,197] or dysarthria–clumsy-hand syndrome,[198] clinical findings that mimic those found in patients with lacunar infarcts in the pons. Lateral basal lesions can spread into the adjacent tegmentum, causing unilateral cranial nerve signs and contralateral hemiparesis. Lateral tegmental hematomas arise from penetrating vessels that course from lateral to medial after branching from the lateral circumferential pontine arteries (see Figure 14.21, arteries labeled C). These lesions involve the rostral pons. Figure 14.22 shows necropsy sections from a patient with a lateral tegmental pontine hemorrhage that extended rostrally into the lower midbrain who died after pulmonary embolism. Findings on neurological examination are those of a predominantly unilateral tegmental lesion.

Most distinctive and diagnostic of lateral tegmental pontine hematomas are the oculomotor abnormalities, which include ipsilateral conjugate gaze paresis, ipsilateral internuclear ophthalmoplegia, or a combination of ipsilateral internuclear ophthalmoplegia and gaze palsy (a "one- and one-half syndrome")[36,183,184,188] in which the only preserved eye motion is abduction of the contralateral eye. Because the sensory lemniscus (joining of the medial lemniscus and spinothalamic tracts) lies in the lateral tegmentum, accompanying loss of pinprick, temperature, and position sense on the opposite side of the body is common. Limb and truncal ataxia are

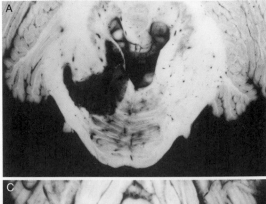

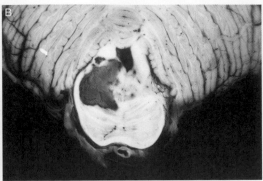

Figure 14.22 A large lateral tegmental pontine hematoma. (A) The largest diameter of the hematoma is in the midpons with extension in a scythe shape into the brachium pontis. (B) Shows the hematoma in the rostral pons where it slightly compresses the rostral IVth ventricle. The hematoma is predominantly tegmental but extends slightly into the basis pontis. (C) Shows extention of the hematoma into the midbrain. From Caplan LR, Goodwin JA. Lateral segmental brainstem hemorrhages. *Neurology* 1982;32:252–260 with permission.

usually present and may be bilateral or predominantly ipsilateral. Unilateral facial numbness or weakness, ipsilateral miosis, and transient deafness may also be present. When contralateral hemiparesis occurs, it is usually slight and transient. Patients with small pontine hematomas generally survive with slight to moderate clinical neurological deficits. Small tegmental hematomas may cause only sensory abnormalities, involving the contralateral limbs and trunk (a pure sensory stroke syndrome)[190,191] or sensory findings limited to the ipsilateral face,[192,193] or ipsilateral VIth nerve or lateral gaze paresis.[200–202]

Cerebellar hemorrhages

Hemorrhage into the cerebellum accounts for about 10% of ICH, approximating the relative percentage of weight of the cerebellum in reference to the entire brain. Anticoagulant usage and bleeding diatheses account for a disproportionate percentage of instances of cerebellar hemorrhage. In a Japanese series, 37 of 327 (11%) consecutive ICHs were cerebellar and 75% of the cerebellar hemorrhages occurred in patients taking anticoagulants.[203] Although the frequency of cerebellar hemorrhage is low, establishing the diagnosis is important because of the potentially serious outcome if not treated and the contrasting good prognosis after surgical treatment.

Cerebellar hemorrhage usually originates in the region of the dentate nucleus, arising from distal branches of the posterior inferior cerebellar artery and the superior cerebellar artery. Hematomas collect around the dentate and spread into the cerebellar hemispheral white matter, frequently extending

into the IVth ventricle. The adjacent brainstem is seldom directly involved, but is compressed from above by the lesion. Occasional cerebellar hemorrhages arise in the vermis in medial branches of the posterior inferior cerebellar artery or the superior cerebellar artery. Figure 14.23 shows a large cerebellar hemorrhage that is compressing the IVth ventricle.

The most consistent symptom is inability to walk.[182,204–207] Some patients even have difficulty remaining in a sitting or standing position, often leaning or tilting toward the side of the hematoma. Patients have been known to crawl, slide, or bump on their bottom to get to the bathroom or phone. Vomiting is also frequent, occurring in 68 (94%) of 72 patients from several series.[182] Headache is also common, usually affecting the occiput, neck, or frontal region. Dysarthria, hiccups, and tinnitus occur, but are less frequent. Loss of consciousness at onset is distinctly unusual, but by the time these patients reach the hospital, approximately one-third are obtunded.[182,204–207]

Neurological signs include: (1) an ipsilateral abducens or gaze palsy toward the side of the hematoma; (2) small pupils, with the ipsilateral pupil slightly smaller; (3) rebound overshoot of the rapidly elevated ipsilateral arm; and (4) gait ataxia. Hemiparesis probably does not occur in cerebellar hemorrhage, but cerebellar lesions do produce an apparent asthenia or slowness of the affected limbs.[204–207] Inferior extremity reflexes are usually symmetrically exaggerated, but plantar responses are flexor. Knee jerks are typically pendular with an increased span of leg motions. Classic cerebellar-type incoordination of the arm on finger-to-nose or toe-to-object testing and frank intention tremor are uncommon. In LRC's

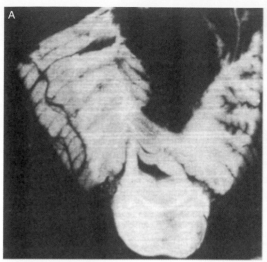
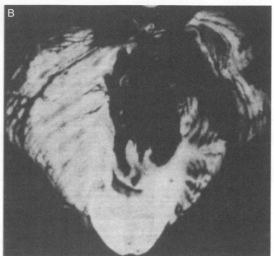

Figure 14.23 Necropsy specimens of two typical cerebellar hematomas that extend into or compress the vermis in the region of the roof of the IVth ventricle. Each distorts and compresses the ventricle. From Caplan LR. *Vertebrobasilar Ischemia and Hemorrhage: Clinical Findings, Diagnosis, and Management of Posterior Circulation Disease.* Cambridge: Cambridge University Press, 2015 with permission.

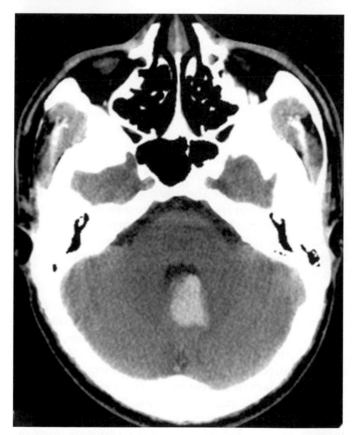

Figure 14.24 CT scan showing a cerebellar hemorrhage centered in the vermis and projecting into the IVth ventricle.

experience with patients with cerebellar infarction and hemorrhage, the single most useful cerebellar sign is elicited when the patient is asked to raise both arms together rapidly, then to brake the ascent quickly. Next, the patient is directed to drop the arms quickly, again braking the descent before the hands hit the bed or table. The arm on the side of the cerebellar lesion lags behind the other arm and overshoots the end-point.

Patients with large cerebellar hematomas often have brainstem compression. They develop increasing stupor, lateral gaze palsy toward the side of the hematoma, and bilateral extensor plantar responses. Among those patients not comatose on admission in one series, only 20% had a smooth, uneventful recovery, 80% deteriorated to coma, with 25% of these becoming comatose within 3 hours after onset.[204] In the series of Fisher et al.,[205] only 2 of 18 patients had a benign course. The other 16 patients developed coma, usually within a few hours. Because the hematoma usually affects the caudal cerebellum, the medulla is the portion of the brainstem compressed, and so vasomotor abnormalities and respiratory arrest may develop. Untreated patients with cerebellar hemorrhage who become comatose invariably die of brainstem compression. CT and MRI not only document the size, locale, and position of the hematoma, but also give considerable information about posterior-fossa pressure. An expanding lesion obliterates the cerebellopontine angle and ambient cisterns, and displaces the IVth ventricle toward the opposite side. Usually, the IVth ventricle compression leads to hydrocephalus, with early dilatation of the temporal horns of the lateral ventricles.

Occasionally, patients with cerebellar hemorrhage have a more indolent course, presenting with symptoms and signs of hydrocephalus. Abulia, dementia, slow-stepped shuffling gait, and incontinence are the characteristic signs of hydrocephalus. The patient and family may fail to emphasize the preceding symptoms of dizziness, headache, and vomiting that had been interpreted as the flu. Other patients have laterally placed cerebellar hematomas that compress the cerebellopontine angle structures. These patients develop dysfunction of the Vth, VIth, VIIth, and VIIIth cranial nerves, in addition to ataxia.

Hemorrhage into the vermis, with headache, vomiting, and sudden coma, is more rare.[207] Figure 14.24 is a CT scan that shows a relatively small cerebellar vermal hemorrhage. Large medially located vermal hemorrhages quickly compress the IVth ventricle and create pressure on the bilateral pontine and medullary tegmentum. Some smaller vermian hemorrhages present with dizziness and gait ataxia.

Because the course of cerebellar hematomas is unpredictable and large lesions frequently cause coma and death, it is probably wise to drain lesions that are 3 cm or larger, especially

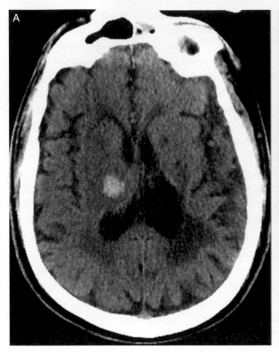 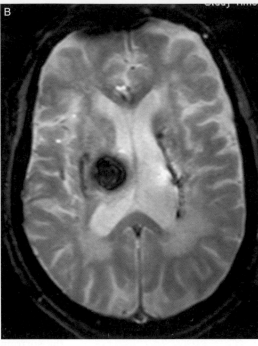

Figure 14.25 (A) CT scan of a patient with a right thalamic hemorrhage. There are many regions of hypointensity near the atrium of the left lateral ventricle and scattered within the cerebral white matter. (B) T2*-weighted MRI showing the acute hematoma as a homogeneous round black lesion abutting on the right lateral ventricle. Older areas of hemosiderin deposition are seen bilaterally appearing as linear slits or microbleeds adjacent to the lateral ventricles and basal ganglia. Kindly submitted by Dr Mark McAllister.

if a decrease in level of alertness develops.[207,208] Some patients have been successfully treated by medical decompression (osmotic diuretic agents) or ventricular drainage.[207,209] Ventricular shunts do not treat brainstem compression and have been followed by delayed deterioration.[210] Ventricular drainage can create a vacuum effect that increases herniation of the cerebellum upwards through the tentorial notch to compress the rostral brainstem.[211,212] Prognosis depends very much on the size of the hematoma and whether the patient has developed stupor or coma before treatment.[213] The outlook for patients with small cerebellar hematomas is excellent. Even patients with large cerebellar hematomas do well if surgically decompressed before they develop decreased consciousness.[204–207,213]

Diagnosis, prognosis, and treatment

Diagnosis

Accurate bedside diagnosis of ICH rests on the presence of an appropriate ecological background, such as hypertension or bleeding diathesis; the non-fluctuating, usually gradually progressive course over minutes or hours; accompanying symptoms, such as headache and vomiting; and neurological signs compatible with a deep lesion. CT has proven to be an excellent instrument for the diagnosis of ICH. Blood provides dense contrast, even acutely. One reported patient with ICH had an abrupt increase in symptoms while in the CT scanner.[214] The initial films had shown a small, round hyperdensity in the lentiform nucleus. A second film of the same area showed a much larger, hyperdense, irregular zone extending laterally from the putamen to the insula.[214] Other investigators have also described enlargement of hematomas on sequential CT scans.[13–16]

Findings on CT and MRI scans can help determine the age of the hematoma. Hematomas are at first regular and smooth.

During the first 48 hours, large hematomas may show fluid blood levels, indicating that the hematoma is partially liquid and has not solidified.[215] During the first 72 hours or longer, edema produces a hypodense area around the lesion and considerable mass effect is noted.[216,217] From 3 to 20 days after bleeding, the dense area becomes smaller, beginning at the periphery. The border develops an irregular contour, which is enhanced with the use of contrast.[216–218] Reduction of edema and mass effect also occurs during this period. Intraventricular blood has usually disappeared by 5 weeks.[219] The absorption coefficient of the hematoma decreases gradually, and the lesion develops a lucent appearance, with absorption characteristics resembling edema fluid or CSF. By 9 weeks, mass effect and enhancement are usually gone, and a local circumscribed region of slight hypodensity remains.[219]

On MRI scans, the zone of altered attenuation or abnormal metabolism is usually much larger than the hypodensity seen on CT. MRI is also effective in imaging acute hematomas[220,221] and is more useful than CT in recognizing hemorrhage in chronic lesions. In Chapter 4, MRI findings in hematomas are discussed in detail. Table 4.2 tabulates the findings depending on various MRI sequences. Acute hematomas are isointense or hypointense on T1-weighted scans, sometimes with a darker hypointense rim, and they are bright and hyperintense on T2-weighted images.[217] Later, the center of the hematoma appears dark on T2 and is surrounded by a bright rim. Chronic hematomas are bright on T2-weighted images. Figure 14.25A is a CT scan of a patient with a recent hypertensive right thalamic hemorrhage. Figure 14.25B is a T2*-weighted MRI that shows the acute hematoma as a homogeneous round lesion. Older areas of hemorrhage are seen on the right as a linear slit and small microbleeds around the left lateral ventricle. These older hemosiderin-containing regions are not visible on CT or other MRI techniques.

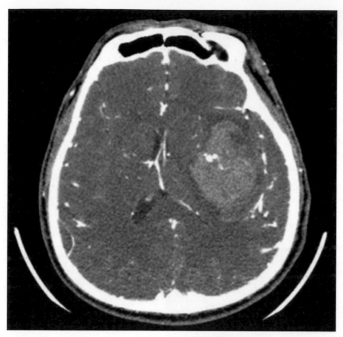

Figure 14.26 CT spot sign. An image from a CT angiogram showing a bright white region of contrast leakage in the medial portion of a large left-hemispheric intracerebral hemorrhage. Kindly submitted by Dr Magdy Selim, Beth Israel Deaconess Medical Center, Boston, MA, USA.

Digital contrast cerebral angiography is usually unnecessary unless the lesion is in an unusual locus or the patient has no risk factors for hemorrhage, such as hypertension or bleeding diathesis. Angiography is used to opacify AVMs or aneurysms that might have caused ICH. When performed acutely, angiography can suggest that the hematoma will likely enlarge. Extravasation of contrast correlates well with subsequent hematoma enlargement, clinical worsening, and poor outcome.[222] The "spot sign" found on CTA of patients with ICH is the CT correlate of contrast extravasation during angiography (Figure 14.26).[21,22]

Prognosis

The three most important predictors of outcome after ICH are the size of the hemorrhage, the location of bleeding, and the state of consciousness of the patient at presentation.[24–26,149,223] The volume of the hematoma is the single most important prognostic factor. Volume is especially important in supratentorial and cerebellar hemorrhages but less dominant a predictor in brainstem hematomas. The volume of a hematoma can be readily calculated by clinicians using the ABC/2 method that measures maximal diameter in 3 planes and divides by 2 to approximate an ellipsoid. In this formula, A is the largest hemorrhage diameter on CT scan, B is the diameter 90° to A, and C is the approximate number of CT slices with hemorrhage multiplied by the slice thickness.[224] Some scanners can provide the volume of a lesion using computer-assisted image analysis. In one study of patients with putaminal hemorrhages, lesions larger than 140 mm^2 in one slice had a poorer outcome.[31] In thalamic hemorrhage, lesions larger than 3.3 cm in maximal diameter had a poor prognosis,[34] as did

cerebellar lesions larger than 3 cm.[225] In seven other studies, large-volume hematomas were associated with a poor outcome.[24,25,149,164,226–228] Pulse pressure, admission blood pressure, and level of consciousness, as measured by the Glasgow Coma Scale, are also important prognostic variables.[24,26,227,229] The presence of hydrocephalus in patients with supratentorial hemorrhages is also an adverse prognostic sign.[228] A large volume of intraventricular blood in basal ganglia (other than caudate nucleus) and lobar hemorrhage patients, adversely affects the prognosis for good recovery.[230]

During the acute phase of ICH, the mass effect of the developing hematoma presents a much greater risk of death than does a comparable-sized cerebral infarct. In the case of ICH, something extra (blood) has been added to the intracranial contents. In cerebral infarction, the already existing contents (brain tissue) are ischemic, but an acute mass has not been added. Later, infarcts and hematomas become edematous, increasing ICP. In the chronic phase, if the patient with ICH has survived, the prognosis for recovery is actually better than cerebral infarcts of similar size and location. Hematomas have dissected and separated the cerebral cortex and other brain parts, but usually the surrounding cortex is preserved. In contrast, infarcts leave dead, non-functioning cortex when they heal. Unlike SAH, recurrence of ICH during the acute illness is rare. These simple facts dictate the approach to ICH treatment – that is, aggressively try to limit the expanding hematoma to prevent death and late morbidity. In patients with ICH, the concern is control of acute mass effect, whereas in SAH the goal is to prevent rebleeding and arterial vasoconstriction.

Treatment

Medical

Careful medical management of patients with ICH may be lifesaving and is important, even in those patients who later have surgical drainage of their hematomas. Increased ICP causes decreased responsiveness and hypoventilation; in turn, hypoventilation causes a low arterial oxygen tension and high carbon dioxide tension, which lead to vasodilatation and further increase in ICP. Maintenance of a good airway and mechanical hyperventilation can reverse this process and quickly lower ICP. Control of systemic blood pressure helps stop intracranial bleeding, but must be done cautiously. In some patients with ICH, systemic blood pressure is further increased to ensure adequate perfusion of the brain. Increased ICP causes increased venous pressure, so elevated arterial pressure is needed to overcome the increased venous pressure to perfuse the tissues. Overzealous lowering of blood pressure could potentially lead to underperfusion and clinical deterioration. Blood pressure should be lowered quickly, but not to hypotensive levels. Patients must be watched carefully during the treatment. The optimum blood pressure goal has been debated. Previous guidelines variously recommended lowering systolic blood pressures to below 180 and 160 mmHg. The Intensive Blood Pressure Reduction in Acute Cerebral Hemorrhage Trial (INTERACT II) showed that lowering the systolic pressure to a target of 140 mmHg or less within an

hour was safe.[231] The most recent Guidelines from the Stroke Council of the American Heart Association suggest, "If the systolic blood pressure is >180 mmHg or the mean arterial pressure (MAP) is >130 mmHg and there is no evidence of elevated ICP, then consider a modest reduction of blood pressure (e.g., MAP of 110 mmHg or target BP of 160/90) using intermittent or continuous intravenous medication to control blood pressure and examine the patient every 15 minutes."[232] A meta-analysis of data from randomized controlled trials concluded that intensive blood pressure lowering to a systolic blood pressure of less than 140 mmHg was safe.[233]

Elevation of the head of the bed, hyperventilation, reducing high body temperatures, and ventricular drainage have been used to control ICP. So-called medical decompression with mannitol, hypertonic saline, or glycerol is widely used in patients with ICH. Because edema develops surrounding hematomas and adds to mass effect, reduction of edema formation is an important therapeutic goal. Few data exist, however, about the effectiveness of osmotic agents in reducing the edema. Concern exists that hypertonic agents could diffuse into the ICH and cause a secondary increase in volume of the hematoma because of ingress of fluid. Langfitt noted that mannitol and forced hyperventilation were effective in reducing ICP in a group of patients with ICH.[234] Poungvarin et al. studied the usefulness of dexamethasone treatment in patients with supratentorial ICH in a double-blind randomized trial. They found that it did not improve mortality, and infections and diabetic complications were more often found in the corticosteroid-treated group.[235] Corticosteroids are not recommended in patients with ICH. Perihematomal edema volume peaks during the third or fourth day after the onset of hemorrhage. The release of iron-containing breakdown products of hemoglobin likely contributes to the development of edema.[236] A trial of the utility of deferoxamine mesylate, an iron-binding agent, in patients with brain hemorrhages is now ongoing.[237]

When intracerebral bleeding develops in patients who are taking a vitamin K antagonist (warfarin and related compounds), replacement of vitamin K and clotting factors is essential and must be performed urgently. Table 14.5 outlines suggestions for reversal of anticoagulation in these patients. The newer anticoagulants function by inhibiting thrombin or factor X. Anticoagulation with these agents does not produce a deficiency of clotting factors but acts by competitively blocking thrombin or preventing activation of factor X. Replacement of clotting factors is posited to be ineffective in reversing bleeding in patients on the newer anticoagulants. These agents, unlike warfarin, have relatively short half-lives necessitating daily or twice daily dosage so that the agents are out of the system faster than warfarin. Much new research now concerns finding antidotes to reverse bleeding in patients taking these agents.[238]

Because hematoma expansion means increased bleeding, it seemed logical to try to limit hematoma expansion even in patients without coagulopathies by administering recombinant activated factor VII (rFVIIa) to patients early in the course of ICHs.[239–242] Two randomized trials of rFVIIa showed that this strategy did reduce hemorrhage expansion but did not substantially improve outcomes. There also was risk related to the induced hypercoagulability. In the first smaller preliminary trial, 399 patients with CT-confirmed intracerebral hematomas were randomly assigned within 3 hours after onset to receive placebo (96 patients), 40 µg of rFVIIa/kg (108 patients), 80 µg/kg (92 patients), or 160 µg/kg (103 patients) within one hour after the initial CT scan.[240,241] The primary outcome measure was the percent change in the volume of the ICH measured at 24 hours. Hematoma volume did increase more in the placebo group than in the rFVIIa groups. The mean increase was 29% in the placebo group, contrasted with 16%, 14%, and 11% in the those given 40 µg, 80 µg, and 160 µg of rFVIIa/kg, respectively ($P = 0.01$ for the comparison of the three rFVIIa groups with the placebo group). Growth in the volume of ICH was reduced by 3.3 ml, 4.5 ml, and 5.8 ml in the three treatment groups, compared with the placebo group ($P = 0.01$).[240,241] Serious thromboembolic adverse events, mainly myocardial or brain infarction, occurred in 7% of rFVIIa-treated patients, compared with 2% of those given placebo ($P = 0.12$).[240]

Because the first preliminary trial showed promise, a larger second trial aimed at assessing clinical outcome was planned and pursued. In this second trial, 841 patients were randomized to placebo, 20 µg of rFVIIa/kg, or 80 µg of rFVIIa/kg within 4 hours after onset.[242] Growth in the volume of the hemorrhage was reduced by 2.6 ml in the 20 µg/kg group and by 3.8 ml in the 80 µg/kg group as compared with the placebo-treated group. Arterial thromboembolic events were more frequent in the high-dose group than controls (9% vs. 4%). There was no difference among the three groups in the rate of poor clinical outcome, 24% in placebo, 26% in the low-dose group, and 29% in the high-dose group.[243] For patients who have severe vascular occlusive disease involving the coronary or peripheral arteries, or past venous thromboembolism, the administration of rFVIIa carries a risk of myocardial infarction or venous occlusion with pulmonary embolism. Given these risks, a promising approach under investigation is to treat with hemostatic agents only those patients at very high risk for hemorrhage expansion, as evidenced by both early presentation and the presence of the CT spot sign.

Surgical considerations

Because hematomas are mass-producing lesions and because, near the time of onset, the contents are liquid, surgical drainage of hematomas seems a very logical and attractive means of decompression. Surgical treatment of ICH has been and remains a very controversial topic with strong supporters and others who feel it is seldom if ever indicated. Unfortunately recent randomized trials have not satisfactorily settled the role of surgery for ICH. The largest randomized trials to date, the Surgical Trials in Intracerebral Hemorrhage (STICH I and STICH II), failed to show a definite superiority of either medical or surgical treatment.[244,245] In the large STICH I trial, 1033 patients from 83 medical centers in 27 countries were randomized to either surgery within 24 hours of randomization or initial conservative management. Among those randomized to early surgery, 26% had a favorable outcome compared with 24% of those

Table 14.5 Reversal of anticoagulation in patients with warfarin-related ICH*¶

Agent	Dose/route administration	Effect	Advantages	Disadvantages
Vitamin K₁	10 mg slow IV injection over 30 min (no faster than 1 mg/min)	Decrease in INR by 0% after 8 h from administration	Widely available Only agent that provides sustained INR reversal	Anaphylactoid reactions, such as hypotension if given too fast Long time to INR reversal (12–24 h)
Fresh frozen plasma	10–15 ml/kg (200 ml/U) Infuse FFP every 45–60 min while checking INR every 4 h Total of 8 U often required	Replaces all four factors (II, VII, IX, X) inhibited by warfarin	Widely available Inexpensive	Time of thawing and infusion (~1 h for each unit) Risk of ICH expansion while INR still prolonged Need large bore IV High fluid volume (~2 L) Risk of CHF Long time to INR reversal INR reversal may not be sustained (requires co-administration of vitamin K₁) Low, variable amounts of factor IX in different batches
Prothrombin complex concentrate	Dose determined by INR Dose (INR): 25 U/kg (2.0–3.9) 35 U/kg (4.0–6.0) 50 U/kg (>6.0) or: fixed dose of 1500–200 U used (center-dependent) Give slowly IV over 10–15 min (~100 U/min) Check INR 30 min post-infusion to ensure reversal	Replaces all 4 factors inhibited by warfarin; also provides the procoagulants protein C and S (3-factor PCC devoid of factor VII also on market)	Given in small volume, without concern for volume overload Rapid INR correction	Thromboembolic complications (~3%) Repeated doses to be avoided b/o increased risk of thromboembolism INR reversal may not be sustained (requires co-administration of vitamin K₁)
Recombinant activated factor VII	IV at dose of 20–40 µg/kg	Replaces warfarin-inhibited factor VII, normalizes INR	Reverses INR rapidly in patients prior to surgical ICH treatment	Thromboembolic complications (~5–10%) High cost May normalize the highly factor VII-dependent INR without fully restoring hemostasis INR reversal may not be sustained (requires co-administration of vitamin K₁)

* The AHA/ASA Guidelines for the Management of Intracerebral Hemorrhage recommend for patients with warfarin-related ICH the routine use of vitamin K₁, the choice of PCC over FFP (depending on availability), and do not recommend the use of rFVIIa based on the lack of sufficient data about effectiveness and safety.
¶ Target INR for reversal <1.4.
b/o, because of; CHF, congestive heart failure; FFP, fresh frozen plasma; ICH, intracerebral hemorrhage; INR, international normalized ratio; IV, intravenous; PCC, prothrombin complex concentrate; rFVIIa, recombinant activated factor VII.

randomized to initial conservative treatment (OR 0.89, 95% CI 0.66–1.19, $P = 0.414$). In this analysis deep and lobar hemorrhages were considered together.[244] Among the 530 patients randomized to initial conservative treatment, 140 crossed over and had surgery, complicating the analysis and interpretation of the results.[246] The investigators concluded that overall "patients with spontaneous supratentorial intracerebral haemorrhage in neurosurgical units show no overall benefit from early surgery when compared with initial conservative treatment."[244] The

STICH I trial did show that the presence of intraventricular bleeding and hydrocephalus adversely affected outcomes.[247]

Clinicians and surgeons posited that the lack of benefit for surgery in STICH I was because of inclusion of deep hemorrhages known to do poorly; lobar hemorrhages might be a better target for drainage. The STICH II trial was limited to lobar hemorrhages.[245] Early surgical hematoma drainage within 12 hours of randomization was compared with early medical management; later hematoma drainage was allowed if

judged necessary. Among the 601 patients, 307 were randomized to early surgery and 294 to early conservative non-surgical management. An unfavorable outcome occurred in 174 (59%) of 297 patients in the early surgery group versus 178 (62%) of 286 patients in the initial conservative treatment group. The conclusion was that early surgery in patients with superficially located lobar hemorrhages did not increase the rate of death or disability at 6 months and might have had "a small but clinically relevant survival advantage for patients with spontaneous superficial intracerebral haemorrhage without intraventricular haemorrhage."[245]

It seemed clear from these two large surgical trials that a policy of generally draining hematomas could not be supported. In the STICH trials almost all surgeries involved craniotomies. During recent decades surgeons have explored stereotactic drainage of hematomas with and without using thrombolytic agents to soften the hematomas to allow better drainage.[248–256] Stereotactic techniques have been used more often in Asian countries than in the west. Drainage is through a small burr hole and no cortisectomy is involved. The drainage instrument is guided stereotactically, using CT or MRI, to the core of the hematoma, which is then evacuated. Fibrinolytic agents also can be instilled to soften and lyse clotted blood.

Stereotactic surgery has been performed with and without using a stereotactic frame and with and without administration of a thrombolytic agent directly into the hematoma. The results show promise and are likely to be better in the hands of experienced surgeons than results from open craniotomy drainage. Endoscopic drainage of hematomas is another promising technique.[257]

The end-point of the surgical STICH trials was function and mortality after a period of 6 months.[244,245] Not studied well was the acute period time in hospital and return to alertness. Drainage of subacute hemorrhages, by reducing increased ICP improves alertness and could reduce the frequency and severity of medical complications that develop in obtunded individuals. The stay in the acute care hospital might also be shortened. Hemicraniectomy is an alternative way of decreasing ICP. Hemicraniectomy after surgery is sometimes performed in patients with sizable hemorrhages that might prove mortal but often the patients are left in a disabled dependent condition.

We believe that an eclectic approach to surgical consideration is still important. Candidates must be selected carefully. When considering surgery and other therapies, hematomas, in practice, can be divided into the following three main groups:

1. Massive, rapidly developing lesions that effectively kill or devastate patients before they reach the hospital. For these lesions, little can or should be done. Surgery is not indicated.
2. Small hematomas, from which the patient will make an excellent spontaneous recovery. Treatment consists of controlling the etiological factors, such as hypertension, to prevent recurrences. Surgery is not indicated.
3. Medium-sized hematomas (hematoma volumes between the two extremes), with developing mass effect after the patient reaches the hospital. Within this third group, medical measures and surgery are potentially most helpful.

Size

Hematomas larger than 3 cm in their widest diameter have a higher mortality and a more delayed recovery rate than smaller lesions. Thus, the larger the lesion on CT, the more logical its drainage would be.

Location

Some hematomas are more accessible surgically, such as those in the cerebellum or cerebral lobes. Although putaminal hemorrhages can be drained through the sylvian fissures and insular cortex, large left basal-ganglionic hemorrhages usually leave patients aphasic and dependent. Thus, treatment should be less aggressive than for right-sided lesions. Cerebellar ICH can cause respiratory arrest without preceding gradual deterioration of neurological function or alertness, and surgical removal of a portion of the cerebellum often leaves no important residual handicap. For these reasons, the threshold for recommending surgery for cerebellar hematomas is lower than other lesions of comparable size. Cerebellar, lobar, and right putaminal hemorrhages are most accessible to surgical drainage. For deeper hemorrhages stereotactic drainage would be preferred.

Mass effect and drainage patterns

Size of the hematoma does not, by itself, solely determine mass effect. Older patients may have sufficient pre-existing atrophy to be able to accommodate a sizable hematoma without a critical rise in ICP or shift in intracranial compartments. Some lesions have a great deal of surrounding edema, whereas others have relatively little. Hydrocephalus can add to the increased mass effect. Does the hematoma compress the third or lateral ventricle? Has a shift of the midline occurred? Is uncal herniation present? In posterior fossa ICH, has displacement of the IVth ventricle been found? Are the ambient, cerebellopontine, and other cisterns effaced? Does the lesion drain into the ventricles or superficially into the subarachnoid space? Entry into the CSF may spontaneously decompress the lesion. Surgical drainage would be indicated more strongly for lesions with greater mass effect and no spontaneous decompression.

Etiology

Even after surgical drainage, hematomas caused by amyloid angiopathy may tend to bleed because of the fragility of the blood vessels.[258] Similarly, hemorrhages in patients with anticoagulant-related or other bleeding disorders can also continue to bleed unless the coagulopathy is reversed before surgery. Ideally, surgeons like to remove the malformations when operating on hematomas caused by vascular malformations while also draining the hematoma. The threshold for surgical treatment should be most favorable for vascular malformations, moderately so for accessible lesions caused by hypertension, and least favorable for CAA or ICH caused by a bleeding diathesis.

Timing

During the first 24–36 hours, hematomas are still at least partly liquid and can be more easily drained. Later, hematomas

solidify and become more difficult to drain. Unfortunately the present CT and MRI technologies do not reliably show the liquidity of hematomas unless there is a fluid level present. Clinicians posited that very early surgery, within 4 hours after symptom onset, might allow drainage of liquid blood and lead to better outcomes than surgery after 12 hours. A planned study to test this hypothesis was stopped prematurely after 11 patients in the 4-hour arm had surgery.[259] The median time to surgery was 180 minutes; median hematoma volume was 40 ml; median baseline National Institutes of Health Stroke Scale (NIHSS) score was 19. Postoperative bleeding developed in 4 patients, four/three of whom died. Rebleeding occurred in 40% of the patients treated within 4 hours compared with 12% of the patients treated within 12 hours. Those that re-bled had a high mortality.[259]

Clearly too early surgery can promote rebleeding which adversely affects outcome. The ideal time to operate is unknown. After 7–10 days, blood begins to be absorbed, and the lesion becomes softer again. Ideally, drainage should occur either early or after 7–10 days for technical reasons. In general, if the patient has survived the first week, improvement occurs as edema subsides. Thus, little argument for late drainage exists except for concurrent removal of a vascular malformation. Some have wondered whether late surgery (1–2 weeks) would speed recovery, but this argument is unsupported by data.

Clinical course

Perhaps the most important factor to consider is whether the patient is improving, stable, or worsening. Patients who deteriorate and show a decrease in level of consciousness to severe lethargy or stupor have a poor outlook for recovery.[24,26,223] In patients with putaminal hemorrhage, other poor prognostic signs include the development of ipsilateral pupillary dilation, an ipsilateral extensor plantar response, or an ipsilateral conjugate gaze paresis. These signs are indicative of midline shift or early brainstem compression. In patients with cerebellar hemorrhage, development of bilateral extensor plantar responses is a poor prognostic sign.[205] In deteriorating patients with accessible lesions, surgery should not be delayed if medical decompression is not quickly beneficial.

> A CT scan in JT showed a large, deep putaminal hemorrhage, with spread to the thalamus and lateral ventricles. At this time, he was comatose; had bilateral horizontal gaze palsies; dilated, unreactive pupils; and bilateral extensor plantar reflexes. LRC judged that nothing could or should be done to reverse his mortal bleed.

Much must be learned regarding therapy for patients with ICH. The technological revolution has made diagnosis easy. More well-designed studies of different modes of treatment in patients with lesions of various etiologies, sizes, locations, and varying levels of consciousness are needed.

References

1. Morgagni GB. *De sedibus, et causis morborum per anatomen indagatis libri quinque.* Vienna: Typographica Remondiana, 1761.

2. Cheyne J. *Cases of Apoplexy and Lethargy with Observations on Comatose Patients.* London: Thomas Underwood, 1812.

3. Gowers W. *A Manual of Diseases of the Nervous System*, Vol **2**. (2nd ed). London: J & A Churchill, 1892;384–421.

4. Osler W. *The Principles and Practices of Medicine* (5th ed). New York: Appleton, 1903;997–1008.

5. Aring C, Merritt H. Differential diagnosis between cerebral hemorrhage and cerebral thrombosis: Clinical and pathological study of 245 cases. *Arch Intern Med* 1935;**56**:435–456.

6. Kunitz S, Gross C, Heyman A, et al. The Pilot Stroke Data Bank: Definition, design, and data. *Stroke* 1984;**15**:740–746.

7. Caplan LR, Hier DB, D'Cruz I. Cerebral embolism in the Michael Reese Stroke Registry. *Stroke* 1983;**14**:530–540.

8. Mohr JP, Caplan LR, Melski J, et al. The Harvard Cooperative Stroke Registry: A prospective registry. *Neurology* 1978;**28**:754–762.

9. Whisnant J, Fitzgibbons J, Kurland L, et al. Natural history of stroke in Rochester, Minnesota, 1945–1954. *Stroke* 1971;**2**:11–22.

10. Matsumoto N, Whisnant J, Kurland L, et al. Natural history of stroke in Rochester, Minnesota, 1955–1969. *Stroke* 1973;**4**:20–29.

11. Caplan LR, Mohr JP. Intracerebral hemorrhage: An update. *Geriatrics* 1978;**33**:42–52.

12. Fisher CM. Pathological observations in hypertensive cerebral hemorrhages. *J Neuropathol Exp Neurol* 1971;**30**:536–550.

13. Kelly R, Bryer JR, Scheinberg P, Stokes IV. Active bleeding in hypertensive intracerebral hemorrhage: Computed tomography. *Neurology* 1982;**32**:852–856.

14. Broderick JP, Brott TG, Tomsick T, et al. Ultra-early evaluation of intracerebral hemorrhage. *J Neurosurg* 1990;**72**:195–199.

15. Fujii Y, Tanaka R, Takeuchi S, et al. Hematoma enlargement in spontaneous intracerebral hemorrhage. *J Neurosurg* 1994;**80**:51–57.

16. Kazui S, Naritomi H, Yamamoto H, et al. Enlargement of spontaneous intracerebral hemorrhage. Incidence and time course. *Stroke* 1996;**27**:1783–1787.

17. Kase C, Robinson K, Stein R, et al. Anticoagulant-related intracerebral hemorrhage. *Neurology* 1985;**35**:943–948.

18. Kase CS. Bleeding disorders. In CS Kase, LR Caplan (eds), *Intracerebral Hemorrhage.* Boston: Butterworth–Heinemann, 1994;117–151.

19. Kornyey S. Rapidly fatal pontile hemorrhage: Clinical and anatomic report. *Arch Neurol Psychiatry* 1939;**41**:793–799.

20. Caplan LR. General symptoms and signs. In CS Kase, LR Caplan (eds), *Intracerebral Hemorrhage.* Boston: Butterworth–Heinemann, 1994;31–43.

21. Wada R, Aviv RI, Fox A, et al. CT angiography "spot sign" predicts hematoma expansion in acute intracerebral hemorrhage. *Stroke* 2007; **38**: 1257–1262.

22. Demchuk AM, Dowlatshahi D, Rodriguez-Luna D, et al. and PREDICT Group. Prediction of haematoma growth and outcome in patients with

intracerebral haemorrhage using the CT-angiography spot sign (PREDICT): A prospective observational study. *Lancet Neurol* 2012;**11**:307–314.

23. Melo TP, Pinto AN, Ferro JM. Headache in intracerebral hematomas. *Neurology* 1996;**47**:494–500.

24. Tuhrim S, Dambrosia JM, Price TR, et al. Prediction of intracerebral hemorrhage survival. *Ann Neurol* 1988;**24**:258–263.

25. Broderick JP, Brott TG, Duldner JE, et al. Volume of intracerebral hemorrhage. *Stroke* 1993;**24**:987–993.

26. Kase CS, Crowell RM. Prognosis and treatment of patients with intracerebral hemorrhage. In CS Kase, LR Caplan (eds), *Intracerebral Hemorrhage.* Boston: Butterworth–Heinemann, 1994;467–489.

27. Borison H, Wang S. Physiology and pharmacology of vomiting. *Pharmacol Rev* 1953;**5**:193–230.

28. Faught E, Peties D, Bartolucci A, et al. Seizures after primary intracerebral hemorrhage. *Neurology* 1989;**39**:1089–1093.

29. Kilpatrick CJ, Davis SM, Tress BM, et al. Epileptic seizures in acute strokes. *Arch Neurol* 1990;**47**:157–160.

30. Berger AR, Lipton RB, Lesser ML, et al. Early seizures following intracerebral hemorrhage. *Neurology* 1988;**38**:1363–1365.

31. Hier DB, Davis K, Richardson EP, et al. Hypertensive putaminal hemorrhage. *Arch Neurol* 1977;**1**:152–159.

32. Claasen J, Jette N, Chum F, et al. Electrographic seizures and periodic discharges after intracerebral hemorrhage. *Neurology* 2007;**69**:1356–1365.

33. Abend NS, Dlugos DJ, Hahn CD, Hirsch LJ, Herman ST. Use of EEG monitoring and management of non-convulsive seizures in critically ill patients: A survey of neurologists. *Neurocrit Care* 2010;**12**:382–389.

34. Walshe T, Davis K, Fisher CM. Thalamic hemorrhage, a computed tomographic-clinical correlation. *Neurology* 1977;**29**:217–222.

35. Hier DB, Babcock DJ, Foulkes MA, et al. Influence of site on course of intracerebral hemorrhage. *J Stroke Cerebrovasc Dis* 1993;**3**:65–74.

36. Fisher CM. Some neuro-ophthalmological observations. *J Neurol Neurosurg Psychiatry* 1967;**30**:383–392.

37. Caplan LR. Intracerebral hemorrhage revisited. *Neurology* 1988;**38**:624–627.

38. Caplan LR. Hypertensive intracerebral hemorrhage. In CS Kase, LR Caplan (eds), *Intracerebral Hemorrhage.* Boston: Butterworth–Heinemann, 1994;99–116.

39. Cole F, Yates P. Intracerebral microaneurysms and small cerebrovascular lesions. *Brain* 1967;**90**:759–768.

40. Rosenblum WI. Miliary aneurysms and "fibrinoid" degeneration of cerebral blood vessels. *Hum Pathol* 1977;**8**:133–139.

41. Fiehler J. Cerebral microbleeds: Old leaks and new haemorrhages. *Int J Stroke* 2006;**1**:122–130.

42. Koennecke HC. Cerebral microbleeds on MRI: Prevalence, associations and potential clinical implications. *Neurology* 2006;**66**:165–171.

43. Greenberg SM, Vernooj MW, Cordonnier C, et al. Cerebral microbleeds: A guide to detection and interpretation. *Lancet Neurol* 2009;**8**:165–174.

44. Green FHK. Miliary aneurysms in the brain. *J Pathol Bacteriol* 1930;**33**:71–77.

45. Santos-Buch CA, Goodhue W, Ewald B. Concurrence of iris aneurysms and cerebral hemorrhage in hypertensive rabbits. *Arch Neurol* 1976;**33**:96–103.

46. Takebayashi S, Kaneko M. Electron microscopic studies of ruptured arteries in hypertensive intracerebral hemorrhage. *Stroke* 1983;**14**:28–36.

47. Takebayashi S, Sakata N, Kawamura K. Re-evaluation of miliary aneurysms in hypertensive brain: Recanalization of small hemorrhage. *Stroke* 1990;**21**(Suppl 1):59–60.

48. Bakemuka M. Primary intracerebral hemorrhage and heart weight: A clinicopathologic case-control review of 218 patients. *Stroke* 1987;**18**:531–536.

49. Brott T, Thalinger K, Hertzberg V. Hypertension as a risk factor for spontaneous intracerebral hemorrhage. *Stroke* 1986;**17**:1078–1083.

50. Caplan LR, Neely S, Gorelick PB. Cold-related intracerebral hemorrhage. *Arch Neurol* 1984;**41**:227.

51. Hines F, Brown G. A standard test for measuring the variability of blood pressure: Its significance as an index of the prehypertensive state. *Ann Intern Med* 1933;**7**:209–217.

52. Barbas N, Caplan LR, Baquis G, et al. Dental chair intracerebral hemorrhage. *Neurology* 1987;**37**:511–512.

53. Cawley CM, Rigamonti D, Trommer B. Dental chair apoplexy. *South Med J* 1991;**84**:907–909.

54. Haines S, Maroon J, Janetta P. Supratentorial intracerebral hemorrhage following posterior fossa surgery. *J Neurosurgery* 1978;**49**:881–886.

55. Waga S, Shimosaka S, Sakakura M. Intracerebral hemorrhage remote from the site of the initial neurosurgical procedure. *Neurosurgery* 1983;**13**:662–665.

56. Sweet WH, Poletti CE. *Complications of Standard Treatment for Trigeminal Neuralgia: Need for Mechanism for Prompt Reporting of Complications (Abstract).* Poster presentation no. 82 in program of the Annual Meeting of the American Association of Neurological Surgeons. Denver, Colorado, 1986:243.

57. Sweet WH, Poletti CE, Roberts JT. Dangerous rises in blood pressure upon heating of trigeminal rootlets: Increased bleeding times in patients with trigeminal neuralgia. *Neurosurgery* 1985;**17**:843–844.

58. Kehler CH, Brodsky JB, Samuels SI, et al. Blood pressure response during percutaneous rhizotomy for trigeminal neuralgia. *Neurosurgery* 1982;**10**:200–202.

59. Norregaard TV, Moskowitz MA. Substance P and sensory innervation of intracranial and extracranial feline cephalic arteries. *Brain* 1985;**108**:517–533.

60. Moskowitz MA. The neurobiology of vascular head pain. *Ann Neurol* 1984;**16**:157–168.

61. Caplan LR, Skillman J, Ojemann R, Fields W. Intracerebral hemorrhage following carotid endarterectomy: A hypertensive complication. *Stroke* 1978;**9**:457–460.

62. Bruetman MF, Fields WS, Crawford ES, DeBakey ME. Cerebral hemorrhage in carotid artery surgery. *Arch Neurol* 1963;**9**:458–467.

63. Wylie EJ, Hein MF, Adams JE. Intracerebral hemorrhage following surgical revascularization for treatment of acute strokes. *J Neurosurg* 1964;**21**:212–215.

64. Humphreys RP, Hoffman JH, Mustard WT, et al. Cerebral hemorrhage

following heart surgery. *J Neurosurg* 1975;**43**:671–675.

65. Sila CA. Spectrum of neurologic events following cardiac transplantation. *Stroke* 1989;**20**:1586–1589.

66. Cole A, Aube M. Migraine with vasospasm and delayed intracerebral hemorrhage. *Arch Neurol* 1990;**47**:53–56.

67. Gokhale S, Ghoshal S, Lahoti SA, Caplan LR. An uncommon cause of intracerebral hemorrhage in a healthy truck driver. *Arch Neurol* 2012;**69**:1500–1503.

68. Fisher CM, Adams RD. Observations on brain embolism with special reference to hemorrhagic infarction. In A Furlan (ed), *The Heart and Stroke*. London: Springer, 1987;17–36.

69. Wilson SAK, Bruce AN. *Neurology* (2nd ed). London: Butterworth, 1955;1367–1383.

70. Veltkamp R, Rizos T, Horstmann S. Intracerebral bleeding in patients on antithrombotic agents. *Semin Thromb Hemost* 2013;**39**:963–971.

71. Cervera A, Amaro S, Chamorro A. Oral anticoagulant-associated intracerebral hemorrhage. *J Neurol* 2012;**259**:212–214.

72. Askey JM. Hemorrhage during long-term anticoagulant drug therapy: Intracranial hemorrhage. *Calif Med* 1966;**104**:6–10.

73. Cucchiara B, Messe S, Sansing L, Kasner S, Lyden P, for the CHANT Investigators. Hematoma growth in oral anticoagulant related intracerebral hemorrhage. *Stroke* 2008;**39**:2993–2996.

74. Connolly SJ, Ezekowitz MD, Yusuf S, et al. Dabigatran versus warfarin in patients with atrial fibrillation. *N Engl J Med* 2009;**361**:1139–1151.

75. Connolly SJ, Eikelboom J, Joyner C, et al. Apixaban in patients with atrial fibrillation. *N Engl J Med* 2011;**364**:806–817.

76. Granger CB, Alexander JH, McMurray JJ, et al. Apixaban versus warfarin in patients with atrial fibrillation. *N Engl J Med* 2011;**365**:981–992.

77. Patel MR, Mahaffey KW, Garg J, et al. Rivaroxaban versus warfarin in nonvalvular atrial fibrillation. *N Engl J Med* 2011;**365**:883–891.

78. Giugliano RP, Ruff CT, Braunwald E, et al. Edoxaban versus warfarin in patients with atrial fibrillation. *N Engl J Med* 2013;**369**:2093–2104.

79. Hacke W. The dilemma of reinstituting anticoagulation for patients with cardioembolic sources and intracranial hemorrhage. How wide is the strait between Skylla and Karybdis? *Arch Neurol* 2000;**57**:1682–1684.

80. Phan TG, Koh M, Wijdicks EFM. Safety of discontinuation of anticoagulation in patients with intracranial hemorrhage at high thromboembolic risk. *Arch Neurol* 2000;**57**:1710–1713.

81. Wijdicks EFM, Schievink W, Brown R, Mullany C The dilemma of discontinuation of anticoagulation therapy for patients with intracranial hemorrhage and mechanical heart valves. *Neurosurgery* 1998;**42**:769–773.

82. Bertram M, Bonsanto M, Hacke W, Schwab S. Managing the therapeutic dilemma: Patients with spontaneous intracerebral hemorrhage and urgent need for anticoagulation. *J Neurol* 2000;**247**:209–214.

83. Qureshi W, Chetan M, Patsias I, et al. Restarting anticoagulation and outcomes after major gastrointestinal bleeding in atrial fibrillation. *Am J Cardiol* 2014;**113**:662–668.

84. Eckman MH, Rosand J, Knudsen K, Singer DE, Greenberg SM. Can patients be anticoagulated after intracerebral hemorrhage? A decision analysis. *Stroke* 2003;**34**:1710–1716.

85. Kase CS, Pessin MS, Zivin JA, et al. Intracranial hemorrhage after coronary thrombolysis with tissue plasminogen activator. *Am J Med* 1992;**92**:384–390.

86. Saver J. Hemorrhage after thrombolytic therapy for stroke. The Clinically Relevant Number Needed to Harm. *Stroke* 2007;**38**:2279–2283.

87. Derex L, Nighoghosian N. Intracerebral haemorrhage after thrombolysis for acute ischaemic stroke: An update. *J Neurol Neurosurg Psychiatry* 2008;**79**:1093–1099.

88. Caplan LR. Drugs. In CS Kase, LR Caplan (eds), *Intracerebral Hemorrhage*. Boston: Butterworth-Heinemann, 1994;201–220.

89. Brust JCM. Stroke and substance abuse. In LR Caplan (ed), *Uncommon Causes of Stroke*, Cambridge: Cambridge University Press, 2008;365–370.

90. Brust JCM. *Neurological Aspects of Substance Abuse* (2nd ed). Boston, Butterworth-Heinemann, 2004.

91. Harrington H, Heller HA, Dawson D, et al. Intracerebral hemorrhage and oral amphetamine. *Arch Neurol* 1983;**40**:503–507.

92. Buxton N, McConachie, NS. Amphetamine abuse and intracranial haemorrhage. *J R Soc Med* 2000;**93**:472–477.

93. Citron B, Halpern M, McCarron M, et al. Necrotizing angiitis associated with drug abuse. *N Engl J Med* 1970;**283**:1003–1011.

94. Rumbaugh C, Bergeron R, Fang H, et al. Cerebral angiographic changes in the drug abuse patient. *Radiology* 1971;**101**:335–344.

95. Rumbaugh C, Bergeron R, Scanlon R, et al. Cerebral vascular changes secondary to amphetamine abuse in the experimental animal. *Radiology* 1971;**101**:345–351.

96. Fisher CM: The arterial lesions underlying lacunes. *Acta Neuropathol* 1969;**12**:1–15.

97. Lukes SA. Intracerebral hemorrhage from an arteriovenous malformation after amphetamine injection. *Arch Neurol* 1983;**40**:60–61.

98. Cahill D, Knipp HJ, Mosser J. Intracranial hemorrhage with amphetamine usage. *Neurology* 1981;**31**:1058–1059.

99. Yu YJ, Cooper DR, Wellenstein DE, Block B. Cerebral and intracerebral hemorrhage associated with methamphetamine abuse: Case report. *J Neurosurg* 1983;**58**:109–111.

100. Levine SR, Welch KMA. Cocaine and stroke. *Stroke* 1988;**19**:779–783.

101. Levine SR, Brust JCM, Futrell N, et al. Cerebrovascular complications of alkaloid cocaine. *N Engl J Med* 1990;**323**:699–704.

102. Eastman J, Cohen S. Hypertensive crisis and death associated with phencyclidine poisoning. *JAMA* 1975;**231**:1270–1271.

103. Bessen H. Intracranial hemorrhage associated with phencyclidine abuse. *JAMA* 1982;**248**:585–586.

104. Stratton M, Witherspoon J, Kirtley T. Hypertensive crisis and phencyclidine abuse. *Va Med* 1978;**105**:569–572.

105. Lasagna L. *Phenylpropanolamine: A Review*. New York: Wiley, 1988.

106. Kernan WN, Viscoli CM, Brass L, et al. Phenylpropanolamine and the risk of hemorrhagic stroke. *N Engl J Med* 2000;**343**:1826–1832.

107. Kikta DG, Devereux MW, Chandar K. Intracranial hemorrhage due to phenylpropanolamine. *Stroke* 1985;**16**:510–512.

108. Kase CS, Foster TE, Reed JE, et al. Intracerebral hemorrhage and phenylpropanolamine use. *Neurology* 1987;**37**:399–404.

109. McDowell JR, Leblanc H. Phenylpropanolamine and cerebral hemorrhage. *West J Med* 1985;**142**:688–691.

110. Glick R, Hoying J, Cerullo L, Perlman S. Phenylpropanolamine: An over-the-counter drug causing cerebral nervous system vasculitis and intracerebral hemorrhage. *Neurosurgery* 1987;**20**:969–974.

111. Mueller S, Muller J, Asdell S. Cerebral hemorrhage associated with phenylpropanolamine in combination with caffeine. *Stroke* 1984;**15**:119–123.

112. Mueller S. Neurologic complications of phenylpropanolamine use. *Neurology* 1983;**33**:650–652.

113. Tark BE, Messe SR, Balcuani C, Levine SR. Intracerebral hemorrhage associated with oral phenylephrine use: A case report and review of the literature. *J Stroke Cerebrovasc Dis* 2014;**23**:2296–2300.

114. Caplan LR, Thomas C, Banks G. Central nervous system complications of addiction to T's and blues. *Neurology* 1982;**32**:623–628.

115. Buxton N, Flannery T, Wild D, Bassi S. Sildenafil (Viagra) induced spontaneous intracerebral hemorrhage. *Br J Neurosurg* 2001;**15**:347–349.

116. McGee HT, Egan RA, Clark WM. Visual field defect and intracerebral hemorrhage associated with use of vardenafil (Levitra). *Neurology* 2005;**64**:1095–1096.

117. Monastero R, Pipia C, Camarda LK, Camarda R. Intracerebral hemorrhage associated with sildenafil citrate. *J Neurol* 2001;**248**:141–142.

118. Gazzeri R, Neroni M, Galarza M, Esposito S. Intracerebral hemorrhage associated with use of tadalafil (Cialis). *Neurology* 2008;**70**:1289–1290.

119. Zenkevich GS. Role of congophilic angiopathy in the genesis of subarachnoid-parenchymatous hemorrhages in middle-aged and elderly persons. *Zh Nevropatol Psikhiatr* 1978;**78**:52–57.

120. Jellinger K. Cerebral hemorrhage in amyloid angiopathy. *Ann Neurol* 1977;**1**:604.

121. Jellinger K. Cerebrovascular amyloidosis with cerebral hemorrhage. *J Neurol* 1977;**214**:195–206.

122. Biffi A, Greenberg S. Cerebral amyloid angiopathy: A systematic review. *J Clin Neurol* 2011;7:1–9.

123. Cordonnier C, Leys D. Cerebral amyloid angiopathies. In LR Caplan (ed), *Uncommon Causes of Stroke* (2nd ed). Cambridge: Cambridge University Press, 2008;455–464.

124. Vinters H, Gilbert J. Cerebral amyloid angiopathy: Incidence and complications in the aging brain: II. The distribution of amyloid vascular changes. *Stroke* 1983;**14**:923–928.

125. Lee S, Stemmerman G. Congophilic angiopathy and cerebral hemorrhage. *Arch Pathol Lab Med* 1978;**102**:317–321.

126. Gilbert J, Vinters H. Cerebral amyloid angiopathy: Incidence and complications in the aging brain: I. Cerebral hemorrhage. *Stroke* 1983;**14**:915–923.

127. Kase CS. Cerebral amyloid angiopathy. In CS Kase, LR Caplan (eds), *Intracerebral Hemorrhage*. Boston: Butterworth–Heinemann, 1994;179–200.

128. Gilles C, Brucher J, Khoubesserian P, et al. Cerebral amyloid angiopathy as a cause of multiple intracerebral hemorrhages. *Neurology* 1984;**34**:730–735.

129. Finelli P, Kessimian N, Bernstein P. Cerebral amyloid angiopathy manifesting as recurrent intracerebral hemorrhage. *Arch Neurol* 1984;**41**:330–333.

130. Caplan LR. Head trauma and related intracerebral hemorrhage. In CS Kase, LR Caplan (eds), *Intracerebral Hemorrhage*. Boston: Butterworth–Heinemann, 1994;221–241.

131. Alvarez-Sabin J, Turon A, Lozano-Sanchez M, et al. Delayed posttraumatic hemorrhage, "spät-apoplexie". *Stroke* 1995;**26**:1531–1535.

132. Kase CS. Intracranial tumors. In CS Kase, LR Caplan (eds), *Intracerebral Hemorrhage*. Boston: Butterworth–Heinemann 1994;243–261.

133. Kase CS. Vasculitis and other angiopathies. In CS Kase, LR Caplan (eds), *Intracerebral Hemorrhage*. Boston: Butterworth–Heinemann 1994;263–303.

134. Caplan LR, Kase CS. Mechanisms of intracerebral hemorrhage. In CS Kase, LR Caplan (eds), *Intracerebral Hemorrhage*. Boston: Butterworth–Heinemann, 1994;95–98.

135. Russell DS. The pathology of spontaneous intracranial hemorrhages. *Proc R Soc Med* 1954;**47**:689–693.

136. Mutlu N, Berry RG, Alpers BJ. Massive cerebral hemorrhage: Clinical and pathological correlations. *Arch Neurol* 1963;**8**:74–91.

137. McCormick WF, Rosenfield DB. Massive brain hemorrhage: A review of 144 cases and an examination of their causes. *Stroke* 1973;**4**:946–954.

138. Schütz H. *Spontane intrazerebrale hamatome: pathophysiologie, klinik, und therapie*. Heidelberg: Springer, 1988.

139. Jellinger K. Zur atiologie und pathogenese der spontanen intrazerebralen blutung. *Therapiewoche* 1972;**22**:1440–1450.

140. Weisberg LA. Computerized tomography in intracranial hemorrhage. *Arch Neurol* 1979;**36**:422–26.

141. Quereshi AI, Suri MAK, Safdar K, et al. Intracerebral hemorrhage in blacks: Risk factors, subtypes, and outcome. *Stroke* 1997;**28**:961–964.

142. Ruiz-Sandoval JL, Cantu C, Barinagarrementeria F. Intracerebral hemorrhage in young people: Analysis of risk factors, locations, causes, and prognosis. *Stroke* 1999;**30**:537–541.

143. Fisher CM. Clinical syndromes in cerebral hemorrhage. In: Pathogenesis and Treatment of Cerebrovascular Disease. In W Fields (ed), *Proceedings of the Annual Meeting of the Houston Neurological Society*. Springfield, IL: Thomas, 1961;318–342.

144. Caplan LR. Putaminal hemorrhage. In CS Kase, LR Caplan (eds), *Intracerebral Hemorrhage*. Boston: Butterworth–Heinemann, 1994;309–327.

145. Chung C-S, Caplan LR, Yamamoto Y, et al. Striatocapsular haemorrhage. *Brain* 2000;**123**:1850–1862.

146. Koba T, Yokoyama T, Kaneko M. Correlation between the location of hematoma and its clinical symptoms in the lateral type of hypertensive intracerebral hemorrhage. *Stroke* 1977;**8**:676–680.

147. Mizukami M, Nishijuma M, Kin H. Computed tomographic findings of good prognosis for hemiplegia in hypertensive putaminal hemorrhage. *Stroke* 1981;**12**:648–652.

148. Stein R, Caplan LR, Hier DB. Intracerebral hemorrhage: Role of blood pressure, location, and size of lesions. *Ann Neurol* 1983;**14**:132–133.

149. LoPresti M, Bruce SS, Camacho E, et al. Hematoma volume as the major determinant of outcomes after intracerebral hemorrhage. *J Neurol Sci* 2014;**345**:3–7.

150. Mizukami M, Kin H, Araki G, et al. Surgical treatment of primary intracerebral hemorrhage: I. New angiographical classification. *Stroke* 1976;**7**:30–36.

151. Metter EJ, Jackson C, Kempler D, et al. Left hemisphere intracerebral hemorrhages studied by (F-18)-fluorodeoxyglucose PET. *Neurology* 1986;**36**:1155–1162.

152. Stein R, Kase C, Hier DB, et al. Caudate hemorrhage. *Neurology* 1984;**34**:1549–1554.

153. Weisberg L. Caudate hemorrhage. *Arch Neurol* 1984;**41**:971–974.

154. Caplan LR. Caudate hemorrhage. In CS Kase, LR Caplan (eds), *Intracerebral Hemorrhage*. Boston: Butterworth–Heinemann, 1994;329–340.

155. Pedrazzi P, Bogousslavsky J, Regli F. Hématomes limités à la tête du Noyau Caudé. *Rev Neurol* 1990;**146**:12:726–738.

156. Caplan LR. Thalamic hemorrhage. In CS Kase, LR Caplan (eds), *Intracerebral Hemorrhage*. Boston: Butterworth–Heinemann, 1994;341–362.

157. Chung, CS, Caplan LR, Han W, et al. Thalamic haemorrhage. *Brain* 1996;**119**:1873–1886.

158. Barraquer-Bordas L, Illa I, Escartin A, et al. Thalamic hemorrhage: A study of 23 patients with diagnosis by computed tomography. *Stroke* 1981;**12**:524–527.

159. Caplan LR. "Top of the basilar" syndrome: Selected clinical aspects. *Neurology* 1980;**30**:72–79.

160. Mohr JP, Walters W, Duncan G. Thalamic hemorrhage and aphasia. *Brain Lang* 1975;**2**:3–17.

161. Ciemins V. Localized thalamic hemorrhage: A cause of aphasia. *Neurology* 1970;**20**:776–782.

162. Samarel A, Wright T, Sergay S, et al. Thalamic hemorrhage with speech disorder. *Trans Am Neurol Assoc* 1975;**101**:283–285.

163. Watson R, Heilman K. Thalamic neglect. *Neurology* 1979;**29**:690–694.

164. Young WB, Lee KP, Pessin MS, et al. Prognostic significance of ventricular blood in supratentorial hemorrhage: A volumetric study. *Neurology* 1990;**40**:616–619.

165. Kawahara N, Sato K, Muraki M, et al. CT classification of small thalamic hemorrhages and their clinical implications. *Neurology* 1986;**35**:165–172.

166. Ikeda K, Yamashima T, Uno E, et al. Clinical manifestations of small thalamic hemorrhages. *Brain Nerve* 1985;**37**:171–179.

167. Gilner L, Avin B. A reversible ocular manifestation of thalamic hemorrhage: A case report. *Arch Neurol* 1977;**34**:715–716.

168. Waga S, Okada M, Yamamoto Y. Reversibility of Parinaud syndrome in thalamic hemorrhage. *Neurology* 1979;**29**:407–409.

169. Kase C, Williams J, Wyatt D, et al. Lobar intracerebral hematomas: Clinical and CT analysis of 22 cases. *Neurology* 1982;**32**:1146–1150.

170. Ropper A, Davis K. Lobar cerebral hemorrhages: Acute clinical syndromes in 26 cases. *Ann Neurol* 1980;**8**:141–147.

171. Kase CS. Lobar Hemorrhage. In CS Kase, LR Caplan (eds), *Intracerebral Hemorrhage*. Boston: Butterworth–Heinemann, 1994;363–382.

172. Kase C. Lobar hemorrhages. In LR Caplan, J van Gijn (eds), *Stroke Syndromes* (3rd ed). Cambridge: Cambridge University Press, 2012;516–525.

173. Zhu XL, Chan MSY, Poon WS. Spontaneous intracranial hemorrhage: Which patients need diagnostic cerebral angiography? A prospective study of 296 cases and review of the literature. *Stroke* 1997;**28**:1406–1409.

174. Caplan LR. Primary intraventricular hemorrhage. In CS Kase, LR Caplan (eds), *Intracerebral Hemorrhage*. Boston: Butterworth–Heinemann, 1994;383–401.

175. Butler A, Partain R, Netsky M. Primary intraventricular hemorrhage in adults. *Surg Neurol* 1977;**8**:143–149.

176. Little JR, Blomquist G, Ethier R. Intraventricular hemorrhage in adults. *Surg Neurol* 1977;**8**:143–149.

177. Ziai WC, Hanley D. Intraventricular hemorrhage. In LR Caplan, J van Gijn (eds), *Stroke Syndromes* (3rd ed). Cambridge: Cambridge University Press, 2012;526–533.

178. Naff NJ, Hanley DF, Keyl PM, et al. Intraventricular thrombolysis speeds blood clot resolution: Results of a pilot prospective, randomized double-blind controlled trial. *Neurosurgery* 2004;**54**:577–584.

179. Steiner T, Diringer MN, Schneider D, et al. Dynamics of intraventricular hemorrhage in patients with spontaneous intracerebral hemorrhage: Risk factors, clinical impact and effect of hemostatic therapy with recombinant factor VII. *Neurosurgery* 2006;**59**:767–773.

180. Bhattathiri PS, Gregson B, Prasad KS, Mendelow AD. Intraventricular hemorrhage and hydrocephalus after spontaneous intracerebral hemorrhage: Results from the STICH trial. *Acta Neurochir Suppl* 2006;**96**:65–68.

181. Zhang Z, Li X, Liu Y, et al. Application of neurendoscopy in the treatment of intraventricular hemorrhage. *Cerebrovasc Dis* 2007;**24**:91–96.

182. Kase CS, Caplan LR. Parenchymatous posterior fossa hemorrhage. In HJM Barnett, JP Mohr, B Stein, F Yatsu (eds), *Stroke: Pathophysiology, Diagnosis and Management*. New York: Churchill Livingstone, 1985;621–641.

183. Caplan LR. Pontine hemorrhage. In CS Kase, LR Caplan (eds), *Intracerebral Hemorrhage*. Boston: Butterworth–Heinemann, 1994;403–423.

184. Chung C-S, Caplan LR. Pontine infarcts and hemorrhages. In LR Caplan, J van Gijn (eds), *Stroke Syndromes* (3rd ed). Cambridge: Cambridge University Press, 2012;448–460.

185. Caplan LR, Zervas N. Survival with permanent midbrain dysfunction after surgical treatment of traumatic subdural hematoma: The clinical picture of a Duret hemorrhage. *Ann Neurol* 1977;**1**:587–589.

186. Steegman T. Primary pontile hemorrhage. *J Nerv Ment Dis* 1951;**114**:35–65.

187. Silverstein A. Primary pontine hemorrhage. In P Vinken, G Bruyn (eds), *Handbook of Clinical Neurology, Vol 12, Part 2. Vascular Diseases of the Nervous System*. Amsterdam: North Holland, 1972;37–53.

188. Caplan LR, Goodwin J. Lateral tegmental brainstem hemorrhage. *Neurology* 1982;**32**:252–260.

189. Kase C, Maulsby G, Mohr JP. Partial pontine hematomas. *Neurology* 1980;**30**:652–655.

190. Graveleau P, DeCroix JP, Samson Y, et al. Déficit sensitive isolé d'un hémicorps par hématome du pont. *Rev Neurol (Paris)* 1986;**142**:788–790.

191. Araga S, Fukada M, Kagimoto H, et al. Pure sensory stroke due to pontine hemorrhage. *J Neurol* 1987;**235**:116–117.

192. Holtzman RNN, Zablozki V, Yang WC, et al. Lateral pontine tegmental hemorrhage presenting as isolated trigeminal sensory neuropathy. *Neurology* 1987;**37**:704–706.

193. Veerapen R. Spontaneous lateral pontine hemorrhage with associated trigeminal nerve root hematoma. *Neurosurgery* 1989;**25**:451–454.

194. Gobernado J, de Molina A, Gimeno A. Pure motor hemiplegia due to hemorrhage in the lower pons. *Arch Neurol* 1980;**37**:393.

195. Kameyama S, Tanaka R, Tsuchida T. Pure motor hemiplegia due to pontine hemorrhage. *Stroke* 1989;**20**:1288.

196. Schnapper R. Pontine hemorrhage presenting as ataxic hemiparesis. *Stroke* 1982;**13**:518–519.

197. Kobatake K, Shinohara Y. Ataxic hemiparesis in patients with primary pontine hemorrhage. *Stroke* 1983;**14**:762–764.

198. Tuhrim S, Yang WC, Rubinowitz H, et al. Primary pontine hemorrhage and the dysarthria-clumsy hand syndrome. *Neurology* 1982;**32**:1027–1028.

199. Nakajima K. Clinicopathological study of pontine hemorrhage. *Stroke* 1983;**14**:485–493.

200. Lhermitte F, Pages M. Abducens nucleus syndrome due to pontine hemorrhage. *Cerebrovasc Dis* 2006;**22**:284–285.

201. Sherman SC, Saadermand B. Pontine hemorrhage and isolated abducens nerve palsy. *Am J Emer Med* 2007;**25**:104–105.

202. Watanabe A, Kobashi T. Lateral gaze disturbance due to cerebral microbleed in the medial lemniscus in the mid-pontine region: A case report. *Neuroradiology* 2005;**47**:908–911.

203. Toyoda K, Okada S, Inoue T, et al. Antithrombotic therapy and predilection for cerebellar hemorrhage. *Cerebrovasc Dis* 2007;**23**:109–116.

204. Brennan R, Berglund R. Acute cerebellar hemorrhage: Analysis of clinical findings and outcome in 12 cases. *Neurology* 1977;**27**:527–532.

205. Fisher CM, Picard E, Polak A, et al. Acute hypertensive cerebellar hemorrhage: Diagnosis and surgical treatment. *J Nerv Ment Dis* 1965;**140**:38–57.

206. Ott K, Kase C, Ojemann R, et al. Cerebellar hemorrhage: Diagnosis and treatment. *Arch Neurol* 1974;**31**:160–167.

207. Kase CS. Cerebellar hemorrhage. In CS Kase, LR Caplan (eds), *Intracerebral Hemorrhage*. Boston: Butterworth–Heinemann, 1994;425–443.

208. Ojemann R, Heros R. Spontaneous brain hemorrhage. *Stroke* 1983;**14**:468–474.

209. Shenkin H, Zavala M. Cerebellar strokes: Mortality, surgical indications and results of ventricular damage. *Lancet* 1982;**2**:429–432.

210. Richardson AE. Spontaneous cerebellar hemorrhage. In P Vinken, G Bruyn (eds), *Handbook of Clinical Neurology*. Amsterdam: North Holland, 1972;54–67.

211. Ecker A. Upward transtentorial herniation of the cerebellum due to tumor in the posterior fossa. *J Neurosurg* 1948;**5**:51–61.

212. Cuneo RA, Caronna JJ, Pitts L, Townsend J, Winestock DP. Upwards transtentorial herniation: Seven cases and a literature review. *Arch Neurol* 1979;**36**:618–623.

213. Dolderer S, Kallenberg K, Aschoff A, et al. Long-term outcome after spontaneous cerebellar haemorrhage. *Eur Neurol* 2004;**52**:112–119.

214. Longo M, Fiumara F, Pandolfo I, et al. CT observation of an ongoing intracerebral hemorrhage. *J Comput Assist Tomogr* 1983;**7**:362–363.

215. Zilkha A. Intraparenchymal fluid-blood level: A CT sign of recent intracerebral hemorrhage. *J Comput Assist Tomogr* 1983;**7**:301–305.

216. Pineda A. Computed tomography in intracerebral hemorrhage. *Surg Neurol* 1977;**8**:55–58.

217. Dul K, Drayer B. CT and MR imaging of intracerebral hemorrhage. In CS Kase, LR Caplan (eds), *Intracerebral Hemorrhage*. Boston: Butterworth–Heinemann, 1994;73–93.

218. Scott W, New P, Davis K, et al. Computerized axial tomography of intracerebral and intraventricular hemorrhage. *Radiology* 1974;**112**:73–80.

219. Herald S, Kummer R, Jaeger C. Follow-up of spontaneous intracerebral hemorrhage by computed tomography. *J Neurology* 1982;**228**:267–276.

220. Schellinger PD, Jansen O, Fiebach JB, et al. A standardized MRI protocol. Comparison with CT in hyperacute intracerebral hemorrhage. *Stroke* 1999;**30**:765–768.

221. Linfante I, Llinas RH, Caplan LR, Warach S. MRI features of intracerebral hemorrhage within 2 hours from symptom onset. *Stroke* 1999;**30**:2263–2267.

222. Yasui T, Kishi H, Komiyama M, et al. Very poor prognosis in cases with extravasation of the contrast medium during angiography. *Surg Neurol* 1996;**45**:560–564.

223. Ruiz-Sandoval JL, Chiquette E, Romero-Vargas S, et al. Grading scale for prediction of outcome in primary cerebral hemorrhages. *Stroke* 2007;**38**:1641–1644.

224. Kothari R, Brott T, Broderick JP, et al. The ABCs of measuring intracerebral hemorrhage volumes. *Stroke* 1996;**27**:1304–1305.

225. Little J, Blomquist G, Ethier R. Cerebellar hemorrhage in adults: Diagnosis by computerized tomography. *J Neurosurg* 1978;**48**:575–579.

226. Rädberg JA, Olsson JE, Radberg CT. Prognostic parameters in spontaneous intracerebral hematomas with special reference to anticoagulant treatment. *Stroke* 1991;**22**:571–576.

227. Terayama Y, Tanahashi N, Fukuuchi Y, Gotoh F. Prognostic value of admission blood pressure in patients with intracerebral hemorrhage. Keio Cooperative Stroke Study. *Stroke* 1997;**28**:1185–1188.

228. Diringer MN, Edwards DF, Zazulia A. Hydrocephalus: A previously unrecognized predictor of poor outcome from supratentorial intracerebral hemorrhage. *Stroke* 1998;**29**:1352–1357.

229. Dandapani B, Suzuki S, Kelley RE, et al. Relation between blood pressure and outcome in intracerebral hemorrhage. *Stroke* 1995;**26**:21–24.

230. Tuhrim S, Horowitz DR, Sacher M, Godbold JH. Volume of intraventricular blood is an important determinant of outcome in supratentorial intracerebral hemorrhage. *Crit Care Med* 1999;**27**:617–621.

231. Anderson CS, Heeley E, Huang Y, et al. Rapid blood pressure lowering in patients with acute intracerebral hemorrhage. *N Engl J Med* 2013;**368**:2355–2365.

232. Morgenstern LB, Hemphill JC III, Anderson C, et al. Guidelines for the management of spontaneous intracerebral hemorrhage: A guideline for healthcare professionals from the American Heart Association/American Stroke Association. *Stroke* 2010;**41**:2108–2129.

233. Tsivgoulis G, Karsanos AH, Butcher KS, et al. Intensive blood pressure reduction in acute intracerebral hemorrhage. *Neurology* 2014;**83**:1523–1529.

234. Langfitt T. Conservative care of intracranial hemorrhage. In R Thompson, J Green (eds), *Advances in Neurology, Vol 11. Stroke*. New York: Raven, 1977;169–180.

235. Poungvarin N, Bhoopat W, Viriyavejakul A, et al. Effects of dexamethasone in primary supratentorial intracerebral hemorrhage. *N Engl J Med* 1987;**316**:1229–1233.

236. Mehdiratta M, Kumar S, Hackney D, et al. Association between serum ferritin level and perihematomal edema volume in patients with spontaneous intracerebral hemorrhage. *Stroke* 2008;**39**:1165–1170.

237. Selim M. Deferoxamine mesylate: A new hope for intracerebral hemorrhage: From bench to clinical trials. *Stroke* 2009;**40**:590–591.

238. Majeed A, Schulman S. Bleeding and antidotes in new oral anticoagulants. *Best Pract Res Clin Haematol* 2009;**49**:1171–1177.

239. Mayer SA. Ultra-early hemostatic therapy for intracerebral hemorrhage. *Stroke*. 2003;**34**:224–229.

240. Mayer SA, Brun NC, Broderick J, et al. Safety and feasibility of recombinant factor VIIa for acute intracerebral hemorrhage. *Stroke* 2005;**36**:74–79.

241. Mayer SA, Brun NC, Begtrup K, et al. Recombinant activated factor VII for acute intracerebral hemorrhage. *N Engl J Med* 2005;**352**:777–785.

242. Mayer SA, Brun NC, Begtrup K, et al. Efficacy and safety of recombinant activated factor VII for acute intracerebral hemorrhage. *N Engl J Med* 2008;**358**:2127–2137.

243. Sugg RM, Gonzales NR, Matherne DE, et al. Myocardial injury in patients with intracerebral hemorrhage treated with recombinant factor VIIa. *Neurology*. 2006;**67**:1053–1055.

244. Mendelow AD, Gregson BA, Fernandes HM, et al. Early surgery versus initial conservative treatment in patients with spontaneous supratentorial intracerebral haematomas in the international surgical trial in intracerebral haemorrhage (STICH): A randomised trial. *Lancet* 2005;**365**:387–397.

245. Mendelow AD, Gregson BA, Rowan EN, Murray GD, Gholkar A, Mitchell PM. Early surgery versus initial conservative treatment in patients with spontaneous supratentorial lobar intracerebral haematomas (STICH II): A randomised trial. *Lancet* 2013;**382**:397–408.

246. Prasad KS, Gregson BA, Bhattathiri PS, Mitchell P, Mendelow AD. The significance of crossovers after randomization in the STICH trial. *Acta Neurochir Suppl* 2006;**96**:61–64.

247. Bhattathiri PS, Gregson B, Prasad KS, Mendelow AD. Intraventricular hemorrhage and hydrocephalus after spontaneous intracerebral hemorrhage: Results from the STICH trial. *Acta Neurochir Suppl* 2006;**96**:65–68.

248. Matsumoto K, Honda H. CT guided stereotaxic evacuation of hypertensive intracerebral hematoma. *J Neurosurg* 1984;**61**:440–448.

249. Kandel EL, Peresadov VV. Stereotactic evacuation of spontaneous intracerebral hematomas. *J Neurosurg* 1985;**62**:206–213.

250. Nizuma H, Suzuki J. Stereotactic aspiration of putaminal hemorrhage using a double track aspiration technique. *Neurosurgery* 1988;**22**:432–436.

251. Nguyen JP, Decq P, Brugieres P, et al. A technique for stereotactic aspiration of deep intracerebral hematomas under computed tomographic control using a new device. *Neurosurgery* 1992;**31**:330–335.

252. Mohadjer M, Eggert R, May J, Mayfrank L. CT-guided stereotactic fibrinolysis of spontaneous and hypertensive cerebellar hemorrhage: Long-term results. *J Neurosurg* 1990;**73**:217–222.

253. Findlay JM, Grace MG, Weir BK. Treatment of intraventricular hemorrhage with tissue plasminogen activator. *Neurosurgery* 1993;**32**:941–947.

254. Schaller C, Rhode V, Meyer B, Hassler W. Stereotactic puncture and lysis of spontaneous intracerebral hemorrhage using recombinant tissue-plasminogen activator (rtPA) after stereotactic aspiration: Initial results. *Neurosurgery* 1995;**36**:328–335.

255. Barnes B, Hanley DF, Carhuapoma JR. Minimally invasive surgery for intracerebral haemorrhage. *Curr Opin Crit Care* 2014;**20**:148–152.

256. Ziai WC, Tuhrim S, Lane K, et al. A multicenter, randomized, double-blinded, placebo-controlled phase III study of Clot Lysis Evaluation of Accelerated Resolution of Intraventricular Hemorrhage (CLEAR III). *Int J Stroke* 2014;**9**:536–542.

257. Cho DY, Chen CC, Chang CS, et al. Endoscopic surgery for spontaneous basal ganglia hemorrhage: Comparing endoscopic surgery, stereotactic aspiration, and craniotomy in noncomatose patients. *Surg Neurol* 2006;**65**:547–556.

258. Tyler K, Poletti C, Heros R. Cerebral amyloid angiopathy with multiple intracerebral hemorrhages. *Neurosurgery* 1982;**577**:286–289.

259. Morgenstern LB, Demchuk AM, Kim DH, et al. Rebleeding leads to poor outcomes in ultra-early craniotomy for intracerebral hemorrhage. *Neurology* 2001;**56**:1294–1299.

Stroke in children and young adults

Gabrielle deVeber, Aneesh B Singhal, and Louis R Caplan

Stroke in children, adolescents, and young adults accounts for approximately 15% of all ischemic strokes, and a higher proportion of all hemorrhagic strokes.[1] Of all strokes among persons 15–44 years of age, approximately 50% are ischemic, 20% are intracerebral hemorrhage (ICH), and 30% are subarachnoid hemorrhage (SAH). When compared to whites, African-Americans have incidence rates twofold higher for ischemic stroke. The clinical features and evaluation strategies of stroke in young individuals (defined as <50 years of age in most published series) are rather different from older adults. In this chapter, we briefly outline some of the key differences, and review the differential diagnoses of strokes in the young. We do not repeat descriptions of stroke syndromes and vascular disorders covered in more depth elsewhere in this book. Chapter 12 includes discussions of many of the conditions that cause stroke in the young.

General features and differences from strokes and cerebrovascular disease in geriatric-age patients

Etiological variations associated with age

Causes of stroke in the young are more heterogeneous than older persons. Young individuals have higher rates of genetic, congenital, metabolic, infectious, and systemic causes. Atherosclerosis and atrial fibrillation are the dominant causes in older adults, although they are now being recognized as significant risk factors even in the young.[2–4] Rates of cryptogenic stroke differ significantly across age groups. This may be partly explained by differences in the extent of diagnostic evaluations. Among the young stroke population, causes of stroke differ considerably with age. For example, the differential diagnosis of stroke in a young baby is quite different from that in a 40-year-old adult, yet both are often referred to as stroke in the young. Three convenient groups can be distinguished: perinatal and neonatal (prenatal to 29 days postnatal age), children including adolescents (ages 1 month to 18 years), and young adults (ages 18–50 years). Each of these groups has different frequencies of various stroke etiologies. Causes also vary considerably, depending on geographical, socioeconomical, and environmental factors. For instance, tuberculous meningitis is an important cause of stroke in India,[5,6] and neurocysticercosis is an important cause of stroke in Mexico

and parts of Central and South America,[7,8] while moyamoya is a common cause of stroke in Japan. These causes of stroke are much less common in the United States.

Several lines of evidence have raised public health concerns about the rising prevalence of traditional vascular risk factors in young individuals, and their potential role in increasing the risk for ischemic stroke, recurrent stroke, and post-stroke mortality.[9–12] These data have started to draw more attention to the problem of stroke in the young[1] and have already stimulated research in the field. An increasing awareness of the frequency and impact of perinatal stroke (minimum frequency 1/2300 live births) and childhood stroke (2/100 000 children per year) has accompanied an accelerated research focus on stroke in pediatric populations.

Prevalence of hemorrhagic stroke

Hemorrhagic strokes, including SAH and ICH, are relatively common in the young. In the geriatric years, the ischemic–hemorrhagic stroke ratio is approximately 4 to 1 (80% of strokes are ischemic), whereas in the young, the ratio is close to 1.0–1.5 (60% are hemorrhagic).[13,14] Among children ischemic strokes may be up to twice as common as hemorrhagic strokes.[15] The ratio also differs according to geography: in a Dutch study of 959 consecutive first-ever stroke or transient ischemic attacks (TIAs), only 91 patients had a hemorrhagic stroke.[12] Accurate comparative statistics are hard to gather because hemorrhagic strokes are often cared for on neurosurgical units, and ischemic strokes are usually admitted to pediatric and adult neurology units.

Prevalence of particular etiologies of stroke

Arteriopathies (including dissection and infectious arteriopathies), and cardiac disease are especially important etiologies in children and young adults. Arteriopathies account for 20–35% of strokes in young adults and up to 50% in children.[16] Drugs and systemic, genetic, and hematological causes are also important in children and young adults. Occlusion of dural venous sinuses and cerebral veins is a more important cause of stroke in the young than in mature adults.

Locations of lesions

Brain and vascular location of lesions are somewhat different in the young due to their different spectrum of etiologies. For example, stroke is often associated with inflammatory/infectious arteriopathies where infarcts are more often distributed

Caplan's Stroke: A Clinical Approach, 5th Edition, ed. Louis R Caplan. Published by Cambridge University Press. © Cambridge University Press, 2016.

in the deep regions of the cerebral hemispheres, especially the striatocapsular region. Also infarcts in patients who have bacterial endocarditis tend to be multiple and widely distributed. Carotid artery dissection usually results in single or multiple unilateral hemispheric infarcts. The reversible cerebral vasoconstriction syndrome typically results in bilateral cortical–subcortical infarcts in arterial watershed regions. Some conditions are associated with highly specific lesion distributions; for example, "transient cerebral arteriopathy" (large unilateral infarcts in the basal ganglia); moyamoya syndrome ("string of pearls" white matter infarcts); Susac syndrome ("snowball" lesions in the corpus callosum); cerebral autosomal dominant arteriopathy with subcortical infarcts and leukoencephalopathy (CADASIL) (external capsule and anterior temporal lobe hyperintense white matter lesions, and small-vessel infarcts). Mitochondrial disorders like mitochondrial encephalopathy, lactic acidosis and stroke (MELAS) usually result in cortical gray matter lesions that cross arterial territories especially in the posterior portions of the cerebral hemispheres.

Vascular-occlusive lesions are more often intracranial, affecting especially the supraclinoid internal carotid artery (ICA), proximal anterior (ACA) and middle (MCA) cerebral arteries, and the basilar artery. Extracranial occlusive disease is much less common. When the occlusive disease occurs at the origin of the MCA, the lenticulostriate branches, the striatum and internal capsule are often involved. Because of the absence of extensive vascular disease in young stroke patients, collateral circulation over the convexity is usually good, in some cases sparing the MCA cortical territory.[17,18] Similarly, proximal posterior cerebral artery occlusion at the origin of the thalamogeniculate branches usually leads to thalamic infarcts, and there may be sparing of the temporal and occipital lobes.[19,20] Vascular malformations are more often periventricular or intraventricular than in adults.

Clinical presentations and features

Young persons are less likely to seek emergency medical care. They are often misdiagnosed even after arrival at the hospital. This is due to atypical presenting symptoms[21] (some of which are shown in Table 15.1), a wider differential diagnosis for focal neurological deficits and a widespread under-appreciation that stroke can affect young individuals. Stroke mimics are common and include: seizures, acute vestibular syndrome, migraine, infections, brain tumors, toxic-metabolic encephalopathy, hypoglycemia, hypertensive encephalopathy, gastroenteritis, conversion disorder, cardiac syncope, herpes-simplex virus encephalitis, demyelinating disease, and myasthenia gravis. In children, seizures at stroke onset are frequent, confounding the diagnosis. In infants and young children focal deficits are less common because the brain is insufficiently mature to demonstrate these. Even cognitive syndromes may be non-specific including agitation and general confusion; specific disorders of higher cognitive function are harder to recognize and less well characterized than in adults. Aphasias in childhood are most often non-fluent, regardless of brain lesion location.[22]

Table 15.1 Atypical stroke presentations

Non-localizing symptoms	Neuropsychiatric symptoms Acute confusional state/delirium Depressed level of consciousness
Abnormal movements	Chorea Hemiballismus Dystonia Unilateral asterixis Hemifacial spasm Alien hand syndrome/deafferentation Limb-shaking transient ischemic attacks Seizures secondary to stroke
Cranial neuropathies	Acute vestibular syndrome Acute hearing loss Ischemic optic neuropathy Horner syndrome Third nerve palsy VIIth-nerve palsy Other cranial neuropathies
Isolated symptoms	Isolated dysarthria Isolated dysphagia/stridor Isolated facial paresis Monoparesis of arm or leg or a part of limb or distal extremity Isolated sensory symptoms Isolated visual loss Isolated headache
Headache	Headache

Adapted from Edlow JA, Selim MH. Atypical presentations of acute cerebrovascular syndromes. *Lancet Neurol* 2011;10:550–560 with permission.

Abnormalities of posture and movement, such as dystonias, chorea, and athetosis, are more frequent features and sequelae of stroke than in adults.[23] These extrapyramidal disorders probably reflect the vulnerability of immature striatocapsular structures to ischemia possibly combined with aberrant rewiring during recovery. In infants with hypoxic ischemic injury, the bilateral basal ganglia and thalami become hypermyelinated, giving them a marbled appearance, referred to as status marmoratus.[24]

Approach to diagnosis

The appropriate diagnosis and management of stroke in young individuals requires a multidisciplinary approach involving neurologists, neuroradiologists, rheumatologists, geneticists, infectious disease specialists, cardiologists, and others. In general, a thorough history combined with detailed examination of the skin, eyes, and organ systems is always warranted. Chronic headaches, cognitive deficits or psychiatric manifestations, with a step-wise accumulation of focal deficits, usually suggests an arteriopathy. Abnormal cerebrospinal fluid (CSF) examination results may suggest cerebral vasculitis or

Table 15.2 Laboratory evaluation: common tests

Complete blood count with differential cell counts

Erythrocyte sedimentation rate

Urinalysis

Prothrombin time (PT with international normalized ratio (INR)), activated partial thromboplastin time (aPTT)

Serum electrolytes, liver and renal function tests

Blood glucose, hemoglobin $A1_C$ level

Lipid panel, lipoprotein (a) level, C-reactive protein level

Pregnancy test

Head computed tomography (CT), brain magnetic resonance imaging (MRI)

Cerebral arterial imaging: CT-, MR-, or digital subtraction angiography of the head and neck, carotid artery Duplex ultrasound, transcranial Doppler (TCD) ultrasound

Brain perfusion imaging; e.g., CT-perfusion or MR-perfusion (optional)

Transthoracic and/or transesophageal echocardiography (ECG)

Cardiac rhythm monitoring

infectious arteriopathies. The skin and eye examination can be particularly informative; for example, ectopia lentis (Marfan's syndrome); iris hamartomas, optic nerve tumors and café-au-lait spots (neurofibromatosis-1); or cataracts, corneal opacities and angiokeratomas (Fabry's disease); atrophic white papules on the skin in Dego's disease, or livedo reticularis in systemic lupus erythematosus. Genetic arteriopathies may be suggested by fundoscopic abnormalities; for example, retinal arteriolar irregularities (CADASIL, retinal vasculopathy with cerebral leukodystrophy (RVCL), or branch retinal artery occlusions (Susac's syndrome)).

Several small-vessel arteriopathies can be confirmed with specialized tests such as skin or brain biopsy, or genetic, immunological, or microbiological tests. Others are diagnosed solely with clinical–imaging correlation; for example, in adults with chronic hypertension, lipohyalinosis and well-defined lacunar strokes, and a corresponding small cerebral infarction in the distribution of a penetrating artery. Careful analysis of the size, location, and distribution of infarcts on brain imaging studies often provides insights into the cause. A thorough evaluation of the cerebral vasculature is important given the high prevalence of cerebral arteriopathies in young stroke patients,

At this time, however, there is no "recommended" battery of tests or guidelines for the etiological evaluation of stroke in the young.[25] In the absence of validated diagnostic criteria or confirmatory tests for many of the causes of stroke in the young, the diagnosis and management remains variable. Table 15.2 contains a list of common laboratory tests available for etiological evaluation.

Prognosis

In youths, the outlook for recovery is better than in adults with comparable brain and vascular lesions. The absence of generalized vascular disease and the presence of good collateral circulation often minimizes the eventual brain damage, making the ultimate infarct smaller than in adults. Also, the developing brain shows more plasticity. Undamaged areas can frequently assume the functions of damaged regions. As a result, focal disorders of cognition and aphasia often improve, leaving no major speech deficit, although general intellectual function may be less than that expected before the stroke. Although the prognosis is better than in the geriatric age group, strokes in the young are far from benign. Among 1040 children with arterial ischemic strokes in the Canadian Pediatric Ischemic Stroke Registry, neurological deficits were found in 61% of children who had neonatal strokes and neurological deficits and recurrent strokes were common in older children.[26] A 1994 study of the prognosis of strokes in patients aged 15–45 years showed that most stroke survivors had emotional, social, or physical impairments that adversely affected employment and reduced their quality of life.[27] Recent data continues to show a significant rate of death, long-term disability, and socioeconomic consequences after stroke in young adults and children. In the Helsinki cohort, mortality was 2.7% at one month, 4.7% at one year, and 10.7% at five years with no gender differences.[28] A prospective Dutch cohort study showed 20-year mortality rates of nearly 25% after TIAs and 27% after ischemic stroke.[12] Traditional vascular risk factors such as diabetes were significant predictors of death. Young adult stroke patients have a 2–3-fold higher risk of remaining unemployed as compared to their peers.[29] These data emphasize the importance of implementing primary and secondary vascular preventive strategies in young individuals, and developing programs that address the long-term psychosocial and economic impact of having stroke at a young age.[30]

Strokes in neonates

Hypoxic-ischemic insults

Hypoxic-ischemic and metabolic injuries are relatively common in neonates. The causes of neonatal brain injury are extremely varied; laboratory and imaging advances are still identifying new etiologies.[31,32] High concentrations of unsaturated fatty acids and free radicals, a high rate of oxygen consumption, and low concentration of antioxidants make the neonatal brain especially vulnerable to oxidative damage.[31,33] Many lesions in premature infants are located in the periventricular white matter. Ischemic cerebral white matter is quite susceptible to free-radical mediated injury to immature oligodendrocytes.[33] These conditions are most often attributable to: (1) intrauterine asphyxia; (2) birth-related problems, such as umbilical cord prolapse, forceps delivery, and breech presentation; (3) uterine and placental abruption; (4) respiratory insufficiency after birth, caused by aspirated meconium; (5) recurrent apnea; (6) hyaline-membrane disease in premature infants; and (7) severe congenital heart disease, with left-to-right shunts in premature and full-term neonates.[34–37] In preterm infants, fetal heart-rate abnormalities,

hypoglycemia, and twin-to-twin transfusion syndrome are other conditions that predispose to brain infarcts.[34] Twin-to-twin transfusion syndrome is due to monochorionic implantation with vascular interconnections or intrauterine death of a co-twin, explaining redistribution of thromboplastic material and potential emboli.[38]

Cerebral blood flow is lower in preterm than in term newborns (20 ml/100 g per min vs. 50–60 ml/100 g per min).[39] The neonatal brain has little autoregulatory capability, so it is much more vulnerable to falls or elevations in blood pressure. Neonatal ischemia is often caused by cardiac disease and sepsis with vascular collapse. Genetic and acquired coagulation abnormalities also may contribute to the development of neonatal strokes and brain ischemia.[26,31,37,40,41]

The most vulnerable areas for hypoxic-ischemic injury are the cerebral white matter and the cerebral cortex, especially the hippocampus, Purkinje cells of the cerebellar cortex, and pontine nuclei in the brainstem.[34–39] Perinatal asphyxia also often causes severe damage to the putamen and thalamus on both sides. More severe hypoxic-ischemic insults damage the caudate nuclei and sensorimotor cortex around the central fissure.[35,42,43] The parasagittal regions, deep periventricular white matter, and basal ganglia-thalami are very common regions injured by hypoxic-ischemic insults.[34–47] The parasagittal cortex between the anterior cerebral artery and MCA, and between the MCA and posterior cerebral artery territories are watershed zones, often selectively damaged by hypotension in the full-term newborn infant.[34,44,45] The most frequent resulting clinical picture is weakness of the proximal limbs, especially the arms. Spastic quadriparesis, which is worse in the arms, is the most characteristic clinical picture.[34,44,45]

Computed tomography (CT), magnetic resonance imaging (MRI), radionuclide studies, and positron emission tomography (PET) scanning can show the parasagittal distribution of ischemic damage.[34,44,45,48]

In premature infants, hypoxic-ischemic injury is often reflected in damage to the white matter around the ventricles, a process usually termed periventricular leukomalacia.[31,39,46,47,49–52] Sometimes, small isolated foci of necrosis exist at the angles of the ventricles. The lesions are often extensive and spread out from the ventricles toward the cortex. The periventricular lesions can be hemorrhagic and are often associated with enlargement of the ventricular system. The predominant clinical finding is spastic weakness of the legs (diplegia), with lesser involvement of the upper limbs. The white matter lesions near the anterior horns intercept the fibers coming from the parasagittal motor cortex, subserving control of the thighs, legs, and feet. CT, MRI, and ultrasound allow diagnosis during the neonatal period and sequential evaluation of the lesions. Figure 15.1 is an MRI that shows periventricular leukomalacia lesions.

Severe, acute hypoxic-ischemic insults during the perinatal period can cause severe damage to the basal ganglia and thalami.[35,42,46,47] The MRI in Figure 15.2 shows these lesions. The clinical findings during the neonatal period include tongue fasciculations and feeding problems, with impaired swallowing, irritability, and tonic posturing of the arms and legs.[35] Many neonates with these lesions die soon after birth. Survivors often have spastic quadriparesis, chorea-athetosis, dystonic postures, and feeding problems with recurrent aspiration and pulmonary infections.[35,47]

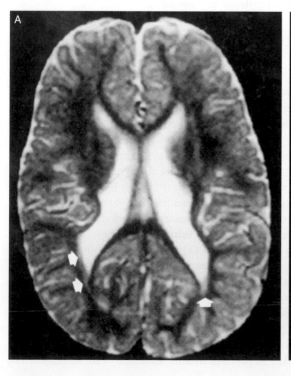
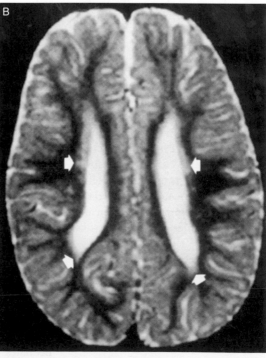

Figure 15.1 T2-weighted MRI scans of a child with spastic diplegia caused by periventricular leukomalacia. (A,B) The scans were taken at 15 months and show irregularity of the ventricular walls, loss of white matter, and T2 prolongation in the periventricular white matter. Arrows point to periventricular abnormalities. From Aida N, Nishimura NA, Hachiya Y, et al. Magnetic resonance imaging of perinatal brain damage: Comparison of clinical outcome with initial and follow-up magnetic resonance findings. *AJNR Am J Neuroradiol* 1998;19:1909–1921 with permission.

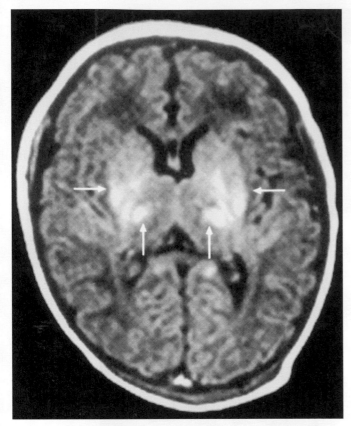

Figure 15.2 T1-weighted MRI scan at 10 days shows abnormal signal intensities (white arrows) in the lenticular nuclei and thalamus in a child who had spastic quadriparesis, seizures, athetoid movements, and developmental delay. From Aida N, Nishimura NA, Hachiya Y, et al. Magnetic resonance imaging of perinatal brain damage: Comparison of clinical outcome with initial and follow-up magnetic resonance findings. *Am J Neuroradiol* 1998;19:1909–1921 with permission.

Arterial and venous strokes in neonates

Focal arterial and venous infarcts often occur in neonates, presenting either with seizures in a newborn at the time of acute infarction, or with hemiparesis presenting gradually during maturation in older infants, many months after the acute infarct (congenital hemiplegia or presumed perinatal ischemic stroke).[34,46,53–56] Most acute neonatal ischemic strokes are located in the territories of the major cerebral arterial distributions, most often affecting the MCA. The lesions may be large and, in the chronic phase, cystic appearing as porencephalic cysts. Some perinatal infarcts presenting in the chronic phase are in the distribution of the terminal vein.[32] Obstruction of an MCA in neonates can cause infarction that predominates in the penetrating artery supply regions with good collaterals preserving the remainder of the cerebral cortex and white matter supplied by the MCA. Arterial infarcts are bilateral in 20% of infants.

The incidence of perinatal arterial ischemic stroke is estimated at one in 3500 live births. Focal infarcts are clearly more common than are now diagnosed. In an autopsy study of 592 neonates, 32 (5.4%) had focal infarcts in a recognized arterial distribution.[53] Full-term neonates more often had focal infarcts than premature infants. Some children with congenital hemiplegia have focal unilateral infarcts on MRI

scans in the corona radiata that are posited to be caused by compression of periventricular veins.[32,56] These periventricular venous infarcts (PVIs) are unilateral and show evidence of hemosiderin deposition related to bleeding into the infarcted territory.[32] Figure 15.3 from Kirton et al.[32] shows MRI scans of 10 infants with PVIs.

Arterial embolization with sepsis and disseminated intravascular coagulation and placental choriamnionitis are common inflammatory/infectious causes of perinatal arterial territorial infarcts. Focal arterial territory infarcts in infants can also result from drugs, especially cocaine use, by the mother.[57] Arterial embolization also can occur due to hypercoagulability and to cardiac disease, when neonates have a 14% risk of stroke recurrence. At least one example has been reported of traumatic occlusion of the carotid artery during delivery.[58] Recurrence after perinatal stroke is otherwise very rare although exceptions do occur.[41] In one series, among 55 infants with presumed perinatal ischemic strokes, 43 were considered arterial (26 main MCA cortical and subcortical, 8 superior division MCA, 5 inferior division MCA, and 4 lenticulostriate), and 12 were thought to represent periventricular venous infarcts.[32]

The perinatal period is a period of very high risk for venous thrombosis: neonates represent approximately 50% of all pediatric patients with cerebral sinovenous thrombosis (CSVT).[59–61] The clinical presentation with seizures and apnea may begin during the first postnatal week although the symptoms can also become evident during the third and fourth weeks. The sagittal sinus is most often involved. Among term infants with intraventricular hemorrhage, 30% have CSVT usually involving the deep venous system (internal cerebral and vein of Galen). Hypoxia at birth, premature rupture of maternal membranes, abruptio placenta, maternal infections, dehydration and infections in the neonate are common associated conditions. Some neonates have prothrombotic findings on laboratory evaluation. The infarcts associated with CSVT are often hemorrhagic.[60] Sinovenous occlusions in neonates is a very serious disorder with a high mortality rate and a high rate of severe neurological disability.[61,62] Recent data suggest that without treatment, neonatal sinovenous occlusion has a 20–30% rate of thrombus propagation, and that the use of anticoagulation in neonates with this condition is safe, with less than 7% risk of major hemorrhage.[63,64]

Primary brain hemorrhages are also an important cause of stroke in the perinatal period. Premature infants are especially susceptible to developing a particular pattern of hemorrhage in the germinal matrix in bilateral periventricular regions, frequently extending to intra-ventricular compartments.[34,39,65–67] Regions of necrosis often surround these hematomas. By full term, the germinal matrix is no longer visible and periventricular and intraventricular hemorrhages arise from residual matrix tissue or directly from the choroid plexus vasculature. Ultrasound and CT are effective ways to diagnose and follow children with intraventricular hemorrhages. Intraventricular hemorrhages can cause temporary hydrocephalus, which resolves itself, or progressive hydrocephalus, requiring ventricular drainage or shunting. Lumbar puncture, with removal of

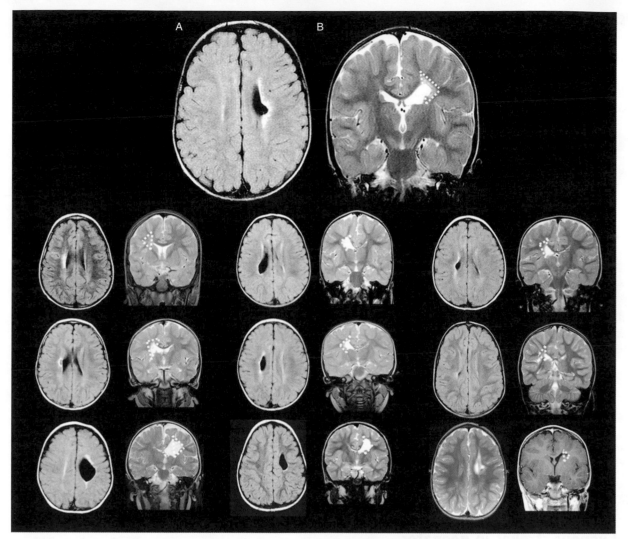

Figure 15.3 Representative pairs of axial fluid-attenuated inversion recovery (A) and coronal T2 (B) MRIs from 10 patients with periventricular venous infarction. Consistent lesion features include focal cystic softening in the periventricular white matter and T2 prolongation in the posterior limb of the internal capsule. A "caudal triangle" in which periventricular white matter is more affected than basal ganglia is diagrammed in the coronal images. Courtesy of Adam Kirton, MD; from Kirton A, deVeber G, Pontigon A-M, et al. Presumed perinatal ischemic stroke: Vascular classification predicts outcome. *Ann Neurol* 2008;63:436–443 with permission.

cerebrospinal fluid, is another effective treatment. Ventricular size should be carefully followed by ultrasound or CT.

Since the mid 1970s, cerebellar hemorrhage has also been recognized to occur in an estimated 15–25% of preterm infants in the early neonatal period.[39,59,68,69] In the late stages of gestation, a cerebellar germinal matrix is present. This probably accounts for the high risk of bleeding in preterm babies. Asphyxia and hyaline-membrane disease are contributing factors.

Parenchymal cerebral hemorrhage in term infants is relatively rare, with a frequency estimated at about 6 per 100 000 live births. Among these, unifocal lobar hemorrhages predominate and 75% are idiopathic. Fetal distress and postmaturity are independent predictors. Seizures, falling hematocrit and bulging anterior fontanelle are signs of hemorrhagic stroke in neonates. Cerebellar hemorrhage in term infants may also present with signs of brainstem compression, such as ocular bobbing or skew deviation; and acute hydrocephalus. Ultrasound, CT, and MRI allow diagnosis. Surgical decompression is often required and can be lifesaving.[59]

Subdural and subarachnoid bleeding are very common in neonates and are related to the normal birth process. Some red blood cells are found in the cerebrospinal fluid of nearly every baby delivered vaginally. Bleeding is most often trivial. More severe birth trauma or coagulation abnormalities can lead to more severe subarachnoid bleeding and diminished alertness in the neonate.[39] Trauma can also cause significant subdural collections of blood.

Strokes in children (1 month to 18 years of age)

Infantile hemiplegia and childhood stroke have been recognized for centuries. In his 1888 textbook on neurology Gowers commented, "Hemiplegia of sudden onset is not uncommon in children, especially in young children."[70] Sigmund Freud observed at the end of the nineteenth century that "a large number of cases of infantile cerebral paralysis are caused by the same factors that bring about cerebral paralysis of adults: by tearing, embolism, and thrombosis of cerebral vessels."[71,72] During the past two decades there have been important advances in knowledge about pediatric stroke. The advent of modern brain imaging, and especially vascular imaging, has identified frequent disorders of the intracranial arteries, now referred to with a non-specific term, *arteriopathy*.[73–77] The present availability of safe, rapid diagnostic technology that provides brain and vascular imaging promises to unlock many aspects of strokes in children concerning etiology, prognosis, and treatment that had been unattainable in the past. Another important recent advance has been the development of registries and databases that are accruing data about childhood stroke. National databases have now linked together to form a multinational collaborative, including the International Pediatric Stroke Study.[26,62,78] Pediatric stroke neurology specialists, a new breed, have sprung up, and begun to collaborate along with other subspecialists to conduct research, accumulate data, and disseminate consensus guidelines for treating pediatric stroke to pediatricians and neurologists who care for children with strokes.

Estimates of the frequency of strokes in neonates and children vary from about 2[26,79,80] to 5.5[81] per 100 000 children-years. Blacks and Hispanic children may have a higher incidence of stroke in North America,[81] and the frequency of strokes may be higher in Asia, although definitive estimates are not available. Between 1979 and 1998, mortality from stroke in children under 20 years of age declined by 58%.[82] The decline in mortality was noted among all ischemic and hemorrhagic stroke types. Mortality was higher in blacks and boys.[82] Although most strokes in children are ischemic, the ratio of ischemia to hemorrhage is lower in children than in adults.

Hemorrhagic strokes in children

Hemorrhagic stroke is a devastating event in children with a similar incidence rate to ischemic stroke.[83] Up to one-third die and 40% have permanent neurological deficits.[84] Intracererebral hemorrhage accounts for the majority of cases (50–75%), and can extend into the intraventricular space. SAH comprises less than 25% and is primarily due to aneurysm. In preadolescent children, vascular malformations are the most common cause of intracranial bleeding.[58,85–87] If all individuals younger than 20 years are included, however, SAH is as common or more common than intracerebral bleeds, and aneurysms are a more common cause of bleeding than vascular malformations. Among 124 young patients with SAH in a 1973 series, 50 patients had aneurysms and 33 had arteriovenous malformations (AVMs).[88] Among 3 series published before 1973, 36% of young patients had aneurysmal bleeding, whereas 27% bled from AVMs.[88] In a series of patients enrolled between 1993 and 2004, among 116 children with non-traumatic hemorrhagic strokes who had structural lesions that caused bleeding, 78% were AVMs, 33% aneurysms, and 37% cavernous malformations.[87]

Aneurysms usually become symptomatic before the age of 2 years or after age 10.[59,89] Aneurysms are more common in individuals with coarctation of the aorta and polycystic renal disease.[59] In childhood, bacterial endocarditis with embolism to the vasa vasorum of intracranial arteries, and mycotic aneurysm formation are especially important causes of intracerebral and subarachnoid hemorrhage. Aneurysms that rupture in childhood have a somewhat different distribution than those found in adults. Shucart and Wolpert analyzed the site of rupture of 100 congenital intracranial aneurysms in children younger than 15 years.[90] Compared with adult series, the intracranial ICA was more often the site of anterior-circulation bleeding in children, whereas the posterior and anterior communicating arteries were less often implicated in children.[90] Posterior-circulation aneurysms were relatively more common in children (23% of the total) than in adults. They especially involved the intracranial vertebral artery and basilar artery apex.[90] Intracranial dissecting aneurysms involving the initial segment of the MCA are increasingly recognized as a cause of stroke in children.[91] Evaluation and treatment of aneurysms is similar in children and adults.

Intracranial vascular malformations are undoubtedly present at birth, but do not become symptomatic in most patients until adulthood. Although AVMs are the most frequent cause of intracranial bleeding in preadolescents, less than 10% of malformations are diagnosed before the age of 10 years.[59] Mackenzie noted in 1953 that 29 of his 50 patients (58%) with brain angiomas developed initial symptoms before age 20 years.[92] The advent of safer and more widely distributed brain imaging means that now cavernous malformations and AVMs are detected earlier and more often than in the past. In adolescents and older children, the most frequent symptoms in patients with vascular malformations are caused by hemorrhage. Most often, bleeding is into the brain (ICH), but superficial lesions and those abutting on ependymal surfaces can cause SAH or primary intraventricular bleeding. Approximately 20% of AVMs in children are infratentorial, equally divided between the cerebellum and brainstem.[93] Supratentorial AVMs are typically superficial and cone-shaped, with the base located on the cortical surface and the apex closer to the ventricle.[94,95] Approximately 10% are deep, involving the basal ganglia and thalamus.[94,95] Focal neurological signs often develop gradually and can be associated with signs of increased intracranial pressure. Epilepsy and headache are other less frequent presentations of vascular malformations.

Neonates and young children often harbor a type of malformation that is rarely, if ever, first discovered in adulthood, a vein of Galen malformation (VGAM). In this condition, the vein of Galen is greatly enlarged, forming a large varix, and the straight sinus is also large and tortuous. The malformation is

517

usually fed by posterior choroidal arteries. The typical CT appearance is that of a round hyperdense mass behind the IIIrd ventricle, connected to a prominent torcula by the dilatated midline straight sinus. Hydrocephalus is present in approximately one-third of patients. The most common presenting syndrome during the neonatal period and infancy is high-output congestive heart failure, caused by the large volume of shunted blood.[59] A loud cranial bruit is usually audible. The combined abnormality in hemodynamics and brain perfusion associated with VGAM is complex, and involves venous hypertension, progressive hydrocephalus and low perfusion pressure due to cardiac failure. This combination can produce a unique form of progressive diffuse brain infarction termed the "melting brain". Older infants and young children may present with SAH or intraventricular hemorrhage, seizures, or signs of hydrocephalus. If left untreated, these malformations are frequently fatal early in life. The outcome of VGAM depends on both the stage of the disorder at diagnosis and the success of early treatment. In older series, infants were treated urgently during the neonatal period.

Cavernous malformations are increasingly recognized with the widespread use of brain imaging. About one-fourth of the patients in the various series of cerebral cavernomas were children.[96–98] Among 172 pediatric patients with cavernomas, Cavalheiro and Braga noted two age peaks – one during the first year of life and the other between the ages of 12 and 16 years.[99] When bleeding does occur, it is invariably within the capsule of the cavernoma.

Intracerebral and subarachnoid hemorrhages occasionally develop in children with various bleeding diatheses, and with acute hypertension as might be found in pheochromocytoma, cocaine and amphetamine use, or acute glomerulonephritis. In one series, recurrent hemorrhages developed in 11 of 116 (10%) of children.[87] Vascular malformations were associated with a high and prolonged risk of recurrent hemorrhage: bleeding diathesis were accompanied by a high recurrence rate but mostly during the first week.[87] Head trauma is another important cause of intracranial hemorrhage in children. Trauma accounted for 24% of 116 hemorrhagic strokes in children in one study.[87] In comparison to older adults with vascular malformations, treatment decisions for pediatric vascular malformations must also consider a risk duration lasting many decades.

Ischemic strokes in children

Differential diagnosis of brain ischemia in children is quite wide (Table 15.3), and up to 15% of patients escape etiological diagnosis, even after full evaluation. Large deep infarcts centered in the basal ganglia, internal capsule, and thalamus are relatively more common in children than in older age groups. Brower and colleagues described the clinical findings, imaging features, and causes among 36 children (newborn to 13 years) with striatocapsular and thalamic infarcts at their medical center during a 6-year period.[100] Most children presented with an acute hemiplegia that usually resolved within a week, leaving minor hemiparesis. Sensory and important cognitive abnormalities were unusual unless infarction

Table 15.3 Differential diagnosis of pediatric brain ischemia (age 1–15 years)

- Migraine
- Trauma: dissection and other vascular injuries; abuse, including whiplash-shake injuries; oral foreign-body; trauma to the internal carotid artery
- Cardiac: congenital heart disease with right-to-left shunts, tetralogy of Fallot, transposition of great vessels, tricuspid atresia, atrial and ventricular septal defects, cardiomyopathies, endocarditis, pulmonary arteriovenous fistula
- Drugs, especially cocaine and heroin
- Infections: bacterial meningitis, especially *Haemophilus influenzae*, pneumonococci, and streptococci; facial, otitic, and sinus infections; acquired immunodeficiency syndrome; dural sinus occlusion and infection; tuberculous meningitis
- Genetic and metabolic: neurofibromatosis, hereditary disorders of connective tissue (Marfan's and Ehlers–Danlos syndromes), pseudoxanthoma elasticum, homocystinuria, Menkes' kinky hair syndrome, hypoalphalipoproteinemia, familial hyperlipidemias, methylmalonic aciduria, MELAS syndrome (mitochondrial, encephalopathy, lactic acidosis, and stroke-like episodes), cytochrome oxidase deficiency
- Hematological and neoplastic: sickle cell anemia, purpuras, leukemia, L-arginase and aminocaproic acid (Amicar) treatment, radiation vasculopathy, hypercoagulable states (e.g., caused by decrease in natural inhibitors, such as antithrombin III, protein C, protein S)
- Systemic disease: rheumatic, gastrointestinal, renal, hepatic, pulmonary, moyamoya syndrome
- Others: arteritis, collagen vascular disease, local infections, Takayasu's syndrome, Behçet's syndrome, venous sinus thrombosis, head and neck infections, dehydration, coagulopathy, paroxysmal nocturnal hemoglobinuria, puerperal or pregnancy-related

was bilateral.[75] A wide variety of vasculopathies was responsible. The deep pattern of infarction is best explained by involvement of the proximal portions of the ICAs or MCAs, or both, and the posterior cerebral artery in the presence of good collateral circulation, which continues to supply adequate blood flow to the cerebral cortex. After pediatric stroke in the basal ganglia, dystonia emerges months to years later in up to 20% of children.

The major causes of brain ischemia in children can be considered as either arterial ischemic stroke (AIS) or cerebral sinovenous thrombosis (CSVT). Causes of AIS include: (1) cardiac-origin embolism; (2) arteriopathy; (3) prothrombotic states; and (4) other acute or chronic childhood disorders. The term *arteriopathy* includes a spectrum of causes that include infection, trauma, migraine, moyamoya, and genetic disorders such as sickle cell disease, Fabry's disease, and mitochondrial disorders. The usual risk factors for the development of ischemic stroke in adults – hypertension, diabetes, hyperlipidemia, and smoking – are not important causes of brain ischemia in children.

About one-fourth of ischemic strokes in young children are attributable to heart disease. A relatively high proportion of

cardiac-related ischemic strokes occur in relation to surgery and other procedures, more than 40% in one study.[26] Brain infarcts in children with cardiac disease are most often caused by embolism. Bacterial endocarditis is an important cause. Congenital heart disease, especially with shunting of blood (atrial and ventricular septal defects and patent ductus arteriosis), and complex congenital defects are frequent.[26,101] Children with stroke and congenital heart disease are often cyanotic and have chronic hypoxia and polycythemia. They may develop venous and arterial occlusions related to the polycythemia. Rheumatic heart disease, endocarditis, cardiomyopathies, and myocarditis are important acquired heart diseases associated with brain embolism.[102] Brain abscess is also common in children with polycythemia and must be distinguished from brain infarction. Diagnostic techniques, especially transesophageal echocardiography and transcranial Doppler (TCD) sonography after intravenous injection of air bubbles, now allow detection of small atrial shunts (atrial septal defects and patent foramen ovale) in children and young adults with otherwise unexplained brain infarcts. Children with cardiogenic stroke are at long-term risk for recurrent stroke. Among 135 children with congenital heart disease studied in the Toronto site of the Canadian Pediatric Ischemic Stroke Registry, 19 had already had recurrent strokes on entry into the Registry.[103] Ten years after their initial stroke, 27% had had a stroke recurrence, 26% had died, and only 47% were alive and free from recurrence.[103] About 50% of these children were receiving anticoagulation at the time of recurrent stroke.[103] Factors associated with recurrence included presence of infection at the sentinel stroke, a mechanical valve, prothrombotic condition, and shorter time from sentinel stroke.

Arterial composition and function in childhood are a bit different from that found in most older adults, since the intracranial arteries are rarely subject to important degenerative atherosclerotic changes. The media is composed of smooth muscle cells, collagen, and elastin. The endothelium is a sensor that can release vasoactive substances, alter the extracellular matrix in the blood vessel wall, and trigger vascular remodeling. Increased vascular elasticity and reactivity contribute to the development of "arteriopathy" in this age group from a variety of different stimuli. Children in whom angiography shows an arteriopathy have a less abrupt, more indolent onset and course than those who do not show an arteriopathy by angiography.[104] The presence of an angiographically confirmed arteriopathy conveys an increased risk for stroke recurrence.[98–102]

The most common arteriopathy in childhood stroke is often termed "transient cerebral arteriopathy (TCA)." This unilateral intracranial arteriopathy occurs spontaneously in toddlers and school-age children, and presents with unilateral basal ganglia infarction. Vascular imaging shows irregularity of the supraclinoid ICA, the M1 and M2 segments of the MCA, and the A1 segment of the ACA. Serial vascular imaging of this arteriopathy typically shows transient increased stenosis in the affected arterial zone during several months, followed by a phase of improvement or stabilization beginning 3–6 months

post-stroke. The pathogenesis of TCA is unknown to date, but is presumed in most cases to represent a transient inflammatory attack on the circle of Willis arteries, a self-resolving focal vasculitis.

An important cause of arteriopathy in childhood is trauma. Direct trauma can lead to arterial occlusion and intense vasoconstriction. Stretching of arteries at locations where they are not anchored can lead to tearing of arterial walls (dissections). Head and neck traumas, even trivial ones, are often mentioned as a predisposing factor by the parents of children with ischemic strokes. Evidence from a recent case-control study supports a 39-fold increased risk of pediatric acute ischemic stroke within a week of head or neck trauma.[105] In another study, 18.5% of Japanese children with ischemic strokes had head trauma in the home within days or a week prior to the stroke.[106] Oral trauma by penetrating objects can cause ICA occlusions.[107,108] Young children may fall while keeping pencils and toothbrushes in their mouths. The pharynx is lacerated or contused, and the ICA is injured during its course behind the faucial pillars. Extracranial carotid and vertebral artery dissection can develop after head or neck injuries, especially involving sudden twisting movements and blunt trauma to the neck. Neck, jaw, or throat pain or headache may be the earliest symptoms. Brain infarction occurs when the blood within the arterial wall dissects into the arterial lumen and embolizes intracranially. At times, the intramural clot occludes the lumen sufficiently that a luminal thrombus forms in situ because of sluggish flow and activation of clotting factors.

LRC has seen several patients in whom seemingly trivial head trauma led to severe intracranial arterial dissections. A young girl developed a fatal intracranial ICA and MCA dissection after her head hit the top of a car when it hit a bump.[109] A young boy fell and hit his head while trick-or-treating on Halloween. Although he appeared uninjured to his mother, he developed a hemiplegia and bilateral motor signs the next day, later shown to be caused by an angiographically documented basilar artery dissection. Dissection was the most common cause of arteriopathy in several modern series that included frequent vascular imaging.[26,79]

Infection was cited as an important predisposing cause of hemiplegia in children in the 1927 report of Ford and Schaffer[72] and in other early writings.[59] Most often, the infections were respiratory or systemic, and the mechanism of stroke was uncertain. In a 1991 study of childhood stroke in the Tohoku district of Japan, 10 of 54 patients (18.5%) had upper respiratory tract infections or fevers of unknown origin.[106] A recent case-control study in the United States reported a fourfold increased rate of infection in the month preceding childhood stroke.[105] Tonsillitis can occasionally lead to occlusive changes in the adjacent pharyngeal portion of the ICA. Influenza and *Mycoplasma pneumoniae* have been occasionally implicated as causes of brain infarction.[59,110,111]

The best studied infectious cause of arteriopathy is infection with the herpes zoster varicella (HZV) virus. In herpes zoster in adults, the virus can be detected in the vascular endothelium, often without an inflammatory response. Virions characteristic of HZV can be found in

the nuclei and cytoplasm of smooth-muscle cells in involved arteries, amplification of HZV viral DNA by polymerase chain reaction (PCR) can show viruses within the endothelium and vessel wall of cranial arteries.[112–114] There are several possible mechanisms for HZV virus to gain access to the cerebral arteries. Virus can access pial arteries by way of the meninges. Second, the virus can reach the unilateral intracranial arteries of the circle of Willis from the trigeminal ganglion via the trigeminovascular bundle. Endothelial viral infection could cause thrombosis by activating platelets and triggering the coagulation cascade. Endothelial perturbation could lead to vasoconstriction compromising distal blood flow and presenting as an "arteriopathy." Systemic infection can lead to changes in circulating globulins, with activation of serine protein coagulation factors, such as factor VIII, and acute-phase reactants such as fibrinogen, promoting thrombosis of involved arteries.

Post-varicella arteriopathy and brain infarction have now been studied extensively in children.[115–117] The course and progression of the arteriopathy was studied in 27 children who had serial vascular imaging.[117] The children in this study acquired varicella infection at age 1.0–10.4 (median 4.4 years) and had their first episode of brain ischemia 4–47 weeks later (median 17 weeks). Arterial imaging abnormalities most often involved the supraclinoid ICA, the M1 and M2 segments of the MCA, and the A1 segment of the ACA.[117] Single regions of focal ring-like stenosis and gradual longer segments of stenosis and multifocal narrowings were found. Brain infarcts were predominantly deep in the basal ganglia, internal capsule, and thalamus. In some patients stenosis was maximal on initial studies, but often later progressed to involve previously uninvolved arteries. The vascular abnormalities improved or completely regressed during follow-up during 6–79 months. Brain ischemic episodes recurred, either acutely or during the 1–33 weeks after symptom onset, often associated with progression of abnormalities on vascular imaging. Symptoms often continued despite antithrombotic treatments. Vasoconstriction may be one mechanism of brain ischemia in the patients with postvaricella brain ischemia.

Migraine is also common in children with brain infarcts. The frequency of its recognition depends on how vigorously physicians have explored the past personal and family history of headache. In 1990, LRC reported a 6-year-old boy with a personal and strong family history of migraine who had severe headache preceding a basilar artery occlusion and no other cause of occlusive disease.[118] In another young boy, a striatocapsular infarct associated with narrowing of the MCA was followed by the development of typical unilateral throbbing migraine headaches, with photophobia, nausea, and vomiting. Migraine probably causes brain infarcts due to prolonged vasoconstriction or the formation of local thrombi related to vascular narrowing and activation of the clotting system.[118,119] A genetically mediated predisposition to migraine may be a contributing factor to heightened vascular reactivity caused by other processes such as trauma and infection. In adults, the reversible cerebral vasoconstriction syndrome (RCVS) of protracted vasoconstriction

(discussed in Chapter 12) may have a counterpart in childhood and explain some instances of arteriopathy. True migrainous infarction diagnosed according to the International Headache Society criteria has been considered uncommon in children,[120] although in LRC's experience many instances of migraine-related brain infarcts are not correctly diagnosed as such.

Sickle cell anemia is an important cause of brain infarction, especially in African-American children and young adults. Sickle cell disease increases the risk of childhood AIS 400-fold. In one study, three-fourths of patients with cerebrovascular complications of sickle cell disease were younger than 15 years.[121] Patients with stroke often have a more severe form of the disease, with frequent sickle crises and lower hematocrits than other patients with the condition. Strokes often occur during a clinical sickle crisis.[59,122] Sickle cell disease is a cause of occlusive changes in large intracranial arteries and small penetrating vessels.[123,124] The walls of intracranial arteries are thickened, and intimal and subintimal proliferation occurs. Subcortical, cortical, and borderzone infarcts are often found on CT and MRI;[124] angiography has shown intracranial occlusions of the major basal arteries. Arteries may become dilated and ectatic even in childhood.[125] Occasionally, veins and dural sinuses thrombose.[126] TCD offers a non-invasive way to detect velocity changes related to intracranial, large-artery narrowing, and allows monitoring of patients with sickle cell disease.[127] Blood transfusions for children whose TCD blood-flow velocities in the ICAs or MCAs, or both, exceed 200 cm/s have been shown in a trial to prevent first strokes from developing.[128] The Stroke Prevention in Sickle Cell Anemia (STOP) trial found that regular transfusions lowering hemoglobin S below 20–30% resulted in a 90% relative risk reduction in stroke and stroke recurrence for children with abnormal velocities.[128]

Various other hematological and coagulation disorders are found in evaluating children with strokes. Thrombocytosis and polycythemia are occasionally found. In a study of 212 children with acute arterial ischemic stroke, abnormalities were found on blood testing in nearly half of the patients.[73] Anemia was the most common finding (40% of children).[73] Anemia, increased platelet and white blood cell counts, are often a reflection of acute or chronic disease. Based on several case-control studies, iron deficiency anemia is a risk factor for AIS and CSVT. Iron deficiency anemia is present in up to 40% of childhood acute ischemic stroke.[129] Anemia especially when severe promotes hypercoagulability. Children with decreased hemoglobin and microcytosis should undergo iron studies. Iron supplementation or even transfusion if severe anemia, are of benefit in correcting this risk factor.

Prothrombotic states defined by laboratory testing are established predisposing factors for initial and recurrent childhood ischemic strokes.[130–132] In a large meta-analysis of published studies, associations were quantified for some of the common prothrombotic disorders.[132] The highest odds ratios (ORs) were for protein C deficiency (11.0/5.13–23.59), antiphospholipid antibodies or lupus anticoagulant (6.95/3.67–13.14), and lipoprotein (a) (6.53/4.46–9.55). Modest

associations were noted for factor V Ledien and prothrombin gene *20210A* mutations while other factors showed minimal or no association (protein S, antithrombin, methylene tetrahydrofolate reductase gene *MTHFR*).[132] Some coagulation abnormalities are a reflection of stimulation of acute phase reactants such as fibrinogen and factors VII and VIII during systemic disease. However congenital deficiency of antithrombin, proteins C and S, and the C2 component of complement are also implicated among the causes of strokes in childhood.[59] Some children have high homocysteine levels often explained by being homozygous for the thermolabile variant of the *MTHFR* gene.[52] Advances in genetics have led to detection of resistance to the anticoagulant function of activated protein C, most often caused by factor V Leiden, and prothrombin gene mutations, in some children and young adults with venous thromboses and strokes.

In some children and young adults, mitochondrial and other metabolic disorders produce stroke-like episodes. These patients develop confusion; visual abnormalities, including hemianopia and visual neglect; and sometimes seizures and headache. Brain imaging often shows white matter abnormalities predominantly, but not exclusively, in the posterior portions of the cerebral hemispheres in the occipital-temporal and parietal regions. Vascular imaging is usually normal. The pathogenesis is related to energy depletion. MELAS syndrome is the best-known disorder that causes stroke-like episodes.[133–136] Autosomal recessive cytochrome oxidase deficiency is also associated with periodic acidosis and stroke-like episodes attributable to metabolic aberrations.[137] These and other mitochondrial disorders are discussed in Chapter 12.

Moyamoya is another very important condition found in childhood. This condition is also discussed in Chapter 12. Although sometimes referred to as a disease, this condition is probably better thought of as a syndrome defined by a characteristic angiographic appearance. The intracranial ICAs show progressive tapering and progressive occlusion at their intracranial bifurcations (the so-called T portion of the ICAs). Basal penetrating branches of the ICAs, ACAs, and MCAs enlarge to provide collateral circulation. These branch arteries form large prominent anastomosing channels, basal telangiectasias, that appear on angiograms as a cloud of smoke; these arteries are especially prominent because of the paucity of MCA sylvian branches. The appearance of these basal telangiectasias led Japanese clinicians to use the term *moyamoya*, which means "something hazy like a puff of cigarette smoke drifting in the air."[138,139] Although first described in Japan,[138] the disease has been reported worldwide.[140–143]

Necropsy studies, although few, have shown severe vascular occlusive abnormalities characterized by endothelial hyperplasia and fibrosis, with intimal thickening and abnormalities of the internal elastic lamina.[144] In contrast, the intracerebral perforating arteries show microaneurysm formation, lipohyalinosis, focal fibrin deposition, and thinning of the elastic laminas and arterial walls.[145] These changes in the perforating arteries are probably the result of greatly increased flow through these small vessels. Inflammatory changes have universally been absent. Ikeda studied the extracranial arteries of 13 Japanese patients with spontaneous occlusions of the circle of Willis at necropsy who met the research definition of moyamoya syndrome.[146] Extracranial arteries showed the same intimal lesions as the intracranial arteries. Characteristically, the proximal pulmonary arteries had fibrous nodular intimal thickening without inflammatory abnormalities.[146] Moyamoya changes have been found in a variety of situations, including sickle cell disease, neurofibromatosis, Takayasu's disease, Down's syndrome, atherosclerosis, and fibromuscular dysplasia, and can be found in young women, especially those who smoke cigarettes and take oral contraceptives.[142,145] A variety of different conditions can probably cause intimal changes, which lead to fibrosis and luminal narrowing.

Moyamoya syndrome is approximately 50 times more common in girls and women than in boys and men.[147] Clinically, the disorder has a bimodal distribution, presenting most often in children younger than 15 years and in adults in their 3rd–5th decades of life. Children usually present with transient episodes of hemiparesis or other focal neurological signs often precipitated by physical exercise or hyperventilation. Several of our young patients have had intermittent choreoathetosis. Other patients have sudden-onset deficits, such as hemiplegia, or the gradual development of intellectual deterioration. Headaches and seizures are common. These symptoms are often accompanied by CT and MRI evidence of brain infarction and cerebral blood flow studies that show regions of hypoperfusion. The abnormal vasculature is often visible on MRI and magnetic resonance angiography (MRA). A variety of surgical procedures have been performed in moyamoya patients to attempt to enhance brain perfusion but surgery has not been studied in randomized therapeutic trials.[142,148–150]

Dural sinus and venous occlusions in children

Cerebral venous occlusive disease is another important consideration in children with acute or subacute brain dysfunction.[151–155] The ratio of venous to arterial causes of brain injury is higher in childhood than in adults. The frequency of cerebral venous thrombosis in children is estimated to be 0.4–0.7 per 100 000 children per year.[62,151–153] Many children are under one year of age;[62] the median age of occurrence was six years in a large German study and boys were involved more than girls.[152]

Most instances, as in adults, involve the superior sagittal or lateral sinus or multiple dural sinuses.[62,151,153,154] The deep venous structures – the internal cerebral vein, the vein of Galen, and the straight sinus – are involved more often in children than in adults. Among 91 children (non-neonates), the most frequent symptoms or signs were headache (59%), focal neurological signs (53%), decreased consciousness (49%), and seizures (48%).[62] Papilledema was detected in 22%.[62] Acute and chronic systemic illnesses and prothrombotic conditions were common causes. The causes were quite varied and included: cancer, dehydration, the use of drugs that had procoagulant effects, liver disease, and nephrotic syndrome

among others.[62] Among toddlers, otitis media and mastoiditis were common associations with CSVT. The nephrotic syndrome is an important cause of childhood sinovenous thrombosis. Trauma is also an important cause of dural sinus thrombosis in children.[153]

Fourteen of 91 patients had recurrent cerebral venous thromboses. The outcome depends on the associated systemic illness; more than a third of children have residual neurological abnormalities. The frequency of detecting an underlying coagulopathy varies. In a Canadian registry of children with sinovenous thrombosis, 39 of 123 patients tested had a prothrombotic risk factor, the most common of which was anticardiolipin antibodies.[62]

Children with dural sinus thrombosis are now frequently anticoagulated as first-line treatment. A number of retrospective analyses indicate that anticoagulation is safe in children and possibly neonates even when a hemorrhagic lesion is shown by brain imaging.[63,153,154] Propagation of the occlusive venous thrombus within days of diagnosis is common in children who do not receive anticoagulation, with frequencies ranging from 20% to 30%.[63] Recurrent cerebral sinovenous thrombosis occurs in about 2% to 8% of pediatric patients.

There is considerably less information about the treatment of strokes in children compared to the data in adults. The only randomized trials concern management of sickle cell disease with transfusions.[128] The available data about treatment of stroke in children has recently been compiled and published.[156] The overall risk of recurrent stroke in children with AIS without antithrombotic treatment is around 50%. The use of either antiplatelet agents (aspirin usually) or anticoagulants (low-molecular-weight heparin or warfarin) is associated with a lowering of the recurrence risk to 10–25%. In the two largest studies that evaluated children with and without antithrombotic treatment, the combined data showed recurrent stroke or TIA in 36 of 163 (22%) children with AIS treated with an antithrombotic agent and in 45 of 119 (38%) children who were not so treated.[156] This represents a 1.7-fold increased rate of recurrence without treatment ($P = 0.005$). Consensus treatment guidelines are now available concerning the treatment of pediatric stroke patients indicating which children should be considered for initial anticoagulation (arterial dissection, cardiac stroke, recurrent stroke) or aspirin (the remainder) for prevention of recurrent stroke.[157–159]

Strokes in young adults (18–50 years of age)

Causes of brain hemorrhage and infarction change as individuals progress from childhood to adulthood. Many causes and risk factors for ischemic stroke in this age group are listed in Table 15.4. The topic of stroke in young adults has received increasing attention, and many series report the relative frequencies of various conditions[5,14,27,160–185] Table 15.5 displays the relative frequency of diagnoses among 20 published reports of young stroke patients in the 1980s and 1990s, and Figure 15.4 shows etiologies in more recent publications.[2,182,183,184,186] The various series are not comparable because of the wide variation in socioeconomic-

environmental factors, including the age, sex, and race/ethnicity of patients; the time of accrual of the series data, with widely varying available technologies for investigation; and the investigations performed to arrive at the stroke etiology. Drug use, tuberculosis, and oral contraceptive use, for example, vary widely among the United States, India, and Japan, accounting for the variability of these specific etiologies. Some compilations focus on risk factors, many on etiologies, and others on outcome. Some series lumped all patients who are between adolescence and mid forties together, while others consider younger adults. Cardiac disease was assiduously sought by some authors using modern echocardiography,[168,169,173,175,178,181–185] but in other series, this technology was not available or was not systematically used. In some series, few patients had angiography, whereas in one series of 148 patients, all patients had angiography.[172] In one series, 234 out of 300 patients (78%) had angiography with abnormalities detected in 130 (56%).[180] Recent series show a similarly high rate of arterial abnormalities detected with less invasive modern imaging techniques such as CTA or MRA.[2,187]

The frequency of detection of the various causes varies, depending on the preliminary hypotheses and biases of the investigators and on whether the series was prospective, allowing the authors to collect the history, or retrospective, gleaned from the charts. Medical records are notoriously poor in historical detail, especially in terms of negative factors. The history in the medical record may not note that the patient did not have migraine, head or neck trauma, a recent infection, and so forth. In some series, various etiologies such as arterial dissections were not considered. In other series, factors, such as oral contraceptive use, migraine, and trauma, were only noted when they were considered etiologically related to the stroke, whereas others simply noted the percentage of subjects in which these risk factors were present.

Clues for specific etiologies

Certain historical features, symptoms, and signs may serve as clues towards specific stroke etiologies.[25] In some diagnoses, the key data come from the history; for example, history of the use of illicit drugs and oral contraceptive agents, historical features suggestive of recurrent thunderclap headaches for the reversible cerebral vasoconstriction syndrome. Clinical clues to an underlying arteriopathy include headache, stereotyped TIAs, associated psychiatric or cognitive disturbances, skin rash, exposure to vasoconstrictive agents, pregnancy, hormonal contraceptive use, head trauma and HIV, tuberculosis, or other infections. Recent minor trauma and sudden neck movements, including chiropractic neck manipulation are associated with arterial dissection, which is the most common arteriopathy in young adults.[188] Patients with cervical artery dissection will frequently report headache and/or neck pain. Painful Horner's syndrome, or coexisting lower cranial neuropathies, should always raise suspicion for dissection. Dissections are discussed in detail in Chapters 7, 8, and 12.

Table 15.4 Selected causes and risk factors for ischemic stroke in young adults and adolescents

A. Frequency of cause of stroke classified by the TOAST (Trial of Org 10172 in Acute Stroke Treatment) criteria

Large-vessel atherosclerosis (2–11%)

Small-vessel disease (7–14%)

Cardiac embolism (20–47%)

Other determined cause (20–34%)

Multiple causes (2–3%)

B. Arterial causes

Cerebral artery dissection

Reversible cerebral vasoconstriction syndromes

Moyamoya disease

Sickle cell disease

Transient cerebral arteriopathy of childhood

Premature atherosclerosis, lipohyalinosis

Radiation-induced arteriopathy

Migraine-induced stroke

Illicit drug abuse (e.g., cocaine, amphetamines, ecstasy)

Infectious arteriopathy (e.g., post-varicella; tuberculosis, fungal or bacterial meningitis; syphilis, HIV)

Inflammatory arteriopathy (e.g., Takayasu arteritis, giant cell arteritis, primary CNS angiitis, polyartertis nodosa, Behcet's disease, Churg–Strauss syndrome, Kohlmeier–Degos disease, cerebral amyloid angiopathy)

Genetic or inherited arteriopathy (e.g., Fabry's disease, fibromuscular dysplasia, dolichoectasia, Susac syndrome, CADASIL, *TREX-1* mutation disorders, MELAS, hyper-homocysteinemia, neurofibromatosis type 1)

C. Cardiac causes

Patent foramen ovale

Congenital heart disease

Infectious and non-bacterial thrombotic endocarditis

Rheumatic valvular heart disease

Post-cardiac surgery or catheter intervention

Arrhythmia (e.g., atrial fibrillation, sick sinus syndrome)

Cardiac tumors (e.g., atrial myxoma, papillary fibroelastoma)

Recent myocardial infarction

Dilated cardiomyopathy

D. Hematological

Heparin-induced thrombocytopenia

Hypercoagulable state due to deficiencies of protein S, protein C, or antithrombin; factor V Leiden mutation, prothrombin gene *G20210A* mutation

Table 15.4 (cont.)

Acquired hypercoagulable state (e.g., cancer, pregnancy, oral contraceptive use, exposure to hormonal treatments such as anabolic steroids and erythropoietin, nephrotic syndrome, antiphospholipid antibody syndrome)

Primary hematological disorders (polycythemia vera, essential thrombocythemia, paroxysmal nocturnal hemoglobinuria, thrombotic thrombocytopenic purpura, leukemia, lymphoma, multiple myeloma)

From Yager Ph, Singhal AB, Nogueira RG. Case records of the Massachusetts General Hospital. Case 31–2012 – An 18-year-old man with blurred vision, dysarthria, and ataxia. *N Engl J Med* 2012;367:1450–1460.

Genetic disorders are suggested by abnormal eye and skin examination findings such as cataracts, corneal opacities, angiokeratomas (Fabry's disease), hyperelastic skin (Ehlers–Danlos type IV), and café-au-lait spots (neurofibromatosis). Stroke lesion topography on brain imaging often provides clues; for example, a unilateral "string-of-pearls" appearance (Figure 15.5) suggests internal carotid or MCA stenosis. Prolonged immobility should raise suspicion for paradoxical embolism through a patent foramen ovale. Fevers, back pain, and joint pain should raise concern for endocarditis. Clues for a hypercoagulable state, a risk factor for cerebral venous sinus thrombosis, include a history of deep venous thrombosis or multiple miscarriages. Skin examination may show underlying coagulation problems, vasculitis, endocarditis, or stigmata of intravenous drug abuse.

In many series, premature atherosclerosis was an important cause of stroke in individuals older than 30 years. Large artery extracranial and intracranial atherosclerosis was a much more common cause in those aged over 40 than in those who were younger. But in all of the series, large-artery atherosclerosis was a much less frequent cause of stroke than that found in series of older adults. Similarly, penetrating artery ("lacunar") disease is not rare in young adults, but it is much less often found under the age of 45 than in the geriatric years. Cardiac-origin embolism is a very important cause of stroke in young adults. The cardiac disorders responsible are somewhat different than those found in childhood and older adult series. Congenital cardiac disease (other than cardiac septal abnormalities), and atrial fibrillation, congestive heart failure, and coronary artery disease-related myocardial dysfunction are not common cardiac sources in patients aged 15–45 years. Rheumatic heart disease, prosthetic valves, infectious endocarditis, and various cardiomyopathies are often mentioned cardiac sources of emboli in this age group. In some recent series, atrial septal defects and patent foramen ovale with or without atrial septal aneurysms are mentioned as the predominant cardiac source of embolism.[181,183–185] Lechat and his French colleagues found that 40% of young patients with ischemic stroke had patent foramen ovale, compared with 10% of controls

Table 15.5 Series of strokes in young adults

Refs[†]	No.	Age/Sex	Hemorrhage	Premature athero-sclerosis (%)	Cardiac emboli (%)	Trauma (%)	Dissection (%)	Oral contraceptive use (%) peripartum (%)	Migraine (%)	Other* Unknown[†] (%)
Hart and Miller,[162] 1983: United States	100 ischemia	<40/NM	–	18	31	2	2	9/5	12	15
Snyder and Ramirez-Lassepas,[161] 1980: United States	61 ischemia	16–49/62% M	–	47	11	NM	NM	11/1	NM	8
Bogousslavsky and Regli,[168] 1987: Switzerland	41 ischemia	<30/27% M	–	5	29/MVP	NM	21	65 NM	15	20
Gautier et al,[169] 1989: France	133 all strokes	9–45/51% M	9	15	12	13	21	34?NM	14	14
Adams et al,[166] 1986: United States	144 ischemia	15–45/51% M	–	27	24	NM	6	4/5	14	42
Hilton-Jones and Warlow,[164] 1985: United Kingdom	75 all strokes	<45/66% M	20	9	7	17	NM	9/NM	13	7
Berlit,[170] 1990: Germany	168 ischemia	<40/46% M	–	32	9	4	2	12/4	10	18
Lisovoski and Rousseaux,[172] 1991: France	148 ischemia	5–40/51% M	–	22	13	NM	10	11	17	–
Baringarrementaria et al,[180] 1996: Mexico	300 ischemia	11–40/46% M	–	4	24	NM	15	NM	3	22
Baringarrementaria et al,[175] 1998: Mexico	130 ischemia	11–40/all F	–	0	36	NM	11	12/2	7	22
Giovannoni and Fritz,[177] 1993: South Africa	75 ischemia	<45/44% M	–	37	38	NM	0	5/NM	9	24
Williams et al,[173] 1997: United States	75 TIA	18–45/52% M	–	16	14	NM	15	NM	NM	32
Kristensen et al,[179] 1997: North Sweden	116 ischemia	11–44/59% M	–	12	33	NM	NM	3/NM	1	30
Carolei et al,[178] 1993: Italy	107 Ischemia	15–44/52% M	–	34	24	NM	0.3	4/NM	1	8
Kappelle et al,[27] 1994: United States	333 Ischemia	15–45/53% M	–	22	21	NM	NM	5 out of 10 patients/NM	NM	42

Note: The percentages in every study do not add to 100. Some authors cite oral contraceptive use, migraine, and trauma, only when thought to cause stroke. Others list all patients with these factors. Some patients have more than one condition (e.g., migraine and oral contraceptives, trauma and dissection).

* Other includes known or probable cause other than those specified in this chart (e.g., moyamoya syndrome, inflammatory diseases, coagulopathy).

† Unknown usually meant the cause was not determined.

F, females; M, males; MVP, mitral valve prolapse; NM, not mentioned; TIA, transient ischemic attack.

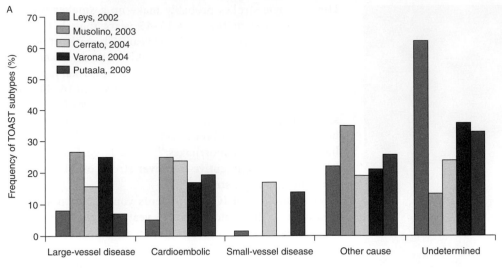

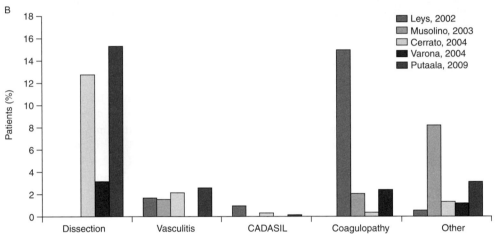

Figure 15.4 Frequency of TOAST (Trial of ORG 10172 in Acute Stroke Treatment) causal subtypes (A) and the frequency of specific conditions under the TOAST subtype "other identified causes" (B) in recent studies of young adults with stroke. From Ferro JM, Massaro A, Mas J-L. Aetiological diagnosis of ischaemic stroke in young adults. *Lancet Neurol* 2010;9:1085–1096.

the same age without stroke.[189,190] Intracardiac shunts can be detected readily by using bubbles introduced intravenously while studying patients with transesophageal echocardiography or TCD ultrasound. Few of the series cited routinely used these techniques.

Many strokes in young women are related to pregnancy, the puerperium, or use of oral contraceptive agents. In countries like India[191] and Mexico,[175,180] puerperal stroke, usually caused by dural venous sinus occlusion, is a very important cause of stroke in young women. Usually, symptoms began during the first three weeks after normal childbirth in multiparous women. In a study of 428 consecutive patients in India, common early findings included seizures (29%), acute focal deficits (29%), and symptoms consistent with benign intracranial hypertension (18%).[191] Good outcome (modified Rankin Scale (mRS) score <2) at 90 days was observed in 71% of 383 patients available for follow-up. The in-hospital mortality rate was 7.7%, and the recurrence rate was 5.1%. Anemia, hyperhomocysteinemia, alcoholism, oral contraceptive use, and postpartum period were the most common risk factors.[191]

Oral contraceptive use was common among young women with strokes, although the relationship to etiology was usually uncertain. Although 34% of young women in the French series of Gautier et al. used oral contraceptives, this was not significantly different from the estimated rate of use in the population of the same age (32%).[169] Lower-dose oral contraceptive agents have less risk of stroke. Published series antedate the widespread use of lower-dose contraceptives or do not report the strength of estrogen and progesterone used. In some series, oral contraceptive use and migraine were combined risk factors. Migraine was mentioned prominently in many series, but the mechanism by which it related to stroke was most often not identified or posited. Some series tabulated all patients that gave a history of migraine, whereas other series listed only patients in whom the authors considered that migraine was the etiology of the brain infarct.

Infections are less important as an etiology of stroke in young adults than in children. Neurosyphilis is an important cause of stroke in young adults in India, as is tuberculous meningitis.[163] Neurocysticercosis was an important cause of stroke in Mexican young adults, accounting for 14 of the 80 cases of non-atherosclerotic vasculopathies found among 300 patients.[180]

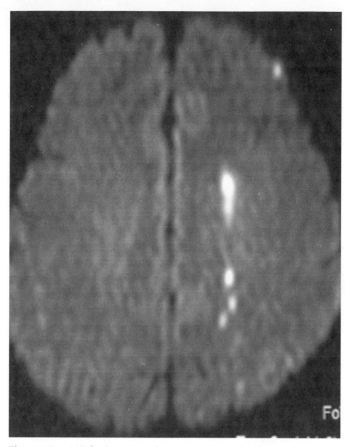

Figure 15.5 MRI fluid-attenuated inversion recovery (FLAIR) image showing a row of small white lesions along the left internal borderzone region and one small lesion on the convexal surface between the anterior and middle cerebrala artery supply zones.

An important factor that may have been unrecognized in the past is the use of drugs. Illicit drugs, especially cocaine, have become an important and frequent cause of ischemia and hemorrhage in young adults.[14] A history of drug use was seldom mentioned in the series reviewed, and was seldom pursued vigorously as a possible etiology. In a case-control study of individuals aged 15–44 years, the estimated overall relative risk for stroke was 6.5 and was 11.2 for patients younger than 35 years.[192] The Baltimore–Washington Young Stroke Study investigators specifically sought data regarding stroke among 422 patients with first ischemic strokes (age range, 17–44 years).[193] Drug use was acknowledged in 94 patients (22%), and 51 individuals (12%) used drugs within the 48 hours before stroke onset.[93] In 20 of these 51 patients (39%) with recent drug use, no other cause of stroke was identified. Strokes were attributed directly to the drug use.[193] Cocaine was the most commonly used drug in this and other series. Drug-related stroke is discussed in more detail in Chapter 12 and 14

Few reports analyze the causes of hemorrhagic stroke in young adults.[167,174,194] Because hemorrhagic stroke patients are often cared for on neurosurgical services and ischemia is usually treated on neurological units, the relative frequencies of the two types of stroke are difficult to determine.

Hemorrhagic strokes probably make up a smaller proportion of strokes in the ages 15–45 years than before age 15 years, and during the geriatric years. The ratio of hemorrhage to ischemia varies considerably with the race/ethnicity, sex, and location of stroke patients. In Osaka, Japan, for example, among 252 young stroke patients aged 16–40 years, 175 had hemorrhagic strokes (70%),[171] whereas in a British series of patients younger than 45 years, only 20% had hemorrhages.[164] In a French series, only 9% of 133 patients had intracranial hemorrhages.[169] In a large Dutch series, 91 out of 959 consecutive first-ever stroke or TIA patients had a hemorrhagic stroke.[12]

The etiology of ICH in patients younger than 45 years is similar to those older than 45 years, except for an over-representation of AVMs, cavernomas, reversible cerebral vasoconstriction syndromes including vasoconstriction associated with drug abuse, and early-life bleeding disorders such as hemophilia. Amyloid angiopathy is not encountered in young adults, and warfarin-related hemorrhages are less frequent than in older patients. Hypertension remains a frequent cause of intraparenchymatous bleeding in both age groups. Toffol and colleagues reviewed the Iowa experience with non-traumatic ICH in patients 15–45 years of age.[167] The most common location was lobar (41/72, 57%), 11 were putaminal (11/72, 15%), and 4 were intraventricular (4/72, 5%). Etiologies included AVMs (21/55, 39%), hypertension (11/72, 15%), aneurysm (7/72, 10%), and drug use with amphetamines or phenyl-propanolamine, or both (5/72, 7%).[167] Among the 15 patients with ICH included in the British series, 6 were caused by AVMs and 2 by hypertension.[164] In a Japanese neurological series among 25 young patients with ICH, 7 had AVMs. In 16 patients, hemorrhages were attributed to hypertension.[171] Aneurysms (51%) accounted for more ICHs than AVMs (19%) among Japanese patients treated on a neurosurgical service.[171] In a Mexican study of 200 patients younger than 40 years with ICHs, AVMs, and cavernous angiomas were the most common causes.[174] In this series, only 22 (11%) hemorrhages were attributed to hypertension. The majority of hemorrhages (55%) were lobar.[174]

Aneurysms in young adults have the same locations and clinical findings as in older patients. SAHs before and after age 40 years are diagnosed and managed in the same fashion.

Differences in evaluation

In young adults and children, clinicians face a dilemma regarding the extensiveness of the evaluation. A patient's youth, with nearly a lifetime remaining of potential risks of future stroke and other vascular diseases, and the vast number of diagnostic possibilities are factors that argue for extensive evaluation. On the other hand, the tendency for young patients to improve dramatically irrespective of treatment, the knowledge that a high proportion of cases go

---

Box 15.1 Selected tests for specific stroke etiologies

Serum and urine toxicology screen

Lower extremity ultrasound, pelvic CT- or MR-venography (in patients with patent foramen ovale)

Advanced brain imaging: axial fat-suppressed T1-weighted MRI, high-resolution (3T) contrast enhanced T1-weighted MRI, PET scan, MR-spectroscopy, TCD ultrasound studies for cerebrovascular "reserve"

Cerebrospinal fluid examination: opening and closing pressure, cell counts, protein and glucose level, oligoclonal bands, cytology, immunoglobulin gene rearrangement analysis, and special tests for viral, fungal, bacterial and parasitic infections, for mitochondrial disease, and for rheumatological diseases

Rheumatological panel blood tests: antinuclear antibody, antibody to double-stranded DNA, rheumatoid factor, anticardiolipin antibodies, complement levels, cryoglobulin level, neutrophil cytoplasm antibody (cANCA and pANCA), Scl-70 antibody, anti-centromere antibody, anti-Ro (SSA) and anti-La (SSB) cytoplasmic antibodies, serum angiotensin-converting enzyme, anti-Proteinase 3 (APR3)

Infectious disease panel tests: for varicella zoster virus, herpes simplex virus, Ebstein–Barr virus, HIV, hepatitis B and C viruses, tuberculosis, syphilis, Lyme, and others

Hypercoagulable panel tests: protein C, protein S, and antithrombin levels, prothrombin gene mutation, factor V Leiden mutation, and others

Hematological panel tests: serum protein electrophoresis, homocysteine level, serum viscosity, Coomb's test, bone marrow aspiration biopsy, and others

Ophthalmological evaluation: e.g., fluorescein retinal angiography, Schirmer's test

Biopsy: brain/leptomeningeal, skin, temporal artery, sural nerve, muscle, etc.

Genetic tests: for conditions like CADASIL, RVCL, *MTHFR 677C-T* pleiomorphism, and others

Adapted from Singhal, AB., Biller J, Elkind M et al. Recognition and management of stroke in young adults and adolescents. *Neurology* 2013;81(12):1089–1097, with permission.

---

undiagnosed despite intensive testing, and the high cost of technology and testing argue for conservatism when ordering tests. Recent information from series that have included vascular imaging show that the presence and nature of an arteriopathy impacts greatly on the future course, outcome, and treatment.[26,73–76,80,81] The finding of cerebral venous occlusive disease also directs evaluation, treatment, prognosis, and outcome. The frequency and importance of cardiac disease, arteriopathy, and venous occlusive disease means that all young patients with strokes and TIAs should have cardiac investigations and imaging of the arteries and veins that supply the brain.

In our opinion, clinicians should spend more time with the clinical encounter. The history should include questions about smoking, headache, trauma, cardiac symptoms, past bleeding, miscarriages, thrombophlebitis, and prior strokes and ischemic attacks. Details are important; for example, was the headache sudden or progressive, what was its duration, is there a background of chronic headaches over the past few weeks, any prior history of migraines, any precipitating factors for headaches? The use of medicines and drugs of any kind (especially cocaine, amphetamines, and other illicit drugs) and oral contraceptive agents is particularly important. The history should include a thorough review of systems, searching for symptoms that might indicate systemic disease. Family history is important. Information about premature atherosclerosis, hypertension, hyperlipidemia, migraine, and metabolic and hereditary diseases in family members should be sought.

The general physical examination should include careful inspection of the skin for rashes and other lesions. Palpation of pulses and cardiac, neck, and cranial auscultation are especially important. Blood tests, including coagulation studies; brain and vascular imaging; and cardiac evaluation are needed in every young person with stroke. Box 15.1 includes suggested testing for specific stroke etiologies. Ultrasound and angiography may be indicated, depending on the findings from the clinical encounter and early investigations. The yield of angiography is high. In one series, two-thirds of angiograms were abnormal, often allowing an etiological diagnosis.[172] MRA, CTA and extracranial and intracranial ultrasound often allow clinicians to non-invasively acquire enough data about the vasculature without risk to the patients. Physicians should order contrast angiography only when preliminary vascular imaging screening suggests a vascular lesion, but does not define it sufficiently to select and monitor treatment.

References

1. Singhal AB, Biller J, Elkind M, et al. Recognition and management of stroke in young adults and adolescents. *Neurology* 2013;**81**:1089–1097.

2. Putaala J, Metso AJ, Metso TM, et al. Analysis of 1008 consecutive patients aged 15 to 49 with first-ever ischemic stroke: The Helsinki Young Stroke Registry. *Stroke* 2009;**40**:1195–1203.

3. Yesilot Barlas N, Putaala J, Waje-Andreassen U, et al. Etiology of first-ever ischaemic stroke in European young adults: The 15 cities Young Stroke Study. *Eur J Neurol* 2013;**20**:1431–1439.

4. Maaijwee NA, Rutten-Jacobs LCA, Schaapsmeerders P, van Dijk EJ, de Leeuw F-E. Ischaemic stroke in young adults: Risk factors and long-term consequences. *Nat Rev Neurol* 2014;**10**:315–325.

5. Chopra JS, Prabhakar S. Clinical features and risk factors in stroke in young. *Acta Neurol Scand* 1979;**60**:289–300.

6. Katrak S. Vasculitis and stroke due to tuberculosis. In Caplan LR (ed): *Uncommon Causes of Stroke*, 2nd ed. Cambridge: Cambridge University Press, 2008, pp 41–45.

7. Del Bruto O. Stroke and vasculitis in patients with cysticercosis. In Caplan LR (ed): *Uncommon Causes of Stroke*, 2nd ed. Cambridge: Cambridge University Press, 2008, pp 53–58.

8. Caplan LR, Estanol B, Mitchell WG. How to manage patients with neurocysticercosis. *Eur Neurol* 1997;**37**:124–131.

9. Putaala J, Haapaniemi E, Metso AJ, et al. Recurrent ischemic events in young adults after first-ever ischemic stroke. *Ann Neurol* 2010;**68**:661–671.

10. George MG, Tong X, Kuklina EV, Labarthe DR. Trends in stroke hospitalizations and associated risk factors among children and young adults, 1995–2008. *Ann Neurol* 2011;**70**:713–721.

11. Kissela BM, Khoury JC, Alwell K, et al. Age at stroke: Temporal trends in stroke incidence in a large, biracial population. *Neurology* 2012;**79**:1781–1787.

12. Rutten-Jacobs LC, Arntz RM, Maaijwee NA, et al. Long-term mortality after stroke among adults aged 18 to 50 years. *JAMA* 2013;**309**:1136–1144.

13. Nencini P, Inzitari D, Baruffi MC, et al. Incidence of stroke in young adults in Florence, Italy. *Stroke* 1988;**19**:977–981.

14. Stern B, Kittmer S, Sloan M, et al. Stroke in the young. *Maryland Med J* 1991;**40**:453–462, 565–571.

15. Agrawal N, Johnston SC, Wu YW, Sidney S, Fullerton HJ. Imaging data reveal a higher pediatric stroke incidence than prior US estimates. *Stroke* 2009;**40**:3415–3421.

16. Mackay MT, Wiznitzer M, Benedict SL, et al. Arterial ischemic stroke risk factors: The International Pediatric Stroke Study. *Ann Neurol* 2011;**69**:130–140.

17. Walsh LE, Garg B. Isolated acute subcortical infarctions in children: Clinical description and radiographic correlation. *Ann Neurol* 1990;**28**:458–459.

18. Caplan LR, Babikian V, Helgason C, et al: Occlusive disease of the middle cerebral artery. *Neurology* 1985;**35**:975–982.

19. Caplan LR, DeWitt LD, Pessin MS, et al. Lateral thalamic infarcts. *Arch Neurol* 1988;**45**:959–964.

20. Caplan LR. Posterior cerebral artery disease. In Caplan LR: *Posterior Circulation Disease*. Boston: Blackwell, 1996, pp 444–491.

21. Edlow JA, Selim MH. Atypical presentations of acute cerebrovascular syndromes. *Lancet Neurol* 2011;**10**:550–560.

22. Ferro JM, Crespo M. Young adult stroke: Neuropsychological dysfunction and recovery. *Stroke* 1988;**19**:982–986.

23. Boardman JP, Ganesan V, Rutherford MA, Saunders DE, Mercuri E, Cowan F. Magnetic resonance image correlates of hemiparesis after neonatal and childhood middle cerebral artery stroke. *Pediatrics* 2005;**115**:321–326.

24. Malamud N. Status marmoratus: A form of cerebral palsy following either birth injury or inflammation of the central nervous system. *J Pediatr* 1950;**37**:610–619.

25. Ferro JM, Massaro A, Mas J-L. Aetological diagnosis of ischaemic stroke in young adults. *Lancet Neurol* 2010;**9**:1085–1096.

26. deVeber G. The Canadian Pediatric Ischemic Stroke Study Group: Canadian pediatric ischemic stroke registry: Analysis of children with arterial ischemic stroke (abstract). *Ann Neurol* 2000;**48**:526.

27. Kappelle LJ, Adams HP, Heffner ML, et al. Prognosis of young adults with ischemic stroke. A long-term follow-up study assessing recurrent vascular events and functional outcome in the Iowa Registry of Stroke in Young Adults. *Stroke* 1994;**25**:1360–1365.

28. Putaala J, Curtze S, Hiltunen S, Toippanen H, Kaste M, Tatlisumak T. Causes of death and predictors of 5-year mortality in young adults after first-ever ischemic stroke: the Helsinki Young Stroke Registry. *Stroke* 2009;**40**:2698–2703.

29. Maaijwee NA, Rutten-Jacobs LC, Arntz R, et al. Long-term increased risk of unemployment after young stroke: A long-term follow-up study *Neurology* 2014;**83**:1132–1138.

30. Singhal AB, Lo W. Life after stroke: Beyond medications. *Neurology* 2014;**83**:1128–1129.

31. Ferriero DM. Neonatal brain injury. *N Engl J Med* 2004;**351**:1985–1995.

32. Kirton A, deVeber G, Pontigon A-M, et al. Presumed perinatal ischemic stroke: Vascular classification predicts outcome. *Ann Neurol* 2008;**63**:436–443.

33. Back SA, Riddle A, McClure MM. Maturation-dependent vulnerability of perinatal white matter in premature birth. *Stroke* 2007;**38**(part 2):724–730.

34. Hill A, Volpe JJ. Stroke and hemorrhage in the premature and term neonate. In Edwards MB, Hoffman HJ (eds): *Cerebral Vascular Diseases in Children and Adolescents*. Baltimore: Williams & Wilkins, 1989, pp 179–194.

35. Roland E, Poskitt K, Rodriguez E, et al. Perinatal hypoxic-ischemic thalamic injury: Clinical features and neuroimaging. *Ann Neurol* 1998;**44**:161–166.

36. Leech RW, Alvord EC Jr. Anoxic-ischemic encephalopathy in the human neonatal period: The significance of brain stem involvement. *Arch Neurol* 1977;**34**:109–113.

37. Golomb MR, MacGregor DL, Domi T, et al. Presumed pre- or perinatal arterial ischemic stroke: Risk factors and outcomes. *Ann Neurol* 2001;**50**:163–168.

38. Benders MJ, Groenendaal F, Uiterwaal CS, et al. Maternal and infant characteristics associated with perinatal arterial stroke in the preterm infant. *Stroke* 2007;**38**:1759–1765.

39. Rorke LB, Zimmerman RA. Prematurity, postmaturity, and destructive lesions in utero. *AJNR Am J Neuroradiol* 1992;**13**:517–536.

40. Nelson KB, Dambrosia JM, Grether JK, Phillips TM. Neonatal cytokines and coagulation factors in children with cerebral palsy. *Ann Neurol* 1998;**44**:665–675.

41. Kurnik K, Kosch A, Strater R. Childhood Stroke Study Group. Recurrent thromboembolism in infants and children suffering from symptomatic neonatal arterial stroke. A prospective follow-up study. *Stroke* 2003;**34**:2887–2893.

42. Johnston MV. Selective vulnerability in the neonatal brain. *Ann Neurol* 1998;**44**:155–156.

43. Martin LJ, Brambrink A, Koehler RC, Traystman RJ. Primary sensory and forebrain motor systems in the newborn brain are preferentially damaged by hypoxia-ischemia. *J Comp Neurol* 1997;**377**:262–285.

44. Volpe JJ. Value of MR in definition of the neuropathology of cerebral palsy in vivo. *AJNR Am J Neuroradiol* 1992;**13**:79–83.

45. Volpe JJ, Pasternak JF. Parasagittal cerebral injury in neonatal hypoxic-ischemic encephalopathy: Clinical and neuroradiologic features. *J Pediatr* 1977;**91**:472–476.

46. Aida N, Nishimura NA, Hachiya Y, et al. MR imaging of perinatal brain damage: Comparison of clinical outcome with initial and follow-up MR findings. *AJNR Am J Neuroradiol* 1998;**19**:1909–1921.

47. Bax M, Tydeman C, Flodmark O. Clinical and MRI correlates of cerebral palsy. The European Cerebral Palsy Study. *JAMA* 2006;**296**:1601–1608.

48. Volpe JJ, Herscovitch P, Perlman JM, et al. Positron emission tomography in the asphyxiated term newborn: Parasagittal impairment of cerebral blood flow. *Ann Neurol* 1985;**17**:287–296.

49. Banker BQ, Larroch JC. Periventricular leukomalacia of infancy: A form of neonatal anoxic encephalopathy. *Arch Neurol* 1962;**7**:386–410.

50. DeReuck J, Chattha AS, Richardson Jr EP. Pathogenesis and evolution of periventricular leukomalacia in infancy. *Arch Neurol* 1972;**27**:229–236.

51. Truwit CL, Barkovich AJ, Koch TK, Ferriero DM. Cerebral palsy: MR findings in 40 patients. *AJNR Am J Neuroradiol* 1992;**13**:67–78.

52. Kuban KC, Leviton A. Cerebral palsy. *N Engl J Med* 1994;**330**:188–195.

53. Barmada MA, Moossy J, Shuman RM. Cerebral infarcts with arterial occlusion in neonates. *Ann Neurol* 1979;**6**:495–502.

54. Mantovani JF, Gerber GJ. "Idiopathic" neonatal cerebral infarction. *Am J Dis Child* 1984;**138**:359–362.

55. Rollins NK, Morris MC, Evans D, et al. The role of early MR in the evaluation of the term infant with seizures. *AJNR Am J Neuroradiol* 1994;**15**:239–248.

56. Takanashi J, Barkovich AJ, Ferriero DM, et al. Widening spectrum of congenital hemiplegia. Periventricular venous infarction in term neonates. *Neurology* 2003;**61**:531–533.

57. Chasnoff IJ, Bussey ME, Savich R, et al. Perinatal cerebral infarction and maternal cocaine use. *J Pediatr* 1986;**108**:456–459.

58. Roessmann CC, Miller RT. Thrombus of the middle cerebral artery associated with birth trauma. *Neurology* 1980;**30**:889–892.

59. Roach ES, Riela AR. *Pediatric Cerebrovascular Disorders*. Mount Kisco, NY: Futura, 1988.

60. Teksama M, Moharirc M, deVeber G, Shroff M. Frequency and topographic distribution of brain lesions in pediatric cerebral venous thrombosis. *AJNR Am J Neuroradiol* 2008;**29**:1961–1965.

61. Fitzgerald KC, Williams LS, Garg BP, et al. Cerebral sinovenous thrombosis in the neonate. *Arch Neurol* 2006;**63**:405–409.

62. deVeber G, Andrew M, Adams C, et al. Canadian Pediatric Ischemic Stroke Study Group. Cerebral sinovenous thrombosis in children. *N Engl J Med* 2001;**345**:417–423.

63. Moharir MD, Shroff M, Stephens D, et al. Anticoagulants in pediatric cerebral sinovenous thrombosis: A safety and outcome study. *Ann Neurol* 2010;**67**:590–599.

64. Jordan LC, Rafay MF, Smith SE, et al. for the Pediatric Stroke Study Group. Antithrombotic treatment in neonatal cerebral sinovenous thrombosis: Results of the International Pediatric Stroke Study. *J Pediatr* 2010;**156**:704–710.

65. Ahmann PA, Lazzara A, Dykes FD, et al. Intraventricular hemorrhage in the high-risk preterm infant: Incidence and outcome. *Ann Neurol* 1980;**7**:118–124.

66. Papile LA, Burstein J, Burstein R, et al. Incidence and evolution of subependymal and intraventricular hemorrhage: A study of infants with birth weights of less than 1500 gm. *Pediatrics* 1978;**92**:529–534.

67. Garcia JH, Pantoni L. Strokes in childhood. *Semin Pediatr Neurol* 1995;**2**:180–191.

68. Grunnet ML, Shields WD. Cerebellar hemorrhage in the premature infant. *J Pediatr* 1976;**88**:605–608.

69. Martin R, Roessmann U, Fanaroff A. Massive intracerebellar hemorrhage in low birth-weight infants. *J Pediatr* 1976;**89**:290–293.

70. Gowers WR. *A Manual of Diseases of the Nervous System*. Philadelphia: P Blakiston, 1888.

71. Freud S. *Die Infantile Cerebrähmung*. Vienna. Hölder, 1897.

72. Ford FR, Schaffer AJ. The etiology of infantile acquired hemiplegia. *AMA Arch Neurol Psychiatry* 1927;**18**:323–347.

73. Ganesan V, Prengler M, McShane MA, et al. Investigation of risk factors in children with arterial ischemic stroke. *Ann Neurol* 2003;**53**:167–173.

74. Lanthier S, Armstrong D, Donni T, deVeber G. Post-varicella arteriopathy of childhood. Natural history of vascular stenosis. *Neurology* 2005;**64**:660–663.

75. Danchaivijitr N, Cox TC, Saunders D, Ganesan V. Evolution of cerebral arteriopathies in childhood arterial ischemic stroke. *Ann Neurol* 2006;**59**:620–626.

76. Kirkham F. Improvement or progression in childhood cerebral arteriopathies: Current difficulties in prediction and suggestions for research. *Ann Neurol* 2006;**580**:582.

77. Sebire G, Fullerton H, Riou E, deVeber G. Toward the definition of cerebral arteriopathies of childhood. *Curr Opin Pediatr* 2004;**16**:617–622.

78. Kuhle S, Mitchell L, Andrew M, et al. Urgent clinical challenges in children with ischemic stroke. Analysis of 1065 patients from the 1-800-NOCLOTS Pediatric Stroke Telephone Consultation Service. *Stroke* 2006;**37**:116–122.

79. Schoenberg BS, Mellinger JF, Schoenberg DG. Cerebrovascular disease in infants and children: A study

of incidence, clinical features, and survival. *Neurology* 1978;**28**:763–768.

80. Fullerton HJ, Wu YW, Sydney S, Johnstone SC. Risk of recurrent stroke in a population-based cohort: The importance of cerebrovascular imaging. *Stroke* 2007;**38**:485.

81. Fullerton HJ, Wu YW, Sydney S, Johnstone SC. Excess stroke risk in black and Hispanic children: A population-based study. *Stroke* 2007;**38**:460.

82. Fullerton HJ, Chetkovich DM, Wu YW, et al. Deaths from strokes in US children 1979–1998. *Neurology* 2002;**59**:34–39.

83. Mallick AA, O'Callaghan FJ. The epidemiology of childhood stroke. *Eur J Paediatr Neurol.* 2010;**14**:197–205.

84. Blom I, De Schryver EL, Kappelle LJ, Rinkel GJ, Jennekens-Schinkel A, Peters AC. Prognosis of haemorrhagic stroke in childhood: a long-term follow-up study. *Dev Med Child Neurol.* 2003;**45**:233–239.

85. So SC. Cerebral arteriovenous malformations in children. *Childs Brain* 1978;**4**:242–250.

86. Ventureyra EC, Herder S. Arteriovenous malformations in children. *Childs Nerv Syst* 1987;**3**:12–18.

87. Fullerton HJ, Wu YW, Sidney S, Johnston SC. Recurrent hemorrhagic stroke in children. A population-based cohort study. *Stroke* 2007;**38**:2658–2662.

88. Sedzimir CB, Robinson J. Intracranial hemorrhages in children and adolescents. *J Neurosurg* 1973;**38**:269–281.

89. Orozco M, Trigueros F, Quintana F, et al. Intracranial aneurysms in early childhood. *Surg Neurol* 1978;**9**:247–252.

90. Shucart WA, Wolpert SM. Intracranial arterial aneurysms in childhood. *Am J Dis Child* 1974;**127**:288–293.

91. Kumar R, Shukla D, Mahapatra AK. Spontaneous intracranial hemorrhage in children. *Pediatr Neurosurg* 2009;**45**:37–45.

92. Mackenzie I. The clinical presentation of the cerebral angioma. *Brain* 1953;**76**:184–213.

93. Humphreys RP. Infratentorial arteriovenous malformations. In Edwards MS, Hoffman HJ (eds): *Cerebral Vascular Disease in Children and Adolescents.* Baltimore: Williams & Wilkins, 1989, pp 309–320.

94. Humphreys RP. Infratentorial arteriovenous malformations. In Edwards MS, Hoffman HJ (eds): *Cerebral Vascular Disease in Children and Adolescents.* Baltimore: Williams & Wilkins, 1989, pp 309–320.

95. Martin NA, Edwards MS. Supratentorial arteriovenous malformations. In Edwards MS, Hoffman HJ (eds): *Cerebral Vascular Diseases in Children and Adolescents.* Baltimore: Williams & Wilkins, 1989, pp 283–308.

96. Metellus P, Kharkar S, Lin D, et al. Cerebral cavernous malformations and developmental venous anomalies. In Caplan LR (ed): *Uncommon Causes of Stroke*, 2nd ed. Cambridge: Cambridge University Press, 2008, pp 189–219.

97. Maraire JN, Awad IA. Intracranial cavernous malformations: Lesion behavior and management strategies. *Neurosurgery* 1995;**37**:591–605.

98. Mottolese C, Hermier M, Stan H, et al. Central nervous system cavernomas in the pediatric age group. *Neurosurg Rev* 2001;**24**:55–71; discussion 72–73.

99. Cavalheiro S, Braga FM. Cavernous hemangiomas. In Choux M, Di Rocco C, Hockley AD, Walker ML (eds): *Pediatric Neurosurgery*. London: Churchill Livingstone, 1999, pp 691–701.

100. Brower MC, Rollins N, Roach ES. Basal ganglia and thalamic infarction in children. Cause and clinical features. *Arch Neurol* 1996;**53**:1252–1256.

101. Terplan AK. Patterns of brain damage in infants and children with congenital heart disease. *Am J Dis Child* 1973;**125**:176–185.

102. Caplan LR, Manning WJ. *Brain Embolism*. New York: Informa Healthcare, 2006.

103. Rodan L, McCrindle BW, Manlhiot C, et al. Stroke recurrence in children with congenital heart disease. *Ann Neurol* 2012;**72**:103–111.

104. Braun KPJ, Rafay M, Uiterwaal CS, Pontigon A-M, deVeber G. Mode of onset predicts etiological diagnosis of arterial ischemic stroke in children. *Stroke* 2007;**38**:298–302.

105. Hills NK, Johnston SC, Sidney S, et al. Recent trauma and acute infection as risk factors for childhood arterial ischemic stroke. *Ann Neurol* 2012;**72**:850–858.

106. Satoh S, Shirane R, Yoshimoto T. Clinical survey of ischemic cerebrovascular disease in children in a district of Japan. *Stroke* 1991;**22**:586–589.

107. Pitner SE. Carotid thrombosis due to intraoral trauma – an unusual complication of a common childhood accident. *N Engl J Med* 1966;**274**:764–767.

108. Pearl PL. Childhood stroke following intraoral trauma. *J Pediatr* 1987;**110**:574–575.

109. Duncan A, Rumbaugh C, Caplan LR. Cerebral embolic disease: A complication of carotid aneurysms. *Radiology* 1979;**133**:379–384.

110. Zilkha A, Mendelsohn F, Borofsky LG. Acute hemiplegia in children complicating upper respiratory infections. *Clin Pediatr* 1976;**15**:1137–1142.

111. Parker P, Puck J, Fernandez F. Cerebral infarction associated with Mycoplasma pneumoniae. *Pediatrics* 1981;**67**:373–375.

112. Doyle PW, Gibson G, Dolman C. Herpes zoster ophthalmicus with contralateral hemiplegia: Identification of cause. *Ann Neurol* 1983;**14**:84–85.

113. Melanson M, Chalk C, Georgevich L, et al. Varicella-zoster virus DNA in CSF and arteries in delayed contralateral hemiplegia: Evidence for viral invasion of cerebral arteries. *Neurology* 1996;**47**:569–570.

114. Ross MH, Abend WK, Schwartz RB, Samuels MA. A case of C2 herpes zoster with delayed bilateral pontine infarction. *Neurology* 1991;**41**:1685–1686.

115. Askalan R, Laughlin S, Mayank S, et al: Chickenpox and stroke in childhood: A study of frequency and causation. *Stroke* 2001;**32**:1257–1262.

116. Hausler MG, Ramaekers VT, Reul J, et al. Early and late onset manifestations of cerebral vasculitis related to varicella zoster. *Neuropediatrics* 1998;**29**:202–207.

117. Lanthier S, Armstrong D, Domi T, deVeber G. Post-varicella arteriopathy of childhood. *Neurology* 2005;**64**:660–663.

118. Caplan LR. Migraine and vertebrobasilar ischemia. *Neurology* 1990;**41**:55–61.

119. Caplan LR. Migraine and posterior circulation stroke. In Caplan LR (ed): *Posterior Circulation Disease: Clinical Findings, Diagnosis, and Management.*

120. Feucht M, Brantner S, Scheidinger H. Migraine and stroke in childhood and adolecence. *Cephalagia* 1995;**15**:26–30.

121. Wood DH. Cerebrovascular complications of sickle-cell anemia. *Stroke* 1978;**9**:73–75.

122. Grotta JC, Manner C, Pettigrew LC, et al. Red blood cell disorders and stroke. *Stroke* 1986;**17**:811–816.

123. Rothman SM, Fulling KH, Nelson JS. Sickle cell anemia and central nervous system infarction: A neuropathological study. *Ann Neurol* 1986;**20**:684–690.

124. Adams RJ, Nichols FT, McKie V, et al. Cerebral infarction in sickle cell anemia: mechanisms based on CT and MRI. *Neurology* 1988;**38**:1012–1017.

125. Steen RG, Langston JW, Ogg RJ, et al. Ectasia of the basilar artery in children with sickle cell disease. Relationship to hematocrit and psychometric measures. *J Stroke Cerebrovasc Dis* 1998;**7**:32–43.

126. Oguz M, Aksungur EH, Soyupak SK, Yildirim AU. Vein of Galen and sinus thrombosis with bilateral thalamic infarcts in sickle cell anemia: CT follow-up and angiographic demonstration. *Neuroradiology* 1994;**36**:155–156.

127. Adams RJ, McKie VC, Nichols F, et al. The use of transcranial ultrasonography to predict stroke in sickle cell disease. *N Engl J Med* 1992;**326**:605–610.

128. Adams RJ, McKie VC, Hsu L, et al. Prevention of a first stroke by transfusions in children with sickle cell anemia and abnormal results on transcranial Doppler ultrasonography. *N Engl J Med* 1998;**339**:5–11.

129. Maguire JL, deVeber G, Parkin PC, et al. Iron deficiency anemia as a risk factor for cerebrovascular events in early childhood: a case-control study. *Ann Hematol* 2014;**93**:571–576.

130. Mackay MT, Monagle P. Perinatal and early childhood stroke and thrombophilia. *Pathology* 2008;**40**:116–123.

131. Barnes C, deVeber G. Prothrombotic abnormalities in childhood ischaemic stroke. *Thromb Res.* 2006;**118**:67–74.

132. Kenet G, Lutkhoff LK, Albisetti M, et al. Impact of thrombophilia on risk of arterial ischemic stroke or cerebral sinovenous thrombosis in neonates and children: A systematic review and meta-analysis of observational studies. *Circulation* 2010;**27**:1838–1847.

133. Koo B, Becker LE, Chuang S, et al: Mitochondrial encephalomyopathy, lactic acidosis, stroke like episodes (MELAS): Clinical, radiological, and genetic observations. *Ann Neurol* 1993;**34**:25–32.

134. Matthews PM, Tampieri D, Berkovic SF, et al. Magnetic resonance imaging shows specific abnormalities in the MELAS syndrome. *Neurology* 1991;**41**:1043–1046.

135. Clark JM, Marks MP, Adalsteinsson E, et al. MELAS: Clinical and pathological correlations with MRI, xenon/CT, and MR spectroscopy. *Neurology* 1996;**46**:223–227.

136. Hirt L. MELAS and other mitochondrial disorders. In Caplan LR (ed): *Uncommon Causes of Stroke*, 2nd ed. Cambridge: Cambridge University Press, 2008, pp 149–154.

137. Morin C, Dube J, Robinson B, et al. Stroke-like episodes in autosomal recessive cytochrome oxidase deficiency. *Ann Neurol* 1999;**45**:389–392.

138. Suzuki J, Kodama N. Moyamoya disease – a review. *Stroke* 1983;**14**:104–109.

139. Suzuki J. *Moyamoya Disease*. Berlin: Springer, 1986.

140. Chiu D, Shedden P, Bratina P, Grotta JC. Clinical features of moyamoya disease in the United States. *Stroke* 1998;**29**:1347–1351.

141. Taveras JM. Multiple progressive intracranial arterial occlusions: A syndrome of children and young adults. *AJR Am J Roentgenol* 1969;**106**:235–268.

142. Scott RM, Smith ER. Moyamoya disease and moyamoya syndrome. *N Engl J Med* 2009;**360**:1226–1237.

143. Ganesan V, Saunders D, Kirkham R, et al. Clinical and radiological features of moyamoya syndrome in British children: Relationship with outcome. *Ann Neurol* 2004;**54**(suppl 7):5–12.

144. Bruno A, Adams HOP, Bilbe J, et al. Cerebral infarction due to moyamoya disease in young adults. *Stroke* 1988;**19**:826–833.

145. Mauro AJ, Johnson ES, Chikos PM, Alvord EC. Lipohyalinosis and miliary microaneurysms causing cerebral hemorrhage in a patient with moyamoya. A clinicopathological study. *Stroke* 1980;**11**:405–412.

146. Ikeda E. Systemic vascular changes in spontaneous occlusion of the circle of Willis. *Stroke* 1991;**22**:1358–1362.

147. Ueki K, Meyer FB, Mellinger JF. Moyamoya disease: The disorder and surgical treatment. *Mayo Clin Proc* 1994;**69**:749–757.

148. Smith ER, Scott RM. Surgical management of moyamoya syndrome. *Skull Base* 2005;**15**:15–26.

149. Scott RM, Smith JL, Roberson RL, et al. Long-term outcome in children with moyamoya syndrome after cranial revascularization by pial synangiosis. *J Neurosurg* 2004;**100**(suppl 2):142–149.

150. Guzman R, Lee M, Achrol A, et al. Clinical outcome after 450 revascularization procedures for moyamoya disease. *J Neurosurg* 2009;**111**;927–935.

151. Lynch JK. Cerebrovascular disorders in children. *Curr Neurol Neurosurg Reports* 2004;**4**:129–138.

152. Heller C, Heinecke A, Junker R, et al. Cerebral venous thrombosis in children: A multifactorial origin. *Circulation* 2003;**108**:1362–1367.

153. Carpenter J, Tsuchida T. Cerebral sinovenous thrombosis in children. *Curr Neurol Neurosci Rep* 2007;**7**:139–146.

154. Sebire G, Tabarki B, Saunders DE, et al. Cerebral venous sinus thrombosis in children: Risk factors, presentation, diagnosis, and outcome. *Brain* 2005;**128**:477–489.

155. Dlamini N, Billinghurst L, Kirkham FJ. Cerebral venous (sinovenous) thrombosis in children. *Neurosurg Clin N Am* 2010;**21**:511–527.

156. Bernard TJ, Goldenberg NA, Armstrong-Wells J, et al. Treatment of childhood arterial ischemic stroke. *Ann Neurol* 2008;**63**:679–696.

157. Paediatric Stroke Working Group. *Royal College of Physicians Guidelines. Stroke in Childhood: Clinical Guidelines For Diagnosis, Management And Rehabilitation*, 2004. http://www.rcpch.ac.uk/sites/default/files/asset_library/Research/Clinical%20Effectiveness/Endorsed%20guidelines/Stroke%20in%20Childhood%20(RCP)/Stroke%20in%20children%20-%20full%20guideline.pdf (accessed November 2015).

Boston: Blackwell Science, 1996, pp 544–568.

158. Monagle P, Chan AK, Goldenberg NA, et al. *American College of Chest Physicians Evidence-Based Clinical Practice Guidelines. Antithrombotic Therapy in Neonates and Children: Antithrombotic Therapy and Prevention Of Thrombosis*, 9th ed. *Chest*. 2012;**141**(2 Suppl): e737S–801S.

159. Roach ES, Golomb MR, Adams R, et al. American Heart Association Stroke Council; Council On Cardiovascular Disease in the Young. Management of stroke in infants and children: A scientific statement from a Special Writing Group of the American Heart Association Stroke Council and the Council on Cardiovascular Disease in the Young. *Stroke* 2008;**39**:2644–2691.

160. Louis S, McDowell F. Stroke in young adults. *Ann Intern Med* 1967;**66**:932–938.

161. Snyder BD, Ramirez-Lassepas M, Cerebral infarction in young adults: Long term prognosis. *Stroke* 1980;**11**:149–153.

162. Hart RG, Miller VT. Cerebral infarction in young adults: A practical approach. *Stroke* 1983;**14**:110–114.

163. Srinivasan K. Ischemic cerebrovascular disease in the young: Two common causes in India. *Stroke* 1984;**15**:733–735.

164. Hilton-Jones D, Warlow CP. The causes of stroke in the young. *J Neurol* 1985;**232**:137–143.

165. Radhakrishnan K, Ashek PP, Sridharan R, Mousa ME. Stroke in the young: Incidence and pattern in Benghazi, Libya. *Acta Neurol Scand* 1986;**73**:434–438.

166. Adams HP, Butler MJ, Biller J, Toffol GJ. Nonhemorrhagic cerebral infarction in young adults. *Arch Neurol* 1986;**43**:793–796.

167. Toffol GJ, Biller J, Adams HP. Nontraumatic intracerebral hemorrhage in young adults. *Arch Neurol* 1987;**44**:483–485.

168. Bogousslavsky J, Regli F. Ischemic stroke in adults younger than 30 years of age. *Arch Neurol* 1987;**44**:479–482.

169. Gautier JC, Pradat-Diehl P, Loron PL, et al. Accidents vasculaires cérébraux des sujets jeunes. Une etude de 133 patients ages de 9 à 45 ans. *Rev Neurol* 1989;**145**:437–442.

170. Berlit P. Cerebral ischemia in young adults. *Ann Neurol* 1990;**28**:258.

171. Yamaguchi T, Yoshinaga M, Yonekawa Y. *Stroke in the Young – Japanese Perspective*. Abstracts International Conference on Stroke. Geneva, May 30–June 1, 1991.

172. Lisovoski F, Rousseaux P. Cerebral infarction in young people: A study of 148 patients with early angiography. *J Neurol Neurosurg Psychiatry* 1991;**54**:576–579.

173. Williams LS, Garg BP, Cohen M, et al. Subtypes of ischemic stroke in children and young adults. *Neurology* 1997;**49**:1541–1545.

174. Ruiz-Sandoval JL, Cantu C, Baringarrementaria F. Intracerebral hemorrhage in young people. Analysis of risk factors, locations, causes, and prognosis. *Stroke* 1999;**30**:537–541.

175. Baringarrementaria F, Gonzalez-Duarte A, Miranda L, Cantu C. Cerebral infarction in young women: Analysis of 130 cases. *Eur Neurol* 1998;**40**:228–233.

176. Kittner SJ, Stern BJ, Wozniak M, et al. Cerebral infarction in young adults. The Baltimore–Washington Cooperative Young Stroke Study. *Neurology* 1998;**50**:890–894.

177. Giovannoni G, Fritz VU. Transient ischemic attacks in younger and older patients. A comparative study of 798 patients in South Africa. *Stroke* 1993;**24**:947–953.

178. Carolei A, Marini C, Ferranti E, et al. A prospective study of cerebral ischemia in the young. Analysis of pathogenic determinants. *Stroke* 1993;**24**:362–367.

179. Kristensen B, Malm J, Carlberg B, et al. Epidemiology and etiology of ischemic stroke in young adults aged 18 to 44 years in Northern Sweden. *Stroke* 1997;**28**:1702–1709.

180. Baringarrementaria F, Figueroa T, Huebe J, Cantu C. Cerebral infarction in people under 40 years. Etiologic analysis of 300 cases prospectively evaluated. *Cerebrovasc Dis* 1996;**6**:75–79.

181. Lee T-H, Hsu W-C, Chen C-J, Chen S-T. Etiologic study of young ischemic stroke in Taiwan. *Stroke* 2002;**33**:1950–1955.

182. Leys D, Bandu L, Henon H, et al. Clinical outcome in 287 consecutive young adults (15–45 years) with ischemic stroke. *Neurology* 2002;**59**:26–33.

183. Musolino R, La Spina P, Granata A, et al. Ischaemic stroke in young people: A prospective and long-term follow-up study. *Cerebrovasc Dis* 2003;**15**:121–128.

184. Cerrato P, Grasso M, Imperiale D, et al. Stroke in young patients: Etiopathogenesis and risk factors in different age classes. *Cerebrovasc Dis* 2004;**18**:154–159.

185. Nedeltchev K, der Maur TA, Georgiadis D, et al. Ischaemic stroke in young adults: Predictors of outcome and recurrence. *J Neurol Neurosurg Psychiatry* 2005;**76**:191–195.

186. Varona JF, Bermejo F, Guerra JM, Molina JA. Long-term prognosis of ischemic stroke in young adults. Study of 272 cases. *J Neurol* 2004;**251**:1507–1514.

187. Ji R, Schwamm LH, Perves MA, Singhal AB. Ischemic stroke and transient ischemic attack in young adults: Risk factors, diagnostic yield, neuroimaging, and thrombolysis. *JAMA Neurol* 2013;**70**:51–57.

188. Debette S, Leys D. Cervical-artery dissections: Predisposing factors, diagnosis, and outcome. *Lancet Neurol* 2009;**8**:668–678.

189. Lechat P, Mas JL, Lescault G, et al. Prevalence of patent foramen ovale in patients with strokes. *N Engl J Med* 1988;**318**:1148–1152.

190. Lechat P, Lascault G, Thomas D, et al. Patent foramen ovale and cerebral embolism. *Circulation* 1985;**72**(suppl 3):134.

191. Narayan D, Kaul S, Ravishankar K, et al. Risk factors, clinical profile, and long-term outcome of 428 patients of cerebral sinus venous thrombosis: Insights from Nizam's Institute Venous Stroke Registry, Hyderabad (India). *Neurol India* 2012;**60**:154–159.

192. Kaku DA, Lowenstein DH. Emergence of recreational drug abuse as a major risk factor for stroke in young adults. *Ann Intern Med* 1990;**113**:821–827.

193. Sloan MA, Kittner SJ, Feeser BR, et al. Illicit drug-associated ischemic stroke in the Baltimore–Washington Young Stroke Study. *Neurology* 1998;**49**:1688–1693.

194. Rutten-Jacobs LC, Maaijwee NA, Arntz RM, et al. Clinical characteristics and outcome of intracerebral hemorrhage in young adults. *J Neurol* 2014;**261**:2143–2149.

Spinal cord vascular disease

Louis R Caplan and Ayrton R Massaro

Stroke located in the spinal region represents a small fraction of all patients with central nervous system vascular disease but continues to present a challenge for diagnosis and treatment. The spinal cord and its vascular system are seldom examined in detail at necropsy. In London, Ontario, Canada, a systematic search for examples of hypoxic myelopathy uncovered 52 cases among 1200 consecutive necropsies (4%).[1,2] Recent advances in diagnostic imaging procedures allows greater accessibility to study the spinal cord and its vascular system during life and has improved the understanding of spinal cord vascular disease.

Unique clinical–anatomical correlations of the spinal cord

The unique anatomy of the spinal cord makes the clinician's approach to spinal lesions quite different from brain lesions. The spinal cord gray matter is located internally in an H-shaped structure, whereas the white matter tracts are located outside. The anterior two-thirds is related to motor and spinothalamic tracts, while the posterior third contains proprioceptive pathways.

Imaging the lesion with magnetic resonance imaging (MRI) or standard angiography requires localization to the craniospinal junction region, cervical cord, thoracic cord, lumbar cord, or *cauda equina*. Rostrocaudal localization depends on the level of findings affecting the long motor and sensory tracts and the presence of local segmental signs.[3] Root or dermatomal distribution of sensory, reflex, or lower motor neuron loss accurately identifies the rostrocaudal level of the process. Local bone tenderness and pain are also usually reliable in pointing to the segment involved. Lesions at different rostrocaudal levels have different likely etiologies.

Dura mater, arachnoid, and pia mater are the membranes that cover the spinal cord. Cerebrospinal fluid is found between the pia and arachnoid layers. The three depths of lesions with clinical importance are: (1) within the epidural space; (2) inside the dura, but outside the spinal cord (intradural extramedullary); and (3) intramedullary. Most epidural lesions reflect disease of the bony fortress and its connective tissue elements that surround the spinal cord. Lesions inside the dura but outside the spinal cord include most benign tumors, hematomas, and abscesses. Intramedullary lesions have a wide differential diagnosis that includes infarcts and hematomas.

Depth localization is more difficult. Epidural lesions usually involve the vertebral column, and bone and root pain usually precede symptoms related to dysfunction of the spinal cord. Intradural lesions cause root pain, but bony findings are absent clinically and by imaging. Intramedullary lesions are most often, but not always, painless. Asymmetric signs, sparing of distal sensory fibers, and dissociated sensory loss are other clues to an intramedullary localization.

Spinal cord vascular system

The spinal cord vascular system was not included in the general discussion of anatomy in Chapter 2. We find it easier to understand and visualize the system by first focusing on a spinal cord segment in axial section (Figure 16.1).

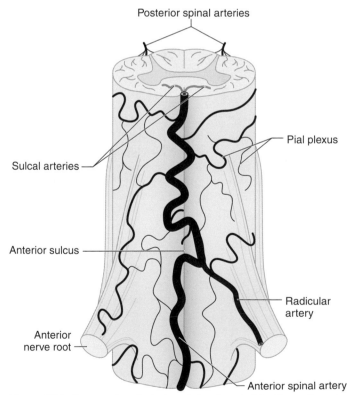

Figure 16.1 Cross-section of spinal cord, showing arterial patterns of supply: The anterior spinal artery is a single midline artery that courses in the anterior fissure. This artery divides into left and right sulcal arteries, which supply the anterior horns and white matter. There are usually two posterior spinal arteries, one on each side, which form an anastomotic rete from which branches emerge to supply the posterior gray horns and the posterior columns.

Spinal cord arterial circulation

A large, single, anterior spinal artery runs in the ventral midline from the rostral beginning of the spinal cord at the spinomedullary junction at the foramen magnum and extends caudally to the tip of the spinal cord, the *filum terminale*. In contrast, paired smaller posterior spinal arteries are located on the dorsal surface, which often form a plexus of small vessels.

The anterior spinal artery supplies the ventral surface of the medulla and also the spinal cord. Rostrally, the anterior spinal artery originates from the intracranial vertebral arteries at the level of the foramen magnum.[4] The anterior spinal supply comes from 5–10 usually single, unpaired radicular arteries, which feed into the anterior spinal artery at various levels (Figure 16.2). Branches from the thyrocervical and costocervical branches of the subclavian arteries and branches of the nuchal vertebral artery feed into the spinal cord at the cervical enlargement. One radicular artery arises from the vertebral arteries and supplies the spinal cord at C3 and another anterior radicular artery originates from ascending cervical arteries supplying the C6, C7 regions.

The thoracic portion of the anterior spinal artery is fed by radicular branches of the deep cervical and intercostal arteries and by branches of the aorta. Blood supply is most marginal in the upper thoracic region (T2–T4). The largest artery usually arises in the lower thoracic or upper lumbar segments, most often between T9 and T12, but can arise as low as L2. This artery is usually referred to as the *artery of Adamkiewicz* or *radiculomedullaris magna*. It usually comes from the left and supplies the lumbar enlargement of the cord. The anterior spinal artery is not continuous and in its midthoracic area there is a critical zone that has often been recognized as a *borderzone* or *watershed region* of the spinal cord.[5] The *conus medullaris* and *cauda equina* are nourished anteriorly from the hypogastric or obturator arteries.

There are differences in the perfusion of the gray and white matter in the spinal cord.[6] The anterior spinal artery gives off deep branches, which course along the ventral sulcus and then branch as they reach the central gray to supply left and right branches to the anterior horn regions on each side.[7,8] Lateral circumferential arteries and their penetrators course laterally from the midline anterior spinal artery to supply the ventral white matter, tips of the anterior horns, and pyramidal tracts.[7,8] This pattern is similar to that found in the brainstem, in which paramedian penetrators and short and long circumferential arteries branch from the vertebral and basilar arteries (see Figure 2.22B).

There are many more posterior radicular arteries that enter along nerve roots from each side at nearly every spinal level to supply the plexus of vessels that lie on the posterior cord surface.[7] Some additional segmental arteries arise from the vertebral, aorta, and iliac arteries to supply the paraspinous structures and then end on the anterior and posterior nerve roots without supplying the spinal cord or penetrating the dura mater. These vessels are often the origin of spinal arteriovenous malformations (AVMs).[9] The posterior spinal artery plexus also gives off penetrating branches to the posterior columns and posterior gray horns.[1,7,8]

The central area of the cord is a watershed region between the anterior and posterior spinal artery supply and it is susceptible for hemodynamic situations. The area between the two zones of supply in the central portion of the cord has often been called the *borderzone* or *watershed* region of supply.[10]

Spinal cord venous circulation

The venous spinal cord anatomy has also been well worked out and studied.[11] Venous drainage of the spinal cord is a complex network of venous structures compartmentalized to intrinsic, extrinsic, and extradural systems.[12] Radicular veins are plentiful and drain into the paravertebral and intravertebral plexus into the pelvic veins. Similar to the arterial supply, anterior and posterior venous drainage systems exist. The posterior portions of the cord drain into a large midline posterior vein. The anterior and posterior venous system forms an extensive network, virtually encircling the spinal cord. Drainage of blood from the spine occurs through the internal and external venous plexus, which is connected to the azygos and hemiazygos venous systems.[12] Venous spinal cord infarction is probably

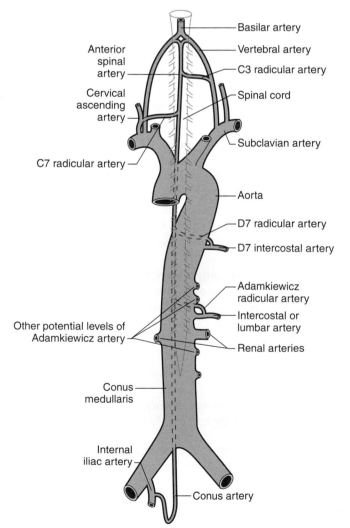

Figure 16.2 Aorta and its branches, showing important feeders at various levels: The cervical feeders come from the vertebral arteries. The others come from the aorta.

more common than venous brain infarcts. This kind of infarction is most often caused by mechanical compression, infection, and inflammation, which obliterate the veins, and to vascular malformations, which cause increased venous pressure. Venous hypertension is an important contributor to spinal cord infarction in patients with spinal dural fistulas.

Spinal cord ischemia and infarction

The history of the development of ideas about spinal cord infarction parallels the evolution of knowledge about the mechanism of brain infarcts. Most of the details of the vascular anatomy of the spinal cord were worked out by Düret, Adamkiewicz, and others in the late nineteenth century.[1,13] Early in the twentieth century, clinicians recognized that most spinal cord infarcts involved the anterior portion of the spinal cord. Clinicians attributed spinal cord infarcts to anterior spinal artery occlusion. The putative cause was intrinsic disease of this artery, especially due to syphilis, diabetes, or atherosclerosis. Recall that during this same era, intracranial anterior circulation infarcts were invariably diagnosed as middle cerebral artery occlusions. Later, it was shown that intracranial arteries were less often the seat of disease than extracranial arteries. Embolism was a more frequent explanation for intracranial arterial occlusion than in-situ atherothrombosis. Similarly, it has become clear that infarction in the distribution of the anterior spinal artery is most often caused by disease of the parent artery (usually the aorta), and less often to embolism. Intrinsic disease of intraspinal arteries is much less common.

Disease of the aorta is undoubtedly the most commonly recognized cause of spinal cord infarction. Interestingly two of the earliest reported examples of spinal cord infarction were related to aortic aneurysms.[14–16] Sir Astley Cooper in 1825 reported the case of a 38-year-old porter who acquired a very large traumatic aneurysm of his iliac artery that extended into the distal aorta.[14,15] Cooper ligated the aorta above the aneurysm and the patient developed urinary retention, fecal incontinence, and loss of sensation below the abdomen and soon died. Necropsy showed that a thrombus had extended above the ligature and blocked much of the distal aorta. Gull, a surgeon at Guy's Hospital in London in 1857 described a patient who developed loss of power and sensation in the lower extremities attributable to an aortic aneurysm.[14,16] When operations on the aorta became common during the last half of the twentieth century, spinal cord infarcts became well known as a complication of the surgery.[14] Surgeons recognized that operations on the aorta both above and below the renal arteries was sometimes associated with spinal paraplegia.[14,17,18]

Most often, paraplegia was recognized after repair of thoracic and abdominal aortic aneurysms.[8,13,19–21] Early reports described infarction after direct open aortic aneurysm surgery but this complication has also been noted after endovascular aortic aneurysm repair (EVAR).[22–25] During repair, flow through radicular supply arteries to the anterior spinal artery is compromised. Fragments of plaque and calcium and or cholesterol can break off and enter spinal cord supply vessels and grafts can partially or completely block the orifices of these branches. When the thoracic cord is involved, usually a flaccid paraplegia is noted directly after surgery, with incontinence and a thoracic sensory level. Later, the lower limbs become spastic. When the lumbar cord is involved, a conus medullaris infarct develops, with hypotonia; wasting and areflexia of the legs; loss of sphincter function; and variable loss of touch and pinprick sensation in the lower limbs, perineum, and lower abdomen.

Similar findings are noted in patients with unruptured aneurysms, dissections of the aorta, traumatic rupture of the aorta, thromboembolic aortic occlusions, and ulcerative aortic plaque disease. Thrombi and plaques can obstruct the orifices of radicular spinal arteries. Dissections can tear or interrupt the orifices of spinal cord feeding arteries, sometimes over a long area. Cholesterol crystals and other plaque materials can embolize into spinal arteries and block branches. In some patients, spinal ischemia develops gradually and insidiously. Spinal ischemia can be misdiagnosed as motor neuron disease or diabetic amyotrophy because of selective ischemia involving the anterior horns and, sometimes, the pyramidal tracts.[26]

In contrast to brain ischemic strokes, spinal transient ischemic attacks (TIAs) are quite unusual, but do occur.[21,27] Infarcts tend to occur in different patterns.[27,28] The regions of spinal cord softening can sometimes be imaged on newer-generation MRI scanners, especially when diffusion-weighted images are included.[27–29] In a French study of 28 consecutive patients with spinal cord infarcts 15 were thoracolumbar, 7 cervical, 3 thoracic, and 3 conus medullaris.[28] Infarcts can be classified as:[27]

1. Bilateral, predominatly anterior (Figure 16.3A): These patients have bilateral motor and spinothalamic type sensory deficits. Posterior column sensory functions (vibration and position sense) are spared.
2. Unilateral, predominantly anterior (Figure 16.3B): The motor deficit is a hemiparesis below the lesion and a contralateral spinothalamic tract sensory loss – Brown–Séquard syndrome.
3. Bilateral, predominantly posterior (Figure 16.3C): Posterior column type of sensory loss below the lesion with variably severe bilateral pyramidal tract signs.
4. Unilateral, mostly posterior (Figure 16.3D): Ipsilateral hemiparesis and posterior column sensory loss.
5. Central (Figure 16.3E): Bilateral pain and temperature loss with spared posterior column and motor functions. Similar to a syrinx.
6. Transverse: Loss of motor, sensory, and sphincter functions below the level of the lesion.

The anterior patterns of infarction and dysfunction are more common than posterior especially after aortic surgery. Transesophageal echocardiography may show aortic plaques in patients who present with acute paraplegia.[30] Other means of imaging the aorta, including MRI are being actively explored.[31,32] Imaging signs of vertebral bone infarction may accompany spinal cord infarction caused by aortic disease.[3,33,34]

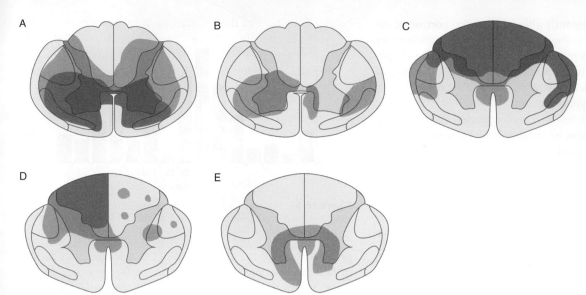

Figure 16.3 Drawings of patterns of spinal cord infarction. Dark gray indicates usual extent while light gray indicates potentially larger area of ischemia. A. Anterior bilateral infarction; B. anterior predominantly unilateral infarction; C. posterior bilateral infarction; D. posterior predominantly unilateral infarction; E. central spinal cord infarction. Based on Novy J, Carruzzo A, Maeder P, Bogousslavsky J. Spinal cord ischemia. Clinical and imaging patterns, pathogenesis, and outcomes in 27 patients. *Arch Neurol* 2006;63:1113–1120 with permission.

Embolism can and does cause spinal cord infarction. LRC has seen several patients with bacterial endocarditis with spinal and brain embolic infarcts, and such have been reported by others.[1,21] Atrial myxoma and non-bacterial thrombotic (marantic) endocarditis are other disorders in which small particles can embolize to the spinal cord.

Since the early 1980s, pathologists and clinicians have become aware that cartilaginous material from intervertebral disks can somehow invade the spinal arteries and veins and cause devastating spinal cord strokes.[3,35–38] Most reported cases are cervical and involve young women. Some patients have been pregnant, puerperal, or on oral contraceptives. Minor trauma, sudden neck motion, or lifting was often mentioned as an immediate precipitant. The first symptoms are usually pain in the neck or upper back, or radicular pain. Then, a rapidly progressive, sometimes asymmetric, spinal cord syndrome with quadriparesis develops. Syringomyelia-like dissociated sensory loss, with loss of pain and temperature (but preserved touch sensation), may be found in the upper limbs or cape region. We found no published reports of reversal of symptoms once paralysis developed. The same syndrome can affect the lumbar spinal cord and cause conus medullaris infarction.[3] MRI, contrast myelography and other studies usually fail to show herniated disks with compression of the cord or nerve roots. Infarction is usually bland, but can be hemorrhagic.[3] Undoubtedly, this syndrome occurs more often than is now diagnosed.

Back or neck pain, often with radicular distribution paresthesias may be noted minutes before signs of spinal cord dysfunction develop. Among 27 spinal cord infarct patients in one series, 16 (59%) had such an onset.[18] The level of spinal cord ischemia was at the level of the pain and paresthesia in these patients. In 13 of these patients, ischemic symptoms developed immediately after a movement of the back, or arm, or after beginning to walk.[27] The spinal infarcts were either anterior or posterior and not central, and were predominantly at the level of acute and chronic vertebral and disk disease. Mechanical stress is posited to impinge on a spinal radicular artery causing localized spinal cord ischemia, although some cases are likely related to cartilaginous disk emboli.

Infarction and inflammation of the meningeal coverings of the spinal cord can spread to the spinal arteries, causing acute spinal cord strokes. The phenomenon is similar to Heubner's arteritis found in the brain in the presence of tuberculosis and syphilis. These two disorders, as well as fungal infections, schistosomiasis, and Lyme borreliosis, probably account for the vast majority of infectious spinal arteritis. Almost invariably, the spinal fluid provides the clue to this problem.

Chronic adhesive arachnoiditis from any cause can also lead to scarring and obliteration of spinal penetrating arteries and ischemic necrosis of the central portion of the spinal cord.[39] The clinical findings are similar to syringomyelia, except that any level of the spinal cord can be involved. Arachnoidal scarring can be caused by trauma, hemorrhage, or infection. The signs and symptoms develop gradually, sometimes years after the spinal injury, bleed, or meningitis.[39] Schistosomiasis especially mansoni is well known to effect the spinal cord.[40–42] This parasite reaches the spinal cord through the blood vessel supply and can cause spinal cord infarction or granulomatous inflammation, most often involving the conus medullaris and the cauda equina. MRI often shows expansion of the thoracic spinal cord with intramedullary regions of nodular enhancement after gadolinium.[42] Spinal cord infarcts are occasionally explained by varicella-zoster virus infection.[43] Rare patients with central nervous system vasculitis develop spinal cord as well as brain infarcts.[44]

Spinal cord ischemia may also develop during severe hypotension, clinical shock and cardiac arrest.[14,21,45–47] Damage is most likely to affect the thoracic spinal cord between the T4 and T8 segments, the most vulnerable region of the spinal

cord.[21] Infarcts predominantly affect the central portion of the cord.[27] Nearly always, spinal cord signs and symptoms are overshadowed by brain hypoxic–ischemic injury. The deeply comatose patient remains hypotonic and areflexic because of accompanying spinal ischemia. A pure spinal syndrome rarely complicates systemic hypoperfusion.

Spinal cord ischemia has also been reported after injection of heroin[48] and inhalation of cocaine.[49] In the case of heroin myelopathy, the spinal cord signs are usually noted after the patient awakens from a stupor. Most often the myelopathy develops when heroin is reintroduced after a period of abstinence. The mechanism of cord damage after drug abuse is most likely prolonged vasoconstriction.

Venous infarction is an important cause of cord ischemia. The infarcts may remain bland[50] or become frankly hemorrhagic.[3,51] Venous infarcts can be attributed to one of three different mechanisms – spinal dural AVMs,[3,9,50–55] coagulopathies with venous thrombosis, or mechanical compression of veins by epidural mass lesions or herniated discs.[50,56] Some patients with acute disk herniations develop the acute onset of severe spinal cord dysfunction and MRI shows a spinal cord lesion at the site of disk herniation. These patients may not show good improvement after decompressive surgery. The spinal cord lesion in these patients is most likely an infarct caused by disk compression of the veins along the surface of the spinal cord.

Spinal vascular malformations

Contrary to the situation within the cranium, spinal vascular malformations often present with ischemia rather than hemorrhage, and some malformations cause bleeding and ischemia. Because of their distinctive characteristics and the fact that many neurologists and stroke experts are inexperienced with the usual findings and diagnosis in such cases, we believe it best to consider spinal vascular malformations separately rather than in relation to the topics of ischemia or hemorrhage.

Spinal malformations should be divided into two large groups, which have differing blood supplies, presentations, and clinical findings (the dural (type l) and intradural (type II) groups).[9,57,58] So-called type I malformations, often referred to as dural, derive their blood supply from arteries located in the dural sleeves of spinal roots.[9,53] The small nidus of arteriovenous communication is fed by dural branches of a radicular artery. These arteriovenous fistulas drain intradurally by one or more arterialized, enlarged, usually tortuous veins, which course on the dorsal surface of the spinal cord, usually above, but occasionally below, the feeding arteries. The dural feeding arteries do not participate in the blood supply of the spinal cord. Spinal dural fistulas occur predominantly in men (4 to 1 ratio) between 40 and 70 years of age – most often in the mid 50s, and involve mostly the lower thoracic and lumbosacral segments.

In one series, 26 of 27 type I malformations were fed by arteries in the thoracic or lumbar regions, and the remaining one malformation was sacral.[58] In another series of 13 dural fistulas, eight were located between T8 and T12, two were at S1, and one each was at L1 and L5.[53] Among 80 patients in a recent Dutch series 49 of 80 were between T5 and T8. Figure 16.4 is a

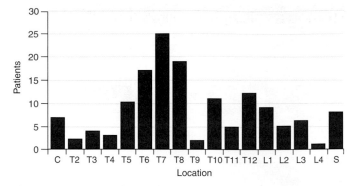

Figure 16.4 Location of spinal dural arteriovenous fistulas among 146 patients. C,cranial; L, lumbar; S, sacral; T, thoracic.

graph that shows the distribution of 146 arteriovenous fistulas in two large series.[45,46] Most often, one feeder exists, but, at times, two or three arterial feeders have been found.[7] Among a series of 27 such lesions, 24 had one feeder and three had two feeders.[58] Usually, this type of AVM is referred to as low flow because angiography results only in slow, low volume filling of the lesions. These lesions are not associated with arterial or venous aneurysms.[9,53] Cutaneous angiomas are not seen, and bruits are not audible.

The most frequent presentation of spinal dural fistulas is that of progressive neurological worsening, often with acute deteriorations.[53] Among a series of 80 patients with documented spinal dural fistulas, 63% had a gradually progressive course.[59] In 21 patients there were episodes of acute transient deterioration superimposed on the gradually progressive loss of function.[59] Five patients had a stepwise deterioration.

These fistulas usually do not cause subarachnoid bleeding, except when the lesions are cervical.[55,60] The cervical fistulas that cause subarachnoid hemorrhage (SAH) are fed by the vertebral artery and are often located near the cervico-medullary junction. Thoracic, lumbar, and sacral fistulas rarely, if ever, present with SAH, but epidural hemorrhage occasionally develops. Pain is present in approximately 40% of patients. Pain can be radicular, sometimes mimicking sciatic pain. Symptoms often worsen after exercise. The most frequent symptoms involve gait, sensory abnormalities in the lower extremities and/or perineum, and lower extremity weakness. Most patients by the time a diagnosis is made have important symptoms and signs that indicate dysfunction of sacral cord segments – loss of sensation in the perineum, and abnormalities of micturition, defecation, and sexual function.[59,61]

Spinal TIAs do occur and are more frequent in patients with spinal dural fistulas than other spinal vascular lesions. One of LRC's patients had two episodes of leg paralysis and numbness that occurred while she was driving a car.[62] Her husband had to grab the wheel and foot controls to avert a crash. Soon, strength and feeling returned. Another patient had a Brown–Séquard distribution attack while in hospital that lasted several hours.[62] Exercise and physical activity worsened symptoms in 19 of 27 patients (70%) in the National Institutes of Health series,[58] and in another large series of patients.[59] Signs usually progress if the lesion is untreated, and most patients become unable to walk within 5 years of

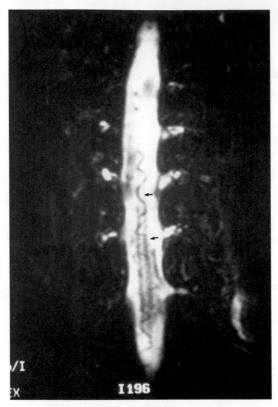

Figure 16.5 Coronal heavily T2-weighted MRI scan of the thoracolumbar spine showing serpiginous vessels (arrows) along the dorsal surface of the spinal cord. From Kleefield J. Magnetic resonance and radiological imaging in the evaluation of back pain. In Aronoff GM (ed), *Evaluation and Treatment of Chronic Pain*, 3rd ed. Baltimore: Williams & Wilkins, 1998, pp 477–504 with permission.

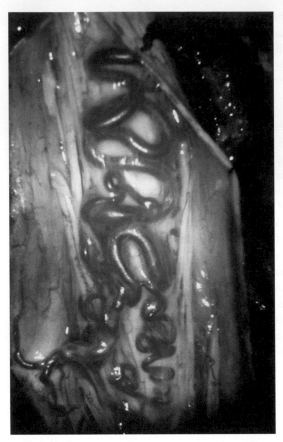

Figure 16.6 Intraoperative view of the surface of the spinal cord after the dura has been opened. Tortuous dilated veins can be seen along the surface of the cord. Kindly submitted by Dr Roberto Heros, University of Miami, FL.

the onset of weakness. These lesions probably cause symptoms because of venous hypertension and occasional thrombosis of the venous drainage system.[9,52–54]

Type I dural lesions are often not well seen in early generation MRI scanning, but newer generation scanners now often do show abnormalities. Diffusion-weighted imaging (DWI) often shows spinal cord infarction and increased T2 signal and spinal cord edema are common.[63–66] The key finding that suggests the possibility of a fistula are serpiginous dilated veins on the surface of the spinal cord. These are often now seen on T2-weighted and gadolinium-enhanced images and on contrast-enhanced MR angiography (MRA).[65–69] Figure 16.5 is an MRI scan that shows these veins. Using MRA techniques, phase display after contrast injection can show the direction of flow within the epidural veins to indicate the likely location of arterial feeders.[66] These coiled, enlarged serpiginous veins are usually visible along the dorsal cord surface during myelography which still has a place in diagnosis.[57,58,63,64] Figure 16.6 is an intraoperative photo that shows these enlarged veins on the surface of the spinal cord. Myelographic films should be taken with the patients lying supine on their backs to show the abnormal veins.

MRA[65–69] and CT angiography (CTA)[69] sometimes shows the supply arteries. Selective spinal angiography in expert, experienced hands often shows the feeding arteries, but occasionally the feeding arteries cannot be opacified. LRC urges

surgical exploration when the clinical findings are typical and abnormal veins are clearly present on myelography or MRA examinations. Ligation of arterial feeders usually prevents worsening, so the venous structures need not be removed.[9] In most patients in whom the fistula has been treated effectively, muscle strength and gait improve although sacral spinal cord dysfunction (urination, defecation, sexual function) often remain unchanged.[70]

Some dural fistulas are located in the spine or paravertebral region, but drain into epidural veins and often into the intradural venous system.[71] The enlarged epidural veins can cause a compressive myelopathy. The venous hypertension that results from these paravertebral fistulas can cause venous hypertension and a congestive myelopathy in the same way as dural AVMs.[71] MRI may show hyperintensity on T2-weighted sequences, spinal cord edema, and prominent perimedullary vessels. Dilatated tortuous epidural veins are often visible on MR sequences and angiography.[71]

The remainder of spinal AVMs are intradural. Type II malformations are usually intramedullary, but can be partially intramedullary, and partially between the dura and the cord. Intradural malformations are divided into various types: (1) glomus, referring to a tightly packed localized nidus of abnormal vessels within the cord; (2) juvenile, in which abnormal vessels occupy the entire spinal cord and are fed by numerous arterial feeding vessels at different levels; (3) direct

arteriovenous fistulas, involving branches of arteries feeding the spinal cord; and (4) cavernous angiomas, which have no major feeding arteries and resemble cavernous angiomas of the brain. Increased availability of MRI leads frequently to identification of spinal cavernous malformations.[9]

Usually, patients with intradural lesions are younger than those with dural lesions, but again, most patients are men. In one series, 65% of patients were younger than 25 years at first presentation.[58] These lesions have high flow, and hemorrhage is relatively common.[9,58] Intradural lesions are more widely distributed along the spinal axis and are often cervical. Spinal aneurysms, extraspinal aneurysms, other AVMs, and arterial bruits are common in patients with intradural AVMs. Most lesions are intramedullary (80% in the National Institutes of Health series)[57] and symptoms and signs are progressive.

Intradural AVMs are usually well-imaged and diagnosed by MRI. Glomus and juvenile lesions and cavernous angiomas have a nidus in the spinal cord parenchyma. The spinal cord is usually enlarged, and multiple serpiginous signal voids are seen.[64] Increased signal on T1-weighted images may represent methemoglobin from a prior hemorrhage. Low, dark signals on T1- and T2-weighted images can represent hemosiderin.[64] Spinal angiography usually readily shows intradural AVMs. Surgical treatment is not as successful for intradural AVMs as for dural ones, but glomus lesions and cavernous angiomas can be removed.

Cavernous angiomas are shown well by MRI.[72–76] Spinal cavernous angiomas usually present during the second to sixth decades and are slightly more common in women.[74] Symptoms can begin abruptly or progress gradually.[74,75] Symptoms may worsen with pregnancy, in the puerperium, and after trauma. As in the cranium, these lesions are angiographically occult. Appearance on MRI is similar to that of brain angiomas – heterogeneous, well-circumscribed, discrete lesions. Cavernous angiomas are well circumscribed and can be removed surgically.[60] When removed surgically, cavernomas appear as well-circumscribed, dark blue-brown, intramedullary, mulberry-shaped lesions that are surrounded by gliosis and hemosiderin staining.[75] In one of the largest series (53 patients: 26 men; 27 women) had a mean age at onset of symptoms at age 40 years (11–80 years).[76] Symptoms were progressive in 32 patients and 20 presented initially as an acute onset myelopathy. Clinical symptoms were caused by spinal cord compression (27) and hemorrhage (22). The lesions were thoracic in 41 patients and cervical in 12. The mean size of the cavernomas was 16.3 mm (3–54 mm). In the 40 surgical patients, long-term follow-up was available in 37 cases for a mean time of 7.3 years (0.4–50.0 years). During the follow-up period, 20 patients improved, 6 remained the same, and 11 worsened. Surgical improvement was more often found in posterior rather than anterior location.[76]

Intradural AVMs can cause chronic arachnoiditis due to bleeding, with subsequent scarring of small cord-feeding arteries and cord ischemia. Veins can thrombose. The so-called Foix–Alajouanine syndrome,[77] a subacute necrotizing ascending myelopathy, probably was, in retrospect, caused by such thrombosed vascular malformations of the dural or intradural variety.[78]

Spinal hemorrhages

Hematomyelia describes bleeding into the substance of the spinal cord parenchyma. The most common cause is trauma. Onset can be immediate or delayed. Usually, the area around the central canal and gray matter are involved, most often in the cervical region. Neck pain, weakness, and areflexia in the arms, associated with a cape-like distribution of pain and temperature loss, are the usual signs. Other causes include AVMs, anticoagulation, hemophilia and other bleeding disorders, and hemorrhage into spinal cord tumors, as well as (rarely) syrinxes. The spinal fluid is bloody, and MRI and myelography reveal a swollen blood-filled cord.

Spinal SAH is unusual. Unlike intracranial SAH, the most common causative lesions are AVMs. Aneurysms on spinal arteries rarely rupture.[79] Localized back pain is often followed by a stiff neck and pain that radiates along a root distribution or down the back or legs. Often, headache ensues, caused by spillage of blood intracranially. Bleeding diatheses and anticoagulants may cause spinal SAH.

Spinal epidural and subdural hematomas are rarer than intracranial hemorrhages in these compartments. Epidural spinal hematomas are approximately four times more common than subdural hematomas. Each most often occurs in patients who are on anticoagulants.[80–85] Some patients have had liver disease and portal hypertension.[80] Lumbar punctures have been known to precipitate these bleeds in patients on anticoagulants. At times, these hemorrhages begin after exertion or straining, and, in some patients, no cause is found, even after full evaluation. Degenerative disk disease could rarely be an etiological factor.[83] The earliest symptom is pain in the back, usually in the neck. This is followed by radicular pain, usually in one or both arms. The earliest symptoms closely mimic disk herniation syndromes. Within hours, or rarely, days, sensory and motor signs develop in the legs, bowel, and bladder, and sexual dysfunction ensues. Usually, weakness and sensory loss are symmetric, but a Brown–Séquard distribution may be found.[80,69]

The diagnosis of spinal epidural or subdural hematoma has in the past usually been made by myelography. A block is most likely found. Computed tomography and MRI show the blood. MRI is superior in defining the location and extent of hematomas. Sagittal T1- and T2-weighted images are usually reliable for diagnosis but hemorrhages and abscesses are difficult to reliably separate by imaging alone. Signs are almost invariably progressive, unless the lesions are decompressed. Anticoagulation should be reversed, using vitamin K, fresh frozen plasma, or prothrombin complex concentrates particularly those enriched with factor VII, factor X, and prothrombin. Decompression is urgent and should be pursued as soon as feasible considering the international normalized ratio (INR). Outcome depends on the severity of the deficit before surgery, the duration of spinal cord compression, and the rapidity of onset of the paraplegia. Chronic spinal subdural hematomas or hygromas are rare and are usually related to prior trauma or small bleeds.[86]

References

1. Buchan AM, Barnett HJM. Infarction of the spinal cord. In Barnett HJM, Mohr JP, Stern B, Yatsu F (eds): *Stroke: Pathophysiology, Diagnosis and Management.* New York: Churchill Livingstone, 1986, pp 707–719.

2. Vinters HV, Gilbert JJ. Hypoxic myelopathy. *Can J Neurol Sci* 1979;6:380.

3. Caplan LR. Case records of the Massachusetts General Hospital: Case 5–1991. *N Engl J Med* 1991;324:322–332.

4. Lazorthes G, Pulhes J Bastide G, Chanchole AR, Zadeh O. Spinal cord vascularization: anatomical and physiological study. *Rev Neurol* 1962;106:535–557.

5. Lazorthes G, Gouaze A, Zadeh O. Arterial vascularization of the spinal cord: Recent studies of the arterial substitution pathways. *J Neurosurg* 1971;35:253–262.

6. Sandler AN, Tator CH. Regional spinal blood flow in primates. *J Neurosurg* 1976;45:647–659.

7. Gillilan L. The arterial blood supply of the human spinal cord. *J Comp Neurol* 1958;110:75–103.

8. Mawad ME, Rivera V, Crawford S, et al. Spinal cord ischemia after resection of thoracoabdominal aortic aneurysms: MR findings in 24 patients. *AJNR Am J Neuroradiol* 1990;11:987–991.

9. Heros R. Arteriovenous malformations of the spinal cord. In Ojemann RG, Heros RC, Crowell RM (eds): *Surgical Management of Cerebrovascular Disease,* 2nd ed. Baltimore: Williams & Wilkins, 1988, pp 451–466.

10. Ishizawa K, Komori T, Shimada T, et al. Hemodynamic infarction of the spinal cord: involvement of the gray matter plus the border-zone between the central and peripheral arteries. *Spinal Cord* 2005;43:306–310.

11. Gillilan L. Veins of the spinal cord. Anatomic details – suggested clinical applications. *Neurology* 1970;20:860–868.

12. Griessenauer CJ, Raborn J, Foreman P, Shoja MM, Loukas M, Tubbs RS. Venous drainage of the spine and spinal cord: a comprehensive review of its history, embryology, anatomy, physiology, and pathology. *Clin Anat* 2015;28:75–87.

13. Hogan EL, Romanul FCA. Spinal cord infarction occurring during insertion of aortic graft. *Neurology* 1966;16:67–74.

14. Silver JR. History of infarction of the spinal cord. *J Hist Neurosci* 2003;12:144–153.

15. Cooper A. *The Lectures of Sir Astley Cooper on the Principles and Practices of Surgery.* London: Thomas and George Underwood, Vol II, 1825, pp 69–72.

16. Gull W. Paraplegia from obstruction of the abdominal aorta. In Wilks S, Poland A (eds): *Guy's Hospital Reports.* London: John Churchill, (3rd series) Vol III.

17. DeBakey ME, Simeone FA. Battle injuries of the arteries in World War II. *Ann Surg* 1946;123:534–536.

18. Picone AL, Green RM, Ricotta JR, May SG, DeWeese JA. Spinal cord ischemia following operations on the abdominal aorta. *J Vasc Surg* 1986;3:94–103.

19. Dodson WE, Landau W. Motor neuron loss due to aortic clamping in repair of coarctation. *Neurology* 1973;23:539–542.

20. Ross RT. Spinal cord infarction in diseases and surgery of the aorta. *Can J Neurol Sci* 1985;12:289–295.

21. Cheshire WP, Santos CC, Massey EW, Howard JF Jr. Spinal cord infarction: etiology and outcome. *Neurology* 1996;47:321–330.

22. Rockman CB, Riles TS, Landis R. Lower extremity paraparesis or paraplegia subsequent to endovascular management of abdominal aortic aneurysms. *J Vasc Surg* 2001;33:178–180.

23. Fortes DL, Atkins BZ, Chiou AC. Delayed paraplegia following infrarenal abdominal aortic endograft placement: case report and literature review. *Vascular* 2004;12:130–135.

24. Acher C, Wynn M. Paraplegia after thoracoabdominal aortic surgery: not just assisted circulation, hypothermic arrest, clamp and sew or TEVAR. *Ann Cardiothorac Surg* 2012;1:365–372.

25. Freyrie A, Testi G, Gargiulo M, Faggioli G, Mauro R, Stella A. Spinal cord ischemia after endovascular treatment of infrarenal aortic aneurysm. Case report and literature review. *J Cardiovasc Surg (Torino)* 2011;52:731–734.

26. Herrick MK, Mills PE. Infarction of spinal cord: Two cases of selective grey matter involvement secondary to asymptomatic aortic disease. *Arch Neurol* 1971;24:228–241.

27. Novy J, Carruzzo A, Maeder P, Bogousslavsky J. Spinal cord ischemia. Clinical and imaging patterns, pathogenesis, and outcomes in 27 patients. *Arch Neurol* 2006;63:1113–1120.

28. Masson C, Pruvo JP, Meder JF, et al. Study Group on Spinal Cord Infarction of the French Neurovascular Society. Spinal cord infarction: Clinical and magnetic resonance imaging and short term outcome. *J Neurol Neurosurg Psychiatry* 2004;75:1431–1435.

29. Shinoyama M, Takahashi T, Shimizu H, Tominaga T, Suzuki M. Spinal cord infarction demonstrated by diffusion-weighted magnetic resonance imaging. *J Clin Neurosci* 2005;12:466–468.

30. Walsh DV, Uppal JA, Karalis DG, Chandrasekaran K. The role of transesophageal echocardiography in the acute onset of paraplegia. *Stroke* 1992;23:1660–1661.

31. Caplan LR. The aorta as a donor source of brain embolism. In Caplan LR, Manning WJ, *Brain Embolism.* New York: Informa Healthcare, 2006, pp 187–201.

32. Amarenco P. Cohen A. Update on imaging aortic atherosclerosis. In Barnett HJM, Bogousslavsky J, Meldrum H (eds) *Ischemic Stroke: Advances in Neurology,* vol 92. Philadelphia: Lippincott, Williams & Wilkins, 2003, pp 75–89.

33. Yuh WT, Marsh EE III, Wang AK, et al. Imaging of spinal cord and vertebral body infarction. *AJNR Am J Neuroradiol* 1992;13:145–154.

34. Faig J, Busse O, Selbeck R. Vertebral body infarction as a confirmatory sign of spinal cord ischemic stroke: report of three cases and review of the literature. *Stroke* 1998;29:239–243.

35. Srigley JR, Lambert CD, Bilbao JM, Pritzker KP. Spinal cord infarction secondary to intervertebral disc embolism. *Ann Neurol* 1981;9:296–301.

36. Raghavan A, Onikul E, Ryan MM, et al. Anterior spinal cord infarction owing to possible fibrocartilaginous embolism. *Pediatr Radiol* 2004;34:503–506.

37. Duprez TP, Danvoye L, Hernalsteen D, Cosnard G, Sindic CJ, Godfraind C. Fibrocartilaginous embolization to the spinal cord: serial MR imaging

monitoring and pathologic study. *AJNR Am J Neuroradiol* 2005;**26**:496–501.

38. Piao YS, Lu DH, Su YY, Yang XP. Anterior spinal cord infarction caused by fibrocartilaginous embolism. *Neuropathol* 2009;**29**:172–175.

39. Caplan LR, Noronha A, Amico L. Syringomyelia and arachnoiditis. *J Neurol Neurosurg Psychiatry* 1990;**53**:106–113.

40. Haribhai HC, Bhigjee AI, Bill PL, et al. Spinal cord schistosomiasis. A clinical, laboratory and radiological study, with a note on therapeutic aspects. *Brain* 1991;**114**:709–726.

41. Saleem S, Belal AI, el-Ghandour NM. Spinal cord schistosomiasis: MR imaging appearance with surgical and pathologic correlation. *AJNR Am J Neuroradiol* 2005;**26**:1646–1654.

42. Van Leusen H, Perquin WV. Spinal cord schistosomiasis. *J Neurol Neurosurg Psychiatry* 2000;**69**:690–691.

43. Orme HT, Smith AG, Nagel MA, et al. Varicella zoster virus spinal cord infarction identified by diffusion-weighted MRI (DWI). *Neurology* 2007;**69**:398–400.

44. Salvarini C, Brown RD Jr, Calamia KT, et al. Primary CNS vasculitis with spinal cord involvement. *Neurology* 2008;**70**:2394–2400.

45. Silver JR, Buxton PH. Spinal stroke. *Brain* 1974;**97**:539–550.

46. Satran R. Spinal cord infarction. Current concepts of cerebrovascular disease. *Stroke* 1987;**22**:13–17.

47. Singh U, Diplomate NB, Silver JR, Weply NC. Hypotensive infarction of the spinal cord. *Paraplegia* 1994;**32**:314–322.

48. Brust JCM. Stroke and substance abuse. In Caplan LR (ed): *Uncommon Causes of Stroke*, 2nd ed. Cambridge: Cambridge University Press, 2008, pp 365–370.

49. Schreiber AL, Formal CS. Spinal cord infarction secondary to cocaine use. *Am J Phy Med Rehab* 2007;**66**:158–160.

50. Kim RC, Smith HR, Henbest ML, Choi BH. Nonhemorrhagic venous infarction of the spinal cord. *Ann Neurol* 1984;**15**:379–385.

51. Hughes JT. Venous infarction of the spinal cord. *Neurology* 1971;**21**:794–800.

52. Larsson EM, Desai P, Hardin CW, et al. Venous infarction of the spinal cord resulting from dural arteriovenous

fistula: MR imaging findings. *AJNR Am J Neuroradiol* 1991;**12**:739–743.

53. Bradac GB, Daniele D, Riva A, et al. Spinal dural arteriovenous fistulas: An underestimated cause of myelopathy. *Eur Neurol* 1993;**34**:87–94.

54. Hurst RW, Kenyon LC, Lavi E, Raps EC, Marcotte P. Spinal dural arteriovenous fistula: The pathology of venous hypertensive myelopathy. *Neurology* 1995;**45**:1309–1313.

55. Hemphill JC III, Smith WS, Halbach VV. Neurologic manifestations of spinal epidural arteriovenous malformations. *Neurology* 1998;**50**:817–819.

56. Roa KR, Donnenfeld H, Chusid JG, Valdez S. Acute myelopathy secondary to spinal venous thrombosis. *J Neurol Sci* 1982;**56**:107–113.

57. DeChiro G, Doppman JL, Ommaya AK. Radiology of spinal cord arteriovenous malformations. *Prog Neurol Surg* 1971;**4**:329–354.

58. Rosenblum B, Oldfield EH, Doppman JL, DiChiro G. Spinal arteriovenous malformations: a comparison of dural arteriovenous fistulas and intradural AVMs in 81 patients. *J Neurosurg* 1987;**67**:795–802.

59. Jellema K, Canta LR, Tijssen CC, et al. Spinal dural arteriovenous fistulas: Clinical features in 80 patients. *J Neurol Neurosurg Psychiatry* 2003;**74**:1438–1440.

60. Do HM, Jensen ME, Cloft HJ, et al. Dural arteriovenous fistula of the cervical spine presenting with subarachnoid hemorrhage. *AJNR Am J Neuroradiol* 1999;**20**:348–350.

61. Strom RG, Derdeyn CP, Moran CJ, et al. Frequency of spinal arteriovenous malformations in patients with unexplained myelopathy. *Neurology* 2006;**66**:928–931.

62. Teal PA, Wityk RJ, Rosengart A, Caplan LR. Spinal TIAs – a clue to the presence of spinal dural AVMs. *Neurology* 1992;**42**(Suppl 3):341.

63. Gilbertson JR, Miller GM, Goldman MS, Marsh WR. Spinal dural arteriovenous fistulas: MR and myelographic findings. *AJNR Am J Neuroradiol* 1995;**16**:2049–2057.

64. Greenberg J. Neuroimaging of the spinal cord. *Neurol Clin* 1991;**9**:696–698.

65. Bowen BC, Fraser K, Kochan JP, et al. Spinal dural arteriovenous fistulas: Evaluation with MR angiography.

AJNR Am J Neuroradiol 1995;**16**:2029–2043.

66. Mascalchi M, Quillici N, Ferrito G, et al. Identification of the feeding arteries of spinal vascular lesions via phase-contrast MR angiography with three-dimensional acquisition and phase display. *AJNR Am J Neuroradiol* 1997;**18**:351–358.

67. Saraf-Lavi E, Bowen BC, Quencer RM, et al. Detection of spinal dural arteriovenous fistulae with MR imaging and contrast-enhanced MR angiography: Sensitivity, specificity, and prediction of vertebral level. *AJNR Am J Neuroradiol* 2002;**23**:858–867.

68. Luetmer PH, Lane JI, Gilbertson JR, Bernstein MA, Huston J, Atkinson JL. Preangiographic evaluation of spinal dural arteriovenous fistulas with elliptic centric contrast-enhanced MR angiography and effect on radiation dose and volume of iodinated contrast material. *AJNR Am J Neuroradiol* 2005;**26**:711–718.

69. Zampakis P, Santosh C, Taylor W, Teasdale E. The role of non-invasive computed tomography in patients with suspected dural fistulas with spinal drainage. *Neurosurgery* 2006;**58**:686–694.

70. Jellema K, Tijssen CC, van Rooiji WJJ, et al. Spinal dural arteriovenous fistulas. Long term follow-up of 44 treated patients. *Neurology* 2004;**62**:1839–1841.

71. Goyal M, Willinsky R, Montanera W, terBrugge K. Paravertebral arteriovenous malformations with epidural drainage: Clinical spectrum, imaging features, and results of treatment. *AJNR Am J Neuroradiol* 1999;**20**:749–755.

72. Lopate G, Black JT, Grubb RL. Cavernous hemangioma of the spinal cord: report of two unusual cases. *Neurology* 1990;**40**:1791–1793.

73. Cosgrove GR, Bertrand G, Fontaine S, et al. Cavernous angiomas of the spinal cord. *J Neurosurg* 1988;**68**:31–36.

74. McCormick PC, Michelson WJ, Post KD, et al. Cavernous malformations of the spinal cord. *Neurosurgery* 1988;**23**:459–463.

75. Ogilvy CS, Louis DN, Ojemann RG. Intramedullary cavernous angiomas of the spinal cord: Clinical presentation, pathological features, and surgical management. *Neurosurgery* 1992;**31**:219–230.

76. Labauge P, Bouly S, Parker F, et al. on behalf of the French Study Group of Spinal Cord Cavernomas. Outcome in

53 patients with spinal cord cavernomas. *Surg Neurol* 2008;**70**:176–181.

77. Foix C, Alajouanine T. La myelite necrotique subaique. *Rev Neurol* 1926;**2**:1–42.

78. Criscuolo GR, Oldfield EH, Doppman JL. Reversible acute and subacute myelopathy in patients with dural arteriovenous fistulas. *J Neurosurgery* 1989;**70**:354–359.

79. Garcia C, Dulcey S, Dulcey J. Ruptured aneurysm of the spinal artery of Adamkiewicz during pregnancy. *Neurology* 1979;**29**:394–398.

80. Mattle H, Sieb JP, Rohner M, Mumenthaler M. Nontraumatic spinal epidural and subdural hematomas. *Neurology* 1987;**37**:1351–1356.

81. Post MJD, Becerra JL, Madsen PW, et al. Acute spinal subdural hematoma: MR and CT findings with pathological correlates. *AJNR Am J Neuroradiol* 1994;**15**:1895–1905.

82. Morandi X, Riffaud L, Chabert E, Brassier G. Acute nontraumatic spinal subdural hematomas in three patients. *Spine* 2001;**26**:e547–551.

83. Cha YH, Chi JH, Barbaro NM. Spontaneous spinal subdural hematoma associated with low-molecular-weight heparin. Case report. *Neurosurg Spine* 2005;**2**:612–613.

84. Gundry CR, Heithoff KB. Epidural hematoma of the lumbar spine: 18 surgically confirmed cases. *Radiology* 1993;**187**:427–431.

85. Russman BS, Kazi K. Spinal epidural hematoma and the Brown–Séquard syndrome. *Neurology* 1971;**21**:1066–1068.

86. Black P, Zervas N, Caplan LR, Ramirez L. Subdural hygroma of the spinal meninges: A case report. *Neurosurgery* 1978;**2**:52–54.

Cerebral venous thrombosis

Louis R Caplan and Marie-Germaine Bousser

Most strokes are caused by occlusion or rupture of brain-supplying arteries. However, brain infarcts, edema, and hemorrhages are sometimes caused by cerebral venous thrombosis (CVT), defined by thrombosis of dural sinuses and cerebral and cerebellar veins. Since the advent of magnetic resonance imaging (MRI), magnetic resonance angiography (MRA), and computed tomography angiography (CTA), the diagnosis of CVT is made much more often than in the past. The anatomy of the venous system is discussed in Chapter 2.

Development of ideas

Occlusions of the veins that drain the brain were first reported in the 1820s. In 1825, Ribes described the first case of dural sinus thrombosis.[1–3] Ribes's patient was a 45-year-old man who developed epilepsy, severe headaches, and delirium. The delirium improved within a month, but headaches persisted and seizures increased in frequency. He died 6 months later. At necropsy, the superior sagittal and left lateral sinuses were thrombosed. The brain was swollen, softened and full of blood. Carcinomatous metastases were present in the brain. Three years later, John Abercrombie described the first case of puerperal dural sinus thrombosis.[4] A 24-year-old woman developed a severe headache after the delivery of her second child. Later, a sense of uneasiness in her head and numb feelings in her occiput and neck were followed by sudden weakness and numbness of her right hand, loss of speech, and twisting of her mouth. Frequent seizures were followed by coma and death. At necropsy, the sagittal sinus was occluded and the draining veins were distended and turgid. The brain showed softening and hemorrhage.[4]

Tonnelle[5] published a review of thrombosis of the dural sinuses in 1829, and Cruveilhier[6] included a chapter on inflammation of the dural sinuses in his popular pathological anatomy atlas. These authors noted that dural sinus thrombosis was common in children, especially those with fever and infections. Tonnelle and Cruveilhier noted that dural sinus thrombosis also tended to develop during the puerperium and in older, ill individuals, so-called "senile cases."[5,6] At the end of the nineteenth century, Quinke, the clinician usually given credit for originating lumbar puncture, described patients who had headache, visual symptoms, papilledema, and evidence of raised intracranial pressure who often recovered and did not have brain tumors.[7,8] At necropsy, one of Quinke's

patients had occlusion of both transverse sinuses and the vein of Galen.

Sir Charles Symonds related the phenomena of benign intracranial hypertension to dural sinus occlusion and, in a series of key papers that spanned a quarter of a century, described the phenomenology of so-called *otitic hydrocephalus* and its relation to lateral sinus thrombosis and disease of the ears and mastoid air cells.[9–12]

In 1967, Kalbag, a neurosurgeon, and Woolf, a neuropathologist, wrote a monograph on the topic of CVT.[1] These physicians reviewed the history of the recognition of this condition, ideas about its pathogenesis, and past contributions. The increased ability to recognize dural sinus and venous occlusions using magnetic resonance technology has led to a dramatic increase in knowledge about venous occlusive disease during the past two decades. This increased knowledge has led investigators and clinicians to publish comprehensive reviews and monographs on the topic of venous and dural sinus occlusions.[2,13–21]

Demography

CVT is a rare variety of venous thromboembolic disease. Its incidence is estimated to be somewhere in the range from 0.2 to 1.32 per 100 000 person-years.[18,21,22] CVT accounts for 0.5% of all strokes.[16,18,21,23] It can occur at any age, including neonates and children with estimated incidences of respectively 1.4–12.0 per 100 000 per year[24] and 0.67 per 100 000 per year.[25] There is a 3 to 1 female preponderance and a peak in incidence in young women because of hormonal factors. The sex and age predominance of patients with CVT contrast dramatically with that found in patients with thromboembolic arterial disease, which has a male predominance and an average age of at least 3 decades older.

Etiologies

Numerous causes and risk factors have been identified in patients who develop CVT.[15,16,18,21] They include all known medical, surgical, and obstetrical causes of deep venous thrombosis in the legs, as well as a number of local causes: infective and non infective such as local infections, head trauma, brain tumors, arteriovenous malformations and fistulas. Some risk factors and causes are complementary. This means that even when an obvious cause is present, a systematic complete

Caplan's Stroke: A Clinical Approach, 5th Edition, ed. Louis R Caplan. Published by Cambridge University Press. © Cambridge University Press, 2016.

etiological evaluation should be performed. For example, a CVT in the puerperium, triggered at least in part by hormonal factors, may be accompanied by a prothrombotic condition.

Infections

In the pre-antibiotic era and until the 1970s, infections were the most common cause of CVT. Otitic and mastoid infections were a common cause of lateral sinus thrombosis, and facial and paranasal sinus infections were a frequent cause of septic cavernous sinus thrombosis. Most infections were pyogenic, but tuberculosis also involved the ear structures and mastoid cells and often spread to the meninges and dural sinuses. During infections of the structures of the middle-third of the face, including the nose, paranasal sinuses, orbits, tonsils, and palate, bacteria entered the facial veins and pterygoid venous plexus to drain into the cavernous sinus via the superior and inferior ophthalmic veins.[26,27]

Dural sinus infection may follow open, direct traumatic injuries when bacteria are introduced into the cranial cavity and after brain and epidural abscesses. Meningitis is also occasionally complicated by dural sinus occlusion. High fever and dehydration, especially in children and the elderly, can also precipitate dural sinus thrombosis. Infections are known to increase the concentrations of acute phase reactants, including serine proteins involved in the coagulation process. The increased coagulability that results also promotes CVT.

Infectious causes were found in 77 (12.3%) patients aged more than 15 years included in the large International Study on Cerebral Vein and Dural Sinus Thrombosis (ISCVT).[28] Infections involving the ears, face, mouth, and neck accounted for 51 of 77 patients, and infections involving the central nervous system were present in 13 patients.[28] An uncommon but important syndrome of tonsillopharyngitis with subsequent thrombophlebitis of the jugular vein was first described by Lemierre and is known as Lemierre's syndrome.[29]

Hormonal factors and pregnancy and the puerperium in women

The female preponderance of CVT is mostly due to occurrences during pregnancy and the postpartum period, oral contraceptives (OC) use, and, to a far lesser extent, to hormone replacement therapy and in-vitro fertilization. The frequency of pregnancy/postpartum-related CVT varies according to location.[30–35] The US National Hospital Discharge Survey (1979–1991) reported 5723 CVT cases among 50 264 631 deliveries, yielding a frequency of 11.4 per 100 000 deliveries.[35] Pregnancy/postpartum–related CVTs are especially common, or at least often reported, in India[32–34] and Mexico.[30–31] They account for 5–20% of all CVTs in high-income countries and up to 60% in some low-income countries.

CVT is far more common in the postpartum period than during pregnancy. In the ICVST study, 53 women developed CVT during the puerperium while 24 had onset during pregnancy.[28] Among a series of 113 patients with non-septic CVT studied in Mexico, 67 women were diagnosed during the puerperium, 5 during pregnancy, and 1 after an abortion.[30]

Most postpartum occurrences are during the first 3 weeks after delivery, whereas most pregnancy instances occur during the third trimester. Postpartum CVT is more common in patients who have had venous thrombosis outside the nervous system during pregnancies (pelvic or lower extremity, venous thrombosis and pulmonary embolism). CVT is more frequent in multiparous women, women from lower socioeconomic strata who have less prenatal care, and after deliveries at home. Explanations for the frequency of CVT in pregnancy and the puerperium include poverty, vegetarian and vitamin-deficient food intake, dehydration, infections, depletion of vitamin and protein stores by multiple pregnancies, and anemia. These factors may cause hyperhomocysteinemia and hypercoagulability, increasing the risk of venous occlusions.[21] Other factors especially situations that promote hypercoagulability often complicate CVTs that develop during pregnancy and soon afterwards. About one-half of the patients in ISCVT[36] and two-thirds of patients in a French series of 286 CVTs that involved young women[37] had at least another prothrombotic cause or risk factor, most frequently congenital thrombophilia.

That OC use can cause CVT was recognized 50 years ago, but for many years, there were controversies about the reality of the association, the size of the risk, the role of hormonal type and dosage and the implication of associated risk factors. There is nowadays no doubt about the reality of the association: in all series of CVT, OC use is the most frequent risk factor for CVT in young women: it was present in 47% in ISCVT[36] and 96% in an Italian study.[38] Other case-control studies[39] and meta-analysis[40] have confirmed that estrogens increase the risk of CVT with an odds ratio (OR) of 5.59 (95% confidence interval (CI), 3.95–7.91, $P < 0.001$). The risk of CVT with estro-progestogens increases with age, and high-dose estrogen content. There are not enough data on CVT to compare the risk associated with all the varieties of hormonal contraception, but cases have also been reported with transdermal patches and vaginal rings[41] in accordance with other data in venous thromboembolic disease. A few CVT cases have also been reported in young women undergoing in-vitro fertilization embryo transfer treatment for infertility, usually in association with signs of the ovarian hyperstimulation syndrome.[42]

Hormonal changes might also be important in males: a healthy 31-year-old man was reported to develop extensive dural sinus occlusions after intramuscular injections of androgens for body building.[43] Among 27 patients with anemia treated with androgen therapy in one series, three patients developed CVT.[44] Among endocrine disorders, some 30 cases of CVT have been reported in patients with thyroid diseases, both hypothyroidism[45] and hyperthyroidism.[46]

Neoplasms

Cancer, with its increase in acute-phase reactants and enhanced coagulability, is another common cause of thrombosis. Adenocarcinomas, especially from the pancreas and gastrointestinal tract, are especially likely to be accompanied by thrombotic complications. Hickey et al. reported three

patients with cancer (two with breast cancer and one with lung adenocarcinoma) who had CVT.[47] They also reviewed 13 prior case reports. All patients had breast cancer, lung cancer, or hematological malignancies, including lymphoma and leukemia. The clinical CVT signs were indistinguishable from non-cancer patients, but coexisting limb venous thrombosis and pulmonary emboli were often present. In some cancer patients, the sinovenous occlusive disease was extensive. One patient with lung cancer at necropsy had occlusion of both renal arteries and veins, both internal carotid arteries, the splenic and portal veins, the pulmonary artery, the superior sagittal sinus, vein of Galen, and numerous cortical veins.[47] In two patients, CVT was the presenting problem occurring before the diagnosis of cancer.

Cranial neoplasms can invade the dura mater and cause occlusions of the adjacent dural sinuses. This probably occurs most often in patients with meningiomas. Metastatic tumors that invade the skull, such as breast cancer and myeloma, may spread to the subjacent dura and dural sinuses and cause thrombosis. Six of the 135 patients (4.5%) in a series of Bousser's had cancer, including 2 with carcinomatous meningitis.[16] Neck tumors and abscesses, which involve the pharynx and occlude the jugular veins, can also cause propagation of clots into the lateral sinuses.[29,48]

Abnormalities of blood and coagulation system

Many acquired and congenital abnormalities of the blood and coagulation system have been reported to cause CVT: thrombocytosis;[49] polycythemia vera;[50] paroxysmal nocturnal hemoglobinuria;[51] antiphospholipid antibody syndrome;[52] severe anemia;[16,24] systemic lupus erythematosus and lupus anticoagulant;[53] sickle cell disease or trait;[54] plasminogen deficiency;[55] elevated levels of factor VIII;[56,57] disseminated intravascular coagulation; and thrombosis associated with heparin-induced thrombocytopenia.[58] The most frequent prothrombotic risk factors for CVT are congenital thrombophilia, particularly the two most frequent ones: factor V Leiden mutation and prothrombin *G20210A* mutations. In a systematic review and meta-analysis, Lauw et al. identified 18 studies evaluating the role of factor V Leiden mutation in 919 CVT cases compared with 3168 healthy controls and found an OR for CVT of 2.89 (95% CI 2.10–3.97, P <0.001).[59] In 15 studies including 776 CVT cases and 2636 controls, the OR for CVT with prothrombin gene mutation was 6.05 (95% CI 4.12–8.90, P <0.001).[60] The OR for other congenital thrombophilia were 3.75 for antithrombin deficiency, 8.35 for prothrombin C deficiency and 6.45 for protein S deficiency, but CIs for these 3 varieties of congenital thrombophilia were extremely wide because of their rarity.[59] The risk of CVT is dramatically increased in women with a congenital thrombophilia using OCs with ORs reaching 30 for factor V Leiden and 79.3 for the prothrombin gene mutation.[37,38]

Two other genetically mediated causes of thrombophilia in patients with CVT have recently been uncovered and are being explored further: promoter polymorphisms in the plasma glutathione peroxidase (*GPx-3*) gene[60] and the factor XII *C46T* gene polymorphism.[61]

Systemic conditions

Numerous systemic conditions predispose to CVT. Patients with the nephrotic syndrome may have renal vein and dural sinus occlusions that are probably related to deficiencies in coagulation proteins caused by the heavy proteinuria.[62] Dehydrated patients probably develop thrombosis because of a relatively high hematocrit and increase in viscosity and coagulability. In ill, cachectic elderly patients, a combination of dehydration and activation of coagulation factors probably cause so-called *senile marantic* venous sinus thrombosis. Congestive heart failure is also an important cause of CVT, presumably because of elevated venous pressure.

Systemic inflammatory diseases are also potential causes of CVT especially inflammatory bowel diseases including both Crohn's disase and ulcerative colitis.[16,63] Behçet's disease is an important cause of CVT in Turkey and Mediterranean countries. Among 250 patients with Behçet's disease followed in Paris, 25 patients (10%) had angiographically confirmed CVT.[64] In a series of patients with CVT studied in Saudi Arabia, Behçet's disease accounted for one-fourth of the cases.[65] In a Turkish series of 26 children with Behçet's disease, 23 had CVT (88.5%), while, by contrast, among the 702 adult patients with Behçet's only 17.2% were diagnosed as having CVT.[66] Other systemic inflammatory disorders which may occasionally cause CVT include Wegener's granulomatous, sarcoidosis, and Sjögren syndrome.[16]

Other causes

Patients with dural arteriovenous fistula may have accompanying thrombosis of dural venous sinuses and draining veins. Conversely, CVT can predispose to the development of arteriovenous fistulas. This topic is discussed in Chapter 13. CVT has also been reported after cranial or systemic surgery, in open or closed head trauma, after lumbar puncture, particularly in multiple sclerosis[67] and in all causes of intracranial hypotension, including spontaneous instances.[68,69]

The cause of CVT remains undetermined at the acute stage in many patients despite extensive investigations. No identifiable cause was found in 12.5% of 624 patients in ISCVT,[28] 21% in a French series of 135 patients,[16,70] 22% in a Mexican series of 113 patients,[30] and in 25% of 40 patients from Saudi Arabia.[65] Table 17.1 tabulates the etiologies of CVT in two large series of patients.[16,28] These results show that in around 20% of patients no cause or risk factor is found, which emphasizes the need for a long follow-up with repeated investigations. In some patients, with CVT initially interpreted as idiopathic, a cause can be discovered, months later, for instance cancer, Behçet's disease or a myeloproliferative disorder.

Pathophysiology

The development of brain pathology in patients with venous occlusions is quite different from arterial occlusive disease.[16,18,71–73] In arterial disease, the delivery of nutrients is directly compromised and brain ischemia and infarction develop. When elements of the venous system are occluded,

Table 17.1 Frequencies of various causes among two large series of patients with cerebral venous occlusions

	Bousser & Ross Russell[16]	Ferro et al.[28]
Thrombophilia	17 (26.6%)	213 (34.1%)
Female hormones	31 (23%)	234 (37.5%)
Puerperium	13 (9.6%)	53 (12.3%)
Pregnancy	4 (3%)	24 (4.3%)
Infections	9 (7%)	77 (12.3%)
Anemia	2 (1.5%)	58 (9.2%)
Malignancy	6 (4.5%)	46 (7.4%)
Surgery	1 (0.75%)	21 (3.3%)
Corticosteroids	3 (2.2%)	10 (1.6%)
Dural fistulas	3 (2.2%)	10 (1.6%)
Behçet's disease	18 (13%)	6 (1%)
Head injury	7 (5%)	7 (1.1%)
Polycythemia	1 (0.75%)	18 (2.8%)
Inflammatory bowel disease	1 (0.75%)	10 (1.6%)
Dehydration	–	12 (1.9%)
Thyroid disease	–	11 (1.7%)
Lumbar puncture	–	12 (1.9%)
Undefined	29 (21%)	78 (12.5%)
Total no. of patients	135	680

drainage of blood is compromised. Pressure increases in the brain tissue drained by the obstructed veins and dural sinuses. Brain edema develops in the involved territory. If tissue pressure increases enough, capillaries and arterioles break and brain hemorrhage occurs. A useful analogy is to visualize draining systems on city streets. When drains become clogged during a rainstorm, water accumulates on the street and may flood nearby land. The major initial findings in patients with CVT are localized brain edema and brain hemorrhage. Bleeding can spill out into the nearby subarachnoid space.

In order to perfuse brain tissue adequately, the blood pressure in the feeding artery must exceed the pressure in the tissue and draining veins. When the venous pressure and intracranial pressure become high enough, arterial perfusion may become inadequate and a true (arterial) brain infarction can ensue. The so called "venous infarct" is completely different and mostly corresponds to brain edema which is potentially reversible while arterial infarct is not. This, together with the capacity of the cerebral veins to develop collateral drainage, explain the remarkable potential for recovery of patients with CVT.

Clinical findings

CVT presents with a remarkably wide spectrum of signs and modes of onset, potentially mimicking numerous neurological conditions. General symptoms are reviewed first followed by the clinical presentations that develop according to the location of the occluded venous structure.

> CD, a 57-year-old man, worked in the anatomy department of a medical school as a repairman. One day, a neuroanatomist working in the laboratory saw him suddenly stop speaking in the midst of a conversation. He repeated, "I can't, I can't" and his right arm briefly shook. He was brought to the emergency room where he was noted to have difficulty speaking. While being examined, he had a grand mal seizure heralded by the turning of his head to the right. Blood pressure was 160/100 mmHg, but it gradually returned to normal (125/80 mmHg). Postictal agitation and aphasia were present. The aphasia was fluent and consisted of paraphasic errors and difficulty naming. He had a right superior quadrantopia. Comprehension and repetition of speech were relatively spared. When he was able to discuss his symptoms, he reported that he had awakened that morning with a headache. He felt well the day before his attack. During the preceding weeks, he had intense headaches. He was being treated for hypertension. A year ago, he had an episode of deep venous thrombosis and was treated with warfarin for 4 months. He was not taking coumadin or aspirin at the time of this attack.

Onset and course

The presentation of patients with CVT may be acute, but, in general, venous occlusions develop and propagate much more slowly than arterial occlusions. In most series, a gradual or stepwise development of symptoms and signs is more common than sudden abrupt onset.[2,16,18] Progression of symptoms after onset is also common and observed more often than in patients with arterial infarcts. The onset can be characterized as acute (sudden onset or development within 48 h), subacute (between 2 days and a month), and chronic (>30 days to evolve).[16]

In the Cantu and Barinagarrementeria series, acute onset was found more often in women who had puerperal venous thrombosis when compared with non-puerperal patients (82% vs. 54%).[30] Subsequent progression was also more common in puerperal thrombosis (72% vs. 52%). Puerperal and infectious cases tend to present more acutely than CVT from other causes.[2,16] Acute onset patients often present with focal signs while chronic cases more often present with headaches. Ameri and Bousser found that the onset of symptoms was acute (<48 h) in 31 (28%) patients, subacute in 46 (42%) patients, and chronic in 33 (30%) patients.[70] Insidious onset, usually without focal neurological signs, has often led to delays in admission to the hospital and presentation to doctors. In ISCVT, the median delay was 7 days. Patients with disturbance of consciousness, seizures and with parenchymal lesions on admission CT or MRI were diagnosed earlier, whereas men and those with isolated intracranial hypertension were diagnosed later.[74] In some

Table 17.2 The frequency of various clinical findings in patients with intracranial venous thromboses in selected series

Clinical finding	Cantu and Barinagarrementeria[30] Puerperium N = 67	Cantu and Barinagarrementeria[30] Non-puerperium N = 46	Ameri and Bousser[70] N = 110	Einhaupl et al.[71] N = 71
Headache	59 (88%)	32 (70%)	83 (75%)	63/69 (91%)
Seizures	40 (60%)	29 (63%)	41 (37%)	34 (48%)
Focal findings	53 (79%)	35 (76%)	57 (52%)	47 (66%)
Altered consciousness	42 (63%)	27 (59%)	33 (30%)	40 (56%)
Pappilledema	27 (40%)	24 (52%)	54 (49%)	19 (27%)

Clinical finding	Tsai et al[81] N = 29	Bousser & Barnett[78] = 76	Daif et al.[65] N = 40	de Bruijn et al.[80] N = 59	Ferro et al.[28] N = 624
Headache	9 (31%)	61(80%)	33 (82%)	56 (95%)	553 (88.1%)
Seizures	3 (10%)	22(29%)	4 (10%)	28 (47%)	245 (39.3)
Focal findings	9 (31%)	34(48%)	11 (27%)	27 (46%)	Not available
Altered consciousness	27(93%)	18(27%)	4 (10%)	32 (54%)	87 (13.9)
Pappilledema	2 (7%)	38(50%)	32 (80%)	23 (41%)	174 (28.3)

patients, symptoms are present for longer than 6 months when the diagnosis is made. Among 102 patients with angiographically proven CVT, 10 % had a history of headache for longer than 6 months before the diagnosis was made.[74]

Necropsy studies sometimes show venous thrombi at different stages of formation and organization.[73,76] Radiologically confirmed extension of thrombosis within the dural sinuses and veins has been noted after anticoagulants are stopped. The slow and gradual onset of symptoms and signs can be explained by the slow evolution and propagation of thrombosis and the potentially broad collateralization potential of the cranial venous and sinus drainage patterns.

Headache

Head discomfort or pain is an extremely common symptom in patients with CVT and is most often the initial one. CD had headaches before and at the onset of his neurological symptoms. Headache is much more common in patients with venous thrombosis than in patients with arterial thromboembolic disease. Table 17.2 lists the symptoms that occurred during the course of illness among various reported series of patients with CVT.[28,30,65,70,71,78–81]

Headache was an important symptom present in at least 949 of the total 1122 patients (85%) in these various series. This frequency of headache is most likely a minimal figure because some obtunded and confused or aphasic patients might not have been able to report the presence of headache. Coutinho et al. discussed the 38 (10%) patients in the ISCVT cohort that did not report headache.[82] These individuals were older, less often female and they had more motor signs and more seizures.[82] Sicker and obtunded individuals are less likely to report headache as a prodromal or onset symptom.

The presence of headache is best explained by two major factors: (1) the local process within the veins and dural sinuses; and (2) the development of increased intracranial pressure. Unlike the brain itself, the dura and overlying skull and venous sinuses are invested with pain-sensitive fibers. Distension of the sinuses, especially when caused by inflammation, activates these pain-sensitive fibers. Thrombosis causes obstruction (at least temporarily) to venous drainage from intracranial structures. The resulting increased venous pressure causes increased intracranial pressure, brain edema, brain hemorrhage and infarction, and decreased absorption of cerebrospinal fluid.

Headache in CVT has no specific diagnostic characteristics. Most often diffuse, it can be unilateral, localized to any region of the head, or even limited to the neck as in jugular vein thrombosis. The severity is also highly variable, ranging from a mild sensation of heaviness to a severe excruciating abrupt headache ("thunderclap" headache).[77–79] In the vast majority of patients, headache is persistent, but it can also be intermittent, particularly initially and it sometimes occurs in attacks.

Headache may be the only symptom of CVT as reported in a series of 17 patients from a prospective series of 123 consecutive patients.[77] These patients had no signs of intracranial hypertension, a normal cerebrospinal fluid and no parenchymal lesion on neuroimaging. The lateral sinus was involved in 15 patients and the most likely mechanism is a distension of the wall of the sinus. In over 90% of cases, headache is associated with any of the symptoms listed in Table 17.2, either in isolation or in combination.

A major pattern of presentation of CVT is isolated intracranial hypertension, present in 25–40% of patients.[70,74,78,79] In this condition, the headache often becomes more severe during days or weeks and is associated with bilateral papilledema and less often with VIth-nerve palsy, tinnitus, and

transient visual obscurations. Neuroimaging shows no parenchymal lesion. This presentation is similar to that of idiopathic intracranial hypertension (previously called pseudotumor cerebri or benign intracranial hypertension), which should never be diagnosed without first excluding thrombosis of dural sinuses.

Headache may sometimes be extremely misleading when presenting for instance as subarachnoid hemorrhage mimicking a ruptured aneurysm,[79] or as a migraine attack with or without aura,[83] or as a mere change in the pattern of headache from a purely orthostatic headache to a persistent one in patients with previous intracranial hypotension.[68]

Focal neurological signs and symptoms

Venous occlusive disease leads to focal parenchymal abnormalities, including edema, hemorrhage, ischemia, and infarction, which cause focal neurological signs and symptoms. A focal neurological sign, aphasia, was the presenting symptom in patient CD. Edema, whether localized or generalized, is the most common brain abnormality in CVT. It can be isolated or associated with hemorrhage and infarcts. The frequency of intracerebral hemorrhage in CVT varies according to diagnostic criteria, from nearly 100% in an old autopsy series to 12.5–46.0% in 7 series reviewed by Crassard and Bousser.[84] The frequency was 39% in ISCVT[28] and 25% in Crassard and Bousser's own series of 234 consecutive cases.[84] Intracerebral hemorrhage was associated in this series with subarachnoid hemorrhage in 5% of patients. Isolated subarachnoid hemorrhage or subdural hemorrhage were also present in 11 other patients (5%).[84]

Focal neurological symptoms and signs are present in approximately one-half of patients with CVT. Focal findings were appreciated in 273 of 498 (55%) patients included in Table 17.2. The signs vary considerably, depending on which dural sinuses are involved and whether the deep venous system is also occluded. Hemiparesis is probably the most common sign. Hemianopia, ataxia, neglect, and aphasia are particularly common when the posterior dural sinuses are occluded.

Seizures

A grand mal seizure developed in CD shortly after onset of aphasia. In contrast to thromboembolic arterial disease in which seizures are rare during the acute period, seizures are quite common in patients with CVT. Seizures are the presenting symptom in about 7–15% of patients, and often occur during the early course of the illness.[85] Seizures were present in 446 of 1122 patients (40%) with intracranial venous thrombosis at some time during the course of illness (see Table 17.2). In ISCVT nearly 40% of patients had seizures at presentation and 7% have seizures within 2 weeks of diagnosis. Seizures were more frequent in hemorrhagic forms of CVT (55%) than in non-hemorrhagic CVT – (28%) in Crassard and Bousser's series of 234 patients.[84] Seizures are approximately equally divided between focal and generalized. Often, the onset of focal seizures or generalized seizures with focal onset is followed by the appearance of residual focal neurological signs. Edematous or partially ischemic nerve cells may have more

potential for discharge than cells rendered non-functional by ischemia. Reversibly injured neurons must be quite common, judging by the high frequency of reversible neurological signs and reversible brain-imaging abnormalities.[73]

Decreased level of consciousness

Although diminished consciousness is not a common presenting symptom, 310 of 1122 (28%) reported patients included in Table 17.2 with CVT had an alteration in their level of alertness at some time during the course of their illness. In one series of patients with CVT diagnosed by neuroimaging techniques, 27 of 29 patients (93%) had some reduction in mentation or level of alertness.[74] This frequency of altered consciousness is much higher than any series of patients with arterial disease except cases of extensive basilar artery thrombosis and pseudotumoral cerebellar infarcts. In patients with CVT, the alteration in level of consciousness is usually reversible (as contrasted with the other two situations). Brain edema and raised intracranial pressure probably account for the decreased level of consciousness found in patients who have dural sinus occlusive disease. In patients with deep venous occlusions, bilateral involvement of the medial thalami also contributes to the occurrence of drowsiness, stupor, and coma. Extensive dural sinus occlusion with involvement of both internal jugular veins is associated with increased intracranial pressure, reduced consciousness, and poor outcomes despite anticoagulation.[86,87]

Distribution of venous structure involvement and findings related to specific locations

Figures 2.25 and 2.26 show the important intracranial dural sinuses. Figure 2.27 shows the major venous structures as they appear in the venous phase of a normal angiogram. In this chapter, the term *lateral sinus* is used to include the transverse and sigmoid sinuses. Some authors use the terms lateral sinus and transverse sinus interchangeably. Table 17.3 lists the distribution of involvement of the various venous structures among reported series of patients.[26,28,30,65,70,78,81] Determination of the sinuses involved should be viewed as approximate estimates because many of the studies are based on incomplete neuroradiological studies. Cortical vein involvement is particularly difficult to assess because these veins, by contrast to the deep venous system, are variable in number and location.

The superior sagittal sinus (SSS) and the lateral sinuses (LS) were the most commonly involved in all of the studies cited. The SSS was involved in 626 of 1171 cases (54%), and the lateral sinuses in 804 of 1171 (69%) (Table 17.3). The isolated involvement of one sinus is rare, less than 30% for SSS and 10% for LS,[16,30,70] but in a recent series of 195 consecutive patients, isolated LS thrombosis (32%) was more frequent than isolated SSS (9%).[87]

Deep venous system thrombosis is much less common than dural sinus thrombosis. Cerebral cortical veins were often involved, but rarely in isolation. Cerebellar cortical veins are very rarely involved. The incidence of multiple venous channel involvement is high. Approximately two-thirds of patients had thrombosis of more than one venous channel (237/368

Table 17.3 Distribution of venous structures involved in various studies

Vein	Cantu & Barinagarrementeria[30] Puerperium N = 67	Cantu & Barinagarrementeria[30] Non-puerperium N = 46	Ameri & Bousser[70] N = 110	Southwick et al.[26] Septic N = 179	Tsai et al.[81] N = 29	Bousser & Barnett[78] N = 76	Daif et al.[65] N = 40	Ferro et al.[28] N = 624
Superior sagittal sinus	60 (22)	45 (11)	79 (14)	23 (7)*	19 (11)	53	34 (22)	313
Lateral sinus	23 (1)	20 (1)	78 (10)	64 (4)*	15 (8)	55	13 (4)	536
Straight sinus	0	0	3 (1)	–	3	10	3	112
Cavernous sinus	0	0	3	92 (8)*	0	2	0	8
Deep venous system	17 (4)	10	9 (1)	–	1	3	4 (1)	68
Cortical or cerebellar superficial veins	13	14	30 (2)	–	0	29	0	110
>1 Venous structure involved	39	34	85	–	9	56	14	–

Note: Numbers in parentheses represent cases that involved structure alone.
* Numbers in parentheses represent personally studied cases. (The remainder derive from literature review.)

patients, 64.5%) among the series that tabulated multiple channel involvement.[30,65,70,78,81] Patency of the jugular veins is not commented on in any of the large series tabulated. Yet the bulk of blood drained from the cranium exits through the two jugular veins in the neck. When these are occluded bilaterally, increased pressure becomes a major problem,[89,90] and may even lead to superficial siderosis of the central nervous system from bleeding of enlarged intrathecal venous collaterals.[91]

The studies cited in Table 17.3 include patients who have had many different etiologies. In puerperal patients, the SSS seems to be involved much more often than in patients with thrombosis unrelated to female hormonal changes. Septic thrombosis involves preferentially the lateral and cavernous sinuses, because of the drainage of the ear and paranasal sinus structures into these dural sinuses.

Cavernous sinus thrombosis

Thrombosis of the cavernous sinus is rare (2.7% in a prospective series of 110 patients).[70] It is a potentially life-threatening complication of local infections. The veins draining the medial portions of the face, orbit, nose, and nasal sinuses lead into the cavernous sinus. The cavernous sinus, in turn, drains via the petrosal sinuses into the LS and ultimately into the jugular vein.

The most common organism implicated in septic cavernous sinus thromboses is *Staphylococcus aureus*.[26,92] Pneumococci, streptococcal species, gram-negative bacteria, and fungi, especially *Aspergillus* species, account for the remainder of cases.[16] The earliest symptoms of septic cavernous sinus thrombosis are headache, facial pain, and fever. The eyelid and eye become red. The eye becomes proptotic. The face may become edematous and red. Orbital and retinal congestion develop, and ophthalmoplegia is found on examination. The oculomotor and trochlear nerves and the ophthalmic and maxillary branches of V course along the lateral wall of the cavernous sinus. The abducens nerve and internal carotid artery with its surrounding sympathetic nerve fibers are located more in the center of the sinus. Any and all of these structures may be involved. Ophthalmoplegia may be complete or partial and is often accompanied by sensory abnormalities in the distribution of V1 and V2. Before the antibiotic era the mortality rate of septic cavernous sinus thrombosis was around 80% with aggressive treatment.[93] It is now less than 30%, but sequelae are present in half the survivors.[92,94,95] Sequelae include oculomotor nerve palsies, trigeminal neuralgia, and visual impairment and blindness due to retinal or optic nerve ischemia.[96]

Head trauma, surgery on facial structures, prothrombotic states, and thrombosis of dural arteriovenous fistulas can cause non-septic cavernous sinus thrombosis.[16] The onset of symptoms and signs in non-septic patients is often gradual and indolent. Proptosis and redness of the eye may be only moderate in severity.

Sagittal sinus thrombosis

The SSS is a very common location of dural venous sinus thrombosis. The sagittal sinus is the favorite location for occlusion during the puerperium. Parasagittal meningiomas, neoplastic disease of the meninges, head trauma, Behçet's disease, and prothrombotic states are other frequent causes. Symptoms and signs depend greatly on the involvement of cerebral veins that drain into the sinus and on involvement of the lateral and other dural sinuses.

When thrombosis is limited to the sagittal sinus, the presentation is that of isolated intracranial hypertension with headache and papilledema.[16] Extension of thrombus into rolandic and parietal veins is common and is often associated with the development of focal motor or sensory signs, or both, and focal or generalized seizures.[16] Sometimes, the neurological signs are transient and closely resemble transient ischemic attacks of arterial origin. The neurological signs are often bilateral, an occurrence that should always bring to mind the possibility of SSS. Edema and hemorrhages are often found on brain imaging in the medial and dorsal portions of the cerebral hemispheres. Reduced consciousness and coma are common when the brain becomes severely edematous and bilateral hemorrhages and hemorrhagic infarcts are present.

Lateral sinus thrombosis

The frequency of LS thrombosis equals or now exceeds that of SSS thrombosis.[88] One or both LS were thrombosed in 69% of 1171 cases included in Table 17.3 and in 80% in a prospective series of 195 patients.[88] Within the posterior circulation, the LS is by far the most commonly occluded dural sinus. A much higher proportion of patients with LS thrombosis than SS thrombosis have an infectious etiology, almost entirely caused by spread of infection from acute or chronic ear and mastoid infections. The infective process within the otological structures often leads to a local thrombophlebitis which spreads into the LS and sometimes into the jugular vein.

LS thrombosis caused by otological infections and mastoiditis have undoubtedly become less common because of the widespread use of antibiotics. The clinical findings in patients with LS thrombosis caused by otitic infections are quite characteristic.[26,97–101] Nearly all patients have had chronically draining ears and show acute infection or perforations of the eardrum. Fever, headache, neck pain, and neck tenderness are important and frequent signs. Pain and tenderness are usually centered along the anterior border of the sternocleidomastoid muscle on one side. The mastoid region is often sensitive and uncomfortable to finger percussion. Pain is usually also felt behind the ear. Headache is common and usually described as severe, persistent, and rather diffuse, located mostly in the frontotemporal and occipital areas of one or both sides.[26] If meningitis develops, bilateral neck stiffness and rigidity develop.

Vertigo, nausea, and vomiting are also often present. Diplopia caused by VIth-nerve palsy and signs of Vth-nerve irritation in the form of temporal and retro-orbital pain are often present. The combination of Vth and VIth nerve involvement, called the Gradenigo's syndrome, indicates involvement of these nerves at the petrous apex in or near Dorello's canal. Decreased alertness may be present and is explained by elevated intracranial pressure when both LS are thrombosed or one LS (most often the right LS) if the other is hypoplastic.[88]

Structures on either side of the tentorium may be involved because both the inferior portions of the temporal lobe and cerebellum drain into the LS. Combined temporal lobe and cerebellar involvement on one side suggests LS thrombosis. Aphasia, agitation, and a right hemianopia or superior quadrantanopia are the most common signs in left temporal lobe involvement. These signs were all present in patient CD, who was found to have left temporal lobe dysfunction related to a left LS occlusion. Right temporal lobe involvement usually causes an agitated state with a left visual field defect. Nystagmus and gait ataxia are the most common signs of cerebellar involvement. Patients with isolated LS thrombosis have a different pattern of presentation. In a series of 62 patients only 5% had a local infectious cause.[88] Clinical symptoms were headache in 95% of patients. Headache was isolated in 45%, associated with signs of intracranial hypertension in 24%, and with other signs such as seizures or dysphasia in 31%. All other signs were present in less than 5% of patients. Acute hearing loss was the presenting symptom in 3%.[88] In a recent series of 38 patients with CVT, 3 had an acute unilateral hearing loss, associated with headache and tinnitus in 2.[102]

Plain x-rays and CT scans of the mastoid regions usually show abnormalities, including increased density with loss of the mastoid air cell trabeculae, bony sclerosis, or lytic lesions of the temporal and parietal bones.[26] Cholesteatomas are common and have sometimes eroded through the temporal bone.[26,100]

Deep venous system thrombosis

Deep venous system thrombosis is much less common than dural sinus thrombosis. Among the series included in Table 17.3, the deep venous system was occluded in 112 of 1171 (9.6%) patients. The straight sinus is also occluded in some patients. The straight sinus and vein of Galen receive venous inflow from both thalami, the basal ganglia, midbrain, geniculate bodies, and the cerebellum. In the past, thrombosis of the deep venous system was thought to be almost exclusively a disorder of babies and young children and uniformly fatal. Since the 1970s, the condition has become recognized in adults, and the course is often much more benign than previously thought.[103–104]

Necropsy studies of patients dying of the deep venous thrombosis system usually show bilateral thalamic and, often, basal ganglionic hemorrhagic infarcts.[103,104] Figure 17.1 is an MRI that shows bilateral basal ganglia and thalamic lesions in a patient with extensive thrombosis of deep veins. Patients with deep venous system thrombosis usually have reduced consciousness and often become stuporous or comatose. Headache may precede other symptoms and may be severe. Stiffness of the limbs with decerebrate postures, coma, and vertical gaze palsy are the most common clinical findings in patients with extensive basal ganglionic and thalamic hemorrhagic infarcts and edema.[2,16] In a recent German/French series of 32 patients with deep venous system thrombosis, the clinical presentation was highly variable with headache (81%) and reduced consciousness (72% including 38% with coma) as the most frequent symptoms.[105] Other main symptoms included motor deficits (44%), confusion (31%), and visual

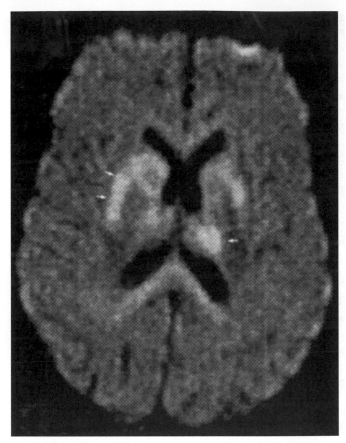

Figure 17.1 Diffusion-weighted MRI showing bilateral basal ganglionic and thalamic abnormalities. The two small white arrows point to the lesion in the putamen on the left of the figure and the small white arrow on the right of the figure points to the lesion in the right thalamus. Courtesy of Rafael Linas, MD.

disturbances (25%). The outcome was much better than in previous series: 75% had an excellent outcome (modified Rankin Scale (mRS) ≤1) including 50% who had no symptoms at all. No patient was severely disabled but two died. This good outcome contrasts with that observed in another recent series of 14 patients among whom 6 (43%) died and 3 (21%) remained severely disabled.[106] This worse outcome was probably due to the far more frequent associated involvement of cortical veins in this series (93%) than in the German/French series (6%).[106]

Cortical vein thrombosis

Isolated thrombosis of cortical veins is rare and possibly still overlooked despite modern neuroimaging techniques.[107–110] Most reported patients have had seizures as a presenting or major symptom. The seizures have most often been focal or have had focal onsets with secondary generalization. Focal neurological signs, such as hemiparesis and aphasia, are common. Headache is less frequent than in dural sinus thrombosis. Reduced consciousness and increased intracranial pressure occur mostly when there is an associated sinus thrombosis, although one of us (M-GB) has seen a patient with bilateral cortical vein thrombosis in the absence of thrombosis of the SSS. The patient presented with headache, hemiplegia, stupor and coma and worsened very rapidly. Bilateral parenchymal

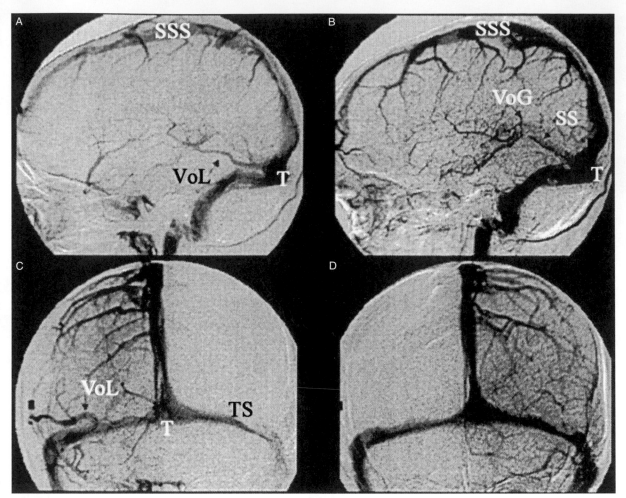

Figure 17.2 Digital subtraction angiogram, venous phase. A and C are shown after right carotid artery injection while B and D are shown after left carotid artery injection. The left vein of Labbé is not opacified. SS, straight sinus; SSS, superior sagittal sinus; TS, transverse sinus; VoG, vein of Galen; VoL, vein of Labbé. From Thomas B, Krishnamurthy T, Purkayastha G. Isolated left vein of Labbé thrombosis. *Neurology* 2005;65:1135 with permission.

lesions and slit ventricles were present on neuroimaging. She recovered almost completely after hemicraniectomy. In unilateral isolated cortical vein thrombosis brain imaging shows a focal region of brain edema often with hemorrhage located along the pial surface of one cerebral hemisphere. In reported cases, occlusion has often involved the vein of Labbé.[111,112] Figure 17.2 is a digital subtraction angiogram that shows an occluded vein of Labbé.[99]

Cerebellar vein thrombosis

Only 14 of the 624 patients (2%) in the ISCVT cohort had involvement of posterior fossa structures, 2 of whom also had supratentorial lesions.[113] The patients who did have parenchymatous posterior fossa lesions tended to have a worse outcome compared to the remainder of the CVT patients.[113] Cerebellar vein thrombosis is rare and most reported cases affect the three major venous drainage systems in the posterior fossa: the superior galenic, the anterior petrosal and the posterior tentorial group.[114–116] In a Mexican series of 230 CVT, 9 (3.9%) had isolated vein thrombosis of the posterior fossa with cerebellar unilateral or bilateral infarcts or hemorrhages.[116] Intracranial hypertension and cerebellar signs were the main

clinical presentation. The outcome was bad with two deaths, two severely disabled and five moderately disabled. A few isolated cases have been reported with a variable outcome. One reported patient had a sudden, severe headache mimicking subarachnoid hemorrhage, and another patient had multiple cranial nerve palsies, cerebellar-type incoordination, and papilledema, a syndrome that mimicked a posterior fossa tumor.[13,16] Another patient had a pseudotumoral syndrome with good recovery after surgery.[116] One reported diabetic patient presented with seizures, coma and death during a severe hyperosmolar state with bilateral large cerebellar hemorrhagic infarcts and hematomas.[115]

Diagnosis

Recognition of CVT depends on a combination of clinical suspicion and neuroimaging confirmation. The demographics and risk factors are quite different from those found in patients with arterial occlusions. Patients with CVT are younger, usually female, and have low frequencies of hypertension, coronary artery disease, diabetes, and smoking when compared with patients with arterial occlusive disease. The conditions, risk factors, and circumstances that should alert

Table 17.4 Situations or findings suggesting that cerebral venous or dural sinus occlusion be strongly considered in differential diagnosis of stroke

Infants and babies with dehydration and sepsis

Puerperal and pregnant women and those taking OCs

Patients with known cancers, especially adenocarcinomas, leukemias, and lymphomas

Meningitis and other intracranial infections

Acute and chronic otitis media and mastoid infections

Acute sinusitis

Presence of inflammatory diseases, such as Behçet's disease, ulcerative colitis, and Crohn's disease

Nephrotic syndrome

Sepsis

Cachexia, malnutrition, and dehydration, especially in the young and old

Known hematological disorders, which predispose to hypercoagulability

Severe anemia

Elevated homocysteine level

Presence of past recurrent leg or other systemic venous thrombosis with or without pulmonary embolism

Intracranial tumors such as meningiomas that involve or abut on dural venous sinuses

Presence of dural arteriovenous fistulas

Penetrating cranial traumatic injuries

clinicians to the possibility of venous occlusive disease are listed in Table 17.4.

Clinical symptoms and signs are helpful clues to the diagnosis. Headache is usually the earliest clinical symptom and often antedates any neurological symptoms or signs. Seizures and decreased alertness are much more common in CVT than in patients with arterial occlusion-related infarcts. Usually, the evolution is slower and more indolent. CVT mimics brain infarction and hemorrhage but also many other conditions such as idiopathic intracranial hypertension, preeclampsia–eclampsia, reversible cerebral vasoconstriction syndrome, vasculitis, encephalitis, brain abscess, meningitis, subdural empyema, brain tumors, all of which are important differential diagnostic considerations.

Imaging and neuroradiological investigations have dramatically improved the ability of clinicians to confirm the diagnosis of CVT. CT scan is probably the most common initial brain imaging test ordered. CT can show abnormalities within the bony structures of the skull, such as evidence of paranasal sinus infection, erosion of the middle ear structures, and changes in the mastoid regions. Mastoid air sinus abnormalities, often thought to be due to a local infection, are frequent in LS thrombosis (39% of cases) in the absence of mastoiditis and

are likely to be due to local venous congestion.[117] Infection-related erosion and thinning of the sinus plate are also sometimes evident. CT also effectively shows parenchymatous brain lesions, especially hemorrhages, and may even show abnormalities within the veins and dural sinuses.[2,16,118–123]

In patient CD, the CT scan showed a hemorrhage in the inferior portion of the left temporal lobe, which extended from the pial surface nearly to the sylvian fissure (Figure 17.3A). The hematoma was surrounded by a rim of lucent brain. A focal region of hyperdensity in the left transverse sinus region was also present. A later CT scan (Figure 17.3B) showed that a large hemorrhagic infarct had developed above the hemorrhage that was previously seen. MRI was unsatisfactory because of motion, but confirmed the temporal lobe hemorrhage, edema, and infarction. Angiography showed early filling of the left basal vein of Rosenthal, non-filling of the left vein of Labbé, and no opacification of the left transverse and sigmoid portions of the left LS (Figure 17.4). The left jugular vein was not filled. In patient CD, the vein of Labbé was occluded in addition to thrombosis of the LS and may have been most responsible for his temporal lobe hemorrhagic infarction.

Visualization of the thrombus within a sinus or a vein is key for the diagnosis of CVT. On non-contrast CT a thrombosed sinus appears as hyperdense, with a round or triangular shape, "the dense triangle" sign.[119] Initially described for SSS, a spontaneous hyperdensity may be seen in thrombosis of other sinuses and veins. In cortical veins, the so-called "cord sign", imaged as a high-density, linear, thin, cylindric structure is specific for cortical vein thrombosis.[109,110] These signs have a low sensitivity with a maximum of 65% in recent series using multidetector-row CT scanners.[124] The specificity is also low because of confounding factors such as high hematocrit, dehydration, subarachnoid hemorrhage which may increase the density of venous structures, mimicking thrombosed vessels.[123] Parenchymatous changes include regions of hypodensity, (representing infarction and edema); hemorrhages; and brain edema with small, compressed ventricles. Often, the distribution of the parenchymal abnormalities, including diffuse edema, bilaterality of infarcts and hemorrhages, predominance of hemorrhagic changes, and the presence of a lesion, which does not conform to a typical arterial distribution, suggests CVT.

More information is usually obtained from contrast-enhanced CT scans than from plain scans.[121] Perhaps most important is the so-called "empty delta sign," first described in patients with SSS.[2,16,118–122] Contrast enhances the smaller collateral veins and walls of the sinus, but not the thrombosed lumen. This may also be seen in LS thrombosis and appears like rails when the slice is parallel to the vessel. Cortical and medullary veins may appear dilated on contrast-enhanced scans because of dilatation of collateral draining channels.[121] Contrast enhancement in a gyral pattern may also occur as it does in arterial disease-related infarcts. The tentorium or other dural structures may enhance in the region of a thrombosed dural sinus.[121,122]

Evidence of brain infarction and edema are more often found on CT scans than direct evidence of venous occlusion.

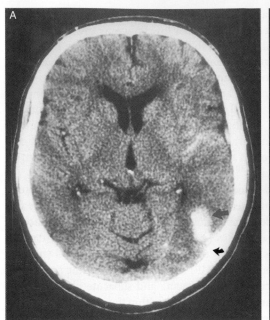

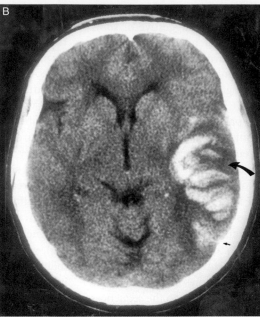

Figure 17.3 CT scans of patient CD. (A) Left temporal-lobe hemorrhage (upper black arrow). Near the surface, the thrombosed LS images as a hyperdensity (lower black arrow). (B) CT scan taken days later shows that a large hemorrhagic zone of infarction (upper black arrow) has developed above the area of hemorrhage that is still seen below (lower black arrow).

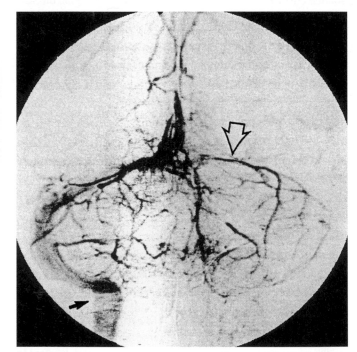

Figure 17.4 Angiogram, venous phase in patient CD. The right LS is well opacified and drains into the right jugular vein (black arrow at bottom left of figure). The left LS (arrow) does not fill, and there is no opacification of the left jugular vein. The left vein of Labbé also did not fill. From Caplan LR. *Posterior Circulation Disease: Clinical Findings, Diagnosis, and Management*. New York: Blackwell Science, 1996, pp 633–685 with permission of Blackwell Publishing Ltd.

In some patients, focal regions of subarachnoid bleeding are found in the vicinity of a cortical vein thrombosis.[110] In patients with cerebellar vein thrombosis, hydrocephalus and compression of the IVth ventricle may be found. In thrombosis of the deep venous system, the characteristic findings are bilateral hypodensities or hemorrhages involving the thalami

and basal ganglia.[105,106] Severe edema with compression of the IIIrd ventricle may occur. The occluded sinuses and deep veins can appear as hyperdense structures on unenhanced CT scans. After contrast, non-opacification of the vein of Galen, straight sinus, and retention of contrast for a prolonged period in the usual draining veins, such as the thalamostriate veins and basal vein of Rosenthal, suggest deep venous system thrombosis.

CT venography (CTV) is now a powerful tool for the detection of CVT.[123–126] Performed on multidetector-row scanners with bolus injection of contrast and imaging acquisition at the venous phase, it allows an excellent visualization of the cerebral venous system. Thrombus appears as a filling defect in a vein or in a sinus that may be seen on native images or after reconstruction. CTV is at least equivalent or even better than magnetic resonance venography two-dimensional time-of-flight (MRV-2D TOF), because it is free of artifacts and has a high resolution.[124,125] Other advantages include its accessibility and rapid acquisition, useful for agitated patients. Disadvantages are the use of iodine contrast and exposure to ionizing radiation.[123–125]

Magnetic resonance imaging is more likely than CT to provide definitive evidence of CVT.[2,16,18,21,108,127] MRI shows a variety of parenchymatous changes, including early infarction, hemorrhage, hemorrhagic infarction, focal edema, and diffuse edema. Gyral enhancement can be shown after gadolinium enhancement. In some patients, mass effect is found without any abnormalities of signal within the edematous regions.[127] A localized subarachnoid hemorrhage is sometimes seen in patients with isolated cortical vein thrombosis.[128] The diagnosis of CVT does not rely on parenchymal brain imaging because, firstly, it may be normal in 10–30% of patients, and, secondly, it mostly shows lesions that are not specific for CVT.[129,130] MRI is extremely useful both to rule out the many conditions that CVT can mimic and to eventually detect

a cause such as a tumor or an abscess. Furthermore, as with CT scan, some patterns of lesions are highly suggestive of some topographic varieties of CVT: bilateral parasagittal hemorrhages suggest SSS and cortical vein thrombosis while bilateral thalamic and basal ganglia lesions point to thrombosis of the deep venous system. Diffusion-weighted imaging has shown that patients with CVT usually have high ADC values (related to vasogenic edema) or a mixed pattern and only rarely low ADC values as found in arterial infarcts.[131–134] These findings again illustrate that so called "venous infarcts" have a much better recovery than arterial infarcts.[21,123]

The most specific finding for the diagnosis of CVT is visualization of the thrombosed vessel and the best tool for such visualization is MRI. Changes in signal within the vessels depend mostly on the presence or absence of flow, and on the transformation of hemoglobin into deoxyhemoglobin. MRI findings heavily depend on the MRI sequences chosen and the stage of the thrombosis. Numerous studies have shown the temporal evolution of MRI findings according to the sequences used. On T1- and T2-weighted images, the thrombus is hyperintense from day 5 to about day 20.[127,135,136] Figure 17.5 is an MRI scan that shows increased signal in SSS on a T2-weighted image. During the first few days the thrombus may be isointense on T1- and hypointense on T2-weighted images, leading to a falsely negative MRI. Later, depending on recanalization, the thrombus signal is decreased on all sequences. The signal becomes inhomogeneous in the late stages. When the sinus completely recanalizes, the signals become normal. Mas and colleagues showed that some patients with dural sinus thrombosis continued to have hyperintensity on T2-weighted images when studied 6 months after symptom onset.[137]

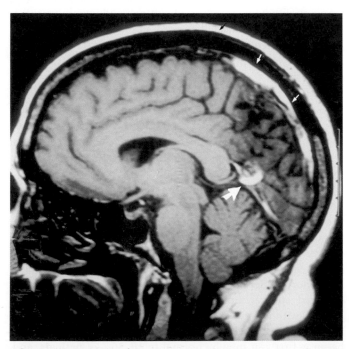

Figure 17.5 MRI of patient with multiple thromboses of dural sinuses. The SSS thrombosis is shown as a hyperintense signal (two small white arrows). The straight sinus is also occluded and shows a hyperintense signal (lower white arrowhead). The non-thrombosed portion of the sagittal sinus appears dark (upper black arrow).

Interpretation of changes on T1- and T2-weighted images is sometimes difficult: slow or low flow may cause artifacts in the sinus that may lead to false positive. This risk is reduced by multiple pulse sequences and multiple orientation acquisitions. Arachnoïd granulations are often quite large, protrude into dural sinuses, and modify the flow mimicking a thrombus. MRI is useful to differentiate LS hypoplasia from LS thrombosis. Hypoplastic sinuses are smaller asymmetric structures on parasagittal images without abnormal signal intensity whereas thrombosed sinuses have increased intraluminal signals.[138]

Decreased blood flow in veins and dural sinuses promotes a local shift in the hemoglobin oxygenation curve toward the formation of deoxyhemoglobin. Deoxyhemoglobin produces a "magnetic susceptibility effect" that images as signal loss (darkening), which is best seen on echo-planar T2*-weighted (susceptibility) images. The T2* MRI sequence can detect the presence of intravenous clot during the acute and subacute phase of CVT, shown as an area of hypointensity within the affected sinus.[108,139] During the first 3 days, the sensitivity of T2*-weighted images is above 90% whereas that of T1-weighted images is about 70%.[138] T2*-weighted images are particularly useful for the diagnosis of isolated cortical vein thrombosis.[110,128] Vessel hyposignal on T2*-weighted images may persist for months or years and should not be misinterpreted as a recurrence of recent thrombosis.[128,139] Susceptibility-weighted imaging is a more recently introduced sequence that further improves thrombus detection.[140,141]

MRA techniques, especially MRV,[140–142] are particularly useful in defining dural sinus and cerebral and cerebellar venous occlusions by abnormalities in the normal flow signals, non-opacification of sinuses, and by showing collateral venous channels. Figure 17.6 illustrates the absence of the deep venous structures on MRV, confirming the diagnosis of deep vein occlusion. MRV has now become the vessel imaging modality most widely used to establish the diagnosis of CVT. MRV can be performed with time-of-flight (TOF) or phase-contrast techniques. TOF relies mainly on flow-related enhancement to produce images of the blood vessels, whereas phase contrast techniques use velocity-induced phase shifts to separate moving blood flow from surrounding stationary tissue. TOF technique has shorter acquisition times and covers more regions. Absence of flow signal within a sinus and its non-opacification suggest intraluminal thrombosis. However, flow gaps in the non-dominant (hypoplastic) transverse sinuses are seen in up to 30% of normal individuals when using TOF MRV, leading to an erroneous diagnosis of sinus thrombosis. These artifactual flow gaps are attributed to slow intrasinus blood flow, in-plane flow, or complex blood flow patterns which can result in intrasinus signal loss mimicking occlusion. Saturation of blood flow when images are parallel to a sinus, especially the anterior portion of the SSS, can result in loss of signal intensity and false diagnosis of sinus occlusion.[140–142]

With the advent of CT and MRV, catheter angiography, once considered the "gold standard," is very rarely used. It can be performed using conventional filming or by digitalized intra-arterial filming techniques. Anteroposterior and lateral films are required with opacification of the entire venous

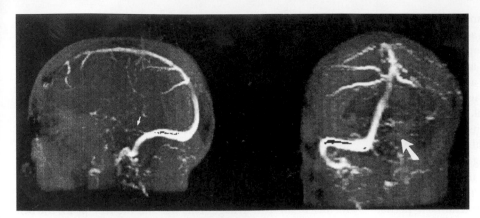

Figure 17.6 MRV in a patient whose MRI is shown in Figure 17.1. The sagittal view on the left shows that the vein of Galen and the straight sinus are not seen. The small white arrow points to their usual location. In the axial view on the right of the figure, the deep veins, straight sinus, and LS on the right of the image are not seen (large white arrow). Courtesy of Rafael Linas, MD.

system. Sometimes, oblique films are also useful, particularly in patients with suspected SSS thrombosis. The partial or complete lack of opacification of venous channels is the primary angiographic evidence of venous occlusion. In patient CD, non-filling of the left LS confirmed the clinical diagnosis (see Figure 17.6). Delayed emptying and dilatation of collateral venous channels are other signs that are often present.[13,16,142] Because of the wide variability in the development of the LS, the entire LS, especially the sigmoid portion, could fail to opacify. Neck films help to show whether the jugular bulb and vein are thrombosed. Delayed venous filling and emptying are common and are found in one-half of the patients with dural sinus occlusions.[13] Dilatated and tortuous cortical veins ("corkscrew veins") are more often seen at angiography than transcerebral collaterals.

Other investigations

Measurement of D-dimer levels can be helpful in diagnosis.[21,143–145] Low levels of D-dimer (<500 ng/ml) have a high negative predictive value in deep vein thrombosis in the legs. The negative predictive value is also high for CVT. In a meta-analysis of 14 studies for a total of 1134 patients the mean sensitivity of D-dimer levels was 93.9% and the specificity 89.7%.[144] However, D-dimers were normal in 13% of patients with deep cerebral venous system thrombosis[105] and in 26% of patients with isolated headache.[145] Normal D-dimers make the diagnosis of CVT less likely but do not exclude the diagnosis. False negatives are explained by patients with isolated headache, a long duration of symptoms, and limited sinus involvement.[143]

Transcranial Doppler (TCD) ultrasonography with or without echo-contrast has been used to diagnose and follow patients with SSS thrombosis particularly at the bedside in intensive care units.[145,146] B-mode ultrasound studies of the neck, usually ordered to study carotid and vertebral artery disease, do show the jugular veins.

Lumbar puncture is still useful and should be performed in some patients with CVT, provided there is no contraindication,[16,28,123] Lumbar puncture is essential in patients presenting with isolated intracranial hypertension both for the diagnosis (raised pressure, possibly raised protein content, presence of red blood cells, and/or pleiocytosis) and

for treatment (lowering intracranial pressure). Lumbar puncture is also required in patients who have fever, if infectious meningitis is suspected, and in patients with CVT of unknown cause to detect rare conditions such as carcinomatous, or inflammatory meningitis.[16] In such cases, provided there is no contraindication, lumbar puncture should preferably be performed before starting anticoagulation.[16,123]

In summary, the diagnosis of CVT is based on neuroimaging. CT scanning remains, in daily clinical practice worldwide, the easiest available method; non-contrast CT rarely shows the thrombosed vessel itself but shows parenchymal changes and may help to differentiate transverse sinus thrombosis from atresia (small sigmoid plate notch).[148] When associated with CTV, CT often allows the diagnosis of CVT, but MRI with its various sequences, particularly T2*-weighted imaging, is much more sensitive than CT to visualize the thrombosed vessel. MRI, coupled with MRV is now considered the gold standard for the diagnosis of CVT. Other investigations have little positive diagnostic value. Normal D-dimers make the diagnostic of CVT less likely but do not exclude it. Lumbar puncture is still useful in some patients, such as those with isolated intracranial hypertension, fever, suspicion of meningitis. Many other investigations are required in patients with CVT as part of the etiological evaluation.[21,123]

Treatment

CVT is an uncommon but potentially life-threatening condition that is probably best managed, at least at the acute stage, in stroke units in order to optimize care and minimize complications.[149,150] The treatment of CVT is based on a combination of etiological, symptomatic, and antithrombotic treatment. Anticoagulation is the mainstay of treatment.

Some etiologies such as malignancies, connective tissue diseases, hematological disorders, and infections may require specific treatments. In patients with septic CVT antibiotics and surgical drainage of infections such as paranasal sinus infections, middle ear and mastoid infections remain the most important treatment.

Symptomatic treatment of headache is based on positioning the patient with head elevated and the use of analgesics. Antiepileptic drugs are usually prescribed only in patients who

present with seizures.[149,150] Some physicians also use them in patients with parenchymal hemorrhage on admission CT scan, as they are at higher risk of seizure. The optimal duration of antiepileptic treatment is unclear, usually at least one year in patients who have had seizures during the acute phase. Raised intracranial pressure can usually be managed with mannitol and acetazolamide. Steroids are not useful, and may even be deleterious.[151] Some patients require intensive care unit care with sedation, hyperventilation, intracranial pressure monitoring, and, sometimes, temporary shunting.[123,149–150] In rare cases, surgery is necessary in patients with massive edematous brain lesions and signs of impending herniation. A specific situation is that of patients with isolated intracranial hypertension and no brain hemorrhage or infarct (pseudo-tumor syndrome). In such patients, particularly if vision is threatened, lumbar puncture with CSF removal is indicated before starting heparin, usually in association with acetazolamide. In the very rare cases of visual failure despite this treatment, shunting procedures should be considered but they require a short cessation of anticoagulant treatment before and during placement of the shunt.[123,149,150]

Despite old controversies and even a recent negative opinion,[152] anticoagulation is, as in other varieties of venous thrombosis, the basis of CVT treatment. Its main goals are to prevent thrombus growth, to facilitate recanalization, and to prevent deep vein thrombosis and pulmonary embolism which is still a major cause of death in CVT.[149,153]

CD was treated with anticonvulsants. Heparin was begun on the sixth hospital day despite the large temporal lobe hematoma. Lupus anticoagulant studies were positive. The platelet count was slightly reduced and the prothrombin time was slightly accelerated. A new phlebothrombosis in the leg was identified and an inferior vena cava filter was placed. CD gradually improved, but remained aphasic.

Anticoagulants were first used to treat patients with puerperal CVT by Stansfield[154] and by Martin and Sheenan[155] in the early 1940s. In their monograph on CVT published in 1967, Kalbag and Woolf favored early anticoagulation before thrombosis spread to cortical veins.[1] In the same year, Krayenbuhl noted that patients treated with anticoagulants and antibiotics had a 7% mortality compared with 37% mortality in those treated only with antibiotics and compared with 70% mortality in those not given antibiotics or anticoagulants.[156] He wrote that he never had a patient who developed intracranial hemorrhage during well-controlled anticoagulant treatment of intracranial venous thrombosis.[156] Despite the opinions of these authorities, most clinicians considered anticoagulants to be too dangerous because of the risk of further brain hemorrhage. This was still the case in 1975 when one of us (M-GB) saw a 69-year-old woman who woke up with a right-arm monoplegia and, who, over the next 3 weeks, worsened gradually with a dense hemiplegia, a massive aphasia, and, finally, a deep coma. The diagnostic of CVT was suspected on conventional angiography. Heparin was not given for fear of hemorrhage until the patient's husband told us: "Look, I had a vein thrombosis in my legs some years ago, I was given heparin and I did well. My wife is getting worse and worse, she is going to die, please give her heparin!" Heparin was then started and the next morning, much to our surprise, the patient was awake! Over the next few days, she made a dramatic improvement and she recovered completely in the next 6 weeks.[157]

During the last 40 years, data have accumulated from case reports, series, registries and randomized clinical trials in favor of the efficacy of anticoagulation[13,16,18,21,28,70,150,156–162] (Table 17.5). A review of 39 studies found a death rate of 9.1% in the 2211 patients treated with heparin and 14% in the 557 not treated ($P < 0.0007$).[152] Among the data reviewed were those of the ISCVT, in which 66 of the 520 anticoagulated patients were dead or dependent at follow-up (12.7%), while 19 of the 104 patients who were not anticoagulated became dependent or died (18.3%).[28] Although these studies cannot prove effectiveness, they do show that anticoagulants are probably seldom harmful, and for most clinicians, they are persuasive.

Table 17.5 Retrospective non-randomized studies of anticoagulation effects in patients with intracranial venous thrombosis

	Anticoagulated		Not anticoagulated	
	Survived/improved	*Died*	*Survived/improved*	*Died*
Krayenbuhl (1954)[142]	16	1	32	24
Bousser et al. (1985)[13]	23	0	11	4
Case reports 1942–1987*	25	3 bled	25	44
Walker (unpublished)*	6	0	7	1
Jacewicz and Plum (1990)[158]	4	1 (veg)	4	5
Totals	**74 (94%)**	**5 (6%)**	**79 (50%)**	**78 (50%)**

* Data from Jacewicz M, Plum F. Aseptic cerebral venous thrombosis. In Einhaupl K, Kempski O, Baethmann A (eds), *Cerebral Sinus Thrombosis: Experimental and Clinical Aspects.* New York: Plenum, 1990, pp 157–170.

A similar beneficial trend came from the two major, but small, placebo-controlled randomized trials.[159,160] The first was a German study stopped after the inclusion of 20 patients because of a dramatic difference between the 2 groups: in the unfractionated heparin (UFH) treated group there was no deaths and 80% of patients had a full recovery, while in the placebo group 30% died and only 10% recovered completely.[159] The second trial was a Dutch study of 59 patients treated with low-molecular-weight heparin (LMWH) or placebo.[160] A poor outcome (death or dependency) was observed in 13% in the LMWH-treated group versus 21% in the placebo group. A meta-analysis of these 2 studies showed that heparin treatment is associated with an absolute risk reduction of poor outcome of 15% and a relative risk reduction of 56%.[160] These results were confirmed in a recent Cochrane review which showed a 13% absolute risk reduction in poor outcome with heparin.[161] Although not statistically significant, these results are clinically very meaningful, particularly since they convincingly show that heparin does not worsen patients with hemorrhagic CVT. In case series as well as in randomized trials, CVT patients with hemorrhagic brain lesions treated with heparin fared even better than those who did not receive heparin. They had less worsening of the hemorrhagic lesion and less new hemorrhages.[159–161] This means that when a patient treated with heparin has an increase in the size of his initial hemorrhage or a new hemorrhage, this is not necessarily due to a deleterious effect of heparin but could as well be due to the insufficient efficacy of the anticoagulation. One must not forget that before the anticoagulation era, CVT patients died of intracerebral hemorrhages.[1,3,16]

In present day practice, it is clear that patients with CVT, even with hemorrhagic brain lesions, have a better chance of good outcome when receiving full early anticoagulation. The European Federation of Neurological Societies guidelines, published in 2006, stated that when there are "no contraindications for anticoagulants – body-weighted subcutaneous low-molecular-weight heparin in full therapeutic dosage or APPT (two times above normal values) dose-adjusted intravenous heparin should be given."[150] A similar recommendation was published by the American Heart Association/American Stroke Association in 2011: "For patients with CVT, initial anticoagulation with adjusted dose UFH or weight-based LMWH in full anticoagulant doses is reasonable, followed by vitamin K antagonist, regardless of the presence of intracranial hemorrhage."[149]

Thrombolytic agents have also been used to treat patients with CVT. Despite numerous case reports and small series, there is no good evidence from systematic reviews that systemic or local thrombolysis gives better results than anticoagulation,[163,164] although recanalization rates might be higher.[149] Thrombolytic therapy and more recently mechanical thrombectomy have been used in patients who deteriorate despite anticoagulation.[149] In a prospective study of 20 patients with severe CVT, managed with endovascular treatment (thrombolysis and/or thrombectomy), 14 patients survived, including 2 with severe handicap, and 6

(30%) died.[165] Large hemorrhagic infarction before treatment was associated with fatal outcome; five patients had increased hemorrhagic lesions after thrombolysis.[165] A randomized clinical trial (TO-ACT) has recently started comparing endovascular thrombolysis with or without mechanical clot removal and heparin at therapeutic dose in patients who have a high probability of poor outcome.

Studies of patients with CVT who died despite acute anticoagulation treatment reveal that a very common cause of failure is occlusion of multiple sinuses and cerebral veins. In a retrospective analysis of 79 patients treated with intravenous heparin, all 8 patients who died had stupor and coma and all had a severe restriction of venous outflow shown angiographically.[166,167] In these patients, increased intracranial pressure and poor brain perfusion proved fatal. In such patients, it is our experience and that of others that endovascular thrombolysis is not effective and does not prevent further brainstem compression.[168] This has led to the development in the last 10 years of decompressive surgery in patients in such "malignant CVT."[169] Several case reports and small series have convincingly shown that decompressive surgery, mostly hemicraniectomy, may be lifesaving and allow a good functional outcome, even in patients with a very severe clinical condition.[168–173] In a review of 69 patients who underwent decompressive surgery (decompressive craniectomy in 45, hematoma evacuation in 7, both interventions in 17), only 12 (17.4%) had an unfavorable outcome (MRS score 5 or death).[172] A complete recovery was observed in 26 (37.7%) including 3 of the 9 patients with bilateral fixed dilated pupils.[172] These results have been confirmed in a recent series from India of 44 patients treated with hemicraniectomy (38) or bifrontal craniectomy (6).[173] Nine patients died (20%) and 27 (77%) of the survivors had a good outcome (mRS ≤2).[173] In practice, the few patients (<5%) who have large brain ischemic or hemorrhagic lesions, massive edema, and clinico-radiological signs of impending herniation and who deteriorate despite heparin are at an extremely high risk of death and should be offered decompressive craniectomy. The chances of survival are over 80%, of complete recovery over 30%, and of good functional outcome over 70%.[168–173]

Outcome

Many studies and reviews have been devoted to the outcome of CVT and to prognostic factors of poor outcome. They all show that CVT has, by contrast to arterial stroke, a remarkable potential for good recovery. Despite worsening after diagnosis in 23% of patients, particularly in those with depressed consciousness on admission,[174] the vast majority of patients improve and have an excellent functional recovery. Among the 624 patients, prospectively recruited in ISCVT, 79% had a MRS ≤1 at last follow-up.[28] Among the 437 patients included prospectively and consecutively in the Lariboisière Neurology department from 1997 to February 2014, 70.5% had a MRS ≤1 when leaving the hospital (M-GB, unpublished observation). A somewhat lower figure (52.8%) was observed among the 428 patients seen in Hyderabad between 2002 and 2010.[34]

The death rate during the acute phase is variable, but is nowadays usually less than 10%: 8.3% in ISCVT,[28] 7.7% in the

Indian series,[34] 4.39% and 2% in 2 large national samples from the United States,[175,176] and 2.1% in the Lariboisière series. The main cause of death is increased intracranial pressure and transtentorial herniation. Other causes include pulmonary embolism, status epilepticus, medical complications, and underlying diseases, such as malignancies and infections. About 5% of survivors remain severely dependent with a MRS ≥4.[28] Prognostic factors of poor outcome include male sex, thrombosis of the deep venous system, intracerebral hemorrhage, hydrocephalus, posterior fossa lesions, decreased level of consciousness, coma, malignancies, infections, and hematological disorders.[28,175–177] Various combinations of these factors have been used to calculate risk scores.[178,179] Despite the interest in these scores, the prognosis remains often unpredictable in individual patients. Interestingly, there is no good correlation between recanalization rates of thrombosed vessels and clinical outcome.[180,181]

Management after the acute phase

After the acute phase, heparin is replaced by oral anticoagulants, presently vitamin K antagonists with an international normalized ratio (INR) of 2–3 since there are no data yet in CVT about the new oral anticoagulants (direct thrombin inhibitors and factor Xa inhibitors). The aim of continuing anticoagulation is to prevent venous thromboembolic events which occur in about 6.5% of patients, mostly during the first year after the cessation of anticoagulation. These events are more frequently deep venous thrombosis in the legs and pulmonary embolism than recurrent CVT.[28,151,182,183] There is no consensus about the duration of anticoagulation: a duration of 3–6 months is recommended in patients with a provoked CVT (associated with a transient risk factor); of 6–12 months in patients with unprovoked CVT; and indefinitely in patients with recurrent venous thromboembolic events or severe thrombophilia, or antiphospholipid antibody syndrome.[149] In patients in whom anticoagulation is stopped, it is important to perform an MRI, in order to evaluate the degree of recanalization and to be able to interpret the eventual occurrence of new neurological symptoms. Following a strategy used in deep venous thrombosis, in the Lariboisière Neurology Department, D-dimers are measured 1 month after discontinuation of anticoagulation. If they are elevated, anticoagulation is resumed for 6 months, and an etiological work up is again performed.[184]

Seizures occur in about 11% of patients, mostly in those who had seizures during the acute stage or had a hemorrhagic brain lesion.[185] Severe visual loss due to optic atrophy is rare (2%).[28,186] Patients with intracranial hypertension should have a close ophthalmological follow-up, including regular evaluation of papilledema, visual acuity, and formal visual field testing. Papilledema may persist and vision may deteriorate even in patients with complete sinus recanalization. Headache is a frequent complaint after CVT, but it is mostly due to migraine and tension-type headache.[186–190] The persistence or recurrence of headache raises suspicion of recurrent CVT or of persistent raised intracranial pressure, and should be addressed accordingly.[149] The occurrence of pulsatile tinnitus may point to a dural arteriovenous fistula usually involving the LS. The exact frequency of dural fistula after CVT is not known, it is estimated at 1–3%.[149] Although the large majority of patients with CVT recover, and are functionally independent, patients may be depressed, have difficulties in concentration and/or fatigue which appear more frequent than in the general population and may have a negative impact on their psychological and employment status.[187,188]

As OC use is a risk factor for CVT, any estrogen-based contraception is contraindicated after CVT. Post-menopausal hormonal therapy is equally contraindicated. By contrast, several studies have shown a low risk of recurrent CVT or new thromboembolic event during future pregnancies so that CVT, even when pregnancy or postpartum related, is not considered a contraindication for future pregnancies.[21,149] A close follow-up is required, but it is debated whether prophylaxis with LMWH should be recommended during pregnancy. There is, however, a consensus in favor of prophylaxis during the postpartum period.[21,149]

References

1. Kalbag RM, Woolf AL: *Cerebral Venous Thrombosis*. London: Oxford University Press, 1967.

2. Caplan LR: *Posterior Circulation Disease: Clinical Findings, Diagnosis, and Management*. Boston: Blackwell Science, 1996.

3. Ribes MF: Des recherches faites sur la phlebite. Revue Medicale Francaise et etrangere et *Jornal de clinique de l'Hotal-Dieu et de la Charite de Paris* 1825;**3**:5–41.

4. Abercrombie J: *Pathological and Practical Researches on Diseases of the Brain and Spinal Cord*. Edinburgh: Waugh & Innes, 1828;83–85.

5. Tonnelle M-L: Memoire sur les maladies des sinus veineux de la dure-mere. *J Hebd Med* 1829;**5**:337–403.

6. Cruveilhier J: *Anatomie pathologique du corps humain: descriptions avec figures lithographiées et caloriées ddes diverses alterations morbides dont le corps humain est susceptible*. Paris: J B Bailliere, 1835–1842.

7. Quinke H: Ueber meningitis serosa. *Inn Med Nr* 1891;**23**:655–694.

8. Quinke H: Ueber meningitis serosa und verwandte Zustande. *Dtsch Z Nervenheilk* 1896;**9**:149–168.

9. Symonds CP: Otitic hydrocephalus. *Brain* 1931;**54**:55–71.

10. Symonds CP: Hydrocephalus and focal cerebral symptoms in relation to thrombophlebitis of dural sinuses and cerebral veins. *Brain* 1937;**60**:531–550.

11. Symonds CP: Cerebral thrombophlebitis. *BMJ* 1940;**2**:348–352.

12. Symonds CP: Otitic hydrocephalus. *Neurology* 1956;**6**:681–685.

13. Bousser M-G, Chiras J, Bories J, Castaigne P: Cerebral venous thrombosis – a review of 38 cases. *Stroke* 1985;**16**:199–213.

14. Einhaupl KM, Kempski O, Baethman A: *Cerebral Sinus Thrombosis: Experimental and Clinical Aspects*. New York: Plenum, 1990.

15. Einhaupl KM, Masuhr F: Cerebral venous and sinus thrombosis. An update. *Eur J Neurol* 1994;**1**:109–126.

16. Bousser M-G, Ross Russell R: *Cerebral Venous Thrombosis*. London: Saunders, 1997.

17. Biousse V, Bousser M-G: Cerebral venous thrombosis. *Neurologist* 1999;**5**:326–349.

18. Stam J: Thrombosis of cerebral veins and sinuses. *N Engl J Med* 2005;**352**:1791–1798.

19. Ehtisham A, Stern BJ: Cerebral venous thrombosis: A review. *Neurologist* 2006;**12**:32–38.

20. Mehdiratta M, Kumar S, Selim M, Caplan LR: Cerebral venous sinus thrombosis: Clinical features, diagnosis and treatment. In Caplan LR (ed): *Uncommon Causes Of Stroke*, 2nd ed. Cambridge: Cambridge University Press, 2008; 497–594.

21. Bousser M-G, Ferro JM: Cerebral venous thrombosis: An update. *Lancet Neurol* 2007;**6**:162–170.

22. Coutinho JM, Zuurbier SM, Aramidch M, Stam J. The incidence of cerebral venous thrombosis: a cross-sectional study. *Stroke* 2012;**43**:3375–3377.

23. Einhäupl K, Stam J, Bousser M-G, et al: European Federation of Neurological Societies. EFNS guideline on the treatment of cerebral venous and sinus thrombosis in adult patients. *Eur J Neurol* 2010;**17**:1229–1235.

24. Berfelo FJ, Kersbergen KJ, Van Ommen CH, et al: Neonatal cerebral sinovenous thrombosis from symptom to outcome. *Stroke* 2010;**41**:1382–1388.

25. deVeber G, Andrew M, Adams C, et al: Canadian pediatric ischemic stroke study group. Cerebral sinovenous thrombosis in children. *N Engl J Med* 2001;**345**:417–423.

26. Southwick FS, Richardson EP, Swartz MN: Septic thrombosis of the dural venous sinuses. *Medicine (Baltimore)* 1986;**65**:82–106.

27. Tveteras K, Kristensen S, Dommerby H: Septic cavernous and lateral sinus thrombosis. *J Laryngol Otol* 1988;**102**:877–882.

28. Ferro JM, Canhao P, Stam J, et al: Prognosis of cerebral vein and dural sinus thrombosis. *Stroke* 2004;**35**:664–670.

29. Bliss SJ, Flanders SA, Saint S: A pain in the neck. *N Engl J Med* 2004;**350**:1037–1042.

30. Cantu C, Barinagarrementeria F: Cerebral venous thrombosis associated with pregnancy and puerperium. Review of 67 cases. *Stroke* 1993;**24**:1880–1884.

31. Estanol B, Rodriguez A, Conte G, et al: Intracranial venous thrombosis in young women. *Stroke* 1979;**10**:680–684.

32. Srinivasan K: Cerebral venous and arterial thrombosis in pregnancy and puerperium, a study of 135 patients. *Angiology* 1983;**34**:733–746.

33. Chopra JS, Banerjee AK: Primary intracranial sinovenous occlusions in youth and pregnancy. In Vinken PJ, Bruyn GW, Klawans HL (eds): *Handbook of Clinical Neurology*, vol **10**. Amsterdam: Elsevier, 1989;425–452.

34. Narayan D, Kaul S, Ravishankar K, Suryaprabha T, Srinivasarao Bandaru VCS: Risk factors, clinical profile, and long-term outcome of 428 patients of cerebral sinus venous thrombosis: Insights from Nizam's Institute Venous Stroke Registry, Hyderabad. *Neurology India* 2012;**60**:154–159.

35. Lanska DJ, Kryscio R: Stroke and intracranial venous thrombosis during pregnancy and puerperium. *Neurology* 1998;**51**:1622–1628.

36. Coutinho JM, Ferro JM, Canhao P, et al: Cerebral venous and sinus thrombosis in women. *Stroke* 2009;**40**:2356–2361.

37. Bousser M-G, Crassard I. Cerebral venous thrombosis, pregnancy and oral contraceptives. *Thrombosis Research* 2012;**130**:19–22.

38. Martinelli I, Sacchi E, Landi G, et al: High risk of cerebral-vein thrombosis in carriers of a prothrombin-gene mutation and in users of oral contraceptives. *N Engl J Med* 1998;**338**:1793–1797.

39. De Bruijn SF, Stam J, Koopman MM, Vandenbroucke JP: The cerebral venous sinus thrombosis study group. Case-control study of risk of cerebral sinus thrombosis in oral contraceptive users and in carriers of hereditary prothrombotic conditions. *BMJ* 1998;**316**:589–592.

40. Dentali F, Crowther M, Ageno W: Thrombophilic abnormalities, oral contraceptives, and risk of cerebral vein thrombosis: A meta-analysis. *Blood* 2006;**107**:2766–2773.

41. Fugate JE, Robinson MT, Rabinstein AA, Wijdicks EF: Cerebral venous sinus thrombosis associated with a combined contraceptive ring. *Neurologist* 2011;**17**:105–106.

42. Man BL, Hui AC: Cerebral venous thrombosis secondary to ovarian hyperstimulation syndrome. *Hong Kong Med J* 2011;**17**:155–156.

43. Jaillard AS, Hommel M, Mallaret M: Venous sinus thrombosis associated with androgens in a healthy young man. *Stroke* 1994;**25**:212–213.

44. Shiozawa Z, Yamada H, Mabuchi C, et al: Superior sagittal sinus thrombosis associated with androgen therapy for hypoplastic anemia. *Ann Neurol* 1982;**12**:578–580.

45. Peralta AR, Canhao P: Hypothyroidism and cerebral vein thrombosis – a possible association. *J Neurol* 2008;**255**:962–966.

46. Squizzato A, Gerdes VE, Brandjes DP, Büller HR, Stam J. Thyroid diseases and cerebrovascular disease. *Stroke* 2005;**36**:2302–2310.

47. Hickey WF, Carnick MB, Henderson IC, Dawson DM: Primary cerebral venous thrombosis in patients with cancer – a rarely diagnosed paraneoplastic syndrome. Report of three cases and review of the literature. *Am J Med* 1982;**73**:740–750.

48. Poe LB, Manzione JV, Wasenko JJ, Kellman RM: Acute internal jugular vein thrombosis associated with pseudoabscess of the retropharyngeal space. *AJNR Am J Neuroradiol* 1995;**16**:892–896.

49. Mitchell D, Fisher J, Irving D, et al: Lateral sinus thrombosis and intracranial hypertension in essential thrombocythaemia. *J Neurol Neurosurg Psychiatry* 1986;**49**:218–219.

50. Haan J, Caebeke JFV, van der Meer FJM, Wintzen AR: Cerebral venous thrombosis as a presenting sign of myeloproliferative disorders. *J Neurol Neurosurg Psychiatry* 1988;**51**:1219–1220.

51. Johnson RV, Kaplan SR, Blailock Z: Cerebral venous thrombosis in paroxysmal nocturnal hemoglobinuria. *Neurology* 1970;**20**:681–686.

52. Agah R, Rice L, Winikates J: Fatal cerebral venous thrombosis as the initial manifestation of the antiphospholipid syndrome. *J Neurol Neurosurg Psychiatry* 1996;**98**:189–191.

53. Vidailhet M, Piette J-C, Wechsler B, et al: Cerebral venous thrombosis in systemic lupus erythematosus. *Stroke* 1990;**21**:1226–1231.

54. Feldenzer JA, Bueche MJ, Venes JL, Gebarski SS: Superior sagittal sinus thrombosis with infarction in sickle cell trait. *Stroke* 1987;**18**:656–660.

55. Schutta HS, Williams EC, Baranski BG, Sutula TP: Cerebral venous thrombosis with plasminogen deficiency. *Stroke* 1991;**22**:401–405.

56. Kim MJ, Cho A-H, No Y-J, et al: Recurrent cerebral venous thrombosis associated with elevated factor VIII. *J Clin Neurol* 2006;**2**:286–289.

57. Anadure RK, Nagaraja D, Christopher R: Plasma factor VIII in non-puerperal cerebral venous thrombosis: A prospective case-control study. *J Neurol Sci* 2014;**339**:140–143.

58. Pohl C, Harbrecht U, Greinacher A, et al: Neurologic complications in immune-mediated heparin-induced thrombocytopenia. *Neurology* 2000;**54**:1240–1245.

59. Lauw MN, Barco S, Coutinho JM, Middeldorp S: Cerebral venous thrombosis and thrombophilia: A systematic review and meta-analysis. *Semin Thromb Hemost* 2013;**39**:913–927.

60. Voetsch B, Jin RC, Bierl C, et al: Role of promotor polymorphisms in the plasma glutathione peroxidase (*GPx-3*) gene as a risk factor for cerebral venous thrombosis. *Stroke* 2008;**39**:303–307.

61. Reuenr KH, Jenetzky E, Aleu A, et al: Factor XII *C46T* gene polymorphism and the risk of cerebral venous thrombosis. *Neurology* 2008;**70**:129–132.

62. Barthelemy M, Bousser M-G, Jacobs C: Thrombose veineuse cerebrale au cours d'un syndrome nephrotique. *Nouv Presse Med* 1980;**9**:367–369.

63. Cognat E, Crassard I, Denier C, Vahedi K, Bousser M-G: Cerebral venous thrombosis in inflammatory bowel diseases: Eight cases and literature review. *Int J Stroke* 2011;**6**:487–549.

64. Wechsler B, Vidailhet M, Piette JC, et al: Cerebral venous thrombosis in Behçet's disease: Clinical study and long-term follow-up of 25 cases. *Neurology* 1992;**42**:614–618.

65. Daif A, Awada A, Al-Rajeh S, et al: Cerebral venous thrombosis in adults. A study of 40 cases from Saudi Arabia. *Stroke* 1995;**26**:1193–1195.

66. Uluduz D, Kürtüncü M, Yapici Z, et al: Clinical characteristics of pediatric-onset neuro-Behçet disease. *Neurology* 2011;**77**:1900–1905.

67. Vandenberghe N, Debouverie M, Anxionnat R, Clavelou P, Bouly S, Weber M: Cerebral venous thrombosis in four patients with multiple sclerosis. *Euro J Neurol* 2003;**10**:63–66.

68. Berroir S, Grabli D, Héran F, Bakouche P, Bousser M-G: Cerebral sinus venous thrombosis in two patients with spontaneous intracranial hypotension. *Cerebrovasc Dis* 2004;**17**:9–12.

69. Schievink WI, Maya MM: Cerebral venous thrombosis in spontaneous intracranial hypotension. *Headache* 2008;**48**:1511–1519.

70. Ameri A, Bousser M-G: Cerebral venous thrombosis. *Neurol Clin* 1992;**10**:87–111.

71. Einhaupl K, Villringer A, Haberl RL, et al: Clinical spectrum of sinus venous thrombosis. In Einhaupl K, Kemski O, Baethmann A (eds): *Cerebral Sinus Thrombosis, Experimental and Clinical Aspects*. New York: Plenum, 1990;149–155.

72. Schaller B, Graf R: Cerebral venous infarction: The pathophysiological concept. *Cerebrovasc Dis* 2004;**18**:179–188.

73. Villringer A, Mehraein S, Einhaupl KM: Pathophysiological aspects of cerebral sinus venous thrombosis (SVT). *J Neuroradiol* 1994;**21**:72–80.

74. Ferro JM, Canhao P, Stam J, et al: Delay in the diagnosis of cerebral vein and dural sinus thrombosis. Influence on outcome. *Stroke* 2009;**40**:3133–3138.

75. Gutschera-Wang L: *Zur klinik von Letalen Hirnvenen – Und Sinus Thrombosen Anhand Von 102 Fallen*. Munich: Erwachsener, 1982.

76. Cervos-Navarro J, Kannuki S: Neuropathological findings in the thromboses of cerebral veins and sinuses: Vascular aspects. In Einhaupl K, Kempski O, Baethmann O (eds): *Cerebral Sinus Thrombosis: Experimental and Clinical Aspects*. New York: Plenum, 1990;15–25.

77. Cumurciuc R, Crassard I, Sarov M, et al: Headache as the only neurological sign of cerebral venous thrombosis: A series of 17 cases. *J Neurol Neurosurg Psychiatry* 2005;**76**:1084–1087.

78. Bousser M-G, Barnett HJM: Cerebral venous thrombosis. In Barnett HJM, Mohr JP, Stein BM, Yatsu F (eds): *Stroke Pathophysiology, Diagnosis, and Management*, 2nd ed. New York: Churchill Livingstone, 1992;517–537.

79. Bousser M-G, Einhäupl K: Cerebral venous thrombosis. In Olesen J,

Tfelt-Hansen P, Welch KMA (eds): *The Headaches*, 2nd ed. Philadelphia: Lippincott Williams & Wilkins, 2000;929–939.

80. de Bruijn SF, de Haan RJ, Stam JF: Clinical features and prognostic factors of cerebral venous sinus thrombosis in a prospective series of 59 patients. Cerebral Venous Sinus Thrombosis Study Group. *J Neurol Neurosurg Psychiatry* 2001;**70**:105–108.

81. Tsai F, Wang A-M, Matovich VB, et al: MR staging of acute dural sinus thrombosis: Correlation with venous pressure measurements and implications for treatment and prognosis. *AJNR Am J Neuroradiol* 1995;**16**:1021–1029.

82. Coutinho JM, Stam J, Canhão P, et al. on behalf of the ISCVT Investigators: Cerebral venous thrombosis in the absence of headache. *Stroke* 2015;**46**:245–247.

83. Newman DS, Levine SR, Curtis VL, Welch KMA: Migraine like visual phenomena associated with cerebral venous thrombosis. *Headache* 1989;**29**:82–85.

84. Crassard I, Bousser M-G. Cerebral venous thrombosis and intracerebral hemorrhage. In Carhuapoma JR, Mayer SA, Hanley DF (eds). *Intracerebral Hemorrhage*. New York: Cambridge University Press, 2009;84–100.

85. Ferro JM, Canhao P, Bousser M-G, et al: Early seizures in cerebral vein and dural sinus thrombosis. Risk factors and role of antiepileptics. *Stroke* 2008;**39**:1152–1158.

86. Mehraein S, Schmidtke K, Villringer A, et al: Heparin treatment in cerebral sinus and venous thrombosis: Patients at risk of fatal outcome. *Cerebrovasc Dis* 2003;**15**:17–21.

87. Masuhr F, Mehraein S: Cerebral venous and sinus thrombosis. Patients with a fatal outcome during intravenous dose-adjusted heparin treatment. *Neurocrit Care* 2004;**1**:355–361.

88. Damak M, Crassard I, Wolff V, Bousser M-G. Isolated lateral sinus thrombosis. A series of 62 patients. *Stroke* 2009;**40**:476–481.

89. Dunsker SB, Torres-Reyes E, Peden JC Jr: Pseudotumor cerebri associated with idiopathic cryofibrinogenemia: Report of a case. *Arch Neurol* 1970;**23**:120–127.

90. Kaplan RE, Springate JE, Feld LG, Cohen ME: Pseudotumor cerebri associated with cerebral venous sinus

thrombosis, internal jugular vein thrombosis, and systemic lupus erythematosus. *J Pediatr* 1985;**107**:266–268.

91. Yavagal DR, Geng D, Akar S, Buonanno F, Kesari S: Superficial siderosis of the central nervous system due to bilateral jugular vein thrombosis. *Arch Neurol* 2010;**67**:1269–1271.

92. DiNubile MJ: Septic thrombosis of the cavernous sinus. *Arch Neurol* 1988;**45**:567–572.

93. Yarington CT Jr: The prognosis and treatment of cavernous sinus thrombosis: Review of 878 cases in the literature. *Ann Otol Rhinol Laryngo* 1961;**70**:263–267.

94. Yarington CT Jr: Cavernous sinus thrombosis revisited. *Proc R Soc Med* 1977;**70**:456–459.

95. Ebright JR, Pace MT, Niazi AF: Septic thrombosis of the cavernous sinuses. *Arch Intern Med* 2001;**161**:2671–2676.

96. Chen JS, Mukherjee, Dillon WP, Wintermark M: Restricted diffusion in bilateral optic nerves and retinas as an indicator of venous ischemia caused by cavernous sinus thrombophlebitis. *AJNR Am J Neuroradiol* 2006;**27**:1815–1816.

97. Samuel J, Fernandes CM: Lateral sinus thrombosis: A review of 45 cases. *J Laryngol Otol* 1987;**101**:1227–1229.

98. Mathews TJ: Lateral sinus pathology: 22 cases managed at Groote Schuur hospital. *J Laryngol Otol* 1988;**102**:118–120.

99. Tveteras K, Kristensen S, Dommerby H: Septic cavernous and lateral sinus thrombosis; modern diagnostic and therapeutic principles. *J Laryngol Otol* 1988;**102**:877–882.

100. Singh B: The management of lateral sinus thrombosis. *J Laryngol Otol* 1993;**107**:803–808.

101. Crassard I, Biousse V, Bousser M-G, Meyer B, Marsot-Dupuch K: Hearing loss and headache revealing lateral sinus thrombosis in a patient with factor V Leiden mutation. *Stroke* 1997;**28**:876–878.

102. Gattringer T, Enzinger C, Birner A, et al: Acute unilateral hearing loss as an early symptom of lateral cerebral sinus venous thrombosis. *Arch Neurol* 2012;**69**:1508–1511.

103. Bots GAM: Thrombosis of the Galenic system veins in the adult. *Acta Neuropathol* 1971;**17**:227–233.

104. Haley EC, Brashear R, Barth JT, et al: Deep cerebral venous thrombosis: Clinical, neuroradiological, and neuropsychological correlates. *Arch Neurol* 1989;**46**:337–340.

105. Pfefferkorn T, Crassard I, Linn J, Dichgans M, Boukobza M, Bousser M-G: Clinical features, course and outcome in deep cerebral venous system thrombosis: An analysis of 32 cases. *J Neurol* 2009;**256**:1839–1845.

106. Sagduyu A, Sirin H, Mulayim S, et al: Cerebral cortical and deep venous thrombosis without sinus thrombosis: Clinical MRI correlates. *Acta Neurol Scand* 2006;**114**:245–260.

107. Jacobs K, Moulin T, Bogousslavsky J, et al: The stroke syndrome of cortical vein thrombosis. *Neurology* 1996;**47**:376–382.

108. Selim M, Fink J, Linfante I, et al: Diagnosis of cerebral venous thrombosis with echo-planar T2*-weighted magnetic resonance imaging. *Arch Neurol* 2002;**59**:1021–1026.

109. Duncan IC, Fourie PA: Imaging of cerebral isolated cortical vein thrombosis. *AJR Am J Roentgenol* 2005;**184**:1317–1319.

110. Urban PP, Müller-Forell W: Clinical and neuroradiological spectrum of isolated cortical vein thrombosis. *J Neurol* 2005;**252**:1476–1481.

111. Dorndorf D, Wessel K, Kessler C, Kompf D: Thrombosis of the right vein of Labbé: Radiological and clinical findings. *Neuroradiology* 1993;**35**:202–204.

112. Thomas B, Krishnamurthy T, Purkayastha G. Isolated left vein of Labbé thrombosis. *Neurology* 2005;**65**:1135.

113. de Sousa DA, Ferro JM, Canhão P, et al. for the ISCVT Investigators: Cerebral venous thrombosis causing posterior fossa lesions: Description of a case series and assessment of safety of anticoagulation. *Cerebrovasc Dis* 2014;**38**:384–388.

114. Rousseaux P, Lesoin F, Barbaste P, Jomin M: Infarctus cerebelleux pseudotumoral d'origine veineuse. *Rev Neurol* 1987;**144**:209–211.

115. Eng LJ, Longstreth WT, Shaw CM, et al: Cerebellar venous infarction: Case report with clinicopathologic correlation. *Neurology* 1990;**40**:837–838.

116. Ruiz-Sandoval JL, Chiquete E, Navarro-Bonnet J, et al: Isolated vein thrombosis of the posterior fossa presenting as localized cerebellar venous infarctions or hemorrhages. *Stroke* 2010;**41**:2358–2361.

117. Fink JN, Mc Auley DL: Mastoid air sinus abnormalities associated with lateral venous sinus thrombosis. Cause or consequence? *Stroke* 2002;**33**:290–292.

118. Singh V, Gress DR: Cerebral venous thrombosis. In Babikian VL, Wechsler LR, Higashida RT (eds): *Imaging Cerebrovascular Disease*. Philadelphia: Butterworth–Heinemann, 2003;209–221.

119. Patronas NJ, Duda EE, Mirfakhraee M, Wollmann RL: Superior sagittal sinus thrombosis diagnosed by computed tomography. *Surg Neurol* 1981;**15**:11–14.

120. Buonanno FS, Moody DM, Ball MR, Laster DW: Computed cranial tomographic findings in cerebral sinovenous occlusions. *J Comput Assist Tomogr* 1978;**2**:281–290.

121. Rao CV, Knipp HC, Wagner EJ: Computed tomographic findings in cerebral sinus and venous thrombosis. *Radiology* 1981;**140**:391–398.

122. Chiras J, Bousser M-G, Meder JF, Koussa A, Bories J: CT in cerebral thrombophlebitis. *Neuroradiology* 1985;**27**:145–154.

123. Mawet J, Crassard I, Bousser M-G: Cerebral venous thrombosis. In Caplan LR, van Gijn J (eds): *Stroke Syndromes*, 3rd ed. Cambridge: Cambridge UniversityPress, 2012;542–553.

124. Linn J, Ertl-Wagner B, Seelos KC, et al: Diagnostic value of mutidetector-row CT angiography in the evaluation of thrombosis of the cerebral venous sinuses. *AJNR Am J Neuroradiol* 2007;**28**:946–952.

125. Ozsvath RR, Casey SO, Lustrin ES, et al. Cerebral venography: Comparison of CT and MR projection venography. *AJR Am J Roentgenol* 1997;**169**:1699–1707.

126. Wetzel SG, Kirsch E, Stock KW, et al: Cerebral veins: Comparative study of CT venography with intraarterial digital subtraction angiography. *AJNR Am J Neuroradiol* 1999;**20**:249–255.

127. Yuh WTC, Simonson TM, Wang A-M, et al: Venous sinus occlusive disease: MR findings. *AJNR Am J Neuroradiol* 1994;**15**:309–316.

128. Boukobza M, Crassard I, Bousser M-G, et al: MR imaging features of isolated cortical vein thrombosis: diagnosis and follow-up. *AJNR Am J Neuroradiol* 2009;**30**:344–348.

129. Leach JL, Fortuna RB, Jones BV, et al: Imaging of cerebral venous thrombosis: current techniques, spectrum of findings, and diagnostic pitfalls. *Radiographics* 2006;**26**:19–41.

130. Poon CS, Chang JK, Swarnkar A, et al: Radiologic diagnosis of cerebral venous thrombosis: Pictorial review. *AJR Am J Roentgenol* 2007;**189**:64–75.

131. Ducreux D, Oppenheim C, Vandamme X, et al: Diffusion-weighted imaging patterns of brain damage associated with cerebral venous thrombosis. *AJNR Am J Neuroradiol* 2001;**22**:261–268.

132. Yoshikawa T, Abe O, Tsuchiya K, et al: Diffusion-weighted magnetic resonance imaging of dural sinus thrombosis. *Neuroradiology* 2002;**44**:481–488.

133. Forbes KP, Pipe JG, Heiserman JE: Evidence for cytotoxic edema in the pathogenesis of cerebral venous infarction. *AJNR Am J Neuroradiol* 2001;**22**:450–455.

134. Mullins ME, Grant PE, Wang B, et al: Parenchymal abnormalities associated with cerebral venous sinus thrombosis: Assessment with diffusion-weighted MR imaging. *AJNR Am J Neuroradiol* 2004;**25**:1666–1675.

135. Dormont D, Axionnat R, Evrard S, et al: IRM des thromboses veineuses cerebrales. *J Neuroradiol* 1994;**21**:81–99.

136. Isensee Ch, Reul J, Thron A: Magnetic resonance imaging of thrombosed dural sinuses. *Stroke* 1994;**25**:29–34.

137. Mas J-L, Meder JF, Meary E: Dural sinus thrombosis: Long-term follow-up by magnetic resonance imaging. *Cerebrovasc Dis* 1992;**2**:137–144.

138. Mas J-L, Meder J-F, Meary E, Bousser M-G: Magnetic resonance imaging in lateral sinus hypoplasia and thrombosis. *Stroke* 1990;**21**:1350–1356.

139. Idbaih A, Boukobza M, Crassard I, et al: MRI of clot in cerebral venous thrombosis: High diagnostic value of susceptibility-weighted images. *Stroke* 2006;**37**:991–995.

140. Ayanzen RH, Bird CR, Keller PJ, et al: Cerebral MR venography: Normal anatomy and potential diagnostic pitfalls. *AJNR Am J Neuroradiol* 2000;**21**:74–78.

141. Ko SB, Kim D-E, Kim SH, Roh J-K: Visualization of venous system by time-of-flight magnetic resonance angiography. *J Neuroimaging* 2006;**16**:353–356.

142. Krayenbuhl H: Cerebral venous thrombosis. The diagnostic value of cerebral angiography. *Schweiz Arch Neurol Neurochir Psychiatry* 1954;**74**:261–287.

143. Kosinski CM, Mull M, Schwartz M, et al: Do normal D-dimer levels reliably exclude cerebral sinus thrombosis? *Stroke* 2004;**35**:2820–2825.

144. Dentali F, Squizzato A, Marchesi C, Bonzini M, Ferro JM, Ageno W: D-dimer testing in the diagnosis of cerebral vein thrombosis: A systematic review and a meta-analysis of the literature. *J Thromb Haemost* 2012;**10**:582–589.

145. Crassard J, Soria C, Tzourio Ch, et al: A negative D-dimer assay does not rule out cerebral venous thrombosis: A series of 73 patients. *Stroke* 2005;**36** 1716–1719.

146. Becker G, Bogdahn U, Gehlberg C, et al: Trans-cranial color-coded real-time sonography of intracranial veins. *J Neuroimaging* 1994;**5**:87–94.

147. Valdueza JM, Schultz M, Harms L, Einhaupl KM: Venous transcranial Doppler ultrasound monitoring in acute dural sinus thrombosis. Report of two cases. *Stroke* 1995;**26**:1196–1199.

148. Chik Y, Gottesman RF, Zeiler SR, Rosenberg J, Llinas RH: Differentiation of transverse sinus thrombosis from congenitally atretic cerebral transverse sinus with CT. *Stroke* 2012;**43**:1968–1970.

149. Saposnik G, Barinagarrementeria F, Brown RD, et al: Diagnosis and management of cerebral venous thrombosis. A statement for healthcare professionals from the American Heart Association/American Stroke Association. *Stroke* 2011;**42**:1158–1192.

150. Einhaupl K, Bousser M-G, de Bruijn SFTM, et al: EFNS guideline on the treatment of cerebral venous and sinus thrombosis. *Eur J Neurol* 2006;**13**:553–559.

151. Canhao P, Cortesao A, Cabral M, et al: Are steroids useful to treat cerebral venous thrombosis? *Stroke* 2008;**39**:105–110.

152. Cundiff DK: Anticoagulants for cerebral venous thrombosis. Harmful to patients? *Stroke* 2014;**45**:298–304.

153. Diaz JM, Schiffman JS, Urban ES: Superior sagittal sinus thrombosis and pulmonary embolism. A syndrome rediscovered. *Acta Neurol Scand* 1992;**86**:390–396.

154. Stansfield FR: Puerperial cerebral thrombophlebitis treated by heparin. *BMJ* 1942;**1**:436–438.

155. Martin JP, Sheenan HL: Primary thrombosis of cerebral veins (following childbirth). *BMJ* 1941;**1**:349.

156. Krayenbuhl H: Cerebral venous and sinus thrombosis. *Clin Neurosurg* 1967;**14**:1–24.

157. Bousser M-G: In a worsening situation, treatment can do more good than harm. *Pratical Neurology* 2003;**3**:112–115.

158. Jacewicz M, Plum F: Aseptic cerebral venous thrombosis. In Einhaupl K, Kempski O, Baethmann A (eds), *Cerebral Sinus Thrombosis: Experimental and Clinical Aspects.* New York: Plenum, 1990, pp 157–170.

159. Einhaupl KM, Villringer A, Meister W, et al: Heparin treatment in sinus venous thrombosis. *Lancet* 1991;**338**:597–600.

160. de Bruijn SF, Stam J: Randomized, placebo-controlled trial of anticoagulant treatment with low-molecular-weight heparin for cerebral sinus thrombosis. *Stroke* 1999;**30**:484–488.

161. Coutinho J, de Bruijn SF, deVeber G, Stam J: Anticoagulation for cerebral venous sinus thrombosis. *Cochrane Database Syst Rev* 2011;**8**:CD002005.

162. Bousser M-G: Cerebral venous thrombosis. Nothing, heparin or local thrombolysis? *Stroke* 1999;**30**:481–483.

163. Canhao P, Falcao F, Ferro JM: Thrombolysis for cerebral sinus thrombosis. A systematic review. *Cerebrovasc Dis* 2003;**15**:159–166.

164. Ciccone A, Canhao P, Falcao F, et al: Thrombolysis for cerebral vein and dural sinus thrombosis. *Cochrane Database Syst Rev* 2004;**1**:CD003693.

165. Stam J, Majoie CB, van Delden OM, et al: Endovascular thrombectomy and thrombolysis for severe cerebral sinus thrombosis: A prospective study. *Stroke* 2008;**39**:1487–1490.

166. Mehraein S, Schmidtke K, Villringer A, et al: Heparin treatment in cerebral sinus and venous thrombosis: patients at risk of fatal outcome. *Cerebrovasc Dis* 2003;**15**:17–21.

167. Masuhr F, Mehraein S: Cerebral venous and sinus thrombosis. Patients with a fatal outcome during intravenous dose-adjusted heparin treatment. *Neurocrit Care* 2004;**1**:355–361.

168. Coutinho JM, Majoie CBLM, Coert BA, Stam J: Decompressive hemicraniectomy in cerebral sinus thrombosis. Consecutive case series and review of the literature. *Stroke* 2009;**40**:2233–2235.

169. Théaudin M, Crassard I, Bresson D, et al: Should decompressive surgery be performed in malignant cerebral venous thrombosis? A series of 12 patients. *Stroke* 2010;**41**:727–731.

170. Weber J, Spring A: Unilateral dekompressive kraniektomie bei thrombose des linken sinus transversus und sigmoideus. *Zentralbl Neurochir* 2004;**65**:135–140.

171. Zuurbier SM, Coutinho JM, Majoie CBLM, Coert BA, van den Munckhof P, Stam J: Decompressive hemicraniectomy in severe cerebral venous thrombosis: A prospective case series. *J Neurol* 2012;**259**:1099–1105.

172. Ferro JM, Crassard I, Coutinho JM, et al: Decompressive surgery in cerebrovenous thrombosis. A multicenter registry and a systematic review of individual patient data. *Stroke* 2011;**42**:2825–2831.

173. Aaron S, Alexander M, Moorthy RK, et al: Decompressive craniectomy in cerebral venous thrombosis: A single centre experience. *J Neurol Neurosurg Psychiatry* 2013;**84**:995–1000.

174. Crassard I, Canhao P, Ferro JM, Bousser M-G, Barinagarrementeria F, Stam J: Neurological worsening in the acute phase of cerebral venous thrombosis in ISCVT (International study on cerebral venous thrombosis). *Cerebrovasc Dis* 2003;**16**:60.

175. Haghighi AB, Edgell RC, Cruz-Flores S, et al: Mortality of cerebral venous-sinus thrombosis in a large national sample. *Stroke* 2012;**43**:262–264.

176. Nasr DM, Brinjikji W, Cloft HJ, Saposnik G, Rabinstein AA: Mortality in cerebral venous thrombosis: Results from the national inpatient sample database. *Cerebrovasc Dis* 2013;**35**:40–44.

177. Canhao P, Ferro JM, Lindgren AG, et al: Causes and predictors of death in cerebral venous thrombosis. *Stroke* 2005;**36**:1720–1725.

178. Ferro JM, Bacelar-Nicolau H, Rodrigues T, et al: ISCVT and VENOPORT Investigators. Risk score to predict the outcome of patients with cerebral vein and dural sinus thrombosis. *Cerebrovasc Dis* 2009;**28**:39–44.

179. Koopman K, Uyttenboogaart M, Vroomen PC, van der Meer J, de Keyser J, Luijckx GJ: Development and validation of a predictive outcome score of cerebral venous thrombosis. *J Neurol Sci* 2009;**276**:66–68.

180. Baumgartner RW, Studer A, Arnold M, Georgiadis D: Recanalisation of cerebral venous thrombosis. *J Neurol Neurosurg Psychiatry* 2003;**74**:459–461.

181. Strupp M, Covi M, Seelos K, Dichgans M, Brandt T: Cerebral venous thrombosis: correlation between recanalization and clinical outcome: A long-term follow-up of 40 patients. *J Neurol* 2002;**249**:1123–1124.

182. Martinelli I, Bucciarelli P, Passamonti SM, Battaglioli T, Previtali E, Mannucci PM: Long-term evaluation of the risk of recurrence after cerebral sinus-venous thrombosis. *Circulation* 2010;**121**:2740–2746.

183. Miranda B, Ferro JM, Canhao P, et al: The ISCVT Investigators. Venous thromboembolic events after cerebral vein thrombosis. *Stroke* 2010;**41**:1901–1906.

184. Palareti G, Cosmi B, Legnani C, et al: PROLONG Investigators. D-dimer testing to determine the duration of anticoagulation therapy. *N Engl J Med* 2006;**355**:1780–1789.

185. Ferro JM, Correia M, Rosas MJ, et al: Seizures in cerebral vein and dural sinus thrombosis. *Cerebrovasc Dis* 2003;**15**:78–83.

186. Ferro JM, Lopez MG, Rosas MJ, Ferro MA, Fontes J: Long-term prognosis of cerebral vein and dural sinus thrombosis: results of the VENOPORT study. *Cerebrovasc Dis* 2002;**13**:272–278.

187. Breteau G, Mounier-Vehier F, Godefroy O, et al: Cerebral venous thrombosis 3-year clinical outcome in 55 consecutive patients. *J Neurol* 2003;**250**:29–35.

188. Koopman K, Uyttenboogaart M, Vroomen PC, et al: Long-term sequelae after cerebral venous thrombosis in functionally independent patients. *J Stroke Cerebrovasc Dis* 2009;**18**:198–202.

189. Madureira S, Canha P, Ferro JM: Cognitive and behavioural outcome of patients with cerebral venous thrombosis. *Cerebrovasc Dis* 2001;**11**:108.

190. de Bruijn, Budde M, Teunisse S, de Haan RJ, Stam J: Long-term outcome of cognition and fuctional health after cerebral venous sinus thrombosis. *Neurology* 2000;**54**:1687–1689.

Stroke prevention

Louis R Caplan and Philip B Gorelick

When meditating over a disease, I never think of finding a remedy for it, but instead a means of preventing it.
Louis Pasteur[1]

Importance of prevention and of public education

Prevention of stroke is much more likely to have a major impact on the health and welfare of the population than even the most effective acute treatments and recurrent stroke preventatives after stroke has occurred. For this reason, much effort should be aimed at identifying and modifying, whenever possible, risk factors for cerebrovascular disease and cardio-vascular disease in general.

Despite these efforts, much of the population is still woefully ignorant about stroke. The medical profession and media have been relatively successful in educating the public about heart attacks, cancer, and acquired immunodeficiency syndrome. Stroke, although the fifth leading cause of death in the United States, has received much less public attention and remains poorly understood by most Americans, and most of the public around the world. Publicity about thrombolysis has increased public awareness about stroke and may increase general knowledge. Surveys and studies show that many individuals throughout the world do not know any of the major symptoms or warning signs of stroke or important stroke risk factors.[2–7] Some do not even know that stroke involves the brain. Many respondents think that strokes are almost invariably permanently disabling.

In the United States, efforts are made to educate the public to call 911 or another specified number if they suspect that they or another person is having a stroke. Sadly, many operators who pick up the phone when 911 is called know little about stroke and do not triage the call as urgent. Furthermore, as few as 1 in 7 adults react properly by electing to call "911" when tested in stroke-related case scenarios, and few are aware that thrombolytic therapy exists, has a time window for treatment from symptom onset of ischemic stroke, and that dialing "911" is indicated.[8,9]

Kothari and colleagues interviewed patients admitted to the emergency room with possible strokes at the University of Cincinnati Medical Center.[4] Their interviews consisted of open-ended questions and were conducted during the first 48 hours after hospital admission. Among 163 patients, 63 (39%) did not know a single symptom or sign of stroke. Unilateral weakness (26%) and numbness (22%) were the most often mentioned symptoms.[4] Persons older than 65 years were less knowledgeable than younger patients.[4] In one study, even when attempts were made to educate patients with transient ischemic attack (TIA) or minor stroke about these conditions, when queried 3 months later, only 15 of 57 (26%) correctly identified the brain as the affected organ and only 21 of 57 (37%) could give a correct description of a TIA or stroke.[6] One study did suggest that gains are being made in public knowledge about stroke. Among 2173 individuals that responded to a survey in Cincinnati, knowledge about stroke warning signs and risk factors improved appreciably between the 1995 and 2000 surveys.[3]

Despite the lack of public knowledge about stroke, an important decline in stroke incidence and mortality occurred during the second half of the twentieth century.[10–13] This fact is probably explained by a number of factors. The public has definitely become more health conscious. Good eating habits; regular exercise; and avoidance of cigarettes, alcohol, and dietary excesses have been an educational and media theme. Reduction in risk factors perceived in the public mind as related to heart attacks has also reduced cerebrovascular disease. Emphasis on check-ups and screenings for high blood pressure, diabetes, and high cholesterol has also had an impact. Physicians' aggressive treatment of hypertension and better technology for assessing vascular disease have also played a role. LRC has tried to do his part in educating the public by writing and publishing four books that are aimed at laymen and primary care physicians.[14–17] Clearly, much more public and physician education are needed for further gains to be made in stroke prevention.

Prevention of stroke is a vast subject. One that we cannot even attempt to do justice to it in this short chapter. Herein we will try to emphasize key topics but will not discuss in any detail specific therapies and treatments. Antithrombotic and other treatments are discussed in detail in Chapter 6.

Prevention strategies

Prevention of stroke and cardiovascular disease has been carried out traditionally by two main approaches.[18] The "high-risk" approach utilizes screening techniques to

Caplan's Stroke: A Clinical Approach, 5th Edition, ed. Louis R Caplan. Published by Cambridge University Press. © Cambridge University Press, 2016.

identify persons at high-risk in the population who besides management of lifestyle factors usually require medication to reduce their stroke and cardiovascular risk factor burden. The "mass" technique, on the other hand, aims to lower the burden of risk factors in the population through legislative and public health measures. An example of the latter approach is the passage of legislation to reduce sodium in the diet of a community to reduce blood pressure and subsequent stroke and cardiovascular disease, and passage of taxes to raise the cost of cigarettes to discourage smoking which is an important cause of stroke and cardiovascular disease. An extreme example of the mass approach was a suggestion offered in the *British Medical Journal* that all individuals 55 and over should take a "polypill."[19] This pill might contain: a statin (e.g., atorvastatin (10 mg daily) or simvastatin (40 mg)); three blood pressure lowering drugs (e.g., a thiazide, a β-blocker, and an angiotensin-converting enzyme inhibitor), each at half the usual dose; folic acid (0.8 mg); and aspirin (75 mg). The authors estimated that this combination would reduce ischemic heart disease events events by 88% and stroke by 80%.[19]

The "mass" approach and the "high risk" approach have limitations and risks, and therefore, both approaches are complementary. The "mass" approach may fail to adequately control risk factors among persons at highest risk who need medication therapy, and the "high-risk" approach may fail to reduce the risk factor burden in those at lower risk as it screens for persons at high risk. Persons at lower risk should not be overlooked as they constitute an important segment of the community because they are so prevalent in the population and account for a high percentage of stroke and cardiovascular events.

Conceptualization of stroke and cardiovascular risk has changed.[20] Rather than explaining risk in relation to a dichotomous category (e.g., hypertension present or not present) or threshold effect (e.g., hypertension as a blood pressure ≥140/90 mmHg), we now address risk based on a continuum. For example, we know that blood pressure is associated with stroke based on a continuous risk relationship which may go down to at least a blood pressure of 115/75 mmHg without evidence of a threshold effect.[21] Therefore, a blood pressure of 190/100 mmHg has a higher relative risk for stroke than a blood pressure of 160/90 mmHg. The risk of stroke in relation to blood pressure remains on a continuum of risk as low as 115/75 mmHg.

In his 2006 Feinberg lecture, Sacco outlined a shift in physician strategy for preventing cerebrovascular disease.[22] Since cardiovascular disease shares most risk factors with cerebrovascular disease, and since cardiac disease poses a risk for brain embolism and hypoperfusion, doctors should evaluate patients for the presence of both cardiovascular and cerebrovascular abnormalities, as well as emphasizing management of treatable risk factors. Optimally the evaluation might include the following:

- Illnesses and behaviors known to increase the risk of vascular disease (for example, smoking, physical inactivity, hypertension, diabetes etc). These are the customary "risk factors" that have long been discussed.

- Subclinical brain lesions (e.g., unexpected infarcts, white matter hyperintensities, microbleeds, etc.)
- Subclinical vascular disease (e.g., carotid artery plaques, arterial intima-media thickness, etc.)
- Biomarkers and genetic findings and conditions known to relate to vascular disease (e.g., fibrinogen, C-reactive protein (CRP), homocysteine levels, etc.)

Extensive information has been accumulated and analyzed regarding risk factors for the general category of stroke[23–33] and brain ischemia.[34–41] With regard to some stroke mechanisms, such as subarachnoid hemorrhage (SAH),[42–46] intracerebral hemorrhage (ICH),[47–50] and brain embolism,[51,52] ample data exist. The causes of hemorrhage are discussed in detail in Chapters 13 and 14. The major risk factors for cardiac-origin embolism are those that predispose to the various cardiac conditions. These are described in Chapter 10. Relatively less information is available about other specific stroke mechanisms, especially within the broad group of patients with brain ischemia. Most analyses of risk factors do not differentiate among patients with stenotic lesions of the extracranial arteries, those with stenosis of the large intracranial vessels, such as the middle cerebral and intracranial vertebral arteries, and those with disease of penetrating arteries, such as the lenticulostriate arteries.

Various risk factors, such as race/ethnicity and sex, have a differential effects on various pathological lesions and on lesions at various loci within the vasculature.[38,53–58] Further data, especially in patients with specific stroke subtypes studied prospectively, are needed. Despite these limitations, the currently identified risk factors are of great significance. These risk factors help identify individuals at risk for stroke in whom modification of lifestyle might reduce the chance of stroke and other cardiovascular diseases. In this section, we only briefly discuss these risk factors. Larger, more detailed reviews of the subject are available.[18,23,25–33] When risk factors are identified, the evidence usually consists of an epidemiological relationship between the factor and the occurrence of stroke; association correlation does not necessarily indicate causation. For example, being female is strikingly associated with becoming pregnant, but clearly this does not cause the condition.

A relatively new concept that Sacco also emphasized in his 2006 Feinberg lecture is the idea of "vascular risk modulators."[22] Doctors and epidemiologists have been accustomed to analyzing various risks as binary variables. For example, an individual is considered to have or not have hypertension if their blood pressure exceeds or falls below a set number such as 140/90 mmHg. Similarly, they are defined as diabetic, or to have hypercholesterolemia if their blood sugar and blood cholesterol levels are above or below arbitrarily designated values. Studies have shown, however, that risk factors are all continuous rather than categorical (yes or no) variables. A systolic blood pressure of 160 carries more risk than 150, and in turn 150 has more risk than 140, and 140 more risk than 130.[22,59] It is simple for clinicians to characterize an individual as hypertensive or not, and obese or not, but this

categorization loses a great deal of information. Risk can often be modulated by reducing blood pressure, blood sugar, weight, and cholesterol levels, even if the present values are considered "within the normal range."

The term "risk factor" refers to factors that heighten risk for a condition and when modified reduce the risk of that condition (e.g., hypertension increases the risk of stroke and treatment of hypertension reduces stroke risk).[59] The term "risk marker," on the other hand, refers to factors that elevate risk for a condition but have not as of yet been shown to reduce that risk because they have either not been tested or efforts at successful modification have failed (e.g.,homocysteine increases the risk of stroke but reduction of homocysteine with B-complex vitamins has not been shown to reduce stroke risk). The two terms are often used interchangeably. In this text, for ease of communication, we will use the two terms interchangeably.

Risk factors (the usual suspects)

Demographic risk factors that are not modifiable

Parents cannot be selected, nor can race/ethnicity and sex. Time cannot be turned back to reverse the aging process. Age, race/ethnicity, sex, and family history of cardiovascular risk factors and disease are among the most important risk factors for stroke.

Age is probably the risk factor best correlated with stroke. The Framingham Study showed that as a person ages, his or her risk of stroke increases, with incidence rates per 10 000 increasing from 22% to 32% to 83% in the age groups 45–55, 55–64, and 65–74 years, respectively.[60] With increasing age, an exponential increase occurs in the frequency of stroke. The great majority of ischemic strokes occur in individuals older than 65 years.[38] The incidence of SAH also rises steadily with age though there is disproportional occurrence of SAH in younger age groups (e.g., women) compared to many other types of stroke.[43] Data on age in patients with ICH also show high frequency in the elderly. Despite the best efforts, aging is inevitable; all of us strive to eventually join the "healthy old aged club." Stroke also occurs in younger patients. In a prior edition of this text we stated that ischemic stroke in patients younger than 45 years is correlated with more frequent cardiac-origin embolism and less common occlusive lesions, whereas in stroke patients older than 65 years, intrinsic large- and small-artery diseases are most common, closely followed by cardiac-origin embolism. Since the fourth edition of this text the International Pediatric Stroke Study Group has reported on arterial ischemic stroke risk factors.[61] Among 676 children aged 29 days to 18 years with stroke who were prospectively enrolled at 30 centers in 10 countries, arteriopathy, defined as any arterial abnormality on vascular imaging other than isolated vessel occlusion, was the most common risk factor (53%) according to age stratified results followed by cardiac disorders (31%), infection (24%), acute head and neck disorders (23%), acute systemic disorders (22%), chronic systemic conditions (19%), and prothrombotic states (13%).

Race/ethnicity and sex also influence the occurrence and subtypes of stroke.[38,53–58] African-Americans and Asians have a higher risk of intracerebral hemorrhage than whites.[47,62] African-Americans, persons of Asian descent, and women may have more intracranial occlusive disease and less extracranial occlusive disease than white men.[53–58] Men have a greater frequency of stroke than women, but because life expectancy is higher in women, overall, more women die of stroke than men and often outnumber men in many stroke studies.[38] Past tradition has taught that during the premenopausal years, women have fewer strokes than men, but the incidence levels off after age 60 years. More recently, however, there has been a substantial rise in rates of stroke among middle-aged women 35–54 years of age that is thought to be accelerated by obesity and factors accompanying obesity such as those that constitute the metabolic syndrome.[63]

The importance of beginning prevention at an early age

A history of stroke or other important cardiovascular disease among first-degree relatives, including coronary artery disease, peripheral vascular disease, and hypertension, is an important risk factor for stroke even after adjustment for other personal stroke risk factors.[64–68] Atherosclerotic lesions often begin at a very young age. Autopsy studies among individuals of varied racial and geographical backgrounds have shown that fatty streaks (yellow lipid deposits that elevate the intima only slightly) are found in the aorta of all groups during infancy and reach a peak in puberty.[69,70] These deposits develop into raised lesions and fibrous plaques in subsequent decades.[69,70] Since familial and genetic factors are quite individual and very important, knowledge of risks and prevention should begin in the young.

One of us (LRC) recalls an informal classroom presentation by a seventh-grade school teacher from the southern part of the United States. During a discussion about health in her classroom, this teacher discovered that few of her students knew about illnesses within their own families. She then gave her students a homework assignment to inquire in detail about the medical conditions that affected close relatives. Doctors volunteered to test the students who were about 12–13 years old for various conditions. Children whose parents both had hypertension had a high frequency of elevated blood pressure themselves. Those with a strong family history of diabetes often had high blood sugars. Children whose family members were overweight, were themselves often far overweight for age and height. Students whose family history included elevated cholesterol levels, frequently had high serum cholesterol levels when tested. In another personal example, a routine examination 30 years ago showed that LRC's cholesterol level was quite high – over 300. When his 6 children (ages 6–18 years at the time) were tested, 5 of them also had abnormally high cholesterol levels. His wife and he then paid careful attention to the children's diets and nutritional behavior.

When neurologists and other physicians care for patients with risk factors and with cardiovascular conditions, such as

myocardial infarcts, strokes, peripheral vascular occlusive disease, high cholesterol, severe hypertension, and diabetes, they should encourage patients to test their children, especially if risk factors have been prevalent in their family histories. It is known that some risk factors are found at relatively early ages, even in children and young adults.[71] In Sweden more than 800 000 young men (18 years of age), evaluated during mandatory military conscription were followed for a median time of 33 years.[72] Risk factors for stroke were often found in these adolescents and these factors highly correlated with the later development of strokes.[72] Finding and modifying risk factors at an early age is far superior to modification only after an index cardiac or cerebrovascular event. The US Department of Health and Human Services in collaboration with the National Heart, Lung and Blood Institute has devised guidelines for cardiovascular health and risk reduction in children and adolescents.[73]

Obesity is a major target for prevention in children and young adults. For example, in young adults, longer duration of overall and abdominal obesity has been associated with subclinical coronary artery disease and its progression in midlife, as measured by coronary artery calcium (CAC) technique. Thus, preventing or delaying the onset of obesity in young adults could lower risk for the development of atherosclerosis later in life.[71,74]

Hypertension

High blood pressure is often referred to as the 'crown jewel' of stroke prevention and the most important modifiable risk factor for stroke. All forms of blood pressure elevation (systolic, diastolic, and combined systolic and diastolic) can raise the risk of stroke. After age, hypertension is the single risk factor that most significantly correlates with stroke. Hypertension plays a role in numerous mechanisms of stroke. Without a prior history of hypertension or cardiomegaly, lacunar infarcts are rarely found at necropsy. The association among hypertension, cardiac disease, and kidney disease is well known. Cardiac and renal pathology contribute to many stroke subtypes. Hypertension plays a role in the degenerative process of atherosclerosis in large blood vessels, resulting in occlusive and artery-to-artery embolic strokes. Hypertension plays a role in the rupture of cerebral aneurysms. Intracerebral hemorrhage in the basal ganglia, thalamus, pons, and cerebellum is most often found in the setting of acute and chronic hypertension.

The literature on hypertension is vast. We hope that some information–opinion short "bites," along with key references that discuss the data in detail, will serve to summarize key points.

1. *Hypertension is extremely common.* Nearly one in three individuals in the United States are estimated to be hyypertensive.[75,76] The prevalence of hypertension increases with age and is more common in blacks than whites, and in women over 65 than in men.[75,76] Figure 18.1 from American Heart Association statistics 2014 displays the prevalence of high blood pressure in men and women by age deciles.[76]

2. *Many individuals with high blood pressure are unaware that they have it; many who are aware are untreated or undertreated.* Awareness and treatment of hypertension are woefully inadequate. The seventh report of the Joint National Committee on Prevention, Detection, Evaluation, and Treatment of High Blood Pressure, issued in 2003, contained the following estimates about individuals in the

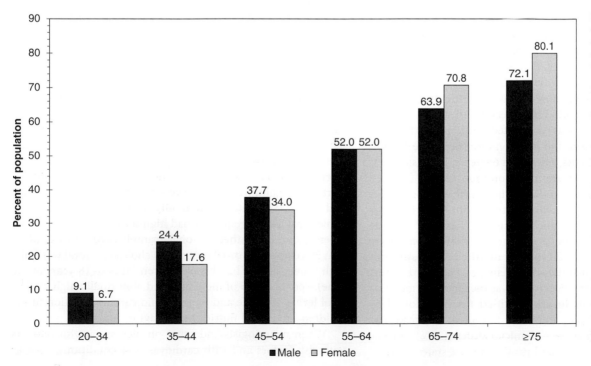

Figure 18.1 Prevalence of high blood pressure in adults aged 20 years or older by age and sex (National Health and Nutrition Examination Survey: 2007–2010). Hypertension is defined as systolic blood pressure ≥140 mmHg or diastolic blood pressure ≥90 mmHg, if the subject said "yes" to taking antihypertensive medication, or if the subject was told on two occasions that he or she had hypertension. Source: National Center for Health Statistics and National Heart, Lung, and Blood Institute: Go AS, Mozaffarian D, Roger VL, et al. Heart diseases and stroke statistics – 2014 update: A report from the American Heart Association. *Circulation* 2014:e28-e92.

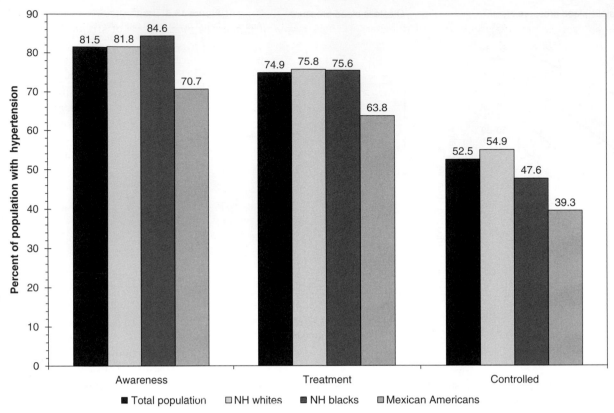

Figure 18.2 Extent of awareness, treatment, and control of high blood pressure by age (National Health and Nutrition Examination Survey: 2007–2010). NH, non-Hispanic. Source: National Center for Health Statistics and National Heart, Lung, and Blood Institute: Go AS, Mozaffarian D, Roger VL, et al. Heart diseases and stroke statistics – 2014 update: A report from the American Heart Association. *Circulation* 2014:e28-e92.

United States: 30% were unaware of hypertension and were untreated, 11% were aware but untreated, 24% were treated but inadequately, and only 35% had blood pressures below the 140/90 mmHg cut-off range.[77] Now, based on more recent data, the estimates of hypertension awareness, treatment and control are 81.5%, 74.9% and 52.5%, respectively.[78] Figure 18.2 has updated figures about hypertension awareness and treatment by age range supplied by the American Heart Association in 2014.[76]

3. *Blood pressure reduction is effective along a range of systolic and diastolic blood pressures, and at all ages, including the elderly.* Figure 18.3 shows the effect of various blood pressures on stroke mortality at various ages.[79] Antihypertensive treatment reduces stroke incidence and mortality in individuals aged over 80 who have high blood pressures.[80–82] In a recent randomized trial, during a mean follow-up period of 1.8 years, among 3845 patients aged 80 or more years (average age 83.6 years), active treatment of hypertension was accompanied by a 30% reduction ($P = 0.06$) in the rate of fatal and non-fatal strokes.[82] The degree of elevation of systolic and diastolic pressure is correlated with the risk of stroke. The risk curve is a continuum without any clear point separating the stroke-prone from the non-stroke-prone individual.

4. *Systolic blood pressure is at least as important and may be more important in promoting stroke and other manifestations of cardiovascular disease as diastolic pressure.*

In the Framingham study, average systolic blood pressure increased by 20 mmHg between ages 30 and 65. Systolic blood pressure continued to rise into the 80s in women and 70s in men.[75] Numerous studies, especially the Systolic Hypertension in the Elderly Program (SHEP)[83–87] show that isolated systolic blood pressure in the elderly is a very important stroke risk factor, and that optimizing systolic blood pressure reduction decreases the risk of stroke.[83–89] An analysis of data from 11 466 men in the Physicians' Health Study concluded that although diastolic blood pressure, pulse pressure, and mean arterial pressure were all significant predictors of stroke risk, none was a significantly better predictor than systolic blood pressure alone.[88]

5. *Blood pressure reduction is as (or more) important in women as it is in men.* For stroke in general and atherothrombotic brain infarction, no evidence exists that shows that women tolerate hypertension better than men. Hypertension is more prevalent in women after age 65 years than in men.[75,90] Women incur as many, if not more, complications of hypertension than men. In women over 65, stroke is the most common vascular event, exceeding myocardial infarction.[91]

6. *Pulse pressure is also very important.* Systolic hypertension is accompanied by increased arterial stiffness and decreased compliance, and as a result diastolic blood pressure often decreases. Pulse pressure is the difference between systolic

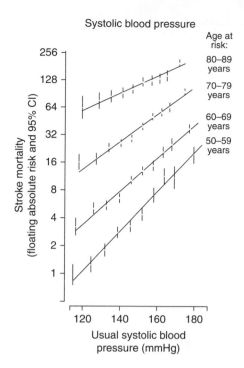

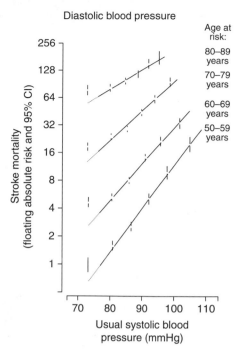

Figure 18.3 The effect of systolic and diastolic blood pressure on mortality from stroke at various ages. Data from Lewington S, Clarke R, Qizilbash N, et al. Prospective studies collaboration. Age-specific relevance of usual blood pressure to vascular mortality: A meta-analysis of individual data for one million adults in 61 prospective studies. *Lancet* 2002;360:1903–1913.

and diastolic pressure. A large pulse pressure may exert its own additional stress on arterial walls. Pulse pressure was an important risk factor for the development of atrial fibrillation in the Framingham study.[92] In one study, mean arterial pressure and pulse pressure were independent predictors of stroke mortality.[93] In other studies pulse pressure was the best predictor of stroke mortality outperforming systolic, diastolic, and mean arterial pressures,[94] and pulse pressure during an acute stroke was an independent predictor of long-term mortality.[95]

7. *Casual blood pressure measurement in a doctor's office are inadequate to quantify the severity of hypertension.* Digital techniques to measure and record blood pressures at home, and at various times and after various circumstances are helpful. The effect of blood pressure on target organs, especially the heart, retina, and kidney are also important in judging the severity and effects of hypertension. Electrocardiograms, echocardiography, measures of renal function, and a careful look at retinal arteries and veins should be part of the evaluation of hypertensive patients. Blood pressure is not a static physiological measure, but rather one that may express variability, a characteristic that is not well tolerated by the brain or brain blood vessels.[96,97]

8. *Twenty-four-hour blood pressure monitoring yields more useful information than casual or even multiple daytime blood pressures.* Blood pressure may not appropriately dip at night (referred to as non-dipping) or often dips too much at night (dipper status). Studies using ambulatory 24-hour blood pressure monitoring have shown that patients with excessively high and abnormally low nocturnal blood pressures and high pulse pressures have a higher frequency of new strokes and hypertension-related white matter damage than patients who have normal nocturnal blood pressures.[98–103]

9. *The type of antihypertensive agent is important.* A variety of different types of antihypertensive agents – diuretics, alpha-blockers, beta-blockers, calcium-channel blockers, angiotensin-converting enzyme (ACE) inhibitors, and angiotensin-receptor binding (ARB) agents – have all proved effective in reducing blood pressure and cardiovascular mortality.[77,104–106] Diuretics are quite effective, especially in African-Americans.[107] Some evidence suggests that ACE inhibitors and ARBs are effective in reversing endothelial dysfunction associated with hypertension, and the combination of an ACE inhibitor and diuretic may be more effective in recurrent stroke reduction than other agents.[108–113] The choice of agent also should consider other comorbidities such as bradycardia, coronary artery disease, renal disease, migraine, and so on because many of the agents that reduce blood pressure also have other cardiovascular effects. Calcium-channel blockers may be a good choice for reducing the risk of a first stroke.[97] Calcium-channel blockers have been shown to be of benefit for stroke reduction in clinical trials and also are known to reduce blood pressure variability as have non-loop thiazide diuretics. Table 18.1 lists recent American College of Cardiology/American Heart Association guidelines recommendations for blood pressure control when there are comorbid conditions.[78]

Heart disease

The incidence of various cardiac diseases is highly correlated with stroke risk. Cardiac disease is a direct cause of stroke when the heart is a donor source of emboli to the brain. Heart disease, usually related to hypertension or coronary artery disease, coexists with hypertensive and atherosclerotic disease

Table 18.1 Recommendations for selection of blood pressure lowering medication according to accompanying cardiovascular comorbidity

1. Coronary artery disease/post-myocardial infarction: BB, ACEI

2. Systolic heart failure: ACEI or ARB, BB, ALDO ANTAG, thiazide diuretic

3. Diastolic heart failure: ACEI or ARB, BB, thiazide diuretic

4. Diabetes: ACEI or ARB, thiazide diuretic, BB, CCB

5. Kidney disease: ACEI or ARB

6. Stroke or TIA: Thiazide diuretic, ACEI

ACEI, angiotensin-converting enzyme inhibitors; ALDO ANTAG, aldosterone antagonist; ARB, angiotensin-receptor blocker; BB, beta blocker; CCB, calcium-channel blocker.

Table 18.2 Components of metabolic syndrome as defined by Proceedings of National Heart, Lung, and Blood Institute and American Heart Association Conference[99]

Abdominal obesity

Atherogenic dyslipidemia

Raised blood pressure

Insulin resistance with or without glucose intolerance

Pro-inflammatory state

Prothrombotic state

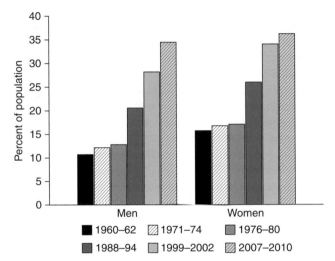

Figure 18.4 Age-adjusted prevalence of obesity in adults ages 20–74 by sex and survey year. (National Health Examination Survey: 1960–1962; National Health and Nutrition Examination Survey: 1971–1974, 1976–1980, 1988–1994, 1999–2002, and 2007–2010). Obesity is defined as body mass index of 30.0 kg/m². Data derived from Health, United States, 2011. Source: National Center for Health Statistics and National Heart, Lung, and Blood Institute: Go AS, Mozaffarian D, Roger VL, et al. Heart diseases and stroke statistics – 2014 update: A report from the American Heart Association. *Circulation* 2014:e28-e92.

of the cervico-cranial arteries in other patients. Cardioembolic stroke occurs in the setting of mitral or aortic valve disease, atrial fibrillation of any cause, prosthetic heart valves, endocarditis, myocardiopathies, akinetic myocardial segments, and ventricular aneurysms. Embolism from cardiac sources is discussed in Chapter 10. Non-valvular atrial fibrillation is the most common cardiac source of brain embolism. Indices of cardiac impairment, such as coronary artery disease, congestive heart failure, and left ventricular hypertrophy as measured by electrocardiography, chest x-ray, and echocardiography, are associated with increased stroke risk. Particularly important is that heart disease is the major cause of death in patients with strokes, TIAs, and carotid artery disease.[114] Stroke is a major risk factor for heart disease even if no overt cardiac disease is observed. Patients with extracranial artery occlusive disease have an especially high frequency of coexistent coronary artery occlusive disease.[115,116] Physicians must carefully consider diligently searching for and treating heart disease in patients with stroke. The treatment of heart disease in association with stroke plays a major role in prolonging life and avoiding significant morbidity.[117]

Obesity, insulin resistance, metabolic syndrome, and diabetes

Doctors, in the past, considered blood glucose levels in a binary fashion – patients were either diabetic or not, and some might be "prediabetic." Now studies show clearly that risk in relation to glucose utilization, like blood pressures, should be considered over a continuum.[118] Glucose metabolism is heavily linked to the secretion and effectiveness of insulin, and to body fat and inflammation. Adipose tissue releases substances that relate to body energy, glucose levels, and insulin effectiveness in controlling glucose utilization. These substances include non-esterified fatty acids, cytokines, and adiponectin.[119] Knowledge of the interrelationship of abdominal obesity to glucose metabolism, insulin sensitivity and resistance, and hypertension has led to definition of a "metabolic syndrome" that represents a very important risk factor for stroke as well as other cardiovascular conditions.[119–126] The components of the metabolic syndrome are listed in Table 18.2. The components of

the metabolic syndrome are also posited to be risk factors for atherosclerosis.

Obesity is an important component of the metabolic syndrome, and data now clearly identifies obesity as a major risk factor for all forms of cardiovascular disease including stroke. There is a major epidemic of overweight, weight gain, and obesity in the United States and many other parts of the world, and now it is estimated that approximately 1 in 3 Americans are obese.[127,128] Figure 18.4 shows changes in the age-adjusted prevalence of obesity in adults between surveys taken from recent surveys in 1960–1962 and 2007–2010.[76] Obesity has often been measured by body mass index (BMI). The BMI is defined as weight in kilograms divided by height in meters squared.[129] A BMI of 30 or higher is a criterion for characterizing someone as obese,[76] and a BMI greater than 30 is an important risk factor for stroke in men and women.[129–131]

The major obesity-related culprit contributing to cardiovascular risk is visceral adipose tissue.[132–134] Visceral adipose tissue can be measured using either modern CT or MRI scanners.[132–134] Although waist circumference is related to both subcutaneous and visceral fat, it correlates quite highly

with the amount of visceral fat and can be used as a convenient surrogate measure of visceral adipose tissue.[132] Some epidemiologists argue that waist circumference should be another vital sign, measured often in those suspected of being overweight. Abdominal obesity as measured by waist circumference is highly associated with an increased risk of developing atherosclerosis and having an ischemic stroke.[131,132,135]

A strong correlation exists between abdominal obesity and insulin resistance. Most obese individuals have postprandial hyperinsulinemia and relatively low insulin sensitivity, although variations are often present within the obese population, and an individual can be insulin resistant and not be obese.[119,120,136,137] Both genetic and fat accumulation contribute to insulin resistance. Obesity also predisposes to an increase in blood markers of inflammation. Inflammation and inflammatory markers are discussed later in this chapter.

Elevation of blood glucose and frank diabetes mellitus have long been known to be associated with an increased risk of atherosclerosis, cardiovascular disease, and ischemic stroke and increased mortality in patients with stroke.[28–39,138–142]

Hypertension is more common among patients with diabetes and in overweight individuals, so that some of the effects attributed to diabetes may be related to accompanying obesity, hypertension, and dyslipidemia. The increased risk of stroke is present in insulin-dependent and non–insulin-dependent diabetic patients and does not diminish with advancing age in either men or women. Diabetes is a risk factor for intracranial and extracranial large artery occlusive disease and penetrating artery disease. Intracranial branch artery atheromatous disease is particularly common among diabetic patients.[143,144] Atheromatous branch disease affects predominantly the paramedian pontine penetrating arteries, anterior choroidal arteries, and anterior inferior cerebellar arteries. Optimizing body weight and glucose metabolism are clearly very important strategies to reduce the risk of stroke. Recent research has identified the endocannabinoid system and the cannabinoid CB_1 receptor as important in determining energy balance and body composition. The CB_1 receptor is an important target for blockade in an attempt to reduce body weight and waist circumference.[145]

Smoking

Convincing epidemiological data strongly relate cigarettes to an increased risk of stroke and extracranial and intracranial atherosclerosis.[146–151] Like blood pressure and blood sugar levels, the exposure to titer of smoking (number of cigarettes/day, number of years of smoking, and current present smoking status) represents a continuum of risk. The increased stroke risk applies to middle-aged and older individuals and men and women, but is especially important in the young. In the Framingham study, smoking was a significant risk factor for atherothrombotic brain infarction only in men younger than 65 years.[152] Paffenbarger and Williams found that smoking was one of the most important risk factors among college students who later had ischemic strokes.[153] Among a series of patients with extracranial carotid artery disease studied at the Mayo Clinic, the total years of cigarette smoking was the single,

most significant, independent predictor of the presence of severe vascular occlusive disease.[148] The duration of cigarette smoking and hypertension were the most important predictors of intracranial internal carotid artery disease in another study.[149]

Stopping smoking mitigates the risk of stroke[154] as it does with other conditions. In a study of Korean men, low cholesterol levels did not confer any lowering of risk against smoking-related atherosclerotic disease.[155] Smoking is an important modifiable risk for ischemic stroke and SAH. In regard to SAH, cigarette smoking seems to be a risk factor in men,[42–46,156] and in women when combined with the use of high-dose estrogen and contraceptive pill use.[43,157] Smoking conveyed the same magnitude of risk for intracerebral hemorrhage as for ischemic stroke among 22 022 men in the Physicians' Health Study.[156]

Genetic factors have recently been found to impact the tendency for tobacco addiction,[158] and the adverse effects of smoking on cardiovascular risks.[159] The risk of stroke begins to revert at about 2 years' time after smoking cessation and reverts to approximately that of a non-smoking population by 5 years after smoking cessation.[160] The posited mechanisms by which smoking increases the risk of stroke include: an increase in blood viscosity and fibrinogen levels, vascular endothelial damage and subsequent formation of atherosclerosis, platelet aggregation, and vasoconstriction.

Elevated blood lipids

Traditionally, abnormalities of blood lipids, especially total cholesterol, triglycerides, and high- and low-density lipoproteins, have been considered less closely correlated with stroke than with coronary heart disease. A possible explanation for the lack of a causal association between dyslipidemia and stroke is the paucity of study by stroke subtype. Intuitively, it is more likely that a lipid-laden extracranial carotid atheromatous plaque would be linked to dyslipidemia than, for example, a stroke caused by a hypercoaguable state or cardiac source embolism from a damaged heart valve. Studies of stroke subtypes that might be influenced by dyslipidemia provides stronger rationale of a causal relationship between lipids and stroke. Some studies do show that elevated low-density lipoprotein cholesterol and low high-density lipoprotein cholesterol levels do increase the risk of stroke.[161–163] Elevated levels of triglycerides are a risk factor for large-artery atherosclerotic stroke.[163] In the Framingham study and others, the risk is primarily shown in patients younger than 55 years old.[164] A relationship between low cholesterol and ICH in Asians has been shown in several reports.[165,166] The risk of ICH is especially high in patients with low cholesterol levels.[167,168] The mechanism of how low cholesterol levels increase the risk for brain infarction and SAH remains obscure. The association has been shown primarily among Asians who have life-long low cholesterol levels. It may not be true for individuals whose cholesterol levels are lowered iatrogenically. Several studies of statin medications have showed that cholesterol lowering can be done effectively and safely.[169–172]

In one large series of more than 350 000 men, a significant relationship existed between morbidity from ischemic stroke

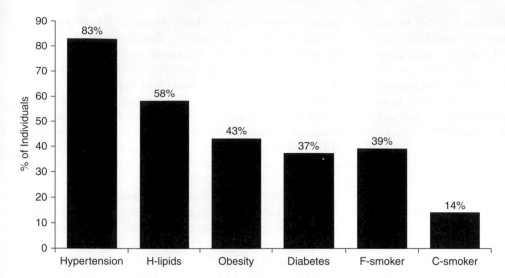

Figure 18.5 Frequency of various risk factors among 18 843 international patients with cerebrovascular disease in the REACH registry. C-smoker, current smoker; F-smoker, former smoker. Data from Bhatt DL, Steg PG, Ohman EM, et al. International prevalence, recognition, and treatment of cardiovascular risk factors in outpatients with atherothrombosis. REACH Registry Investigators. *JAMA* 2006;295:180–189.

and high serum cholesterol levels.[166] Among 27 937 US women in the Women's Health Study, total cholesterol, low-density lipoprotein cholesterol, total cholesterol/high-density lipoprotein cholesterol, and non–high-density lipoprotein cholesterol levels were significantly associated with an increased risk of ischemic stroke.[173] In a study of ischemic stroke mortality among 8586 Israeli men, low high-density lipoprotein cholesterol levels were related to an increased risk of death caused by stroke.[174] Elevated levels of low-density lipoproteins, a decrease in concentrations of high-density lipoproteins, and the presence of lipoprotein(a) correlate better with coronary and extracranial atherosclerosis than do total cholesterol levels.[175,176] Patients with ischemic cerebrovascular disease have an increased frequency of elevated levels of lipoprotein(a).[177] Low levels of high-density lipoprotein cholesterol correlate with carotid atherosclerosis in men,[178] but serum lipids and lipoprotein levels are not as powerful predictors of extracranial internal carotid artery disease as are hypertension and cigarette smoking.[179]

A recently published meta-analysis of trials supports the use of statins for stroke prevention as there is a 22% relative risk reduction for stroke.[180] One of the strongest indicators that cholesterol may have an important role in extracranial and intracranial atherosclerosis and ischemic stroke is the effectiveness of hydroxyl-methyglutaryl-coenzyme A reductase inhibitors (statins) in decreasing the growth of atherosclerotic plaques in the carotid arteries and reducing the incidence of stroke.[181–184] Although these drugs may have effects on plaques and vascular endothelia in addition to their cholesterol-lowering effects, reduction of low-density lipoprotein cholesterol is their predominant action.

Alcohol use

The amount of alcohol that an individual consumes affects his or her stroke risk.[185] Excess alcohol intake increases the risk of brain hemorrhage. Finnish studies, although not well controlled, clearly linked heavy alcohol consumption and recent alcohol use to the occurrence of SAH.[186] ICH can be caused by

the hypoprothrombinemia accompanying cirrhosis of the liver. In the Honolulu Heart Study, alcohol consumption was associated with intracranial hemorrhage, not with ischemic stroke.[165,187]

Most epidemiologists describe a J-shaped curve in relation to alcohol consumption and the risk of ischemic stroke. Light-to-moderate regular consumption of alcohol seems to be inversely related to carotid artery and systemic atherosclerosis, yet acute and chronic heavy use of alcohol increases ischemic stroke risk.[188–190] The effect of alcohol as a stroke risk factor is at least partially explained by the frequent coexistence of hypertension and cigarette smoking.[191,192] The effect of the type of alcohol consumed has not been well studied. In a study performed in Copenhagen, regular wine consumption did confer a protective effect, whereas intake of beer and other spirits did not.[193] The salutary effects of wine have been attributed to its non-alcoholic contents, especially to antioxidant flavonoids and tannins, which are posited to have a protective effect against atherosclerosis.[193–195] Grape juice might have the same effects as alcohol, although this remains a controversial hypothesis that has not been systematically studied. Acute alcohol intoxication may precipitate ischemic strokes and amongst a number of possible mechanisms, temporary myocardial dysfunction (which can eventually become permanent – alcoholic cardiomyopathy) and cardiac rhythm disturbances such as atrial fibrillation ("holiday heart" syndrome) can promote occurrence of ischemic stroke.[196–200]

Figure 18.5 shows the relative frequency of the various risk factors discussed so far in the REduction of Atherothrombosis for Continued Health (REACH) registry.

Symptomatic atherosclerosis of coronary and peripheral limb arteries

Peripheral vascular arterial occlusive disease is a strong predictor of extracranial cerebrovascular and coronary artery disease. Patients with claudication and peripheral arterial disease have a high frequency of stroke and cardiovascular

mortality.[201–203] We have already commented earlier in this chapter on the close association between coronary artery and extracranial arterial disease and stroke. An old plumber's adage may hold true here; "rotten in the basement, rotten in the attic." When the plumbing pipes (i.e., large peripheral arteries) are blocked in the basement (i.e., legs), they are likely to be blocked in the attic (i.e., coronary and cerebral circulations). Peripheral vascular disease serves as a marker of risk for cerebral and coronary atherosclerosis.

Transient ischemic attacks

When properly diagnosed, TIAs are an indication that occlusive cerebrovascular disease has already become established. With development of CT and MRI scanning in the 1970s and 1980s, it became evident that many patients with clinical TIAs have brain imaging evidence of infarction in regions that correlate with the symptoms.[204–206]

When modern advanced MRI technology became available in the 1990s, the frequency of positive diffusion-weighted MRI images in patients with clinical TIAs was even higher than that seen previously.[207,208] Inatomi and colleagues studied 129 consecutive TIA patients. among whom 57 patients (44%) had positive diffusion-weighted image lesions appropriate to the neurological symptoms.[208] When the TIAs lasted more than 30 minutes and contained a higher cortical function abnormality, the likelihood of a positive diffusion-weighted image lesion was high.[208]

Risk factors and prognosis are similar for patients with TIAs and those with minor strokes because the underlying vascular diseases are the same.[209] Many studies in varied populations have shown that TIAs carry a very substantial risk of imminent brain infarction and should be handled emergently.[210–218] Johnston et al. analyzed the outcomes among 1707 patients with TIAs who presented to emergency departments in 16 California hospitals.[210] During the 90 days after the emergency room visit, 180 patients (10.5%) returned with a stroke, occurring in half the patients within the first 2 days.[210] Daffertshofer and colleagues collected data from 82 German hospitals.[211] Among 1380 TIA patients seen during a 6-month period, stroke frequency during the hospital stay was 8% and another 5% of TIA patients had a stroke within the first half-year.[211] Kleindorfer et al. performed a population-based study of 1023 TIA events among 927 individuals occurring in the Cincinnati-northern Kentucky region during 1 year.[212] Within 6 months of the index TIA, 144 patients had an ischemic stroke and 77 died. The median time for stroke to develop was 12 days.[212] Hill et al. reviewed data from Alberta, Canada during a 1-year period.[213] Stroke occurred in 15.1% of TIA patients within 1 year; half of the risk at 1 year was accrued within the first 38 days.[213] Rothwell and Warlow used a different approach.[214] A retrospective review of 2146 stroke admissions in the United Kingdom showed that a preceding TIA was present in 23%; 17% of TIAs occurred on the day of the stroke, 9% on the preceding day, and 43% during the preceding week.[214]

The largest data bank of TIA patients has recently been collected as part of a TIA registry.[215] Sixty one sites in 21 countries across Europe, South America, the Middle East, and Asia enrolled 4789 patients during a 2½ year period. Among these patients 90% were examined within 24 hours in a location dedicated to rapidly evaluating individuals who had a TIA. Many had brain infarcts and cardiac and vascular lesions that needed urgent management. Overall 33.2% of patients had an acute infarct, 23.2% had 1 or more extra-or intracranial stenosis at 50% or greater, or occlusion, and 10.4% had atrial fibrillation or flutter. At 1 year, a total of 257 patients had at least 1 primary outcome (event rate of 6.1% (95%CI, 5.4–6.9%)).[215]

The data are quite clear and consistent. A TIA is a major risk factor for imminent stroke and is a true medical emergency.[217] Patients with clinical TIAs who have infarcts on brain imaging may have an especially high risk of stroke soon after the TIA.[218]

For the individual patient, failure to recognize that a TIA has occurred and failure to diagnose and treat potentially remediable abnormalities can be a great personal and family tragedy. All too often, patients do not understand the importance of temporary focal nervous system and ocular symptoms (fallacy: if it is temporary, it must be benign). Patients often do not report these transient symptoms to their physicians. In our experience, general physicians often reassure patients that the spells are not important. When the nature of the spells is correctly identified, treatment often involves automatic prescription of the latest panacea for ischemic stroke (i.e., oral anticoagulation warfarin, vasodilators, and aspirin). Thoughtful and thorough evaluation of the cause in the individual patient followed by treatment of the specific TIA mechanism is essential.

The definition of TIA has changed over time and now emphasizes the typical short nature of the spells (often times <1 h in duration) and the importance of neuroimaging to define any tissue-based component of brain ischemia.[219,220]

Clinical (ABCD2)[221] and clinical plus neuroimaging (ABCD3-I)[222] scores have been developed to predict stroke risk, especially early stroke risk, after TIA but in our opinion the ABCD scores should not be used to exclude patients from thorough evaluation by physicians experienced and knowledgeable about stroke.[223] The ABCD2 score was generated to screen patients who present with TIAs. The statistics derive from the frequency of the later development of strokes. Individuals with a low score are posited to have a low frequency of stroke in the ensuing days after a TIA. Admission to hospital or rapid evaluation by stroke specialists is often recommended for an ABCD2 score of 4 or more. The components of the score are all general risk factors. One analysis found that TIA patients with an ABCD2 score of less than 4 had similar 90-day stroke risks as those with scores of greater than 4.[224] My colleagues and I (LRC) analyzed the predictive use of the ABCD2 score among 121 consecutive TIA patients.[225] Those with an ABCD2 score of 3 or less had an equal chance of requiring urgent in-hospital interventions as those with a score of 4 to 7.[225] Omitted entirely in the score is the etiology and mechanism of the transient brain ischemia. Very divergent causes – atrial fibrillation, carotid artery

stenosis and occlusion, basilar artery occlusion, arterial dissection, penetrating artery disease, and even brain aneurysms – can cause TIAs as well as important brain injury in the ensuing hours and days after a TIA. Preventive treatment is often available that is relatively specific for etiology. Early diagnosis and treatment soon after TIA has been shown to substantially reduce the risk of stroke after TIA.[215,223,226]

Hormones and oral contraceptive use

Most of the data that attributed a risk of stroke to the use of oral contraceptives were acquired in patients who used pills with a relatively high estrogen content (50 μg of ethinyl estradiol or estranes).[227–230] In these studies, hypertension, migraine, diabetes, hyperlipidemia, cigarette smoking, age older than 35 years, and prolonged use of oral contraceptive pills compounded the risk of ischemic stroke in oral contraceptive users. Lower-dose estrogen (20–40 μg of ethinyl estradiol) combined with newer progestational drugs are now usually prescribed as oral contraceptive agents. Studies show that young women who take these lower-dose pills do not have an important increased risk of stroke.[231–234] Contraceptive patches that contain 35 μg of ethinyl estradiol did not increase the risk of ischemic stroke or myocardial infarction in one study.[235] Among users of low-dose contraceptives, strokes most often occur in older women who have other stroke risk factors, such as hypertension and cigarette smoking.[236] Genetics also play a role, but this has been inadequately explored. Patients with prothrombin gene mutations have an increased risk of stroke when they take oral contraceptives.[237] The presence of factor V Leiden; prothrombin gene mutations; other causes of resistance to activated protein C; abnormalities of antithrombin, protein C, and protein S; and other genetic-related disorders of coagulation proteins might make women who take oral contraceptives or smoke cigarettes especially susceptible to thrombosis.

In a 2012 publication on hormonal contraceptive use and cardiovascular outcomes from a 15-year Danish cohort study of women 15–49 years old, the absolute risks of thrombotic stroke and myocardial infarction associated with hormonal contraception were low.[238] The risk increased depending on the dose of ethinyl estradiol, but there were relatively small differences based on progestin type. Risk increased by a factor of 0.9–1.7 with ethinyl estradiol at a dose of 20 μg but by a factor of 1.3–2.3 with ethinyl estradiol at a dose of 30–40 μg.[238]

The influence of female hormones on stroke frequency and subtypes has also been explored by studies on pregnancy and stroke.[230] Women with six or more pregnancies are at a higher risk for stroke and cerebral infarction than women who have had fewer pregnancies.[239] One study showed that the risk of stroke was not increased during pregnancy, but the risk of brain infarction and brain hemorrhage were significantly increased during the 6 weeks after delivery.[240] The risk of cerebral venous thrombosis is especially high during the puerperium.

The most controversial hormone-related topic relates to the risk of stroke in postmenopausal women who were prescribed hormone replacement therapy.[230] Four published

cohort studies revealed a neutral or minor effect of hormonal replacement. One study, National Health and Nutrition Examination Survey (NHANES), showed a protective effect on stroke, a relative risk of 0.69,[241] while the others – the Nurses Health Study,[242] Danish Nurse Study,[243] and Framingham study[244] – showed a small relative risk of stroke.

Randomized controlled trials showed that hormone replacement therapy did increase the risk of stroke.[245–250] The Heart and Estrogen/Progestin Replacement Study (HERS) studied women who were given conjugated equine estrogen (Premarin)/medroxyprogesterone (Provera) or placebo and had one or more cardiovascular risk factors.[245,246] Overall there was no significant difference in strokes, but a 1.6 relative risk for fatal strokes. The Women's Estrogen Stroke Trial (WEST) studied 1 mg of 17-beta estradiol (Estrace) versus placebo as hormonal replacement in postmenopausal women.[247] There was no overall difference in strokes or deaths between groups, but there was an increased incidence of strokes during the first 6 months in the Estrace replacement group (relative risk of 2.3; 95% confidence interval, 1.1–5.0).[247] The Women's Health Initiative (WHI), which included 162 000 post-menopausal women aged 50–79, was the largest study.[248,249] The cumulative hazards for stroke were 1.3 in an intention-to-treat analysis and 1.5 in an on-treatment analysis.[248,249] Another study within the WHI studied 10 739 post-menopausal women who had hysterectomies and were treated with either conjugated equine estrogen (Premarin) or placebo.[250] There was no impact on heart disease, but there was an increased frequency of venous thrombosis and stroke in the Premarin-treated group.[250]

Under the umbrella of the US Preventive Services Task Force a systematic review was carried out on menopausal hormone therapy for primary prevention of chronic conditions.[251] The reviewers concluded that menopausal hormone therapy with estrogen plus progestin and estrogen therapy alone decreased the risk of fractures but increased the risk for stroke, thromboembolic events, gallbladder disease, and urinary incontinence. Combined estrogen–progesterone therapy increased the risk for breast cancer and dementia, but estrogen alone decreased the risk of breast cancer.[251] The timing of the introduction of hormonal replacement therapy is posited to be potentially important. Hormonal replacement therapy may be indicated in a critical time window whereby early post-menopausal therapy for a limited period of time may be beneficial.[252] The North American Menopause Society has previously supported initiation of hormone therapy (estrogen therapy alone is favored by virtue of its safety profile) around the time of menopause for the treatment of menopause-related symptoms and to prevent osteoporosis in women at high risk of fractures for up to 3–5 years.[253] The US Preventive Services Task Force, however, has recommended against the use of combined estrogen–progesterone and estrogen therapy alone for the prevention of chronic conditions, respectively, in women who are post-menopausal or who have had a hysterectomy.[254] In a 2013 publication from the Women's Health Initiative Memory Study in Younger Women (WHIMSY), among those who were 50–55 years of

age at the time of assignment of hormone therapy or placebo and followed for a mean of 7.2 years after treatment was halted, there was no evidence of key worsening of cognitive function related to hormonal use suggesting no ill effect of hormonal therapy on cognition in these relatively younger women treated in an early time window.[255]

Sedentary lifestyle and lack of exercise

The effect of physical activity and exercise on health and disease has been the focus of much attention. In a study of 7735 British middle-aged men, regular, moderate-degree physical activity reduced the risk of stroke and heart attacks, but more vigorous physical activity did not confer any further protection.[256] Similarly, in the North Manhattan Stroke Study,[257] Copenhagen City Heart Study,[258] Reykjavik (Iceland) Study,[259] and in patients in Seoul, Korea,[260] participation in at least moderate-degree physical activity had a protective effect against stroke when compared with individuals who did not exercise regularly. This finding was true for men and women. Lee and Paffenbarger studied the relationship between physical activity (walking, climbing stairs, sports participation, and recreational physical activities) and stroke risk among 11 130 men who were Harvard University alumni.[261] They found that decreased stroke risk was found at energy expenditures of 1000–1999 kcal per week, with further decrements found at 2000–2999 kcal per week. Higher rates of exercise did not further decrease the risk of stroke.[261] In the Physicians Health Study among 21 823 male physicians, regular exercise that was vigorous enough to produce a sweat was associated with decreased stroke risk.[262] In the Nurses Health Study, among 72 488 female nurses, physical activity including moderate-intensive exercise such as walking was associated with substantial reduction in risk of total and ischemic stroke.[263] A meta-analysis of 23 studies concluded that there was strong evidence that moderate and high levels of physical activity were associated with reduced risk of total, ischemic, and hemorrhagic stroke.[264] The mechanism by which exercise decreases stroke risk is likely multifactorial, reducing hypertension,[265–267] weight, and lipids, and increasing cerebral blood flow by a salutary effect on cerebral endothelial activity.[268]

A 2013 guideline statement from the American College of Cardiology/American Heart Association recommended moderate to vigorous physical activity for about 40 minutes per session at a frequency of 3–4 sessions on average per week to reduce LDL-cholesterol and non-HDL cholesterol and to lower blood pressure.[269] Through exercise it is estimated that one must burn 3500 calories to lose 1 pound. The target heart rate during exercise is 60–85% of the maximum for age or about 220 minus one's age. Working up sweat may be an alternate and practical target to assure adequacy of exercise, but breathing so hard that one cannot sing a tune, may be considered overdoing exercise. One must be cautious when exercising as there is risk of bodily injuries or other complications if exercise is too vigorous for an individual's ability.

Geographical location

In the United States, physicians and epidemiologists have long been aware of a so-called "stroke belt." This region of high incidence of stroke and stroke mortality is located within the southeastern portion of the United States, with extreme mortality rates in Georgia and the Carolinas.[270–272] Clusters of regions with high stroke mortality rates also exist along the Mississippi and Ohio river valleys.[270] Residence in these regions conveys to men and women of all races/ethnicities a strikingly higher rate of stroke than in other locations within the United States.[271] The excess stroke risk for individuals living in the stroke belt seems limited to those who were there during childhood and not those who moved there as adults.[272] Hypertension is very common in these regions, especially among blacks.[273]

The reason for the presence of such a stroke belt has remained mostly obscure, but many factors, such as the genetic makeup of the people; distribution of stroke risk factors, including hypertension and cigarette smoking; dietary habits; and even constituents of the water have been posited.[274] A US National Institutes of Health study called Reasons for Geographical and Racial Differences in Stroke (REGARDS) is seeking explanations for these phenomena. The reader is referred to the REGARDS website where there is a posting of numerous publications emanating from the study that attempt to elucidate why there are geographical and racial differences in stroke in the US (www.regardsstudy.org).

Subclinical brain, eye, and systemic lesions and vascular and hematological findings that indicate the presence of vascular disease and vascular risks

Modern brain imaging often reveals abnormalities related to vascular diseases even when an individual has not had a known stroke. The most important vascular-related abnormalities are unexpected brain infarcts, white matter lesions, and cerebral microbleeds. Any of these findings indicate that a vascular process is biologically active despite the fact that there is no history of a stroke.

Unexpected brain infarcts

CT and MRI scans very often reveal definite brain infarcts even when the patient gives no history of stroke. In the Rotterdam Scan Study, a population-based cohort study of 1077 individuals aged 60–90, "silent brain infarcts" were five times more common than symptomatic brain infarcts.[275] Although these have traditionally been called "silent infarcts," we prefer the term *unexpected infarcts*. Often these infarcts were not truly silent but were not suspected by the individual who ordered the brain image. In our experience, even though the patient may not give a history of having had a stroke, a wife or other accompanying person will remind the patient of an incident (e.g., "Don't you remember at Ms X's house, you stumbled and had difficulty walking for a few days, and then got better.").

Often symptoms had been present but were misinterpreted as arthritis, the flu, too much alcohol, and so on. In other patients, findings on neurological examination give strong evidence of past brain vascular-related damage, but the patient and his or her family relate no history of one or more acute events. Whether brain infarcts are truly silent depends very much on the zeal and time spent by the examiner in taking a detailed history from the patient and significant others and careful examination of the patient as well as the size and location of the brain infarcts. The importance of questioning the patient and family about possible past stroke symptoms was emphasized by the REGARDS study group under the clinical rubric "whispering" stroke symptoms.[276] So-called "silent strokes" are not always silent and they are associated with an elevated risk of cognitive impairment and subsequent clinically manifest stroke.[276]

Unexpected brain infarcts are seen more often on T2-weighted and FLAIR MRI scans than on brain CT scans.[276,277] These infarcts fall into two large groups with varying significance: small deep infarcts (lacunes), and cortical or cortical and subcortical infarcts. Lacunes are often accompanied by white matter hyperintensities. These lesions give evidence that the patient has a biologically active process that has already damaged the brain. Usually this means inadequately controlled hypertension, diabetes, or polycythemia. Cortical–subcortical infarcts mean that the individual must harbor a source of embolism or hypoperfusion in the cardiac–aortic–extracranial–intracranial pathway that supplies the infarct. This should lead to a search for one or more culprit vascular lesions along this vascular pathway. The many manifestations of small vessel disease as captured by modern neuroimaging techniques have been operationalized and are discussed by a distinguished study group elsewhere.[278]

White matter lesions

Abnormal intensity of the white matter is often found on brain imaging scans of elderly individuals. CT often shows periventricular hypodensities. On MRI, the findings are more obvious and dramatic, with zones of periventricular increased density on T2-weighted images and patchy white matter abnormalities.[279] Often these periventricular abnormalities are related to Alzheimer's disease, especially if the lesions are uniform and surround the ventricles. In some other patients, the periventricular lesions represent transependymal flow of CSF and not active vascular disease. When the white matter abnormalities are irregular and are located in the corona radiata or centrum semi-ovale and jut out from the periventricular area into these regions, then active vascular disease is present. Most often the underlying condition is one that predisposes to penetrating artery disease – hypertension, diabetes, or hyperviscosity.[280–283] In some patients, these white matter lesions are attributable to cerebral amyloid angiopathy, especially when small hemorrhages are also evident on T2*-weighted MRI images.[284–286] White matter abnormalities are often seen before clinical symptoms in patients with CADASIL.[287–289] These white matter abnormalities and conditions that cause them are discussed in more detail in Chapter 9 on penetrating artery disease.

Brain microbleeds

Echo planar MRI scans often show small old lesions that image as discrete, black, usually round abnormalities. These black regions indicate that hemosiderin or blood is present. Some of these discrete black images are small blood vessels cut transversely. These abnormalities are often referred to as *microbleeds*. Some likely represent hemosiderin within or adjacent to small infarcts and are not truly bleeds in the strict sense. Others are tiny dot hemorrhages.[290–292] The two most common conditions that produce small hemorrhages are hypertension and cerebral amyloid angiopathy. Hypertension usually causes deep microbleeds and cerebral amyloid angiopathy causes mostly cortically-based ones. Microbleeds are often accompanied by white matter abnormalities in patients with cerebral amyloid angiopathy and are likely predictive of future hemorrhages.[290] Bacterial endocarditis is another condition known to cause microbleeds that are scattered.[293] Some lesions that appear black on echo planar MRI represent cavernous angiomas. These are usually larger than the average microbleed.

Other target organ vascular damage

The retina provides ready access to view blood vessels, and, is supplied by the internal carotid artery that also supplies the brain. Old retinal infarcts, Hollenhorst plaques and other retinal emboli,[294,295] and the presence of venous stasis retinopathy[296,297] provide evidence of a potential embolic source or severe occlusive disease in the heart-aorta-carotid-ophthalmic artery pathway. These and other ocular signs of carotid artery disease are discussed and illustrated in Chapters 3 and 7.

Recently one of us (LRC) was surprised to find on abdominal imaging (often done for belly pain and not neurological reasons) discrete infarcts in the spleen, kidneys, or other visceral organs. One such patient had bacterial endocarditis, and another had intermittent atrial fibrillation that was not suspected until after the abdominal scans were interpreted. We know that systemic embolisms to peripheral and visceral locations are often present but difficult to diagnose clinically. In one study, among 27 consecutive patients with non-valvular atrial fibrillation, 6 had subdiaphragmatic visceral infarcts on diffusion-weighted abdominal MRI imaging (3 recent renal, 1 recent splenic, and 3 old splenic infarction).[298] The median time between onset of ischemic stroke and abdominal MRI was 8 days (range 3–15 days).[298] The presence of visceral infarcts gives strong evidence of a source of embolism in the heart or aorta. Abdominal imaging has often been useful in seeking such evidence of systemic embolization in puzzling cases.

Subclinical cardio-cervico-cranial-hematological lesions

Physicians are now able to detect many different cardio-vascular-hematological lesions that, although not known to have caused strokes, pose risks for causing brain damage. We list some of these in Table 18.3.

Table 18.3 Subclinical cardiac-cervico-cranial-hematological lesions

Cardiac valvular lesions
Myocardial infarcts
Myocardiopathies with poor ejection fractions
Atrial fibrillation
Aortic atheromas
Plaques or stenosis of carotid and/or vertebral arteries in neck
Carotid intima-media thickness
Stenosis of intracranial arteries
Dolichoectasia of intracranial arteries
Unruptured aneurysms
Polycythemia or anemia
Thrombocytosis or thrombocytopenia
Hypercoagulability

Cardiac and aortic lesions

Many cardiac conditions pose a risk for stroke. The heart often serves as an embolic source. Furthermore, coronary artery disease often parallels extracranial vascular occlusive disease and itself poses strong health and mortality risks for patients. Electrocardiogram (ECG) can detect regions of myocardial hypertrophy and ischemic damage and identify arrhythmias. In patients suspected of having an arrhythmia, ambulatory cardiac rhythm monitoring can document atrial fibrillation, sick-sinus syndrome, and other important rhythm disturbances. Transthoracic echocardiography yields a good image of the cardiac valves and ventricles and can show areas of akinesis, hypokinesis, and generalized cardiac dysfunction with a low ejection fraction. Transesophageal echocardiography (TEE) shows the atria, and is useful in identifying cardiac septal abnormalities as well as providing a view of the aortic arch and ascending aorta. Large aortic plaques are readily visible on TEE. CT angiography (CTA) can show the aortic arch in more detail than TEE and can identify calcifications and plaques.[299]

Non-invasive coronary artery imaging using modern electron-beam CT or MRI can show coronary artery calcifications that correlate well with coronary artery occlusive disease. Coronary angiography is sometimes useful even in asymptomatic patients in whom the ECG, echocardiography, stress testing, or non-invasive vascular imaging gives rise to a strong suspicion of important coronary artery disease. Cardiac evaluation is discussed in more detail in Chapter 4 on diagnosis and Chapter 10 on brain embolism.

Abnormalities in cervico-cranial and intracranial arteries that supply the brain

Patients with extracranial carotid and vertebral artery plaques and thickened arterial walls have atherosclerosis, and thus have a higher risk of ischemic strokes and brain and retinal infarcts.[300–302] The risk increases proportionally to the severity of arterial stenosis and also correlates with the presence of ulcerated carotid artery plaques. Narrowing and plaques within the proximal portion of the vertebral artery also correlate with the presence of carotid artery and coronary artery disease.[301,302] The availability of duplex carotid and vertebral artery ultrasound scanning makes it possible to objectively detect and measure the severity of atherosclerotic abnormalities within the neck arteries. The intima-media thickness of the carotid artery is also an important parameter to study since increased thickness correlates with atherosclerotic disease. The progression or regression of these abnormalities during and after treatment gives clinicians a means of monitoring the atherosclerotic process in the arteries studied. Although epidemiological studies have shown an association between neck bruit and risk of stroke, which may be caused by a mechanism other than ipsilateral carotid occlusive disease, and myocardial infarction, the presence of a neck bruit may be caused by other factors (e.g., hyperdynamic flow state, transmitted heart murmur) and, thus, should not be used as a risk factor because some bruits are not associated with carotid or vertebral artery disease. Ultrasound studies should be performed in patients who have bruits thought to indicate atherosclerotic narrowing to identify and quantify the disease. MRA and CTA are other relatively non-invasive techniques able to provide useful images of the cervical brain-supplying arteries. The strategy to study asymptomatic carotid stenosis either in various populations or in those with audible cervical bruits, is not recommended as the yield is low and would lead to false positive findings and unnecessary diagnostic testing and treatments.

The intracranial arteries can also be studied effectively using Doppler techniques (transcranial Doppler (TCD)) and CTA and MRA. Occlusive lesions, vasoconstriction, and dolichoectasia can all be identified and monitored, often before a stroke develops. At times these diagnostic techniques also show aneurysms that have not ruptured, yielding an opportunity to prevent devastating subarachnoid hemorrhage. Vascular imaging is discussed in detail in Chapter 4.

Hematological abnormalities

Polycythemia and severe anemia both predispose to stroke and cerebral venous occlusions. Thrombocytosis and thrombocytopenia also convey important stroke risks. A complete blood count including a platelet count and a prothrombin time reported as an international normalized ratio (INR) should be part of the routine evaluation for stroke risk. Hematological and other blood screening testing is discussed at length in Chapter 4.

Biomarkers and genetic findings and conditions known to relate to vascular disease

Results of blood and urine tests of certain factors also correlate with the probability of an individual developing a stroke. These

Table 18.4 Biomarkers that correlate with cardiovascular and cerebrovascular disease

Hematocrit
White blood count
C-reactive protein (CRP)
Homocysteine
Erythrocyte sedimentation rate (ESR)
Fibrinogen
Albuminuria
Lipoprotein-associated phospholipase A$_2$ (LpPLA2)

are listed in Table 18.4. These biomarkers have also been discussed in Chapter 4. Pathologically elevated and high normal hematocrits have been associated with increased stroke and TIA risk even when hypertension and cigarette smoking are accounted for in the analysis.[303,304] High hemoglobin levels are also correlated with the presence of brain infarction[305] and larger brain infarcts.[306] This correlation might be partly caused by the fact that chronic hypoxemia, pulmonary disease, and smoking may have caused high hematocrits. The adverse effect of high hematocrits could also relate to increased whole-blood viscosity.[306,307] Cerebral blood flow nearly doubles when a hematocrit of 45 is lowered to 35.

The white blood cell (WBC) count is often elevated in patients with myocardial infarction and is also often slightly high in patients with brain infarcts. In the Northern Manhattan Study, there was an increased risk of ischemic stroke with each quartile of WBC even after adjusting for other stroke risk factors.[308] A high WBC count has been correlated with the severity of carotid atherosclerosis[309] and carotid[310] and aortic arch plaque thickness,[311] but interpretation of this finding is clouded by the fact that cigarette smoking is one cause of a high WBC count. A high WBC at entry into the Warfarin-Aspirin Symptomatic Intracranial Disease (WASID) trial was associated with an increased risk of stroke and vascular death when compared with patients with the lowest quartile of WBC counts.[312] Patients with elevated WBC counts also have reduced endothelial reactivity.[313] A high WBC count is also a marker of inflammatory activity in the body and inflammation is an important cause of blood vessel damage.[314]

Both acute and chronic infection have been linked to elevated stroke risk. Acute infections, particularly respiratory ones, may precipitate stroke by hypercoaguable mechanisms, and chronic infections have been linked to formation of atherosclerotic plaques.[315] By capturing the number of exposures to infection over time an infectious burden scale can be created and may be a better metric to capture risk of stroke related to infection.[315]

Elevated, high-sensitivity C-reactive protein levels correlate with a risk of stroke, cardiovascular disease, and carotid and intracranial large-artery atherosclerosis.[316–318] Some patients with significant atherosclerotic lesions have normal lipids but high CRP levels, indicating the likely importance of inflammation in contributing to their vascular disease. An inflammatory marker that is specific to blood vessel inflammation, lipoprotein-associated phospholipase A2 (LpPLA2), is a useful marker to determine risk of stroke and myocardial infarction.[319]

The plasma level of fibrinogen is also an important determinant of stroke risk. Individuals with high levels of fibrinogen have an increased risk of developing myocardial infarction and stroke.[320–322] Fibrinogen levels relate to age, sex, female hormone status, smoking, body weight, alcohol intake, and the presence of vascular and inflammatory diseases.[321] Fibrinogen is an important participant in the development of red and white thrombi. Along with the hematocrit, fibrinogen is an important determinant of whole-blood viscosity.[322,323]

Elevated levels of plasma homocysteine increase the risk of developing myocardial infarction and stroke.[324–327] The risk is important especially when the homocysteine level is very high. High plasma homocysteine levels and low concentrations of folic acid and vitamin B$_6$ (probably because of their role in homocysteine metabolism) are associated with increased risk of large artery atherosclerosis.[328,329] There is also an association with penetrating artery disease.[329] We have seen several patients with very high homocysteine levels (>40) that had repeated penetrating artery-related lacunar strokes. Unfortunately, reduction of homocysteine level by B-complex vitamins has not been shown to reduce risk of recurrent stroke, but most patients in these studies had no or modestly elevated homocysteine levels.[330,331]

Glycosuria and heavy proteinuria predispose to stroke. Even relatively small amounts of protein in the urine (microalbuminuria) and reduced glomerular filtration rate are risk factors for stroke.[331–335] Chronic kidney disease is also associated with brain white matter hyperintensities.[336] In a study of 186 older men and women (average age, 65 years), the presence of microalbuminuria (20–200 mg/l) was three times more prevalent in patients with recent stroke when compared with normal, healthy individuals and individuals with risk factors for stroke who did not have a recent stroke.[332] Tight control of blood glucose has been associated with reduction of microvascular complications such as retinopathy, nephropathy, and peripheral neuropathy, but not macrovascular disease such as stroke or myocardial infarction, One study, however, showed that intensive, multifactorial, therapeutic interventions in patients with non-insulin-dependent diabetes and microalbuminuria did decrease the incidence of macrovascular events (myocardial infarcts and stroke).[333]

Genetic conditions

Some genetic disorders, such as Fabry's disease, homocystinuria, Ehlers–Danlos syndrome, and pseudoxanthoma elasticum, are recognized to confer increased stroke risk. Various genetically-related disorders affect blood coagulability including factor V Leiden and a prothrombin gene mutation. Research on genetic determinants of atherosclerosis, hypertension, stroke, and other vascular disease is progressing at a rapid rate. This research gives promise for unlocking some of the present mysteries and uncertainties about stroke development,

especially among the young and offers prospects for personalized medicine.[337–344] Genetic disorders are considered in Chapters 5 and 12.

Primary and secondary stroke prevention

Prevention is customarily separated into primary prevention (strategies to prevent stroke in patients who have never had a stroke) and secondary prevention (strategies to prevent a stroke recurrence).

Primary (first) prevention

For primary prevention, public education must be improved, especially in underdeveloped countries. Improvement in general health practices in the population undoubtedly decreases modifiable stroke risk factors in many patients. Educating the public to implement good general health measures probably would have a large impact on the frequency of stroke and other cardiovascular disease. The public should be encouraged to stop smoking, avoid excessive alcohol intake, exercise regularly, make time for leisure activities, avoid becoming overweight, and decrease intake of foods high in sodium, fat and cholesterol.

The risk of stroke varies greatly among individuals and depends heavily on individual factors present in each person. For example, some individuals can eat large quantities of eggs, milk, ice cream, and red meat and still have quite normal serum cholesterol and lipid values, whereas in others, genetic and environment factors lead to excessively high cholesterol levels; simply smelling foods high in cholesterol seems to send their cholesterol levels skyrocketing. We have already emphasized the importance of hereditary diseases in the family and beginning awareness of these early in life. We believe that each individual should become aware of the cardiovascular disorders and stroke and heart disease risk factors prevalent in their families. Periodic check-ups with physicians who monitor blood pressure, weight, blood sugar and lipid levels, and who inquire about habits and health practices are important. This strategy is especially important for the children of patients who have had a myocardial infarct, stroke, or important stroke risk factors, such as hypertension, diabetes, and hypercholesterolemia.

When multiple risk factors are considered together, patients at particular risk for stroke can be identified. When systolic hypertension, elevated serum cholesterol, glucose intolerance, cigarette smoking, and electrocardiogram findings of left ventricular hypertrophy are combined, a population accounting for one-third of all strokes can be identified.[152] Wolf and his colleagues created a stroke risk-factor score based on data obtained from the Framingham Study, which reflects an individual's 10-year probability of having a stroke.[345,346]

Recent guidance on primary prevention of cardiovascular disease from the US National Heart, Lung, and Blood Institute in collaboration with the American Heart Association and American College of Cardiology published in 2013 emphasizes the following: lifestyle modification; a risk-based strategy for

cholesterol lowering; reduction of not only coronary heart disease but also stroke as the major atherosclerotic cardiovascular disease (ASCVD) outcomes of interest.[347] Based on clinical trial study results, the target goal for blood pressure lowering has been changed from the traditional target of less than 140/90 mmHg to less than 150/90 mmHg for persons 60 years of age and older.[128,269,347–349] Stroke reduction substantially tracks with blood pressure lowering; however, the new guidance statements do not specifically address a target for blood pressure lowering for stroke reduction alone. Based on the available literature and the possible absence of a J-shaped curve for the relationship between hypertension and stroke with usual lowering of blood pressure, it is reasonable to aim for a systolic blood pressure lowering target for stroke prevention in the 130–139 mmHg range and a diastolic target in the 80–85 mmHg range.[350]

According to the new guidance statements, in relation to cholesterol lowering, statins are the primary treatment modality, and the following four groups of persons are to be targeted for statin therapy including those with: 1. ASCVD; 2. elevation of LDL-cholesterol ≥190 mg/dL; and individuals 40–75 years and LDL-C 70–189 mg/dL with: 3. a history of diabetes but no clinical ASCVD or 4. an estimated 10-year ASCVD risk of 7.5% or greater but no history of clinical ASCVD or diabetes.[348] The American Heart Association and American Stroke Association published detailed guidelines for primary stroke prevention in 1994 that were also approved by Neurological and Neurosurgical organizations.[351]

Secondary (recurrent) prevention

For secondary stroke prevention, identification of the mechanism of the initial stroke is most important. In patients who have lacunar infarcts caused by penetrating artery disease due to hypertension and in patients who have hypertensive ICHs, control of blood pressure is the most important strategy. In patients with severe carotid artery stenosis, surgery or angioplasty of the involved carotid artery may be the best strategy for secondary prevention. In patients with non-stenosing plaques, statins, and an agent that decreases platelet functions, such as aspirin, clopidogrel, cilostazole, or combined low-dose aspirin and modified-release dipyridamole, are probably most effective. In patients who have had brain embolism caused by atrial fibrillation, anticoagulation with warfarin or one of the newer oral anticoagulant agents (e.g., direct thrombin inhibitor, factor Xa inhibitor) represents the best strategy for secondary stroke prevention unless contraindications to the use of oral anticoagulants are present.

In most patients, recurrent strokes are caused by the same mechanism as the initial stroke.[352] Sometimes, second and third strokes, however, have a different stroke mechanism than the initial stroke.[352,353] For example, some patients with atrial fibrillation also have hypertension and carotid artery disease. Their initial stroke may have been caused by their carotid artery disease, but atrial fibrillation poses a threat for brain embolism. The results of the North American Symptomatic Carotid Endarterectomy Trial, which included patients with various severities of carotid artery occlusive

disease and excluded patients with cardiac lesions thought to carry high risk of cardioembolism, found that a significant number of subsequent strokes were caused by cardioembolism and penetrating artery disease.[354] Identification of all stroke risk factors by thorough cardiac, cerebrovascular, and blood evaluations at the time of the initial stroke allows factors and lesions present in the individual to be recognized and creates a database for the logical selection of strategies for secondary prevention of stroke and myocardial infarction.[352] Even when stroke has already occurred, treatment of identifiable stroke risk factors, such as hypertension, was shown in one study to decrease the expected mortality and stroke recurrence rate during the 5 years after the first stroke.[355] Several studies show that the optimal opportunity to begin secondary stroke prevention is when the patient is still in the hospital.[356,357] Computerized programs can ensure that, upon discharge, key preventive strategies are addressed and appropriate follow-up care is arranged. Doctors and nurses or other non-physician providers who have treated the patient in the hospital must communicate with the patient's primary physician the findings, recommendations, medications, instructions, and treatment plan. Otherwise, lack of continuity of care can lead to recurrent stroke and early post-stroke re-admissions to the hospital.

The incidence of stroke is declining, but much more can be done. Advances will probably involve the following:

- Improved general health measures initiated by individuals concerned about their cognitive and functional status as they age.
- Education for patients regarding the symptoms and significance of hypertension, excess weight, exercise, and TIAs. Patients should become educated consumers who recognize and seek the most competent care.
- Education for the public about the brain and symptoms that might indicate stroke and other brain diseases.
- Education of general physicians. Physicians should know about the warning signs of stroke, stroke risk factors, and how to manage patients with cerebrovascular disease.
- Education of neurologists, vascular surgeons, neurosurgeons, and other stroke specialists. These specialists should know when and how to manage risk factors, as well as how to treat the presenting stroke problem.
- Basic and clinical research. This will surely advance the present capabilities for diagnosing and treating stroke patients and stroke-prone individuals.

References

1. Pasteur L: *Address to the Fraternal Association of Former Students of the École Centrale des Arts et Manufactures.* Paris, May 15, 1884.

2. Sug YS, Heller RF, Levi C, et al: Knowledge of stroke risk factors, warning symptoms, and treatment among an Australian urban population. *Stroke* 2001;**32**:1926–1930.

3. Schneider AT, Pancioli AM, Khoury JC, et al: Trends in community knowledge of the warning signs and risk factors for stroke. *JAMA* 2003;**289**:343–346.

4. Kothari R, Sauerbeck L, Jauch E, et al: Patients' awareness of stroke signs, symptoms, and risk factors. *Stroke* 1997;**28**:1871–1875.

5. Pandian JD, Jaison A, Deepak SS, et al: Public awareness of warning symptoms, risk factors, and treatment of stroke in northwest India. *Stroke* 2005;**36**:644–648.

6. Maasland L, Koudstaal PJ, Habbema JD, Dippel DW: Knowledge and understanding of disease process, risk factors and treatment modalities in patients with a recent TIA or minor ischemic stroke. *Cerebrovasc Dis* 2007;**23**:435–440.

7. Nedeltchev K, Fischer U, Arnold M, et al: Low awareness of transient ischemic attacks and risk factors for stroke in a Swiss urban community. *J Neurol* 2007;**254**:179–184.

8. Anderson BE, Rafferty AP, Lyon-Callo S, Fussman C, Reeves MJ: Knowledge of tissue plasminogen activator for acute stroke among Michigan adults. *Stroke* 2009;**40**:2564–2567.

9. Fussman C, Rafferty AP, Lyon-Callo, Morgenstern LB, Reeves MJ: Lack of association between stroke symptom knowledge and intent to call 911. A population-based study. *Stroke* 2010;**41**:1501–1507

10. Garraway WM, Whisnant JP, Furlan AJ, et al: The declining incidence of stroke. *N Engl J Med* 1979;**300**:449–452.

11. Bonita R, Stewart A, Beaglehole R: International trends in stroke mortality: 1970–1985. *Stroke* 1990;**21**:989–992.

12. Sytkowski PA, Kannel WB, D'Agostino RB: Changes in risk factors and the decline in mortality from cardiovascular disease. *N Engl J Med* 1990;**322**:1635–1641.

13. Lackland DT, Roccella E, Deutsch AF, et al: Factors influencing the decline in stroke mortality. A Statement From the American Heart Association/American Stroke Association. *Stroke* 2013; published online before print Dec. 5, 2013, doi: 10.1161/01. str.0000437068.30550.cf.

14. Caplan LR, Dyken ML, Easton JD: *American Heart Association Family Guide to Stroke Treatment, Recovery, and Prevention.* New York: Random House–Times Books, 1994.

15. Hutton C, Caplan LR: *Striking Back at Stroke: A Doctor–Patient Journal.* New York: Dana Press, 2003.

16. Caplan LR: *Stroke.* New York: Demos–American Academy of Neurology, 2005.

17. Caplan LR: *Navigating the Complexities of Stroke.* New York, Oxford University Press, 2013.

18. Gorelick PB: The future of stroke prevention by risk factor modification. *Handb Clin Neurol* 2009;**94**:1261–1276.

19. Wald NJ, Law MR: A strategy to reduce cardiovascular disease by more than 80%. *BMJ* 2003;**326**:1419.

20. Gorelick PB: New horizons for stroke prevention: PROGRESS and HOPE. *Lancet Neurol* 2002;**1**:149–156.

21. Lawes CMM, Bennett DA, Feigin VL, Rogers A: Blood pressure and stroke. An overview of published reviews. *Stroke* 2004;**35**:1024–1033.

22. Sacco RL: The 2006 William Feinberg lecture. Shifting the paradigm from stroke to global vascular risk estimation. *Stroke* 2007;**38**:1980–1987.

23. Wolf P, Dyken M, Barnett HJM, et al: Risk factors in stroke. *Stroke* 1984;**15**:1105–1111.

24. Shaper AG, Phillips AN, Pocock SJ, et al: Risk factors for stroke in middle-aged British men. *BMJ* 1991;**302**:1111–1115.

25. Matchar DB, McCrory DC, Barnett HJM, Feussner JR: Medical treatment for stroke prevention. *Ann Intern Med* 1994;**121**:41–53.

26. Bronner LL, Kanter DS, Manson JE: Primary prevention of stroke. *N Engl J Med* 1995;**333**:1392–1400.

27. Kalra L, Perez I, Melbourn A: Stroke risk management. Change in mainstream practice. *Stroke* 1998;**29**:53–57.

28. Gorelick PB, Sacco RL, Smith DB, et al: Prevention of a first stroke. A review of guidelines and a multidisciplinary consensus statement from the National Stroke Association. *JAMA* 1999;**281**:1112–1120.

29. Whisnant JP: *Stroke Populations, Cohorts, and Clinical Trials*. Boston: Butterworth–Heinemann, 1993.

30. Dorndorf W, Marx P: *Stroke Prevention*. Basel: Karger, 1994.

31. Norris JW, Hachinski VC: *Prevention of Stroke*. New York: Springer, 1991.

32. Gorelick PB, Alter M: *The Prevention of Stroke*. Boca Raton, FL: Parthenon Publishing Group, 2002.

33. Go AS, Mozaffarian D, Roger VL, et al: Heart disease and stroke statistics – 2014 update. A report from the American Heart Association. *Circulation* 2014;**129**:e28–e292.

34. Sobel E, Altu M, Davanipour Z, et al: Stroke in the Lehigh Valley: Combined risk factors for recurrent ischemic stroke. *Neurology* 1989;**39**:669–672.

35. Davis PH, Dambrosia JM, Schoenberg BS, et al: Risk factors for ischemic stroke: A prospective study in Rochester, Minnesota. *Ann Neurol* 1987;**22**:319–327.

36. Simons LA, McCallum J, Friedlander Y, Simons J: Risk factors for ischemic stroke. Dubbo study of the elderly. *Stroke* 1998;**29**:1341–1346.

37. Whisnant JP, Wiebers DO, O'Fallon WM, et al: A population-based model of risk factors for ischemic stroke: Rochester, Minnesota. *Neurology* 1996;**47**:1420–1428.

38. Sacco RL: Risk factors, outcomes, and stroke subtypes for ischemic stroke. *Neurology* 1997;**49**(suppl 4):S39–S44.

39. Goldstein LB, Adams R, Becker K, et al: Primary prevention of ischemic stroke: A statement for healthcare professionals from the Stroke Council of the American Heart Association. *Stroke* 2001;**32**:280–299.

40. Johnson P, Rosewell M, James MA: How good is the management of vascular risk after stroke, transient ischemic attack, or carotid endarterectomy? *Cerebrovasc Dis* 2007;**32**:156–161.

41. Romero JR: Prevention of ischemic stroke: Overview of traditional risk factors. *Curr Drug Targets* 2007;**8**:794–801.

42. Longstreth WT, Koepsell T, Yerby M, et al: Risk factors for subarachnoid hemorrhage. *Stroke* 1985;**16**:377–385.

43. Teunissen LL, Rinkel GJE, Algra A, van Gijn J: Risk factors for subarachnoid hemorrhage. A systematic review. *Stroke* 1996;**27**:544–549.

44. Qureshi AI, Suri MF, Yahia AM, et al: Risk factors for subarachnoid hemorrhage. *Neurosurgery* 2001;**49**:607–612.

45. Isaksen J, Egge A, Waterloo K, et al: Risk factors for aneurysmal subarachnoid haemorrhage: The Tromso study. *J Neurol Neurosurg Psychiatry* 2002;**73**:185–187.

46. Ohkuma H, Tabata H, Suzuki S, Islam S: Risk factors for aneurysmal subarachnoid hemorrhage in Aomori, Japan. *Stroke* 2003;**34**:96–100.

47. Broderick JP: Intracerebral hemorrhage. In Gorelick PB, Alter M (eds): *Handbook of Neuroepidemiology*. New York: Marcel Dekker, 1994, pp 141–167.

48. Qureshi AI, Suri MA, Safdar K, et al: Intracerebral hemorrhage in blacks: Risk factors, subtypes, and outcome. *Stroke* 1997;**28**:961–964.

49. Bateman BT, Schumacher HC, Bushnell CD, et al: Intracerebral hemorrhage in pregnancy: Frequency, risk factors, and outcome. *Neurology* 2006;**67**:424–429.

50. Mitchell P, Mitra D, Gregson BA, Mendelow AD: Prevention of intracerebral haemorrhage. *Curr Drug Targets* 2007;**8**:832–838.

51. Caplan LR: Brain embolism. In Caplan LR, Hurst JW, Chimowitz M (eds): *Clinical Neurocardiology*. New York: Marcel Dekker, 1999, pp 35–185.

52. Caplan LR, Manning WJ: *Brain Embolism*. New York: Informa Healthcare, 2006.

53. Gorelick PB, Caplan LR, Hier DB, et al: Racial differences in the distribution of anterior circulation occlusive cerebrovascular disease. *Neurology* 1984;**34**:54–59.

54. Gorelick PB, Caplan LR, Hier DB, et al: Racial differences in the distribution of posterior circulation occlusive disease. *Stroke* 1985;**16**:785–790.

55. Caplan LR: Race, sex, and occlusive cerebrovascular disease: A review. *Stroke* 1986;**17**:648–655.

56. Caplan LR: Cerebral ischemia and infarction in blacks. Clinical, autopsy, and angiographic studies. In Gillum RF, Gorelick PB, Cooper ES (eds): *Stroke in Blacks*. Basel: Karger, 1999, pp 7–18.

57. White H, Boden-Albala B, Wang C, et al: Ischemic stroke subtype incidence among whites, blacks, and Hispanics: The Northern Manhattan Study. *Circulation* 2005;**111**:1327–1331.

58. Sacco RL, Kargman DE, Gu Q, Zamanillo MC: Race-ethnicity and determinants of intracranial atherosclerotic cerebral infarction. The Northern Manhattan Stroke Study. *Stroke* 1995;**26**:14–20.

59. Lewington S, Clarke R, Qizilbash N, et al: Age-specific relevance of usual blood pressure to vascular mortality: A meta-analysis of individual data for one million adults in 61 prospective studies. *Lancet* 2002;**360**:1903–1913.

60. Kannel WB: Current status of the epidemiology of brain infarction associated with occlusive vascular disease. *Stroke* 1971;**2**:295–318.

61. Mackay MT, Wiznitzer M, Benedict SL, et al: Arterial ischemic stroke risk factors: The International Pediatric Stroke Study. *Ann Neurol* 2011;**69**:130–140.

62. Gebel J, Broderick J: Primary intracerebral hemorrhage and subarachnoid hemorrhage in black patients: Risk factors, diagnosis, and prognosis. In Gillum RF, Gorelick PB, Cooper ES (eds): *Stroke in Blacks*. Basel: Karger, 1999, pp 29–35.

63. Towfighi A, Zheng L, Obviagele B: Weight of the obesity epidemic. Rising stroke rates among middle-aged women in the United States. *Stroke* 2010;**41**:1371–1375.

64. Kiely DK, Wolf PA, Cupples LA, et al: Family aggregation of stroke: The Framingham Study. *Stroke* 1993;**24**:1366–1371.

65. Liao D, Myers R, Hunt S, et al: Family history of stroke and stroke risk. The

Family Heart Study. *Stroke* 1997;**28**:1908–1912.

66. Wannamethee SG, Shaper AG, Ebrahim S: History of parental death from stroke or heart trouble and the risk of stroke in middle-aged men. *Stroke* 1996;**27**:1492–1498.

67. Jousilahri P, Rastenyte D, Tuomilehto J, et al: Parental history of cardiovascular disease and risk of stroke. A prospective follow-up of 14,371 middle-aged men and women in Finland. *Stroke* 1997;**28**:1361–1366.

68. Meschia JF, Case LD, Worrall BB, et al: Ischemic Stroke Genetics Study Group. Family history of stroke and severity of neurologic deficit after stroke. *Neurology* 2006;**67**:1396–1402.

69. McGill HC, Arias-Stella J, Carbonell LM, et al: General findings of the International Atherosclerosis Project. *Lab Invest* 1968;**18**:498–502.

70. Solberg LA, McGarry PA, Moosy J, et al: Distribution of cerebral atherosclerosis by geographic location, race, and sex. *Lab Invest* 1968;**158**:604–612.

71. Freedman DS, Khan LK, Dietz WH, Srinivasan SR, Berenson G: Relationship of obesity in childhood to coronary heart disease risk factors in adulthood: The Bogalusa Heart Study. *Pediatrics* 2001;**108**:712–718.

72. Högström G, Nordström A, Eriksson M, Nordström P: Risk factors assessed in adolescence and the later risk of stroke in men: a 33-year follow-up study. *Cerebrovasc Dis* 2015;**39**:63–71.

73. Expert Panel. *Summary Report on Integrated Guidelines of Cardiovascular Health and Risk Reduction in Children and Adolescents.* Bethesda, MD: US Department of Health and Human Services, National Heart, Lung and Blood Institute, NIH Publication No. 12-7486A, October 2012, pp 1–72.

74. Reis JP, Loria CM, Lewis CE, et al: Association between duration of overall and abdominal obesity beginning in young adulthood and coronary artery calcification in middle age. *JAMA* 2013;**310**:280–288.

75. Kannel WB: Blood pressure as a cardiovascular risk factor. *JAMA* 1996;**275**:1571–1576.

76. National Heart, Lung, and Blood Institute: *Working Group Report on Primary Prevention of Hypertension: National High Blood Pressure Education Program.* NHLBI Doc 93-2669. Bethesda, MD: National Institutes of Health, 1993.

77. Chobanian AV, Bakris GL, Black HR, et al: The seventh report of the Joint National Committee on Prevention, Detection, Evaluation, and Treatment of High Blood Pressure. *JAMA* 2003;**289**:2560–2572.

78. Go AS, Mozaffarinan D, Roger VL, et al. on behalf of the American Heart Association Statistics Committee and Stroke Statistics Subcommittee. Heart disease and stroke statistics – 2013 update, a report from the American Heart Association. *Circulation* 2013;**127**:e6–e245.

79. Prospective Studies Collaboration: Age-specific relevance of usual blood pressure to vascular mortality: A meta-analysis of individual data for one million adults in 61 prospective studies. *Lancet* 2002;**360**:1903–1913.

80. Gueyffier F, Bulpitt C, Boissel J-P, et al: Antihypertensive drugs in very old people: A subgroup meta-analysis of randomized controlled trials. *Lancet* 1999;**353**:793–796.

81. Howard G, Manolio TA, Burke GL, et al: Does the association of risk factors and atherosclerosis change with age? *Stroke* 1997;**28**:1693–1701.

82. Beckett NS, Peters R, Fletcher AE, et al: Treatment of hypertension in patients 80 years of age or older. HYVET Study Group. *N Engl J Med* 2008;**358**:1887–1898.

83. SHEP Cooperative Research Group: Prevention of stroke by antihypertensive drug treatment in older persons with isolated systolic hypertension. *JAMA* 1991;**265**:3255–3264.

84. Sutton-Tyrrell K, Alcorn HG, Herzog H, et al: Morbidity, mortality, and antihypertensive treatment effects by extent of atherosclerosis in older adults with isolated systolic hypertension. *Stroke* 1995;**26**:1319–1324.

85. Davis BR, Vogt T, Frost PH, et al: Risk factors for stroke and type of stroke in persons with isolated systolic hypertension. The Systolic Hypertension in the Elderly Program (SHEP) Research Group. *Stroke* 1998;**29**:1333–1340.

86. Perry HM, Davis BR, Price TR, et al: Effect of treating isolated systolic hypertension on the risk of developing various types and subtypes of stroke. Systolic Hypertension in the Elderly Program (SHEP) Cooperative Research Group. *JAMA* 2000;**284**:465–471.

87. Staessen JA, Gasowski J, Wang JG, et al: Risks of untreated and treated isolated systolic hypertension in the elderly: Meta-analysis of outcome trials. *Lancet* 2000;**355**:865–872.

88. Bowman TS, Gaziano JM, Kase CS, et al: Blood pressure measures and risk of total, ischemic, and hemorrhagic stroke in men. *Neurology* 2006;**67**:820–823.

89. Chobanian AV: Isolated systolic hypertension in the elderly. *N Engl J Med* 2007;**357**:789–796.

90. Wenger NK: Hypertension and other cardiovascular risk factors in women. *Am J Hypertens* 1995;**8**:94S–99S.

91. Rothwell PM, Coull AJ, Silver LE, et al: Population-based study of event-rate, incidence, case fatality, and mortality for all acute vascular events in all arterial territories (Oxford Vascular Study). *Lancet* 2005;**366**:1773–1783.

92. Mitchell GF, Ramachandran SV, Keyes MJ, et al: Pulse-pressure and risk of new-onset atrial fibrillation. *JAMA* 2007;**297**:709–715.

93. Weitzman D, Goldbourt U: The significance of various blood pressure indices for long-term stroke, coronary heart disease, and all-cause mortality in men. The Israeli Ischemic Heart Disease Study. *Stroke* 2006;**37**:358–363.

94. Paultre F, Mosca L: Association of blood pressure indices and stroke mortality in isolated systolic hypertension. *Stroke* 2005;**36**:1288–1290.

95. Vemmos KN, Tsivgoulis G, Spengos K, et al: Pulse pressure in acute stroke is an independent predictor of long-term mortality. *Cerebrovasc Dis* 2004;**18**:30–36.

96. Rothwell PM: Limitations of the usual blood pressure hypothesis and importance of variability, instability, and episodic hypertension. *Lancet* 2010;**375**:938–948.

97. Gorelick PB: Reducing blood pressure variability to prevent stroke? *Lancet Neurol* 2010;**9**:448–449.

98. Watanabe N, Imai Y, Nagai K, et al: Nocturnal blood pressure and silent cerebrovascular lesions in elderly Japanese. *Stroke* 1996;**27**:1319–1327.

99. Yamamoto Y, Akiguchi I, Oiwa K, et al: Adverse effect of nighttime blood pressure on the outcome of lacunar infarct patients. *Stroke* 1998;**29**:570–576.

100. Lip GY, Zarifis J, Farooqi S, et al: Ambulatory blood pressure monitoring in acute stroke. The West Birmingham Stroke Project. *Stroke* 1997;**28**:31–35.

101. Staessen JA, Thijs L, Fagard R, et al: Predicting cardiovascular risk using

conventional vs. ambulatory blood pressure in older patients with systolic hypertension. Systolic Hypertension in the Europe Trial Investigators. *JAMA* 1999;**282**:539–546.

102. Goldstein IB, Bartzokis G, Guthrie D, Shapiro D: Ambulatory blood pressure and the brain. A 5-year follow-up. *Neurology* 2005;**64**:1846–1852.

103. Tsivgoulis G, Spengos K, Zakopoulos N, et al: Twenty-four-hour pulse pressure predicts long-term recurrence in acute stroke patients. *J Neurol Neurosurg Psychiatry* 2005;**76**:1360–1365.

104. Rashid P, Leonardi-Bee J, Bath P: Blood pressure reduction and secondary prevention of stroke and other vascular events. A systematic review. *Stroke* 2003;**34**:2741–2749.

105. Psaty BM, Lumley T, Furberg CD, et al: Health outcomes associated with various antihypertensive therapies used as first-line agents. *JAMA* 2003;**289**:2534–2544.

106. Blood Pressure Lowering Treatment Trialists' Collaboration: Effects of different blood-pressure-lowering regimens on major cardiovascular events: Results of prospectively-designed overviews of randomized trials. *Lancet* 2003;**362**:1527–1535.

107. Hall WD, Kong W: Hypertension in blacks: Nonpharmacologic and pharmacologic therapy. In Saunders E (ed): *Cardiovascular Disease in Blacks.* Philadelphia: FA Davis, 1991, pp 157–169.

108. Rajagopalan S, Harrison D: Reversing endothelial dysfunction with ACE inhibitors. A new trend? *Circulation* 1996;**94**:240–243.

109. Bosch J, Yusuf S, Pogue J, et al: Use of ramipril in preventing stroke: Double blind randomized trial. HOPE Investigators. *BMJ* 2002;**324**:1–5.

110. van Gijn J: The PROGRESS Trial: Preventing strokes by lowering blood pressure in patients with cerebral ischemia. *Stroke* 2002;**33**:319–320.

111. Hankey GJ: Angiotensin-converting enzyme inhibitors for stroke prevention. Is there HOPE for PROGRESS after LIFE? *Stroke* 2003; **34**:354–356.

112. Chapman N, Huxley R, Anderson C, et al: Effects of a perendopril-based blood pressure-lowering regimen on the risk of recurrent stroke according to stroke subtype and medical history.

The PROGRESS Trial. *Stroke* 2004;**35**:116–121.

113. Iadecola C, Gorelick PB: Hypertension, angiotensin, and stroke: Beyond blood pressure. *Stroke* 2004;**35**:348–350.

114. Toole FJ, Janeway R, Choi K, et al: Transient ischemic attacks due to atherosclerosis: A prospective study of 160 patients. *Arch Neurol* 1975;**32**:5–12.

115. Chimowitz MI, Weiss DG, Cohen SL, et al: Veterans Affairs Cooperative Study Group 167. Cardiac prognosis of patients with carotid stenosis and no history of coronary artery disease. *Stroke* 1994;**25**:759–765.

116. Chimowitz MI: Asymptomatic coronary artery disease in patients with carotid artery stenosis: Incidence, prognosis, and treatment. In Caplan LR, Hurst JW, Chimowitz M (eds): *Clinical Neurocardiology.* New York: Marcel Dekker, 1999, pp 287–295.

117. Adams R, Chimowitz MI, Alpert JS, et al. Coronary risk evaluation in patients with transient ischemic attack and ischemic stroke: a scientific statement for healthcare professionals from the Stroke Council and the Council on Clinical Cardiology of the American Heart Association/ American Stroke Association. *Stroke* 2003;**34**:2310–2322.

118. DECODE Study Group, European Diabetes Epidemiology Group: Glucose tolerance and mortality: Comparison of WHO and American Diabetes Association diagnostic criteria. *Lancet* 1999;**354**:617–621.

119. Grundy SM, Brewer Jr B, Cleeman JI, et al: NHLBI/AHA Conference proceedings. Definition of metabolic syndrome. *Circulation* 2004;**109**:433–438.

120. Grundy S, Cleeman JI, Daniels SR, et al: Diagnosis and management of the metabolic syndrome. An American Heart Association/National Heart Lung, and Blood Institute Scientific Statement. *Circulation* 2005;**112**:2735–2752.

121. Bang OY, Kim JW, Lee JH, et al: Association of the metabolic syndrome with intracranial atherosclerotic stroke. *Neurology* 2005;**65**:296–298.

122. Mak KH, Ma S, Heng D, et al: Impact of sex, metabolic syndrome, and diabetes mellitus on cardiovascular events. *Am J Cardiol* 2007;**100**:227–233.

123. Arenillas JF, Moro MA, Dávalos A: The metabolic syndrome and stroke: Potential treatment approaches. *Stroke* 2007;**38**:2196–2203.

124. Kurl S, Laukkanen JA, Niskanen L, et al: Metabolic syndrome and the risk of stroke in middle-aged men. *Stroke* 2006;**37**:806–811.

125. Boden-Albala B, Sacco RL, Lee H-S, et al: Metabolic syndrome and ischemic stroke risk. Northern Manhattan Study. *Stroke* 2008;**39**:30–35.

126. Li W, Ma D, Liu M, et al: Association between metabolic syndrome and risk of stroke: A meta-analysis of cohort studies. *Cerebrovasc Dis* 2008;**25**:539–547.

127. Mokdad AH, Bowman BA, Ford ES, et al: The continuing epidemics of obesity and diabetes in the United States. *JAMA* 2001;**286**:1195–1200.

128. Jensen MD, Ryan DH, Apovian CM, et al. 2013 AHA/ACC/TOS Guideline for the Management of Overweight and Obesity in Adults. A Report of the American College of Cardiology/ American Heart Association Task Force on Practice Guidelines and The Obesity Society. *J Am Coll Cardiol* 2014;014;63(25_PA):doi:10.1016/j.jacc.2013.11.004.

129. Kurth T, Gaziano JM, Berger K, et al: Body mass index and the risk of stroke in men. *Arch Intern Med* 2002;**162**:2557–2562.

130. Kurth T, Gaziano JM, Rexrode KM, et al: Prospective study of body mass index and risk of stroke in apparently healthy women. *Circulation* 2005;**111**:1992–1998.

131. Hu G, Tuomilehto J, Silventoinen K, et al: Body mass index, waist circumference, and waist–hip ratio on the risk of total and type-specific stroke. *Arch Intern Med* 2007;**167**:1420–1427.

132. Depres J-P, Lemieux I, Prud'homme D: Treatment of obesity: Need to focus on high risk abdominally obese subjects. *BMJ* 2001;**322**:716–720.

133. Fox CS, Massaro JM, Hoffmann U, et al: Abdominal visceral and subcutaneous adipose tissue compartments: Association with metabolic risk factors in the Framingham Heart Study. *Circulation* 2007;**116**:39–48.

134. Lear SA, Humphries KH, Kohli S, et al: Visceral adipose tissue, a potential risk factor for carotid atherosclerosis.

Results of the Multicultural Community Health Assessment Trial (M-CHAT). *Stroke* 2007;**38**:2422–2429.

135. Suk SH, Sacco RL, Boden-Albala B, et al: Abdominal obesity and risk of ischemic stroke: The Northern Manhattan Stroke Study. *Stroke* 2003;**34**:1586–1592.

136. Ruderman N, Chisholm D, Pi-Sunyer X, Schneider S: The metabolically obese, normal weight individual revisited. *Diabetes* 1998;**47**:699–713.

137. McLaughlin T, Allison G, Abbasi F, et al: Prevalence of insulin resistance and associated cardiovascular risk factors among normal weight, overweight, and obese individuals. *Metabolism* 2004;**53**:495–499.

138. Schoenberg BS, Schoenberg DG, Pritchard DA, et al: Differential risk factors for completed stroke and transient ischemic attack (TIA): Study of vascular disease (hypertension, cardiac disease, peripheral vascular disease) and diabetes mellitus. *Trans Am Neurol Assoc* 1980;**105**:165–167.

139. Burchfiel CM, Curb D, Rodriguez B, et al: Glucose intolerance and 22-year stroke incidence. The Honolulu Heart Program. *Stroke* 1994;**25**:951–957.

140. Jorgenson H, Nakayama H, Raaschou HO, Olsen TS: Stroke in patients with diabetes. The Copenhagen Stroke Study. *Stroke* 1994;**25**:1977–1984.

141. Karapanayiotides TH, Piechowski-Jozwiak B, van Melle G, et al: Stroke patterns, etiology, and prognosis in patients with diabetes mellitus. *Neurology* 2004;**62**:1558–1562.

142. Fox C, Coady S, Sorlie P, et al: Increased cardiovascular disease burden due to diabetes mellitus. The Framingham Heart Study. *Circulation* 2007;**115**:1544–1550.

143. Caplan LR: Intracranial branch atheromatous disease: A neglected, understudied, and underused concept. *Neurology* 1989;**39**:1246–1250.

144. Caplan LR: Diabetes and brain ischemia. *Diabetes* 1996;**45**(suppl 3):595–597.

145. Depres J-P, Golay A, Sjostrom L: Effects of rimonabant on metabolic risk factors in overweight patients with dyslipidemia. Rimonabant in Obesity–Lipids Study Group. *N Engl J Med* 353:2121–2134.

146. Higa M, Davanipour Z: Smoking and stroke. *Neuroepidemiology* 1991;**10**:211–222.

147. Love BB, Biller J, Jones MP, et al: Cigarette smoking: A risk factor for cerebral infarction in young adults. *Arch Neurol* 1990;**47**:693–698.

148. Whisnant JP, Homer D, Ingall TJ, et al: Duration of cigarette smoking is the strongest predictor of severe extracranial carotid artery atherosclerosis. *Stroke* 1990;**21**:707–714.

149. Ingall TJ, Homer D, Baker HL, et al: Predictors of intracranial carotid artery atherosclerosis: Duration of cigarette smoking and hypertension are more powerful than serum lipid levels. *Arch Neurol* 1991;**48**:687–691.

150. Colditz GA, Bonita R, Stampfer MJ, et al: Cigarette smoking and risk of stroke in middle-aged women. *N Engl J Med* 1988;**318**:937–941.

151. Donnan GA, You R, Thrift A, McNeil JJ: Smoking as a risk factor for stroke. *Cerebrovasc Dis* 1993;**3**:129–138.

152. Wolf P, Kannel WB, Verter J: Current status of risk factors for stroke. In Barnett HJM (ed): *Neurologic Clinics, vol 1. Cerebrovascular Disease*. Philadelphia: Saunders, 1983, pp 317–343.

153. Paffenbarger R, Williams J: Chronic disease in former college students: V. Early precursors of fatal stroke. *Am J Public Health* 1967;**57**:1290–1299.

154. Kawachi I, Colditz GA: Smoking cessation and decreased risk of stroke in women. *JAMA* 1993;**269**:232–236.

155. Jee SH, Suh I, Kim IS, Appel LJ: Smoking and atherosclerotic cardiovascular disease in men with low levels of serum cholesterol. *JAMA* 1999;**282**:2149–2155.

156. Kurth T, Kase CS, Berger K, et al: Smoking and the risk of hemorrhagic stroke in men. *Stroke* 2003;**34**:1151–1155.

157. Collaborative Group for the Study of Stroke in Young Women: Oral contraceptives and stroke in young women: Associated risk factors. *JAMA* 1975;**231**:718–722.

158. Fust G, Arason GJ, Kramer J, et al: Genetic basis of tobacco smoking: Strong association of a specific major histocompatibility complex haplotype on chromosome 6 with smoking behavior. *Int Immunol* 2004;**16**:1507–1514.

159. Arason GJ, Kramer J, Blasko B, et al: Smoking and a complement gene polymorphism interact in promoting cardiovascular disease morbidity and mortality. *Clin Exp Immunol* 2007;**149**:132–138.

160. Gorelick PB: Burden of stroke and risk factors. In Bornstein NM (ed): *Stroke*. Basel: Karger, 2009, pp 9–23.

161. Tell GS, Crouse JR, Furberg CD: Relation between blood lipids, lipoproteins, and cerebrovascular atherosclerosis. A review. *Stroke* 1988;**19**:423–430.

162. Kurth T, Everett BM, Buring JE, et al: Lipid levels and the risk of ischemic stroke in women. *Neurology* 2007;**68**:556–562.

163. Bang OY, Saver JL, Liebeskind DS, et al: Association of serum lipid indices with large artery atherosclerotic stroke. *Neurology* 2008;**70**:841–847.

164. Kannel WB: Epidemiology of cerebrovascular disease. In Ross-Russel RW (ed): *Cerebral Arterial Disease*. New York: Churchill Livingstone, 1976, pp 1–23.

165. Kagan A, Popper J, Rhoads G: Factors related to stroke incidence in Hawaiian Japanese men: The Honolulu Heart Study. *Stroke* 1980;**11**:14–21.

166. Stemmerman G, Hayashi T, Resch J, et al: Risk factors related to ischemic and hemorrhagic cerebrovascular disease at autopsy: The Honolulu Heart Study. *Stroke* 1984;**15**:23–28.

167. Iso H, Jacobs DR, Wentworth D, et al: Serum cholesterol levels and six year mortality from stroke in 350,977 men screened for the Multiple Risk Factor Intervention Trial. *N Engl J Med* 1989;**320**:904–910.

168. Yano K, Reed DM, Maclean CJ: Serum cholesterol and hemorrhagic stroke in the Honolulu Heart Program. *Stroke* 1989;**20**:1460–1465.

169. Goldstein LB, Amarenco P, Szarak M, et al: SPARCL Investigators. Hemorrhagic stroke in the Stroke Prevention by Aggressive Reduction in Cholesterol Levels study. *Neurology* 2008;**70**:2364–70.

170. Heart Protection Study Collaborative Group: MRC/BHF Heart Protection Study of cholesterol lowering with simvastatin in 20,536 high-risk individuals: A randomized placebo-controlled trial. *Lancet* 2002;**360**:7–22.

171. Hackam DG, Austin PC, Huang A, et al: Statins and intracerebral

hemorrhage: A retrospective cohort study. *Arch Neurol* 2012;**69**:39–45.

172. Nakamura H, Arakawa A, Itakura H, et al: Primary prevention of cardiovascular events with pravastatin in Japanese (MEGA) study: A prospectively randomized controlled trial. *Lancet* 2006;**30**:1155–1163.

173. Kurth T, Everett BM, Buring JE, et al: Lipid levels and the risk of ischemic stroke in women. *Neurology* 2007;**68**:556–562.

174. Tanne D, Yaari S, Goldbourt U: High-density lipoprotein cholesterol and risk of ischemic stroke mortality. A 21-year follow-up of 8586 men from Israeli Ischemic Heart Disease Study. *Stroke* 1997;**28**:83–87.

175. Steinberg D, Parthasarthy S, Carcio TE, et al: Beyond cholesterol: Modification of low-density lipoprotein that increases its atherogenicity. *N Engl J Med* 1989;**320**:915.

176. Scanu A, Lawn RM, Berg K: Lipoprotein (a) and atherosclerosis. *Ann Intern Med* 1991;**115**:209–218.

177. Pedro-Botet J, Senti M, Nogues X, et al: Lipoprotein and apolipoprotein profile in men with ischemic stroke. Role of lipoprotein (a), triglyceride-rich lipoproteins, and apolipoprotein E polymorphism. *Stroke* 1992;**23**:1556–1562.

178. Wilt TJ, Rubins HB, Robins SJ, et al: Carotid atherosclerosis in men with low levels of HDL cholesterol. *Stroke* 1997;**28**:1919–1925.

179. Homer D, Ingall TJ, Baber HL, et al: Serum lipids and lipoproteins are less powerful predictors of extracranial carotid artery atherosclerosis than are cigarette smoking and hypertension. *Mayo Clin Proc* 1991;**66**:259–267.

180. Taylor FC, Huffman M, Ebrahim S: Statin therapy for primary prevention of cardiovascular disease. *JAMA* 2013;**310**:2451–2452.

181. Bucher HC, Griffith LE, Guyatt GH: Effect of HMGCoA reductase inhibitors on stroke. A meta-analysis of randomized controlled trials. *Ann Intern Med* 1998;**128**:89–95.

182. Amarenco P, Lavallee P, Touboul P-J: Stroke prevention, blood cholesterol, and statins. *Lancet Neurol* 2004;**3**:271–278.

183. SPARCL Investigators: High-dose atorvastatin after stroke or transient ischemic attack. *N Engl J Med* 2006;**355**:549–559.

184. Paciaroni M, Hennerici M, Agnelli G, Bogousslavsky J: Statins and stroke prevention. *Cerebrovasc Dis* 2007;**24**:170–182.

185. Gorelick PB: The status of alcohol as a risk factor for stroke. *Stroke* 1989;**20**:1607–1610.

186. Hillborn M, Kaste M: Alcohol intoxication: A risk factor for primary subarachnoid hemorrhage. *Neurology* 1982;**32**:706–711.

187. Kagan A, Yano K, Rhoads G, et al: Alcohol and cardiovascular disease: The Hawaiian experience. *Circulation* 1981;**64**(suppl 3):27–31.

188. Bogousslausky J, Van Melle G, Despland PA, Regli F: Alcohol consumption and carotid atherosclerosis in the Lausanne stroke registry. *Stroke* 1990;**21**:715–720.

189. Palomaki H, Kaste M: Regular light-to-moderate intake of alcohol and the risk of ischemic stroke. *Stroke* 1993;**24**:1828–1832.

190. Kiechi S, Willeit J, Rungger G, et al: Alcohol consumption and atherosclerosis: What is the relation. Prospective results from the Bruneck Study. *Stroke* 1998;**29**:900–907.

191. Gorelick PB, Rodin MB, Langenberg P, et al: Is acute alcohol ingestion a risk factor for ischemic stroke? *Stroke* 1987;**18**:359–364.

192. Gorelick PB, Rodin MB, Langengerg P, et al: Weekly alcohol consumption, cigarette smoking, and the risk of ischemic stroke. *Neurology* 1989;**39**:339–343.

193. Truelsen T, Gronbaek M, Schnohr P, Boysen G: Intake of beer, wine, and spirits and risk of stroke. The Copenhagen Heart Study. *Stroke* 1998;**29**:2467–2472.

194. Hertog MG, Feskens EJ, Hollman PC, et al: Dietary antioxidant flavonoids and risk of coronary heart disease. *Lancet* 1993;**342**:1007–1011.

195. Frankel EN, Kanner J, German JB, et al: Inhibition of oxidation of human low-density lipoproteins by phenolic substances in red wine. *Lancet* 1993;**341**:454–457.

196. Hillbom M, Haapaniemi H, Juvela S, et al: Recent alcohol consumption, cigarette smoking, and cerebral infarction in young adults. *Stroke* 1995;**26**:40–45.

197. Mostofsky E, Burgern MR, Schlaug G, et al: Alcohol and acute ischemic stroke onset. The Stroke Onset Study. *Stroke* 2010;**41**:1845–1849.

198. Conen D, Tedrow UB, Cook NR, et al: Alcohol consumption and risk of incident atrial fibrillation in women. *JAMA* 2008;**300**:2489–2496.

199. Sull JW, Yi S-W, Nam CM, Ohrr H: Binge drinking and mortality from all causes and cerebrovascular diseases in Korean men and women. A Kangwha cohort study. *Stroke* 2009;**40**:2953–2958.

200. Sundell L, Salomaa V, Vartiainen E, et al: Increased stroke risk is related to a binge drinking habit. *Stroke* 2008;**39**:3179–3184.

201. Criqui MH: Peripheral arterial disease and subsequent cardiovascular mortality: A strong and consistent association. *Circulation* 1990;**82**:2246–2247.

202. Criqui MH, Langer RD, Fronek A, et al: Mortality over a period of 10 years in patients with peripheral arterial disease. *N Engl J Med* 1992;**326**:381–386.

203. Bhatt DL, Steg PG, Ohman EM, et al: International prevalence, recognition, and treatment of cardiovascular risk factors in outpatients with atherothrombosis. REACH Registry Investigators. *JAMA* 2006;**295**:180–189.

204. Bogousslavsky J, Regli F: Cerebral infarct in apparent transient ischemic attack. *Neurology* 1985;**35**:1501–1503.

205. Awad I, Modic M, Little JR, et al: Focal parenchymal lesions in transient ischemic attacks: Correlation of computed tomography and magnetic resonance imaging. *Stroke* 1986;**17**:399–403.

206. Caplan LR: TIAs: We need to return to the question, "What is wrong with Mr Jones?" *Neurology* 1988;**39**:791–793.

207. Fazekas F, Fazekas G, Schmidt R, et al: Magnetic resonance imaging correlates of transient cerebral ischemic attacks. *Stroke* 1996;**27**:607–611.

208. Inatomi Y, Kimura K, Yonehara T, et al: DWI abnormalities and clinical characteristics in TIA patients. *Neurology* 2004;**62**:376–380.

209. Dennis MS, Bamford JM, Sandercock PA, Warlow CD: A comparison of risk factors and prognosis for transient ischemic attacks and minor ischemic strokes. *Stroke* 1989;**20**:1494–1499.

210. Johnston SC, Gress DR, Browner WS, Sidney S: Short-term prognosis after

emergency department diagnosis of TIA. *JAMA* 2000;**284**:2901–2906.

211. Daffertshofer M, Mielke O, Pullwitt A, et al: Transient ischemic attacks are more than "ministrokes." *Stroke* 2004;**35**:2453–2458.

212. Kleindorfer D, Pangos P, Pancoli A, et al: Incidence and short-term prognosis of transient ischemic attack in a population-based study. *Stroke* 2005;**36**:720–724.

213. Hill MD, Yiannakoulias N, Jeerakathil T, et al: The high risk of stroke immediately after transient ischemic attack. A population-based study. *Neurology* 2004;**62**:2015–2020.

214. Rothwell PM, Warlow CP: Timing of TIAs preceding stroke. Time window for prevention is very short. *Neurology* 2005;**64**;817–820.

215. Amarenco P, Lavallée P, Labreuche J, et al: Contemporary profile and prognosis of transient ischemic attacks in the era of urgent management. *N Engl J Med*, 2016;in press.

216. Touze E, Varenne O, Chatellier G, et al: Risk of myocardial infarction and vascular death after transient ischemic attack and ischemic stroke. *Stroke* 2005;**36**:2748–2755.

217. Nguyen-Huynh MN, Johnston SC: Transient ischemic attack: A neurologic emergency. *Curr Neurol Neurosci Rep* 2005;**5**:13–20.

218. Ay H, Koroshetz WJ, Benner T, et al: Transient ischemic attack with infarction: A unique syndrome. *Ann Neurol* 2005;**57**:679–686.

219. Albers GW, Caplan LR, Easton JD, et al., for the TIA Working Group: Transient ischemic attack: proposal for a new definition. *N Engl J Med* 2002;**347**:1713–1716.

220. Easton JD, Saver JL, Albers GA, et al: Definition and evaluation of transient ischemic attack: A scientific statement for healthcare professionals from the American Heart Association/American Stroke Council, Council on Cardiovascular Surgery and Anesthesia, Council on Cardiovascular Radiology and Intervention, Council on Cardiovascular Nursing, and the Interdisciplinary Council on Peripheral Vascular Disease: The American Academy of Neurology affirms the value of this statement as an educational tool for neurologists. *Stroke* 2009;**40**:2276–2293.

221. Johnston SC, Rothwell PM, Nguyen-Huynh MN, et al: Validation and refinement of scores to predict very early stroke risk after transient ischaemic attack. *Lancet* 2007;**369**:283–292.

222. Merwick A, Albers GW, Amarenco P, et al: Addition of brain and carotid imaging to the ABCD2 score to identify patients at early risk of stroke after transient ischemic attack: a multicenter observational study. *Lancet Neurol* 2010;**9**:1060–1069.

223. Caplan LR: Scores of scores. *JAMA Neurol* 2013;**70**:252–253.

224. Amarenco P, Labreuche J, Lavallée PC: Patients with transient ischemic attacks with ABCD2 ≤4 can have similar 90-day stroke risks as patients with transient ischemic attacks with ABCD2 ≥4. *Stroke* 2012;**43**:863–865.

225. Lou M, Safdar A, Edlow JA, et al: Can ABCD score predict the need for in-hospital intervention in patients with transient ischemic attacks? *Int J Emerg Med* 2010;**3**:75–80.

226. Rothwell PM, Giles MF, Chandratheva A, et al: for the Early Use of Existing Preventive Strategies for Stroke (EXPRESS) Study. Effect of urgent treatment of transient ischaemic attack and minor stroke on early recurrent stroke (EXPRESS Study): A prospective population-based sequential comparison. *Lancet* 2007;**370**:1432–1442.

227. Collaborative Group for the Study of Stroke in Young Women: Oral contraception and increased risk of cerebral ischemia or thrombosis. *N Engl J Med* 1973;**288**:871–878.

228. Handin R: Thromboembolic complications of pregnancy and oral contraceptives. *Prog Cardiovasc Dis* 1974;**16**:395–405.

229. Layde P, Beral V, Kay C: Further analyses of mortality in oral contraceptive users. *Lancet* 1981;**1**:541–546.

230. Bushnell CD: Stroke and the female brain. *Nat Clin Pract Neurol* 2008;**4**:22–33.

231. Lidegaard O, Kreiner S: Cerebral thrombosis and oral contraceptives: A case-control study. *Contraception* 1998;**57**:303–314.

232. Schwartz SM, Siscovick DS, Longstreth WT Jr, et al: Use of low-dose oral contraceptives and stroke in young women. *Ann Intern Med* 1997;**127**:596–603.

233. Schwartz SM, Petitti DB, Siscovick DS, et al: Stroke and use of low-dose oral contraceptives in young women. A pooled analysis of two US studies. *Stroke* 1998;**29**:2277–2284.

234. Siritho S, Thrift A, McNeil JJ, et al: Risk of ischemic stroke among users of the oral contracveptive pill. The Melbourne Risk Factor Study (MERFS) Group. *Stroke* 2003;**34**:1575–1580.

235. Jick SS, Jick H: The contraceptive patch in relation to ischemic stroke and acute myocardial infarction. *Pharmacotherapy* 2007;**27**:218–220.

236. Chasan-Taber L, Stampfer MJ: Epidemiology of oral contraceptives and cardiovascular disease. *Ann Intern Med* 1998;**128**:467–477.

237. Martinelli I, Sacchi E, Landi G, et al: High risk of cerebral-vein thrombosis in carriers of a prothrombin-gene mutation and in users of oral contraceptives. *N Engl J Med* 1998;**338**:1793–1797.

238. Lidegaard O, Lokkegaard E, Jensen A, Skovlund CW, Keiding N: Thrombotic stroke and myocardial infarction with hormonal contraception. *N Engl J Med* 2012;**366**:2257–2266.

239. Qureshi A, Giles WH, Croft JB, Stern BJ: Number of pregnancies and risk for stroke and stroke subtypes. *Arch Neurol* 1997;**54**:203–206.

240. Kittner SJ, Stern BJ, Feeser BR, et al: Pregnancy and the risk of stroke. *N Engl J Med* 1996;**335**:768–774.

241. Finucane FF, Madans JH, Bush TL, et al: Decreased risk of stroke among postmenopausal hormone users. *Arch Intern Med* 1993;**153**:73–79.

242. Grodstein F, Manson JE, Colditz GA, et al: A prospective observational study of postmenopausal hormone therapy and primary prevention of cardiovascular disease. *Ann Intern Med* 2000;**133**:933–941.

243. Lokkegaard E, Jovanovic Z, Heitemann BL, et al: Increased risk of stroke in hypertensive women using hormone therapy. Analysis based on the Danish Nurse Study. *Arch Neurol* 2003;**60**:1379–1384.

244. Wilson PW, Garrison RJ, Castelli WP: Postmenopausal estrogen use, cigarette smoking, and cardiovascular morbidity in women over 50. The Framingham Study. *N Engl J Med* 1985;**313**:1038–1043.

245. Simon JA, Hsia J, Cawley JA, et al: Postmenopausal hormone therapy and risk of stroke. The Heart and Estrogen/Progestin Replacement Study (HERS). *Circulation* 2001;**103**:638–642.

246. Grady D, Harrington D, Bittner V, et al: For the HERS Research Group. Cardiovascular disease outcomes during 6–8 years of hormone therapy. The Heart and Estrogen/Progestin Replacement Study (HERS II). *JAMA* 2002;**288**:49–57.

247. Viscoli CM, Brass LM, Kernan WN, et al: A clinical trial of estrogen-replacement therapy after ischemic stroke. *N Engl J Med* 2001;**345**:1243–1249.

248. Rossouw JE, Anderson GL, Prentice RL, et al: Risks and benefits of estrogen plus progestin in healthy postmenopausal women: Principal results from the Women's Health Initiative randomized controlled trial. *JAMA* 2002;**288**:321–333.

249. Wassertheil-Smoller S, Hendrix SL, Mimacher M, et al: Effect of estrogen plus progestins on stroke in postmenopausal women. The Women's Health Initiative: A randomized controlled trial. *JAMA* 2003;**289**:2673–2684.

250. The Women's Health Initiative Steering Committee: Effects of conjugated equine estrogen in postmenopausal women with hysterectomy. The Women's Health Initiative: A randomized controlled trial. *JAMA* 2004;**291**:1701–1712.

251. Nelson H, Walker M, Zakher B, Mitchell J: Menopausal hormone therapy for the primary prevention of chronic conditions: a systematic review to update the US Preventive Serices Task Force recommendations. *Ann Intern Med* 2012; **157**: 104–113.

252. Whitmer RA, Quesenberry CP, Zhou J, Yaffe K: Timing of hormone therapy and dementia: the critical window theory revisted. *Ann Neurol* 2011;**69**:163–169.

253. The 2012 Hormone Therapy Position Statement of the North American Menopause Society. *Menopause* 2012;**19**:257–271.

254. Moyer VA, on behalf of the US Preventive Services Task Force: Menopausal hormone therapy for the primary prevention of chronic conditions: US Preventive Services Task Force recommendation statement. *Ann Intern Med* 2013;**158**:47–54.

255. Espeland MA, Shumaker SA, Leng I, et al: Long-term effects on cognitive function of postmenopausal hormone therapy presecribed to women aged 50 to 55 years. *JAMA Intern Med* 2013;**173**:1429–1236.

256. Wannamethee G, Shaper AG: Physical activity and stroke in middle-aged men. *BMJ* 1992;**304**:597–601.

257. Sacco RL, Gan R, Boden-Albala B, et al: Leisure-time physical activity and ischemic stroke risk. The Northern Manhattan Stroke Study. *Stroke* 1998;**29**:380–387.

258. Lindenstrom E, Boysen G, Nyboe J: Lifestyle factors and risk of cerebrovascular disease in women. The Copenhagen City Heart Study. *Stroke* 1993;**24**:1468–1472.

259. Agnarsson U, Thorgeirsson G, Sigvaldson H, Sigfusson N: Effects of leisure-time physical activity and ventilatory function on risk for stroke in men: The Reykjavik Study. *Ann Intern Med* 1999;**130**:987–990.

260. Choi-Kwon S, Kim JS: Lifestyle factors and risk of stroke in Seoul, South Korea. *J Stroke Cerebrovasc Dis* 1998;**7**:414–420.

261. Lee I-M, Paffenbarger Jr RS: Physical activity and stroke incidence. The Harvard Alumni Health Study. *Stroke* 1998;**29**:2049–2054.

262. Lee I-M, Hennekens CH, Berger K, et al: Exercise and risk of stroke in male physicians. *Stroke* 1999;**30**:1–6.

263. Hu FB, Stampfer MJ, Colditz G, et al: Physical activity and risk of stroke in women. *JAMA* 2000;**283**:2961–2967.

264. Lee CD, Folsom AR, Blair SN: Physical activity and stroke risk. A meta-analysis. *Stroke* 2003;**34**:2475–2482.

265. Paffenbarger Jr RS, Wing AL, Hyde RT, Jung DL: Physical activity and incidence of hypertension in college alumni. *Am J Epidemiol* 1983;**117**:245–257.

266. Paffenbarger Jr RS, Jung DL, Leung RW, Hyde RT: Physical activity and hypertension: An epidemiological view. *Ann Med* 1991;**23**:319–327.

267. Hayashi T, Tsumura K, Suematsu C, et al: Walking to work and the risk of hypertension in men: The Osaka Health Survey. *Ann Intern Med* 1999;**130**:21–26.

268. Endres M, Gertz K, Lindauer U, et al: Mechanisms of stroke protection by physical activity. *Ann Neurol* 2003;**54**:582 590.

269. Eckel RH, Jakicic JM, Ard JD, et al: 2013 AHA/ACC guideline on lifestyle management to reduce cardiovascular risk. *Circulation* 2014;**129**:S76–S99.

270. Wing S, Casper M, Davis WB, et al: Stroke mortality maps. *Stroke* 1988;**19**:1507–1513.

271. Lanska DJ: Geographic distribution of stroke mortality in the United States: 1939–1941 to 1979–1981. *Neurology* 1993;**43**:1839–1851.

272. Lanska DJ, Kryscio R: Geographic distribution of hospitalization rates, case fatality, and mortality from stroke in the United States. *Neurology* 1994;**44**:1541–1550.

273. Glymour WM, Avendano M, Berkman LF: Is the "stroke belt" worn from childhood? Risk of first stroke and state of residence in childhood and adulthood. *Stroke* 2007;**38**:2415–2421.

274. Howard G, Prineas R, Moy C, et al: Racial and geographic differences in awareness, treatment, and control of hypertension: The Reasons for Geographic and Racial Differences in Stroke Study. *Stroke* 2006;**37**:1171–1178.

275. Vermeer SE, Koudstaal PJ, Oudkerk M, et al: Prevalence and risk factors of silent brain infarcts in the population-based Rotterdam Scan Study. *Stroke* 2002;**33**:21–25.

276. Howard G, Safford MM, Meschia JF, et al. Stroke symptoms in individuals reporting no prior stroke or transient ischemic attack are associated with decreased indices of mental and physical functioning. *Stroke* 2007; **38**: 2446–2452.

277. Caplan LR: Significance of unexpected (silent) brain infarcts. In Caplan LR, Shifrin EG, Nicolaides AN, Moore WS (eds): *Cerebrovascular Ischaemia. Investigation and Management.* London: Med-Orion, 1996, pp 423–433.

278. Wardlaw JM, Smith EE, Biessels GJ, et al: Neuroimaging standards for research into small vessel disease and its contribution to aging and neurodegeneration. *Lancet Neurol* 2013;**12**:822–838.

279. Ward NS, Brown MM: Leukoaraiosis. In Donnan G, Norrving B, Bamford J, Bogousslavsky J (eds):*Subcortical Stroke*, 2nd ed. Oxford: Oxford University Press, 2002, pp 47–66.

280. Caplan LR, Schoene WC: Clinical features of subcortical arteriosclerotic encephalopathy (Binswanger's disease). *Neurology* 1978;**28**:1206–1215.

281. Caplan LR: Binswanger's disease – revisited. *Neurology* 1995;**45**:626–633.

282. Babikian V, Ropper AH: Binswanger disease: A review. *Stroke* 1987;**18**:1–12.

283. Fisher CM: Binswanger's encephalopathy: A review. *J Neurol* 1989;**236**:65–79.

284. Gray F, Dubas F, Roullet E, Escourolle R: Leukoencephalopathy in diffuse hemorrhagic cerebral amyloid angiopathy. *Ann Neurol* 1985;**18**:54–59.

285. Dubas F, Gray F, Roullet E, Escourolle R: Leukoencephalopathies arteriopathiques. *Rev Neurol* 1985;**141**:93–108.

286. Loes D, Biller J, Yuh WT, et al: Leukoencephalopathy in cerebral amyloid angiopathy: MR imaging in four cases. *AJNR Am J Neuroradiol* 1990;**11**:485–488.

287. Baudrimont M, Dubas F, Joutel A, et al: Autosomal dominant leukoencephalopathy and subcortical ischemic stroke: A clinicopathological study. *Stroke* 1993;**24**:122–125.

288. Davous P: CADASIL: A review with proposed diagnostic criteria. *Eur J Neurology* 1998;**5**:219–233.

289. Chabriat H, Levy C, Taillia H, et al: Patterns of MRI lesions in CADACIL. Neurology 1998;**51**:452–457.

290. Chen YW, Gurol ME, Rosand J, et al: Progression of white matter lesions and hemorrhages in cerebral amyloid angiopathy. *Neurology* 2006;**67**:83–87.

291. Imaizumi T, Honma T, Horita Y, et al: Hematoma size in deep intracerebral hemorrhage and its correlation with dot-like hemosiderin spots on gradient echo T2*-weighted MRI. *J Neuroimaging* 2006;**16**:236–242.

292. Imaizumi T, Horita Y, Hashimoto Y, Niwa J: Dotlike hemosiderin spots on T2*-weighted magnetic resonance imaging as a predictor of stroke recurrence: A prospective study. *J Neurosurg* 2004;**101**:915–920.

293. Klein I, Iung B, Labreuche J, et al. and the IMAGE Study Group: Cerebral microbleeds are frequent in infective endocarditis. *Stroke* 2009;**40**:3461–3465.

294. Hollenhorst R: Ocular manifestations of insufficiency or thrombosis of the internal carotid artery. *Am J Ophthalmol* 1959;**47**:753–767.

295. Fisher CM: Observations of the fundus oculi in transient monocular blindness. *Neurology* 1959;**9**:333–347.

296. Kearns T, Hollenhorst R: Venous stasis retinopathy of occlusive disease of the carotid artery. *Mayo Clin Proc* 1963;**38**:304–312.

297. Carter JE: Chronic ocular ischemia and carotid vascular disease. In Bernstein EF (ed): *Amaurosis Fugax*. New York: Springer, 1988, pp 118–134.

298. Slaoui T, Klein IF, Guidoux C, et al: Prevalence of subdiaphragmatic visceral infarction in cardioembolic stroke. *Neurology* 2010;**74**:1030–1032.

299. Chatzikonstantinou A, Krissak R, Fluchter S, et al: CT angiography of the aorta is superior to transesophageal echocardiography for determining stroke subtypes in patients with cryptogenic ischemic stroke. *Cerebrovasc Dis* 2012;**33**:322–328.

300. Nicolaides AN: Asymptomatic carotid stenosis and the risk of stroke (the ACSRS Study): Identification of a high-risk group. In Caplan LR, Shifrin EG, Nicolaides AN, Moore WS (eds): *Cerebrovascular Ischaemia: Investigation and Management*. London: Med-Orion, 1996, pp 435–441.

301. Wityk RJ, Chang H-M, Rosengart A, et al: Proximal extracranial vertebral artery disease in the New England Medical Center Posterior Circulation Registry. *Arch Neurol* 1998;**55**:470–478.

302. Caplan LR: *Posterior Circulation Disease: Clinical Findings, Diagnosis, and Management*. Boston: Blackwell, 1996.

303. Toghi H, Yamanouchi H, Murakami M, et al: Importance of the hematocrit as a risk factor in cerebral infarction. *Stroke* 1978;**9**:369–374.

304. Harrison MJG, Pollock S, Thomas D, et al: Hematocrit, hypertension, and smoking in patients with transient ischemic attack and in age and sex matched controls. *J Neurol Neurosurg Psychiatry* 1982;**45**:550–551.

305. Di Mascio R, Marchioli R, Vitullo F, Tognoni G: A positive relation between high hemoglobin values and the risk of ischemic stroke. Progetto 3A Investigators. *Eur Neurol* 1996;**36**:85–88.

306. Harrison MJG, Pollock S, Kendall B, et al: Effect of hematocrit on carotid stenosis and cerebral infarction. *Lancet* 1981;**2**:114–115.

307. Thomas DJ, Marshall J, Ross-Russel RW, et al: Effects of hematocrit on cerebral blood flow in man. *Lancet* 1977;**2**:940–943.

308. Elkind MS, Sciacca RR, Boden-Albala B, et al: Relative elevation in baseline leukocyte count predicts first cerebral infarction. *Neurology* 2005;**64**:2121–2125.

309. Mercuri M, Bond MG, Evans G, et al: Leukocyte count and carotid atherosclerosis. *Stroke* 1991;**22**:134.

310. Elkind MS, Cheng I, Boden-Albala B, et al: Elevated white blood cell count and carotid plaque thickness: The Northern Manhattan Stroke Study. *Stroke* 2001;**32**:842–849.

311. Elkind MS, Sciacca R, Boden-Albala B, et al: Leukocyte count is associated with aortic arch plaque thickness. *Stroke* 2002;**33**:2587–2592.

312. Ovbiagele B, Lynn MJ, Saver JL, et al: Leukocyte count and vascular risk in symptomatic intracranial atherosclerosis. WASID Study Group. *Cerebrovasc Dis* 2007;**24**:283–288.

313. Elkind MS, Sciacca RR, Boden-Albala B, et al: Leukocyte count is associated with reduced endothelial reactivity. *Atherosclerosis* 2005;**181**:329–338.

314. Elkind MS: Inflammation, atherosclerosis, and stroke. *Neurologist* 2006;**12**:140–148.

315. Elkind MSV: Impact of innate inflammation in population studies. *Ann NY Acad Sci* 2010;**1207**:97–106.

316. Eikelboom JW, Hankey GJ, Baker RI, et al: C-reactive protein in ischemic stroke and its etiologic subtypes. *J Stroke Cerebrovasc Dis* 2003;**12**:74–81.

317. Arenillas JF, Alvarez-Sabin J, Molina CA, et al: C-reactive protein predicts further ischemic events in first-ever transient ischemic attack or stroke patients with intracranial large-artery occlusive disease. *Stroke* 2003;**34**:2463–2470.

318. Wakugawa Y, Kiyohara Y, Tanizaki Y, et al: C-reactive protein and risk of first-ever ischemic and hemorrhagic stroke in general Japanese population. The Hisayama Study. *Stroke* 2006;**37**:27–32.

319. Gorelick PB: Lipoprotein-associated phospholipase A2 and risk of stroke. *Am J Cardiol* 2008;**101**(suppl):34F–40F.

320. Wilhelmsen L, Svarrdsudd K, Korsan-Bengtsen K, et al: Fibrinogen as a risk factor for stroke and myocardial infarction. *N Engl J Med* 1984;**311**:501–505.

321. Drouet L: Fibrinogen: A treatable risk factor. *Cerebrovasc Dis* 1996;**6**(suppl 1):2–6.

322. Kristensen B, Malm J, Nilsson T, et al: Increased fibrinogen levels and acquired hypofibrinolysis in young adults with ischemic stroke. *Stroke* 1998;**29**:2261–2267.

323. Grotta J, Ackerman R, Correia J, et al: Whole-blood viscosity parameters and cerebral blood flow. *Stroke* 1982;**13**:296–298.

324. Graham IM, Daly LE, Refsum HM, et al: Plasma homocysteine as a risk factor for vascular disease. The European Concerted Action Project. *JAMA* 1997;**277**:1775–1781.

325. Welch GN, Loscalzo J: Homocysteine and atherothrombosis. *N Engl J Med* 1998;**338**:1042–1050.

326. Giles WH, Croft JB, Greenlund KJ, et al: Total homocyst(e)ine concentration and the likelihood of nonfatal stroke. Results from the Third National Health and Nutrition Examination Survey, 1988–1994. *Stroke* 1998;**29**:2473–2477.

327. Sacco RL, Ananad K, Lee H-S, et al: Homocysteine and the risk of ischemic stroke in a triethnic cohort. The Northern Manhattan Study. *Stroke* 2004;**35**:2263–2269.

328. Selhub J, Jacques PF, Bostom AG, et al: Association between plasma homocysteine concentrations and extracranial carotid-artery stenosis. *N Engl J Med* 1995;**332**:286–291.

329. Eikelboom JW, Hankey GJ, Ananad S, et al: Association between high homocyst(e)ine and ischemic stroke due to large and small-artery disease but not other etiologic subtypes of ischemic stroke. *Stroke* 2000;**31**:1069–1075.

330. Toole JF, Malinow MR, Chambless LE, et al: Lowering homocysteine in patients with ischemic stroke to reduce recurrent stroke, myocardial infarction and death. The Vitamin Intervention for Stroke Prevention (VISP) randomized controlled trial *JAMA* 2004;**291**:565–575.

331. VITATOPS Trial Study Group. B vitamins in patients with recent transient ischaemic attack or stroke in the VITAmins TO Prevent Stroke (VITATOPS) trial: A randomised, double-blind, parallel, placebo-controlled trial. *Lancet Neurol* 2010;**9**:855–865.

332. Beamer NB, Coull BM, Clark WM, Wynn M: Microalbuminuria in ischemic stroke. *Arch Neurol* 1999;**56**:699–702.

333. Gaede P, Vedel P, Parving H-H, Pederson O: Intensified multifactorial intervention in patients with type 2 diabetes mellitus and micro-albuminuria: The Steno type 2 randomized study. *Lancet* 1999;**353**:617–622.

334. Gerstein H, Mann JFE, Yi Q, et al: F Albuminuria and risk of cardiovascular events, death, and heart failure in diabetic and nondiabetic individuals. HOPE Study Investigators. *JAMA* 2001;**286**:421–426.

335. Ovbiagele B: Impairment in glomerular filtration rate or glomerular filtration barrier and occurrence of stroke. *Arch Neurol* 2008;**65**:934–938.

336. Khatri M, Wright CB, Nickolas TL, et al: Chronic kidney disease is associated with white matter hyperintensity volume. The Northern Manhattan Study (NOMAS). *Stroke* 2007;**38**:3121–3126.

337. Alberts MJ: *Genetics of Cerebrovascular Disease*. Armonk, NY: Futura, 1999.

338. Meschia JF, Worrall BB: New advances in identifying genetic anomalies in stroke-prone probands. *Curr Neurol Neurosci Rep* 2004;**4**:420–426.

339. Gretarsdottir S, Thorleifsson G, Reynisdottir ST, et al: The gene encoding phosphodiesterase 4D confers risk of ischemic stroke. *Nat Genet* 2003;**35**:131–138.

340. Yee RYL, Brophy VH, Cheng S, et al: Polymorphisms of the phosphodiesterase 4D, camp-specific (*PDE4D*) gene and risk of ischemic stroke. A prospective, nested case-control evaluation. *Stroke* 2006;**37**:2012–2017.

341. Worrall BB, Mychaleckyj JC: *PDE4D* and stroke. A real advance or a case of the emperor's new clothes? *Stroke* 2006;**37**:1955–1957.

342. Ruigrok YM, Rinkel GJE, Wijmenga C: Genetics of intracranial aneurysms. *Lancet Neurol* 2005;**4**:179–189.

343. Ruigrok YM, Rinkel GJ, Wijmenga C: The versican gene and the risk of intracranial aneurysms. *Stroke* 2006;**37**:2372–2374.

344. Markus H: Stroke genetics: prospects for personalized medicine. *BMC Med* 2012;**10**:113, accessed at http://www.biomedcentral.com/1741-7015/10/113.

345. Wolf PA, D'Agostino RB, Belanger AJ, Kannel WB: Probability of stroke: A risk profile from the Framingham Study. *Stroke* 1991;**22**:312–318.

346. Wolf PA, Belanger AJ, D'Agostino RB: Quantifying stroke risk factors and potentials for risk reduction. *Cerebrovasc Dis* 1993;**3**(suppl 1):7–14.

347. Goff DC, Lloyd-Jones DM, Bennet G, et al: 2013 ACC/AHA guideline on the assessment of cardiovascular risk: A report of the American College of Cardiology/American Heart Association Task Force on Practice Guidelines. *J Am Coll Cardiol* 2014;**63**:2935–2959.

348. Stone NJ, Robinson JG, Lichtenstein AH, et al: 2013 ACC/AHA guideline on the treatment of blood cholesterol to reduce atherosclerotic cardiovascular risk in adults: A report of the American College of Cardiology/American Heart Association Task Force on Practice Guidelines. *J Am Coll Cardiol* 2014;**63**:2889–2934.

349. James PA, Oparil S, Carter BL, et al: 2014 evidence-based guideline for the management of high blood pressure in adults: Report from the panel members appointed to the Eight Joint National Committee (JNC 8). *JAMA* 2014;**311**:507–520, erratum 7;311:1809.

350. Banach M, Aronow WS: Blood pressure J-curve: Current concepts. *Curr Hypertens Rep* 2012;**14**:556–566.

351. Meschia JF, Bushnell C, Bodsen-Albala B, et al. on behalf of the American Heart Association Stroke Council, Council on Cardiovascular and Stroke Nursing, Council on Clinical Cardiology, Council on Functional Genomics and Translational Biology, and Council on Hypertension: Guidelines for the primary prevention of stroke. A statement for healthcare professionals from the American Heart Association/American Stroke Association. *Stroke* 2014;**45**:3754–3832.

352. Yamamoto H, Bogousslavsky J: Mechanisms of second and further strokes. *J Neurol Neurosurg Psychiatry* 1998;**64**:771–776.

353. Caplan LR: Editorial. *J Neurol Neurosurg Psychiatry* 1998;**64**:716.

354. Inzitari D, Eliasziw M, Gates P, et al: The causes and risk of stroke in patients with asymptomatic internal-carotid-artery stenosis. North American Symptomatic Carotid Endarterectomy Trial Collaborators. *N Engl J Med* 2000;**342**:1693–1700.

355. Leonberg SC, Elliot FA: Prevention of recurrent stroke. *Stroke* 1981;**12**:731–735.

356. Ovbiagele B, Saver JL, Fredieu A, et al: In-hospital initiation of secondary stroke prevention therapies yields high rates of adherence at follow-up. *Stroke* 2004;**35**:2879–2883.

357. Touze E, Coste J, Voicu M, et al: Importance of in-hospital initiation of therapies and therapeutic inertia in secondary stroke prevention. Implemetation of prevention after a cerebrovascular event (IMPACT) study. *Stroke* 2008;**39**:1834–1843.

Complications in stroke patients

Louis R Caplan and Sandeep Kumar

Sometimes, the brain injury that develops during a stroke is not the only medical problem the patient, family, and doctor must battle. Strokes, like many other serious medical illnesses, can be followed by a host of other problems. These complications can sometimes cause neurological deterioration; in other instances, the patient feels worse and the deterioration is falsely attributed to worsening of the stroke. Most of the complications that occur after stroke are medical and not neurological. Complications are extremely common. In the Randomized Trial of Tirilazad Mesylate in Acute Stroke (RANTTAS) trial, 95% of the 279 stroke patients had at least one complication.[1] Complications may occur during hospitalization for acute stroke or may develop during rehabilitation and neurological recovery. A number of reports and reviews discuss the various complications of stroke, frequencies of occurrence, and prevention and management.[1–11] Tables 19.1 and 19.2 list the frequency of various medical complications found in four series of stroke patients.[1,7–9] Although medical errors such as giving wrong medications, omitting medications and treatments, and wrong dosing also occur all too often,[12] these problems are not unique to stroke patients and, therefore, will not be discussed here.

Complications can be serious and cause death. The most common causes of death in patients with stroke are shown in Table 19.3. Brain edema, cardiac abnormalities, and pulmonary embolism dominate during the first week.[13] Pneumonia, urinary tract infections, bed sores, phlebothrombosis and pulmonary embolism, gastrointestinal bleeding, contractures, falls, osteopenia, and depression also occur during the first week. These problems may continue during recovery and even after patients return home. Randomized trials, analyses, and meta-analyses have all shown that units dedicated solely to the care of stroke patients decrease mortality and morbidity among stroke patients.[14–19] One important function of stroke units and stroke teams is to systematically pursue measures to monitor complications and prevent their occurrence.

Neurological complications

Stroke progression or recurrence

Deterioration of neurological functions, including a decrease in the level of consciousness or progression of focal neurological signs, develops in more than 25% of stroke patients.[6] In most patients, this progression occurs during the first 24–72 hours

and is much less common thereafter.[6,20,21] In patients with intracerebral hemorrhages, the deterioration is often caused by continued bleeding.[22–25] In patients with aneurysmal subarachnoid hemorrhage, rebleeding and vasoconstriction with delayed brain ischemia are most often responsible for neurological deterioration during the 2 weeks after the initial bleed. Progression of brain ischemia is most common in patients with occlusions of large extracranial and intracranial arteries and those with lacunar infarcts. In patients with ischemic strokes, progression of brain ischemia is often related to propagation of thrombi, embolism, and failure of collateral circulation to develop adequately.

Table 19.1 Most frequent important medical events among 279 stroke patients in the control limb of the randomized trial of tirilazad mesylate in acute stroke

Event	Serious	Total
Sepsis	3 (1%)	3 (1%)
Cellulitis	2 (1%)	5 (2%)
Congestive heart failure	7 (3%)	30 (11%)
Cardiac arrest	5 (2%)	5 (2%)
Angina, myocardial infarct	4 (1%)	16 (6%)
Deep vein thrombosis	3 (1%)	6 (2%)
Pulmonary embolism	3 (1%)	4 (1%)
Peripheral vascular disease	2 (1%)	2 (1%)
Pneumonia (all)	13 (5%)	27 (10%)
Aspiration pneumonia	8 (3%)	16 (6%)
Dyspnea	3 (1%)	11 (4%)
Pulmonary edema	3 (1%)	9 (3%)
Gastrointestinal bleed	7 (3%)	15 (5%)
Dehydration	3 (1%)	6 (2%)
Hypoxia	2 (1%)	8 (3%)
Urinary tract infection	3 (1%)	30 (11%)

Source: Johnston KC, Li JY, Lyden PD, et al. Medical and neurological complications of ischemic stroke. Experience from the RANTTAS trial. *Stroke* 1998;29:447–453, Table 4.

Table 19.2 Number of observed medical complications among 100 consecutive stroke patients during rehabilitation

Medical complication	No.
Urinary tract infection	44
Musculoskeletal pain	31
Urinary retention	25
Falls	25
Fungal rash	24
Hypotension	19
Diabetes mellitus	16
Hypertension	15
Cardiac arrhythmia	8
Pneumonia	7
Congestive heart failure	6
Angina pectoris	4
Myocardial infarct	0
Thrombophlebitis	4
Pulmonary embolism	0
Other miscellaneous complications	135
Total	**363**

From Dromerick A, Reding M. Medical and neurological complications during in-patient stroke rehabilitation. *Stroke* 1994;25:358(361) with permission.

Table 19.3 Causes of death in stroke patients with supratentorial lesions

Cause of death	Infarction		Hemorrhage	
	Week 1	Week 2–4	Week 1	Week 2–4
Transtentorial herniation	36	6	42	2
Pneumonia	0	28	1	2
Cardiac	7	17	0	2
Pulmonary embolism	0	4	0	0
Sudden death	2	8	0	0
Septicemia	1	4	0	0
Unknown	0	12	1	3
Brainstem extension of hematoma			1	1
Total	**46**	**79**	**45**	**10**

Reprinted with permission from Silver F, Norris JW, Lewis A, Hachinsky V. Early mortality following stroke: a prospective review. *Stroke* 1984;15:494.

A second stroke may develop in the days and weeks after the initial stroke. This may occur while the patient is still in the acute hospital or during rehabilitation. Among 1273 patients with brain infarcts entered in the Stroke Data Bank, 40 had a stroke recurrence during the 30 days after the index stroke.[26] The likelihood of recurrence depends heavily on the mechanism of the first stroke and treatment. Recurrences are most likely to be caused by the same stroke mechanism as the index stroke.[27] Patients with cardiac-origin embolism are at the highest risk for having a second stroke, but different sources of emboli have different rates of recurrence.[28,29]

Brain edema

The most lethal complication of stroke is brain edema that develops after large ischemic and hemorrhagic strokes. In stroke units, brain edema, pulmonary embolism, and cardiac abnormalities are the major cause of early death.[6,14,30] Brain infarcts evolve rapidly, whereas brain edema not only varies with time but also varies in severity in different areas within and surrounding the lesion.[31] The two main components of the edema are: (1) intracellular (cytotoxic) edema, which results from damage to the sodium-potassium pump with failure of the cell to maintain the normal osmotic gradient across its membrane; and (2) extracellular (vasogenic) edema with fluid occupying the interstitial spaces, especially at the edge of infarcts and hemorrhages.

Brain edema may begin within hours but usually does not become clinically obvious until 1–4 days after the stroke. Some patients, especially those with distal internal carotid artery (ICA) and proximal middle cerebral artery (MCA) occlusions can develop massive brain swelling, which can start within the first 24 hours after a stroke. This condition, called malignant MCA infarction, carries a very high mortality in untreated patients, estimated at between 40% and 80%.[32,33] Ropper and Shafran analyzed the fluctuating clinical course of patients with stroke and brain edema.[34] During the acute initial presentation, patients were often drowsy. Usually, a subsequent improvement in the level of consciousness occurred, and by the second or third day, patients were usually more alert. As brain edema increased, patients again became drowsy. In the series of Ropper and Shafran, drowsiness was not the only sign and was accompanied by one or more of the following:[34]

1. Pupillary asymmetry or lack of pupillary response to light. In most patients, the larger pupil was on the side ipsilateral to the brain infarct; pupillary asymmetry varied from 0.5 to 2.0 mm.
2. Periodic breathing patterns.
3. VIth nerve paresis.
4. Extensor plantar responses on the previously spared side.
5. Papilledema.
6. Headache or vomiting.
7. Bilateral spontaneous extensor posturing.

The clinical findings clearly need not follow the typical "central" or "uncal" herniation syndromes described originally by Plum and Posner.[35]

Computed tomography (CT) and magnetic resonance imaging (MRI) show mass effect from the edema with compression of the lateral ventricles and shift of midline structures. Barber and colleagues found that early CT scan signs (within first 48 h of stroke) including anteroseptal shift ≥5 mm, pineal shift ≥2 mm, hydrocephalus, temporal lobe infarction, and other vascular territory involvement were associated with a fatal outcome in large MCA territory infarction.[36] When intracranial pressure (ICP) monitoring is performed, pressures consistently greater than 15 mmHg as determined by subarachnoid screw devices are usually fatal.[34]

In patients with large cerebellar infarcts and hemorrhages, small amounts of swelling can compress the brainstem, injure its vital structures, and cause a rapidly progressive obstructive hydrocephalus.[37,38] CT may show crowding of the perimesencephalic, ambient, and cerebellopontine-angle cisterns and lack of visibility or displacement of the IVth ventricle. The typical syndrome of cerebellar infarction and hemorrhages includes headache, vertigo, nausea, vomiting, and ataxia. Patients with significant cerebellar edema may subsequently develop signs of tegmental brainstem compression over the next 12 hours to 4 days, including gaze palsies, diplopia, facial numbness and weakness. Drowsiness and ipsilateral limb paresis usually indicate significant brainstem compression. It is not unusual for a patient with cerebellar infarction to be sent home from the emergency room with the diagnosis of labyrinthitis only to return in 24–48 hours in a coma.[39] This serious mistake can be avoided if the patient's gait is tested at the time of the initial evaluation. Patients with sizable cerebellar hemorrhages and infarcts nearly always cannot walk or have abnormal gaits with veering or leaning to one side. In the presence of increased posterior fossa pressure, suboccipital decompressive surgery or draining cerebrospinal fluid by a shunt can be life saving.[39,40]

In supratentorial lesions, the therapy for increased pressure is twofold. First, physicians avoid factors that can further increase ICP and promote fluid retention. These include unusual head and neck positions, fever, increased central venous pressure, overhydration, hypoxia, hypercapnia, increased mean airway pressure, and agitation. Second, specific measures can be attempted to decrease pressure. Hyperventilation with reduction of the arterial carbon-dioxide tension to between 20 and 34 mmHg reduces ICP during the short term, but ICP usually returns to pretreatment levels. Infusion of mannitol, glycerol, or hypertonic saline,[41,42] to maintain blood osmolality between 300 and 310 Osm/l, also decreases intracranial pressure. This osmotic therapy is effective only when the cell endothelium and membranes are intact. Thus, this therapy is not effective within the core of the infarct or for cytotoxic edema, but it helps reduce the extracellular edema that surrounds infarcts.[31]

Steroids have also been used. The effectiveness and mechanism of action of steroids in decreasing ICP is obscure. Steroids may ameliorate the extracellular edema that surrounds the infarct (as they do in brain tumors) or in areas where the cell membrane is not severely damaged. Steroids may also protect against free-radical generation. The efficacy of steroids is in doubt. Increased risk of gastrointestinal bleeding, infections, and exacerbation of diabetes are reported when steroids are used in stroke patients.[43–45] We rarely use steroids after ischemic infarction. In occasional patients, especially young individuals, an impressive edema exists despite a relatively small zone of infarction. Similarly in young patients with small subdural hematomas, edema in the ipsilateral hemisphere may develop and cause important intracranial pressure shifts. In these rare situation, steroids can be helpful. In patients with brain hematomas, we use steroids and osmotic agents to reduce pressure. In patients with large infarcts, although steroids occasionally allow survival for the short term, most such patients remain in disabled states and succumb later from pneumonia or other complications. We rarely use steroids in patients with massive infarcts. Craniectomy is another important consideration, especially in young patients with swollen cerebral hemispheres and incipient brain herniation.[46,47] Craniectomy as a decompressive strategy is discussed in Chapter 6.

Seizures

Seizures may also follow strokes. As early as 1864, Jackson recognized seizures as a complication that frequently occurred during the recovery phase of stroke.[48] Among 1000 patients in a data bank collected in Girona, Spain, 50 (5%) patients had epileptic seizures during the first 48 hours after stroke.[49] Patients with brain hemorrhages have seizures more often than those with infarcts. In the Lausanne Stroke Registry, 7% of intracerebral hemorrhage patients had seizures during acute strokes compared with less than 1% of patients with ischemic strokes.[50] In the Harvard Stroke Registry, 6% of patients with hematomas had seizures during acute hospitalization.[51] Subcortical "slit" hemorrhages are most often accompanied by seizures.[52] Among patients with brain infarcts, those patients who have large and hemorrhagic infarcts are most likely to develop seizures.[49,53,54] Patients with lesions that include the cerebral cortex have a much higher frequency of seizures than those whose lesions are only subcortical.[49,53–55] Patients with embolic brain infarcts of cardiac-origin have a much higher frequency of seizures than those who have large artery occlusive disease. Among 770 patients with supratentorial brain infarcts in one series, the presence of cardiac-origin brain embolism meant that the patient had a relative risk of 5.14 of developing early seizures compared with patients without cardiac-origin embolism.[54] Post-stroke seizures can occasionally cause worsening of neurological deficits.[56] Patients who develop early seizures after stroke have a higher in-hospital mortality than those without seizures, probably reflecting the observation that patients with large infarcts are more likely to develop seizures.[57]

Approximately 10% of patients with strokes have seizures at some time after their stroke. In the Seizures after Stroke Study, a prospective, multicenter study among university hospitals in Canada, Australia, Israel, and Italy, 8.3% of stroke patients had seizures.[58] In this series, more than one-half of seizures occurred on the first day. Eighty percent of seizures occurred by the first month.[58] Gupta and colleagues analyzed

the timing of post-infarction seizures.[59] In their series of 70 patients with seizures after ischemic strokes, one-third occurred within the first 2 weeks. Ninety percent of the 30 early seizures occurred within the first 24 hours.[59] Nearly three-fourths of seizures occurred within the first year. Only 2% developed more than 2 years after stroke.[59]

The electroencephalogram (EEG) may have some prognostic value concerning the likelihood of a stroke patient developing a seizure.[60] Patients with periodic, lateralizing, epileptiform discharges are particularly likely to develop seizures. Patients who have focal spikes are also at increased risk, with 78% developing seizures. In patients with focal slowing, diffuse slowing, or normal EEG records, only 20%, 10%, and 5%, respectively, had seizures.[60] Early seizures are usually focal spells with secondary generalization. Late-onset seizures are more often generalized.[49,59] Patients with cortical infarcts, especially large infarcts with persistent hemiplegia, are most susceptible to postinfarction epilepsy.[55,59] Usually, post-stroke seizures are readily controlled with one anticonvulsant.[59] We do not prescribe prophylactic anticonvulsants in stroke patients. The vast minority of stroke patients develop seizures. Potential side effects and toxicity of anticonvulsants complicates the care of patients. We use anticonvulsants only after the patient has had a well-documented seizure.

Now in many academic medical centers in the United States, very sick patients with brain hemorrhages and infarcts who are being managed in neurological intensive care units have continuous EEG monitoring. These EEGs may show very abnormal focal discharges that are interpreted as being compatible with "non-convulsive status epilepticus." It is not certain if these discharges represent true seizures or are merely representative of the residual activity of a very injured brain. It is also not clear if anticonvulsant treatment of these patients with already reduced alertness improves neurological outcome.

Medical complications

Deep vein thrombosis and pulmonary embolism

Pulmonary embolism is the most feared and lethal medical complication in stroke patients. Pulmonary embolism occurs in about 1% of stroke patients and accounts for up to 15% of deaths.[8] Most of the patients who develop pulmonary embolism have deep vein thrombi in their lower extremities. Thrombi tend to develop mostly in paretic limbs in patients who are not yet walking. Some venous thrombi are located in pelvic structures. Very rarely the primary venous occlusion is in the intracranial dural sinuses and has extended into the jugular vein.[61] Stasis of blood and an increase in acute phase reactants that follows brain ischemia increase blood coagulability and combine to promote venous thrombosis and thromboembolism. Among patients in 8 trials that studied the effect of treatment with heparin given within the first 3 weeks after ischemic stroke, 54% of control patients developed deep vein thrombosis as detected by systematic iodine (I^{125}) fibrinogen scanning or venography.[6,62] Prophylactic administration of heparin, low-molecular-weight heparin, or

heparinoids in these patients led to an 81% reduction in deep vein thrombosis as detected by I^{125} fibrinogen scanning and venography.[62]

Patients who harbor deep vein thrombi detected by non-invasive techniques and venography often do not have abnormal physical signs or symptoms.[63,64] Patients with severe leg weakness,[65] and those with congestive heart failure and atrial fibrillation,[66] are most likely to develop deep vein thrombosis. Venous occlusions most often involve the paretic leg in patients with hemiparesis. The true frequency of pulmonary emboli is unknown because many are silent. In necropsy series of patients who die during the first week after stroke, pulmonary emboli, although not always the cause of death, are frequently noted by the pathologist. Wijdicks and Scott reviewed the patient records of 33 patients who had pulmonary emboli after strokes during 2 decades (1976–1995) at the Mayo Clinic.[67] In three patients who died of progressive brain swelling, pulmonary emboli were found in small pulmonary arteries at necropsy. Among the remaining 30 patients, 15 patients had brain infarcts and 15 patients had intracerebral hemorrhages. None received heparin.[67] Pulmonary embolism occurred from days 3–120 (median day, 20) after stroke. Pulmonary embolism resulted in sudden death in 15 of the 30 patients.[67] Small peripheral located pulmonary emboli can cause pleuritic chest pain, dyspnea or hemoptysis whereas larger emboli are more likely to produce hypoxia, hypotension and syncope.

Physical measures such as compression stockings and devices that produce intermittent pneumatic compression are in common use to prevent the development of phlebothrombosis, but their effectiveness is marginal at best.[68–72] Unfractionated heparin and low-molecular-weight heparin are more effective than aspirin or physical measures.[73,74] Some studies indicate that relatively low doses of low-molecular-weight heparin have a better benefit–risk ratio than use of unfractionated heparin.

We consider all stroke patients at risk for the development of deep venous thrombosis. We pay particular attention to patients who are immobile. Obesity, obtundation, congestive heart failure, paralysis of one or both legs, hypercoagulability, dehydration, malignancy, abulia, and severity of stroke are risk factors for phlebothrombosis. We keep some patients with acute cerebral ischemia at bed rest to maximize cerebral blood flow. We mobilize all other patients as soon as possible. Physical therapy is started at the bedside. We encourage patients to flex and extend the knees and ankles throughout the day. Support hose or special inflated stockings are often used. Patients who have not had a hemorrhagic stroke and are not on anticoagulants are given low-dose subcutaneous heparin (5000 U ("mini" heparin) twice per day) or low-molecular-weight heparin.

Patients who have sudden shortness of breath, chest pain, hypotension, hemoptysis, change in respiratory pattern, hypoxemia, agitation, confusion, or other worsening are suspected of having pulmonary embolism. Depending on the index of suspicion, evaluation should include the following tests:

1. Examination of arterial blood gases.
2. Chest x-ray.

3. Electrocardiogram.
4. Non-invasive studies of the venous circulation in the legs.
5. Venography, nuclear lung ventilation, and perfusion scans.
6. Pulmonary CT angiography or dye-contrast angiography.

Patients who develop phlebothrombosis or pulmonary embolism, or both, are treated urgently with intravenous full-dose heparin or low-molecular-weight heparin.

A recent brain hemorrhage contraindicates the acute use of full-dose anticoagulation. Antifibrinolytic therapy with urokinase or streptokinase therapy is also contraindicated in the presence of a recent stroke. If the pulmonary emboli were multiple and life threatening, the patient might require placement of a venous umbrella or other procedure to occlude the venous circulation. Pulmonary embolism remains a vexing problem throughout the rehabilitation process in patients who remain paretic.

Cardiac abnormalities

Cardiac dysfunction is another frequent accompaniment of stroke. The dysfunctioning heart may be the source of stroke, coexist with stroke, or be the result of stroke.[29,75] Cardiac-related mortality is the second most common cause of death in the acute stroke population, second only to neurological complications.[76] In the VistA data compilation, among 846 ischemic stroke patients, 35 (4.1%) died of cardiac causes and 161 (19%) had at least one serious cardiac adverse event.[76] Serious cardiac events are common in the acute stroke patients and usually peak 2–3 days after a stroke.[76] Death from cardiac-related events is highest during the first month after stroke and declines in frequency thereafter.

Patients with ischemic and hemorrhagic stroke have been shown at necropsy to have subendocardial hemorrhages and focal regions of necrosis of cardiac muscle cells.[75,77–80] Electrocardiogram (ECG) changes consistent with ischemia, elevated creatine–phosphokinase–myoglobin levels, troponin levels, and various cardiac arrhythmias are found in stroke patients even without known previous heart disease.[75,81–83] In some series, one-third to one-half of patients with strokes have serious cardiac rhythm disturbances, including ventricular tachycardia, salvos or couplets of premature ventricular beats greater than 10 premature beats per minute, second- or third-degree heart block, or asystole.[75,81,83,84] In control populations matched for age and history of cardiac disease, such arrhythmias are found in only 15%. Mortality has rarely been related to these arrhythmias. Atrial fibrillation can also develop as a sequel to stroke.[85]

Lesions of particular regions of the brain are most likely to be associated with cardiac abnormalities.[75,86] Three ways that strokes cause secondary cardiac, cardiovascular, and respiratory changes are as follows:

1. Direct involvement of critical structures, such as the cortex of the insula of Reil, hypothalamus, and brainstem nuclei that make up the central autonomic network,[79] which activate autonomic descending fiber pathways to the heart, blood vessels, and lungs.
2. Mass effect with compression of the hypothalamus or brainstem, or both, also activates autonomic pathways.

3. The acute brain lesion and its stress effects stimulate the hypothalamic-pituitary axis triggering the release of catecholamines and corticosteroids.

Electrical stimulation of the anterior part of the brain, including the frontal pole, premotor and motor cortex, cingulate gyri, orbital frontal gyri, insular cortex, anterior part of the temporal lobe, amygdala, and hippocampus are all known to produce pressor or depressor effects on blood pressure or atrial and ventricular arrhythmias.[75,80,86–90] Stimulation of some of these regions may cause cardiovascular effects because of a non-specific activation of limbic cortex, which has secondary effects on the hypothalamus, autonomic nervous system, and hypothalamic–pituitary–endocrine axis. Stimulation of the insula has a more specific relation to cardiac and cardiovascular functions. After showing that stimulation of the posterior portions of the rat insular cortex had reproducible effects on heart rate and rhythm, Oppenheimer and colleagues stimulated the insular cortex of human epileptic patients.[89,90] They found that electrical stimulation of areas within the left human insular cortex produced bradycardia and reduced blood pressure, whereas stimulation of the right insular cortex elicited tachycardia and increased blood pressure.[90] Strokes that involve the insular cortex may be accompanied by arrhythmias and other cardiovascular effects. The insular cortex is very commonly involved in patients with acute non-lacunar middle cerebral artery territory infarcts.[91]

Projections from the cerebral cortex of the frontal lobe sometimes passing through the temporal lobes and thalami are relayed to the hypothalamus and brainstem nuclei, which then project directly to the intermediolateral cell columns of the thoracic spinal cord that control sympathetic nervous system output to the heart. Stimulation of the lateral and posterior portions of the hypothalamus cause the release of large amounts of catecholamines from the adrenal medulla.[80] Sympathetic stimulation mostly increases the rate and force of the heartbeat and dilates coronary arteries, whereas parasympathetic stimulation slows the atrial rate and force of contractions and constricts the coronary arteries.[75] Brainstem compression and direct involvement of the medulla oblongata can lead to vagal discharges, which can cause sinus bradycardia, cardiac arrhythmias, and even cardiac arrest, as well as elevation of systolic blood pressure and a fall in diastolic blood pressure. This train of events is the likely explanation of the blood pressure and pulse changes found in patients with increased ICP and brain herniations that were discovered and emphasized by Harvey Cushing. These changes are usually called the *Cushing response*.

When these changes occur during strokes, creatine-phosphokinase and troponin elevations tend to be longer lasting than those associated with primary cardiac disease. Elevations may peak at the fifth day and persist until the twelfth day.[82] When levels of norepinephrine, epinephrine, and dopamine are measured in patients with stroke, patients with transient ischemic attacks, and non-stroke controls, the highest levels are found in stroke patients.[75] The next highest levels are found in transient disorders. Normal values occur in the control population.[75,92] Those

patients with stroke and the highest cardiac enzyme values have the highest levels of norepinephrine. This information suggests that stroke causes an increase in sympathetic tone elevating levels of catecholamines, which in turn cause focal myocardial damage and subsequent arrhythmias.

Patients who have subarachnoid hemorrhage and vertebrobasilar-territory ischemia and hemorrhages sometimes develop acute pulmonary edema, which is often sudden in onset and sometimes fatal.[75,93] Pulmonary edema is most likely to develop when a sudden-onset and severe increase in ICP occurs. Weir studied the occurrence of pulmonary edema in patients with fatal subarachnoid hemorrhages.[93] The sudden onset of coma was present in 70% of his fatal cases of patients with ruptured aneurysms who developed pulmonary edema. Respiratory symptoms were noted within a short time period after the onset of headache and neurological symptoms.[93] Weir attributed the occurrence of pulmonary edema to a sudden, severe increase in ICP, which in turn caused massive autonomic stimulation. Experimental data from studies in cats confirm this hypothesis.[94] Myocardial enzyme release and electrocardiogram changes that indicate abnormal wall motion are often accompanied by decreased left ventricular performance in patients with subarachnoid hemorrhage.[95] Decreased cardiac output often results from the impaired left ventricular function.[95]

Myocardial infarction is also common after stroke, especially in patients with pre-existent ischemic heart disease. The increase in acute phase reactants that accompanies stroke can promote coronary thrombosis. Gongora-Rivera and his French colleagues examined the frequency of cardiac-related ischemic lesions among 341 stroke patients that came to necropsy at the Salpetriere hospital in Paris.[96] The frequency of coronary atherosclerotic plaques in these patients was 26.8%, while coronary artery stenosis was found in 37.5% and myocardial infarcts in 40.8%.[96] Two-thirds of the myocardial infarcts were not recognized during life and were found only at autopsy.[96] Significant coronary artery disease was especially common in patients with occlusive lesions in the cervical-cranial arteries. It may be difficult in individual patients, especially those with large strokes, to differentiate the changes related to myocytolysis from those caused by coronary artery thrombosis without echocardiography and coronary angiography.

Older patients with cerebral hemispheric infarction have the highest risk for cardiac arrhythmias.[84] Heart rate variability is common in patients with cerebral hemispheric and medullary infarcts.[97] All stroke patients require careful attention to the cardiovascular system by clinical examination and laboratory tests. In addition to surveillance for symptoms, clinicians should carefully monitor vital signs, regular cardiovascular examinations, echocardiography, and routine electrocardiograms. In some patients, continuous cardiac rhythm monitoring may be needed. Although its efficacy is unproved, propranolol or other beta-blockers are theoretically useful in patients with neurogenic cardiac arrhythmias, treating both the arrhythmia and its cause.[84] Propranolol could, however, worsen sinus bradycardia, heart block, and episodes of asystole. In experimental animals, the cardiac rhythm abnormalities secondary to cerebral ischemia can be effectively treated with propranolol and atropine.[98] If rhythm disturbances occur, we treat with standard antiarrhythmics according to suggestions of cardiology consultants.

Swallowing abnormalities, aspiration, and pneumonia

Dysphagia and aspiration are common after stroke. Symptomatic dysphagia is noted in approximately one-fourth to one-third of stroke patients.[99,100] Dysphagia and aspiration are especially common in patients who have had bilateral hemispheric strokes or strokes that involve the brainstem.[101] Severe strokes and patients with reduced consciousness and dementia are also conditions in which dysphagia and aspiration are common. So-called silent aspiration is also common when clinicians look for it.

Clinical bedside testing of swallowing ability should be a part of the early assessment of each stroke patient. Examination of the pharynx and palate as they move on saying "ah" and watching the patient swallow some water should be part of the routine examination. Dysphonia, dysarthria, abnormal cough to extricate food from the oropharynx, and voice change after swallowing are highly predictive of a heightened risk of aspiration.[102] A change in pulse oximetry after swallowing has also been used to detect potential for aspiration.[102] Videofluoroscopic examination and fiberoptic endoscopic evaluation of swallowing detects more patients with dysphagia and aspiration than the clinical examination. Videofluoroscopic studies can detect abnormalities of swallowing in approximately 50% of stroke patients.[102–107] In one study among 128 patients hospitalized for first strokes, 65 (51%) had swallowing abnormalities detected clinically and 82 (64%) had swallowing abnormalities shown by videofluoroscopy.[105] During the next 6 months, 26 patients (20%) had pulmonary infections, among whom 24 had videofluoroscopic swallowing abnormalities when studied during their acute stroke.[105] Physical therapy with guidance in positioning of food within the oral cavity and pharynx, choice of foods, the use of thermal stimulation, and instructions to the patient can help prevent aspiration. Most patients are able to resume oral feeding within months, although feeding tubes may be needed temporarily.

Pneumonia is common after stroke during the immediate and late periods. The frequency of pneumonia has varied between 4–22% in different stroke studies.[106,107] The cause of pneumonia in patients with stroke is multifactorial. Decreased alertness, severe neurological deficits, and dysphagia are highly associated with the development of pneumonia during hospitalization.[108] In a recumbent position, atelectasis and poor mobilization of secretions often occur. Difficulty in swallowing may also lead to aspiration. Coughing and deep breathing may not be done or may be only poorly performed. Chest movements are also decreased on the hemiplegic side.[109,110] Kaldor and Berlin noted that pneumonia is more likely to exist on the hemiparetic side because of the decreased thoracic movements and impaired pulmonary

circulation.[111] Respiratory drive and the function of interstitial muscles are often abnormal on the hemiplegic side.[111] Recently, investigators have found evidence that strokes create an immunodepressed state, and this also can contribute to the development of pneumonia and other infections while in the hospital and afterward.[112–114]

Although many dysphagic patients are fed through nasogastric tubes, this does not seem to prevent pneumonia.[115] Among 100 acute stroke patients given tube feedings because of dysphagia, pneumonia developed in 44.[115] Swallowing function should be tested before giving patients oral feedings. Physiotherapy or nursing techniques probably help to prevent pneumonia after stroke. We encourage oral hygiene, deep breathing, coughing, frequent turning, and early mobilization of patients. If fever develops despite these measures, the lung should be aggressively evaluated as the potential source of infection.

Metabolic and nutritional disorders

Prolonged undernutrition is an important but seldom recognized complication of stroke, especially in elderly patients whose nutritional intake was poor or marginal before their stroke. Undernutrition is an important predictor of poor outcome.[116] Finestone and colleagues evaluated the nutritional state of 49 consecutive stroke patients admitted to a rehabilitation unit and found that approximately one-half were malnourished.[117] In another study, the authors correlated serum albumin concentration, an index of nutritional state, and the presence of chronic disease with the frequency of medical complications and found that 79% of patients with an albumin less than 2.9 g/dl had at least one medical complication during rehabilitation.[118] A high serum albumin correlated with good gains in neurological functional status.[119] Malnutrition can contribute to diminished immune functions, cardiac and gastrointestinal dysfunction, and abnormal bone metabolism. Malnutrition is a factor in the formation and repair of decubitus ulcers.

To help maintain an adequate nutritional state, we give multivitamins and especially thiamine orally, if the patient is able, or parenterally. If the patient is unable to eat by the fourth or fifth day, we insert a small nasogastric feeding tube through which nutritional supplements can be given. Prolonged inability to swallow may require the placement of gastric feeding tubes. The use of percutaneous endoscopic gastrostomy (PEG) tubes with maintenance of nutrition has undoubtedly helped many stroke patients maintain reasonable nutritional balance despite dysphagia. However, early PEG placement after stroke has been shown to worsen outcomes in a large multicenter trial.[120] Routine early PEG placement is therefore discouraged in the early phases of stroke recovery and nasogastric tube feeding is preferred during this time. Nutrition can be better maintained using PEGs than with nasogastric tube feedings.[117] PEG placement can be usually managed with few complications, such as wound infection and gastrointestinal bleeding. In approximately 25% or more of patients, PEGs can be removed when swallowing improves.[121]

Fluid, electrolyte, and nutritional abnormalities may also occur during the acute stroke and recovery periods. Approximately 15% of patients with acute stroke develop hyponatremia. Hyponatremia can cause nausea, vomiting, weakness, confusion, and seizures. Joynt et al. posited that post-stroke hyponatremia is usually related to inappropriate secretion of antidiuretic hormone (ADH).[122] They showed that stroke patients often had excess ADH even in the presence of normal serum sodium levels. Although the mechanism of the inappropriate ADH secretion is unknown, Joynt et al. reviewed some of the potential mechanisms, including damage to the anterior hypothalamus, effects on ADH secretion related to recumbency, resetting of osmoreceptors, damage to a more widespread vasopressin neuronal system, increased release of ADH, and secondary stroke-related elevations in serum catecholamines and cortisol.[122] Changes in the levels of atrial natriuretic factor have also been posited to cause abnormalities of serum sodium concentrations.

In hyponatremic patients, volume depletion and overload must be excluded as contributing factors. To assess this problem, remember that fluid may accumulate in the sacral regions during prolonged bed rest. If volume status is normal, the syndrome of inappropriate ADH secretion can be diagnosed if symptoms, including decreased serum osmolality, continued urinary excretion of sodium, urine less than maximally dilute, normal renal function, and normal thyroid function, exist in addition to hyponatremia. During the acute stroke period, we advise carefully following the patient's volume status by clinical examination; uniform charting of input, output, and daily weights; and monitoring of renal function and electrolytes.

Urinary tract infections and urinary incontinence

Urinary tract infections are also a common complication of stroke. The reported frequency of urinary tract infections in stroke patients has varied between 6% and 30%.[11] The high frequency of urinary tract infections is probably caused by the following two factors. First, an indwelling catheter is often placed to empty the urinary bladder. This foreign body allows for the introduction and growth of bacteria. Whenever possible, continuous catheter drainage should be avoided. Intermittent catheterization using strict sterile techniques is preferable. In some men, condom catheters suffice. A Foley catheter should never be used as a convenience for the staff. Second, the functioning of the urinary bladder and external sphincter can be compromised by the stroke. Urinary symptoms are common even in patients with uninfected bladders and include urinary urgency, frequency, and retention. Tsuchida et al. documented these symptoms and attempted to establish their relationship to brain lesions.[123] Patients with frontal and internal-capsular lesions showed a hyperactive bladder or uninhibited sphincter relaxation with subsequent urinary frequency or incontinence. Patients with putaminal lesions had hyperactive bladders with usually normal sphincter function. Patients who had urinary retention showed an inactive or hypoactive bladder with an uncoordinated or normal sphincter; localization of the offending lesion could not be

accomplished in these patients. Men in the stroke age group are often geriatric and also have large prostates, which can contribute to the obstructive uropathy.

When confronted with patients with abnormal micturition, we survey for and treat bacterial urinary tract infections when present. In addition, we consider other mechanisms that may be causing symptoms, such as inability to reach the commode or urinal because of gait or limb abnormalities, communication difficulty that may make it hard to signal the nurse, and unavailable nursing personnel. Measurement of post-voided residual urine may be all that is needed, but at times, cystometrics and imaging of the kidneys and urinary tract are required to define the problem. We encourage frequent voiding during the day and night in an effort to train the bladder. Pharmacotherapy can be used if these maneuvers fail to help alleviate the problem.

Gastrointestinal bleeding and other complications

Physicians have long realized that some patients with stroke and other brain diseases develop gastrointestinal hemorrhage. This problem, usually called *Cushing's ulcers, stress ulcers*, or *hemorrhagic gastritis*, can be life threatening when severe. Davenport and colleagues reported that 18 of 607 (3%) stroke patients at their hospital in Edinburgh had gastrointestinal hemorrhages.[124] One-half of the hemorrhages were severe.[124] Most patients had hematemesis or melena, but one patient suddenly developed abdominal pain and hemodynamic shock.[124] Older patients with severe strokes and decreased levels of consciousness are most likely to develop gastrointestinal bleeding. Corticosteroids given for brain edema also increase the risk of stress ulceration in the stomach. However, indiscriminate use of proton-pump inhibitors and H2-blockers can predispose to pneumonia in these patients.[125]

Obstipation and altered gastrointestinal motility are other important complications found in stroke patients.[126]

Immobility and its complications

Pressure decubitus ulcers

The development of bed sores is an iatrogenic and preventable complication of stroke that significantly hinders the rehabilitation process. Patients who are immobilized, have limited ability to reposition themselves, and do not sense the need to change positions; they are at risk of developing bedsores if they are not frequently turned and repositioned.[127] Incontinence also increases the risk of developing skin breakdown. The skin should be kept clean and dry, and the patient should be turned frequently. Adequate nutrition should be given. Pressure on anesthetic or immobilized limbs must be avoided. The use of padded heel boots can spare the heels from ulcers. Egg-crate mattresses, waterbeds, or soft cotton padding may help retard the development of sacral pressure sores. Physicians and nursing personnel should periodically examine the entire skin surface looking for any area of early breakdown. Particular attention should be paid to susceptible areas, such as the sacrum, buttocks, heels, elbows, wrists, toes, and occiput.

If an ulcer develops, pressure on that area should be totally avoided, special mattresses should be used, and the wound should be dressed and, if necessary, debrided and the skin grafted.

Contractures and shoulder pain

Limb immobility and maintenance in fixed, usually flexed positions can lead to fixed contractures at the knees and elbows. Decreased shoulder movement can lead to shoulder pain, frozen shoulders, and the so-called shoulder–hand syndrome. In the Lund Stroke Register, 22% of over 300 patients developed significant shoulder pain within 4 months after stroke.[128] In one study, 36 of 132 (27%) hemiplegic stroke patients developed the shoulder–hand syndrome.[129] The shoulder–hand syndrome is characterized by pain and tenderness when abducting, flexing, and externally rotating the upper arm; pain and swelling over the carpal bones; and edema of the distal hand joints. Severe shoulder weakness, spasticity, and subluxation of the shoulder increase the likelihood of developing shoulder pain and swelling of the upper extremity. Early full range of movement of the shoulder joint is important in preventing this unpleasant and disabling stroke complication. Non-steroidal anti-inflammatory drugs, such as indomethacin and low-dose corticosteroids, may be helpful in patients who develop shoulder pain. The most important treatment, however, is vigorous physical therapy.[129] Subluxation of the shoulders is another complication of hemiparesis. The weak arm should not be left to hang without support.

Peripheral nerve injuries

Peripheral nerve compression is also a hazard in limbs with weakness and reduced sensation. The peroneal nerve is most commonly involved; its compression causes a foot drop. Ulnar palsy caused by compression of the nerve at the elbow is also common, especially in wheelchair-bound patients. Occasionally, patients compress their femoral nerve in relation to local pressure on the groin region while consciousness is reduced. The femoral nerve can also be compressed by retroperitoneal hemorrhages that involve the iliopsoas muscles. The most common cause of these hematomas is anticoagulation. The earliest sign is often a dropped knee jerk on the side of the retroperitoneal hematoma.

Osteopenia and osteoporosis

Studies of bone mineral densities after stroke have shown that a significant reduction in bone mineral density occurs on the hemiplegic side.[130–133] The causes are multifactoral but include immobilization-induced calcium resorption from bone, sometimes with hypercalcemia; lack of sunlight exposure; poor nutrition with inadequate vitamin D stores; and osteoporosis before the stroke. The hemiosteoporosis is most severe in those patients with severe hemiplegia, especially those that have prolonged immobilization. Use of anticoagulants can further contribute to bone loss. The reduced bone density predisposes to hip and other fractures, which tend to occur predominantly

on the hemiplegic side. Calcium and vitamin D supplements are important prophylactically in patients at risk for this complication. Early mobilization and exposure to sunlight are also important. In one small study, Zoledronate, given within 35 days after stroke in a single intravenous infusion of 4 mg, prevented hip osteopenia on the hemiplegic side.[134]

Fatigue

Stroke patients often complain of fatigue, even long after their stroke. Fatigue is a well-known problem after other neurological illnesses, especially multiple sclerosis. Although some causative factors are evident, they do not always explain the extreme fatigue that develops in some stroke patients. Patients with neurological deficits may need to use more energy to do the same activities that they were able to perform easily before their strokes. The stroke and post-stroke period may have led to a prolonged decrease in physical activity and deconditioning likely developed and persisted. Fatigue correlates with the severity of the neurological deficit.[135] Fatigue should be separated from apathy and disinterest in performing activities. Fatigue is also quite different from depression. Several studies have noted that fatigue is quite common and underappreciated after stroke, can persist for an extended and even indefinite period, and is not explained by depression.[135,136] Patients and their caregivers should be encouraged to gradually increase the physical activity level to potentially increase the stroke patient's stamina.

Depression and other psychological effects of stroke

One of the most important and yet often overlooked complications of stroke is depression. New personality traits can emerge or old ones become accentuated. The patient may become apathetic, inflexible, rigid, impulsive, insensitive, or indifferent to others; adopt a poor perception of self; or become guilt-ridden, paranoid, or suicidal.

Depression is reported to occur in 26–60% of stroke patients.[137–141] Approximately 20–25% of patients have a major depressive disorder.[140–142] Astrom and colleagues analyzed the prevalence of major depression at various time intervals after stroke and their most important correlations and determinants.[140] Approximately 25% of their stroke patients had a major depression during the acute post-stroke period, and 31% were depressed at 3 months. Acute depression was most frequent in patients with anterior lesions in the left hemisphere, aphasic patients, and those who lived alone. At one year, 16% of patients were depressed. Two- and 3-year depression rates were 19% and 29%, respectively. Dependency and lack of social contacts were important determinants of late depression.[140] In another study, among 202 stroke patients, depressive symptoms were present in 43% at 6 months, 36% at 1 year, 24% at 2 years, and 18% at 3 years.[143]

Patients who have a history of depression before their stroke are also prone to become depressed after a stroke.[141] Six months after a stroke, there is an increased prevalence of symptoms of both major and minor depressive symptoms, increasing from 23% and 20%, respectively, immediately after the stroke to 35% and 26% at 6 months.[142,144] Diagnosis of depression is often difficult because functional psychogenic reactions are hard to separate from organic behavioral changes related to the stroke, such as abulia, apathy, aprosodia, impersistence, and anosognosia.[145]

Facial expression, gestures, pauses, loudness, emphasis, and other non-linguistic aspects give verbal communication an emotive context. Aprosodia is the inability to express or understand the emotive content of spoken language. Patients with right perisylvian strokes may be unable to communicate emotion in spoken language. An observer might erroneously believe that they are depressed. Binder noted additional factors complicating the recognition of depression.[146] An accurate history may not be available because of aphasia or slowed responses. Vegetative and autonomic signs may also be difficult to interpret. Stroke may suppress appetite, change sleep patterns, or create a pseudobulbar state with rapid shifts from laughing to crying. To complicate matters, persistent depressive symptoms are more common in patients with cognitive and behavioral abnormalities.[143] Neurological and psychological effects often coexist and augment each other. Loss of function makes individuals sad, and depressive patients cannot perform up to their potential.

Often, sexual function in patients with stroke is ignored. For some patients, stroke may make sexual relations cumbersome and decrease their frequency. The patient and family should be reassured that for most mechanisms of stroke, sex is unlikely to cause a recurrent stroke. Sexual activity should be encouraged in those couples who were sexually active before the stroke, although it may require some creativity on the part of the participants.

Ross and Rush proposed guidelines for the diagnosis of depression.[147] Depression should be considered in patients who are not making expected recovery, are uncooperative in rehabilitation, or lose previously achieved milestones. Emotional outbursts, inflexibility, irritability, insensitivity to others, and suicidal ideations may occur. A flat affect must be distinguished from a depressed affect. Collateral history from friends and caregivers are also often needed.

In some studies, depression was more common after left- than right-hemisphere strokes.[138,140,143,148–151] In the left hemisphere, the more anteriorly placed infarctions are correlated with a higher frequency of depression.[149,150] When cortical and basal ganglia lesions, infarcts, and hemorrhages affect the left hemisphere anteriorly, they are more likely to be associated with depression than similarly placed right-cerebral lesions.

Finkelstein et al. used the dexamethasone-suppression test to assess patients with mood and vegetative disturbances after stroke.[139] An abnormal test is defined as failure to suppress cortisol secretion in response to exogenously administered dexamethasone. This test is reported to be abnormal in 60–80% of psychiatric patients with endogenous depression. Abnormal dexamethasone suppression tests in patients with stroke were associated with occurrence of moderate to severe mood, sleep, and appetite disturbances.[139]

Box 19.1 Prevention of complications

1. Care for patients in stroke units of the hospital where physicians and nurses have protocols to protect against complications
2. Evaluate swallowing function. The water swallow test is a useful screen. Do not give oral liquids, or foods to patients with dysphagia
3. Consider prophylactic measures to prevent deep vein thrombosis in limbs that are not active
4. Mobilize patients as soon as appropriate. Passive range of motion should be performed often in paralyzed upper and lower limbs
5. Evaluate cardiac and respiratory function
6. Pay attention to urinary function, and prevent overdistention of the bladder
7. Monitor for infection, especially pneumonia and urinary tract infections, and treat early with appropriate antibiotics
8. Pay attention to the nutritional state of the patient
9. Protect pressure points on the patient's body, and turn and move patients often to avoid pressure sores
10. Be alert for the development of depressive symptoms and treat early
11. Involve potential caregivers early in procedures to prevent complications once the patient is home

From Silver F, Norris JW, Lewis A, Hachinski V. Early mortality following stroke: a prospective review. *Stroke* 1984;15:494 with permission.

The causes of late depressive reaction are often unknown. Whether it is a reaction to the loss the patient feels or a result of brain injury is unclear. Injury may result in depletion of noradrenergic neurotransmitters resulting in depression. Nortriptyline, trazodone, and serotonin re-uptake inhibitors are reported to be effective in ameliorating significantly the symptoms of depression in patients with stroke.[145,152–154]

Beyond pharmacological therapy, clinicians should try to adopt a hopeful and fighting attitude. We encourage activity and independence for the family and patient. Physicians should attempt to promote continued affection, understanding, and respect between the family and patient. We suggest that physicians reassure all involved that efforts are intended to maximize rehabilitation and prevent recurrent stroke. We recommend that physicians promote the patient's self-confidence and emphasize the old adage, "When the going gets tough, the tough get going!"

Box 19.1 summarizes suggestions for prevention of stroke complications.

Caregivers and their reactions to the stroke patient

Strokes and stroke patients do not live in a vacuum. Strokes cause important ramifications that affect all those who interact with the individual stroke survivor, but most of the burden falls on the family and principal caregiver. Stroke is a condition that hits the whole family constellation, not merely the stroke patient.

Stroke patients who have severe deficits often become dependent on caregivers for daily activities and physical and emotional support. Members of the family must deal with the physical handicaps and, often, new personality traits. If the patient is dependent on family members for care, the main caregiver can develop feelings of entrapment, isolation, anger, and depression. In some families, it seems as if a new dependent child has been thrust on them. Physicians should remember that caregivers are often old and sick and have their own physical and emotional problems.

Researchers have begun to analyze and quantitate burdens perceived by those caring for stroke patients. Researchers have also begun to describe and quantify the emotional and physical consequences of caregiving.[155–159] A Dutch study analyzed the burden of caregiving among 121 partners of patients who were living at home.[157] The investigators interviewed the caregivers 3 years after stroke had affected their loved ones. Caregivers reported feeling overwhelmed with responsibility, uncertainty, and worry. They found it difficult to handle the restraints placed on their own social lives and interests.[157] Analysis showed that higher levels of burden were attributable to the stroke patient's degree of disability and the amount of care needed. The caregiver's emotional distress, loneliness, and perception of his or her ability to care for the stroke patient shaped the burden the caregiver felt.[157]

The emotional outcome of stroke on care-givers was analyzed in a Scottish study of 231 stroke patients and their caregivers.[158] Severe emotional distress and depression were common among caregivers. Caregivers were more likely to be depressed if the stroke patient was dependent or emotionally distressed. The caregivers' emotional state in terms of anxiety and depression highly correlated with the emotional state of the stroke patient. Women who cared for male stroke patients had more anxiety and depression than male caregivers. Older caregivers were more depressed than young caregivers.[158] In another study, the proportion of caregivers that were depressed did not diminish over time.[155]

Clearly, care, education, and concern must be addressed to the caregivers and their families, as well as the stroke patients.

References

1. Johnston KC, Li JY, Lyden PD, et al: Medical and neurological complications of ischemic stroke: Experience from the RANTTAS trial. RANTTAS Investigators. *Stroke* 1998;**29**:447–453.

2. Davenport RJ, Dennis MS, Wellwood I, Warlow CP: Complications after acute stroke. *Stroke* 1996;**27**:415–420.

3. Smithard DG, O'Neill PA, Park C, et al: Complications and outcome after acute stroke. *Stroke* 1996;**27**:1200–1204.

4. Biller J, Patrick JT: Management of medical complications of stroke. *J Stroke Cerebrovasc Dis* 1997;**6**:217–220.

5. Zorowitz RD, Tietjen GE: Medical complications after stroke. *J Stroke Cerebrovasc Dis* 1999;**8**:192–196.

6. van der Worp HB, Kappelle LJ: Complications of acute ischaemic stroke. *Cerebrovasc Dis* 1998;**8**:124–132.

7. Dromerick A, Reding M: Medical and neurological complications during inpatient stroke rehabilitation. *Stroke* 1994;**25**:358–361.

8. Langhorne P, Stott DJ, Robertson L, et al: Medical complications after stroke. *Stroke* 2000;**31**:1223–1228.

9. Weimar C, Roth M, Zillessen G, et al: Complications following acute ischaemic stroke. On behalf of the German Stroke Data Bank Collaborators. *Eur Neurol* 2002;**48**:133–140.

10. Kappelle LJ, van der Worp HB: Treatment and prevention of complications of acute ischemic stroke. *Curr Neurol Neurosci Rep* 2004;**4**:36–41.

11. Kumar S, Selim M, Caplan LR: Medical complications after stroke. *Lancet Neurol* 2010;**9**:105–118.

12. Holloway RG, Tuttle D, Baird T, Skeleton WK: The safety of hospital care. *Neurology* 2007;**68**:550–555.

13. Silver F, Norris JW, Lewis A, Hachinski V: Early mortality following stroke: A prospective review. *Stroke* 1984;**15**:494.

14. Kaste M, Palmomaki H, Sarna S: Where and how should elderly stroke patients be treated? A randomized trial. *Stroke* 1995;**26**:249–253.

15. Indredavik B, Slordahl SA, Bakke F, et al: Stroke unit treatment. Long term effects. *Stroke* 1997;**28**:1861–1866.

16. Stroke Unit Trialists' Collaboration: Collaborative systematic review of the randomized trials of organised in-patient (stroke unit) care after stroke. *BMJ* 1997;**314**:1151–1159.

17. Stroke Unit Trialists' Collaboration: How do stroke units improve patient outcomes? A collaborative systematic review of the randomized trials. *Stroke* 1997;**28**:2139–2144.

18. Diez-Tejedor E, Fuentes B: Acute care in stroke: Do stroke units make the difference? *Cerebrovasc Dis* 2001;**11** (suppl 1):31–39.

19. Birbeck GL, Zingmond DS, Cui X, Vickrey BG: Multispecialty stroke services in California hospitals are associated with reduced mortality. *Neurology* 2006;**66**:1527–1532.

20. Toni D, Fiorelli M, Gentile M, et al: Progressing neurological deficit secondary to acute ischemic stroke: a study on predictability, pathogenesis, and prognosis. *Arch Neurol* 1995;**52**:670–675.

21. Davalos A, Cendra E, Teruel J, et al: Deteriorating ischemic stroke: risk factors and prognosis. *Neurology* 1990;**40**:1865–1869.

22. Kelly R, Bryer JR, Scheinberg P, Stokes IV: Active bleeding in hypertensive intracerebral hemorrhage: Computed tomography. *Neurology* 1982;**32**:852–856.

23. Broderick JP, Brott TG, Tomsick T, et al: Ultra-early evaluation of intracerebral hemorrhage. *J Neurosurg* 1990;**72**:195–199.

24. Fujii Y, Tanaka R, Takeuchi S, et al: Hematoma enlargement in spontaneous intracerebral hemorrhage. *J Neurosurg* 1994;**80**:51–57.

25. Kazui S, Naritomi H, Yamamoto H, et al: Enlargement of spontaneous intracerebral hemorrhage. Incidence and time course. *Stroke* 1996;**27**:1783–1787.

26. Sacco RL, Foulkes MA, Mohr JP, et al: Determinants of early recurrence of cerebral infarction. The Stroke Data Bank. *Stroke* 1989;**20**:983–989.

27. Yamamoto H, Bogousslavsky J: Mechanisms of second and further strokes. *J Neurol Neurosurg Psychiatry* 1998;**64**:771–776.

28. Caplan LR: Brain embolism. In Caplan LR, Hurst JW, Chimowitz MI (eds): *Clinical Neurocardiology*. New York: Marcel Dekker, 1999, pp 35–185.

29. Caplan LR, Manning W (eds): *Brain Embolism*. New York: Informa Healthcare, 2006, pp 129–186.

30. White DB, Norris JW, Hachinski VC, et al: Death in early stroke: Causes and mechanisms. *Stroke* 1979;**10**:743.

31. O'Brien MD: Ischemic cerebral edema. In Caplan LR (ed): *Brain Ischemia. Basic Concepts and Clinical Relevance*. London: Springer, 1995, pp 43–50.

32. Hacke W, Schwab S, Horn M, et al: "Malignant" middle cerebral artery territory infarction: Clinical course and prognostic signs. *Arch Neurol* 1996;**53**:309–315.

33. Huttner HB, Schwab S: Malignant middle cerebral artery infarction: Clinical characteristics, treatment strategies, and future perspectives. *Lancet Neurol* 2009;**8**:949–958.

34. Ropper AH, Shafran B: Brain edema after stroke. *Arch Neurol* 1984;**41**:26–29.

35. Plum F, Posner JB: *Diagnosis of Stupor and Coma* (3rd ed). Philadelphia: Davis, 1980.

36. Barber PA, Demchuk AM, Zhang J, et al: Computed tomographic parameters predicting fatal outcome in large middle cerebral artery infarction. *Cerebrovasc Dis* 2003;**16**:230–235.

37. Caplan LR: *Posterior Circulation Disease: Clinical findings, Diagnosis, and Management*. Boston: Blackwell, 1996.

38. Caplan LR: Cerebellar infarcts. Key features. *Rev Neurol Dis* 2005;**2**:51–60.

39. Savitz SI, Caplan LR, Edlow JA: Pitfalls in the diagnosis of cerebellar infarction. *Acad Emerg Med* 2007;**14**:63–68.

40. Rieke K, Krieger D, Adams H-P, et al: Therapeutic strategies in space-occupying cerebellar infarction based on clinical, neuroradiological, and neurophysiological data. *Cerebrovasc Dis* 1993;**3**:45–55.

41. Mortazavi MM, Romeo AK, Deep A, et al: Hypertonic saline for treating raised intracranial pressure: Literature review and meta-analysis. *J Neurosurg* 2012:**116**:210–221.

42. Ropper A: Hyperosmolar therapy for raised intracranial pressure. *N Engl J Med* 2012;**367**:746–752.

43. von Rosen F, Guazzo EP: Increased intracranial pressure. In Brandt T, Caplan LR, Dichgans J, et al. (eds): *Neurological Disorders: Course and Treatment*. San Diego: Academic, 1996, pp 521–529.

44. Norris JW: Steroid therapy in acute cerebral infarction. *Arch Neurol* 1976;**33**:69–71.

45. Ottonello GA, Primavera A: Gastrointestinal complications of high dose corticosteroid therapy in acute

cerebrovascular patients. *Stroke* 1979;**10**:208–210.

46. Gupta R, Connolly ES, Mayer S, Elkind MS: Hemicraniectomy for massive middle cerebral artery territory infarction: a systematic review. *Stroke* 2004; **35**: 539–43.

47. Vahedi K, Hofmeijer J, Juettler E, et al. Early decompressive surgery in malignant infarction of the middle cerebral artery: A pooled analysis of three randomised controlled trials. *Lancet Neurol* 2007;**6**:215–222.

48. Taylor J: *Selected Writings of John Hughlings Jackson on Epilepsy and Epileptiform Convulsions,* Vol. **1.** London: Hodder & Stoughton, 1931, pp 230–235.

49. Davalos A, de Cendra E, Molins A, et al: Epileptic seizures at the onset of stroke. *Cerebrovasc Dis* 1992;**2**:327–331.

50. Bogousslavsky J, van Melle G, Regli F: The Lausanne Stroke Registry: Analysis of 1000 consecutive patients with first stroke. *Stroke* 1988;**19**:1083–1092.

51. Mohr JP, Caplan LR, Melski JW, et al: The Harvard Cooperative Stroke Registry: A prospective registry. *Neurology* 1978;**28**:754–762.

52. Caplan LR: General symptoms and signs. In Kase CS, Caplan LR (eds): *Intracerebral Hemorrhage.* Boston: Butterworth–Heinemann, 1994, pp 31–43.

53. Bladin CF: *Seizures after Stroke,* MD thesis. University of Melbourne, Australia, 1997.

54. Heuts-van Rank EPM: *Seizures Following a First Cerebral Infarct. Risk Factors and Prognosis,* thesis. Rijksuniversiteit Limberg, Maastricht, the Netherlands, 1996.

55. Olsen TS, Hogenhaven H, Thage O: Epilepsy after stroke. *Neurology* 1987;**37**:1209–1211.

56. Bogousslavsky J, Martin R, Regli F, et al: Persistent worsening of stroke sequelae after delayed seizures. *Arch Neurol* 1992;**49**:385–388.

57. Arboix A, Comes E, Massons J, et al: Relevance of early seizures for in-hospital mortality in acute cerebrovascular disease. *Neurology* 1996;**47**:1429–1435.

58. Bladin CF, Johnston PJ, Smuraloska L, et al: What causes seizures after stroke? *Stroke* 1994;**25**:245.

59. Gupta SR, Naheedey MH, Elias D, Rubino F: Postinfarction seizures: A clinical study. *Stroke* 1988;**19**:1477–1481.

60. Holmes GL: The electroencephalogram as a predictor of seizures following cerebral infarction. *Clin Electroencephalogr* 1980;**11**:83–86.

61. Diaz JM, Schiffman JS, Urban ES: Superior sagittal sinus thrombosis and pulmonary embolism: a syndrome rediscovered. *Acta Neurol Scand* 1992;**86**:390–396.

62. Sandercock PAG, van den Belt AGM, Lindley RI, Slattery J: Antithrombotic therapy in acute ischaemic stroke: an overview of the completed randomised trials. *J Neurol Neurosurg Psychiatry* 1993;**56**:17–25.

63. Warlow C, Ogston D, Douglas AS: Deep venous thrombosis of the legs after stroke. *BMJ* 1976;**1**:1178–1183.

64. Kearon C, Julian JA, Math JM, et al: Noninvasive diagnosis of deep venous thrombosis. *Ann Intern Med* 1998;**128**:663–677.

65. Landi G, D'Angelo A, Boccardi E, Candelise L, et al: Venous thromboembolism in acute stroke: prognostic importance of hypercoagulability. *Arch Neurol* 1992;**49**:279–283.

66. Noel P, Gregoire F, Capon A, Lehrert P: Atrial fibrillation as a risk factor for deep venous thrombosis and pulmonary emboli in stroke patients. *Stroke* 1991;**22**:760–762.

67. Wijdicks EFM, Scott JP: Pulmonary embolism associated with acute stroke. *Mayo Clin Proc* 1997;**72**:297–300.

68. Kamran SI, Downey D, Ruff RL: Pneumatic sequential compression reduces the risk of deep vein thrombosis in stroke patients. *Neurology* 1998;**50**:1683–1688.

69. Kamphulsen PW, Agnelli G, Sebastianelli M: Prevention of venous thromboembolism after acute ischemic stroke. *J Thromb Haemost* 2005;**3**:1187–1194.

70. Mazzone C, Chiodo GF, Sandercock P, Miccio M, Salvi R: Physical methods for preventing deep vein thrombosis in stroke. *Cochrane Database Syst Rev* 2004;**18**:CD001922.

71. Andre C, de Freitas GR, Fukujima MM: Prevention of deep vein thrombosis and pulmonary embolism following stroke: A systematic review of published articles. *Eur J Neurol* 2007;**14**:21–32.

72. Muir KW, Baxter G, Grosset DG, Lees KR: Randomized trial of graded compression stockings for prevention of deep-vein thrombosis after acute stroke. *Quart J Med* 2000;**93**:359–364.

73. Kamphulsen PW, Agnelli G: What is the optimal pharmacological prophylaxis for the prevention of deep-vein thrombosis and pulmonary embolism in patients with acute ischemic stroke? *Thromb Res* 2007;**119**:265–274.

74. Sherman DG, Albers GW, Bladin C, et al. for the PREVAIL Investigators: The efficacy and safety of enoxyparin versus unfractionated heparin for the prevention of venous thromboembolism after acute ischaemic stroke (PREVAIL study): An open-label randomized comparison. *Lancet* 2007;**369**:1347–1355.

75. Caplan LR, Hurst JW: Cardiac and cardiovascular findings in patients with nervous system diseases–brain diseases–stroke. In Caplan LR, Hurst JW, Chimowitz MI (eds): *Clinical Neurocardiology.* New York: Marcel Dekker, 1999, pp 303–312.

76. Prosser J, MacGregor L, Lees KR et al. on behalf of the VISTA Investigators: Predictors of early cardiac morbidity and mortality after ischemic stroke. *Stroke* 2007;**38**:2295–2302.

77. Norris JW, Kolin A, Hachinski VC: Focal myocardial lesions in stroke. *Stroke* 1980;**11**:130.

78. Connor RC: Focal myocytolysis and fuchsinophilic degeneration of the myocardium of patients dying with various brain lesions. *Ann N Y Acad Sci* 1969;**156**:261–270.

79. Samuels M: "Voodoo" death revisited: The modern lessons of neurocardiology. *Neurologist* 1997;**3**:293–304.

80. Ali AS, Levine SR: Heart and brain relationships. In Caplan LR (ed): *Brain Ischemia, Basic Concepts and Clinical Relevance.* London: Springer, 1995, pp 317–328.

81. Rolak LA, Rokey R: Electrocardiographic features. In Rolak LA, Rokey R (eds): *Coronary and Cerebrovascular Disease. A Practical Guide.* Mt Kisco, NY: Futura, 1990, pp 139–197.

82. Puleo P: Cardiac enzyme assessment. In Rolak LA, Rokey R (eds): *Coronary and Cerebrovascular Disease. A Practical Guide.* Mt Kisco, NY: Futura, 1990, pp 199–216.

83. Myers MG, Norris JW, Hachinski VC, et al: Cardiac sequelae of acute stroke. *Stroke* 1982;**13**:838–842.

84. Mikolich JR, Jacobs WC, Fletcher GF: Cardiac arrhythmias in patients with

acute cerebrovascular accidents. *JAMA* 1981;**246**:1314–1317.

85. Vingerhoets F, Bogousslavsky J, Regli F, Van Melle G: Atrial fibrillation after acute stroke. *Stroke* 1993;**24**:26–30.

86. Oppenheimer SM, Gelb A, Given JP, Hachinski VC: Cardiovascular effects of human insular cortex stimulation. *Neurology* 1992;**42**:1727–1732.

87. Benarroch EE: The central autonomic network: Functional organization, dysfunction, and perspective. *Mayo Clin Proc* 1993;**68**:988–1001.

88. Talman WT: Cardiovascular regulation and lesions of the central nervous system. *Ann Neurol* 1985;**18**:1–12.

89. Oppenheimer SM, Cechetto DF, Hachinski VC: Cerebrogenic cardiac arrhythmias. Cerebral electrocardiographic influences and their role in sudden death. *Arch Neurol* 1990;**47**:513–519.

90. Oppenheimer SM, Hopkins DA: Suprabulbar neural regulation of the heart. In Armour JA, Ardell JL (eds): *Neurocardiology*. New York: Oxford University Press, 1994, pp 309–341.

91. Fink JN, Selim MH, Kumar S, Voetsch B, Fong WC, Caplan LR: Insular cortex infarction in acute middle cerebral artery territory stroke: predictor of stroke severity and vascular lesion. *Arch Neurol* 2005;**62**:1081–1085.

92. Myers MS, Norris JW, Hachinski VC, et al: Plasma norepinephrine in stroke. *Stroke* 1981;**12**:200–204.

93. Weir BK: Pulmonary edema following fatal aneurysmal rupture. *J Neurosurg* 1978;**49**:502–507.

94. Hoff JT, Nishimura M: Experimental neurogenic pulmonary edema in cats. *J Neurosurg* 1978;**18**:383–389.

95. Mayer SA, Lin J, Homma S, et al: Myocardial injury and left ventricular performance after subarachnoid hemorrhage. *Stroke* 1999;**30**:780–786.

96. Gongora-Rivera F, Labreuche J, Jaramillo A, et al: Autopsy prevalence of coronary atherosclerosis in patients with fatal stroke. *Stroke* 2007;**38**:1203–1210.

97. Korpelainen JT, Sotaniemi KA, Makkallio A, et al: Dynamic behavior of heart rate in ischemic stroke. *Stroke* 1999;**30**:1008–1013.

98. Weidler DJ, Das SK, Sodeman TM: Cardiac arrhythmias secondary to acute cerebral ischemia: Prevention by autonomic blockade. *Circulation* 1976;**53**(Suppl 2):102.

99. Horner J, Massey EW: Silent aspiration following stroke. *Neurology* 1988;**38**:317–319.

100. Groher ME, Bukatman R: The prevalence of swallowing disorders in two teaching hospitals. *Dysphagia* 1986;**1**:3–6.

101. Horner J, Massey EW, Brazer SR: Aspiration in bilateral stroke patients. *Neurology* 1990;**40**:1686–1688.

102. Alberts MJ, Horner J: Dysphagia and aspiration syndromes. In Bogousslavsky J, Caplan LR (eds): *Stroke Syndromes*. Cambridge: Cambridge University Press, 1995, pp 213–222.

103. Ramsey DJ, Smithard DG, Kaira L: Can pulse oximetry or a bedside swallowing assessment be used to detect aspiration after stroke? *Stroke* 2006;**37**:2984–2988.

104. Leder SB, Espinosa JF: Aspiration risk after stroke: comparison of clinical examination and fiberoptic endoscopic evaluation of swallowing. *Dysphagia* 2002;**17**:214–218.

105. Horner J, Massey EW, Risler JE, et al: Aspiration following stroke: Clinical correlates and outcome. *Neurology* 1988;**38**:1359–1362.

106. Mann G, Dip PG, Hankey GJ, Cameron D: Swallowing function after stroke. Prognosis and prognostic factors at 6 months. *Stroke* 1999;**30**:744–748.

107. Ramsey DJ, Smithard DG, Kaira L: Early assessment of dysphagia and aspiration risk in acute stroke patients. *Stroke* 2003;**34**:1252–1257.

108. Sellars C, Bowie L, Bagg J et al: Risk factors for chest infection in acute stroke: A prospective cohort study. *Stroke* 2007;**38**:2284–2291.

109. Fluck DC: Chest movements in hemiplegia. *Clin Sci* 1966;**31**:383–388.

110. Przedborski S, Brunko E, Hubert M, et al: The effect of acute hemiplegia on intercostal muscle activity. *Neurology* 1988;**38**:1882–1884.

111. Kaldor A, Berlin I: Pneumonia, stroke, and laterality. *Lancet* 1981;**1**:843.

112. Dirnagl U, Klehmet J, Braun, et al: Stroke-induced immunodepression. Experimental evidence and clinical relevance. *Stroke* 2007;**38**(part 2):770–773.

113. Chamorro A, Urra X, Planas AM: Infection after acute ischemic stroke. A manifestation of brain-induced immunodepression. *Stroke* 2007;**38**:1097–1103.

114. Emsley HCA, Hopkins SJ: Acute ischaemic stroke and infection: Recent and emerging concepts. *Lancet Neurol* 2008;**7**:341–353.

115. Dziewas R, Ritter M, Schilling M, et al: Pneumonia in acute stroke patients fed by nasogastric tube. *J Neurol Neurosurg Psychiatry* 2004;**75**:852–856.

116. Yoo S-H, Kim JS, Kwon SU, et al: Undernutrition as a predictor of poor clinical outcomes in acute ischemic stroke patients. *Arch Neurol* 2008;**65**:39–43.

117. Finestone HM, Green-Finestone LS, Wilson ES, Teasell RW: Malnutrition in stroke patients on the rehabilitation service and at follow-up. Prevalence and predictors. *Arch Phys Med Rehabil* 1995;**76**:310–316.

118. Aptaker RI, Roth EJ, Reichhardt G, et al: Serum albumin level as a predictor of geriatric stroke rehabilitation outcome. *Arch Phys Med Rehabil* 1994;**75**:80–84.

119. Dennis MS, Lewis SC, Warlow C; FOOD Trial Collaboration: Effect of timing and method of enteral tube feeding for dysphagic stroke patients (FOOD): A multicentre randomised controlled trial. *Lancet* 2005;**365**:764–772.

120. Norton B, Homer-Ward M, Donnelly MT, et al: A randomized prospective comparison of percutaneous endoscopic gastrostomy and nasogastric tube feedings after acute dysphagic stroke. *BMJ* 1996;**312**:13–16.

121. Wijdicks EFM, McMahon MM: Percutaneous endoscopic gastrostomy after acute stroke: complications and outcome. *Cerebrovasc Dis* 1999;**9**:109–111.

122. Joynt RJ, Feibel JH, Sladek CM: Antidiuretic hormone levels in stroke patients. *Ann Neurol* 1981;**9**:182–184.

123. Tsuchida S, Noto H, Yamaguchi D, et al: Urodynamic studies on hemiplegia patients after cerebrovascular accident. *Urology* 1983;**21**:315–318.

124. Davenport RJ, Dennis MS, Warlow CP: Gastrointestinal hemorrhage after acute stroke. *Stroke* 1996;**27**:421–424.

125. Herzig SJ, Howell MD, Ngo LH, Marcantonio ER: Acid-suppressive medication use and the risk for hospital-acquired pneumonia. *JAMA* 2009;**301**:2120–2128.

126. Camara-Lemarroy CR, Ibarra-Yruegas BE, Gongora-Rivera F: Gastrointestinal

complications after ischemic stroke. *J Neurol Sci* 2014;**346**:20–25.

127. Smith DM: Pressure ulcers in the nursing home. *Ann Intern Med* 1995;**123**:433–442.

128. Lindgren I, Jonsson A-C, Norrving B, Lindgren A: Shoulder pain after stroke. *Stroke* 2007;**38**:343–348.

129. Braus DF, Krauss JK, Strobel J: The shoulder-hand syndrome after stroke: A prospective clinical trial. *Ann Neurol* 1994;**36**:728–733.

130. Sato Y, Kuno H, Kaji M, et al: Increased bone resorption during the first year after stroke. *Stroke* 1998;**29**:1373–1377.

131. Sato Y, Maruoka H, Oizumi K: Amelioration of hemiplegia-associated osteopenia more than 4 years after stroke by 1 alpha-hydroxyvitamin D3 and calcium supplementation. *Stroke* 1997;**28**:736–739.

132. Sato Y, Fujimatsu Y, Honda Y, et al: Accelerated bone remodeling in patients with poststroke hemiplegia. *J Stroke Cerebrovasc Dis* 1998;**7**:58–62.

133. Ramnemark A, Nyberg L, Lorentzon R, et al: Hemiosteoporosis after severe stroke, independent of changes in body composition and weight. *Stroke* 1999;**30**:755–760.

134. Poole KES, Loveridge N, Rose CM, Warburton EA, Reeve J: A single infusion of Zoledronate prevents bone loss after stroke. *Stroke* 2007;**38**:1519–1525.

135. van der Werf SP, van den Broek HLP, Anten HWM, Bleijenberg G: Experience of severe fatigue long after stroke and its relation to depressive symptoms and disease characteristics. *Eur Neurol* 2001;**45**:28–33.

136. Ingles JL, Eskes GA, Phillips SJ: Fatigue after stroke. *Arch Phys Med Rehabil* 1999;**80**:173–178.

137. Feibel JH, Springer CJ: Depression and failure to resume social activities after stroke. *Arch Phys Med Rehabil* 1982;**63**:276–277.

138. Robinson RG, Szetela B: Mood change following left hemisphere brain injury. *Ann Neurol* 1981;**9**:447–453.

139. Finkelstein S, Benowitz LI, Baldessarini RJ, et al: Mood, vegetative disturbances, and dexamethasone suppression test after stroke. *Ann Neurol* 1982;**12**:463–468.

140. Astrom M, Adolfdon R, Asplund K: Major depression in stroke patients. A 3-year longitudinal study. *Stroke* 1993;**24**:976–982.

141. Pohjasvaara T, Leppavuori A, Siira I, et al: Frequency and clinical determinants of post-stroke depression. *Stroke* 1998;**29**:2311–2317.

142. Robinson RG, Price TR: Post-stroke depressive disorders: A follow-up study of 103 patients. *Stroke* 1982;**13**:635–641.

143. Verdelho A, Henon H, Lebert F, Pasquier F, Leys D: Depressive symptoms after stroke and relationship with dementia. A three-year follow-up study. *Neurology* 2004;**62**:905–911.

144. Robinson RG, Starr LB, Price TR: A two-year longitudinal study of mood disorders following stroke. *Br J Psychiatry* 1984;**144**:256–262.

145. Ghika-Schmid F, Bogousslavsky J: Affective disorders following stroke. *Eur Neurol* 1997;**38**:75–81.

146. Binder LM: Emotional problems after stroke. *Stroke* 1984;**15**:174–177.

147. Ross ED, Rush AJ: Diagnosis and neuroanatomical correlates of depression in brain-damaged patients. *Arch Gen Psychiatry* 1981;**38**:1344–1354.

148. Robinson RG, Starr LB, Kubos K, et al: A two-year longitudinal study of post-stroke mood disorders: findings during the initial evaluation. *Stroke* 1983;**14**:736–741.

149. Robinson RG, Kubos KL, Starr LB, et al: Mood disorders in stroke patients: Importance of location of lesion. *Brain* 1984;**107**:81–93.

150. Robinson RG, Kubos KL, Starr LB, et al: Mood changes in stroke patients: Relationship to lesion location. *Compr Psychiatry* 1983;**24**:555–566.

151. Herrmann M, Bartels C, Schumacher M, Wallesch C-W: Poststroke depression. Is there a pathoanatomic correlate for depression in the postacute stage of stroke? *Stroke* 1995;**26**:850–856.

152. Lipsey JR, Robinson RG, Pearlson GD, et al: Nortriptyline treatment of poststroke depression: A double-blind study. *Lancet* 1984;**1**:297–300.

153. Reding JJ, Orto LA, Winter SW, et al: Antidepressant therapy after stroke: A double blind trial. *Arch Neurol* 1986;**43**:763–765.

154. Andersen G, Vestergaard K, Lauritzen L: Effective treatment of post-stroke depression with the selective reuptake inhibitor citalopram. *Stroke* 1994;**25**:1099–1104.

155. Wade DT, Legh-Smith J, Langton-Hewer R: Effects of living with and looking after survivors of a stroke. *BMJ* 1986;**293**:418–420.

156. Anderson CS, Linto J, Stewart-Wynne EG: A population-based assessment of the impact and burden of caregiving for long-term stroke survivors. *Stroke* 1995;**26**:843–849.

157. Scholte OP, Reimer WJ, de Haan RJ, Rijnders PT, Limburg M, van den Bos GA: The burden of caregiving in partners of long-term stroke survivors. *Stroke* 1998;**29**:1605–1611.

158. Dennis M, O'Rourke S, Lewis S, et al: A quantitative study of the emotional outcome of people caring for stroke survivors. *Stroke* 1998;**29**:1867–1872.

159. van Exel NJ, Koopmanschap MA, van den Berg B, Brouwer WB, van den Bos GA: Burden of informal caregiving for stroke patients. Identification of caregivers at risk of adverse health effects. *Cerebrovasc Dis* 2005;**19**:11–17.

Recovery, rehabilitation, and repair

Steven C Cramer and Louis R Caplan

Recovery

The human brain is in many ways a coalition of many different systems and structures. Consistent with this, a stroke can manifest with innumerable patterns of behavioral deficits, with motor deficit being the most common.[1,2] When a stroke occurs, numerous biological pathways are set into motion. These include acute injury cascades and a series of immunological events, as well as a sequence of restorative events that support behavioral recovery.

Some degree of behavioral recovery is seen in nearly all patients after stroke, although this recovery is incomplete in most instances, and, as a result, stroke is perennially the most common cause of acquired adult disability in developed countries.[3] Some principles are apparent. For example, patients with milder deficits tend to recover faster and achieve a higher level of function as compared to patients with more severe deficits. Recovery after stroke is complex[4] and depends on many factors.[5,6] Some of these factors relate to the nature and severity of the stroke mechanism. Some tissues are temporarily deprived of blood and nutrition. When the circulation is restored these tissues regain function. Neuroanatomical factors play a major role; the location and size of infarcts and hemorrhages are important, as are the lobes and brain regions that are spared.[5,7–14] Some functions are localized to single brain regions; for example, vision is localized in the occipital lobes, while other functions are more widely distributed. Recovery can occur when other brain regions subserve the functions of infarcted damaged regions.

Patient age is also among the key determinants of recovery after stroke.[15,16] Social, economic, and environmental factors are also very important such as the presence of a caregiver[17] and nutritional status.[18] Safety of the home environment can be a critical factor in some patient's recovery:[19] Are sufficient economic resources available? What floor does the patient live on? Is an elevator available in the building? Are stores, restaurants, movie theaters, and recreational and social activities within easy access for the patient and the caregivers? Are family members and friends nearby? Are they supportive and helpful? The answers to these queries are seldom noted in hospital charts – and are little considered in rodent models of stroke – but are just as important for meaningful recovery as the extent of brain injury and the nature and severity of the neurological signs. Individual patient characteristics also heavily influence recovery. Some individuals are "survivors" and have the intelligence, determination, and character to succeed under adverse circumstances. Past personal accomplishments, flexibility, and attitudes are important determinants of functional recovery and ability to adapt to a disability. Medical comorbidities such as cardiopulmonary disease, obesity, and arthritis also impact a patient's recovery.

Considerable heterogeneity across patients characterizes recovery of motor functions. While studies find that overall, maximum arm function is achieved by 95% of patients within 9 weeks of stroke onset,[20] the first voluntary movements can be noticable anywhere from 6–33 days after a hemiplegic stroke.[21] Similar findings have also been described in studies of recovery of language function after stroke. Pedersen et al. found that the final level of language function is achieved in 95% of patients at 10 weeks when aphasia is severe, but in only 2 weeks when aphasia is mild.[22] Language recovery, in contrast to motor recovery, can develop with continued gains for months or years after stroke onset.[23,24] This pattern of persistent recovery has been reported for many types of cognitive deficits after stroke. Among patients whose stroke was accompanied by cognitive impairment, 36% continued to show recovery of cognitive function beyond the first 3 months post-stroke.[25] Similar results have been reported for recovery of memory[26] and constructional apraxia after stroke.[27] While recovery of neglect symptoms after right hemisphere stroke often resolves within 3 months of stroke onset,[7,28] improvement can continue for months beyond this in patients who have more severe deficits.[29]

Another key point regarding behavioral recovery after stroke is that when a patient has multiple neurological deficits, these often recover with varying and separate temporal trajectories – different neural systems recover at different rates within the same patient.[7,30–32] For example, during recovery from a middle cerebral artery (MCA) territory infarct, patients often regain the ability to walk, whereas recovery of contralateral arm function may remain minimal.[33] Similarly, following a dominant hemisphere MCA territory infarct with aphasia, an auditory comprehension deficit may clear considerably, whereas spontaneous speech may remain severely dysarthric and non-fluent.[34] Visual neglect may clear over time, whereas a dense visual field cut may not, and different aspects of neglect such as anosognosia and motor impersistence can have different rates of recovery.[7]

Since damaged brain tissue does not fully regenerate in adult humans, these functional gains most likely occur on the basis of reorganization or proliferation of surviving cellular

Caplan's Stroke: A Clinical Approach, 5th Edition, ed. Louis R Caplan. Published by Cambridge University Press. © Cambridge University Press, 2016.

elements.[35–37] Animal models and preclinical studies have characterized the cellular and molecular underpinnings of spontaneous stroke recovery. After an experimental infarct, brain regions become excitable, in some cases showing gamma-aminobutyric acid (GABA) receptor down-regulation and increased N-methyl-D-aspartate (NMDA) receptor binding. Expression changes for a number of genes resulting, at times, in increased levels of several growth factors. Angiogenesis is accompanied by structural changes in axons, dendrites, and synapses, and in both white matter and gray matter. These changes are often preferentially seen in the area surrounding an infarct, and in areas with network connections to injured zones. In many instances, recovery shares changes that are characteristic of normal development and learning.[38–41]

Direct cellular and molecular measures are difficult to obtain in human subjects. New technologies that can non-invasively localize and quantify changes in brain anatomy and function have enabled a biological approach to stroke rehabilitation and recovery.[6,42–47] Examples include functional magnetic resonance imaging (fMRI), positron emission tomography (PET), and transcranial magnetic stimulation. MRI techniques can be used to study the integrity of selected white matter tracts, Wallerian degeneration, and the degree of network connectivity across the human brain.[44,46,48–50]

These studies have provided insights into stroke recovery in humans, results of which have generally been concordant with findings in animal studies. Overall, results indicate that a focal injury such as stroke not only reduces local tissue function, but also has distant effects on activity in a number of brain areas connected within a distributed network. Recent studies emphasize the importance of network interactions after stroke.[51–55] After a single unilateral supratentorial stroke, multiple changes can be seen within multiple brain areas of the affected hemisphere. These changes develop in patients with subcortical strokes and with cortical strokes. Diaschisis refers to a depression in activity seen in areas that are not injured but which share a connection with injured zones.[56,57] Over time, resolution of diaschisis can be followed by over-activation of network nodes, a pattern reminiscent of the brain during increased effort in healthy subjects. Changes in cortical map representations are also seen in relation to behavioral recovery, with numerous patterns having been described.[45,58–60] Changes in the function of brain networks can also be seen within the contralesional cerebral hemisphere.[61] The contribution of the contralesional hemisphere to spontaneous behavioral recovery after stroke seems largest in subjects with the greatest injury and deficits.[62–64]

In many western countries, spontaneous recovery after stroke is supported by a host of rehabilitation therapies. Access is sometimes sharply reduced in third world countries.[65] Scientific aspects of stroke recovery are receiving increased emphasis, with the molecular events underlying stroke recovery studied as therapeutic targets. With this, an increasing body of evidence supports the potential for repair-based therapies to improve outcomes in patients with stroke.

Rehabilitation

In the preceding chapters of this volume, care by physicians was generally centered either in outpatient facilities, or in acute care hospitals. A unique feature in relation to recovery and the after-effects of stroke is that much care occurs in rehabilitation units. Systems of stroke rehabilitation therapy are a core component of recovery in western countries, and emerging strategies targeting brain repair (below) are prescribed within this setting.

Rehabilitation services are quite different from most traditional medical and surgical units and the process is unfamiliar to many physicians. Rehabilitation has a different emphasis and goal than traditional medicine. Stroke rehabilitation focuses on recovery of, and adaptation to, loss of neurological function, along with preventative efforts. In contrast, traditional medicine has a pathological and pathophysiological emphasis, and is more focused on treating and preventing disease. Rehabilitation units have a slower pace, longer patient stays, and, at times, different reimbursement rules for third-party payers. Rehabilitation is usually performed in buildings or units separated from acute-care hospitals and other neurological facilities. Parts of rehabilitation units look more like gymnasiums, exercise areas, workshops, or schools than standard medical wards, and these units use a lot of equipment such as braces, walking aids, and parallel bars that is foreign to most medical units.

Rehabilitation units often have a high ratio of non-physician to physician staff members. Although a physician usually captains the team, the role of other allied health professionals is more important than in most acute-care medical and surgical units. The physician in-charge is often a physical medicine specialist. Internists, cardiologists, geriatricians, orthopedists, and neurologists may also be involved, as rehabilitation facilities typically house patients recovering from a variety of medical and orthopedic conditions and surgeries. In the past and at present, few neurologists in the United States have chosen to specialize in rehabilitation or to work full time in rehabilitation units. These differences underscore discontinuities in care that may be seen when a patient with stroke is cared for by a neurology team acutely and is then transferred to a rehabilitation medicine team subacutely. The issue is further compounded when the patient's long-term care is led by a primary care physician who was not involved in the acute care hospital or during the stay in the rehabilitation unit. The primary care physician is then charged with continuing strategies and practices that he had no part in carrying forward or prescribing.

Stroke outcomes can be classified in relation to several dimensions along the World Health Organization's (WHO's) International Classification of Functioning, Disability, and Health (ICF).[66] Loss of body functions and structures, formerly referred to as impairments, includes deficits that are a consequence of stroke. Activities limitations, formerly referred to as disabilities, reflect difficulties patients with stroke notice in the performance of functional tasks. Participation restrictions, formerly referred to as handicaps, refer to difficulties patients with stroke encounter in societal roles.

Strong evidence indicates that interdisciplinary stroke rehabilitation can improve outcomes, across WHO ICF dimensions., including reduced death and dependency.[67,68] Rehabilitation has been studied in a number of trials.[67–79] Some trials considered units within the hospital and others relate to separate units. These trials suggest that the milieu and greater frequency and intensity of rehabilitation services in dedicated stroke and rehabilitation units lead to better outcomes. Mortality is reduced. More patients return home and less patients are transferred to chronic hospitals and nursing homes. Short- and long-term functional outcomes are also improved. Doubt that stroke units work no longer exists. Some trials have studied the use of various techniques and strategies for specific functions, such as recovery of hemiplegic gait,[80–82] improvement in upper-extremity function,[20] recovery from aphasia,[83,84] and management of spatial neglect.[85] Other trials study the effects of specific strategies on general functional outcome (e.g., the effect of sensory stimulation on outcome of patients with severe stroke-related hemiparesis).[86]

Ottenbacher and Jannell performed a meta-analysis of trials and studies conducted between 1960 and 1990.[75] The analysis included patients who had a stroke-related hemiparesis who were given rehabilitation services in a design that compared at least two groups or conditions for change in a quantifiable functional measure. Outcomes studied included gait, hand functions, activities of daily living, response times, and visual perceptual functions. From 173 statistical evaluations performed on 3717 patients studied in these trials, the meta-analysis showed that the average patient who received a program that included focused stroke rehabilitation or a particular procedure performed better than approximately 65% of patients in the comparison groups.[69,75] Greater effects of treatment were obtained when rehabilitation was performed early. Younger patients tended to do better than older patients.

Unfortunately, the high cost of in-patient rehabilitation programs has led managed-care payers to offer therapy programs in the patients' homes, nursing homes, or as outpatients instead of at rehabilitation facilities.[69] The push from managed-care personnel to get patients out of acute care hospitals sicker and quicker means that many patients who are transferred to rehabilitation units require more acute care than they did in the past, and recent trends for shorter inpatient rehabilitation stays means less time for therapists to effectively promote recovery.[87] The issue takes on greater significance when one considers that some treatment approaches are focused on compensation, whereby function returns by any pattern of behavior, whereas other approaches are focused on true recovery of the original pre-stroke behavioral pattern. The distinction between compensation and recovery has deep implications; for example, regarding promoting neural plasticity, and maximum level of attainable function, and so is an area of active research.[88–92]

Functioning in rehabilitation units

Rehabilitation should be considered in terms of the general process of stroke recovery. Rehabilitation occurs during the first weeks and months after stroke onset. Natural recovery mechanisms occur at the same time, especially if patients remain active. Much of the recovery is natural, although most patients are inclined to give complete credit for their improvement to various therapies that they receive during rehabilitation.

Strategies and methods of rehabilitation vary greatly between units and have changed over time.[93] Descriptions of the methods, techniques, and aids used during rehabilitation are far beyond the scope of this book and beyond the knowledge and expertise of the authors. Excellent chapters and monographs devoted entirely to this subject exist elsewhere.[2,69,70,94–98] Stroke units and rehabilitation services exist in different locations, some within acute-care hospitals, others in free-standing chronic care hospitals apart from acute-care facilities, and some in out-patient facilities in the community.

In excellent rehabilitation facilities, a number of goals are pursued concurrently.[2,69,70,94,95,97,99,100] Methods used to treat acute stroke and preventive strategies emphasized at the acute-care facility should be continued. This means that physicians and nurses at the rehabilitation facility should become fully knowledgeable about the causative stroke mechanism and treatments used to minimize the deficit and prevent worsening and stroke recurrence. In some instances, patients are sent to rehabilitation units with incomplete evaluations at acute-care facilities. Investigations of the causative cardio-cerebrovascular-hematological causes of stroke in these patients must be pursued further while the patient is being rehabilitated. Control of stroke risk factors, such as cessation of smoking and appropriate diet, should be continued at the rehabilitation unit.

The process of evaluating the nature and severity of various neurological, medical, and psychological dysfunctions and disabilities should begin shortly after the patient is transferred to the rehabilitation unit.[100,101] Motor functions of the limbs, micturition, swallowing, gait, speech, perception, cognitive and behavioral abilities, psychological reactions, and intelligence should be assessed. Recognition of impairments and disabilities is the first step in devising strategies and programs to train the stroke patient to overcome and adapt to any dysfunctions found and prevent the development of further disability. Exercise training improves functional capacity, the ability to perform activities of daily living, and quality of life, and it reduces the risk for subsequent cardiovascular events. Physical activity goals and exercise prescription for stroke survivors need to be customized for the individual to maximize long-term adherence.[102] Secondary stroke prevention is of paramount importance to the patient recovering from stroke;[103] such efforts also reduce the risk of myocardial infarction, the leading cause of death after stroke.

During rehabilitation, strategies are devised to safely reintegrate the patient back to his or her home. This often entails evaluation of the home and suggestions to make the home environment safer for the patient. For example, if the patient customarily slept on the second floor and the kitchen, television, and living and dining rooms are on the first floor, it might

be simpler to create a sleeping area for the patient on the first floor to facilitate eating and daily activities. Showers may need to be made safer and more readily usable. Social agencies may need to be mobilized for the care and support of the patient. Visiting nurses, therapists, homemakers, and food delivery services may need to be consulted when patients return to their homes.

Although rehabilitation is important, not all stroke patients benefit from treatment within a rehabilitation unit. Selection of appropriate patients is important. On one end of the spectrum, patients who are already ambulatory and have only slight or temporary deficits are not likely to derive substantial gain from admission to a rehabilitation unit, and do well with outpatient therapy as needed. On the other end of the spectrum is a patient who is stuporous, or who has severe right-hemisphere dysfunction, and so is unlikely to be able to derive benefit from rehabilitation unit admission. Most observers agree that the middle group between these two extremes is the appropriate target for inpatient rehabilitative care post-stroke.

How should this target subgroup of patients with stroke be identified? Which factors are most important for making this critical triage decision? Historically this issue has been addressed using clinical measures; however, an increasing body of research (below) suggests the added utility of biologically based approaches. Response to inpatient rehabilitation therapy after stroke can to some extent be predicted using a number of clinical and neurological variables.[16,101] Neurological findings such as paralysis are prognostically important.[2,70,100,104] Patients who have substantial cognitive impairments or who have severe medical comorbid illness may be unable to participate effectively given the higher demands of an inpatient rehabilitation program, as such patients are likely to be unable to learn compensatory techniques or unable to tolerate the physical demands. The mere presence of aphasia does not preclude stroke rehabilitation. When outcome is measured in terms of activities of daily living, ability to walk, or discharge disposition, no difference has been found between aphasic and non-aphasic patients referred for rehabilitation.[105–108] Higher cortical-function abnormalities other than aphasia, such as perceptual abnormalities, anosognosia, aprosodia, neglect, impersistence, reduplicative paramnesia, and prosopagnosia, may make rehabilitation more difficult, but not impossible. These cognitive abnormalities tend to improve with time, allowing the stroke rehabilitation process to proceed.[5,7] Patients of all ages can be offered rehabilitation. Although younger age may be associated with better outcome after stroke rehabilitation,[109] substantial recovery is noted in all age groups.[2,70,105,110]

A number of seemingly mundane factors also apply when deciding on treatment for a stroke patient.[111–114] What was the patient's pre-stroke level of function? Does the patient have financial support to help with special equipment, transportation, and so forth? Does the patient have a car or access to other transportation? Does the patient have someone at home who is motivated, capable, and available to help and encourage recovery? Does the home have stairs or a bathroom on every floor? Is a meals-on-wheels program or a store that delivers and takes telephone orders accessible to the patient? What community services are available? These prognostic factors and others must be considered to offer rehabilitation to those who will benefit most. When prognosis is uncertain, physicians should err on the side of offering a trial period of rehabilitation given the stakes at hand.

The general theme of stroke rehabilitation is a disability-oriented, multidisciplinary team approach. Team members include the patient, patient's family, primary care physician, neurologist, physical therapist, occupational therapist, speech therapist, social worker, and rehabilitation nurse. Members of the team should meet regularly to identify specific rehabilitation goals, strategies for their attainment, and methods of implementation. These team members educate and train patients and family members in their areas of expertise. Ideally, the team rehabilitation process should begin early in the course of the acute stroke so that improvement in quality of life can be achieved as early as possible.

Nurses and physicians in rehabilitation units must monitor the occurrence of stroke complications and use strategies to prevent them.[67,115–117] Chapter 19 is devoted to stroke complications. Probably one of the major explanations for the success of stroke units is their focus on systematically watching for and treating complications that develop. Mobilization and physical therapy help prevent complications such as urinary tract infections and urosepsis, aspiration pneumonia, deep venous thrombosis, pulmonary embolism, malnutrition, limb contractures, falls, and bedsores.

The role of physicians differs within rehabilitation units from the traditional role of doctors in an acute-care facility.[70] Physicians direct the team. They evaluate and prognosticate. These physicians interact with the team of therapists about compensatory physical and cognitive strategies and assist devices. They try various drug interventions to treat pain, spasticity, and cognitive and mood disorders. These physicians serve as administrative brokers to gather the resources and services that the patients and their families need.

Rehabilitation nurses are key members of the team. Often, one nurse acts to coordinate physician orders and integrate the various strategies used in the rehabilitation process. Nurses must often pursue an attitude unusual in the nursing profession. A nurse is usually the provider of direct care. On a rehabilitation unit, however, the nurse must often sit back and let the patient accomplish tasks at hand, providing teaching, encouragement, and help as needed. Extreme patience is required. Nurses must synthesize the recommendations of other team members and directly apply these ideas to the everyday care of patients. Nurses also monitor and direct treatment for medical complications that might occur during rehabilitation.

The physical therapist's main function is training the patient for ambulation. Balancing, weight-shifting techniques, parallel bars, various orthotics, and quad canes are used. Severe weakness in a lower extremity does not preclude ambulation. Often, a patient is unable to lift his or her leg from the bed yet eventually becomes ambulatory. Increased extensor tone combined with minimal bracing

permits walking. Even before ambulation training begins, physical therapists perform range-of-motion, strengthening, and endurance exercises. Physical therapists also can help provide appropriate supporting apparatus, such as lapboards, chair-arm supports, and swings. Range-of-motion exercises are passive and active and should be performed at least four times daily. Patients can use the normal arm to passively move the paralyzed extremity through a full range of motion. These exercises help prevent deconditioning, excessive spasticity, joint contractures, and peripheral edema. Range-of-motion exercises combined with upper-extremity support are the keys to preventing a painful shoulder caused by subluxation or spasticity. Both the family and nursing staff should take active roles using the recommendations of the physical therapist for remobilization throughout the day.

Occupational therapists perform upper-extremity retraining with particular attention to teaching practical activities of daily living. Patients and therapists work on improving fine-motor skills so that activities such as feeding, dressing, personal hygiene, and cooking can be accomplished. These skills allow the development of independent function. Often, special devices, including a reacher, utensil holder, specially placed rails or handles, commodes, tub benches, or hand-held showers, are used. An occupational therapist can customize these techniques and physical changes in the home to adapt to the patient's deficits.

Speech therapists work to improve communication skills. The goal is to facilitate communication early in the patient's rehabilitation. The methods may be verbal or non-verbal, using spoken or written words, gestures, or word boards. The boards may contain letters that patients point to for spelling words or may contain words or pictures to designate needs or wishes. Computer programs are often helpful for facilitating communication skills. Often, therapists can develop techniques of non-verbal communication for severely aphasic patients so their needs can be met and feelings of isolation eliminated. During the first 3 months after a stroke, much spontaneous language recovery occurs. Beyond 3 months, the therapist's role is to enhance further recovery of language function. Physicians should not accept a nihilistic attitude toward speech therapy. We advise physicians to start aphasic patients on a comprehensive program of speech therapy early during the course of treatment. Physicians should continue to pursue a vigorous course of treatment in most patients, withholding treatment only in patients who are demented or severely globally aphasic. Speech therapists also help evaluate and treat dysarthria and dysphagia, breath control, and articulation. Speech therapists can often suggest types of foods, liquids, and eating techniques that might be best tolerated by patients.

Strokes do not only affect the individual stroke patient. Stroke is a disease that affects the patient's family, friends, and environment. The caregiver, family, and friends play a major role in rehabilitation. Educating and training caregivers are important tasks during the rehabilitation process.

Caregivers should be instructed about the nature of the stroke patient's dysfunctions and strategies used to deal with these impairments.

Next to the patient, family members have the most difficult task. Usually medically unsophisticated, they must learn new skills from rehabilitation team members and directly supervise the care of the stroke patient. The family's questions and concerns should be carefully addressed by each team member. It is often useful for the family member most directly involved in home care to spend a few days at the hospital to effectively acquire the necessary skills. Once patients return home, continued contact with the team is crucial so progress can be monitored, new problems identified, and solutions implemented. This contact may be in the form of visits to the home or appointments at the rehabilitation unit with individual team members.

Perhaps most important are the spirit and milieu of the unit. Personnel must possess an optimistic outlook accompanied by understanding. Planning should be practical, and goals must be realistic. The use of equipment, strategies, and programs that help patients and caregivers recognize and deal with disabilities is helpful.

Coordination of acute and long-term care

To be optimally successful, rehabilitation should be fully integrated with traditional medical care. Therapy should begin as early as possible while the patient is still on the acute medical or neurological unit. Physicians, nurses, and other personnel must be involved. Therapy should not be completely delegated to physical and occupational therapists. Consultations should not be limited to the 30 minutes or so that patients typically spend each day with therapists. Passive and active range-of-motion exercises and other physical therapy should be encouraged by ward personnel. If the patient goes to a rehabilitation unit, the acute-care team should continue to follow the patient whenever possible. Acute medical problems do not suddenly disappear when the patient is transferred. Subsequent strokes and medical complications are common among recuperating patients.

The patient receives mixed signals if treatment and advice begun on the acute-care unit are not followed through at the rehabilitation unit. The patient may have been persuaded by a doctor on the acute-care unit who advised the need for a low-salt, low-cholesterol diet, only to be served butter, cream, and eggs on the rehabilitation unit. Medical treatment and surveillance should be continued during rehabilitation and afterward. Similarly, when the patient leaves the rehabilitation unit, physicians must continue to emphasize the need to carry out various rehabilitation techniques. After treatment in the acute-care center and rehabilitation facilities, patients usually return to the care of their primary care physician, most likely an internist or family practitioner. The primary care physician must be kept up-to-date with the patient's findings, current treatment decisions, and recommendations so they can continue medical treatment and retraining procedures and strategies. Rehabilitation and traditional medical care should be

intertwined and overlapped, not seen by the patient as unrelated phases with one consultation succeeding the other.

Repair

An emerging family of therapies is focused on neural repair. Unlike acute stroke reperfusion and neuroprotection therapies, which aim to limit injury, repair-based therapies focus on promoting favorable neural plasticity to improve outcomes.[118,119] As such, brain repair therapies often have a time window measured in days–weeks, which emphasizes their complementary value to acute stroke therapies, many of which can only be offered to a minority of patients with stroke. Increasing evidence suggests the potential for such restorative therapies to favorably modify patient outcomes by targeting the cellular and molecular events (see above) that underlie recovery from stroke. Many of these newer strategies remain unproven; however, positive phase III trial evidence exists in some instances.

Brain repair strategies for augmenting recovery after stroke

Activity-based therapies

Activity-based therapies achieve their effects by promoting plasticity in the brain, and perhaps spinal cord and muscle as well. Activity-based interventions are important to brain repair after stroke for at least two reasons. First, activity-based therapies have proven utility as a stand-alone approach, including many forms of standard of care rehabilitation therapy. Second, activity-based therapies serve a critical role as adjuvant for many pharmacological and biological therapies, as discussed below. Many types of activity-based therapy have been introduced, but it remains uncertain whether important differences exist across the most common schools of post-stroke rehabilitation.[120]

Researchers have explored the effectiveness of forcing use of a hemiparetic arm by constraining the good arm, an approach known as constraint-induced movement therapy (CIMT). This approach is a form of activity-based therapy that focuses on overcoming learned disuse of a stroke-affected hand to improve motor function and has been found useful in selected subpopulations of patients with unilateral hemiparesis.[121] With CIMT, the non-affected hand is restrained while the affected hand undergoes a very intense course of therapy. The long-term efficacy of CIMT for patients with moderate arm motor deficits was supported by the Extremity Constraint Induced Therapy Evaluation (EXCITE) study,[122] a prospective, single-blind, randomized, multisite phase III clinical trial that enrolled 222 patients 3–9 months after stroke at 7 US academic centers between January 2001 and January 2003. In order to qualify for the study, individuals must have had some wrist and finger extension in their hemiparetic hand. Participants were assigned to receive either constraint-induced movement therapy wearing a restraining mitt on the less-affected hand while engaging in therapy on the

weak arm and hand (N = 106) or usual and customary care that ranged from no treatment after formal acute stroke rehabilitation to pharmacological or physiotherapeutic interventions (N = 116). Restraint with accompanying physical therapy on the hemiparetic hand produced statistically significant and clinically relevant improvements in arm motor function that persisted for at least one year.[122] Simplified forms of CIMT may also be useful,[123] and the overall approach has been extended to other domains such as language.[124,125] It remains uncertain whether this approach can be directly extended to patients at early time points after stroke.[126]

Substantial evidence indicates that greater amount, duration, and intensity of activity-based therapy after stroke are associated with improved outcome.[127–134] Unfortunately, many patients do not receive high-dose/high-intensity therapy in clinical practice.[135–139] For example, in a recent US study, patients receiving inpatient stroke rehabilitation received on average only 23 functional arm repetitions per treatment session.[135]

Gait training

Gait training is a specific type of activity-based therapy but its importance is underscored by the critical role that walking unaided plays in a person's life. Gait is commonly affected by stroke and is ranked as the top priority by hemiplegic patients,[140] and although a measure of impairment (loss of body function and structure) it is directly linked to quality of life[141] and social participation.[142] After stroke, walking can be the difference between becoming ambulatory and mobile without help and remaining dependent. Animal experiments show that forced locomotion activates spinal and supraspinal automatic systems active during gait.[143] A number of studies suggest the utility of body-weight supported treadmill training (BWSTT).[82,143–148] In the Locomotor Experience Applied Post-Stroke (LEAPS) trial[149] enrollees had leg weakness plus gait velocity less than 0.8 m/s, and each was randomized to 36 sessions of 90 minutes duration of either BWSTT starting 2 months post-stroke, BWSTT starting 6 months post-stroke, or home exercises starting 2 months post-stroke. The primary outcome, the proportion of patients who at one year post-stroke improved functional walking ability, was found in 52% of enrollees, with no significant difference between treatment groups. The LEAPS trial emphasizes that in many if not most patients, the CNS retains the potential to undergo clinically relevant plasticity even 6 months after stroke onset.

Robot-based therapies

A robot is a mechanical device, guided by a computer, that senses or moves within its environment.[150,151] Robots can be viewed as devices that perform repetitive movements and measurements according to their design and programming. Robotic devices have potential advantages such as consistent output, programmability, utility for gaming applications, ability to precisely measure patient behavior, and the potential for an improved therapist-to-patient ratio.[152]

Clinical experience with robotic devices has been variable but generally favorable.[153–159] In a large stroke recovery trial of

a robotic device, Lo et al.[160] used a multicenter, controlled randomized design to recruit 127 patients with severe baseline motor deficits, who were on average 4.6 years after stroke onset. Enrollees were randomized to robot-assisted upper extremity rehabilitation, which used high-intensity, repetitive proximal and distal arm movements (36 1-hour sessions over 12 weeks), a dose- and intensity-matched conventional rehabilitation therapy, or usual care. No significant difference was found in the primary end-point, change in arm motor status, although in some secondary analyses robot-assisted therapy appeared favorable.

Many different robotic devices have been designed.[151,161,162] Potential applications include lower extremity deficits and sensory deficits.[163] Challenges for robotic therapy include identifying optimal protocols, consideration of object affordance and task ecology, and identifying the optimal forms of robotic assistance.[150,151,161,162,164]

Telerehabilitation

Telerehabilitation has been defined as "the delivery of rehabilitation services via information and communication technologies."[165] Like robotic therapy, some components of telerehabilitation represent a specific form of activity-based therapy, useful for increasing the dose and intensity of stroke rehabilitation. However, telerehabilitation also encompasses other services including patient assessment, stroke prevention, and counseling and so may have specific advantages.

A major potential use of telerehabilitation is to provide high doses of therapy to a large fraction of patients. Despite a massive body of evidence indicating that many benefits of rehabilitation therapy are dose-dependent, many patients do not receive post-stroke motor therapy of high duration, frequency, and intensity. For some patients this is due to financial constraints.[128,166] In other cases, patients (e.g., in rural areas) cannot get to a rehabilitation therapy provider because it is too far from their home. This is exacerbated by the fact that in some regions a shortage of rehabilitation care has limited provision of adequate services to stroke survivors.[167] Telerehabilitation might represent a cost-effective approach to provide more rehabilitation therapy, at higher intensities, to patients wherever they live. Telehealth systems readily integrate with a new generation of sensors, including body-worn sensors, which could have a high impact on health care performance; for example, by facilitating patient monitoring, feedback, and therapeutic intervention with varied levels of medical supervision.[168]

Increasing evidence supports the potential of a telerehabilitation approach for reducing neurological deficits.[169–175] A major component of this may be derived from promoting patient participation in health care via use of games,[176–180] which can motivate patients to engage in enjoyable play behavior that involves useful therapy-related movements.[181,182] Additional research is needed to optimize prescription of emerging telehealth approaches.[165,183–188]

Sensory stimulation

Sensory stimulation might potentially be a critical component of activity-based therapies. One study examined the effect of repetitive sensorimotor training of the arm after stroke by having the hemiplegic arm perform rocking movements.[189] One hundred consecutive stroke patients who were 2–5 weeks post-stroke were randomly assigned to an experimental group that received daily additional sensorimotor stimulation of the arm or to a control group. The treatment period was 6 weeks. Assessments of the patients were made before and after treatment and at 6 and 12 months after stroke, and in 62 patients, 5 years after stroke. At the 5-year follow-up, there was a statistically significant difference in function tests favoring the treatment group that received early, repetitive, and targeted stimulation of the paretic arm. Extra stimulation of the arm during the acute phase after a stroke resulted in a clinically meaningful and long-lasting salutary effect on motor function.[189] Another study showed that 100-Hz current applied to finger surfaces in patients with chronic post-stroke deficits improved the use of utensils with the involved hand.[69] Passive arm movement prior to active motor therapy may be superior to active motor therapy alone in patients with chronic stroke, and may provide this advantage by promoting brain plasticity by rebalancing cortical excitability.[190] Many different types of sensory input – musical, optokinetic, neck proprioceptive, vestibular, and somatosensory – show improvement in neglect in stroke patients.[137,191,192]

Brain stimulation

The brain is an electrical organ and so modulation of brain function can be achieved via electromagnetic approaches. It must be remembered that brain stimulation, in the form of electroconvulsive therapy has long been used to treat depression.[193] Many types of brain stimulation have been examined to improve outcome after stroke, most non-invasive but some requiring an invasive neurosurgical procedure.[194]

Transcranial magnetic stimulation (TMS) can be used to focally stimulate the brain. During TMS, an insulated stimulator is placed atop the scalp, and issues a magnetic pulse that induces action potentials upon reaching neurons in the cerebral cortex. A single TMS pulse over the motor cortex produces a brief contralateral muscle twitch. Repetitive delivery of TMS pulses can have enduring effects on cortical function. At lower frequencies (e.g., 1 Hz), the effect is usually to decrease cortical excitability. This effect is of potential interest if overactivity within a particular cortical region is seen as an impediment to stroke recovery.[195–197] At higher frequencies, the effect of repetitive TMS (e.g., 5–20 Hz) is to increase cortical excitability, which could increase activity in dormant cortical regions; high frequency TMS carries potential risks and must be administered according to safety guidelines.[198] A number of positive small, studies have been reported. For example, low frequency repetitive TMS applied to the motor cortex on the side opposite a brain infarct can improve function in the hand that was weakened by stroke.[199–202] This approach is based on the assumption that inhibition of pathological activity contralateral to an infarct facilitates favorable activity in the ipsilesional hemisphere. Other studies showed that high frequency repetitive TMS (at 3 Hz[203] or at 10 Hz[204]) administered to the ipsilesional

motor cortex improves function of the contralateral weak hand. A recent Cochrane review concluded that current evidence does not support routine use of repetitive TMS to improve overall function after stroke, possibly due to heterogeneity between trials and small sample sizes;[205] however, meta-analysis of repetitive TMS studies that focused specifically on arm motor recovery did identify a significant benefit.[206]

Direct current can also be applied transcranially. During transcranial direct current stimulation (tDCS), a low-amplitude (1–2 mA) DC current is directed at the underlying cerebral cortex using simple electrodes on the scalp.[207,208] The current is not sufficient to generate action potentials but instead alters neuronal resting membrane potentials. Anodal stimulation generally increases brain activity and excitability, while cathodal stimulation is generally inhibitory. Preliminary studies suggest that tDCS can facilitate motor recovery after stroke.[207,209,210] In patients with stroke, tDCS has been found safe, and a number of studies suggest the potential to improve certain behaviors.[211–213] Direct current stimulation has also been used in the treatment of aphasia. One study analyzed the effect of direct current stimulation on aphasia recovery in patients treated with melodic intonation therapy.[84] They compared the effect of anodal transcranial direct current stimulation and sham treatment over the right inferior frontal gyrus (a region they had previously shown to be activated by therapy) during melodic intonation therapy sessions. The direct current stimulation group performed better on expressive speech tests.[84] A recent Cochrane review that combined wide-ranging tDCS methods found limited evidence that tDCS improves overall function after stroke,[214] but a meta-analysis of studies that focused on arm motor recovery did find significant benefit of tDCS.[215]

Pharmacological therapies

Many drugs have been tried in the past, mostly in an attempt to enhance recovery regarding motor and cognitive and behavioral sequelae of strokes. The effectiveness of most attempts at pharmacological manipulation have been disappointing. However, administering pharmacological agents as an adjunct to other therapies has shown some promise. The most frequently used agents are noradrenergic or dopaminergic.[69,216–220] The most frequently reported agents used include amphetamine, methylphenidate, amantidine, memantine, bromcriptine, and carbidopa/levodopa.[219]

Some pharmacological agents can retard recovery. Haloperidol has a definite negative effect on recovery.[221,222] Drugs that enhance GABA transmission, such as diazepam, might increase inhibition of function and also delay recovery.[219,223] Stroke patients are often exposed to polypharmacy.[224–226] Some drugs were prescribed before the stroke and others are given after the stroke to treat various symptoms and general medical conditions. The acute and chronic effects of concurrent drugs on recovery have been poorly studied but are definitely important. Sedatives, anticonvulsants, haloperidol, and opiates should be avoided when possible.

The Subacute Therapy with Amphetamine and Rehabilitation for Stroke (STARS) study was a randomized, double-blind, placebo-controlled trial that found no benefit from amphetamine administered twice-weekly for 5 weeks in 71 patients enrolled 5–10 days post-stroke; the drug was safe but did not improve the primary outcome, motor recovery during 3 months.[227]

A randomized, double-blind, placebo-controlled trial of 53 patients within 6 months of stroke found that levodopa (Sinemet) 100 mg per day combined with physical therapy was significantly better than placebo combined with physical therapy for improving motor status.[228] Measures of genetic variability may help predict inter-subject differences in treatment response to dopaminergic drugs.[229] This study awaits replication.

The largest body of favorable data for drugs to enhance stroke recovery is in relation to serotonin. Robinson et al. in a multisite randomized controlled trial enrolled 176 non-depressed patients within 3 months of stroke onset.[230] Patients who were randomized to placebo were significantly ($P <0.001$) more likely to reach the primary outcome, development of major or minor depression compared to patients in either of the two active study arms: the selective serotonin reuptake inhibitor (SSRI) escitalopram or problem-solving therapy.[230] A sub-study from this trial reported that cognitive outcomes at 12 months were significantly better among those randomized to escitalopram, independent of depression.[231] In the Fluoxetine for Motor Recovery After Acute Ischemic Stroke (FLAME) study, Chollet et al. used a double-blind, placebo-controlled trial design.[232] Patients with weakness but no depression were randomized within 10 days of ischemic stroke onset to 3 months of oral fluoxetine (20 mg/day) or placebo. Those randomized to fluoxetine showed significantly greater gains on the primary end-point, change in arm and leg motor status at day 90 ($P = 0.003$).

Stem cells

Stem cell research has greatly stimulated an interest in the plasticity of the nervous system and regeneration. Numerous cell-based therapies are under study to improve stroke recovery.[233,234] Different donor cells include transformed tumor cells, adult stem cells such as mesenchymal stromal cells, umbilical cord cells, placental cells, fetal stem cells, embryonic stem cells, and induced pluripotent cells. Cells can be autologous, allogeneic, or xenogeneic; introduced with a bioscaffold; cultured using conditions such as hypoxia or an enriched cell environment; contain modified genes; and can be introduced through various routes including intracerebral, intra-arterial, and intravenous.

One of the most exciting new research strategies to promote recovery involves introducing primitive pluripotential stem cells into patients with stroke.[235–238] Early transplantation experiments that involved introducing primitive cells into the brains of animals showed that grafted neurons survive and remain viable only if they are immature before they have elaborated axonal connections. Preliminary studies in humans that used post-mitotic human neuron-like cells, derived

originally from a human testicular germ cell tumor, showed the feasibility of implanting cells into humans after striato-capsular infarcts and hemorrhages.[239,240] Cyclosporine immunosuppression was given to the transplanted patients. Some patients seemed to improve.[239,240] There were no major complications. Transplantation of fetal porcine cells derived from the lateral ganglionic eminence have also been transplanted into five patients with basal ganglionic infarct cavities.[235,241] To prevent rejection in this study, the cells were pretreated with an anti-MHC1 antibody and the patients were not given immunosuppressive agents.[241]

Stem cell research in stroke patients is clearly very preliminary. When primitive embryonal cells are used, the transplants often also contain abundant growth factors that could stimulate endogenous proliferation of neural elements. Researchers are exploring the potential for using bone-marrow stromal cells[235,237,238,242–245] and blood from the human umbilical cord[235,237,246,247] as potential donor sources of cells and accompanying growth factors. Endothelial progenitor cells are also potential donor type cells. Researchers are actively exploring different ways to introduce cells and growth factors: directly into or near the lesion, intra-arterially into the ipsilateral carotid artery, and intravenously. A meta-analysis of preclinical mesenchymal stem cells found large effect sizes for improving stroke outcomes with effects being consistent across routes of administration.[248] The discovery that animals and humans have a reservoir of primitive cells within brain regions has led to research into means of stimulating these endogenous cells to proliferate and migrate into injured areas. Initial results from small human studies suggest safety and the need for larger clinical trials,[245] while other studies suggest mechanisms of action in humans.[249]

Key questions remain in the application of stem cells:[234,238] (1) When should cells be introduced? If too early, ischemia may reduce the potential for the implants to take, and cytokines and leukocytes could impair implantation. In addition, prognosis is often less evident during the acute period, making it less likely that patients and physicians would accept an experimental procedure soon after stroke onset. Transplantation weeks or months after stroke may be too late. (2) Which cells should be chosen as a donor source and how many? Both neurogenesis and angiogenesis are important for recovery. (3) Should growth factors be introduced with, or instead of, cells? (4) Which strokes? Should only patients with infarcts limited to one area, such as the putamen, be chosen? Would transplants be effective if a number of divergent neuronal cells are infarcted (cortical, putaminal, hippocampal, etc.)? What about size? What if the infarct involves mostly white matter or involves important white matter tracts such as those that travel in the internal capsule? Are patients with intracerebral hemorrhages also candidates for cell or growth factor treatment? (5) What route of administration should be used to introduce the cells? Intravenous, intra-arterial or directly into the brain? If into the brain, where should the cells be implanted? Directly into the infarct or in the presumed penumbra? Multisite injections or one large implant? Hopefully, ongoing research will answer these queries.

Growth factors

Growth factors are polypeptide proteins that influence cell growth, maturation, and division, and have an important role in the response to stroke.[97,250] Brain levels of many growth factors increase after stroke.[251] These play a critical role in neural repair through mechanisms that include angiogenesis, reduced apoptosis, stem cell proliferation, and immunomodulation.[252] Basic fibroblastic growth factor (bFGF),[253] brain-derived neurotrophic factor (BDNF),[254] vascular endothelial growth factor (VEGF),[255] erythropoietin (EPO),[256,257] and granulocyte-colony stimulating factor (G-CSF),[258] have all shown promise in experimental studies of brain ischemia. Some growth factors seem able to penetrate through the normal blood–brain barrier while others do not, so that the access route for their introduction will vary.

Human studies of growth factors to date have focused on hematopoietic factors, some of which have extensive human experience targeting other diagnoses. The AX200 for Ischemic Stroke (AXIS) study[259] found that G-CSF given within 12 hours of stroke was safe and well-tolerated in 44 patients, a finding echoed in a separate study of 60 patients.[260] The AXIS-2 study[261] compared the middle G-CSF dose from the AXIS study (135 µg/kg) with placebo in 328 patients less than 9 hours post-stroke using a multicenter, randomized, placebo-controlled design and found that G-CSF was not different from placebo on the primary end-point, disability at day 90.

Preclinical studies suggest that systemically administered erythropoietin can enter the brain and improve outcome when introduced up to 24 hours after stroke onset.[262] Sequential growth factor administration – e.g., epidermal growth factor[263] or beta-human chorionic gonadotropin (hCG)[264] followed by erythropoietin, beginning up to 7 days after stroke – might also improve outcomes. This approach was translated to humans in the Beta hCG + Erythropoietin in Acute Stroke (BETAS) study, a single dose, multisite, open-label, uncontrolled safety trial that gave 3 hCG doses beginning 1–2 days post-stroke followed by 3 erythropoietin doses beginning 7–8 days after stroke. No safety concerns were identified.[265] The BETAS study was followed by the REGENESIS study,[266] which was intended to be a randomized, placebo-controlled, double-blind proof of concept study of sequential hCG and erythropoietin using the BETAS study treatment schedule, but which was modified to be a dose-ranging safety study and, due to financial constraints, largely moved to India; enrollment was terminated early by the sponsor, and treatment groups did not differ in safety or in the primary end-point, National Institutes of Health Stroke Scale (NIHSS) score change to Day 90.[266]

Delivering growth factors across the blood–brain barrier presents challenges.[267] Alternate approaches under study include intranasal or intracerebral delivery, a Trojan horse strategy involving conjugation of a growth factor with a molecule that can cross the blood–brain barrier, delivery via gene-modified stem cells, and development of small ligands.[268–270]

Mental activity, movement observation and other cognitive strategies

A relatively new concept that is driving rehabilitation strategies is based on the discovery of so-called "mirror neurons" by Rizzolatti and colleagues.[271,272] These nerve cells discharge during various hand-directed actions and also while observing others performing the same actions. Mirror neurons also are likely activated during face and lower extremity goal-directed actions and almost surely in relation to emotional activities. This system is important in understanding actions, during learning to imitate novel complex actions, and in internal rehearsal of actions.[273,274] Mental practice (cognitive rehearsal),[275] and observing others performing a task,[276] when combined with standard physical therapy in which the task is actively performed, may facilitate a patient's ability to perform.[277] Other cognitive strategies include those focused on mirror visual feedback to overcome hemi-inattention,[278] computerized delivery of stimuli target activity in selected neural circuits,[279] real-time neural feedback,[280–282] and techniques focused on virtual reality and augmented reality.[283,284]

Aphasia, other cognitive deficits, and visual field loss

The effectiveness of various strategies on recovery from motor deficits has been easier to study than cognitive and behavioral abnormalities. Weakness and gait disorders can be quantified in a variety of ways, such as time, power, and duration of a specific activity with specific body parts. The clinical manifestations of higher cortical functions and their neuroanatomical correlations are much more diverse and less easily quantified and homogenized than weakness. Speech therapists have used various strategies and modalities to improve language function.[69,148,285,286] Some researchers have begun to apply a strategy used in treating motor abnormalities – that is, combining stimulation (magnetic, direct current, pharmacological) with physical therapy in order to augment use-related improvement. In one study, direct current stimulation with melodic intonation therapy seemed to complement each other.[84]

Visual field defects, especially if accompanied by visual neglect or difficulty reading, can be quite disabling for many stroke patients. Visual field defects most often involve one side of visual space (hemianopia) and vary considerably in their configuration – some involving only one superior or inferior quadrant, some sparing macular vision, and some involving only a hole in vision (scotoma).[287] Strokes, both ischemic and hemorrhagic, are by far the most common cause of persistent visual field defects.[288] Most physicians considered that visual field defects were usually permanent and immutable. Until recently, there was little enthusiasm for available remedial techniques to promote visual recovery.

Experimentalists have shown that plasticity does occur in the human adult central nervous system, even after strokes, a recurrent theme and emphasis in this chapter.[36] Research in mammals and humans shows that the human striate and peristriate visual cortex is also plastic and able to adopt and change after injury.[289–291] Studies of patients with stroke-related hemianopia show that recovery is quite common.[292]

Renewed interest and novel strategies are now being studied to restore visual function in patients with visual field defects.[293]

One of the most promising treatments involves a computer-based training program that patients with visual field defects perform at home, with periodic supervision.[294] In this visual restoration training program, while fixating on a central point, patients press keys in response to repetitive visual stimuli presented in the transition zone between their intact and damaged visual field sectors.[293–297] Their responses are monitored by a computer and stimulus patterns are sequentially changed in accord with the responses. The results show promise in enlarging the visual field, especially the parafoveal portion, allowing important practically useful gains in visual function.[293–297] The visual field improvement persists years after the training period ends.[297] The visual restoration training program takes months of regular hour-long sessions, and so patients must be highly motivated and compulsive enough to sustain the training. The aim of this therapy is to stimulate plasticity in neurons adjacent to the damaged visual cortex.

Others have tried to restore visual function in hemianopic visual fields by directing attention and gaze into the previously blind field.[293,298] One promising approach takes advantage of optokinetic reflexes to expand attention to visual field defects.[298] When hemianopic individuals read, they produce many more saccadic eye movements than normal individuals. Their hemianopia diminishes their appreciation of key visual information about words that will appear next in their blind field.[298] Training patients with visual field defects by scanning moving text can train involuntary saccades and so improve reading and other visual perception in the previously blind visual field.[298]

Principles of brain repair

A number of principles of brain repair have emerged from preclinical and human studies of therapies aiming to improve stroke recovery.[98,299,300]

First, brain repair is time-sensitive. Some biological targets are only relevant during a specific time period after stroke. Some therapies have different effects depending on when they are administered in relation to the time of stroke onset: GABA agonists or NMDA-receptor blockers can be favorable if administered in the early hours after stroke[301,302] but deleterious if initiated days later;[303–305] while the reverse may be true for VEGF,[306] α-amino-3-hydroxy-5-methyl-4-isoxazolepropionic acid (AMPA) receptor signaling,[307] matrix metalloproteinases,[308] and immune modulators.[309,310]

Second, brain repair is experience-dependent. The classic study by Feeney et al. showed that a stimulant promoted improved motor outcome only when its exposure was paired with training.[221] Increasing evidence suggests that a restorative therapy needs the right kind of experience to produce best results, with subsequent studies confirming this principle across numerous classes of restorative therapy.[311–315]

Third, patient stratification is likely important to post-stroke brain repair.[316] Numerous variables have been found to be potential predictors of stroke outcome (see above). Such

measures may be of pivotal value in defining the population most likely to benefit from a given therapy.

Fourth, human preferences might have a sharp effect on therapeutic efficacy in ways that are not apparent in rodent studies. Rehabilitation therapy effects are greatest when a therapy is challenging, repeated many times, task-specific, motivating, interesting, and intensive.[157,299,317,318]

Fifth, domain-specific measures are useful to measure treatment effects.[319] Improvement in global clinical status is of course a goal of paramount importance, but a treatment that provides gains by promoting neuroplasticity might demonstrate maximum effect in brain networks that have subtotal injury. A behavior whose underlying brain regions are destroyed is less likely to improve than a behavior whose underlying regions are accessible to a restorative therapy. A domain whose neural underpinnings are partially spared, such as arm motor function or language, might show substantial gains in response to a restorative therapy, with only modest effects on global measures of post-stroke outcome, and this might be considered worthwhile by many patients and so worthy of measuring in clinical trials. Global outcome measures might lack the granularity to detect improvements in specific neural systems.

References

1. Rathore S, Hinn A, Cooper L, Tyroler H, Rosamond W. Characterization of incident stroke signs and symptoms: Findings from the atherosclerosis risk in communities study. *Stroke.* 2002;**33**:2718–2721

2. Gresham G, Duncan P, Stason W, et al. *Post-stroke Rehabilitation.* Rockville, MD: US Department of Health and Human Services. Public Health Service, Agency for Health Care Policy and Research; 1995

3. World Health Organization. *World Health Report 2003.* Geneva: World Health Organization; 2003

4. Luria A. *Restoration of Function After Brain Injury.* New York: Macmillan Company; 1963

5. Caplan LR, Hier DB. Recovery from right hemisphere stroke. In: Courbier R, ed. *Basis for a Classification of Cerebral Arterial Diseases.* Amsterdam: Excerpta Medica; 1985:163–171

6. Cramer S. Repairing the human brain after stroke. I. Mechanisms of spontaneous recovery. *Ann Neurol.* 2008;**63**:272–287

7. Hier D, Mondlock J, Caplan LR. Recovery of behavioral abnormalities after right hemisphere stroke. *Neurology.* 1983;**33**:345–350

8. Fries W, Danek A, Scheidtmann K, Hamburger C. Motor recovery following capsular stroke. Role of descending pathways from multiple motor areas. *Brain.* 1993;**116**:369–382

9. Binkofski F, Seitz R, Arnold S, Classen J, Benecke R, Freund H. Thalamic metbolism and corticospinal tract integrity determine motor recovery in stroke. *Ann Neurol.* 1996;**39**:460–470

10. Shelton F, Reding M. Effect of lesion location on upper limb motor recovery after stroke. *Stroke.* 2001;**32**:107–112

11. Crafton K, Mark A, Cramer S. Improved understanding of cortical injury by incorporating measures of functional anatomy. *Brain.* 2003;**126**:1650–1659

12. Hillis A, Barker P, Wityk R, et al. Variability in subcortical aphasia is due to variable sites of cortical hypoperfusion. *Brain Lang.* 2004;**89**:524–530

13. Lindenberg R, Renga V, Zhu LL, Betzler F, Alsop D, Schlaug G. Structural integrity of corticospinal motor fibers predicts motor impairment in chronic stroke. *Neurology.* 2010;**74**:280–287

14. Riley JD, Le V, Der-Yeghiaian L, et al. Anatomy of stroke injury predicts gains from therapy. *Stroke.* 2011;**42**:421–426

15. Ween JE, Alexander MP, D'Esposito M, Roberts M. Factors predictive of stroke outcome in a rehabilitation setting. *Neurology.* 1996;**47**:388–392

16. Chang E, Chang E, Cragg S, Cramer S. Predictors of gains during inpatient rehabilitation in patients with stroke: A review. *Crit Rev Phys Rehabil Med.* 2013;**25**:55–73

17. Mayo NE, Wood-Dauphinee S, Cote R, Durcan L, Carlton J. Activity, participation, and quality of life 6 months poststroke. *Arch Phys Med Rehabil.* 2002;**83**:1035–1042

18. Ottenbacher KJ, Karmarkar A, Graham JE, et al. Thirty-day hospital readmission following discharge from postacute rehabilitation in fee-for-service medicare patients. *JAMA.* 2014;**311**:604–614

19. Baker CM, Miller I, Sitterding M, Hajewski CJ. Acute stroke patients comparing outcomes with and without case management. *Nurs Case Manag.* 1998;**3**:196–203

20. Nakayama H, Jorgensen H, Raaschou H, Olsen T. Recovery of upper extremity function in stroke patients: The Copenhagen Stroke Study. *Arch Phys Med Rehabil.* 1994;**75**:394–398

21. Twitchell T. Restoration of motor function following hemiplegia in man. *Brain.* 1951;**74**:443–480

22. Pedersen P, Jorgensen H, Nakayama H, Raaschou H, Olsen T. Aphasia in acute stroke: Incidence, determinants, and recovery. *Ann Neurol.* 1995;**38**:659–666

23. Kertesz A. What do we learn from recovery from aphasia? *Adv Neurol.* 1988;**47**:277–292

24. Kertesz A, McCabe P. Recovery patterns and prognosis in aphasia. *Brain.* 1977;**100** Pt 1:1–18

25. Desmond D, Moroney J, Sano M, Stern Y. Recovery of cognitive function after stroke. *Stroke.* 1996;**27**:1798–1803

26. Wade D, Parker V, Langton Hewer R. Memory disturbance after stroke: Frequency and associated losses. *Int Rehabil Med.* 1986;**8**:60–64

27. Sunderland A, Tinson D, Bradley L. Differences in recovery from constructional apraxia after right and left hemisphere stroke? *J Clin Exp Neuropsychol.* 1994;**16**:916–920

28. Cassidy T, Lewis S, Gray C. Recovery from visuospatial neglect in stroke patients. *J Neurol Neurosurg Psychiatry.* 1998;**64**:555–557

29. Levine D, Warach J, Benowitz L, Calvanio R. Left spatial neglect: Effects of lesion size and premorbid brain atrophy on severity and recovery following right cerebral infarction. *Neurology.* 1986;**36**:362–366

30. Marshall J, Cross A, Jackson D, Green A, Baker H, Ridley R. Clomethiazole protects against hemineglect in a primate model of stroke. *Brain Res Bull.* 2000;**52**:21–29

31. Markgraf C, Green E, Hurwitz B, et al. Sensorimotor and cognitive consequences of middle cerebral artery

occlusion in rats. *Brain Res.* 1992;**575**:238–246

32. Nys GM, Van Zandvoort MJ, De Kort PL, et al. Domain-specific cognitive recovery after first-ever stroke: A follow-up study of 111 cases. *J Int Neuropsychol Soc.* 2005;**11**:795–806

33. Jorgensen H, Nakayama H, Raaschou H, Vive-Larsen J, Stoier M, Olsen T. Outcome and time course of recovery in stroke. Part I: Outcome. The Copenhagen Stroke Study. *Arch Phys Med Rehabil.* 1995;**76**:399–405

34. Mohr J, Pessin M, Finkelstein S, Funkenstein H, Duncan G, Davis K. Broca aphasia: Pathologic and clinical. *Neurology.* 1978;**28**:311–324

35. Cramer S, Nelles G, Benson R, et al. A functional MRI study of subjects recovered from hemiparetic stroke. *Stroke.* 1997;**28**:2518–2527

36. Carmichael ST. Cellular and molecular mechanisms of neural repair after stroke: Making waves. *Ann Neurol.* 2006;**59**:735–742

37. Dancause N, Barbay S, Frost SB, et al. Extensive cortical rewiring after brain injury. *J Neurosci.* 2005;**25**:10167–10179

38. Cramer S, Chopp M. Recovery recapitulates ontogeny. *Trends Neurosci.* 2000;**23**:265–271

39. Hermann DM, Chopp M. Promoting brain remodelling and plasticity for stroke recovery: Therapeutic promise and potential pitfalls of clinical translation. *Lancet Neurol.* 2012;**11**:369–380

40. Overman JJ, Carmichael ST. Plasticity in the injured brain: More than molecules matter. *Neuroscientist.* 2014;**20**:15–28

41. Nudo RJ. Neural bases of recovery after brain injury. *J Commun Disord.* 2011;**44**:515–520

42. Weiller C, Chollet F, Frackowaik RSJ. Physiological aspects of recovery from stroke. In Ginsberg M, Bogousslavsky J, eds. *Cerebrovascular disease: Pathophysiology, Diagnosis, and Management.* Malden, MA: Blackwell Science; 1998:2057–2067

43. Binkofski F, Seitz RJ, Hacklander T, Pawelec D, Mau J, Freund HJ. Recovery of motor functions following hemiparetic stroke: A clinical and magnetic resonance-morphometric study. *Cerebrovas Dis.* 2001;**11**:273–281

44. Feydy A, Carlier R, Roby-Brami A, et al. Longitudinal study of motor recovery after stroke: Recruitment and focusing of brain activation. *Stroke.* 2002;**33**:1610–1617

45. Ward NS, Cohen LG. Mechanisms underlying recovery of motor function after stroke. *Arch Neurol.* 2004;**61**:1844–1848

46. Han BS, Kim SH, Kim OL, Cho SH, Kim YH, Jang SH. Recovery of corticospinal tract with diffuse axonal injury: A diffusion tensor image study. *NeuroRehabilitation.* 2007;**22**:151–155

47. Cramer S. Functional imaging in stroke recovery. *Stroke.* 2004;**35**:2695–2698

48. Burke E, Cramer SC. Biomarkers and predictors of restorative therapy effects after stroke. *Curr Neurol Neurosci Rep.* 2013;**13**:329

49. Stinear C. Prediction of recovery of motor function after stroke. *Lancet Neurol.* 2010;**9**:1228–1232

50. Stinear CM, Ward NS. How useful is imaging in predicting outcomes in stroke rehabilitation? *Int J Stroke.* 2013;**8**:33–37

51. Sharma N, Baron JC, Rowe JB. Motor imagery after stroke: Relating outcome to motor network connectivity. *Ann Neurol.* 2009;**66**:604–616

52. Grefkes C, Nowak DA, Eickhoff SB, et al. Cortical connectivity after subcortical stroke assessed with functional magnetic resonance imaging. *Ann Neurol.* 2008;**63**:236–246

53. Carter AR, Astafiev SV, Lang CE, et al. Resting interhemispheric functional magnetic resonance imaging connectivity predicts performance after stroke. *Ann Neurol.* 2010;**67**:365–375

54. Grefkes C, Fink GR. Reorganization of cerebral networks after stroke: New insights from neuroimaging with connectivity approaches. *Brain.* 2011;**135**:1264–1276

55. Burke Quinlan E, Dodakian L, See J, et al. Neural function, injury, and stroke subtype predict treatment gains after stroke. *Ann Neurol.* 2014;**77**:132–145

56. von Monakow C. Diaschisis, 1914. In Pribram K, ed. *Brain and Behavior 1. Mood, States and Mind.* Baltimore: Penguin Books; 1969:26–34

57. Feeney D, Baron J. Diaschisis. *Stroke.* 1986;**17**:817–830

58. Weiller C, Ramsay S, Wise R, Friston K, Frackowiak R. Individual patterns of functional reorganization in the human cerebral cortex after capsular infarction. *Ann Neurol.* 1993;**33**:181–189

59. Cramer S, Moore C, Finklestein S, Rosen B. A pilot study of somatotopic mapping after cortical infarct. *Stroke.* 2000;**31**:668–671

60. Cramer S, Crafton K. Changes in lateralization and somatotopic organization after cortical stroke. *Stroke.* 2004;**35**:240

61. Murase N, Duque J, Mazzocchio R, Cohen L. Influence of interhemispheric interactions on motor function in chronic stroke. *Ann Neurol.* 2004;**55**:400–409

62. Netz J, Lammers T, Homberg V. Reorganization of motor output in the non-affected hemisphere after stroke. *Brain.* 1997;**120**:1579–1586

63. Turton A, Wroe S, Trepte N, Fraser C, Lemon R. Contralateral and ipsilateral EMG responses to transcranial magnetic stimulation during recovery of arm and hand function after stroke. *Electroencephalogr Clin Neurophysiol.* 1996;**101**:316–328

64. Heiss WD, Thiel A. A proposed regional hierarchy in recovery of post-stroke aphasia. *Brain Lang.* 2006;**98**:118–123

65. Teasell R, Meyer MJ, McClure A, et al. Stroke rehabilitation: An international perspective. *Top Stroke Rehabil.* 2009;**16**:44–56

66. World Health Organization. *International Classification of Functioning, Disability and Health (ICF).* Geneva, Switzerland: World Health Organization; 2008.

67. Miller EL, Murray L, Richards L, et al. Comprehensive overview of nursing and interdisciplinary rehabilitation care of the stroke patient: A scientific statement from the American Heart Association. *Stroke.* 2010;**41**:2402–2448

68. Foley N, Teasell R, Bhogal S, Speechley M, Hussein N. *The Efficacy of Stroke Rehabilitation.* Available from http://www.ebrsr.com/evidence-review/5-efficacy-stroke-rehabilitation. Last updated November, 2013

69. Dobkin B. *Neurologic Rehabilitation.* Philadelphia, PA: F A Davis; 1996

70. Dobkin BH. Clinical practice. Rehabilitation after stroke. *New Engl J Med.* 2005;**352**:1677–1684

71. Wood-Dauphinee S, Shapiro S, Bass E, et al. A randomized trial of team care following stroke. *Stroke.* 1984;**15**:864–872

72. Strand T, Asplund K, Eriksson S, Hagg E, Lithner F, Wester PO.

A non-intensive stroke unit reduces functional disability and the need for long-term hospitalization. *Stroke.* 1985;**16**:29–34

73. Indredavik B, Bakke F, Solberg R, Rokseth R, Haaheim LL, Holme I. Benefit of a stroke unit: A randomized controlled trial. *Stroke.* 1991;**22**:1026–1031

74. Kalra L, Dale P, Crome P. Improving stroke rehabilitation. A controlled study. *Stroke.* 1993;**24**:1462–1467

75. Ottenbacher KJ, Jannell S. The results of clinical trials in stroke rehabilitation research. *Arch Neurol.* 1993;**50**:37–44

76. Kaste M, Palomaki H, Sarna S. Where and how should elderly stroke patients be treated? A randomized trial. *Stroke.* 1995;**26**:249–253

77. Indredavik B, Slordahl SA, Bakke F, Rokseth R, Haheim LL. Stroke unit treatment. Long-term effects. *Stroke.* 1997;**28**:1861–1866

78. Stroke Unit Trialists Collaboration. Collaborative systematic review of the randomized trials of organized in-patient (stroke unit) care after stroke. *BMJ.* 1997;**314**:1151–1159

79. Stroke Unit Trialists Collaboration. How do stroke units improve patient outcomes? A collaborative systematic review of the randomized trials. *Stroke.* 1997;**28**:2139–2144

80. Colborne GR, Olney SJ, Griffin MP. Feedback of ankle joint angle and soleus electromyography in the rehabilitation of hemiplegic gait. *Arch Phys Med Rehabil.* 1993;**74**:1100–1106

81. da Cunha-IT Jr, Lim PA, Qureshy H, Henson H, Monga T, Protas EJ. Gait outcomes after acute stroke rehabilitation with supported treadmill ambulation training: A randomized controlled pilot study. *Arch Phys Med Rehabil.* 2002;**83**:1258–1265

82. Maple FW, Tong RKY, Li LSW. A pilot study of randomized clinical controlled trial of gait training in subacute stroke patients with partial body-weight support electromechanical gait trainer and functional electrical stimulation. *Stroke.* 2008;**39**:154–160

83. Shewan CM, Kertesz A. Effects of speech and language treatment on recovery from aphasia. *Brain Lang.* 1984;**23**:272–299

84. Vines BW, Norton AC, Schlaug G. Applying transcranial direct current stimulation in combination with melodic intonation therapy facilitates language recovery for Broca's aphasic patients. *Stroke.* 2007;**38**:519

85. Halligan P, Marshall JC. Spatial neglect. Position papers on theory and practise. *Neuropsych Rehabil.* 1994;**4**:103–230

86. Johansson K, Lindgren I, Widner H, Wiklund I, Johansson BB. Can sensory stimulation improve the functional outcome in stroke patients? *Neurology.* 1993;**43**:2189–2192

87. Ottenbacher KJ, Smith PM, Illig SB, Linn RT, Ostir GV, Granger CV. Trends in length of stay, living setting, functional outcome, and mortality following medical rehabilitation. *JAMA.* 2004;**292**:1687–1695

88. McKenna JE, Whishaw IQ. Complete compensation in skilled reaching success with associated impairments in limb synergies, after dorsal column lesion in the rat. *J Neurosci.* 1999;**19**:1885–1894

89. Nakayama H, Jorgensen HS, Raaschou HO, Olsen TS. Compensation in recovery of upper extremity function after stroke: The Copenhagen stroke study. *Arch Phys Med Rehabil.* 1994;**75**:852–857

90. Cirstea MC, Levin MF. Improvement of arm movement patterns and endpoint control depends on type of feedback during practice in stroke survivors. *Neurorehabil Neural Repair.* 2007;**21**:398–411

91. Friel K, Nudo R. Recovery of motor function after focal cortical injury in primates: Compensatory movement patterns used during rehabilitative training. *Somatosens Mot Res.* 1998;**15**:173–189

92. Levin MF, Kleim JA, Wolf SL. What do motor "recovery" and "compensation" mean in patients following stroke? *Neurorehabil Neural Repair.* 2009;**23**:313–319

93. Pollock A, Baer G, Campbell P, et al. Physical rehabilitation approaches for the recovery of function and mobility following stroke. *Cochrane Database Syst Rev.* 2014;**4**:CD001920

94. Miyai I, Reding MJ. Stroke recovery and rehabilitation. In Ginsberg M, Bogousslavsky J, eds. *Cerebrovascular Disease: Pathophysiology, Diagnosis, and Management.* Malden, MA: Blackwell Science; 1998:2043–2056

95. Bates B, Choi JY, Duncan PW, et al. Veterans affairs/Department of Defense clinical practice guideline for the management of adult stroke rehabilitation care: Executive summary. *Stroke.* 2005;**36**:2049–2056

96. Duncan PW, Zorowitz R, Bates B, et al. Management of adult stroke rehabilitation care: A clinical practice guideline. *Stroke.* 2005;**36**:e100–143

97. Cramer SC. Repairing the human brain after stroke. II. Restorative therapies. *Ann Neurol.* 2008;**63**:549–560

98. Langhorne P, Bernhardt J, Kwakkel G. Stroke rehabilitation. *Lancet.* 2011;**377**:1693–1702

99. Dobkin BH. Training and exercise to drive poststroke recovery. *Nature Clin Pract.* 2008;**4**:76–85

100. Alexander MP. Stroke rehabilitation outcome. A potential use of predictive variables to establish levels of care. *Stroke.* 1994;**25**:128–134

101. Caplan LR. Neurologic management plan. In Ozer MN, Materson RS, Caplan LR, eds. *Management of Persons with Stroke.* St Louis, MI: Mosby; 1994:61–113.

102. Billinger SA, Arena R, Bernhardt J, et al. Physical activity and exercise recommendations for stroke survivors: A statement for healthcare professionals from the American Heart Association/ American Stroke Association. *Stroke.* 2014;**45**:2532–2553

103. Kernan WN, Ovbiagele B, Black HR, et al. Guidelines for the prevention of stroke in patients with stroke and transient ischemic attack: A guideline for healthcare professionals from the American Heart Association/ American Stroke Association. *Stroke.* 2014;**45**:2160–2236

104. Taub NA, Wolfe CD, Richardson E, Burney PG. Predicting the disability of first-time stroke sufferers at 1 year. 12-month follow-up of a population-based cohort in Southeast England. *Stroke.* 1994;**25**:352–357

105. Feigenson JS, McDowell FH, Meese P, McCarthy ML, Greenberg SD. Factors influencing outcome and length of stay in a stroke rehabilitation unit. Part 1. Analysis of 248 unscreened patients – medical and functional prognostic indicators. *Stroke.* 1977;**8**:651–656

106. Feigenson JS, McCarthy ML, Greenberg SD, Feigenson WD. Factors influencing outcome and length of stay in a stroke rehabilitation unit. Part 2. Comparison of 318 screened and 248 unscreened patients. *Stroke.* 1977;**8**:657–662

107. Feigenson JS, McCarthy ML, Meese PD, et al. Stroke rehabilitation I. Factors predicting outcome and length of stay – an overview. *N Y State J Med.* 1977;77:1426–1430

108. Nicholas ML, Helm-Estabrooks N, Ward-Lonergan J, Morgan AR. Evolution of severe aphasia in the first two years post onset. *Arch Phys Med Rehabil.* 1993;74:830–836

109. Kelly PJ, Furie KL, Shafqat S, Rallis N, Chang Y, Stein J. Functional recovery following rehabilitation after hemorrhagic and ischemic stroke. *Arch Phys Med Rehabil.* 2003;84:968–972

110. Feigenson JS. Neurological rehabilitation. In Baker AB, ed. *Clinical Neurology.* New York: Harper and Row; 1983:1–66

111. DeJong G, Branch LG. Predicting the stroke patient's ability to live independently. *Stroke.* 1982;13:648–655

112. Hakkennes S, Hill KD, Brock K, Bernhardt J, Churilov L. Selection for inpatient rehabilitation after severe stroke: What factors influence rehabilitation assessor decision-making? *J Rehab Med.* 2013;45:24–31

113. Hakkennes SJ, Brock K, Hill KD. Selection for inpatient rehabilitation after acute stroke: A systematic review of the literature. *Arch Phys Med Rehabil.* 2011;92:2057–2070

114. Li CC, Chen YM, Tsay SL, Hu GC, Lin KC. Predicting functional outcomes in patients suffering from ischaemic stroke using initial admission variables and physiological data: A comparison between tree model and multivariate regression analysis. *Disabil Rehab.* 2010;32:2088–2096

115. Fregni F, Boggio PS, Valle AC, et al. A sham-controlled trial of a 5-day course of repetitive transcranial magnetic stimulation of the unaffected hemisphere in stroke patients. *Stroke.* 2006;37:2115–2122

116. Kreisel SH, Hennerici MG, Bazner H. Pathophysiology of stroke rehabilitation: The natural course of clinical recovery, use-dependent plasticity and rehabilitative outcome. *Cerebrovasc Dis.* 2007;23:243–255

117. Katz S, Ford AB, Chinn AB, et al. Prognosis after stroke: Part II long-term course of 159 patients. *Medicine.* 1966;45:236–246

118. Cramer SC, Sur M, Dobkin BH, et al. Harnessing neuroplasticity for clinical applications. *Brain.* 2011;134:1591–1609

119. Corbett D, Nguemeni C, Gomez-Smith M. How can you mend a broken brain? Neurorestorative approaches to stroke recovery. *Cerebrovasc Dis* 2014;38:233–239

120. Teasell R, Foley N, Salter K, Bhogal S, Jutai J, Speechley M. Evidence-based review of stroke rehabilitation: Executive summary, 12th edition. *Top Stroke Rehab.* 2009;16:463–488

121. Taub E, Uswatte G, Mark VW, Morris DM. The learned nonuse phenomenon: Implications for rehabilitation. *Eura Medicophys.* 2006;42:241–256

122. Wolf SL, Winstein CJ, Miller JP, et al. Effect of constraint-induced movement therapy on upper extremity function 3 to 9 months after stroke: The EXCITE randomized clinical trial. *JAMA.* 2006;296:2095–2104

123. Page SJ, Levine P. Back from the brink: Electromyography-triggered stimulation combined with modified constraint-induced movement therapy in chronic stroke. *Arch Phys Med Rehabil.* 2006;87:27–31

124. Meinzer M, Elbert T, Djundja D, Taub E, Rockstroh B. Extending the constraint-induced movement therapy (CIMT) approach to cognitive functions: Constraint-induced aphasia therapy (CIAT) of chronic aphasia. *Neuro Rehabilitation.* 2007;22:311–318

125. Berthier ML, Pulvermuller F. Neuroscience insights improve neurorehabilitation of poststroke aphasia. *Nat Rev Neurol.* 2011;7:86–97

126. Dromerick AW, Lang CE, Birkenmeier RL, et al. Very early constraint-induced movement during stroke rehabilitation (VECTORS): A single-center RCT. *Neurology.* 2009;73:195–201

127. Kwakkel G, Wagenaar R, Twisk J, Lankhorst G, Koetsier J. Intensity of leg and arm training after primary middle-cerebral-artery stroke: A randomised trial. *Lancet.* 1999;354:191–196

128. Galvin R, Cusack T, O'Grady E, Murphy TB, Stokes E. Family-mediated exercise intervention (FAME): Evaluation of a novel form of exercise delivery after stroke. *Stroke.* 2011;42:681–686

129. Kwakkel G, van Peppen R, Wagenaar RC, et al. Effects of augmented exercise therapy time after stroke: A meta-analysis. *Stroke.* 2004;35:2529–2539

130. Outpatient Service Trialists. Rehabilitation therapy services for stroke patients living at home: Systematic review of randomised trials. *Lancet.* 2004;363:352–356

131. Bhogal S, Teasell R, Speechley M. Intensity of aphasia therapy, impact on recovery. *Stroke.* 2003;34:987–993

132. Van Peppen RP, Kwakkel G, Wood-Dauphinee S, Hendriks HJ, Van der Wees PJ, Dekker J. The impact of physical therapy on functional outcomes after stroke: What's the evidence? *Clin Rehab.* 2004;18:833–862

133. Galvin R, Murphy B, Cusack T, Stokes E. The impact of increased duration of exercise therapy on functional recovery following stroke – what is the evidence? *Top Stroke Rehab.* 2008;15:365–377

134. Cauraugh JH, Naik SK, Lodha N, Coombes SA, Summers JJ. Long-term rehabilitation for chronic stroke arm movements: A randomized controlled trial. *Clin Rehab.* 2011;25:1086–1096

135. Lang CE, Macdonald JR, Reisman DS, et al. Observation of amounts of movement practice provided during stroke rehabilitation. *Arch Phys Med Rehabil.* 2009;90:1692–1698

136. Bernhardt J, Chan J, Nicola I, Collier JM. Little therapy, little physical activity: Rehabilitation within the first 14 days of organized stroke unit care. *J Rehab Med.* 2007;39:43–48

137. Sarkamo T, Tervaniemi M, Laitinen S, et al. Music listening enhances cognitive recovery and mood after middle cerebral artery stroke. *Brain.* 2008;131:866–876

138. Wade DT, Skilbeck CE, Hewer RL, Wood VA. Therapy after stroke: Amounts, determinants and effects. *Int Rehabil Med.* 1984;6:105–110

139. Kimberley TJ, Samargia S, Moore LG, Shakya JK, Lang CE. Comparison of amounts and types of practice during rehabilitation for traumatic brain injury and stroke. *J Rehab Res Develop.* 2010;47:851–862

140. Bohannon R, Andrews A, Smith M. Rehabilitation goals of patients with hemiplegia. *Int J Rehab Research.* 1988;11:181–183

141. Salbach NM, Mayo NE, Higgins J, Ahmed S, Finch LE, Richards CL. Responsiveness and predictability of gait speed and other disability measures in acute stroke. *Arch Phys Med Rehabil.* 2001;82:1204–1212

142. Perry J, Garrett M, Gronley J, Mulroy S. Classification of walking

handicap in the stroke population. *Stroke*. 1995;**26**:982–989

143. Lovely RG, Gregor RJ, Roy RR, Edgerton VR. Effects of training on the recovery of full-weight-bearing stepping in the adult spinal cat. *Exp Neurol*. 1986;**92**:421–435

144. Hesse S, Bertelt C, Jahnke MT, et al. Treadmill training with partial body weight support compared with physiotherapy in nonambulatory hemiparetic patients. *Stroke*. 1995;**26**:976–981

145. Visintin M, Barbeau H, Korner-Bitensky N, Mayo NE. A new approach to retrain gait in stroke patients through body weight support and treadmill stimulation. *Stroke*. 1998;**29**:1122–1128

146. Kosak MC, Reding MJ. Comparison of partial body weight-supported treadmill gait training versus aggressive bracing assisted walking post stroke. *Neurorehabil Neural Repair*. 2000;**14**:13–19

147. da Cunha-Filho IT, Lim PA, Qurey H, et al. A comparison of regular rehabilitation and regular rehabilitation with supported treadmill ambulation training for acute stroke patients. *J Rehabil Res Develop*. 2001;**3**:37–47

148. Breen JC, Baker B, Thibault K, Snyder DE. Body weight support treadmill training improves walking in subacute and chronic severely disabled stroke patients. *Stroke*. 2007;**38**:571

149. Duncan PW, Sullivan KJ, Behrman AL, et al. Body-weight-supported treadmill rehabilitation after stroke. *N Engl J Med*. 2011;**364**:2026–2036

150. Reinkensmeyer DJ. Robotic approaches to stroke recovery. In Cramer SC, Nudo RJ, eds. *Brain Repair After Stroke*. Cambridge, UK: Cambridge University Press; 2010:195–205

151. Volpe BT, Huerta PT, Zipse JL, et al. Robotic devices as therapeutic and diagnostic tools for stroke recovery. *Arch Neurol*. 2009;**66**:1086–1090

152. Cramer SC. Brain repair after stroke. *N Engl J Med*. 2010;**362**:1827–1829

153. Aisen M, Krebs H, Hogan N, McDowell F, Volpe B. The effect of robot-assisted therapy and rehabilitative training on motor recovery following stroke. *Arch Neurol*. 1997;**54**:443–446

154. Volpe B, Krebs H, Hogan N, Edelsteinn L, Diels C, Aisen M. Robot

training enhanced motor outcome in patients with stroke maintained over 3 years. *Neurology*. 1999;**53**:1874–1876

155. Volpe BT, Krebs HI, Hogan N. Robot-aided sensorimotor training in stroke rehabilitation. *Adv Neurol*. 2003;**92**:429–433

156. Krebs HI, Volpe BT, Ferraro M, et al. Robot-aided neurorehabilitation: From evidence-based to science-based rehabilitation. *Top Stroke Rehabil*. 2002;**8**:54–70

157. Takahashi CD, Der-Yeghiaian L, Le V, Motiwala RR, Cramer SC. Robot-based hand motor therapy after stroke. *Brain*. 2008;**131**:425–437

158. Modo M, Ambrosio F, Friedlander RM, Badylak SF, Wechsler LR. Bioengineering solutions for neural repair and recovery in stroke. *Curr Opin Neurol*. 2013;**26**:626–631

159. Norouzi-Gheidari N, Archambault PS, Fung J. Effects of robot-assisted therapy on stroke rehabilitation in upper limbs: Systematic review and meta-analysis of the literature. *J Rehabil Res Dev*. 2012;**49**:479–496

160. Lo AC, Guarino PD, Richards LG, et al. Robot-assisted therapy for long-term upper-limb impairment after stroke. *N Engl J Med*. 2010;**362**:1772–1783

161. Brewer BR, McDowell SK, Worthen-Chaudhari LC. Poststroke upper extremity rehabilitation: A review of robotic systems and clinical results. *Top Stroke Rehabil*. 2007;**14**:22–44

162. Reinkensmeyer D, Emken J, Cramer S. Robotics, motor learning, and neurologic recovery. *Annu Rev Biomed Eng*. 2004;**6**:497–525

163. Semrau JA, Herter TM, Scott SH, Dukelow SP. Robotic identification of kinesthetic deficits after stroke. *Stroke*. 2013;**44**:3414–3421

164. Reinkensmeyer DJ, Wolbrecht ET, Chan V, Chou C, Cramer SC, Bobrow JE. Comparison of three-dimensional, assist-as-needed robotic arm/hand movement training provided with Pneu-WREX to conventional tabletop therapy after chronic stroke. *Am J Phys Med Rehabil*. 2012;**91**:S232–241

165. Brennan D, Tindall L, Theodoros D, et al. A blueprint for telerehabilitation guidelines – October 2010. *Telemed J E Health* 2011;**17**:1–4

166. Langhorne P, Coupar F, Pollock A. Motor recovery after stroke: A

systematic review. *Lancet Neurol*. 2009;**8**:741–754

167. Teasell RW, Foley NC, Salter KL, Jutai JW. A blueprint for transforming stroke rehabilitation care in Canada: The case for change. *Arch Phys Med Rehabil*. 2008;**89**:575–578

168. Steins D, Dawes H, Esser P, Collett J. Wearable accelerometry-based technology capable of assessing functional activities in neurological populations in community settings: A systematic review. *J Neuroeng Rehabil*. 2014;**11**:36

169. Reinkensmeyer DJ, Pang CT, Nessler JA, Painter CC. Web-based telerehabilitation for the upper extremity after stroke. *IEEE Trans Neural Syst Rehabil Eng*. 2002;**10**:102–108

170. Lai JC, Woo J, Hui E, Chan WM. Telerehabilitation – a new model for community-based stroke rehabilitation. *J Telemed Telecare*. 2004;**10**:199–205

171. Lum PS, Uswatte G, Taub E, Hardin P, Mark VW. A telerehabilitation approach to delivery of constraint-induced movement therapy. *J Rehabil Res Dev*. 2006;**43**:391–400

172. Sanford JA, Griffiths PC, Richardson P, Hargraves K, Butterfield T, Hoenig H. The effects of in-home rehabilitation on task self-efficacy in mobility-impaired adults: A randomized clinical trial. *J Am Geriatr Soc*. 2006;**54**:1641–1648

173. Carey JR, Durfee WK, Bhatt E, et al. Comparison of finger tracking versus simple movement training via telerehabilitation to alter hand function and cortical reorganization after stroke. *Neurorehabil Neural Repair*. 2007;**21**:216–232

174. Deutsch JE, Lewis JA, Burdea G. Technical and patient performance using a virtual reality-integrated telerehabilitation system: Preliminary finding. *IEEE Trans Neural Syst Rehabil Eng*. 2007;**15**:30–35

175. Dallolio L, Menarini M, China S, et al. Functional and clinical outcomes of telemedicine in patients with spinal cord injury. *Arch Phys Med Rehabil*. 2008;**89**:2332–2341

176. Baranowski T, Buday R, Thompson DI, Baranowski J. Playing for real: Video games and stories for health-related behavior change. *Am J Prev Med*. 2008;**34**:74–82

177. Brox, E, Fernandez-Luque L, Tøllefsen T. Healthy gaming – video game

design to promote health. *Appl Clin Inform*. 2011;2:128–142

178. Hansen MM. Versatile, immersive, creative and dynamic virtual 3-D healthcare learning environments: A review of the literature. *J Med Internet Res*. 2008;10:e26

179. Lieberman D. Designing serious games for learning and health in informal and formal settings. In Ritterfeld M, Vorderer P, eds. *Serious Games: Mechanisms and Effects*. New York: Routledge; 2009:117–130

180. Thompson D, Baranowski T, Buday R, et al. Serious video games for health; how behavioral science guided the development of a serious video game. *Simul Gaming*. 2010;41:587–606

181. Robert Wood Johnson Foundation. Games for health: Connecting the worlds of video games and health, with positive results. Available at www.rwjf.org/pr/product.jsp?id=29171. May 6, 2008.

182. Parker SG for the Robert Wood Johnson Foundation. Health games research: Advancing effectiveness of interactive games for health. Available at www.rwjf.org/content/rwjf/en/research-publications/find-rwjf-research/2011/03/advancing-the-field-of-health-games.html. September 18, 2015.

183. Kaplan SH, Billimek J, Sorkin DH, Ngo-Metzger Q, Greenfield S. Who can respond to treatment? Identifying patient characteristics related to heterogeneity of treatment effects. *Med Care*. 2010;48:S9–16

184. Hersh W, Hickam D, Severance S, Dana T, Krages K, Helfand M. *Telemedicine for the Medicare Population: Update. Evidence Report/ Technology Assessment No. 131*. AHRQ publication no. 06–e007. Rockville, MD: Agency for Healthcare Research and Quality; 2006

185. Institute of Medicine of the National Academies. *Initial National Priorities for Comparative Effectiveness Research*. Washington, DC: Institute of Medicine of the National Academies; 2009

186. Jimison H, Gorman P, Woods S, et al. *Barriers and Drivers of Health Information Technology Use for the Elderly, Chronically Ill, and Underserved. Evidence Report/ Technology Assessment No. 175*. AHRQ publication no. 09–e004. Rockville, MD: Agency for Healthcare Research and Quality; 2008

187. Clifford GD, Clifton D. Wireless technology in disease management and medicine. *Annu Rev Med*. 2012;63:479–492

188. Topol E. *The Creative Destruction of Medicine. How the Digital Revolution Will Create Better Health Care*. New York: Basic Books; 2012

189. Feys H, De Weerdt W, Verbeke G, et al. Early and repetitive stimulation of the arm can substantially improve the long-term outcome after stroke: A 5-year follow-up study of a randomized trial. *Stroke*. 2004;35:924–929

190. Stinear CM, Barber PA, Coxon JP, Fleming MK, Byblow WD. Priming the motor system enhances the effects of upper limb therapy in chronic stroke. *Brain*. 2008;131:1381–1390

191. Teasell RW, Kalra L. What's new in stroke rehabilitation. *Stroke*. 2004;35:383–385

192. Kerkhoff G. Modulation and rehabilitation of spatial neglect by sensory stimulation. *Prog Brain Res*. 2003;142:257–271

193. American Psychiatric Association. *Practice Guideline for the Treatment of Patients With Major Depressive Disorder*, 3rd ed. Arlington, VA: American Psychiatric Association; 2010

194. Plow EB, Carey JR, Nudo RJ, Pascual-Leone A. Invasive cortical stimulation to promote recovery of function after stroke: A critical appraisal. *Stroke*. 2009;40:1926–1931

195. Naeser MA, Martin PI, Nicholas M, et al. Improved picture naming in chronic aphasia after TMS to part of right Broca's area: An open-protocol study. *Brain Lang*. 2005;93:95–105

196. Liew SL, Santarnecchi E, Buch ER, Cohen LG. Non-invasive brain stimulation in neurorehabilitation: Local and distant effects for motor recovery. *Front Hum Neurosci*. 2014;8:378

197. Dayan E, Cohen LG. Neuroplasticity subserving motor skill learning. *Neuron*. 2011;72:443–454

198. Rossi S, Hallett M, Rossini PM, Pascual-Leone A. Safety, ethical considerations, and application guidelines for the use of transcranial magnetic stimulation in clinical practice and research. *Clin Neurophysiol*. 2009;120:2008–2039

199. Fregni F, Boggio PS, Lima MC, et al. A sham-controlled, phase II trial of transcranial direct current stimulation for the treatment of central pain in traumatic spinal cord injury. *Pain*. 2006;122:197–209

200. Takeuchi N, Chuma T, Matsuo Y, Watanabe I, Ikoma K. Repetitive transcranial magnetic stimulation of contralesional primary motor cortex improves hand function after stroke. *Stroke*. 2005;36:2681–2686

201. Kobayashi M, Hutchinson S, Theoret H, Schlaug G, Pascual-Leone A. Repetitive TMS of the motor cortex improves ipsilateral sequential simple finger movements. *Neurology*. 2004;62:91–98

202. Nowak DA, Grefkes C, Dafotakis M, et al. Effects of low-frequency repetitive transcranial magnetic stimulation of the contralesional primary motor cortex on movement kinematics and neural activity in subcortical stroke. *Arch Neurol*. 2008;65:741–747

203. Khedr EM, Ahmed MA, Fathy N, Rothwell JC. Therapeutic trial of repetitive transcranial magnetic stimulation after acute ischemic stroke. *Neurology*. 2005;65:466–468

204. Kim YH, You SH, Ko MH, et al. Repetitive transcranial magnetic stimulation-induced corticomotor excitability and associated motor skill acquisition in chronic stroke. *Stroke*. 2006;37:1471–1476

205. Hao Z, Wang D, Zeng Y, Liu M. Repetitive transcranial magnetic stimulation for improving function after stroke. *Cochrane Database Syst Rev*. 2013;5:CD008862

206. Hsu WY, Cheng CH, Liao KK, Lee IH, Lin YY. Effects of repetitive transcranial magnetic stimulation on motor functions in patients with stroke: A meta-analysis. *Stroke*. 2012;43:1849–1857

207. Hummel F, Celnik P, Giraux P, et al. Effects of non-invasive cortical stimulation on skilled motor function in chronic stroke. *Brain*. 2005;128:490–499

208. Webster BR, Celnik PA, Cohen LG. Noninvasive brain stimulation in stroke rehabilitation. *NeuroRx*. 2006;3:474–481

209. Hummel F, Cohen LG. Improvement of motor function with noninvasive cortical stimulation in a patient with chronic stroke. *Neurorehabil Neural Repair*. 2005;19:14–19

210. Alonso-Alonso M, Fregni F, Pascual-Leone A. Brain stimulation in post-stroke rehabilitation. *Cerebrovasc Dis*. 2007;24(supp 1):157–166

211. Nair DG, Pascual-Leone A, Schlaug G. Transcranial direct current

stimulation in combination with occupational therapy for 5 consecutive days improves motor function in chronic stroke patients. *Stroke.* 2007;**38**:518

212. Shah PP, Szaflarski JP, Allendorfer J, Hamilton RH. Induction of neuroplasticity and recovery in post-stroke aphasia by non-invasive brain stimulation. *Front Hum Neurosci.* 2013;**7**:888

213. Lindenberg R, Renga V, Zhu LL, Nair D, Schlaug G. Bihemispheric brain stimulation facilitates motor recovery in chronic stroke patients. *Neurology.* 2010;**75**:2176–2184

214. Elsner B, Kugler J, Pohl M, Mehrholz J. Transcranial direct current stimulation (TDCS) for improving function and activities of daily living in patients after stroke. *Cochrane Database Syst Rev.* 2013;**11**:CD009645

215. Butler AJ, Shuster M, O'Hara E, Hurley K, Middlebrooks D, Guilkey K. A meta-analysis of the efficacy of anodal transcranial direct current stimulation for upper limb motor recovery in stroke survivors. *J Hand Ther.* 2013;**26**:162–170;quiz 171

216. Davis JN, Crisostomo EA, Duncan P, Propst M, Feeney DM. Amphetamine and physical therapy facilitate recovery of function from stroke: Correlative animal and human studies. In: Raichle ME, Powers WJ, eds. *Cerebrovascular Diseases.* New York: Raven Press; 1987:297–304

217. Goldstein LB. Amphetamine-facilitated functional recovery after stroke. In Ginsberg MD, Dietric WD, eds. *Cerebrovascular Diseases.* New York: Raven Press; 1989:303–308

218. Sawaki L, Cohen LG, Classen J, Davis BC, Butefisch CM. Enhancement of use-dependent plasticity by d-amphetamine. *Neurology.* 2002;**59**:1262–1264

219. Dombovy ML. Understanding stroke recovery and rehabilitation: Current and emerging approaches. *Curr Neurol Neurosci Rep.* 2004;**4**:31–35

220. Goldstein LB. Effects of amphetamines and small related molecules on recovery after stroke in animals and man. *Neuropharmacology.* 2000;**39**:852–859

221. Feeney D, Gonzalez A, Law W. Amphetamine, haloperidol, and experience interact to affect the rate of recovery after motor cortex injury. *Science.* 1982;**217**:855–857

222. Houda DA, Feeney DM. Haldoperidol blocks amphetamine induced recovery of binocular depth perception after bilateral visual cortex abilities in the cat. *Proc West Pharmacol Soc.* 1985;**28**:209–211

223. Schallert T, Hernandez TD. GABAergic drugs and neuroplasticity after brain injury. In Goldstein L, ed. *Restorative Neurology: Advances in Pharmacotherapy of Recovery After Stroke.* Armonk, NY: Futura Publishing; 1998:91–120

224. Goldstein LB, Davis JN. Physician prescribing patterns following hospital admission for ischemic cerebrovascular disease. *Neurology.* 1988;**38**:1806–1809

225. Goldstein LB. Potential effects of common drugs on stroke recovery. *Arch Neurol.* 1998;**55**:454–456

226. Goldstein LB. Common drugs may influence motor recovery after stroke. The Sygen in acute stroke study investigators. *Neurology.* 1995;**45**:865–871

227. Gladstone DJ, Danells CJ, Armesto A, et al. Physiotherapy coupled with dextroamphetamine for rehabilitation after hemiparetic stroke: A randomized, double-blind, placebo-controlled trial. *Stroke.* 2006;**37**:179–185

228. Scheidtmann K, Fries W, Muller F, Koenig E. Effect of levodopa in combination with physiotherapy on functional motor recovery after stroke: A prospective, randomised, double-blind study. *Lancet.* 2001;**358**:787–790

229. Pearson-Fuhrhop KM, Minton B, Acevedo D, Shahbaba B, Cramer SC. Genetic variation in the human brain dopamine system influences motor learning and its modulation by L-dopa. *PloS One.* 2013;**8**:e61197

230. Robinson RG, Jorge RE, Moser DJ, et al. Escitalopram and problem-solving therapy for prevention of poststroke depression: A randomized controlled trial. *JAMA.* 2008;**299**:2391–2400

231. Mikami K, Jorge RE, Moser DJ, et al. Prevention of post-stroke generalized anxiety disorder, using escitalopram or problem-solving therapy. *J Neuropsychiatry Clin Neurosci.* 2014;**26**:323–328

232. Chollet F, Tardy J, Albucher JF et al. Fluoxetine for motor recovery after acute ischaemic stroke (FLAME): A randomised placebo-controlled trial. *Lancet Neurol.* 2011;**10**:123–130

233. Lindvall O, Kokaia Z. Stem cell research in stroke: How far from the clinic? *Stroke.* 2011;**42**:2369–2375

234. Savitz SI, Cramer SC, Wechsler L. Stem cells as an emerging paradigm in Stroke 3: Enhancing the development of clinical trials. *Stroke.* 2014;**45**:634–639

235. Savitz S, Rosenbaum D, Dinsmore J, Wechsler L, Caplan LR. Cell transplantation for stroke. *Ann Neurol.* 2002;**52**:266–275

236. Roitberg B. Transplantation for stroke. *Neurol Res.* 2004;**26**:256–264

237. Bliss T, Guzman R, Daadi M, Steinberg GK. Cell transplantation therapy for stroke. *Stroke.* 2007;**38**:817–826

238. Savitz SI, Rosenbaum DM. *Stroke Recovery With Cellular Therapies.* Totowa, NJ: Humana Press; 2008

239. Kondziolka D, Wechsler L, Goldstein S, et al. Transplantation of cultured human neuronal cells for patients with stroke. *Neurology.* 2000;**55**:565–569

240. Kondziolka D, Steinberg GK, Wechsler L, et al. Neurotransplantation for patients with subcortical motor stroke: A phase 2 randomized trial. *J Neurosurg.* 2005;**103**:38–45

241. Savitz SI, Dinsmore J, Wu J, Henderson GV, Stieg P, Caplan LR. Neurotransplantation of fetal porcine cells in patients with basal ganglia infarcts: A preliminary safety and feasibility study. *Cerebrovasc Dis.* 2005;**20**:101–107

242. Chen J, Li Y, Wang L, et al. Therapeutic benefit of intravenous administration of bone marrow stromal cells after cerebral ischemia in rats. *Stroke.* 2001;**32**:1005–1011

243. Chopp M, Li Y. Transplantation of bone marrow stromal cells for treatment of central nervous system diseases. *Adv Exp Med Biol.* 2006;**585**:49–64

244. Tang Y, Yasuhara T, Hara K, et al. Transplantation of bone marrow-derived stem cells: A promising therapy for stroke. *Cell Transplant.* 2007;**16**:159–169

245. Eckert MA, Vu Q, Xie K, et al. Evidence for high translational potential of mesenchymal stromal cell therapy to improve recovery from ischemic stroke. *J Cereb Blood Flow Metab.* 2013;**33**:1322–1334

246. Chen J, Sanberg PR, Li Y, et al. Intravenous administration of human

umbilical cord blood reduces behavioral deficits after stroke in rats. *Stroke.* 2001;**32**:2682–2688

247. Newman MB, Emerich DF, Borlongan CV, Sanberg CD, Sanberg PR. Use of human umbilical cord blood (HUCB) cells to repair the damaged brain. *Curr Neurovasc Res.* 2004;**1**:269–281

248. Vu Q, Xie K, Eckert M, Zhao W, Cramer SC. Meta-analysis of preclinical studies of mesenchymal stromal cells for ischemic stroke. *Neurology.* 2014;**82**:1277–1286

249. Honmou O, Houkin K, Matsunaga T, et al. Intravenous administration of auto serum-expanded autologous mesenchymal stem cells in stroke. *Brain.* 2011;**134**:1790–1807

250. Ren JM, Finklestein SP. Growth factor treatment of stroke. *Curr Drug Targets CNS Neurol Disord.* 2005;**4**:121–125

251. Finklestein SP, Caday CG, Kano M, et al. Growth factor expression after stroke. *Stroke.* 1990;**21**:III122–124

252. Lanfranconi S, Locatelli F, Corti S, et al. Growth factors in ischemic stroke. *J Cell Mol Med.* 2011;**15**:1645–1687

253. Kawamata T, Dietrich W, Schallert T, et al. Intracisternal basic fibroblast growth factor (bFGF) enhances functional recovery and upregulates the expression of a molecular marker of neuronal sprouting following focal cerebral infarction. *Proc. Natl Acad Sci U S A* 1997;**94**:8179–8184

254. Schabitz WR, Berger C, Kollmar R, et al. Effect of brain-derived neurotrophic factor treatment and forced arm use on functional motor recovery after small cortical ischemia. *Stroke.* 2004;**35**:992–997

255. Zheng GZ, Li Z, Quan J, et al. VEGF enhances angiogenesis and promotes blood–brain barrier leakage in the ischemic brain. *J Clin Invest.* 2000;**106**:829–838

256. Wang L, Zhang Z, Wang Y, Zhang R, Chopp M. Treatment of stroke with erythropoietin enhances neurogenesis and angiogenesis and improves neurological function in rats. *Stroke.* 2004;**35**:1732–1737

257. Tsai PT, Ohab JJ, Kertesz N, et al. A critical role of erythropoietin receptor in neurogenesis and post-stroke recovery. *J Neurosci.* 2006;**26**:1269–1274

258. Schneider UC, Schilling L, Schroeck H, Nebe CT, Vajkoczy P, Woitzik J. Granulocyte-macrophage colony-stimulating factor-induced vessel growth restores cerebral blood supply after bilateral carotid artery occlusion. *Stroke.* 2007;**38**:1320–1328

259. Schabitz WR, Laage R, Vogt G, et al. AXIS: A trial of intravenous granulocyte colony-stimulating factor in acute ischemic stroke. *Stroke.* 2010;**41**:2545–2551

260. England TJ, Abaei M, Auer DP, et al. Granulocyte-colony stimulating factor for mobilizing bone marrow stem cells in subacute stroke: The stem cell trial of recovery enhancement after Stroke 2 randomized controlled trial. *Stroke.* 2012;**43**:405–411

261. Ringelstein EB, Thijs V, Norrving B, et al. Granulocyte colony-stimulating factor in patients with acute ischemic stroke: Results of the AX200 for ischemic stroke trial. *Stroke.* 2013;**44**:2681–2687

262. Jerndal M, Forsberg K, Sena ES, et al. A systematic review and meta-analysis of erythropoietin in experimental stroke. *J Cereb Blood Flow Metab.* 2010;**30**:961–968

263. Kolb B, Morshead C, Gonzalez C, et al. Growth factor-stimulated generation of new cortical tissue and functional recovery after stroke damage to the motor cortex of rats. *J Cereb Blood Flow Metab.* 2007;**27**:983–997

264. Belayev L, Khoutorova L, Zhao KL, Davidoff AW, Moore AF, Cramer SC. A novel neurotrophic therapeutic strategy for experimental stroke. *Brain Res.* 2009;**1280**:117–123

265. Cramer SC, Fitzpatrick C, Warren M, et al. The beta-hCG + erythropoietin in acute stroke (BETAS) study: A three-center, single-dose, open-label, noncontrolled, phase IIa safety trial. *Stroke.* 2010;**41**:927–931

266. Cramer SC, Hill MD. Human choriogonadotropin and epoetin alfa in acute ischemic stroke patients (REGENESIS-LED trial). *Int J Stroke.* 2014;**9**:321–327

267. Pardridge WM. Drug transport across the blood–brain barrier. *J Cereb Blood Flow Metab.* 2012;**32**:1959–1972

268. Hermann DM. Enhancing the delivery of erythropoietin and its variants into the ischemic brain. *Sci World J.* 2009;**9**:967–969

269. Zhang Y, Pardridge WM. Conjugation of brain-derived neurotrophic factor to a blood–brain barrier drug targeting system enables neuroprotection in regional brain ischemia following intravenous injection of the neurotrophin. *Brain Res.* 2001;**889**:49–56

270. Yasuhara T, Borlongan C, Date I. Ex vivo gene therapy: Transplantation of neurotrophic factor-secreting cells for cerebral ischemia. *Front Biosci.* 2006;**11**:760–775

271. Gallese V, Fadiga L, Fogassi L, Rizzolatti G. Action recognition in the premotor cortex. *Brain.* 1996;**119**:593–609

272. Fogassi L, Ferrari PF, Gesierich B, Rozzi S, Chersi F, Rizzolatti G. Parietal lobe: From action organization to intention understanding. *Science.* 2005;**308**:662–667

273. Kalra L, Ratan R. Recent advances in stroke rehabilitation 2006. *Stroke.* 2007;**38**:235–237

274. Small SL, Buccino G, Solodkin A. The mirror neuron system and treatment of stroke. *Dev Psychobiol.* 2012;**54**:293–310

275. Page SJ, Levine P, Leonard A. Mental practice in chronic stroke: Results of a randomized, placebo-controlled trial. *Stroke.* 2007;**38**:1293–1297

276. Celnik P, Webster B, Glasser DM, Cohen LG. Effects of action observation on physical training after stroke. *Stroke.* 2008;**39**:1814–1820

277. Kho AY, Liu KP, Chung RC. Meta-analysis on the effect of mental imagery on motor recovery of the hemiplegic upper extremity function. *Aust Occup Ther J.* 2014;**61**:38–48

278. Ramachandran VS, Altschuler EL. The use of visual feedback, in particular mirror visual feedback, in restoring brain function. *Brain.* 2009;**132**:1693–1710

279. Dodakian L, Sharp K, See J, et al. Targeted engagement of a dorsal premotor circuit in the treatment of post-stroke paresis. *NeuroRehabilitation.* 2013;**33**:13–24

280. Berman BD, Horovitz SG, Venkataraman G, Hallett M. Self-modulation of primary motor cortex activity with motor and motor imagery tasks using real-time fMRI-based neurofeedback. *NeuroImage.* 2012;**59**:917–925

281. Sitaram R, Veit R, Stevens B, et al. Acquired control of ventral premotor cortex activity by feedback training: An exploratory real-time fMRI and TMS study. *Neurorehabil Neural Repair.* 2012;**26**:256–265

282. Sulzer J, Haller S, Scharnowski F, et al. Real-time fMRI neurofeedback: Progress and challenges. *NeuroImage*. 2013;76:386–399

283. Fasotti L, van Kessel M. Novel insights in the rehabilitation of neglect. *Front Hum Neurosci*. 2013;7:780

284. Hondori HM, Khademi M, McKenzie A, Dodakian L, Lopes C, Cramer S. Utility of augmented reality in relation to virtual reality in stroke rehabilitation. *Stroke*. 2014;45:ATMP43

285. Hillis AE. Aphasia: Progress in the last quarter of a century. *Neurology*. 2007;69:200–213

286. Hillis AE. Pharmacological, surgical, and neurovascular interventions to augment acute aphasia recovery. *Amer J Phys Med Rehabil*. 2007;86:426–434

287. Zhang X, Kedar S, Lynn MJ, Newman NJ, Biousse V. Homonymous hemianopias: Clinical–anatomic correlations in 904 cases. *Neurology*. 2006;66:906–910

288. Zhang X, Kedar S, Lynn MJ, Newman NJ, Biousse V. Homonymous hemianopia in stroke. *J Neuroophthalmol*. 2006;26:180–183

289. Gilbert CD, Wiesel TN. Intrinsic connectivity and receptive field properties in visual cortex. *Vision Res*. 1985;25:365–374

290. Gilbert CD, Wiesel TN. Receptive field dynamics in adult primary visual cortex. *Nature*. 1992;356:150–152

291. Kaas JH, Krubitzer LA, Chino YM, Langston AL, Polley EH, Blair N. Reorganization of retinotopic cortical maps in adult mammals after lesions of the retina. *Science*. 1990;248:229–231

292. Zhang X, Kedar S, Lynn MJ, Newman NJ, Biousse V. Natural history of homonymous hemianopia. *Neurology*. 2006;66:901–905

293. Pambakian A, Currie J, Kennard C. Rehabilitation strategies for patients with homonymous visual field defects. *J Neuroophthalmol*. 2005;25:136–142

294. Kasten E, Wust S, Behrens-Baumann W, Sabel BA. Computer-based training for the treatment of partial blindness. *Nature Med*. 1998;4:1083–1087

295. Kasten E, Poggel DA, Sabel BA. Computer-based training of stimulus detection improves color and simple pattern recognition in the defective field of hemianopic subjects. *J Cogn Neurosci*. 2000;12:1001–1012

296. Poggel DA, Kasten E, Sabel BA. Attentional cueing improves vision restoration therapy in patients with visual field defects. *Neurology*. 2004;63:2069–2076

297. Kasten E, Muller-Oehring E, Sabel BA. Stability of visual field enlargements following computer-based restitution training – results of a follow-up. *J Clin Exp Neuropsychol*. 2001;23:297–305

298. Spitzyna GA, Wise RJ, McDonald SA, et al. Optokinetic therapy improves text reading in patients with hemianopic alexia: A controlled trial. *Neurology*. 2007;68:1922–1930

299. Kleim JA, Jones TA. Principles of experience-dependent neural plasticity: Implications for rehabilitation after brain damage. *J Speech Lang Hear Res*. 2008;51: S225–S239

300. Cramer SC. Issues in clinical trial methodology for brain repair after stroke. In Cramer SC, Nudo RJ, eds. *Brain Repair After Stroke*. Cambridge, UK: Cambridge University Press; 2010:173–182

301. Green AR, Hainsworth AH, Jackson DM. GABA potentiation: A logical pharmacological approach for the treatment of acute ischaemic stroke. *Neuropharmacology*. 2000;39:1483–1494

302. Ovbiagele B, Kidwell CS, Starkman S, Saver JL. Neuroprotective agents for the treatment of acute ischemic stroke. *Curr Neurol Neurosci Rep*. 2003;3:9–20

303. Kozlowski D, Jones T, Schallert T. Pruning of dendrites and restoration of function after brain damage: Role of the NMDA receptor. *Restor Neurol Neurosci*. 1994;7:119–126

304. Wahlgren N, Martinsson L. New concepts for drug therapy after stroke. Can we enhance recovery? *Cerebrovasc Dis*. 1998;8 Suppl 5:33–38

305. Barth T, Hoane M, Barbay S, Saponjic R. Effects of glutamate antagonists on the recovery and maintenance of behavioral function after brain injury. In Goldstein L, ed. *Restorative Neurology: Advances in Pharmacotherapy for Recovery After Stroke*. Armonk, NY: Futura Publishing; 1998:79–90

306. Narasimhan P, Liu J, Song YS, Massengale JL, Chan PH. VEGF stimulates the ERK 1/2 signaling pathway and apoptosis in cerebral endothelial cells after ischemic conditions. *Stroke*. 2009;40:1467–1473

307. Clarkson AN, Overman JJ, Zhong S, Mueller R, Lynch G, Carmichael ST. AMPA receptor-induced local brain-derived neurotrophic factor signaling mediates motor recovery after stroke. *J Neurosci*. 2011;31:3766–3775

308. Zhao BQ, Tejima E, Lo EH. Neurovascular proteases in brain injury, hemorrhage and remodeling after stroke. *Stroke*. 2007;38:748–752

309. Allan SM, Rothwell NJ. Inflammation in central nervous system injury. *Philos Trans R Soc Lond B Biol Sci*. 2003;358:1669–1677

310. Lucas SM, Rothwell NJ, Gibson RM. The role of inflammation in CNS injury and disease. *Br J Pharmacol*. 2006;147 Suppl 1:S232–240

311. Fang PC, Barbay S, Plautz EJ, Hoover E, Strittmatter SM, Nudo RJ. Combination of NEP 1–40 treatment and motor training enhances behavioral recovery after a focal cortical infarct in rats. *Stroke*. 2010;41:544–549

312. Starkey ML, Schwab ME. Anti-Nogo-A and training: Can one plus one equal three? *Exp Neurol*. 2012;235:53–61

313. Hovda D, Feeney D. Amphetamine with experience promotes recovery of locomotor function after unilateral frontal cortex injury in the cat. *Brain Res*. 1984;298:358–361

314. Adkins-Muir D, Jones T. Cortical electrical stimulation combined with rehabilitative training: Enhanced functional recovery and dendritic plasticity following focal cortical ischemia in rats. *Neurol Res*. 2003;25:780–788

315. Adkins DL, Hsu JE, Jones TA. Motor cortical stimulation promotes synaptic plasticity and behavioral improvements following sensorimotor cortex lesions. *Exp Neurol*. 2008;212:14–28

316. Cramer SC. Stratifying patients with stroke in trials that target brain repair. *Stroke*. 2010;41:S114–S116

317. Woldag H, Hummelsheim H. Evidence-based physiotherapeutic concepts for improving arm and hand function in stroke patients: A review. *J Neurol*. 2002;249:518–528

318. Cramer SC. Repairing the human brain after stroke: I. Mechanisms of spontaneous recovery. *Ann Neurol*. 2008;63:272–287

319. Cramer SC, Koroshetz WJ, Finklestein SP. The case for modality-specific outcome measures in clinical trials of stroke recovery-promoting agents. *Stroke*. 2007;38:1393–1395

Index

Caplan's Stroke